EMERGENCY DEPARTMENT MANAGEMENT

PRINCIPLES AND APPLICATIONS

EMERGENCY DEPARTMENT MANAGEMENT
PRINCIPLES AND APPLICATIONS

Editors-in-Chief

RICHARD F. SALLUZZO, M.D., F.A.C.E.P.
Chairman, Department of Emergency Medicine
Albany Medical Center and
Associate Professor, Department of Emergency Medicine
Albany Medical College, Albany, New York

THOM A. MAYER, M.D., F.A.C.E.P., F.A.A.P.
Chairman, Department of Emergency Medicine
Medical Director, Flight Services
Fairfax Hospital, Falls Church, Virginia and
Professor of Emergency Medicine
Georgetown University School of Medicine
George Washington University School of Medicine, Washington, D.C.

ROBERT W. STRAUSS, M.D., F.A.C.E.P.
Chairman, Emergency Treatment Associates
Associate Chairman, Department of Emergency Medicine
St. Francis Hospital, Poughkeepsie, New York

PAMELA KIDD, R.N., Ph.D., A.R.N.P., C.E.N.
Associate Professor
College of Nursing, University of Kentucky
Family Nurse Practitioner, V.A. Hospital
Manager, Motor Vehicle Injury Prevention Program
Kentucky Injury Prevention and Research Center
Lexington, Kentucky

Editors

STEPHEN J. DRESNICK, M.D., F.A.C.E.P.
President/CEO, The Sterling Healthcare Group, Coral Gables, Florida;
Clinical Associate Professor of Emergency Medicine
University of Florida School of Medicine, Gainesville, Florida

JOHN G. KEENE, M.D., F.A.C.E.P.
President and CEO, Emergency Treatment Associates
President and CEO, New York Occupational Medicine
CEO, Health Link Partners
Emergency Treatment Associates
Poughkeepsie, New York

VINCENT P. VERDILE, M.D., F.A.C.E.P.
Vice-Chairman, Department of Emergency Medicine
Albany Medical Center and
Associate Professor, Department of Emergency Medicine
Albany Medical College, Albany, New York

Mosby

St. Louis Baltimore Boston Carlsbad Chicago Naples New York Philadelphia Portland
London Madrid Mexico City Singapore Sydney Tokyo Toronto Wiesbaden

Mosby
Dedicated to Publishing Excellence

A Times Mirror
Company

Vice President and Publisher: Anne Patterson
Editor: Kathryn H. Falk
Project Manager: Patricia Tannian
Production Editor: Melissa Mraz Lastarria
Book Design Manager: Gail Morey Hudson
Manufacturing Manager: Karen Lewis
Cover Designer: Teresa Breckwoldt

Printed in the United States of America
Composition by Clarinda Company
Printing/binding by Maple-Vail Book Mfg Group

Mosby–Year Book, Inc.
11830 Westline Industrial Drive
St. Louis, Missouri 63146

Library of Congress Cataloging in Publication Data

Emergency department management : principles and application / editors -in-chief, Richard F. Salluzzo . . . [et al.].
p. cm.
Includes bibliographical references and index.
ISBN 0-8151-7751-8
1. Hospitals—Emergency service—Administration. I. Salluzzo, Richard F.
[DNLM: 1. Emergency Service, Hospital—organization & administration—United States. 2. Emergency Medical Services—organization & administration—United States. WX 215 E5298 1997]
RA975.5.E5E398 1997
362.18′068--dc21
DNLM/DLC 96-37038
for Library of Congress CIP

96 97 98 99 00 / 9 8 7 6 5 4 3 2 1

Contributors

RICHARD V. AGHABABIAN, M.D., F.A.C.E.P.
Chairman
Department of Emergency Medicine
University of Massachusetts Medical Center
Worcester, Massachusetts

E. JACKSON ALLISON, Jr., M.D./M.P.H., F.A.C.E.P.
Sterling Distinguished Professor
Department of Emergency Medicine
East Carolina University School of Medicine
Greenville, North Carolina

MICHAEL F. ALTIERI, M.D.
Pediatric Section Chief
Department of Emergency Medicine
Fairfax Hospital
Falls Church, Virginia

PAUL S. AUERBACH, M.D.
Chief Operating Officer
Sterling Healthcare Group
Coral Gables, Florida

JOEL M. BARTFIELD, M.D.
Assistant Professor
Department of Emergency Medicine
Albany Medical Center
Albany, New York

JEAN G. BRANNON, B.A.
Group Practice Manager
Van Meter and Associates
New Orleans, Louisiana

ROBERT B. BURLEIGH
President
Brandywine Healthcare Services
Malvern, Pennsylvania

DON B. COHEN, M.D., C.P.A., F.A.C.E.P.
Associate Director
Division of Emergency Medicine
Evanston Hospital
Evanston, Illinois

STEPHEN A. COLUCCIELLO, M.D.
Clinical Services Director and Trauma Coordinator
Department of Emergency Medicine
Carolinas Medical Center
Charlotte, North Carolina;
Assistant Professor of Emergency Medicine
University of North Carolina
Chapel Hill, North Carolina

STEPHEN CUMBIE
Chairman, Fairfax Hospital Board
President, NV Commercial Inc.
Vienna, Virginia

LLOYD M. DeBOER
Chairman Emeritus
Inova Health System Board;
Professor Emeritus of Management
George Mason University
Fairfax, Virginia

KENNETH L. DeHART, M.D., F.A.C.E.P.
President/CEO
Strand Physician Specialists
Grand Strand Regional Medical Center
Myrtle Beach, South Carolina

EDWARD T. DICKINSON, M.D., NREMT-P
Assistant Professor and Director of EMS
Department of Emergency Medicine
Albany Medical College
Albany, New York;
Medical Director
Town of Colonie EMS Department
Colonie, New York

CELIA H. DOVER, R.N., M.S.N., C.E.N.
Head Nurse/Trauma Coordinator
Emergency Department
Carraway Methodist Medical Center
Birmingham, Alabama

STEPHEN J. DRESNICK, M.D., F.A.C.E.P.
President/CEO, The Sterling Healthcare Group
Coral Gables, Florida;
Clinical Professor
Department of Emergency Medicine
University of North Carolina School of Medicine
Chapel Hill, North Carolina

JOHN DALE DUNN, M.D., J.D., F.A.C.E.P., F.A.C.L.M., F.A.A.F.P.
Director
Emergency Services
Brownwood Regional Medical Center
Brownwood, Texas

CARAL LYNNE EDELBERG
President
Medical Management Resources, Inc.
Jacksonville, Florida

JAY W. EDELBERG, M.D., F.A.C.E.P.
President
Emergency Physicians Group, Inc.
Jacksonville, Florida

LUIS F. ELJAIEK, Jr., M.D., F.A.C.E.P.
Operational Medical Director
Inova Medical AirCare and
Attending Physician
Department of Emergency Medicine
Fairfax Hospital
Falls Church, Virginia;
Clinical Instructor
Department of Emergency Medicine
George Washington University School of Medicine and
Assistant Clinical Professor of Emergency Medicine
Georgetown University School of Medicine
Washington, D.C.;
Medical Director
Choice American Ambulance
Alexandria, Virginia

JAMES M. ELLIS, Jr., M.D., F.A.C.E.P.
Vice President
Pinnacle Emergency Consultants;
Co-Chair, Olympic Medical Support Group
Atlanta Committee for the Olympic Games
Venue Medical Director, Olympic Stadium
1996 Summer Olympic Games;
Consultant with Medical Sports Group to the NFL for Super Bowl
Morrow, Georgia

HOWARD A. FREED, M.D.

Associate Professor
Department of Emergency Medicine
Albany Medical College
Albany, New York;
Medical Director, Emergency Department
Director of Emergency Services
Nathan Littauer Hospital
Gloversville, New York

GUS M. GARMEL, M.D., F.A.C.E.P.

Associate Residency Director
Stanford/Kaiser Emergency Medicine Residency Program
Department of Emergency Medicine
Stanford University Hospital/Kaiser Permanente Medical Center
Palo Alto, California;
Senior Emergency Medicine Physician
Department of Emergency Medicine
Kaiser Permanente Medical Center
Santa Clara, California

JAMES E. GEORGE, M.D., J.D., F.A.C.E.P.

President, Emergency Physician Associates, P.A.;
Partner, Law Firm of George, Korin, Quattrone and Blumberg;
Attending Physician
Department of Emergency Medicine
Underwood-Memorial Hospital
Woodbury, New Jersey;
Director
Department of Liability Control
Medical Society of New Jersey
Lawrenceville, New Jersey

WILLIAM H. GINSBURG, J.D.

Senior Partner
Ginsburg, Stephan, Oringher, and Richman
Los Angeles, California

LOUIS G. GRAFF, M.D., F.A.C.E.P.

Associate Chief
Emergency Medicine
New Britain General Hospital
New Britain, Connecticut;
Associate Professor of Clinical Medicine
Associate Professor of Clinical Surgery
University of Connecticut Medical School
Farmington, Connecticut

LINDA GREENBERG, R.N., B.S.N., M.S., C.E.N.

Former Director
Emergency, Trauma, and Air Ambulance Services
Sacred Heart Medical Center
Spokane, Washington;
Former Chief Clinical Officer
Columbia-Willamette
Valley Medical Center
McMinnville, Oregon

LLOYD E. GREENE, Ed.D.

Vice President
Human Resources
Organization Development
Seton Health Network
Austin, Texas

REGINA M. HEISER, R.N., B.S.N., M.S.N., C.E.N.

Case Manager, Operating Room Services and Emergency Department
University of Kentucky Hospital
Lexington, Kentucky

GREGORY L. HENRY, M.D., F.A.C.E.P.

Chief
Department of Emergency Medicine
Oakwood Hospital—Beyer Center
Ypsilanti, Michigan;
Clinical Associate Professor
Department of Surgery
Section of Emergency Services
University of Michigan
Ann Arbor, Michigan;
President
American College of Emergency Physicians
Dallas, Texas;
Vice President, Emergency Physicians Medical Group, PC
Ann Arbor, Michigan

JAMES JAY HOELZ, R.N., M.S., M.B.A., C.E.N.

Director
Quality Management
Mercer Medical Center
Trenton, New Jersey

ROBERT S. HOFFMAN, M.D.

Director
New York City Poison Center
Assistant Professor of Clinical Surgery
Department of Emergency Medicine
New York University School of Medicine
New York, New York

KAREN SUE HOYT, R.N., M.N., C.E.N.

NP Clinical Placement Coordinator
Philip Y Hahn School of Nursing
University of San Diego
San Diego, California;
Clinical Consultant
Emtek, A Motorola Company
Phoeniz, Arizona

GEORGE M. INNES, Jr., EMT-P, M.D., F.A.C.E.P.

Associate Director and
Emergency Medical Services Director
Albany Memorial Hospital;
Clinical Instructor
Department of Emergency Medicine
Albany Medical College
Albany, New York

BRUCE D. JANIAK, M.D.

Medical Director
Department of Emergency Medicine
The Toledo Hospital
Toledo, Ohio

JOHN C. JOHNSON, M.D., F.A.C.E.P.

Regional Medical Director
Unity Physician Group, P.C.
EMS Medical Director
Porter Memorial Hospital Health System
Valparaiso, Indiana;
Clinical Associate Professor
Division of Emergency Medicine
Department of Medicine
University of Chicago Hospitals
Chicago, Illinois;
Clinical Assistant Professor of Medicine
Department of Emergency Medicine
Indiana University School of Medicine
Indianapolis, Indiana;
Associate Professor
School of Public and Environmental Affairs
Indiana University
Bloomington, Indiana

DAVID KALIFON, M.D., J.D., F.A.C.E.P., F.C.L.M.

OF Counsel
Jeffer, Mangels, Butler & Marmaro, LLP
Los Angeles, California

JOHN G. KEENE

President and CEO, Emergency Treatment Associates
President and CEO, New York Occupational Medicine
CEO, Health Link Partners
Emergency Treatment Associates
Poughkeepsie, New York

CATHERINE T. KELLY, R.N., M.S.N., C.E.N., C.C.R.N.

Assistant Professor
Mount Saint Mary College
Division of Nursing
Newburgh, New York;
Past President
Board of Certification for Emergency Nursing
Park Ridge, Illinois

PAMELA KIDD, R.N., Ph.D., A.R.N.P., C.E.N.

Associate Professor
College of Nursing
University of Kentucky;
Family Nurse Practitioner V.A. Hospital;
Manager
Motor Vehicle Injury Prevention Program
Kentucky Injury Prevention and Research Center
Lexington, Kentucky

SAMUEL J. KIEHL, M.D., F.A.C.E.P.

Director, Department of Emergency Medicine
Riverside Methodist Hospital;
Assistant Clinical Professor
Department of Emergency Medicine
The Ohio State University College of Medicine;
President, Olentangy Emergency Physicians
Columbus, Ohio

ELEANORE R. KIRSCH, R.N., M.S., C.E.N.

Deputy Executive Director
Nursing Services
Emergency Nurses Association
Park Ridge, Illinois

RICHARD M. KNAPP, Ph.D.

Executive Vice President
American Association of Medical Colleges
Washington, D.C.

JON R. KROHMER, M.D., F.A.C.E.P.

EMS Director
Emergency Medicine Residency Program
Butterworth Hospital
Grand Rapids, Michigan;
Medical Director
Kent County EMS
Grand Rapids, Michigan;
Associate Professor
College of Human Medicine
Michigan State University
East Lansing, Michigan

BARBARA A. KYES, R.N.

Kyes Kreative Consulting
Tampa, Florida

FORD N. KYES, R.N., M.P.M.

Vice President, Operations
St. Anthony's Hospital
St. Petersburg, Florida

DIETER A. LEHNORTT, M.A.

Executive Director
MedTrust Healthcare Services Company
Dallas, Texas

NEAL LITTLE, M.D., F.A.C.E.P.

Emergency Physician
St. Joseph Mercy Hospital;
Clinical Assistant Professor of Internal Medicine
Department of Surgery
University of Michigan Medical School
Ann Arbor, Michigan

KEITH E. LORING, M.D., M.P.H.

Assistant Director of Medical Education
Department of Emergency Medicine
Johns Hopkins Hospital;
Instructor
Department of Emergency Medicine
Johns Hopkins University School of Medicine
Baltimore, Maryland

STEPHAN G. LYNN, M.D., F.A.C.E.P.

Director
Department of Emergency Medicine
St. Luke's-Roosevelt Hospital Center;
Assistant Professor of Clinical Surgery
The College of Physicians and Surgeons at Columbia University
New York, New York;
ACEP Representative
Guidelines Revision Committee
American Institute of Architects;
Chairman
National ACEP Task Force on Hospital and ED Overcrowding 1988-1991

VINCENT MARKOVCHICK, M.D., F.A.C.E.P.

Director
Emergency Medical Services
Denver Health Hospitals;
Professor of Surgery
Division of Emergency Medicine
University of Colorado Health Sciences Center;
Department of Emergency Medicine
Denver General Hospital
Denver, Colorado

DAN M. MAYER, M.D.

Attending Physician
Department of Emergency Medicine
Albany Medical College Hospital;
Associate Professor
Theme Leader Comprehensive Care Case Studies Course
Department of Emergency Medicine
Albany Medical College
Albany, New York

THOM A. MAYER, M.D., F.A.C.E.P., F.A.A.P.

Chairman, Department of Emergency Medicine
Medical Director, Flight Services
Fairfax Hospital
Falls Church, Virginia;
Professor of Emergency Medicine
Georgetown University School of Medicine
George Washington University School of Medicine
Washington, D.C.

RICHARD M. McDOWELL, M.D., F.A.C.E.P.

Chairman, Department of Emergency Medicine
Medical Director, Crozer EMS
Crozer-Chester Medical Center
Upland, Pennsylvania

DAVID T. OVERTON, M.D., M.B.A., F.A.C.E.P., F.A.C.P.

Program Director
Department of Emergency Medicine
Michigan State University Kalamazoo Center for Medical Studies;
Associate Professor of Emergency Medicine
Michigan State University College of Human Medicine
Kalamazoo, Michigan

DIGHTON C. PACKARD, M.D., F.A.C.E.P.

Medical Director
Emergency Department
Baylor University Medical Center
Chief Medical Officer
EMCARE
Dallas, Texas

JANET GREN PARKER, M.S., R.N.

Vice President, Nursing
St. Mary's Medical Center
Saginaw, Michigan

MARK B. PARSHALL, R.N., M.S.N., C.N.S., C.E.N.

Doctoral Student
University of Kentucky
College of Nursing
Lexington, Kentucky

MICHAEL J. PEIKERT, M.D., F.A.C.E.P.

Associate Clinical Professor
Department of Emergency Medicine
Michigan State University Kalamazoo Center for Medical Studies;
Past Chief of Staff
Borgess Medical Center
Kalamazoo, Michigan

DAVID J. PILLOW, M.D., F.A.C.E.P.

Chairman, Department of Emergency Medicine
Saint Paul Medical Center
Director of Training and Development
Metroplex Emergency Physician Associates
Dallas, Texas

PETER T. PONS, M.D., F.A.C.E.P.

Attending Physician
Emergency Department
Denver General Hospital
Associate Professor
Division of Emergency Medicine
Department of Surgery
University of Colorado Health Sciences Center
Denver, Colorado

KELVIN P. QUAN, J.D., M.P.H.

Associate
Cooley, Godward, Castro, Huddleston, & Tatum
Palo Alto, California

JAN RICH, R.N., M.S.N., M.B.A., C.E.N., C.N.A.

Administrator
Northwest Emergency Physicians
Seattle, Washington

KATHLEEN M. RICHMOND, R.N., F.S., C.E.N., T.N.S.

Clinical Supervisor
Department of Infirmary
Sisters of St. Casimir
Chicago, Illinois;
Clinical Manger/Pre-Hospital Coordinator
Emergency Department
Olympia Fields Osteopathic Medical Center
Olympia Fields, Illinois

SUZANNE RITA, R.N., M.S.N., C.E.N., C.N.S.

Clinical Specialist
Emergency Department
Sentara Norfolk General Hospital
Norfolk, Virginia

EDGARDO J. RIVERA-RIVERA, M.D.

Major, USAF, MC, FS
Chief Emergency Services
82nd Medical Group;
EMS/Prehospital Care Consultant
Air Education and Training Command, USAF;
Medical Director, EMS Programs
Sheppard Air Force Base, Texas

NORMAN ROSENFELD, F.A.I.A.

Bachelor of Architecture
Pratt Institute 1956
Principle
Norman Rosenfeld Architects
New York, New York

RICHARD F. SALLUZZO, M.D., F.A.C.E.P.

Chairman
Department of Emergency Medicine
Albany Medical Center;
Associate Professor
Department of Emergency Medicine
Albany Medical College
Albany, New York

MAUREEN SCAHILL, R.N., M.S., C.S.

Nurse Practitioner
Emergency Department
Strong Memorial Hospital of the University of Rochester
Rochester, New York

THOMAS A. SCALETTA, M.D.

Associate Director
Department of Emergency Medicine
Cook County Hospital;
Associate Professor of Emergency Medicine
Rush Medical College
Chicago, Illinois

LAURA R. SEFF, M.B.A.

President, Emesco Inc.
Miami, Florida

REBECCA SMITH-COGGINS, M.D., F.A.C.E.P.

Assistant Professor
Emergency Medicine
Stanford University
Stanford, California

SUSAN W. SOMERSON, M.S.N., R.N., C.S., A.R.N.P., C.E.N.

Nurse Practitioner
Urgent Care Center
Mercer Medical Center
Trenton, New Jersey

PETER L. SOSNOW, M.D., F.A.C.E.P.

Director
Emergency and Outpatient Services
Department of Emergency Medicine
Albany Memorial Hospital;
Adjunct Assistant Professor
Department of Emergency Medicine
Albany Medical College
Albany, New York

ROXANE SPITZER-LEHMANN, Ph.D., R.N., M.B.A., F.A.A.N.

Professor and Associate Dean for Practice Management
School of Nursing
Vanderbilt University Medical Center
Nashville, Tennessee

JOEL A. STETTNER, M.D., F.A.C.E.P.

Assistant Chairman
Department of Emergency Medicine
Summit Medical Center;
Managing Partner
California Emergency Physicians Medical Group;
President, MedAmerica, Inc.
Oakland, California

ROBERT W. STRAUSS, M.D., F.A.C.E.P.

Chairman
Emergency Treatment Associates
Associate Chairman
Department of Emergency Medicine
St. Francis Hospital
Poughkeepsie, New York

SUSAN F. STRAUSS, R.N., C.E.N.

Clinical Nurse
Emergency Department
St. Luke Hospital
Newburgh, New York

DANIEL J. SULLIVAN, M.D., J.D., F.A.C.E.P.

Chairman
Department of Emergency Medicine
Ingalls Memorial Hospital
Harvey, Illinois;
Assistant Professor
Department of Emergency Medicine
Cook County Hospital
Chicago, Illinois;
President
Illinois College of Emergency Physicians
Oak Brook Terrace, Illinois;
President
Midwest Emergency Associates, Ltd.
Oak Brook, Illinois;
Executive Editor
ED Legal Letter
Atlanta, Georgia

COLLEEN H. SWARTZ, R.N., M.S.N., C.C.R.N.

Trauma Coordinator/Chief Flight Nurse
University of Kentucky Hospital
Lexington, Kentucky

MARILYN P. SWINFORD, R.N., B.S.N., C.E.N.

Clinical Coordinator
Emergency Department
Saint Joseph Hospital
Lexington, Kentucky

ROBERT A. SWOR, M.D., F.A.C.E.P.

Clinical Instructor of Emergency Medicine
University of Michigan
Ann Arbor, Michigan;
Director, EMS Fellowship Program
William Beaumont Hospital
Royal Oak, Michigan

ELLEN TALIAFERRO, M.D.

Associate Professor
Division of Emergency Medicine
Department of Surgery
University of Texas Southwestern Medical School
Dallas, Texas

PAULA TANABE, R.N., Ph.D.(C), C.E.N., C.C.R.N.

Clinical Nurse Specialist
Trauma Coordinator
Northwest Community Hospital
Arlington Heights, Illinois

WILLIAMS S. TENNANT

Chairman, Inova Health System Board
Attorney-at-Law, Krooth & Altman
Washington, D.C.

GEORGE TERRANOVA, M.D., F.A.C.E.P.

Chairman
Department of Emergency Medicine and Primary Care
Danbury Hospital
Danbury, Connecticut;
Lecturer
Department of Medicine
Yale School of Medicine
New Haven, Connecticut

RICHARD C. TOBEY, M.D., M.P.H., F.A.C.E.P., A.B.P.M.

Department of Emergency Medicine
St. Francis Hospital
Poughkeepsie, New York

KEITH W. VAN METER, M.D., F.A.C.E.P.

Clinical Associate Professor of Medicine
Louisiana State University School of Medicine
New Orleans, Louisiana

JEFFREY W. VAWTER, M.H.A.

Senior Consultant
Premier
Charlotte, North Carolina

TENER GOODWIN VEENEMA, M.S., R.N., P.N.P.

Education Coordinator and Coordinator for Clinical Pathway Development, Emergency Services
Emergency Department
Strong Memorial Hospital
University of Rochester Medical Center
Rochester, New York

VINCENT VERDILE, M.D., F.A.C.E.P.

Vice-Chairman
Department of Emergency Medicine
Albany Medical Center Hospital;
Associate Professor
Department of Emergency Medicine
Albany Medical College
Albany, New York

GREGORY A. VOLTURO, M.D., F.A.C.E.P.

Director
Department of Emergency Medicine
Assistant Professor
Departments of Emergency Medicine and Medicine
University of Massachusetts Medical School
Worcester, Massachusetts

JOHN H. WALES, M.D., F.A.C.E.P.

Medical Director
Department of Emergency Medicine
East Jefferson General Hospital
Metairie, Louisiana;
President
John Wales Associates, Inc.
Albany, New York;
Clinical Assistant Professor
Department of Medicine
Louisiana State University School of Medicine
New Orleans, Louisiana

SUZANNE M. WALL, R.N.C., M.S., C.E.N.

Supervisory Nurse Practitioner
Emergency Department
Rochester General Hospital
Rochester, New York

DANIEL P. WALSH, D.O., F.A.C.E.P.

Regional Vice President and Director of Customer Service
InPhyNet Medical Management
Fort Lauderdale, Florida

PAUL M. WAX, M.D., F.A.C.E.P.

Assistant Professor
Department of Emergency Medicine
Assistant Director
Finger Lakes Poison Control Center
Department of Emergency Medicine
University of Rochester School of Medicine and Dentistry
Rochester, New York

MARC V. WEINER, F.A.C.H.E., M.H.A.

Senior Vice President
Chief Operating Officer
Barnert Hospital
Patterson, New York

LARRY D. WEISS, M.D., F.A.C.E.P.

Clinical Associate Professor of Medicine
Section of Emergency Medicine
Louisiana State University School of Medicine
New Orleans, Louisiana

DENNIS C. WHITEHEAD, M.D., F.A.C.E.P.

Associate Clinical Professor
Department of Emergency Medicine
Michigan State University
Lansing, Michigan;
Chief of Emergency Medicine
Dickinson County Memorial Hospital
Iron Mountain, Michigan

JAMES B. WIELAND, J.D.

Partner
Health Case Group
Cooley Godward Castro Huddleson & Tatum
Palo Alto, California

WALTER PAGE YOUNG, B.S.N., R.N., C.E.N.

Nurse Manager
Emergency Center
St. Joseph's Hospital
Tampa, Florida

CHARLES L. ZELLER, Jr., M.D., F.A.C.E.P.

Associate Clinical Professor of Medicine
Michigan State University College of Human Medicine
Division of Emergency Medicine;
Corporate President
Southwestern Michigan Emergency Services, P.C.;
Program Director
Continuing Medical Education
Michigan State University Kalamazoo Center for Medical Studies
Kalamazoo, Michigan

LESLIE S. ZUN, M.D., M.B.A., F.A.C.E.P.

Chairman
Department of Emergency Medicine
Mount Sinai Hospital Medical Center
Associate Professor of Emergency Medicine
Finch University/Chicago Medical School
Chicago, Illinois

To

Nancy, Jennifer, Jody, and Karen

for their forbearance and support

RICHARD F. SALLUZZO

To my beautiful and brilliant wife,

Maureen,

our sons **Josh, Kevin, and Gregory**

and to my father, affectionately known to everyone as

Grandpa Jim

their love and support have sustained me in this and all other work

THOM A. MAYER

To

Susan, Bo, and Shelby

for their support and patience and for being my anchor

ROBERT STRAUSS

To all of my **students**, *past, present, and future*

to my **parents**

who instilled in me the sense of responsibility to share my knowledge

and to my wife

Abby

who endured lonely days and nights while I pursued my dreams

STEPHEN J. DRESNICK

To my wonderful wife

Mimi Dunne

and our delightful daughter

Catharine

for their love and guidance in all things

JACK KEENE

To my wife

Lou-Ann

who provides me with unwavering love and support

and to my **parents**

who by example, taught me the fundamentals of management

VINCENT P. VERDILE

Preface

"There is nothing more difficult to take in hand, more perilous to conduct, or more uncertain in its success than to take the lead in the introduction of a new order."

Machiavelli

Healthcare now occupies a central place in our society and is an important part of the public policy debate regarding the future of our nation. Expenditures for health-related expenses have only recently begun to stabilize, although there is a serious question whether this can be continued, particularly in the face of an aging population. Faced with these issues, it has become clear that clinical care of the patient is only one part of healthcare's responsibility to the public: leadership and management of the resources entrusted to healthcare are an equally important part of the responsibility of medicine, nursing, and healthcare administration to the patients we serve. This textbook represents an ambitious step in the direction of providing a unified body of knowledge regarding the management of the emergency department. The intent of the textbook is to provide a broad view of the tools, techniques, and philosophic basis for comprehensive management of the emergency department and the personnel comprising it.

The text is divided into ten parts, representing the essential competencies necessary for effective emergency department management:

- Management Principles
- Operations
- Contract Management
- Financial Management and Reimbursement Issues
- Quality
- Risk Management/Legal Issues
- Human Resource Management
- Practice Diversification
- Professional Relations
- Prehospital Care

The editors have carefully chosen the Table of Contents and have made every effort to identify the best possible author for each of the subjects presented. We believe the choice of a large number of knowledgeable experts gives the text the needed diversity and depth to be relevant to all emergency department managers.

Emergency healthcare is by nature a "team sport" involving the integration of efforts of emergency physicians, nurses, technicians, support personnel, as well as hospital administrators. For that reason, the textbook is designed to appeal not only to emergency physicians and physician-leaders, but also to nurses, nurse managers, and administrators responsible for managing the 90 million patients who present to emergency departments in this country each year. The subjects chosen and the instructions to authors reflected a strong bias on the part of the editors to assure that the chapters were written in a practical and straightforward fashion. Each chapter is intended to assure that a practical, pragmatic approach is taken to each subject, which is of benefit to leaders and managers of emergency departments throughout the country in continuing to improve services. It is our sincere hope that the textbook is one that is heavily underlined, dog-eared, and referred to as a frequent resource in facing the substantial challenges of managing the emergency department.

In addressing the comprehensive aspects of emergency department management, including practical applications, the editors have attempted to introduce a resource that is currently not available in the literature. In that sense, we are aware of Machiavelli's warning regarding "the introduction of a new order." Any errors of omission or commission in this textbook are the responsibility of the editors; any praise for the quality of the manuscript should go to the authors, all of whom are extremely busy practitioners of the art and science of emergency department service. Finally, the editors strongly feel that emergency departments represent both a health and a social safety net for our society, delivering care to patients without regard to ability to pay, social status, level of patient acuity, or time of day or night. All who care for such patients are privileged to serve them, and it is our privilege as editors to attempt to provide a resource to assist the providers in that care.

The editors gratefully acknowledge the following faculties, staffs, and individuals without whose support and encouragement this textbook would not have been completed: Albany Medical Center Department of Emergency Medicine, especially Rosemarie Lupoli; Fairfax Hospital Department of Emergency Medicine, especially Joy Sparks-Gaviria, who patiently produced thousands of pages of manuscript and offered many helpful suggestions to the textbook; Kaye Wear, Drs. Robert Cates, Michael Altieri, Luis Eljaiek, Jr., Peter Paganussi, Glenn Druckenbrod, and George Colson, all of whom provided their insights to the textbook; Mary Jane Mastorovich and Dr. Keith Ghezzi, who provided invaluable support and substantial insight; Drs. David Sabiston, Madison Spach, Dale G. Johnson, and Michael E. Matlak, who served as mentors to Dr. Mayer and instilled the idea of physician leadership many years ago; and Emergency Treatment Associates, in particular, Vickie Clewell and Pam Smith. A special thanks to all of the authors who met the first deadline of this book. We appreciate your revisions and patience.

Richard F. Salluzzo, M.D., F.A.C.E.P.
Thom A. Mayer, M.D., F.A.C.E.P., F.A.A.P.
Robert W. Strauss, M.D., F.A.C.E.P.
Pamela Kidd, R.N., Ph.D., C.E.N.
Stephen J. Dresnick, M.D., F.A.C.E.P.
Jack Keene, M.D., F.A.C.E.P.
Vincent Verdile, M.D., F.A.C.E.P.

Contents

PART ONE
Management Principles

1 Leadership, Management, Stewardship, and Motivation

Thom A. Mayer

"The first responsibility of the leader is to define reality. The last is to say thank you. In between, the leader is a servant."
Max DePree, *Leadership is an Art*[1]

"Leadership requires the courage to resist the pressures of immediate situations."
Joseph Badaracco, Jr., and Richard Ellsworth, *Leadership and the Quest for Integrity*[2]

"Management is doing things right; leadership is doing the right things."
Warren Bennis, *On Becoming a Leader*[3]

"There is nothing inconsistent between practicing stewardship and partnership and being a boss. Stewardship is the willingness to hold power, without using reward and punishment and directive authority to get things done. Leadership performs much the same duties, but is simultaneously concerned with the acquisition and centralization of power."
Peter Block, *Stewardship: Choosing Service over Self Interest*[4]

OUTLINE

Traditional physician perceptions of management
Leadership and management: general principles
Leadership styles
Why is leadership rare?
Stewardship
  Choosing partnership over patriarchy
  Choosing adventure (empowerment) over safety (entitlement)
  Choosing service over self-interest
  Defining the stewardship contract
  The emotional work of stewardship
Leadership, management, and stewardship in the emergency department
  Creating a learning organization in the emergency department
  Practical emergency department application
Motivation
Summary

Regardless of the size or sophistication of the hospital, the emergency department is an area of complex interactions involving multiple providers involved in numerous, interrelated processes with disparate resources. The impact of an emergency department on the healthcare community is staggering in its reach, confusing in its complexity, and intimidating in its scope. Because of its complexity, a patient encounter requires that multiple jobs are provided in a smooth, coordinated fashion for the patient to receive the best possible care. However, if a thousand sequential functions must be performed correctly, doing 999 of those things right is a formula for failure, not success. From the standpoint of the patient, the family, and the healthcare provider, all 1000 functions must be coordinated in a timely fashion, or the patient and the system that serves the patient will both suffer.

The emergency department constitutes a substantial business entity in any hospital, accounting for no less than 25%, and often up to 50%, of the total hospital admissions.[5] Of these, a disproportionate number are intensive care unit admissions because nearly two thirds of all intensive care stays in this country are generated through emergency department admissions.[6] Even small emergency departments are businesses approaching or exceeding $1 million in annual revenue, and large emergency departments can account for literally tens of millions of dollars of revenue.

For all these reasons, success in the emergency department requires effective management because it is impossible to deliver effective clinical care without appropriate leadership skills that coordinate emergency department processes. These skills are necessary to allow the clinician and all the members of the emergency department team to have the training, resources, facilities, staff attributes, and sense of mission that are required for appropriate clinical care.

Despite the complexity, sophistication, and financial importance of the emergency department, the degree to which formal management and leadership training are applied varies widely. One of the central functions of this textbook is to ensure that the principles of emergency department management are available to those entrusted with the care of emergency patients. Since its beginnings as a defined specialty in the late 1960s, emergency medicine has depended on a body of knowledge that comprises effective emergency department management and leadership. This chapter, and the others that follow, seek to distill the best available resources to assist the emergency department team in delivering the best possible clinical care in environments that are conducive to long-term practice of emergency medicine.

Specifically, the goals of this chapter are:

- To define and distinguish leadership and management.
- To define stewardship as a management model.
- To address the concept of creating "learning organizations."
- To provide specific emergency department examples of such principles.
- To address basic concepts of motivation.

TRADITIONAL PHYSICIAN PERCEPTIONS OF MANAGEMENT

Certain traditional biases have influenced physicians' views of management in general, and hospital administration in particular. In many extremely successful organizations, these traditional views have been surpassed by the concept of effective teamwork between physicians and their colleagues in the management and delivery of healthcare. Nonetheless, because there are still individuals in organizations who hold these outmoded attitudes, it is important to address them, at least briefly.

Some physicians traditionally viewed medicine as an art and a science, but have been somewhat less enthusiastic in embracing it as a business. It is quite clear that healthcare reform and economic pressures will require a businesslike approach to the management of the healthcare dollar, as well as to the individual patient encounters that generate the expenditure of such healthcare dollars. Medicine is thus an art, a science, *and* a business. To neglect any of the three weakens the whole.

In past decades, physicians often viewed their role in medicine as primarily an active, proactive, full-time job with a clearly specified and defined body of knowledge comprising the elements of patient care delivery. In contradistinction, administration was viewed as a passive, reactive position, clearly secondary and less important than the role of the primary patient caregiver. In addition, instead of a clearly defined body of knowledge, many physicians perceived that administration and management was more of an evanescent, ill-defined aspect of healthcare. This resulted in the paradox summarized in Box 1-1, in which physicians viewed themselves as autonomous, patient oriented, emphatic scientists involved in the "real" business of providing patient care. This image was in contrast to administrators, who were viewed more as cost-efficiency experts, delegators, "bean-counters," and business men and women, primarily responsible for ensuring that the facility, staff, and tools were available for the clinician to provide clinical care.

These stereotypes are important to recognize because they provide an attitude that must be transcended if effective healthcare is to be delivered into the next century. The majority of healthcare institutions now recognize that effective delivery of clinical care in a cost-efficient fashion *requires* a team approach between clinicians and managers. Indeed, as indicated in Chapter 9, the role of the physician manager is critical for the success of American medicine in general and emergency medicine in particular. Although the specific difficulties of making the transition from a physician to physician manager are addressed in that chapter, it has become increasingly obvious that effective clinical care can be provided only when there is a collegial and cooperative approach between clinicians and healthcare managers.

LEADERSHIP AND MANAGEMENT: GENERAL PRINCIPLES

Hundreds of books address, in both specific and general terms, the distinctions between leadership and management. The quotations at the beginning of this chapter help delineate some of those differences, but the following discussion will help summarize and clarify current management theory with regard to these issues. As John Kotter noted,

> Leadership and management are two distinctive and complementary systems of action. Each has its own function and characteristic activities. Both are necessary for success in an increasingly complex and volatile. . . environment. Most U.S. corporations today are overmanaged and underled.[7]

In the business environment, and certainly in the emergency department, both leadership and management are essential features for success. How do these two entities differ? Several seminal thinkers on leadership and management can assist us in answering this question. The simplest definitions hold that management is involved in the day-to-day details of moving an organization through its assigned tasks to achieve its desired goals. It is an activity of maintenance, control, short-range thinking, bottom-line focus, not unlike progressing persistently along a defined path. It conjures the expected images of control, perseverance, and, unfortunately,

BOX 1-1

ZALEZNIK'S DISTINCTIONS BETWEEN MANAGERS AND LEADERS

Manager		Leader
Reactive	Attitudes towards goals	Active
Arise as necessities		Personal vision
Narrow variability	Conception of work	New approaches, options
Low risk		High risk
Enabling process		Mundane affliction
Perpetuates existing order		Seeks change
Prefer working with people	Relationship to others	Prefer some solitude
Relate to others as roles they play		Intuitive, empathetic
Relates to *how* things are done		Relates to what it means
Feels order	Sense of self	Tolerates (enjoys?) chaos
Belonger, joiner		Apart, distance
Problem solver		Innovator

Adapted from Zaleznik A: *Harvard Business Review* 70:126-135, 1992.

drudgery. In contradistinction, leadership connotes motivation, vision, empowerment, long-range focus, and the ability to envision new and potentially exciting ways of performing. Not surprisingly, this conjures a more appealing image in which the leader has the view from the bridge and the manager has the view from the trenches. Bennis,[3] Block,[4] Drucker,[8] Zaleznik,[11] and Kotter,[7] each in their unique way, have contributed to our understanding of these definitions. Box 1-2 summarizes many of these distinctions and is drawn from the works of each of the authors. It should be referred to during the course of the following discussion.

Zaleznik[11] noted that leadership involves using power to influence the thoughts and actions of others in the organization. He pointed out that a crucial difference between managers and leaders is their conception of chaos and order. Whereas leaders tolerate and to some extent enjoy chaos, disorder, and lack of structure, managers are nearly compulsively drawn to seek order and control, with a focus on disposing of problems in a timely fashion, sometimes even before the natural consequences are understood. Managers therefore emphasize *rationality* and *control* and envision themselves primarily as *problem solvers.* The questions that a manager asks are:

- What problems need to be solved?
- In what order should they be solved?
- What are the best ways to deploy resources to solve such problems?

The key attributes for a manager are not genius, heroism, or innovation, but rather persistence, tough mindedness, adherence to detail, analytical ability, and, perhaps more important, tolerance and endurance.

Zaleznik was perhaps the first to recognize that managers tend to adopt fairly impersonal and impassive *attitudes toward goals,* which are seen to arise out of the necessities of the environment, as opposed to any clear sense of vision about where the organization is or should be going. Leaders, on the other hand, have a much clearer focus on where the organization should be headed and therefore have active, personal, often impassioned attitudes towards goals and objectives. Leaders play an active role in shaping ideas and conceptions, but much less attention to specific detail in ensuring that the tasks necessary to achieve such goals are carried out. Zaleznik also notes that managers and leaders differ in their *conceptions of work.* Managers tend to view work as an enabling process wherein the goals and objectives of the organization and the workers entrusted in reaching them interact in ways that maximize output. The manager uses certain rules and tactics by which to negotiate, bargain, reward, or otherwise coerce suppliers to provide maximum output. As pointed out in Chapter 51, this view is a classic traditional management strategy that is not part of more recent continuous quality improvement models.

Managers are continually balancing and coordinating resources to ensure the best possible outcome in attaining specified goals and objectives. Leaders work in nearly the opposite fashion. Whereas managers act to limit choices, leaders work to expand them in substantial ways and open issues to new perspectives and options. Leaders tend to view mundane, day-to-day work as an affliction, focusing instead on the more high-risk conceptions of how the work could be done in a totally different fashion.

Managers and leaders also differ from each other in their *relationships with other individuals within the organization.* Because of their direct involvement, managers almost instinctively prefer to work with other people and avoid most forms of solitary activity. The manager depends heavily on the people in the organization to the extent that they are actively involved in events and processes. Leaders view their relationship with others differently and often prefer solitary activity to being enmeshed in day-to-day detail with other providers. The primary relationship of the leader to others in the organization is certainly empathetic, but focuses more on ideas and conceptions as opposed to specific process interactions. The manager focuses on how and when specific tasks are taken care of; the leader focuses on the what and why.

One of the most important ways that Zaleznik distinguished between managers and leaders is the *inherent self-image* of each type of person. Managers inherently seek order and instinctively attempt to place order where it may not necessarily exist. In many senses, managers are seen as the regulators and conservators of the existing order or status quo, gaining an inherent sense of self-worth in complicity with order. For a manager, problems exist to be solved, and to the extent that they can be solved with satisfactory results equanimity exists. To the extent that they cannot be solved, dissonance reigns. Leaders, on the other hand, are much closer to what William James described in *The Varieties of Religious Experience* as "twice born personalities."[12] These people have an inherent sense of separateness from their environment and, far from having a constant, peaceful transition from stage to stage in their lives, have had much more of an inner sense of continual struggle for meaning and order. They are in some respects similar to the description that St. Paul gave of early Christians; they are "in but not of the world." Leaders certainly work *in* organizations, but in some respects never fully belong to such organizations. Instead of attempting to enforce order and solve problems, leaders tend not only to tolerate chaos, but in some sense to draw sustenance and life force from it. Chapter 13 discusses in more detail the philosophy of change management and chaos

BOX 1-2

CONTRAST BETWEEN MANAGEMENT AND LEADERSHIP

Management	Leadership
Administers	Innovates
Maintains	Develops
Systems/structure	People
Control	Empowerment
Focus on short term	Long range
How? When?	What? Why?
Eyes to the ground	Eyes on horizon
Imitates	Originates
Status quo	Change
Good soldier	Individual
Does things right	Does the right thing

Adapted from Bennis W: *On becoming a leader,* Reading, Mass, 1989, Addison-Wesley.

theory, but leaders tend to follow more of a path of personal mastery in their development, as opposed to the inherent sense of socialization that one would expect from a peer or manager. Box 1-1 summarizes Zaleznik's distinction between managers and leaders in the four areas listed previously.

In a classic *Harvard Business Review* article, Kotter[7] further delineated the dimensions of management and leadership. One of his important contributions was to recognize that all organizations require *both* leadership and management, simply because the two concepts are complementary, not competitive. As he indicated, "The real challenge is to combine strong leadership and strong management and to use each to balance the other."[7] An additional challenge is to recognize which individual's talents best lend themselves to either leadership or management. He also expanded some of the concepts described by Zaleznik in relation to management's focus in dealing with complexity by bringing about order and consistency versus leadership's focus in coping with change. With the massive changes occurring in healthcare, it has become increasingly clear that improving performance by 10% to 15% can no longer be considered a formula for success, either in healthcare or any other industry. Instead successful organizations, and emergency departments in particular, will have to deal effectively with major changes.

Kotter also delineated differences in management and leadership in the following areas:

- Setting a direction versus planning and budgeting.
- Aligning people versus organizing and staffing.
- Motivating people versus controlling and problem solving.

Box 1-3 summarizes these differences. Planning is a primarily deductive management process that brings about orderly results through the analysis of data. The results of the planning process are usually quite detailed and specify clearly how and when things will be accomplished. In contrast, leaders have the task of setting an overall direction or vision for an organization, a primarily inductive process. Rather than producing plans, the leader produces visions or overall strategies for an organization as it relates to what it should become. Nonetheless, this process should not be perceived to be somehow mystical in nature, but should simply combine effective use of data with the inductive process. As Kotter pointed out, "What is crucial about a vision is not its originality, but how well it serves the interests of important constituencies. . . and how easily it can be translated into a realistic competitive strategy. Planning works best not as a substitute for direction setting, but as a complement to it."[7]

All emergency departments share a common feature of the necessity of interdependence; multiple and diverse providers must cooperate for the good of the patient, and no one has complete autonomy in the process. In such a setting, traditional managers make every effort to organize providers to implement plans as precisely and efficiently as possible. Their work focuses on organizing and staffing through job design, job descriptions, motivation, training, and other aspects of the overall process.

The leader's role of aligning people is more communicative in nature, as opposed to design and implementation. Put simply, aligning staff leads to a form of empowerment and enfranchisement in a way that organizing is rarely able to. Aligning the staff involves ensuring that there is a clear sense of direction, as well as the freedom to initiate appropriate actions to achieve desired goals. In such organizations, because the vision is clear, the inherent energy of the organization tends to stall less when different initiatives collide with each other.

Kotter's final distinction between leadership and management involves motivating people versus controlling and problem solving. Traditional management approaches are similar in some respects to quality control efforts in continuous quality improvement. Controlling and problem solving ensure that people do their jobs in a prescribed way to produce a defined product, with ongoing meticulous measurement of the results of their work. As in quality control, mechanisms are put in place to ensure that the system is performing according to previously described control limits. Leadership is much more involved in motivating and inspiring the work force, as opposed to controlling and prescribing how, what, and when things will be done. Leadership focuses more on basic human needs for achievement, belonging, self-control and therefore is a much more powerful response than would be expected from more controlling aspects of behavior. Over time, appropriate blending of these aspects of leadership and management can help create organizations that are much more intrinsically motivating.

The vast majority of leaders have faced early challenges during which their skills and expertise are brought to bear in times of extreme difficulty in relatively early stages of their career. Leaders have usually been faced with extreme challenges that have broadened their personal scope; yet they have usually taken on such challenges both voluntarily and enthusiastically. Again, change is not particularly threatening to leaders, but it is much more so to managers. Finally, in

BOX 1-3

MANAGERS' AND LEADERS' ROLES: ESSENTIAL DIFFERENCES

Managers' roles	Leaders' roles
1. Planning and budgeting • Deductive • Produces plans	1. Setting a vision • Inducive • Produces strategies
2. Organizing and staffing • Design • Implementing present goals • Focus on full-time equivalents, job descriptions • Compliance	2. Aligning people/teams • Communication • Comprehending a vision • Focus on path, direction • Focus on capability
3. Controlling and problem solving • Control mechanisms, reduce variance • Accountability • Focus on roles and results	3. Motivating people • Aligning needs with vision • Motivation • Focus on capability

Adapted from: Kotter JP: *Harvard Business Review* 68:103-111, 1990.

addition to having such early challenges, most leaders have developed appropriate skills and attained education, which allows them to further their leadership potential.

One of the most telling comments about leadership, management, and their application as it applies to the emergency department is attributed to Napoleon, who was reported to have said that he had to be present personally on the battlefield if his army was to win. As the battlefields on which his soldiers fought became larger, more complex, and more diverse, he simply could not be everywhere at once. His subsequent losses and ignominy were thus predictable. In the emergency department setting, neither a leader nor a manager can be present 24 hours a day, 7 days a week. Instead, it is essential to combine leadership and management skills to ensure that those who provide the service on a day-to-day basis have the motivation, tools, and inherent management and leadership attributes to ensure that high quality patient care occurs at all times.

LEADERSHIP STYLES

In their terse and tightly reasoned treatise *Leadership and the Quest for Integrity,* Badaracco and Ellsworth[2] present important insights for those who wish to understand the essential principles of leadership. The ideal organization has clear goals and expectations, has well-defined duties and responsibilities, has high-quality talent and clear-cut standards, promotes people on merit, is immune to bureaucracy, produces high level financial performance, and is ethical and principled in its internal and external approaches. The question is, how can such an organization be put into place? The answers are extremely difficult, but Badaracco and Ellsworth argue that successful leaders are able to do so only by approaching their organizations with certain prejudices, the most important of which is a quest for integrity, that spans moral, philosophic, and practical dimensions.

The authors argue that there are three extant attitudes about leadership, all of which fail to encompass the qualities needed for creation and maintenance of a successful organization, and which therefore are *leadership dilemmas*. The first dilemma holds that leadership is essentially due to *charisma* and is therefore rare, illusive, and cannot be taught. This school holds that "leaders are born, not made." This dilemma is not false; it is simply inadequate and misleading because it ignores the practical experience of leadership development from all walks of life, including the business community, the military, political realms, and certainly major leaders in the field of medicine. Although charisma can be important to a leader, this dilemma ignores the roles of experience, judgment, boldness, tenacity, and simple hard work on the part of those entrusted with leading organizations.

No less satisfying is the second dilemma, which holds that *training* is the main element necessary to produce leaders. This doctrine holds that management and leadership are quantifiable and can be transmitted in a scholarly and predictable manner to those who would pick up the leadership gauntlet. Training is certainly a necessary, but hardly a sufficient, condition to produce effective managers and leaders. Professional management knowledge is extremely important, but skills and techniques alone are not sufficient to produce progress, much less deal with the substantial amount of change that faces organizations at the present time. In addition, the *training dilemma* often leads to the *paralysis of analysis,* in which leaders and managers are often unable to act in clear and decisive fashions when faced with critical, time-dependent problems.

The third vision of leadership that presents a dilemma holds that the proper response to leadership and management challenges varies widely among situations. This *situational leadership* or *style* philosophy basically indicates that the appropriate response comes down to this: "It all depends." In its simplest form this simply means that the leader's style should vary with each situation and that the style should change as the circumstances dictate. The style dilemma has strong analogies to the development of situational ethics by Joseph Fletcher and his colleagues, but is subject to the same substantial and penetrating criticisms that greeted situation ethics.

Badaracco and Ellsworth indicate that all of these approaches are ultimately unable to account for the breadth and depth of leadership styles for an important and fundamental reason:

> In the end, there is a single powerful reason why charisma, professional management, and style are inadequate ways for managers to approach and resolve the dilemmas they face. Resolving dilemmas involves a person's philosophy of management. Whether they believe it or not, all managers have them. These philosophies are tacit, not explicit. The philosophies involve fundamental assumptions about human nature, about people and organizations, about the work of managers, and the kind of activities that lead to outstanding results. . . A few managers stop, reflect on, and make explicit philosophies of management and leadership. But these deep assumptions influence almost everything they do.[2]

After careful study of leaders and managers in a broad range of organizations, they classify three philosophies of leadership and management: (1) political leadership (2) directive leadership, and (3) values-driven leadership.

Political leadership is defined as a philosophy that human beings are essentially motivated by self-interest in a search for wealth, power, and coherence, while facing the similarly self-interested behavior of others, both within the organization and in other organizations. Like Machiavelli's Prince, the political leader is astute, but essentially selfish and manipulative. Political leadership is practiced by many well-intentioned leaders who nearly religiously promote the interests of their organizations or companies. The philosophy of political leadership holds that there are several *splintering forces* that detract from a company's efforts, including self-interest (the dominant motivator of human behavior), a zero-sum mentality (which requires clear winners and losers), increased specialization resulting from intense competition outside and complexity inside organizations, and local, focused interests of identified subunits.

In addition, certain inertial forces within organizations tend to cause them to drift toward inflexibility and excessive bureaucracy. The political leadership philosophy assumes that people seek security and resist change, which could increase their uncertainty or jeopardize their self-interest. These inertial forces include resistance to change, standard operating procedures, and "satisficing."[2] Resistance to change is addressed in some detail in Chapter 13, but it is well recognized that restraining forces can easily overpower enabling forces, as is classically demonstrated in the concept of force field analysis by Kurt Lewin. Inherent systems and standard operating procedures can often become inertial forces because they suppress initiative, cooperation, and improvement. "Satisficing" refers to behaviors that occur in organizations where workers and management combine to do "just enough" (and not one bit more) to meet goals, objectives, or specifications.

The central tenet of political leadership is that strong leaders must be adept at moving forward in small, incremental steps and at orchestrating their work astutely behind the scenes. This includes setting and communicating company goals, managing formal systems and structures, resolving conflicts, and managing day-to-day business. In summary, the political leadership philosophy recognizes self-interest as a primary motivating factor that relies on precise, carefully reasoned maneuvers to position the individual and the organization.

The *directive leadership* philosophy does not reject the realities of political leadership, but simply argues that they are too limited for explaining all of human motivation, because people are also driven by a competitive desire to achieve. Individuals desire personal responsibility for their decisions and clearly want the satisfaction of knowing that they have won through efforts that they have placed in action for the good of themselves and for the organization. This strong, innate desire to reach potential is described by Maslow as *self-actualization*.[13] In this analogy, as individuals strive for the ability to reach their potential, they marry their self-interest with corporate interest under the direction of strong leadership. In distinction to political leadership, directive leadership places primary importance on quantifiable facts, strategic substance, and the direct, personal, and individual involvement of the leader in guiding the organization to improve performance. The directive leader makes three essential assumptions:

- People are motivated far more by internal forces than external forces.
- Coherence comes to organizations with great difficulty.
- Both coherence and substance are more important than the methods used to attain them.

Thus the central concept of directive leadership is that the manager/leader must of necessity have a clear, direct, and forceful vision of the organization and provide "unremitting personal determination and direct, personal action."[2]

The *values-driven* leadership philosophy ratchets the directive leader's philosophy even further, adding the dimension that people need to find meaning in life through their experience at work, such meaning being derived from the ability to use creativity in the service of broader, more worthwhile purposes. This philosophy holds that creativity, commitment, compassion, and energy can be unleashed from individuals collectively working toward broader motives. In this regard, the values-driven leader has as a primary purpose the need to shape an organization so that its values and ideals are strongly tied to its individual members. Badaracco and Ellsworth offer a substantially deeper vision of leadership in that the philosophy of values-driven leadership is not simply an alternative to political and directive leadership, but actually transcends it. They concur with Phillip Selznick, who indicated that a leader is "primarily an expert in the promotion and protection of values."[13] The concept of values-driven or principle-centered leadership has a rich but incompletely articulated heritage. For example, leaders such as James McGregor Burns[14] had stressed the moral character of leadership and emphasized its "transforming" and "transcending" qualities, as opposed to "transactional" leadership, in which exchanges of money, status, power, and authority occur for the actions that they want their workers to take. As Burns indicated:

> Transforming leadership ultimately becomes moral in that it raises the level of human conduct and ethical aspirations of both leader and led, and thus it has a transforming effect on both. . . Transcending leadership is dynamic leadership in the sense that the leaders throw themselves into a relationship with followers, who will feel singly "elevated" by it and often become more active themselves, thereby creating new cadres of leaders.[14]

The concept of transcending and transforming leadership is particularly applicable to settings in which the "real work" of the business occurs in settings of autonomy. In such situations, excessive top-down intervention can undermine appropriate values, whereas autonomy without appropriate standards and accountability can result in substandard and lackadaisical performance. In that regard, values-driven leadership would seem to apply particularly to the emergency department, inasmuch as the activity of seeing patients on the day-to-day basis requires substantial degrees of autonomy at multiple levels of the emergency department team.

Much of the current literature on transformational leadership[15-17] owes a significant philosophic debt to the work of Burns[14] and Badaracco and Ellsworth.[2] Nonetheless, transformational leadership adds specific dimensions of change management and delineates three areas that must be addressed: (1) reorganizing the need for revitalization and awakening, (2) creating a new vision or envisioning, and (3) institutionalizing or rearchitecting the change.[15]

In the analysis of Badaracco and Ellsworth, individuals need to look at each of these leadership styles and help determine, in each individual situation, the extent to which their decisions and actions reflect these philosophies. They conclude that the most effective managers and leaders avoid the difficulties of the three dilemmas of charisma, professional management, and style and instead argue that successful managers and leaders are consistent across situations in their behaviors, which, at its bedrock, reflect their philosophy of management. They also argue that, in and of themselves, none of the three philosophies of leadership are completely sufficient. However, they do note, through careful analysis of practical examples of leadership and management, that a combination of directive and values-driven management philosophies are most likely to succeed in the current environment. This does not ignore the tough minded realism of the political management philosophy, but simply recognizes that it is hazardous for the long term and less successful than a balance of directive and values-driven approaches.

WHY IS LEADERSHIP RARE?

Despite the numerous distinctions and delineations made between leadership and management in this chapter, why is leadership found so rarely in our organizations, in our educational institutions, and in our day-to-day practices of emergency medicine? Although the issue is admittedly complex, it can be understood. One reason that leadership is rare is the lack of understanding of the distinctions between leadership and management detailed earlier in this chapter. As we are able to have a more complete and widely shared understanding of these distinctions, it is likely that we will find a clearer path toward leadership. Some of the fault clearly lies within ourselves. We have many misguided assumptions about human behavior and how best to motivate and channel individuals toward desired outcomes. As Shakespeare said in *Julius Caesar,* "The fault, dear Brutus, lies not in the stars, but in ourselves, that we are underlings." Too often we reduce human motivation only to the self-interest and pursuit of power, money, and authority, and ignore the legitimate place that serving worthwhile ends plays in human motivation.

An additional reason for rarity of leadership is our societal and educational structure. Bluntly, that structure has stressed conformity, consistency, and rigidity, often at the expense of primary leadership traits of individuality, vision, and uniqueness. If we take seriously James Burns' concept of leadership as transforming and transcending, we would expect leaders to raise the level of human conduct within their organization. This is often difficult to do when the educational and societal structures excessively resist change and enforce uniformity.

Finally, although it may be unpleasant to consider, the rarity of leadership is often a simple lack of courage. As Bismarck once noted, "Courage on the battlefield is common among us. But you will frequently find very respectable people lacking in civil courage." This lack of courage often boils down to a simple inability to exert pressure to accede to the demands of the particular situations, accepting a convenient solution to a problem that requires far more understanding and complexity. If the leader's role is to transform and transcend common levels of human conduct, the leader must have the courage to act clearly and decisively on the actions required for enacting the vision of the organization. Courage and integrity therefore lie at the center of what leadership must be. Courage and integrity imply a level of intellectual, personal, professional, and ethical honesty that are indeed rare in isolation, and exceedingly so in combination. In fact, the path to personal leadership requires consistent dedication to such goals, which can result in leadership of extraordinary capability.

STEWARDSHIP

Although traditional concepts of leadership and management are deeply ingrained and would seem to have served business and industry well, Block[4] has pointed out that there is an "underbelly of leadership," which has largely been unrecognized. He argues persuasively that our present concepts of leadership lead to patriarchy, colonialism, and excessively dependent workers and middle managers. Most organizations have an essentially patriarchal structure in which leadership attempts to create accountability through the centralization of power, privilege, and position. Top managers and leaders are responsible for strategy and vision, middle management is responsible for defining tactics, and the providers simply implement. Too often there is little interchange between these levels of the organization, resulting in disenfranchisement of those who provide the service and inability of those at the top of the organization to understand how work is done, much less what the interface with the customer feels like. In such organizations, managers and leaders attempt to create accountability by giving order to the centralization of power, which creates a hierarchy in which leaders and managers:

- Are central to meaningful change
- Prescribe what change is best for others
- Define desired organizational behaviors
- Appraise and pay to ensure alignment
- Provide parenting with a human touch

Such organizations and their entirely well-intentioned leaders are born out of rich traditions in education, parenting, and organizational dynamics. Block observes that such structures and the organizations that produce them have certain inherent, inexorable but largely unintended consequences. Chief among these is the development of a system that essentially subjugates the provider, specifically because of the assumption that leadership is responsible for the control and direction of the organization and its people. The provider therefore becomes dependent, relying on the belief that those in power know what is best both for the organization and those who work within it. This can be a subtly seductive concept for the provider in some ways, because it is a short logical step to conclude that the leader is therefore responsible for creating an environment structured not only for business success, but also for provider happiness and career stability. Too often staff blame leadership and management for the place in which they find themselves, generating such comments as, "Staff morale is at an all time low. Leadership and management are failing us."

Although dependency and paternalism are inherent in management and leadership concepts as they have been developed, it should not be assumed that leaders and managers desire dominance. Rather, the structures themselves are based on an autocratic, hierarchical governance system that understandably withers the spirit of those in the system. Further, providers themselves lay their autonomy at the feet of the leader in the quest for order, the desire to be taken care of, and the safety of defined boundaries in which the provider is responsible only for limited tasks, not the totality of the product or service. This concept of leadership, while it has had great appeal, simply will not carry us the distance we need to go in creating organizations in which providers are fully empowered to deliver quality service, in addition to creating a vision for further improvement. Block notes that, in our focus on leadership, we have given over to patriarchy, paternalism, and an "intimate colonialism" in which consistency, control, and predictability are valued above all else. As he notes:

> To state it bluntly, strong leadership does not have within itself the capability to create the fundamental changes our organizations require. It is not the fault of the people in these positions. It is the fault of the way we have all framed the role. Our search for strong leadership in others expresses a desire for others to assume the ownership and responsibility for our group, our organization, our society. The effect is to localize power, purpose, and privilege in the one we call the leader. Focusing power and purpose at one point in

organization, usually the top, has over time the impact of destroying the culture and very outcomes we sincerely intend to create.[4]

How do we avoid this outcome? According to Block, three choices must be made:

- Choosing partnership over patriarchy
- Choosing adventure (empowerment) over safety (entitlement)
- Choosing service over self-interest

Choosing Partnership Over Patriarchy

Patriarchy constitutes the belief that, to reach a common goal, there must be centralization of control, consistency, predictability, and power. In relying too heavily on these aspects, the purpose and vision of the organization and its people become displaced. If ownership, responsibility, and accountability are needed from core workers, the model of patriarchy simply cannot go the distance to deliver them, because accountability is stolen from the middle of the organization. In patriarchal organizations, too much of the focus of the provider is on the boss or the hierarchical structure of the organization itself. In such circumstances, those who actually provide services have a difficult time being accountable because the focus of control is at the top of the organization. Perhaps one of the most telling questions to determine if an organization is patriarchal, is "Who is your most important customer?" If your boss is your most important customer and decisions regarding how to make changes within the organization and its processes are focused on the response of those in power, the organization is patriarchal by nature, with all of its attendant limitations.

Even when patriarchal organizations are dressed in the attractive, finely spun cloth of "leadership," these limitations still exist. In many circumstances, entirely well-intentioned leaders have made cosmetic calls for *empowerment, entrepreneurism,* or, far worse, *intrapreneurism* for those in the middle and bottom of the organization. However, unless serious thought and effort are given to changing the structure and operations of the organization to a partnership mentality, such exhortations remain cosmetic in nature and do not change the essential foundation of the organization. More important, such initiatives invariably result in embitterment and disenfranchisement because they collapse under the weight of their own self-created limitations, with managers, leaders, and providers each blaming the other for the failure of the grand experiment in cosmetic change. As Block notes, "When patriarchy asks its own organization to be more entrepreneurial and empowered, it is asking people to break the rules that patriarchy itself has created and enforces."[4]

Partnership is diametrically opposed to the concept of patriarchy and occurs when control goes from managers to core workers, from suppliers to customers, from doctors to patients, from teachers to students, and from community agencies to citizens. Block delineates four requirements for the partnership equation: (1) Exchange of purpose, (2) The right to say no, (3) Joint accountability, and (4) absolute honesty.

Exchange of purpose and partnership involves a clear definition of purpose and vision at all levels of the organization. Although it is fine for leadership and management to have a vision statement, the vision should define *their* piece of the organization, but should not legislate strictly the boundaries and parameters of the vision for the entire organization. Rather, a dialogue must occur at each level of the organization, which can be guided by the principles of the vision and mission of leadership and management, but which does not totally constrain the organization's creativity in further defining the mission and vision as it relates to the whole. Genuine dialogue is essential to such an endeavor because individuals truly discover their own sense of purpose through dialogue both between themselves and the individuals in the other layers of the organization. Each level of the organization therefore should be responsible for defining mission, values, and levels of control through the discovery of dialogue. In too many organizations, mission and vision are established centrally, and the staff are "enrolled" into the organization. This is, as Block wryly notes, "soft core colonialism" and should be avoided at all costs. The very term "enrollment" strongly implies forcing those at the middle and lower levels of the organization to get on board, get motivated, get with the plan, get focused—all with the real intent of ensuring compliance to an externally applied vision. When genuine dialogue begins at each level of the organization, true exchange of purpose has begun. Equally important, most organizations that have begun this journey have found well-trained and articulate providers who are capable of a level of creativity and confidence that pays substantial rewards not only to the customer, but also to the organization and its leadership.

The *right to say no* is not a right to be obstructive or obstreperous. It is simply an acknowledgment that, although you may lose the argument, you never lose your voice. The concept of exchange of purpose ensures that each voice is heard, not that the end result is simply the lowest common denominator of those voices. Instead, the right to say no is an acknowledgment of the value of the provider's skills, talents, abilities, and opinions. However, a call to dialogue is not a call to anarchy.

The third requirement of partnership is *joint accountability.* This simply means that bosses are no longer caretakers, coaches, or associates because the price of the freedom of dialogue is to take personal accountability on an ongoing basis for that part of the organization or process in which one is involved. Many organizations, particularly those in the healthcare setting, seem to have a deep wish for a benevolent monarch, on whose doorstep all of our burdens, troubles, frustrations, and hostilities toward the inequities of the system can be laid. Leadership and management often accept this burden, incorrectly assuming that it is their job to ensure that all of the providers are happy, stimulated, and proud of a job that is essentially demoralizing by its very nature. This is a dangerous and, frankly, deeply troubled view of the relationship between leadership/management and the providers. As stated previously the complaint that, "Morale is at an all time low" is often heard. The unstated, but clearly intended corollary is, "And it is your fault!" The concept of joint accountability inherent in partnership recognizes that morale, as well as purpose, vision, operational processes, protocols, etc, are truly a joint responsibility that arises out of the ongoing dialogue between the providers and their leadership.

The requirement for *absolute honesty* in partnership may seem both obvious and odd. In traditional hierarchical and patriarchal structures, however, one of the guiding principles is that knowledge is power. The unstated, but clearly palpable result is that knowledge is therefore hoarded and kept to oneself, rather than shared. Concepts such as information control, managing the message, and guiding perceptions all reek of obfuscation and unclear communication, guided by an essentially patriarchal structure that is not truly intellectually honest.

Is commitment to these four principles of partnership enough? Bluntly, no. Although these principles begin to change both the structure and the relationship of a patriarchal organization, the hard work of ongoing commitment to these principles is essential. Over time, the needs of the customers and providers become more important than the needs of those responsible for leading the organization, which in itself further assists in the transition from a patriarchal to a partnership environment.

Nonetheless, essential changes are still necessary in the role of the boss. How does the role of the boss change in a partnership model? First of all, in the spirit of being deeply committed to cosmetic change, many organizations have used terms such as *associate, coach,* and *facilitator,* to describe the new role for bosses (leaders, managers, etc.) in an organization. Although there certainly may be elements of these terms in the new role for bosses, it would be extremely difficult in the current fiscal environment to justify a layer in the organization that simply provides vision statements, coordinates training, and cheers on the providers. The concept of the leader as coach is particularly disturbing, connoting substantial degrees of control and manipulation on the part of the coach compared with the players. As Block indicates, people wearing shorts are not in power positions. (The same might be said of those who wear scrubs.)

Instead, the nature of the boss changes substantially to that of a broker and banker. The banking functions are particularly important, as management and leadership are responsible for providing the financial underpinnings in negotiating with others both within and outside of the organization to ensure that there is appropriate financial support. In addition, leaders, managers, and bosses also have a substantial brokering function, handling a series of issues including boundary management and negotiation with others both within and outside the organization to ensure that nonfinancial resources are also provided to those who deliver the service on a daily basis.

A strong analogy exists here between Block's work and the work of healthcare. In an emergency department setting, the roles of the chair and nursing director of the emergency department can often be stated in extraordinarily succinct terms:

1. To deliver the best possible patient care and customer service available.
2. To provide an environment in which providers have the resources, training, and technical support available to deliver patient care.

It is important to note that it is *not* the role of the leader or manager in these circumstances to ensure the entitlement of each provider, but rather to ensure that the tools, financial support, and other resources are available for the patient and the providers. This is an important distinction in moving from a patriarchal to a partnership model. Caring should be a human act, not a supervisory act. Patriarchy is sustained by our love of leadership, which creates accountability by giving order to the centralization of power. Typically, this means that the top creates changes, prescribes what is best for others, defines desired behaviors, appraises and pays for such behaviors, and constitutes parenting with a human touch in the best of circumstances and dictatorial control in the worst.

Partnership on the other hand is sustained by seeking stewardship, which creates accountability by giving order through a thoughtful, reasoned dispersion of power in appropriate fashions to those who provide the service on a day-to-day basis. Stewardship or partnership organizations have core work teams that are essential to change and that are chosen with a focus on the customer, not the boss. In such organizations, the end of caretaking has been signaled and the beginning of citizenship has occurred. Entitlement is ending and is being replaced by genuine empowerment, which is discussed in the next section.

In essence, stewardship offers a choice in exchange for a promise. The choice is a chance to accept the challenge of partnership, empowerment, and service. The promise is a commitment to an invitation to the playing field in which four questions are asked and answered through genuine dialogue throughout the organization.

1. What is the nature of the choice/invitation?
    - What is the playing field? (see later)
    - Who are the members involved?
    - What is the nature of the social contract? (patriarchy? partnership?)
2. What are core elements of the playing field?
    - What compelling value does our organization bring to the marketplace?
    - What outcomes are essential?
        - Customer
        - Employee
        - Economic
3. What are the constraints, the elements that are "untouchables?" List them and make them known.
4. What is the basic governing strategy of the organization?

Attention should be focused on this dialogue throughout the organization.

In summary, the first choice in developing stewardship is choosing partnership over patriarchy by addressing the questions discussed here. There should be no inconsistency between practicing stewardship, and continuing to be a boss. Stewardship is simply the willingness to use power without using reward, punishment, and directive authority as the primary means of getting things done. Leadership essentially performs the same functions, but is simultaneously concerned with the acquisition and centralization of power, privilege, and control.

Choosing Adventure (Empowerment) Over Safety (Entitlement)

To begin to choose adventure or empowerment over the safety of our well-recognized entitlement mentality is the second choice, which is as difficult as the first. In most organizations a deep cynicism surrounds the concept of *empowerment* largely because the word empowerment has been spoken, when in fact *entitlement* is what has been meant. To begin to address this issue is to understand how to deal with people's deep wish to be taken care of, to maintain the status quo, and to recognize the deep wish for a benevolent monarch, which is inherent in all of us. Entitlement is largely built on years of experience in which people truly believe that their interests are more important than that of the organization and that the business exists largely for the individual's sake. Loyalty is the prime value of entitlement and is rewarded with safety and stability as an implied bond. As limiting as this concept of entitlement is, it involves a high degree of safety, because loyalty, even when it is grudging, has often been mustered.

Many leaders and managers have taken their organizations on an absurd journey of empowerment, giving verbal assurances that empowerment is the goal, while maintaining a structure that totally precludes it. In such organizations, empowerment is measured, appraised, and rewarded. Training is provided to ensure that everyone has the prescribed core competencies of empowerment, but the training occurs in an environment of deep commitment to cosmetic change, resulting in providers who are constrained, not empowered. Most management training is designed to make patriarchy palatable and therefore helps feed the entitlement mentality.

To begin to make the choice of empowerment over entitlement requires individuals to make the decision to reclaim their own sovereignty, which begins by answering several questions. What kind of place will we work in? What kind of culture will we create? What kind of people will we be? How will we define our organization and ourselves on a daily basis? Block astutely notes that our consciousness is where the revolution begins because 50% of the work must be on ourselves. This is a difficult transition because we love the current system (and its safety) because we were born, raised, and trained in it; because we have succeeded quite well in it; and because we know its borders and its boundaries. Although it is not an essentially deeply satisfying system, it is nonetheless palatable and well known to us. Further, professionals have a long and glorious history of celebrating the defeat of others in this system, inasmuch as most successful people have gotten where they are by rising to the top.

How then do we acknowledge that accountability comes through acts of choice? How do we begin to engage people in acts of choice in which safety and entitlement are given up for adventure and empowerment? First, it is important to recognize that for most people this is a step into uncertainty. Although patriarchy has its limitations, those are largely known limitations. Partnership is frightening because it is unknown, uncharted territory. Second, people must begin to accept the reality that the answer to the question, "Are you here to build a career or to build an organization?" must be clear and without hesitation: We are here first to build the organization. Third, instead of expecting our leaders or managers to give us direction and purpose, our job becomes teaching those above us how an effective community can be created in which the patient and customer interact with the providers in ways that are substantially more satisfying to both because their needs are first sought and acknowledged and then met. Partnership and empowerment are thus a commitment to a dialogue concerning these issues, not an act of concession. Finally, lest this seem too much of a revolution from within, it must be made clear that, with rare exceptions, the leaders we have are just fine; new ones do not need to be recruited. What does need to occur is a redefinition of leaders as stewards, moving away from reward, punishment, and directive authority toward service, empowerment, and partnership.

Choosing Service Over Self-Interest

Choosing service over self-interest is the third choice in the stewardship equation. This choice involves ensuring that leaders, managers, and providers hold in trust the well-being of the organization, not their individual self-interest. Most organizations have sought compliance with management's dictates, exhibited largely through directive authority, all in the name of predictability, control, and power. In fact, compliance is the antithesis of true accountability, simply because it undermines emotional ownership, investment, and empowerment. It is not surprising therefore that compliance is often grudging in nature.

Much of the reason for the dissonance between desired accountability and grudging compliance is that leaders, managers, and providers recognize that the organization has separated those who manage from those who do. What is necessary is a reintegration of the management of work with doing the work, which can only occur through the genuine dialogue among leaders, managers, and providers outlined previously. Without this dialogue, calling for the choice of service over self-interest is in itself hollow, self-serving, and protective of essentially patriarchal structures.

Drawing from the work of Gandhi, Block outlines three important features of stewardship regarding the concept of service. First, power is granted from those we lead. Traditional concepts of leadership in which the leader is the central focus of power and control are largely inadequate for leading organizations in turbulent times of change. Instead, it has become increasingly clear that power is truly granted from the center of the organization. Second, our contribution is primarily our humanity; it is impossible to be a good leader without being a good person. This contrasts with formulations in which the leader is considered to be the repository of knowledge, power, control, finances, etc. Third, what is true and important is known to each of us. What distinguishes the leader is in many cases the courage to state what is true and the integrity to act on it. Each of these three tenets contributes to the concept of choosing service over self-interest.

Because of these features, and because of the necessity of reintegrating managing the work with doing the work, Block's concept of stewardship has been described as "teaching revolution to the ruling class."[4] The description is accurate in that stewardship depends on a willingness to be accountable for results without using control or caretaking as the means to reach them. This involves several components. First, choosing service over self-interest is an essential affirmation of the spirit and helps address essential needs, as outlined in numerous formulations, including that of Maslow.[13] Second, many of our fundamental beliefs on how to use power and accountability to organize work fail to produce intended results. Third, the dominant belief that leaders lead and followers follow is responsible for both low morale and dependency within our organizations. Fourth, the separation of managing the work from doing the work has resulted in deep and persistent customer service failures in many businesses and industries, with many businesses offering services and products that do not answer essential customer needs. Healthcare in particular has been subject to this problem. Fifth, our existing organizational dynamics and work structures reflect the primacy of consistency, control, and predictability, instead of focusing on the needs of our most essential customers, including the internal customer—the provider. Finally, all of this results in an increasing awareness that change is needed; however, the actions of our organizations in response to the need for change uniformly disappoint. In essence, although patriarchy is a root cause of the malaise and service failure, we attempt to use patriarchial means to solve the problem.

It is essential therefore that a choice be made between service and self-interest. Until meaningful dialogue begins with regard to recreating the organization around concepts of partnership, empowerment, and service, the transition cannot be accomplished, no matter how much activity we may place into cosmetic reform.

Defining the Stewardship Contract

In beginning the transition toward stewardship, it is important to recognize that both the journey and destination are important. It is impossible to choose between them because the destination is not a predetermined place, nor can a prescribed pathway be followed in a cookie-cutter fashion—"Do this and everything will be fine." Such an approach reeks of the inherent patriarchy and paternalism that stewardship seeks to surmount in the first place. Defining the stewardship contract is work and always begins with the dialogue concerning partnership over patriarchy, empowerment over entitlement, and service over self-interest. It is hard work because of the degree to which patriarchy has permeated educational structures, child rearing, organizational dynamics, and even, one might argue, religion. Further, most of us have not been educated to any substantial degree in some of what might be considered the "discovery tools" necessary for the journey from patriarchy to stewardship, including conflict-resolution, negotiation skills, change management skills, and essential communication skills necessary for the dialogue itself. Nonetheless, all of these issues can and should be answered in the course of the transition, and the necessary skills can be readily acquired.

In beginning to define the stewardship contract, it is also somewhat discouraging that simply trying to copy others results in mimicry, not the learning and discovery that are necessary for the organization to redefine itself. The popular emergence of benchmarking is fine for establishing hope that organizations can make the transition and is certainly beneficial in raising aspirations. However, benchmarking should never be confused as an answer to the question, "How?" This has to be discovered through the process itself.

How then can we begin to define the initial work of the journey? To begin with, as Block has indicated, more than 50% of the work must be done on ourselves, which is why stewardship constitutes a revolution of the ruling class. Once that step has been taken, several others follow. First, maximize choice for those who are closest to the work. Use the provider to answer two important questions, "Who is the customer?" and "What do I need to have available to me to serve the customer?" Second, reintegrate managing and doing. This requires partially dismantling essential hierarchical and patriarchal structures within the organization. Does this constitute downsizing? Not necessarily. Although downsizing may be one of the results, it should never be one of the original intentions. Instead, this is simply a recommitment to what Zaleznik[39] called the "real work" of the organization. Third, to the extent that measurements and controls are necessary within the organization, those measurements and controls should serve core workers and providers, as well as the customers they serve. Measurements and controls should not be primarily for the purpose of providing information to managers and leaders who are constantly appraising and reappraising the provider.

Fourth, leaders should support local solutions to the problems that are unearthed through this process. There is a natural tendency to lay difficult problems at the doorstep of leaders and managers because that is the way that organizations have been run for years. Resist the temptation to step in by providing solutions. Rather, rededicate the providers and support their efforts at determining their own solutions to these problems. As broker and banker, bosses should be willing to commit resources and support and should avoid any "magic wand" resolutions. Fifth, there should be a clarion call that "service is everything" both within the realms of management and the providers. The concept of service should permeate the organization, including service to the customer, and to those who provide that service. Sixth, secrecy within the organization should be ended. Knowledge *is* power and therefore should be shared as widely within the organization as possible. In many cases, disseminating this information may require changes in management information systems. Seventh, leaders and managers should make clear to the providers that the stewardship contract constitutes both a redefinition of the organization and the requirement of a promise for the providers to commit themselves completely to the process and to the organization. Finally, the stewardship contract involves an essential redistribution of the power and, in most cases, the wealth of the organization.

Unless there is an essential commitment to this redistribution of both power and privilege, the call for commitment to the process will ring hollow. As mentioned previously, the contract itself involves defining the core mission of the unit, ensuring that there is financial accountability, clearly describing the existing structure and the constraints it entails, discussing basic governance strategy and its changes, and focusing appropriate attention and resources on the difficult journey this transition represents.

Defining the stewardship contract is difficult, primarily because of an essential paradox that develops. Patriarchy, using a mixture of leadership, consistency, control, and predictability attempts to implement a new system of empowerment, partnership, and self-management. Understandably, patriarchy most often simply reinvents itself by living out the promise of its own demise. Further, the transition to a culture of stewardship is often difficult for the providers themselves, inasmuch as all of us have some degree of longing for a benevolent monarch. One of the most common symptoms of a deep longing for parenting is providers' disgruntlement during the course of the transition, which is often a symptom that they either want a better parent or to be the parent themselves. Although the transition is daunting, it is one well worth the physical, intellectual, and emotional price.

The Emotional Work of Stewardship

At its essence, the transition to stewardship involves a personal choice to be of service and to be accountable without having to be in charge. It should not occur out of a desire to please or to change the circumstances of dependency and dominance to a structure in which power, control, and consistency are simply redistributed to another level of the organization. Until we are able to take back ownership of accountability, we cannot hope to extend it to those with whom we work. Many emergency department managers find themselves in a position where the staff want to be empowered. The staff thus think that leaders and managers have the power and simply will not give it up. Part of the paradox is that the leaders and managers of emergency departments often want to give up power, but that feel the staff are unready, unwilling, or unable to take it. Thus continues the crazy spiral of the patriarchal structure, which demands an answer to the question, "Who is in charge here?" Shouldn't the answer be, "We are"? Until the organization can renegotiate the internal transaction wherein our expectations are reformed, beginning with the needs of those we serve, we cannot hope to have all levels of the organization say "We are!"

In making this transition of our expectations, it is important to recognize that it is not an either/or equation. There are both dependent and autonomous parts in each of us, often on a single issue. Accepting this paradox simply means that, first, the problem is in our control, and second, for those who choose to resist partnership and empowerment, there is always something within them we can reach because it is within ourselves as well. When that resistance is encountered, using our understanding of our own resistance therefore can be invaluable in assuring them that the difficult process of the transition is worthwhile.

At the same time, when leaders and managers make clear that they no longer can act as caretakers or controllers, it is imperative that something real, palpable, and meaningful be given in return. What should be given is the assurance that there is both a real choice and a real promise. The real choice is participation in defining and creating an organization's purpose and in which partnership, empowerment, and service have genuine meaning. The real promise is that, through this process, control over the ways in which work gets done and managed will be an essential function of the providers and that the results of their hard work will be put into place within the organization. A sure sign of genuine progress is a provider who is skillful at both articulating the principles, purposes, mission, and vision of the organization, as well as insisting that others construct their own pathways to this destination.

The goals of stewardship are to choose partnership over patriarchy, empowerment over entitlement, and service over self-interest. More specifically, leaders and managers define the playing field and make the invitation, but the specific vision and mission are defined through the dialogue that occurs among those who provide the service itself. Second, the organization must be committed to widespread business literacy that involves the use of a common language, so that both the choice and the promise have a shared meaning. Third, specific implementation should be designed by each unit of the organization, with a structure focused on the customers and their needs, using unique learning events, and qualitative measures designed by those being measured, rather than those doing the measuring. Fourth, managers and providers should work together responsibly in core work teams that are close to the customer and do the difficult work of redesigning the processes to meet their needs. Finally, the transition to stewardship involves the distinct and palpable redistribution of power and privilege within the organization to make work more self-directed, so that "manager" and "leader" are tasks, not levels within the organization, and so that there is full disclosure of information.

In many respects, Block's work is a radical assessment of the inherent limitations of our commitment to placing power, privilege, and control in the hands of leaders and managers, as opposed to deeper within the organization. Properly viewed, the work does not refute the importance of the leadership and management skills listed previously, but in fact complements them. Although the choice of partnership, empowerment, and service seem both attractive and simple, Block rightly notes that this transition runs directly counter to much of our societal emphasis on patriarchy, hierarchical structure, and the need for directive authority. Rather than presenting a prescribed detailed format, Block argues that such a format defeats the purpose by denying the essential and necessary dialogue that must occur during the course of the organization's discovery and rediscovery of itself. Perhaps his own words best summarize the essence of the stewardship concept.

> If we took responsibility for freedom, commited ourselves to service, and had faith that our security lay in ourselves, you could stop asking the question, "How?" You would see that we have the answer. In every case the answer to the question "How?" is "Yes." It places the location of the solution in the right place. With the questioner.[4]

LEADERSHIP, MANAGEMENT, AND STEWARDSHIP IN THE EMERGENCY DEPARTMENT

Taken as a whole, the preceding discussion might seem to indicate that the role of a leader is preferable to that of a manager. Who would not aspire to be thought of as the individual responsible for setting the vision and direction of the organization, as opposed to slugging it out on the day-to-day details of emergency department operations? It is essential to recognize, however, that the practical nature of emergency department operations is such that skills of leadership, management, and stewardship must be present in all of those who are charged with responsibility. Why is this the case? First, the nature of emergency department organizational structures (addressed in more detail in Chapters 3 and 4) is such that, with rare exceptions, the leaders and managers of an emergency department are not stratified into multiple layers, as are most business organizations. Second, most emergency department managers or leaders also provide day-to-day clinical service to the patient and to the other members of the department. Thus roles of the manager and leader are far less distinct in an emergency department setting than in many other areas of the hospital. The leader and manager must also work on a day-to-day basis to provide the services they are responsible for managing. Third, one of the most important aspects of gaining respect as a leader and manager in the emergency department setting is to ensure a high level of clinical competence on the part of the manager and leader. Particularly among members of the medical staff, regardless of how effective an individual's leadership and management skills may be, it is also critical that he or she be respected as a competent clinician in the day-to-day evaluation and treatment of emergency department patients. This may be less true for nurse-managers, who in some cases are not involved in day-to-day clinical care on an ongoing basis. Nonetheless, for emergency department physicians, there are few circumstances in which leaders and managers are not also providers of daily clinical service. Finally, practical emergency department management experience has generally shown the limitations of a patriarchal, directive authority model. Rather, emergency department management, by its very nature, lends itself to the concepts of empowerment, service, and collaboration as developed in the stewardship model. By nature, the practice of emergency medicine is a participative, collaborative approach among emergency physicians, emergency nurses, and multiple other healthcare providers cooperating in delivering service to their patients.

Distinct management, leadership, and stewardship skills *must* be developed in those who are responsible for providing supervision for the emergency department. Not surprisingly, some will find a mantle of leadership easier to assume than that of day-to-day, "in the trenches" management. It is highly unlikely, however, that an individual can aspire to or attain the position as a leader in the emergency department without establishing basic competencies at the management level because both management and leadership skills are necessary for the department to succeed. Sadly, the majority of formal educational training for physicians in management and leadership skills has been lacking, consisting largely of on-the-job training. Successful emergency departments need to ensure that their educational structure is one that addresses not only clinical needs, but also the personal and professional development of leaders and managers within the emergency department. This approach should always be handled in a collaborative fashion, wherein the physician and nursing staff are provided similar, if not identical, training and exposure to similar types of philosophies with regard to leadership and management development.

Management focuses on complexity and dealing with it in an effective fashion to reach the organization's goals; leadership focuses on establishing vision, aligning people, and managing change in an effective fashion. An emergency department without leadership has no rudder and drifts aimlessly without any clear sense of purpose. An emergency department without effective management has no engine to drive the organization through the difficult seas of change toward some recognizable and attainable goal. Both leadership and management are clearly essential to effective emergency department operations and are particularly necessary for the organization to progress toward fully recognizing its potential and that of its team members.

Creating a Learning Organization in the Emergency Department

In a classic treatise, Senge[18] argued persuasively for creating *learning organizations* to help manage through the dramatic changes currently facing business, industry, and healthcare. Senge defined the learning organization thusly:

> Learning organizations are places where people continually expand their ability to create the results they truly desire, where new and expansive patterns of thinking are nurtured, where collective aspiration is set free, and where people are continually learning to learn together.[18]

Basing his work partly on the theories of organizational learning of Argyris,[19] Stata,[20] and Kauffman,[21] Senge indicated that what primarily distinguishes a learning organization from a traditional, authoritarian organization is a mastery of certain basic disciplines:

- Systems thinking
- Personal mastery
- Mental models
- Shared vision
- Team learning

Focusing on these five disciplines requires a fairly dramatic paradigm shift or, as Senge refers to it, *metanoia*. Much of this need for a paradigm shift or change in the way we perceive things is because of a lack of training in dealing with systems thinking, which Senge describes as *the fifth discipline,* which is the title of his book. His primary reasoning is that the core learning dilemma is that "we learn best from experience, but we never directly experience the consequences of many of our most important decisions." This is similar to the Jewish philosopher Elie Wiesel's insight that the fundamental injustice of the human situation is that we accept or reject situations that only develop fully later, when it is already too late.

The elements of systems thinking were pioneered by Ackoff,[22] Hardin,[23] and Forrester.[24] One of the central tenets of systems thinking is viewing an organization and its processes with a view toward *integration,* viewing the whole of the entity, as opposed to the separate parts. The focus therefore is on the dynamic complexity of the whole, instead of the individual component parts. The analogy often used is that one can have a complete understanding of each of the component parts of an automobile, but if the automobile is broken apart and understood only in terms of the functions of its component parts, there can be no true sense of understanding of the interrelationship of the parts to form the meaningful whole that constitutes the automobile itself. Thus despite a complete understanding of the parts, or even the systems comprising parts of the automobile (e.g., electrical system, mechanical system, drive train), the overall function of the automobile cannot be truly understood, managed, much less driven toward its destination.

A second key precept of systems thinking is attention to interdependent processes over time, as opposed to snapshots or one-time events. The failure of nonsystems thinking to recognize, much less focus on these interdependent processes, has been a major failing of organizations and institutions and is particularly pertinent to healthcare institutions. Although the origins of systems thinking are tentacular in nature, two essential origins are the feedback concept, first developed in cybernetics, and the concept of servomechanisms, derived from engineering theory that has been extant since the early twentieth century. Systems theory combines these concepts in a way that allows a vision of interrelationships that creates a discipline for seeing wholes as more than the sum of their parts. Systems theory recognizes both the common place and commonly recognized aspect of *detail complexity,* which is what most people think about when they entertain the concept of complexity. Detail complexity simply recognizes that there is often a high degree of variability in the output of work processes, but fails to quantify and act on the complexity. Systems theory recognizes a far more important aspect of *dynamic complexity,* which indicates that substantial cause-and-effect relationships exist such that the effects of intervention over time are often subtle and incompletely recognized. Most solutions in the past have dealt with detail complexity, but this simply results in a situation in which complexity is fraught with further complexity, resulting in confusion and increased waste, instead of improved outcomes. System theory recognizes that the best hope for improvement deals with acting on areas of dynamic complexity, in which the interrelationships between the parts of the system are operational.

Focusing on the application of systems theory to areas of dynamic complexity results in what Senge describes as maximal *leverage*. Leverage simply refers to strategic interventions guided by careful statistical study that result in maximal changes, often seemingly disproportionate to the interventions themselves. Because changes focus on areas of dynamic complexity, as opposed to detail complexity, the potential for improvement of the system is greatly increased. The concept can be demonstrated with the analogy of the trim tab. Turning a large ship or sailboat can often be a difficult venture because the rudder is pushing against a substantial amount of mass and force. Recognizing this dilemma in changing the course of a large ship or sailboat, R. Buckminster Fuller designed the concept of the trim tab, which is essentially a small tab attached to the rudder, which helps initiate movement of a rudder more energy-efficiently. Because of the application of a trim tab, the rudder can be moved much more easily and the ship or sailboat's course can be altered in a much more rapid and radical fashion.

Senge summarizes the essence of the discipline of systems thinking as a *metanoia* or paradigm shift from:

- Seeing interrelationships rather than linear, cause-effect relationships.
- Seeing processes of change and recognizing recurrent structures rather than viewing as isolated problems in time.

In many respects, systems thinking involves the transition from seeing multiple isolated problems as straight lines in time to the recognition that, when the interrelationships between these lines are recognized, they actually form a circle of influence in which the lines are interconnected in meaningful ways. As Senge notes, "Eventually, systems thinking forms a rich language for describing a vast array in interrelationships and patterns of change. Ultimately, it *simplifies life* by helping us see the deeper patterns lying behind the events and the details."[18]

Systems thinking is far more than an abstract theory; however, it involves specific tools and techniques to help benefit those who embrace its concepts. The four most commonly used tools are (1) idealized design, (2) mapping, (3) diagraming, and (4) computer simulation. Idealized design is the concept that was first developed by Ackoff[22] and involves a specific planning method requiring stakeholders to work backwards from an "ideal present" as opposed to planning forward from the present toward a prospective future. Ackoff persuasively argues that it is far more practical and effective to design the idealized system that we envision would best meet the needs of the patient and the provider, and then work backwards from that state to determine what must be done to put the structure and processes in place to allow its realization. This requires creating a common vision among diverse stakeholders and sustaining a customer focus that fully recognizes linkages and interdependencies often ignored by nonsystems approaches. Such a concept of design or redesign of the system relies on the inherent assumption that it is what the designers would like to have *right now,* not at some future date, inasmuch as this eliminates the need to forecast future technologies or future desired states, and instead concentrates on existing situations. Ackoff[22] indicates that an idealized design system should be technologically feasible, operationally viable, and capable of rapid learning and adaptation. He further delineates the benefits derived from this form of planning and design:[22]

- **Participation:** facilitates participation in the planning process.
- **Aesthetics:** enables the stakeholders to incorporate their values into the process.
- **Consensus:** forms a consensus among those who participate.
- **Commitment:** idealized design and the consensus emerging from it generate a commitment to help the project succeed.
- **Creativity:** stimulates creativity for both the organization and the individuals.
- **Implementability:** enlarges the designer's conceptions of what can and should be implemented.

The systems thinking tool of *mapping* lays out the scope of the system and defines its boundaries. This includes both external boundaries with the environment and internal boundaries among functions, processes, or players within the system. The mapping process looks for high leverage places, which are often found just outside what are considered to be the traditional boundaries of the organization or its processes. Because traditional management structures tend not to look at the interrelationships and boundaries, (particularly those that are outside of traditional management systems) they are unable to find such high leverage places for interventions. Examples of mapping tools include stock and flow diagrams, cich picturing, interrelationship diagraphs, and macroflow charting.

Diagraming describes causal relationships and interdependencies. It takes a closer look at the interrelationship between structures than does mapping. This often involves the use of causal loop diagrams, microflow charts, and system archetypes. *Computer simulation* is a relatively recent yet rich source of tools used to analyze system structure and the outcome performance the structure can generate. Within the next decade, it is likely that computer simulation and modeling will be widely used by most organizations as they attempt to adopt process of systems thinking.

What is needed to help apply systems thinking to create a learning organization, which as Garvin defines it as "an organization skilled at creating, acquiring, and transferring knowledge, and at modifying its behavior to reflect new knowledge and insights[25]"? Garvin indicates the need for three essential features to create a learning organization:

- **Meaning:** a clear, precise, and practical definition that can be easily applied is necessary.
- **Management:** precise guidelines for practicing within learning organizations need to be developed, full of operational advice as opposed to platitudes.
- **Measurement:** tools must be available to assess the organization's rate and level of learning to quantify gains.

The necessary *meaning* can begin with the definitions of Senge and Garvin. Senge details the concepts of the five component disciplines that a learning organization must master, including systems thinking, personal mastery, mental models, clear vision, and team learning. An alternate formulation of learning organizations was offered by Ikujiro Nonaka, who described them as places where "inventing new knowledge is not a specialized activity. . .it is a way of behaving, indeed, a way of being, in which everyone is a knowledge worker."[25] Such organizations draw sustenance from converting new ideas into processes and structures that allow for better performance. Unless such changes are made practical, only the *potential* for improvement exists; to the extent that learning remains an abstraction, no organization can be successful.

A beginning at creating clear-cut guidelines that help *manage* the transition to a learning organization is offered by Garvin, who focuses on the fact that learning organizations are skilled at five main activities: (1) systematic problem solving, (2) experimentation with new approaches, (3) learning from experience and history, (4) learning from the experiences and best practices of others, and (5) transferring knowledge efficiently.

Systematic problem solving begins with a heavy reliance on the scientific method, as opposed to guesswork. The work of Deming,[26] Juran,[27,28] and Shewhart[29] is essential to understanding the need for statistical process control (see Chapter 51). Insisting on data and using simple statistical tools (Pareto diagrams, cause-and-effect diagrams, flowcharts, etc.) can help ensure that accuracy and precision are present within the organization to assist learning. A constant focus of both the providers and management on answering the question "How do we know this is true?" is essential, as are the skills necessary for correctly answering that question. It is also important to ensure, at the earliest stages of the creation of the learning organization, that the problems are small enough to be practically solved. Early success in adopting the principles of statistical process control and the scientific method is best assured by addressing problems of a scope and magnitude that can be reasonably addressed. For example, beginning the transition by focusing on "reducing waiting time" is far less likely to be successful than addressing the related, but more circumscribed issues of component aspects of triage, registration, laboratory, radiology, or other specific components of waiting time.

Experimentation requires a systematic search for testing new knowledge in a practical setting. Learning organizations should create a culture and/or incentive program that favors, rewards, and encourages risk taking in the creation of new processes. The skills for experimentation include statistical analysis tools, process analysis, creativity techniques, and concepts such as idealized design. All of the forms of experimentation evolve from superficial, incomplete levels of knowledge to deeper understandings of the processes and services required within an organization. As Garvin aptly notes, "Knowing *how* is partial knowledge; it is rooted in norms of behavior, standards of practice, and settings of equipment. Knowing *why* is more fundamental: it captures underlying cause-and-effect relationships and accommodates exceptions, adaptations, and unforeseen events."[25] (Emphasis added.) Learning from past experience is also an essential feature of the practicality of learning organizations. The philosopher George Santayana is best remembered for his dictum, "Progress, far from consisting of change, depends upon retentiveness. Those that cannot remember the past are condemned to fulfill it."[30] Any organizational failure should be regarded as a potential source of insight into organizational learning, behaviors, and cultures, that help empower teams to move forward to better design in the present. IBM's legendary founder, Thomas Watson, Sr, understood this concept well. The story is told that a young manager enthusiastically created a venture for IBM that ended up losing ten million dollars. He was called into Watson's office, certain that he was about to be fired. As soon as he entered the office, the young man offered his resignation. Watson's legendary reply is telling in this regard: "You can't be serious. We just spent ten million dollars educating you."[3] This sense of learning from one's mistakes must be systematically built into the organization and into its culture, including specific educational programs that help assist in this regard.

Learning from others, particularly best industry practices, is also commonly known as benchmarking, which is addressed in Chapter 51. Benchmarking should include not only similar organizations, but also investigation of companies and processes outside one's immediate environment. For example, in looking at process times for patients admitted to the hospital, it is instructional to look at reservation systems for hotel chains. The concept of learning from others is also typified by the classic remark about the difference between plagiarism and research: If you steal from one person, it is plagiarism; if you steal from several people, it is research. Finally, one of the richest sources of learning from others is to listen carefully to the voice of the customer through personal contact, interviews, and statistically designed surveys.

Transferring knowledge is also an essential feature of a learning organization; knowledge must be moved through the organization as quickly and efficiently as possible. To do so, organizations must overcome the conception that knowledge is power and that power should be protected, rather than shared. In a learning organization, knowledge *is* power, but power is only effective when it is shared throughout multiple levels of the organization. The more incentives can be designed to ensure that team learning will be applied outside of the specific team's area of influence, the more successful a learning organization can be.

The final area is a process of *measuring* learning. Those organizations that have the shortest cycle time for learning processes are most likely to have the most improved performance. Nonetheless, caution should be exercised to ensure there is recognition that some types of learning take years to complete, but result in dramatic and important changes. The measuring process put into place should account for both short- and long-term learning.

Most organizational learning progresses through three distinct but overlapping stages. *Cognitive* organizational learning involves a phase in which the members of the organization are exposed to new ideas, begin to expand their knowledge, and approach the process of thinking differently about products, services, and issues. The second stage of organizational learning is *behavioral*. In this stage, staff begin to internalize their insights and approach the process of altering their behavior. Finally, the third step in organizational learning is *performance improvement,* in which behavioral changes result in changes in performance.

How does an individual begin to create a learning organization in the emergency department? What is perhaps telling about the intersection between learning organizations, systems theory, and the emergency department is that the primary introductory learning tool for systems theory and process management is a game called "Friday night at the ER (sic)." This game simulates conditions to which a busy emergency department might be exposed on a Friday evening and involves the intersection of multiple areas of interdependency of various processes. The game is used in many conferences on systems thinking, even those outside the healthcare setting. What could offer more telling testimony to the applicability of systems thinking to the emergency department than the fact that consultants and philosophers have recognized that an emergency department is a classic area where complex systems link in interdependent fashions?

Moving the emergency department toward systems thinking and the transformation to a learning organization involves several steps. First, a philosophic environment must be created that is conducive to learning across traditional boundaries. A premium must be placed on learning; and time for reflection, analysis, and reading must be not only encouraged, but also reserved. Concepts of visioning, development of strategic plans and mission statements, and development of organizational goals and objectives must be important parts of the organization. Second, it is important to ensure in a practical fashion that learning occurs across traditional boundaries. For example, learning must occur not just with the physician staff in the emergency department, but with the nursing staff, technicians, registration personnel, and ancillary services. Equally important these processes should be shared with other areas of the hospital that deeply affect the emergency department, particularly the admissions process, trauma service, and critical care units. Development of boundaryless or seamless organizations is an important concept of Senge and many other thinkers. Third, to create a seamless learning organization, learning forums and teams should be developed within the organization, with the primary focus on recognizing cross-functional interdependencies. For example, there should be a routine meeting of the emergency department team members (management, physicians, nurses, technicians, laboratory, radiography, registration) during which the overall operations of the emergency department are examined. This strategy provides an excellent forum in which to introduce these concepts, at first in an educational context, and later as a routine manner of functioning. Finally, all the members of the organization should be exposed to the tools and techniques necessary to help ensure that new processes are responsive to the needs of the patient, staff, and other emergency department customers.

To the extent that such a philosophy and the tools and techniques that represent it are implemented, the emergency department can be made into an environment that is more professionally and personally stimulating to those who are responsible for delivering patient care. Therefore such precepts not only result in better outcomes for patients, medical staff, and families, but also help create a more satisfying environment for the staff themselves, the primary resource of any emergency department.

Practical Emergency Department Application

This chapter has presented principles common to industrial and service industries, many of which have been applied in the healthcare setting. We have seen that leaders look at new ways of working together to achieve common visions, whereas managers help ensure compliance with the way processes are designed to work. Organizations that have a shared common vision and have created the elements that allow it to learn to apply systems thinking within a framework of a learning organization have great potential for success. Both leadership and management are required in the emergency department for the many reasons described previously. How are these principles applied in an emergency department setting? This discussion provides several examples designed to provide practical aspects of the application of these principles in the emergency department setting.

The Emergency Department at Fairfax Hospital reports more than 60,000 emergency visits a year in a space designed to accommodate 48,000 patients. The hospital is a level I trauma center and also has a highly developed pediatric emergency medicine service, comprising nine physicians, board certified or prepared in both adult and pediatric emergency medicine. More than 13,000 patients a year are admitted from the emergency department, accounting for nearly 40% of the hospital's total admissions. Emergency department visits account for nearly two thirds of all intensive care unit admissions. The hospital has undergone substantial downsizing, and additional space or staff will not be available to deal with the increasing numbers of patients seen in the emergency department. Like most other emergency departments, the care of the patients is increasingly complex, owing to their increased level of acuity, the effect of managed care, language barriers, increased customer expectations, and many other factors.

The emergency department thus finds itself with a burgeoning need for its services and a setting of increased acuity, complexity, and customer expectations, but stable or declining resources. The department has committed itself to concepts of continuous quality improvement, systems thinking, and the precepts of creating a learning organization. Surveying internal and external customers has resulted in a large amount of data, which when statistically analyzed reveals the following situations. First, the physician and nursing staff are recognized as delivering high-quality acute care to ill and injured patients in the adult and pediatric population. It is widely recognized that the trauma center function is disruptive to general emergency department operations, but the medical staff, administration, and board are supportive of maintaining this area of the department. Second, the quality of care delivered to patients with minor illnesses and injuries is also perceived as excellent, but is subject to substantial delays and a wide degree of variability in timeliness because of the large number of critically ill and injured patients who move through the department. Third, although previous surveys indicated pediatricians were happier with the pediatric emergency medicine service than family practice and internists were with the adult service, this is no longer true, because the adult service has been substantially improved. Fourth, despite its reputation for excellent service to critical care patients, the department was widely perceived to communicate both with the community and with the internal customer in a less than completely satisfying manner. The terms *trench warfare, MASH-unit atmosphere* and *burnout* appeared in various forms in the surveys, indicating the high degree of stress that the staff was experiencing.

Based on results from these surveys, the primary problems facing the emergency department are waiting times, communication, and the development of a customer service philosophy and a complaint management system. What do the precepts of leadership, management, motivation, systems thinking, and learning organizations have to offer in solving these problems?

The emergency department physician group had a mission statement that was intended to help focus the group on its overall goals and objectives. Box 1-4 lists the mission statement itself. In addition, a business planning effort is also used in the emergency department, which identified several areas of focus (Box 1-5). Unfortunately, because of several changes in management personnel, the business plan had not been carefully followed or specified in terms of precise statistical areas of improvement. One area the department needed to address is the concept of having a clear vision with about the overall purpose of the emergency department. The department was meeting community needs pertaining to critical care services, but was much less highly rated for treating more minor illnesses and injuries. The leadership and management structure began addressing these issues by ensuring that the respective management teams agreed on a common sense of purpose. Thus the Physician Management Team and the Emergency Department Management Team (which comprises nursing, physicians, registration, laboratory, radiography, ED technician, and EMS components) agreed on a common need for a shared vision of the emergency department's operations and services.

Although mission statements and business plans had been devised in the past, there was a widely recognized need for updating this information and ensuring that it truly met a sense of shared common vision of the members of the emergency department team. Once the vision statement clearly reflected the department's commitment to *all* aspects of emergency department services (including acute and nonacute care), it was easier to help ensure that the staff was committed philosophically and practically to meeting this goal. Next, specific strategic goals and objectives were laid out, some of which were adapted from the previous mission statement and business plan.

By using an adaptation of the concept of idealized design, the staff recognized areas of interdependence and cross relationships that impeded patient flow through the emergency department. The department was designed along classic lines of triage, registration, and waiting room. Patients were called to the treatment area by a primary care nurse who made a preliminary evaluation. The chart was placed on the deck to await the physician/resident evaluation and entry of pertinent orders. Diagnostic and/or therapeutic interventions were obtained, reevaluated, and disposed by either discharge or admission to the hospital. In evaluating the current system, multiple areas of potential intervention were identified when viewed in an interdependent fashion. For example, expansion of the previously existing standing orders and development of an Advanced Triage/Advanced Initiatives system allowed for earlier input of specific orders (patients with abdominal pain, neutropenic patients with fever, extremity injuries, patients with acute nontraumatic chest pain, minor head injuries, asthma treatment guidelines) and helped obviate the need for waiting for physician evaluation before order entry. This innovation reduced waiting time and improved patient satisfaction. A somewhat less expected result was improve-

BOX 1-4

ED Mission Statement: All emergency departments should have a clearly defined and articulated mission statement jointly developed and committed to by the ED staff.

MISSION STATEMENT
EMERGENCY PHYSICIANS OF NORTHERN VIRGINIA, LTD.
DEPARTMENT OF EMERGENCY MEDICINE
FAIRFAX HOSPITAL

Emergency Physicians of Northern Virginia, Ltd.—and the Department of Emergency Medicine at Fairfax Hospital is a professional group of career emergency physicians which exists to:

1. Provide comprehensive, quality emergency care in a timely fashion.
2. Provide an environment which promotes the interests of emergency medicine and emergency physicians and which is:
   - Professionally Satisfying
   - Conducive to Long Term Stability
   - Economically Sound
   - Intellectually Stimulating
   - Educationally Productive
   - Clinically Efficient and Cost Effective
   - Open to Career Development Opportunities
   - Commensurate in Matching Responsibility and Authority for Department Operations
3. Provide for professional educational resources and commitment matched to those of Fairfax Hospital and its Medical Staff for the growth, training, and educational needs of:
   - Emergency Medicine Residents
   - Resident Physicians
   - EMS Personnel
   - Nurses
   - Medical Students
   - Other Health Care Providers
   - Community

Courtesy of Emergency Physicians of Northern Virginia, Ltd., Falls Church, Va.

BOX 1-5

FAIRFAX HOSPITAL—EMERGENCY DEPARTMENT BUSINESS PLAN

Overall Goal: Maintain Emergency Department volume while increasing profitability.

Objective 1: Decrease patient turnaround time by 15% among non-monitored patients through improved system efficiencies and patient flow.

Objective 2: Increased ED staff (physicians and employees) satisfaction by 20% within six months.

Objective 3: Increase satisfaction among non-monitored patients by 15% within six months.

Objective 4: Improve the working relationship between the ED staff and private (referring) physicians by 20% as measured by staff surveys.

Courtesy of Fairfax Hospital Emergency, Fall Church, Va.

ment in staff satisfaction, probably as a result of feelings of empowerment.

One of the most critical areas identified through the idealized design process was a desire for less delay in obtaining patient rooms for patients with moderate or minor illnesses and injuries. Pareto diagrams clearly established that the longest areas of delays were for patients who had been registered, but were awaiting room assignment. Team members recognized that part of the problem was that, "The emergency department was digesting like a snake, instead of a person." This simply meant that, once a bolus of patients occurred, the problem of inadequate beds created a delay that marched sequentially through the system, often creating further delays.

As a result of the idealized design process and application of systems thinking, a system was implemented wherein several changes occurred. First, one of the physicians or physician assistants previously deployed in the treatment area could now be deployed to the triage area itself, as dictated by patient flow needs. This physician or physician assistant was not intended to *replace* the nurse at triage, but simply to ensure that certain patients could be moved through the system more rapidly by providing initial evaluation and treatment at the triage area when no patient rooms were available. Second, the actual use of the treatment rooms was reconsidered and analyzed for value added to the patient's evaluation and treatment. For many patients with minor or moderate illnesses or injuries, it was determined that the treatment rooms could be used as "staging areas" in which initial evaluation and therapy could occur, after which the patient could be moved to another area to await results. This allowed the rooms to be used more frequently, reducing waiting times for evaluation and treatment. The issue of moving patients out of rooms was addressed prospectively by creating "service fail-safes"[31] consisting of prescribed explanations to the patient and family for moving them out of the room, thereby minimizing customer dissatisfaction.

Many patients with extremely minor illnesses and injuries who had previously been cared for in a separate Fast Track area of the emergency department could now be seen and undergo diagnostic and therapeutic interventions almost as soon as their arrival at the hospital. Although it was necessary to have a registration number to enter diagnostic tests (because of limitations of the computer system), the patient was already seen by the physician or physician assistant, and in some cases had appropriate therapeutic interventions ordered before registration itself. The second group of patients in whom time-to-treatment was dramatically decreased were those with more intermediate level problems. For example, patients with acute abdominal pain, who required laboratory and radiographic studies and often intravenous fluids or other therapies, could undergo their initial evaluation with the physician or physician's assistant at the triage area. Diagnostic tests and response to therapy could be reviewed by either the same or a second physician in the treatment area itself (depending on flow patterns) once space had been cleared for the patient. This concept resulted in dramatic decreases in waiting times; it had an even more important effect on the perception of the patient and family with regard to the *responsiveness* of emergency department care.

This innovation required accentuation of the computer system at the triage area, deployment of technician and nursing resources in unusual ways, and a substantial amount of financial investment by the emergency department group. Nonetheless, by using systems thinking and idealized design, dramatic improvement occurred in the service in the emergency department. Financial analysis indicated that return of emergency department patients who had previously gone elsewhere more than offset the up-front investment costs of converting to the new system. Thus by using concepts of leadership, management, systems thinking, and idealized design, the emergency department was able to radically reform the way in which care was provided to a specific segment of patients. This target population had been identified by surveys as least likely to be satisfied under the "old system." The precepts of a learning organization were required to ensure that the staff could make the transition to this new system, despite the fact that it ran against many of the traditional concepts of emergency department design and management.

Implementation of a customer service philosophy and complaint management system also offers important insights into the application of such principles. By using benchmarking techniques, it was determined that the level of complaints voiced by medical staff and patients were actually already below benchmark hospitals of similar size, scope, and sophistication. Nonetheless, as a part of the vision, mission statement, and strategic planning process, common goals of reducing patient and medical staff complaints and developing a specific customer service philosophy were adopted.

An educational session titled Emergency Department Survival Skills© was developed for all emergency department staff. This 1-day course consisted of elements of customer service philosophy, stress recognition and management, conflict resolution, negotiation skills, customer fail-safes, and Point of Impact Intervention (see Chapter 8). In effect, the course both raised the staff's customer service awareness and skills and developed a sense of accountability, partnership, empowerment, and stewardship. One of the essential insights from the course is identifying the elements of power, control, and expectations as the locus of much of the provider-patient (customer) interaction. It emphasizes specific skills that can be used in the practical emergency department setting to assist in this transition.

In the past patient complaints were viewed as a source of problems rather than an opportunity to hear more clearly the customer's expectations for the services. Through participative interaction with the staff, a philosophy that viewed customer dissatisfaction as a failure to meet prepurchase expectations was developed. The entire staff committed itself to a philosophy of ensuring that patients, families, medical staff, and other stakeholders in the emergency department encounter were satisfied with the outcome of the service, in both acute care and minor illness and injury segments. Educational sessions were held to help disseminate the philosophy that had been developed in the committee, which had been handled in a collaborative and participative fashion. Concepts of personal mastery were used to ensure that ownership of this philosophy occurred on an individual basis throughout the department. Ongoing statistical summaries of patient complaints were compiled, and the complaint management system was radically changed.

In the past management responded to patient and/or medical staff complaints. In the new system, the staff members responsible for the patient encounter not only provided input before the response to the patient, but also guided the actual response to customer dissatisfaction itself. In most cases, the emergency department team members themselves responded directly to the person concerned about the service. In other cases, at the direction of the staff members, management compiled and delivered the response to the patient, family, or medical staff member. These changes in the philosophic and practical ways of handling customer service and patient complaints resulted in statistically demonstrable changes in satisfaction with the emergency department. Patient complaints dropped from 2.6/1000 to 0.6/1000 ($P < .001$). Customer satisfaction similarly increased.

These examples indicate in a practical fashion the ways in which the concepts described in this chapter can be of benefit in the radically changing milieu of emergency department practice in the 1990s and beyond. Although they apply specifically to a fairly large and complex emergency department setting, similar models could easily be developed for different emergency department practices. There is ample reason to believe that the application of leadership and management principles, coupled with concepts of systems thinking and the creation of learning organizations, can have a dramatic impact in the delivery of emergency department care.

MOTIVATION

It is impossible for a busy, complex emergency department to function without ensuring that its staff is motivated. The stresses of day-to-day practice in emergency medicine preclude the ability to function properly without highly motivated providers. Although this seems obvious, what does *motivation* mean to emergency physicians, emergency nurses, and other members of the emergency department team?

The word *motivate* comes from French and Latin roots, which in their earliest derivations simply referred to "moving" or "movement". This etymologic distinction is interesting given the more modern meanings of motivation. Specifically, motivation has come to be recognized as a complex array of factors that influence individuals to act in certain ways. However, as we shall see, an important distinction in motivational theory is that negative, extrinsic motivators do not actually lead to motivation itself, but rather to simple "movement."

What factors motivate emergency department personnel to do their jobs on a daily basis? From a theoretic standpoint, motivating factors have been classified as both positive and negative, as well as internal and external. Negative motivating factors have been well described by Herzberg,[31] who showed that such factors, whether physical or psychologic, are at best poor, incomplete, and unsatisfying. However, he also makes the important distinction that what he refers to as "positive KITA" (which he wryly describes as "kick in the pants") is also a recipe for failure in most settings in which motivation is needed. For example, an owner has a dog that he wishes to teach to move. Negative motivation would be to kick the dog in the rear, which, depending on the velocity and aim, has a variable chance of inducing movement. Positive motivation might involve the use of treats as a reward for when the dog moves. When properly viewed, however, it is the owner who is *motivated* and the dog who *moves,* through the mechanism of the dog biscuit. For decades, industry and manufacturing firms have applied various forms of dog biscuits to attempt to get their managers and providers to "move." Herzberg points out, however, that while negative motivation is a form of coercion, positive motivation is co-option, "but in fact, it is worse to be co-opted than to be coerced because coercion is externally imposed, whereas co-option means that you give your compliance. The organization does not have to kick you; you kick yourself."[31] According to Herzberg's formulation, true motivation, is a function of growth resulting from intrinsic rewards offered from work that is inherently challenging and stimulating. Because it is based on personal growth, it is an "internal engine" and therefore much more likely to succeed.

An alternate formulation for classifying motivations is to describe them as internal or external. Internal motivating factors derive from the basic and inherent aspects of the job itself, including the sense of satisfaction gained from the work, the sense of contribution to a meaningful whole, cooperation among talented professionals, and the sense that one is answering a certain "calling" or vision to which the individual and the organization are committed. Extrinsic motivation is generally classified as various forms of rewards or punishments that are meted out and returned for positive or negative results. For decades most businesses and industries, as well as many medical practices, have assumed that there is some power of redemption in reward systems, under the assumption that people will do a better (or at least a faster) job if there is a built-in incentive.

The concepts of incentive plans and external motivation arise out of behaviorist theory that has been responsible for programs such as piece work in factory settings, stock options for executives, commissions for sales people, and strict fee-for-service arrangements in medicine. These reward programs derive from operant conditioning theory, which holds that behavior is a direct function of its consequences.[32]

Given the extensive experience with external motivators, can we provide any evidence that reward systems work? A vast amount of research and experience indicates that rewards largely work in one relatively narrow aspect—temporary compliance with the dictates of the system.[33-35] Indeed, virtually any external motivation system can be manipulated in such a way that intelligent participants can "game the system" by using the details of the various pay-for-performance plans to maximize their personal benefit, which may or may not be in accord with the overall goals and visions of the organization. Thus they do not produce commitment, but rather result in compliance.

Even more important, a surprisingly large amount of data indicate that reward systems also do not significantly increase productivity, but simply result in increased "compensation" for those who are already productive.[33-36] This distinction is important because all such pay-for-performance plans involve a significant amount of complexity in their design, monitoring, and compensation mechanisms. If all they produce is a higher reward for those who were known to produce quality productivity, isn't it far simpler and wiser to devise a compensation system that recognizes this without the need for complex pay-for-performance schemes? Further, in treating and evaluating emergency department patients, the distinction between quality of work and turnaround times or cycle times is extremely difficult and complex. Both from theoretic and practical standpoints, it is difficult to design an external motivational system in an emergency department setting that can effectively consider both of these factors and result in *both* compliance and commitment.

Why do external motivators and reward systems usually fail? Although popular wisdom holds that such systems have a benefit, it is rarely noted that significant harm can result from them. Because rewards do "buy" temporary compliance, on the surface it would seem that performance is addressed, at least superficially. Even more difficult, our society has placed such reward systems in virtually every form of educational and family unit. "Be good and I will buy you a toy" in essence is quite similar to "If you see the patients very quickly, I will pay you more money." Just as the flaws of behaviorist theory and operant conditioning have been increasingly noted, so too have the limitations of rewards and punishment systems been noted.[36]

Deming noted long ago that pay is not the primary motivator for quality work.[36] In surveys of factors influencing job satisfaction, pay typically ranks between fourth and sixth on the scale of what matters most to professional workers. Herzberg made the extremely important observation that too little money can irritate and demotivate people. It is also categorically true, however, that more and more money does not necessarily result in increased satisfaction, and can bring about decreased motivation. One of the fundamental arguments against reward systems is that they constitute a form of "positive punishment," and therefore are no less a form of coercion than negative motivations. Thus such reward systems can have a negative and punitive effect because they are at their essence highly manipulative. In addition, if the reward system is competitive, it can result in substantial divisiveness among workers, including highly trained professionals. As Kohn[37] noted in a classic work on incentive plans, "The surest way to destroy cooperation and, therefore organizational excellence, is to force people to compete for rewards or recognition or to rank them against each other."

There are even more persuasive reasons that extrinsic or external motivation systems are counterproductive. Many studies support the concept that successful organizations have a shared common purpose in which the employees are strongly committed to the overarching vision of that organization.[33-37] Such systems succeed because there is high degree of cooperation and accommodation of a diversity of opinions. As Scholtes[38] noted, "Reward systems are at stark cross purposes with this philosophy, since everyone is pressuring the system for individual gain. No one is improving the system for collective gain. This system will inevitably crash." This is certainly true in the emergency department setting, where the talents of multiple individuals must be harnessed so that service to the patient is at its highest quality.

An additional problem with motivational systems relying on extrinsic factors is that they often result in a situation where neither the managers nor the providers have a clear sense of how the fundamental work of the organization gets done. Because of the complexity of reward systems, it becomes extremely easy to confuse the end points of the reward system with an understanding of how the system works. However, more fundamental concentration on what Zaleznik[39] calls the "real work of organizations" would greatly benefit both the providers and the patient. As Pearce[40] noted, "Pay-for-performance schemes actually impede the abilities of managers to manage."

Examples of such performance plans are common in emergency medicine. Many groups base their extrinsic motivational structure on some form of fee-for-service or pay-for-performance basis. Whether based on actual billings, collections, numbers of patients seen, net contribution to group revenue, or other factors, such schemes are widely used in emergency medicine. Do they work? On close examination, the problem would seem to be that too much faith is placed on such systems to ensure that the "real work" of seeing the patients in a timely and quality fashion is done. Such systems may motivate people, but probably motivate them only to get the rewards of the system. For example, in a strict fee-for-service environment, numerous emergency department physician groups have noted that uncompensated patients or patients who have a poor reimbursement profile can languish while patients with highly paying commercial insurance are seen in a more timely fashion. Such systems can also have an odd, but common psychologic effect on emergency department staff, which can be characterized as follows. "If they are having to pay me highly and provide external motivation for me to want to see these patients, there must be something inherently wrong or less desirable about seeing these patients in the first place. If they have to bribe me to do it, there must be something I shouldn't want to do, and therefore I must be given a reward to take the 'bitter pill'." Although this psychologic effect has never been studied systematically, personal experience with numerous emergency department groups indicates that it may have an impact on the so-called "burnout" in emergency medicine. Similarly, emergency physicians may be motivated by modified fee-for-service systems to move patients at an extremely rapid rate. Nonetheless, if the rate is too fast, it can result in substantial risk management problems, so that the group's overall goals are not well served.

In contradistinction to extrinsic motivation or reward punishment systems, intrinsic motivation is far more subtle, but in many ways more powerful. Intrinsic motivation includes factors such as sense of personal and professional worth, internal recognition for doing a difficult job, personal and professional growth and advancement, and contributing to the overall well-being of the community and the healthcare environment. Although in its simplest formulations, intrinsic motivation can sound like an advertisement for the power of positive thinking, careful study by management theorists like Badaracco and Ellsworth,[2] Covey,[9-10] Argyris,[19] and Senge[18] indicates that a principle-centered or *values driven* approach results in professionals and organizations whose goals are clear, whose processes are innovative, who attract high-caliber talent to perform in ethical and inspiring ways, and who remain with the organization on a long-term basis. Such formulations can seem naive unless backed up by a strong commitment by the organization to a clear understanding of the "real work" done in the organization, as well as the tools, education, and infrastructure to make these declarations meaningful. The leadership of such organizations usually has a clear vision of leadership with regard to the reasons for the organization's existence, as well as a cooperative and meaningful interaction about the future of the organization between leadership and providers.

What do motivational systems mean for emergency department groups? First, it is important to understand the limitations of negative motivation and reward and punishment systems. When taken alone, they are too often assumed to provide both necessary and sufficient conditions for success in the practice of emergency medicine. Second, although there are substantial limitations to reward and punishment systems, there is reason to believe that *limited* reliance on compensation packages based on ability to evaluate patients in a quality and timely fashion could form *part* of a motivational structure for an emergency department group. However, such systems must be simple, fair, openly communicated, and designed to operate as a simple baseline way in which to ensure that the purposes of the organization are met. Finally, such a system is still subject to all of the limitations discussed previously and therefore should be used *only* in conjunction with a strong intrinsic motivation process within the organization. This ensures that members of the emergency department team are deeply committed not only to the care of their patients, but also to the growth and development of the organization and of the team members who comprise that organization. Given all of the stressors on the practice of emergency medicine, this is a difficult and complex task, which requires ongoing dialogue between the leaders and managers of the organization and the physicians, nurses, technicians, and other team members who provide the "real work." To the extent that emergency departments align the purposes of the organization with the changing needs of their patients and providers, they stand a reasonable chance of assuring that all members of the organization are motivated appropriately. Without attention to these theoretic and practical concerns, most emergency departments will find themselves far short of their capabilities, stuck in stagnation, and facing high degrees of turnover and burnout in their staff. From a practical standpoint, several areas of motivation should be addressed by all emergency department teams and physician groups.

To begin with, there needs to be a clear-cut, collaboratively derived mission/vision statement, which concisely states the values and objectives of the emergency team and of the emergency department physician group. Chapter 5 addresses the mission/vision statement in more detail, but it is often necessary to ensure that there is a mission/vision statement for both the emergency department team and the physician group specifically, recognizing that there will be considerable overlap, but some areas of divergence. In formulating such a statement of values, leadership and management play a key role, but the provider's active input should always be sought to ensure that it truly reflects the desires and motivations of the staff themselves. Second, the mission statement should be updated and reviewed at least yearly, to ensure that it is responsive to the changing needs of the emergency department environment. Third, the organization must address the needs for personal and professional growth of the team members. Training in the acquisition of skills required for dealing with a changing environment need to be included among the clinical training offered to members of the emergency department team. Fourth, the organization should offer an environment that balances purpose, values, and compensation in a reasonable fashion.

Kohn offers the advice of balancing the "three Cs": choice, collaboration, and content. Choice simply means that the emergency department team members should be able to participate in decisions that will affect the processes and services delivered in that department. (The precepts of continuous quality improvement are instructive in this regard, as is detailed in Part 5: Quality.) Collaboration refers to the need to structure teams to facilitate change, to open exchange of ideas, and to create a climate of support and encouragement. Content refers to the jobs that we ask members of the emergency department team to perform on a day-to-day basis. It also refers to assisting in refining both those jobs and the processes that they entail and to creating an environment that sustains personal and professional growth. As Herzberg[31] noted: "If you want people motivated to do a good job, give them a good job to do."

SUMMARY

Understanding the concepts of leadership, management, stewardship, learning organizations, and motivation is essential for those charged with leading the emergency department. Yet these skills are not formally taught in medical schools, nursing schools, residencies, or, except in some circumstances, inservice training. Far from being abstract, theoretic constructs, these principles form the strata on which practical management applications can be built. For this reason, it may be helpful to refer to this chapter during the course of implementation of specific strategies in the emergency department.

REFERENCES

1. DePree M: *Leadership is an art,* Ann Arbor, 1988, University of Michigan Press.
2. Badaracco JL Jr, Ellsworth RR: *Leadership and the quest for integrity,* Boston, 1989, Harvard Business School Press.
3. Bennis W: *On becoming a leader,* Reading, Mass, 1989, Addison-Wellsley.
4. Block P: *Stewardship: choosing service over self interest,* San Francisco, 1993, Berrett-Kochle-Publishing.

5. Mayer T: The emergency department medical director, *Emerg Med Clin North Am* 5:1-29, 1987.
6. Mayer T: Emergency department staffing. In Schwartz GR Cayten CG, Mayer T et al, editors: *Principles and practice of emergency medicine,* ed 3, Philadelphia, 1993, Lea & Febiger.
7. Kotter JP: What leaders really do, *Harvard Business Review* 68:103-111, 1990.
8. Drucker P: The new society of organizations, *Harvard Business Review* 70:95-104, 1992.
9. Deleted in proofs.
10. Deleted in proofs.
11. Zaleznik A: Managers and leaders: Are they different? *Harvard Business Review* 70:126-135, 1992.
12. James W: *The varieties of religious experience,* New York, 1967, Doubleday.
13. Maslow A: *Motivation and personality,* New York, 1954, Harper & Row.
14. Burns JM: *Leadership,* New York, 1978, Harper & Row.
15. Tichy N, Devanna MA: *The transformational leader.* New York, 1986, John Wiley & Sons.
16. Adams JD: *Transforming leadership: from vision to results,* Alexandria, Va, 1987, Miles Review Press.
17. Atcheson TA: *Turning health care leadership around,* San Francisco, 1990, Jossey-Bass.
18. Senge PM: *The fifth discipline: The art and practice of the learning organization,* New York, 1990, Doubleday.
19. Argyris C: *On organizational learning,* Cambridge, 1992, Blackwell Publishing.
20. Stata R: Organizational learning: The key to management innovation, *Sloan Management Review* 30:63-64, 1989.
21. Kauffman D Jr: *Systems I: An introduction to systems thinking,* Minneapolis, 1980, Future Systems.
22. Ackoff R: *Creating the corporate future,* New York, 1981, John Wiley & Sons.
23. Hardin G: *Nature and man's fate,* New York, 1961, New American Library.
24. Forrester J: *The counter intuitive behavior of social systems,* Technology Review 21:52-68, 1971.
25. Garvin DA: Building a learning organization, *Harvard Business Review* 71:78-91, 1993.
26. Deming EW: *Out of crises,* Cambridge, 1989, Massachusetts Institute of Technology Press, Center for Advanced Engineering Study.
27. Juran JM: *Juran on planning for quality,* New York, 1988, The Free Press.
28. Juran JM: *Juran on leadership for quality: Executive handbook,* New York, 1989, The Free Press.
29. Shewhart WA: *Economic control of quality manufactured products,* New York, 1931, Van Nostrand.
30. Santayana G: *The logic of reason,* New York, 1912, Harper & Rowe.
31. Herzberg F: One more time: how do you motivate employees? *Harvard Business Review* 46:53-62, 1968.
32. Rich JT, Larsen JA: Why some long-term incentives fail. In Nalbantian HR, editor: *Incentives, cooperation, and risk sharing,* Totowa NJ, 1987, Rowman & Littlefield.
33. Deci EL, Ryan RM: *Intrinsic motivation in self-determination in human behavior,* New York, 1985, Plenum Press.
34. Lepper MR, Greene D: *The hidden costs of reward: new perspectives on the psychology of human motivation,* Hillsdale NJ, 1978, Erlbaum Associates.
35. Halachmi A, Holzer M: Merit pay, performance targeting, and productivity. *Review of Public Personnel Administration* 7:80-91, 1987.
36. Kohn A: *Punished by rewards: the trouble with goal stars, incentive plans, A's, praise, and other bribes,* Boston, 1993, Houghton Mifflin.
37. Kohn A: Why incentive plans cannot work, *Harvard Business Review* 71:54-62, 1993.
38. Scholtes PR: An elaboration on Deming's teachings on performance appraisal. In McLean GN, (editor): *Performance appraisal: perspectives on a quality management approach,* Alexandria, Va, 1990, University of Minnesota Training and Development Research Center.
39. Zaleznik A: Real work, *Harvard Business Review* 67:31-38, 1989.
40. Pearce: Why merit pay doesn't work: implications from organization theory. In Balkin DB, Gomez-Mejiah LR, (editors): *New perspectives on compensation,* Englewood Cliffs, NJ, 1987, Prentice Hall.

2 Effective Use of Administrative Power:

A VIEW FROM THE RANK AND FILE

Gregory Henry

"Be not afraid of greatness: some men are born great, some achieve greatness, and some have greatness thrust upon them."

William Shakespeare, *Twelve Night, Act II, Scene 5*

Power is an unusual commodity for many reasons, not the least of which is that you first have to decide what it is. The ability to influence events and outcomes in one's favor is one definition of power. Physicians have held a common misconception that if they do the right thing consistently for the patient, ignoring everything else, their good works will speak for themselves, and they will not have to worry about the outside world. This is both naive and wrong. We live and work in a political environment; everything we do is political to some extent. When patients paid their own bills, they reached in their pockets and they took out their wallets. Doctors had to ask them for the money and they had to give it to them. Patients had the ultimate control in this system because they would ask questions such as, "Doctor, do I really need that? Doctor, do I really have to have this done?" The doctor had to sit there and think, "You know I bet there is a less expensive way to do this for this person or family." Since the end of World War II, however, we have concentrated money for healthcare in larger and larger entities. At least half the hospital bills in the United States today are paid by the federal government. This means that doctors are no longer able to negotiate with each patient or each small payor for fees. It is done en masse. Whenever money is concentrated, money and power run together, but they are not the same thing. Lots of people have money but little power. Some people have little money but some power.

If you think you have power, you probably do. If you don't think you have it, you don't. Real power, the only power that actually exists in the world, is getting people committed to your ideas. How do you do that? Rule number one:

"Absolute power corrupts absolutely."

Lord Acton

Lord Acton is right, but don't worry about it because in emergency medicine, we don't have absolute power, despite the fact that we have absolute liability.

An important lesson that follows this rule of power is rule number two:

When you use power for yourself, you lose it.

When you use power for others or for the cause, you gain power. The great Oxford dons have a power that is can be both transferred and manipulated because of their understanding that they only have power if they give it away or share it. Only the person who has true power can actually share it. Thus you gain power by taking whatever you have gained and putting it back into the cause.

Our real power in emergency medicine is what we can do for others. Keeping the patient as central focus is everything. Emergency physicians are presented daily with the reality of customer service and the expectations it entails. Emergency medicine evokes so much emotion in other specialties, and at times generates anger, because it represents the conscience of medicine; it is the naked underbelly of American medicine and society. When our fellow physicians bemoan our calls in the middle of the night, they are actually looking at a defect in themselves. After all, the reason that emergency physicians are the focal point, why they sit at the bottom of the societal birdcage so to speak, is that emergency physicians have taken on the traditional role of "the doctor." No group of physicians in this country deserve more to carry the staff of Aesculapius than the emergency physician. Who is there at 2 o'clock in the morning to take care of the children on Christmas Eve? Who is there to comfort the homeless? Who is there to look after the alcoholics whom no one else will see? When emergency physicians interact with physicians in other specialties, they show them the ugly side of what American medicine has become. It has become more important to charge for a procedure than to take care of people. Power is shifting to those who care for patients on a regular basis because forces outside of medicine recognize that emergency physicians have done and will continue to do yeoman's service to our communities, to society, and to maintaining high standards of care to *all* patients they care for. Emergency medicine residencies are growing. The number of outstanding people coming out of medical schools who want to practice emergency medicine is rapidly increasing. The specialty is growing stronger because it has looked after patients' interests. This fact should be considered when the hospital complains about the emergency department; it is critical for the hospital to understand the origins of such feelings.

Rule number three:

It is a strange rule of power to begin by seeking power and end by losing liberty. Power only goes to those who are committed.

If a doctor is a free, ethereal spirit, if he or she expects to just float in and float out, that doctor will never have power. Power goes to those who are committed to the cause. It never goes to those who want to pick and choose when they will be committed to an idea. "Power without responsibility, the prerogative of the harlot throughout the ages." Who is this? This is the attending at the end of the phone who wants to decide whether somebody ought to go home without seeing the patient. This is the doctor who wants to Monday morning quarterback, to decide how medical care *should* have been given in the emergency department. This type of person is too often the type of physician that emergency medicine must deal with.

The next lesson coming out of rule number three is the most important one of the discussion. If anyone wants real power, they must get it the old fashion way—earn it. Some emergency departments have tremendous strength in their hospitals and have fewer problems with attending physicians. In such departments, when the emergency physician says "admit!" the attendings say, "Thank you!" In these situations, emergency physicians have "saved" the attending physician so many times that their credibility and integrity are well known. That credibility and integrity is only earned through constant, ongoing clinical contact that results from a well-managed emergency department in conjunction with articulate and well-trained emergency physicians. These emergency departments often play a substantial role in continuing medical education programs at the hospital, particularly in training physicians and nurses in resuscitation courses. They have emergency physicians who sit on every major committee of the hospital, investing time, energy, effort, and political capital in the future of their group. Respect and integrity earn power in any institution, regardless of its location. As the old adage goes, "Excellence is what we strive for, but consistency is what we demand." You've got to *be there* to do things. As Woody Allen said, "90% of success is showing up." Certainly 90% of power is showing up and doing the job consistently.

Loyalty and integrity are recognized and admired by friend and foe alike. If you stand up for principles, even those who do not always like you will respect you. The medical staff do not have to love an emergency physician as an individual, but it is important for them to understand the physician's thought process and a goal and an aim toward which he or she is working. An emergency physician who views himself or herself as less qualified than the attending physicians will be treated that way. Earn, demand, and therefore attain respect.

The backpacker emergency physician is a thing of the past. Gone are the days when an emergency physician can wander in and say, "I'm skiing at Aspen for six weeks. I'm in for two months and I'm gone again." This gets no respect from physicians on the staff who are running practices and working hard, much less from the nursing and administrative staffs. Any credibility as an active member of the medical staff is completely lost unless there is active, ongoing, deep commitment for the workings of the hospital and its medical staff, including committee work. Emergency physicians need an action plan and mission statement for their department. They should know and be represented on all strategically important committees of the hospital. Ensuring that discussions include the perspective of the emergency department is essential to ensuring that small problems do not get blown out of proportion.

In addition, the emergency physician can usually mention other cases that attending physicians on the medical staff have handled in a way that have created problems. An emergency physician may manage cases from other physicians' offices that were not optimally managed. It is never wise to talk indiscriminately about such cases, but it is important to recall, document, and remember them because they often resurface at politically important times. Over time, this power becomes implicitly understood by the important political players in the hospital. Great walls crumble one block at a time, in the same way that they were built. Whenever you think things are going well in the department, when you stop paying attention to detail, and start thinking about missing a few committee meetings, it is important to recognize that you are slowly eroding your base of power one block at a time. Understand what you need to maintain a power base so that your department is well represented and stick to that plan. Finally, timing is everything. In any power relationship, the emergency department will come head-to-head with other departments or people at certain moments. Even at times of conflict there will be an issue on which the two departments can agree, and when the two of you agree on any issue, the possibility of further agreement becomes more likely. Rule number four:

"Political power grows out of the barrel of a gun - and the Joint Commission." There is nothing as useful to success as being right. You gain power when your goals and desires are aligned with those of the institution and regulatory agencies. The point is, always reference your desires and aims with a higher authority. The rules and regulations of the Joint Commission are clear. If the hospital has a practice that contradicts the rules of the Joint Commission, it needs to be pointed out. It is important to talk to the people who have the power to make decisions. There are often low level administrators, who are often the victims of ongoing restructuring; these people may be involved in policy discussions but lack decision-making authority. For an emergency department director to carry out policy discussions with people who are not in the position to make policy is not only a waste of time, but a dangerous practice. Physicians must carry out policy discussions with people who can influence and change policy, which may vary according to the organizational structure of an institution. Emergency physicians are the master of doing two things: complaining to the wrong people (usually their partner or the nurses in the department) and taking the problems of the world on their shoulders. Why do emergency physicians assume the problems of the hospital and society? Why don't radiologists figure out who should be taking the patients who don't have doctors? Why don't anesthesiologists set up a follow-up clinic? Why don't pathologists run the in-house codes for free? The political milieu, not common sense, dictates the current answer to these questions.

There are different types of power. It is essential for emergency physicians to understand what kind of power they have. The first type of power is the *power to reward.* This is the best power to have. Never fail to reward loyal co-workers. Remember that loyalty and integrity are prized above all other values, and those who have been loyal to the cause need to be commended. Use the power to reward freely and it will certainly come back to you. This power to reward can be verbal, written, monetary, or any other form that appropriately recognizes a job well done.

There is also the *power to punish.* The power to punish is the last power a leader ever wants to use. Punishment power can be used to do unusual things in unusual settings. In a public forum, an emergency physician has the power to embarrass the chief of staff or the hospital administrator. It is also quite likely the last time the physician would exercise either the power to punish or any other sort of power, because those in leadership positions often have not only their own powers, but also long memories. The power to punish is the last sword a leader should ever use. The power to punish is a sword that causes other people to harden their positions and to develop long-term memory for all the real or perceived slights that have ever come their way.

The *power of authority* is another type of power. The age of hierarchy is over. As soon as you have to say to the patient, "I'm the doctor—you're not," you are no longer wielding power; you are yielding power. The *power of expertise* is a variant of authority. Physicians have more of this kind of power than any other kind. Do you realize how often a doctor is put on a committee or invited to do something simply because he or she is a physician? Physicians bring with them an aura of a certain competence. The power of expertise is used to obtain information from people. Physicians talk to families and ask them extremely personal and sometimes intimate questions. They expect answers and they receive them because of the confidence and trust engendered by the physician-patient relationship. Appropriate use of the power of expertise therefore can be helpful. Expertise is a useful tool in all power relationships and one of the basic tools by which to positively influence people.

The last important issue is the *power of reference* itself. Control is an illusion. It comes from people who possess similar values and allow such control. History is replete with examples of conquering forces that were vastly outnumbered by the societies they were charged with governing. Their span of control was vast. How did the British, located 8000 miles from India control the then most populous nation in the world? It occurred in part because people were willing to be controlled. Ghandi confronted the populace with that fact and showed them that "The Emperor had no clothes." They could not control people 8000 miles away who truly wanted to control themselves. All power has an element of illusion to it.

Communication is the most important source of power. Organizations are fond of drawing organizational charts, but no organization functions solely according to these plans. The real job of the chief executive is to move among the people, saying, "How are you doing? Is there something I can get for you? How can we redesign the system to work better for you and the patient?" The job is to share power in a way that empowers everybody else because power carries with it responsibility. An expert leader is able to get others to feel responsible for what goes on. That is real political power and influence.

What are the legitimate sources of power? Let's apply some of these principles of power to medicine as it is currently practiced in this country. The first source of power is money. It represents a potential reserve to influence the outcome of any situation. For example, if the problem is laboratory turnaround time, then the laboratory has to recognize potential power. The advent of hand-held, whole blood analyzers provides rapid results for numerous studies, with 2% variance. If that information is made available to the pathologist with a note that says, "We're coming!" you are likely to see laboratory turnaround times improve. Financial interests therefore have a legitimate source of power. Such power cannot be arbitrary or capricious. For example, we negotiated an interesting contract at one hospital in which the laboratory had to guarantee quality and turnaround times or substantial financial penalties had to be paid. The first month of the contract the pathology department owed the emergency department $5000. They did not wait until the second month to say, "You know, at the end of the year that's $60,000. We can hire an extra technician for that and have the equipment ready to support them." This sounded reasonable to all parties involved and represents the type of arrangement that can happen when financial interests and logical, not capricious, planning occurs. The goal is always to improve patient care and throughput time.

Emergency physicians are often faced with the *power of knowledge*. This power is most often used against emergency physicians. The classic argument from authority using the power of knowledge comes from specialty groups that imply that the emergency department knows nothing about their subspecialty interest. "I'm the cardiologist—I know." For example, in many hospitals, when there are cocaine-related cardiac problems, the cardiologist often calls the emergency department for consultation because emergency physicians see more of these problems than cardiologists. Orthopedic surgeons are used to the concept of using the emergency physician to assist them in conscious sedation of patients for manipulation for painful procedures. The decision to use thrombolytic agents in the emergency department is almost universally made by emergency physicians because cardiologists, internists, and other healthcare providers have clearly recognized that delays in administration of therapy to contact specialty care are both impractical and inhumane.

Emergency physicians should remember the *power of official recognition*. When emergency physicians become fellows and board certified in that, they should send out cards to announce the enlargement of their roles. They should have practice brochures that describe the training and expertise of their members, along with pictures so that new medical staff members can easily recognize them. When emergency physicians publish articles, they should mail them to members of the medical staff, administration, and the board. When members of the emergency department write textbooks, copies of the books should be given to the hospital, with pictures in the medical staff or board mailouts. Official recognition outside of the institution of both the specialty and the individual physician is extremely important.

The *power of clinical ability* is an essential type of power. Private physicians have a certain sense of security when they turn their patients over to another physician who cares for them appropriately. Most attending physicians want to provide good patient care and greatly respect an emergency physician who can manage clinical care issues.

Finally, we live in a political world. No matter how difficult it is to do the right thing, someone will ensure that the right action occurs. You need to make sure that person is you. Friends and allies are critical. Reward loyalty and integrity, not just in your own members, but with hospital staff as well. Give positive reinforcement. An experienced gynecologist on our staff has assumed responsibility for difficult cases. The emergency department sent her a card with a dozen roses simply saying, "You are a great person to work with." Does a card like that generate power? You bet it does.

How is power translated into policy? Organizations, like people, need a core set of values and principles. People need to have a statement that clarifies what it is they stand for—a value statement or mission statement, around which the organization is centered. All successful policy must then be technically feasible, have cost-benefit analysis, and also be related to either stated or implied values or missions.

Policy is a science, but science often takes a back seat to political expediency. No matter how correct a solution may be, if the politics aren't right at the time, the solution won't be accepted. Policy is in its most powerful form when it is in its simplest form. Policy must be stated succinctly, procedures can be explained in more detail if necessary. All emergency departments have a policy on transfers and on the admission of drug addiction patients to the hospital. These policies should be stated simply and in accord with the values of the organization. In fact, the real challenge to emergency departments is to relate policy to the value or mission statement of the organization. Policy based on values is strongest and lasts the longest. Good policy ideas can come from anywhere. Everyone in an organization should have equal access to the policy chain.

In power relationships, the quality of mercy is not strained, but is pureed frequently. The lesson is always to set up a "win-win" situation. Establish criteria early and remember it is not what you want at the moment, it is where you are going. The problem of dictated emergency department medical records illustrates how a win-win situation can resolve a discussion or negotiation. There are two ways to approach this situation. One can walk into the administrator's office and say, "The emergency department demands dictated medical records!" The administrator may well say, "That costs money. When can we expect your check?" You can also approach the problem by stating, "I think I have an idea that can save the hospital a substantial amount of money." This approach always gets an administrator's undivided attention, particularly in today's healthcare environment. If your approach is, "I've got a way of saving you money. We are spending too much time doing Quality Assurance; we are having poor communication with our doctors. This is probably why we aren't getting enough outside referrals, particularly from paying patients. I have a way that we can improve this and here's the system." This is a true win-win situation in which both parties can relate to a common goal. In such situations real progress is far less difficult. The ultimate reward in power sharing is to have the other person present the idea as if it were his or her own at Executive Committee. At one of our hospitals, one physician typed his records for a week, simply as a trial. At the next Executive Committee, the Chief of Medicine said, "I've never had anything as good in my whole life. I now know what my patients had when they went to the emergency department." The Chief of Medicine proposed at Executive Committee that the hospital type all emergency department medical records. The Emergency Department Chairman did not have to present the idea and the hospital ended up recouping about 15% more in reimbursement.

An important rule of power is that small areas of agreement can lead to big areas of agreement. The process is often more important than the outcome. You need to be eternally optimistic in power situations because your mood and attitude are infectious. Edison once said, "There are two kinds of people, those who think they can and those who think they can't. Both groups are correct."

Decoys and red herrings rule the world. People set up all kinds of "straw men" in power situations and in negotiations to try to divert attention away from the goal. Learn how to use that situation to your advantage. When a physician says that she needs an emergency department dictation system and new furniture for the office, and it would also be good to recarpet the waiting room, the hospital administrator would say, "We can't do all that." The next response should be, "Okay I can live without the furniture in my office, but can we get the waiting room recarpeted this week?" We often set up a red herring as a negotiating ploy. Hospitals, physicians, and others also use this strategy. Don't let it divert you from your goals. A classic mistake of emergency physicians in power situations arises when an administrator comes in and says, "Well, you have to start doing X now. It is really important, and there are only about 20 forms that you will have to fill out now with patients who have X." This is a classic "tyranny of the immediate." Someone comes to you in a crisis situation expecting you to solve that crisis, often by an incredibly complex action or series of actions. Analyze these situations carefully. Decide when you are and when you are not in a crisis situation. Do not make policy in a crisis mode unless it is absolutely necessary. Even then, such policy should be in effect only for the duration of the crisis.

The principle rule of all power and policy in the emergency department is that it begins and ends with patient care. Regardless of the issue for which you are negotiating or the subject under discussion, always frame it in terms of what is best for the patient. The extent to which emergency medicine is true to its calling is the extent to which it does not deviate from doing what is best for the patient. That is the truest, purest, and most complete definition of power that emergency medicine can hope to attain.

3 Emergency Department Organizational Structure: THE ACADEMIC SETTING

Keith E. Loring, Gus M. Garmel, and Paul S. Auerbach

OUTLINE

Evolution of academic emergency medicine
Overall structure of the academic emergency department
Administration of academic emergency clinical practice
  Emergency department director
  Clinical director
  Nurse manager
Administration of emergency medicine residency training
  Residency program director
  Education director
  Research director
  Chief resident and housestaff
  Emergency medicine fellow
Additional administration coordination
  Administrative assistant
Summary

We have chosen the defining characteristic of an academic emergency department (ED) to be primary responsibility for an emergency medicine residency training program within a university teaching hospital. The methods by which an academic ED balances clinical teaching and research with patient care distinguish it from nonacademic community clinical departments. This chapter focuses on the additional administrative roles required to achieve the academic mission.

EVOLUTION OF ACADEMIC EMERGENCY MEDICINE

Emergency medicine evolved differently from other medical specialties. In the broadest sense, it began in the community and then gradually broached academia. The specialty was not conceived out of a need to narrow the focus of an existing discipline; rather it evolved because of a need for better care in a specific clinical setting. The "emergency room" had rapidly become the center for medical emergencies, primary care of the uninsured, and continued care of persons who had no regular medical care. Recognizing these needs, part-time physicians began devoting a full-time commitment to emergency medical care. They subsequently developed the specialty of emergency medicine and stimulated the development of departments of emergency medicine.

These pioneer physicians saw the need to refine the science of emergency medical care and establish standards that could come only from a disciplined approach. This necessitated the organization of emergency medicine residency training, which began in a handful of academic medical centers (AMCs) in the early 1970s. There was some degree of philosophic and bureaucratic opposition to this training from the traditional specialties of internal medicine, surgery, and pediatrics, because housestaff physicians in training from these specialties provided the majority of patient care in the ED. Few academic institutions saw a need for direct supervision of these residents. Even fewer saw a need to establish independent residency training in emergency medicine. However, concern for patient welfare, unattended educational opportunities, litigation cost containment, an emerging sensitivity to healthcare consumers, and reimbursement pressures surfaced in the EDs of university hospitals nationwide. To adapt, institutions engaged attending physicians to supervise and teach trainees.

It became clear that emergency medicine residencies were vital. Increasingly, AMCs began incorporating emergency medicine as an integral part of their academic mission. In 1972, the first emergency medicine residency graduate completed his training in Cincinnati, Ohio. By 1975, 23 residency programs were endorsed by the newly formed Liaison Residency Endorsement Committee of the American College of Emergency Physicians. Residency refinement and standardization progressed rapidly within participating AMCs through the early 1990s. By 1996, the number of programs grew to 114, providing training for more than 2800 residents annually.

Institutional politics and placement of the specialty within the organization of individual AMCs (division, department, service) have contributed to variations in the specialty's influence among institutions. This variation by necessity reflects the manner in which the specialty entered the academic medical scene, but standardization is anticipated. Presently, some of the most prestigious AMCs in the United States do not fully embrace emergency medicine as an integral component of medical education. Nonetheless, the specialty is blossoming in the many participating AMCs, evidenced by increasing numbers of essential clinical and laboratory investigations that come from academic EDs. Academic emergency medicine programs are involved in social issues and investigate such areas as violence, injury prevention, disaster management, access to medical care, and outcomes research.

OVERALL STRUCTURE OF THE ACADEMIC EMERGENCY DEPARTMENT

Although the majority of emergency medicine residency programs use several emergency departments affiliated with the university, it is usually the ED in the central institution that requires a markedly different organizational structure. Therefore this discussion focuses primarily on the department recognized as the administrative hub of an emergency medicine residency program.

The underlying mission of the academic ED is the same nationwide: the advancement of emergency medicine in concert with rigorous training of future clinicians, researchers, and teachers. This training and associated research, educational, and clinical programs set the academic ED apart from all other EDs. Differences among academic EDs reflect the size of the hospital and its community, the institution's attitude toward emergency medicine, and the enthusiasm with which the specialty has been developed in a particular institution. The clinical and financial challenges facing an inner city academic ED usually differ from those of a suburban academic ED. Larger hospitals generally have higher volume EDs, which may require more expanded administrative efforts divided among a larger number of individuals.

Many AMCs do not have emergency medicine residency programs. Although the EDs within these centers provide patient care through housestaff physicians, often including emergency medicine housestaff from external emergency medicine residency programs, these departments' organizational structures usually do not deviate from traditional ED structures outlined here and expanded on in other chapters (Figures 3-1 and 3-2). Additionally, some academic EDs are preparing to launch emergency medicine residency programs. These departments find themselves in transition toward an academic organizational structure.

Many academic EDs are divisions of other departments within the AMC. The implications of divisional status vary. Without independent departmental status, an ED program faces potential disadvantages, particularly with regard to issues of resource allocation. In addition, nontenure track faculty may not be eligible to participate in democratic decision-making bodies within the AMC, its affiliated medical school, and/or university. Nontenure status may preclude lead investigator status on grant applications. However, national trends are toward parity with other academic departments within the institution. *Clinical professorate* status in many institutions addresses the realities of meeting the needs of essential university clinicians, educators, and program managers. As the significance of emergency medicine's contributions to both individual AMCs and medical education are fully appreciated, the specialty may become one of the best models in this regard. Increasingly, academic department status is being accorded nationwide, with 49 academic departments of emergency medicine now recognized.

With or without department status, the core administrative challenges of an academic ED are essentially the same. The activities of patient care and professional training must progress in concert. Patient care, however, should be the primary focus. The added responsibility of supervising housestaff challenges daily activities. Academic EDs must be more creative and vigilant to remain efficient when faced with the trust of training residents (within and outside the specialty), medical students, nursing students, and other emergency healthcare providers.

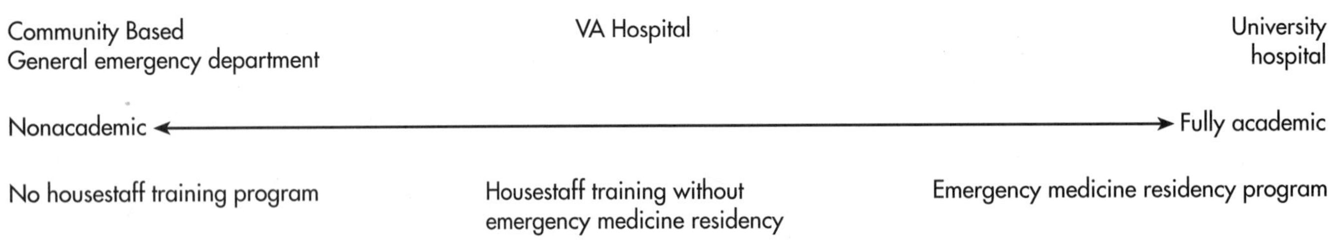

FIGURE 3-1 The academic spectrum in emergency medicine.

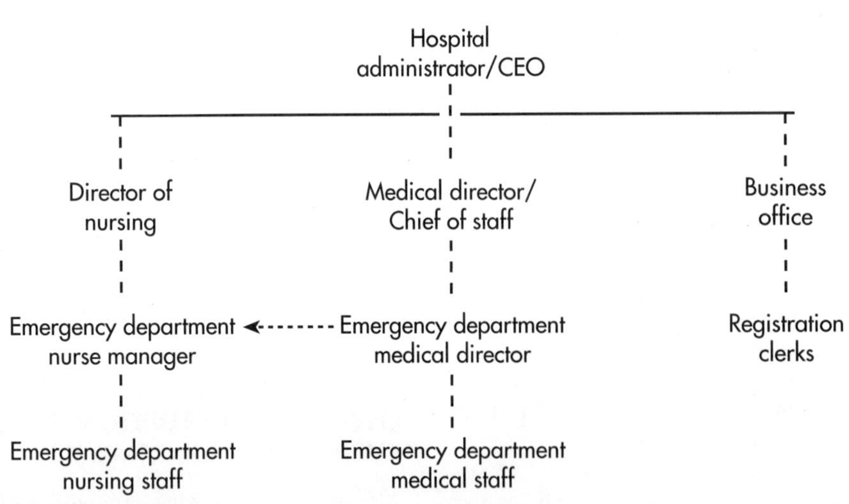

FIGURE 3-2 Nonacademic emergency department organization structure.

(Modified from Ramsey FE: Emergency department organizational structure. In Hellstern RA, editor: ***Managing the emergency department: a team approach,*** Dallas, 1992, American College of Emergency Physicians.)

Administrators of academic EDs therefore face the formidable challenge of balancing patient needs against the myriad intrainstitutional and extrainstitutional demands associated with an AMC and multiple residency programs. The added responsibilities are typically carried out by expanding some traditional administrative roles and by creating new roles as needed. The manner in which these modifications occur depends on the lead individuals within the ED and the emphasis of the ED's residency training program (Figure 3-3).

ADMINISTRATION OF ACADEMIC EMERGENCY CLINICAL PRACTICE

Emergency Department Director

Demands on the academic ED director are great; therefore the director must have outstanding abilities. The position requires a leader with confidence, ambition, and vision. The ability to compromise, and thus to resolve conflict, is just as important as the ability to be decisive, particularly in the face of limited information. The importance of the mission demands that an ED director have proven credibility in his or her field before assuming the position. Therefore intensive familiarity with the workings of an AMC is critical. A background in management and/or finances is certainly helpful.

The responsibilities of an academic ED director are greater than those of a nonacademic ED director. Not only does the director oversee emergency patient care, but he or she must ensure quality management in a setting where clinical teaching is ongoing. Often, the goals of clinical teaching and patient care are at odds. For instance, a delicate balance must be struck between a patient's desire for privacy and the need of a teacher to instruct a student or demonstrate physical findings at the bedside. The ultimate challenge arises with regard to patient flow. A medical student or intern progressing methodically through a workup significantly extends the length of stay of a patient who would otherwise receive a timely disposition from an experienced clinician. It is the medical director's responsibility to provide mechanisms that control this problem. Engaging competent and dedicated faculty, nurses, technicians, social workers, and other ancillary personnel is critical to buffering the delays caused by placing students and residents on the front lines in the ED. Depending on the total administrative load of the director, these functions are often facilitated through a separately designated clinical director.

Clinical Director

Because of the magnitude of an academic ED director's responsibilities, he or she may appoint a clinical director. The clinical director reviews and approves all protocols for care in the ED, including those that originate from other clinical

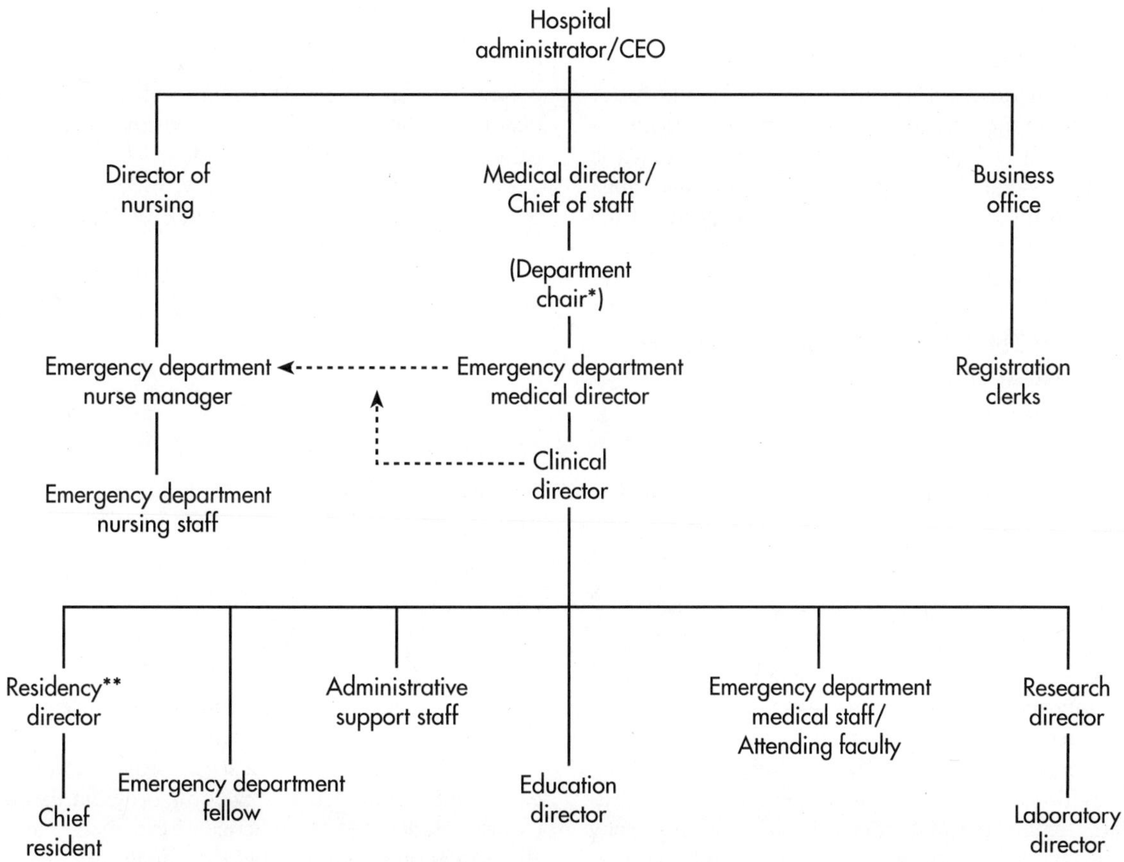

FIGURE 3-3 Academic emergency department organizational structure. *Only of significance in an academic emergency department recognized as a division of another department within the AMC. **Assisted by an associate director and others in larger programs.

(Modified from Ramsey FE: Emergency department organizational structure. In Hellstern RA, editor: ***Managing the emergency department: a team approach,*** Dallas, 1992, American College of Emergency Physicians.)

services. This individual manages the clinical faculty practice and coordinates housestaff practice with the emergency medicine residency director. Additionally, if nurse practitioners, physician assistants, or other physician extenders are present, the clinical director supervises their activities.

Usually, emergency medicine faculty have trained and practiced in many disparate institutions. As a result, the faculty often advocate widely differing approaches to clinical practice. This provides both an opportunity and a challenge. The opportunity is to synthesize the best features of clinical care; however, perceived advisory chaos can create a poor educational environment. Success depends on the clinical director's ability to focus on problems and attain consensus when possible.

The clinical director establishes practice standards in coordination with the department nurse manager. This involves ongoing quality review of emergency medical care by attending physicians, housestaff, nurses, and clinical support staff. Ideally, the clinical director will be an outstanding clinician, a respected motivator, and a facilitator in consensus building among ego-directed healthcare professionals. Teamwork cannot be overemphasized, especially true in the academic setting, where medical students and residents from all disciplines seek guidance from emergency medicine attendings.

Nurse Manager

The nurse manager is an important leader of the administrative and clinical teams. In the academic ED, the nurse manager must coordinate nursing care closely with the needs of housestaff and medical student training. Nursing staff must work with physicians who often possess marginal clinical judgment and experience. The nurse manager should foster an environment among nursing staff that promotes patient advocacy in a setting where the least experienced physician is often the first to evaluate the patient. The nurse manager must recruit the best clinical nurses possible who understand the importance of housestaff training and are willing to provide positive contributions in that effort.

ADMINISTRATION OF EMERGENCY MEDICINE RESIDENCY TRAINING

Residency Program Director

The abilities of a suitable emergency medicine residency director generally match those of the department director. The greatest strengths must be in education and motivation. Clearly, the residency director holds a position unique to the academic ED. This individual is primarily responsible for the content and quality of housestaff education. He or she must provide a smooth transition for residents from medical school to independent practice in emergency medicine. The administrative relationship between the residency director and the department director is an important key to the success of the department's academic mission. The ED director depends on the residency director for information about required teaching standards within the department. In turn, the residency director relies on the department director to ensure appropriate clinical facilities for teaching and to maintain a culture among the healthcare staff that is conducive to professional training.

The residency director has direct responsibility for planning and overseeing clinical rotations, scheduling housestaff, and providing didactic conferences covering the established Core Content for Emergency Medicine. Additionally, the residency director is responsible for housestaff well-being, including discipline. The program director may also be involved in guiding resident research and educational activities. These challenging responsibilities may be achieved by the program director alone, in conjunction with an associate director, and/or through integration of a chief resident or other administrative housestaff positions. Additional positions of education director, research director, and direct administrative support staff may be warranted.

Coordinating clinical rotations must occur with the cooperation of nearly every department within the AMC and often involves other affiliated institutions. The residency director must consider the requirements of different specialty training programs within an institution and work to mutually benefit everyone while not detracting from the residency experience in emergency medicine. In this regard, the residency director needs to establish strong relationships with other specialty heads to negotiate effectively.

The residency program director completes all responsibilities commensurate with the standards set forth by the Accreditation Council for Graduate Medical Education (ACGME). This council develops rules by which a residency (and therefore an academic ED) must operate. The ACGME regulates residency programs through Residency Review Committees (RRC). The RRC for emergency medicine is composed of emergency physicians to ensure strong educational standards geared toward current practice. The accreditation process necessitates close coordination of department policy between the department director and the residency director, emphasizing that this relationship is one of the administrative cornerstones of the academic ED.

Emergency medicine residency directors nationally have the opportunity to join the Council of Residency Directors within the Society for Academic Emergency Medicine. In this forum, residency directors address concerns that arise as a direct result of the policies set forth by the RRC. Through this exchange, residency directors strive to provide their own programs and associated emergency departments with the positive experiences of others nationwide.

Education Director

The education director has the task of organizing medical student education. Medical students are a distinct group in academic EDs. Medical students make up the pool from which future residents will be selected. Moreover, they are the future medical specialists and generalists who will serve as consultants or admitting physicians and whose patients will present to the ED. Therefore the importance of providing medical students with an optimal experience in emergency medicine cannot be understated.

The education director must coordinate between the medical school and the ED to develop a program that adequately exposes students to the practice of emergency medicine. An ED education program should stimulate medical students to pursue careers in this specialty. Simultaneously, it should foster an appreciation for emergency medicine among students who enter other fields. This position requires an individual with enthusiasm for teaching, who can establish good rapport with students, and who can enhance the teaching efforts of others.

Research Director

In the academic ED, an active program of research should be ongoing. These activities may be coordinated by the research director. This person must have a solid background in scientific methodology and the art of grantsmanship. He or she needs to be a source of independent ideas, as well as a facilitator for the ideas of others.

The research director should have a method for directing housestaff and medical students through the endeavors of research. This effort should extend to other faculty as well, either through a formal didactic program or on an individual project basis. Key areas that should be emphasized are study design, funding, human subjects approval, study implementation, data acquisition, and statistical analysis with interpretation. Furthermore, the research director should provide assistance with preparation of oral/poster presentations and manuscripts for peer-review publication. A research program may require a laboratory director to manage nonclinical investigations.

Departmental commitment to ongoing research is often difficult to maintain, but it is essential to the progress of emergency medicine in general and the academic ED specifically. Funding for this activity depends largely on the faculty's ability to procure grants. Institutional financial support usually hinges on grant support.

Chief Resident and Housestaff

Many residency programs select a chief resident(s) each year. This position allows development of leadership, administrative, and teaching skills. The chief resident devotes varying amounts of time to educational activities, administrative tasks, research projects, clinical teaching, and practice. These efforts are focused primarily on the emergency medicine residency program and are directly supervised by the residency director. Typically, a residency will tailor the chief resident position based on the particular needs of the program. Ideally, the position can be given enough latitude to promote the individual interests of the chief resident(s) as well.

Emergency Medicine Fellow

Although fellowship training is not generally essential to the functioning of an academic ED, an emergency medicine fellow can greatly enhance the research, educational, and clinical aspects of a residency training program. Currently, fellowship programs exist in the areas of academic emergency medicine, emergency medicine administration, emergency medical systems, pediatric emergency medicine, emergency medical research, and toxicology.

ADDITIONAL ADMINISTRATIVE COORDINATION

Administrative Assistant

Many general administrative tasks become particularly complex in academic EDs. Funding sources come not only from patient billing, but also from the hospital, health plan, medical school, grants, contracts, and gifts. Office space and facility support for faculty, residents, nursing management, researchers, billing staff, and others require detailed coordination that should not distract the director from other crucial functions. Therefore some directors employ an administrative assistant. The assistant often prepares budgets, supervises business operations, assists with grant writing, procures capital equipment acquisition and supervises maintenance, and provides personnel management.

SUMMARY

The practice of emergency medicine has undergone substantial development since the inception of dedicated residency training almost two decades ago. Leaders in academic EDs have played a crucial role in the success of emergency medicine. As seen through the eyes of patients and healthcare providers alike, the future of emergency medicine depends on continued education, determination, and foresight by academic specialists who direct their departments well.

Were Abraham Flexner alive today, he might again be reporting on the need to refocus medical education in the United States. He might no longer see an urgent need to improve the quality of education; his original report ensured the development of today's strong academic standards. Rather, he might conclude that the emphasis of medical training should change so that medical professionals are trained in primary care specialties to address the general medical needs of the American people. An established academic ED ought to serve as one model in this regard.

Although some may argue that there should be a clear delineation between *emergency, urgent,* and *primary* care, the trend toward national healthcare and efficient use of resources suggests that the ED will continue to serve many masters. Nowhere is this more true than in the academic health center. Administrative support for this enterprise is crucial.

BIBLIOGRAPHY

Allison JE: Academic emergency medicine: past, present, and future trends, *Ann Emerg Med* 18:772-773, 1989.

American College of Emergency Physicians, American Board of Emergency Medicine, and the Society for Academic Emergency Medicine Joint Policy Statement: Core content for emergency medicine, *Ann Emerg Med* 20:920-934, 1991.

Association of Academic Chairs of Emergency Medicine: Academic departments of emergency medicine, *The Society For Academic Emergency Medicine Newsletter.* 5:5, 1993.

Chernow SM, Emerman CL, Langdorf M et al: Academic emergency medicine: a national profile with and without emergency medicine residency programs, *Ann Emerg Med* 21:947-951, 1992.

Dailey RH: Approach to administration in the emergency department. In Rosen P, editor: *Emergency medicine: principles and practice,* ed 3, St Louis, 1992, Mosby.

Darr K, Longest BB, Rakich JS: *Managing health services organizations,* Philadelphia, 1977, WB Saunders.

Ebert RH: Flexner's model and the future of medical education, *Acad Med* 67:737-742, 1992.

Flexner A: *Medical education in the United States and Canada. A report to the Carnegie Foundation for the Advancement of Teaching,* Bulletin No. 4, Boston, 1910, Updyke.

Gallagher EJ, Goldfrank LR, Anderson GV et al: Role of emergency medicine residency programs in determining emergency medicine career choice among medical students, *Ann Emerg Med* 22:904-907, 1993.

Gallagher EJ, Goldfrank LR, Anderson GV et al: Current status of academic emergency medicine in the United States, *Acad Emerg Med* 1:41-46, 1994.

Graduate Medical Education, Appendix II, Tables 1-4, *JAMA* 270:1116-1120, 1993.

Hamilton GC: Content listings for consistency of policies and procedures in an academic department, *Ann Emerg Med* 18:673-677, 1989.

Hamilton GC: Reorganizing academic emergency medicine: Who? Why? How? *Am J Emerg Med* 6:416-423, 1988.

Henneman PL, Hockberger RS, Chiu C: Attending coverage in academic emergency medicine: a national survey, *Ann Emerg Med* 18:34-41, 1989.

Holliman CJ, Wuerz RC, Kimak MJ et al: Documentation of the need for attending supervision of residents in the emergency department, *Ann Emerg Med* 22:904-908, 1993.

Jenkins AL: *Emergency department organization and management,* ed 2, St Louis, 1978, Mosby.

King C, Nilsen GJ, Henretig FM et al: Proposed fellowship training program in pediatric emergency medicine for emergency medicine graduates, *Ann Emerg Med* 22:542-546, 1993.

Kroboth FJ, Brown FH, Stewart R et al: Impact of attending level supervision of the emergency department experience, *Ann Emerg Med* 11:192-196, 1982.

McNamara RM, Kelly JJ: Impact of an emergency medicine residency program on the quality of care in an urban community hospital ED, *Ann Emerg Med* 21:528-533, 1992.

McNamara RM, Kelly JJ: Cost of care in the emergency department: impact of an emergency medicine residency program, *Ann Emerg Med* 21:956-962, 1992.

Managazzi JJ, Wolfson AB, Yealy DM: A model of a residency research design and statistics curriculum, *Ann Emerg Med* 20:472-475, 1991.

Martini CJM, Grenholm G: Institutional responsibility in graduate medical education and highlights of historical data, *JAMA* 270:1053-1060, 1993.

Menegazzi JJ, Wolfson AB, Yealy DM: A model of a residency research design and statistics curriculum, *Ann Emerg Med* 20:472-475, 1991.

Miller M: *The nurse manager in the emergency department,* St Louis, 1983, Mosby.

Nilsen GJ, Neiman L: An educational fellowship in emergency medicine, *Ann Emerg Med* 20:469-471, 1991.

Panacek EA, Rutherford WF, Jouriles NJ: The effect of varying levels of attending supervision of housestaff on emergency department patient disposition decisions, *Ann Emerg Med* 21:616-619, 1992.

Podolsky SM et al: Characteristics of emergency medicine fellowships, *Ann Emerg Med* 17:1-5, 1988.

Ramsey FE: Emergency department organizational structure. In Hellstern RA, editor: *Managing the emergency department: a team approach,* Dallas, 1992, American College of Emergency Physicians.

Riggs LM: A vigorous new specialty, *N Engl J Med* 304:480-483, 1981.

Rosen P, Markovchick V: Attending coverage, *Ann Emerg Med* 14:897-899, 1985.

Rupke JA: *Twenty-five years on the front line,* Dallas, 1993, American College of Emergency Physicians.

Rusnak RA, Hamilton GC, Allison EJ: Autonomous departments of emergency medicine in contemporary academic medical centers, *Ann Emerg Med* 20:680-687, 1991.

Sacchetti A, Carraccio C, Harris R: Resident management of emergency department patients: is closer attending supervision needed? *Ann Emerg Med* 21:749-752, 1992.

Schwab RA, Kuhlman TP, Fau YH: Impact of emergency medicine residency program on rotators' emergency medicine education, *Ann Emerg Med* 21:614-615, 1992.

Schwartz A, Ginsburg PB, LeRoy LB: Reforming graduate medical education: summary report of the Physician Payment Review Commission, *JAMA* 270:1079-1082, 1993.

Tachakra SS: Outpatient undergraduate education: our pivotal role, *Ann Emerg Med* 21:456-457, 1992.

Trott A, Blackwell T: Academic emergency medicine in United States medical schools, *Ann Emerg Med* 21:952-955, 1992.

Tydman RJ, Zalenski RJ, Fagan JK: An evaluation of research training from a large residency program, *Ann Emerg Med* 21:612-613, 1992.

van de Leuv JH: *Management of emergency services,* Rockville, 1987, Aspen Publishers.

Weigand JV, Kuhn G, Gerson LW: Directing an emergency medicine residency: The problems and their solutions, *Ann Emerg Med* 22:904 (abstract) 1993.

Whitley TW, Spivey WH, Abramson NS et al: A basic resource guide for emergency medicine research, *Ann Emerg Med* 19:1306-1309, 1990.

4 Emergency Department Organizational Structure in the Community Hospital

Bruce D. Janiak

OUTLINE

Perhaps at no time in the last few decades has the future of emergency medicine, indeed of all medical practice in the United States been harder to predict. Medical futurists, especially the pessimists, do not lack for material to fuel their negativism. Yet in every threat there is opportunity, and emergency medicine should be well positioned to analyze choices and take full advantage of change.

Community hospitals will be major players in healthcare alliances, and the formation of these alliances seems to be taking place in advance of any government mandates. Hospital administrators have become aware that the emergency department is responsible for a large part of the institution's community image. Thus the organization of the emergency department is crucial to the institution's efficient operation and its ability to deliver high-quality care in a financially restricted environment.

THE NEED FOR DEPARTMENTALIZATION

Departmentalization allows parity with other departments, a voice and vote in hospital governance, an advocacy position for patients' needs, a focus for marketing efforts, a structure for new lines of business, and a chair of responsibility that answers to medical staff, administration, the board, and the patients served in the community.

When the emergency department (or "emergency room" in this case) is not an autonomous unit with attendant rights and responsibilities, emergency leadership flounders without a structure to effect change. Thus criticisms are left unsaid and the department leadership may become narrowly focused into a "don't rock the boat" operational philosophy. Policies and procedures tend to be written in response to needs of individual medical staff members or administration rather than in response to needs of the emergency patients. In sum, the patients and the emergency department team are left out of the picture.

The emergency department needs to be a department. The physician director should be a voting member of the executive committee. He or she should have a line of communication to the board of trustees. The director should be responsible for the department budget and have the task of justifying expenditures for capital and staff. Support for this responsibility should be provided by a full-time secretarial staff and attendant office space in larger institutions; smaller hospitals may be adequately served by shared staff or part-time secretarial support.

Nursing and all other personnel can report directly to the emergency physician leader or to the director of nursing for the emergency area. There are many variations, although the principle of physician leadership should not be subverted. Many departments are "secretly" led by the emergency department nursing director because of a physician leadership vacuum. This situation must change before the emergency department can achieve an appropriate level of respect and responsibility within those institutions.

USE OF THE EXECUTIVE COMMITTEE

From the emergency department's viewpoint, the executive committee should function both as a platform for communication and as an instrument for change. An emergency department director who passively attends the meetings only to listen and vote on generic medical staff issues is not getting full value from the membership position. Emergency department statistics should be reported frequently, especially those that represent problems. For example, if emergency department radiographs are read first by the radiologist because of a radiography department policy, and resultant through-put times are needlessly prolonged, then those facts should be reported. The best outcome would be a policy change; the worst would be to have the executive committee accept the responsibility for the negative public relations effect of continuing the old practice.

Many medical staff members in primary care still view the emergency department and emergency physicians as a necessary evil. The emergency department still "competes" for their patients. One way to counter this way of thinking is to calculate the number of new, unassigned patients seen in the emergency department every year and present this information to the executive committee and medical staff. In many emergency departments, the insurance mix for this group of patients is surprisingly good. Members of the executive committee should then understand that the emergency department can be a significant source of new business, a fact already understood by surgical and medical specialists.

The message here is to *use* the executive committee, rather than let it use you.

INTERDEPARTMENTAL AND INTRADEPARTMENTAL ORGANIZATION

Every community-based hospital emergency department should have a physician director who functions as both the administrative and clinical leader. Many emergency department nursing leaders also carry the title of *emergency department director.* Therefore to avoid confusion it is reasonable to have a nursing director and a physician medical director, as long as the overall leadership responsibility rests with the physician. The relationship of these two individuals must be respectful, congenial, and symbiotic. *Any* friction, mistrust, or ego problems tend to promote dysfunctional leadership—a situation easily detected by all emergency department staff.

The larger the department, the greater the need for delegation of leader/director functions on both the physician and nursing levels. A vice-chairperson should be named to cover for the physician director when he or she is unavailable. High-volume departments may need to delegate specific administrative responsibilities to many of the emergency physicians. For instance, one could consider placing an emergency physician in charge of continuing medical education (CME), disaster management, graduate and medical education, nursing relations, policy development, new equipment/product evaluations, observation unit, fast tracks, hospital committee representations, and quality improvement.

DEPARTMENTAL MEETINGS

Although Joint Commission on Accreditation of Healthcare Organizations (JCAHO) requirements are changing, I believe regular meetings are essential. There should be a written agenda in the regular format (Box 4-1). Minutes should be kept to allow any interested department member to view the "paper trail" of issue resolution. Emergency department meetings are typically longer than those of non–hospital-based departments, probably because departmental clinical issues and group business issues are intermingled. (It may be convenient to keep separate minutes; it certainly is not necessary to record group business for the hospital or JCAHO.) Another reason for longer meetings is simply the multiple functional interrelationships of the emergency department.

It makes good sense to allow emergency department nursing regular time on the emergency department physician meeting agenda. I find it helpful to have some time allotted at each meeting, although it is used only about half the time. In our situation, the majority of physician-nurse communication issues are dealt with in weekly "Progress and Planning" meetings, attended by physician and nursing leadership. The agenda for this "briefing" session includes a review of the most recent minutes of the physician's group and the nursing staff meetings. Issues that the nurses wish the physicians would respond to are communicated (and recorded) and vice-versa (Box 4-2). This format prevents us from "dropping the ball," and helps to focus on high priority projects. Communication is an important part of leadership; no one is likely to follow you without knowing the direction in which you are headed.

BOX 4-1

AGENDA EMERGENCY PHYSICIANS' MEETING
(DATE OF MEETING)
(LOCATION)

Invited Guest(s):

1. Call to Order/Approval of Minutes
2. Report of the Medical Director
3. Report of Director, Pediatric Emerg. Med.
4. Report of the Asst Med Director
5. Report of DME
6. MICU/LCEMS Report
7. New Equipment/Products
8. Risk Management
9. Express Care
10. Nursing Issues
11. Observation Area

Old Business:
New Business:
Case Situation/Issues:
Correspondence:

BOX 4-2

PROGRESS AND PLANNING MEETING
One Hour/Week

Objective: Communication—To keep us on track of projects and work toward goals and objectives.
Attendees:
Agenda:

1. Review appropriate minutes of physicians' meeting(s)
2. Review appropriate minutes of unit meetings
3. Review policy and procedures previous minutes and discuss each item
4. JCAHO Manual
5. Add new items if indicated

Methods:

1. Follow each area to completion
2. Assistant care managers to report to staff at shift meetings
3. Minutes created—secretary to attend—sent to administration
4. Establish priorities for items and projects

A MISSION STATEMENT

All hospital departments must have a reason to exist, a mission. The *development* of a mission statement is an essential first step in creating a cohesive emergency department team, so that all personnel can share the same goals and objectives. The content of the statement and the process of its creation are equally important. Everyone who works in the emergency department should be given the opportunity to contribute, either as part of the initial development team, or by virtue of everyone's right to comment, approve, or suggest revisions. This statement need not be overlong, but should outline the responsibilities of the department to the institution and the community. It should appear in the nursing and physician departmental meeting minutes and thus be available for review and approval by the executive committee. At that time, everyone should be "on board" with regard to the most basic aspects of department philosophy.

The mission statement should not be a static document. Communities and hospitals can change. Emergency departments develop new product lines and new focuses. If the mission statement is gathering dust somewhere, set up a group to review it. It is a healthy and worthwhile exercise.

DELEGATION OF RESPONSIBILITIES

Depending on the size of the department and the interest of the physician leader, administrative responsibilities vary greatly. The trend, however, is distinctly away from the old-fashioned limited approach of "you do the schedule and I'll pay some lip service to QA." The delivery of adequate or even excellent emergency health care is no longer enough to ensure job security in our competitive environment. A successfully organized emergency department will be an active contributor to the institution's reputation. The emergency department should provide leadership in marketing, public relations, and innovation. New ideas should be encouraged, presented, evaluated, and explored. Mistakes, even expensive ones, should be thought of as opportunities to learn rather than excuses for punishment.

If department size and volume justify it, every member of the physician group should have an opportunity to lead some area of the department. It is the department director's job to match skills and interest to areas of responsibility. Further, there is always a need to motivate interest in certain more passive individuals, and eventually, to identify those who just "want to work." Meeting agendas will then be composed of reports from various members on their areas of expertise and/or responsibility. Ideally, this approach should allow for more focused energy on certain areas, while promoting professional development of group physicians. Compensations arrangements can be made to ensure appropriate rewards for these extra efforts.

ENABLING OBJECTIVES

How can all these objectives be realized? How can people be arranged so that meetings can occur, tasks accomplished, goals achieved? On one end of the spectrum lies a department and group devoted to working shifts and patient care only. On the other end lies an administrative hydra, each head worried about other heads, with no consideration for the body. The current pathologic obsession with quality improvement (QI) is a case in point: great gangs of middle managers professing their QI faith, but rendered impotent by lack of time to do good administrative works. A balance must be achieved.

First, the emergency department physician leader must have time to lead. Continuous patient care duties sap energy. Administrative efforts will be limited to the "must be dones" and the "should be dones" will be ignored. Because leadership time and patient volume are roughly related, a 20,000-visit department needs at least a 10-hour/week effort, a 30,000-visit department needs 20 hours/week, a 40,000-visit department needs 30 hours/week, and a 50,000-visit or greater department needs a full-time effort. Failure by the director to work any clinical shifts will erode clinical skills, then clinical credibility, then leadership credibility. Thus no matter how busy the department, the director must see patients regularly.

Second, the director must be compensated for the administrative effort by compensating for administrative hours and clinical hours equally, by placing the director on salary, or by a combination of approaches. It should *not* be accomplished by "rotating" the department directorship among the group. This will provide a fragmented, chaotic leadership that would, at best, have the department running in circles, and at worst, leave the department dead in the water while all hands wait for the changing of the guard rather than accomplish anything that might later be undone.

Third, adequate support services, in the form of a secretary and office, are necessary. Show me a physician who types his or her own letters and I will show you a $100/hour typist (and probably a bad one, at that).

Fourth, no one can lead without being given a license to do so. The group must feel that the dollars they are using to support the leader, or the hours they are working to fill in for the leader, are well spent. Conversely, the leader's job is to improve the lot of the group member either financially, or by reducing stress by improving the working environment. A one-word biologic definition for this relationship would be *symbiotic*.

Fifth, nothing can occur if the hospital administration does not believe in emergency medicine. It must understand that the emergency department exists not to serve the medical staff but to serve the patients in the hospital's catchment area. Some of these patients may have private physicians, but those physicians do not "own them" as some private physician behaviors would indicate. They must understand that the emergency department is not an overpriced necessary evil, but an institutional image-maker, providing thousands of opportunities yearly to educate the community about the talents and the heart of the institution.

Finally, the administration must be willing to risk some capital on new ideas, *if* those ideas are well thought out and provide a situation in which the institution, the medical staff members, and the emergency department all stand a good chance for a positive outcome.

RELATIONSHIPS WITH ADMINISTRATION

A sound working relationship with the hospital president, vice presidents, and others in administration is essential and should be built on a foundation of mutual respect. The goal of the emergency department director should be to exhibit such leadership skill to ensure the group's longevity. Job security in emergency medicine is related to performance and productivity. We do not have tenure. Emergency physicians, like all hospital-based physicians, live with a certain degree of job uncertainty. Rather than lament our vulnerability we should focus our energies into making ourselves and, by association, our groups and departments indispensable. This cannot be accomplished passively. We cannot expect immunity from change if our only two virtues are good clinical care and willingness to respond administratively when asked.

Constant interaction with the president's office is necessary. I have seen several departments in which the emergency department director sees the president only at executive committee meetings. This behavior should be replaced by a proactive approach. The emergency department director needs to informally "drop in" to the president's office on a regular basis. He or she should know the president's secretary well enough to be connected to the informal informational pipeline that exists in all businesses. This is not to say that all visits should be frivolous. Frequent reports to the president or designee on census changes, failures, and successes will heighten administrative awareness of the emergency department. New ideas, such as physician triage described in the next section, are great fodder for such brief discussions. In every consultation I have made in which the emergency department group contract was in jeopardy, the administrator reported minimal or *no* interactions with the emergency department leader.

Improved interaction with hospital administration should be paralleled by efforts to communicate with the board of trustees. To most members of boards of trustees, hospital-based physicians are faceless entities. Perhaps one or two are known to them, but the rest are merely names without personalities. Further, most members of boards of trustees are not aware of the day-to-day activities in emergency medicine. The emergency director should make every effort to be appointed to a board of trustee committee. The medical staff should encourage the hospital administrator to have annual "retreats" or events in which the medical staff leadership and executive committee intermingle.

I have described a political process that promotes strong advocacy for the emergency department and that is essential for its survival. This process should not be limited to the chief executive officer or the board of trustees alone, but needs to be repeated with at least every vice president. Strong relationships with the director of nursing, risk management, marketing, public relations, pharmacy, maintenance, security, etc, will pay many dividends over the years. For example, our worn out ENT examination chair was in need of replacement, but the expenditures did not make the budgetary "short list." When I explained a recent problem with short-circuited wiring in the chair to our risk manager, he intervened with the budget committee on our behalf and we got the new chair.

The emergency department director must make the hospital view the emergency department as indispensable. This department advocacy role must be linked to a constant search for win-win situations.

FAST TRACK MANAGEMENT

The existence of a fast track is justification for assigning a group member to lead that area. If fast track staffing is accomplished by family practice, or pediatrics, or both, those specialties should be in the management loop as long as control remains with the emergency physician leadership. Interdepartmental issues, quality assurance, marketing, policies, and other areas require an element of on-line management. If no other specialties are involved, matters of staffing, quality assurance, nurse relations, and triage will remain.

OBSERVATION AREA

Books have been written on clinical observation issues. The groundwork laid before the observation area opens will spell the difference between success and failure. Control issues can be the number one stumbling block. Can private physicians admit patients to observation? Can emergency physicians admit patients to observation without the concurrence or knowledge of the primary physician? When a patient has been admitted to observation, which doctor is responsible for ongoing care? Which doctor is responsible for discharge? Is the discharge responsibility shared? Does a cardiologist have to be assigned to all chest pain patients? How will billing be managed? Are current emergency nurses (or physicians, for that matter) qualified to "observe" these patients? How are observation patients transferred at change-of-shift? Finally, perhaps the most important question: What type of patients are to be observed? Those with chest pain only? Anyone in a gray clinical zone? Or is the criterion something between these two extremes?

There are probably more questions than answers, but it should be clear by now that careful planning is essential. Any emergency physicians planning an observation area should either visit an ongoing operation and/or hire an experienced consultant to help them through the process or both.

5 Strategic Planning and Mission Statements

E. Jackson Allison, Jr and Jeffrey W. Vawter

OUTLINE

To be effective in today's dynamic healthcare arena, healthcare professionals must constantly assess the reason for their organizations' existence by monitoring the internal and external environments; and they must plan accordingly. The political, social, economic, regulatory, and competitive factors that surround the healthcare industry are manifested in the emergency department. The persistence of violent crimes, the spread of acquired immune deficiency syndrome (AIDS), and the primary needs of the uninsured population deliver outside factors into emergency departments every day. In addition, agencies such as the Joint Commission on Accreditation of Healthcare Organizations (JCAHO) set and survey care standards.

The nature of the business in emergency departments produces staff concerned with critical, life-and-death episodes that demand immediate, tactical decision making. These people must also deal with security issues and the stress brought on by such daily concerns. The resulting, understandable frame of mind can sometimes pose a barrier to strategic, or long-term, thinking. On the other hand, the teamwork and collaboration that are imperative in emergency departments are a strategic planning advantage. Thus the emergent atmosphere does have potential to be tapped for strategic planning efforts.

At the University Medical Center of Eastern Carolina–Pitt County, in Greenville, North Carolina (population approximately 50,000), emergency department staff are confronting environmental challenges proactively. As the medical hub of eastern North Carolina (serving 29 counties), the Medical Center is made up of three constituents: Pitt County Memorial Hospital (PCMH), the Eastern Carolina University School of Medicine (ECU SOM), and the associated private practice physicians. ECU SOM was founded in 1975 to promote family medicine and primary care. It graduated its first class in 1981. Graduating class size has averaged 70 students. The Department of Emergency Medicine (founded in 1980) is a fully autonomous academic department. It established its residency program in 1983. The medical staff consists of 15 MD faculty, 1 fellow, 2 researchers (1 MD, 1 PhD), and 30 residents. With the completion of a new bed tower for critical care and support services in late 1993, PCMH expanded from 609 to 725 beds. An upcoming 20-bed expansion of the rehabilitation center will increase licensed bed capacity to 745.

This chapter draws from several models of strategic planning and from examples at the University Medical Center of Eastern Carolina–Pitt County. To begin with the end in mind, we predict your expanded knowledge on the following topics on completion of the chapter:

- Strategic planning terminology
- An organizational strategic planning framework
- The importance of mission statements and other components of a strategic plan
- The relevance of strategic planning for individual departments like the emergency department

STRATEGIC THINKING

To anticipate events to any degree, a strategic mind set is required. *Strategic thinking* is a continuous state of mind in which creative ideas flow freely and where internal and external environments merge with present and future concerns to set forth models for decision making. Before effective planning can occur, staff at all levels of the organization must begin thinking strategically. In many organizations, a recent embrace of the *continuous quality improvement* philosophy has helped promote the level of staff participation necessary to bring creative ideas to the forefront of organizational planning. After all, "Treating everybody in the organization as planners increases the number of creative ideas."[2] When managers and their staff are thinking strategically together, communication of organizational agendas shows everybody where they fit in the big picture.

Strategic planning for an organization, a department, or an individual, is a means to acknowledge the current situation, determine the desired situation, and plan to narrow the gap between the two. Effective healthcare strategic planning demands a team approach to predict what will happen with regard to external environmental variables such as the following:[3]

- What new laws and reimbursement mechanisms will affect the healthcare field?
- What new competitive healthcare delivery forms will evolve, and how will they affect existing healthcare organizations?
- How will the economy react, and what impact will it have on healthcare usage?

Answers to these questions lead to others such as: How will internal variables including culture, staffing, education, finances, and planning efforts position the organization for coping with environmental fluctuations?

Strategic management is an "externally oriented philosophy of managing an organization" that links strategic planning to operational planning (specific short-term action).[4] Strategic managers continuously "attempt to achieve a fit between the organization's external environment (political, regulatory, economic, technologic, social, and competitive forces) and its internal situation (vision, values, culture, finance, organization, human resources, marketing, information systems, etc)."[4] Adapting to the practice of strategic management does not require a bombardment of policies and forms. In other words, "It is an attitude, not a series of documents."[4]

STAGES OF STRATEGIC MANAGEMENT

Capturing the facets of a managerial attitude in a conceptual model can be rather difficult. However, the approach taken by Duncan et al.[4] supports a malleable model for making decisions through strategic management. This model (Figure 5-1) groups planning processes into four interrelated and evolving stages: (1) situational analysis, (2) strategic formulation, (3) strategic implementation, and (4) strategic control.

During these stages of strategic management, strategic plans and operational plans may be developed. The *situational analysis* and *strategic formulation* stages supply all necessary information to write a strategic plan. A strategic plan is the document that provides "a framework for carrying out strategic thinking, direction, and action leading to the achievement of consistent and planned results."[5] The document should be used to communicate the organization's mission and direction to the staff and community. Below et al.[5] advise planners to use seven integrated elements in a strategic plan[5] (Box 5-1).

The *strategic implementation* stage is facilitated by operational plans. *Operational (tactical) planning* is short-term action planning resulting in a plan to achieve incrementally goals set in the strategic plan. Whereas strategic planning broadly addresses what business you should be in and the direction you should be going, operational planning focuses specifically on how the organization is going to get there.[5] *Strategic control* mechanisms continuously check the congruence of actions with plans and allow adjustments when necessary. Although planning does not adhere to a strict, orderly protocol, each of these stages is described separately. The elements of the written plan are mentioned within the most appropriate stage for their development.

Stage 1: Situational Analysis

Situational analysis is the process of examining the organization's environmental position. These activities provide the material for the strategic analysis section (the database) and the organizational mission section of the strategic plan. Situational analysis is accomplished by three processes: (1) external environmental analysis to identify external opportunities and threats facing the organization, (2) internal environmental analysis to identify internal strengths and weaknesses,

BOX 5-1

COMPONENTS OF A STRATEGIC PLAN

Organizational mission	*addresses*	What?
Strategic analysis	*addresses*	Why?
Strategy	*addresses*	Where?
Long-term objectives	*address*	When? and How?
Integrated programs	*address*	When? and How?
Financial projections	*incorporate*	Portions of each of the first five elements
Executive summary (last)	*incorporates*	Portions of each of the first five elements

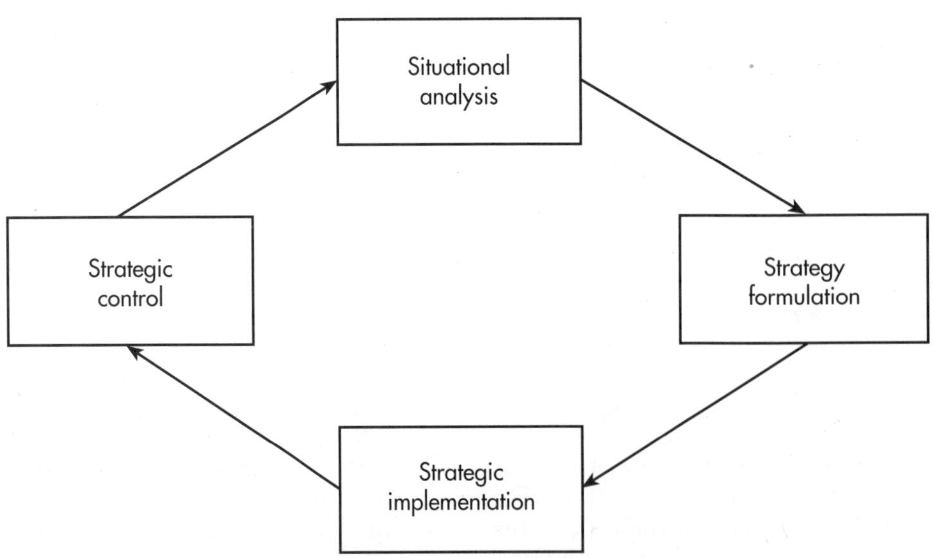

FIGURE 5-1 Stages of strategic management.

(From Duncan WJ, Gunter PM, Swayne LE: ***Strategic management of health care organizations,*** Boston, 1992, PWS-KENT.)

and (3) the development of the organization's purpose, vision, mission, and objectives.[4]

External Environmental Analyses. Four fundamental processes are common to all external environmental analyses: (1) scanning, the process of viewing and organizing external information in an attempt to detect relevant issues that will affect the organization; (2) monitoring, the process of searching for additional information to confirm or disprove the trend, development, dilemma, or likelihood of the occurrence of the event; (3) forecasting, the process of extending issues, identifying their interrelationships and developing alternative projections; and (4) assessing, the process of evaluating the significance of the issues.[4]

Identified issues are usually classified as either technologic, social, political, regulatory, economic, or competitive; and then labeled either an "opportunity" or a "threat."[4] Possible threats could be location, competition, and the aging population. Possible opportunities could be diversification, recruitment, and regional networking. Of course, opportunities and threats are relative to the unique positions of different healthcare organizations.

There are a number of techniques for determining the significance of identified opportunities and threats. Two are stakeholder analysis and solicitation of expert opinions.[4] Stakeholders are organizations, groups, and individuals that have an interest in the success of the organization. Examples of external stakeholders in healthcare organizations are suppliers, third-party payers, competitors, regulatory agencies, the media, and the local community. The stakeholder analysis requires a determination of the nature, positive or negative, of the relationship between each stakeholder and the organization. This process can be followed by discussion of the best communication strategies to foster desired relationships. Healthcare reform could pose threats or opportunities depending on the type of institution and its location.

Multidisciplinary experts may be asked to judge the importance of various issues. Methods for stimulating unbiased idea generation (the Delphi technique, the nominal group technique, brainstorming, and focus groups) are described in the section *Preparing to Plan*.

Internal Environmental Analyses. The internal environmental analysis inspects the organizational culture, management practices, and factors such as staffing and location to identify strengths and weaknesses. This analysis comes after the external environment has been examined because "We can only identify internal strengths and weaknesses in relation to the external environment."[4]

Culture can be defined as "something that characterizes a healthcare organization's customary way of doing things, the values that most members of the organization share, and the things that must be learned and subscribed to by new members if they are to be satisfied and productive in their jobs."[4] An organization's culture is a powerful force that often sets the tone for interactions. For example, a hospital can be inherently conservative, risk-taking, team oriented, or internally competitive. Culture can either help or hinder response to external opportunities and threats.

An internal audit may be performed to determine strengths and weaknesses. In an audit, planners determine functional subsystems such as clinical, administrative services, marketing, financial, and general management. A list of questions is developed to evaluate each subsystem on key factors such as staff, information and intelligence, and technical capabilities.[4] Possible strengths could be low cost, team work, reputation, nurse/patient ratio, and strategic planning. Possible weaknesses could be payer mix, old equipment, financial inefficiency, and land shortage for expansion.

Identifying strengths manages the consequences of risk, because "Internal strength succeeds even in the face of extraordinary turbulence because knowing who you are, what you can do, and what you cannot do gives the organization the confidence and stability to know when to adapt to an external stimulus (opportunity or threat) or not."[2]

Mission Statements. Once the organization is aware of its environmental position, it is able to determine its mission. Duncan et al.[4] define a mission as "the consensus and articulation of the organization's understanding of the external opportunities and threats, the internal strengths and weaknesses, and the organizational purpose and vision. It is a general statement of what distinguishes the organization from all others of its type." In other words, the mission answers the *what* questions. What business should the organization be in? What is the basic nature and concept of the organization? What is the philosophic basis for its existence?[5] Reasons for having a mission include the following: (1) to ensure consistency and clarity of purpose throughout the organization, (2) to provide a point of reference for all major planning decisions, (3) to gain commitment from those within the organization through clear communication of the nature and concept of the organization's business, and (4) to gain understanding and support from those people outside the organization who are important to its success.[5]

Mission statements are visible organizational communicators. Therefore content and substance are worth careful consideration. Although organizational philosophy is included in mission statements, a statement consisting only of a broad philosophy is just a "platitudinous obeisance to motherhood and apple pie."[2] Statements like "We strive to provide high quality care to all the members of the community," without including elements to differentiate the organization from others, are much too general. Box 5-2 shows an original mission (general) and the revised mission with better detail.[4]

To form a mission statement, a multidisciplinary planning group meeting may be convened. Participation is the key to successful adherence to a mission because an organization "does not have inherent values; it takes on the values of the people who run it." Furthermore, "if the organization wants to do well, its values match as closely as possible those of its customers."[2] The participants should consider the following questions: (1) Are we not doing anything new that we should be doing? (2) Are we doing some things now that we should not be doing? (3) Are we doing some things now that we should continue to do, but in a different way?[4]

Mission statements are of various lengths, depending on the type of organization and its affiliations. A typical mission statement has any combination of the following components:[4]

- target customers and markets
- principal services delivered by the organization
- geographic area within which the organization intends to concentrate
- the organization's philosophy
- confirmations of the organization's preferred self-image
- specification of the organization's desired public image.

BOX 5-2

SPARKMAN CENTER MISSION STATEMENT: OLD AND NEW

Original mission	Recommended mission
The mission of the John Sparkman Center is to be the leader in public health education training.	The mission of the John Sparkman Center is to provide medium-term, graduate and professional education programs, on-site, utilizing available expertise with the ultimate intent of improving the quality, quantity, and delivery of public health services to people in less-developed nations.

From Duncan WJ, Ginter PM, Swayne LE; *Strategic management of health care organizations,* Boston, 1992, PWS-KENT.

Missions may start with an umbrella statement followed by a series of statements of specific philosophy and overall operation.[5] Some missions may be divided into several interdependent sections. For instance, an academic medical center may have a general mission, a service mission, an educational mission, and a research mission. The American College of Emergency Physicians developed a Statement of Direction that includes a mission statement, preamble, and value statements (Appendix A).[6] Pitt County Memorial Hospital uses a statement of mission describing the structure and type of organization, followed by more concise operational mission statement describing the type of care given (Box 5-3).

Mission statements should be reviewed formally at least once a year. Although they should stand the test of time to a certain extent, changes are periodically necessary. To keep the mission current and in the minds of the stakeholders, the mission (or an excerpt) may be printed as a footer on organizational stationary. Managers may also ask employees at random (in a nonthreatening way) if they know and understand the mission.

> "An organizational mission statement—one that truly reflects the deep shared vision and values of everyone within the organization—creates a great unity and tremendous commitment. It creates in people's hearts and minds a frame of reference, a set of criteria or guidelines, by which they will govern themselves. They don't need someone else directing, controlling, criticizing, or taking cheap shots. They have bought into the changeless core of what the organization is about."[1]

Stage 2: Strategic Formulation

Based on the results of the situational analysis, *strategy formulation* is "the process of generating strategic alternatives, evaluating the alternatives, and formulating a strategy for the organization."[4] Strategic formulation supplies the strategy, long-term objectives, integrated programs, and financial projections for the strategic plan. The strategy determines the overall direction of the organization. It requires the chief executive officer and the planning team to think strategically in terms of *where* the organization should be going rather than *how* it should get there.[5] Currently, vertical integration is a popular strategy to position for healthcare reform. Long-term objectives describe what the organization wants to have or become at some point in the future, usually within 3 to 5 years. Because long-term objectives are strategic in nature, they focus more on a position to be attained than on specific

BOX 5-3

PITT COUNTY MEMORIAL HOSPITAL

Statement of mission

Pitt County Memorial Hospital is a voluntary not-for-profit hospital owned by the County of Pitt and operated by a nonstock, non-profit corporation with Board members being appointed by the Pitt County Board of Commissioners and the University of North Carolina Board of Governors. The Hospital is established to maintain and operate hospitals, clinics, nursing homes and other related facilities to provide for the care and treatment of persons suffering from illnesses, injuries, or disabilities which require outpatient or inpatient hospital care; and,

To carry on any educational activities related to the care of the sick and disabled and the promotion of health and preventive medicine, which in the opinion of the Board of Trustees, may be justified by the facilities, personnel, funds or other resources that are or can be made available; and,

To use the revenues of this corporation and the profits, if any, for the purposes of affording hospital care to those unable to pay for the same, promoting better health, to maintain its hospitals and equipment in good repair and modern condition, and in general, to use, invest and hold all revenues and the profits, if any, for the purposes for which this corporation is organized.

Operational mission statement

The mission of Pitt County Memorial Hospital is to provide excellent patient care services to Pitt County citizens who require community hospital care and also to provide excellent tertiary care services to all of the citizens of Eastern North Carolina. This service will be provided in a caring and compassionate environment with attention to holistic needs of the patient and family. In fulfilling this mission, Pitt County Memorial Hospital will be the primary teaching/research site for the East Carolina University School of Medicine and for other schools of nursing and allied health and will contribute to the future health care of Eastern North Carolina by participating in clinical research.

From: University Medical Center of Eastern Carolina–Pitt County Strategic Plan, April 1992.

accomplishments. For example, an emergency department may state that it wants to open by 1995 a Fast Track component to triage the least acute patients and to open by 1996 a freestanding urgent care center in a local shopping center to attract paying episodic patients. Strategic objectives should (1) be as explicit and as measurable as possible, (2) be attainable, and (3) relate to the key performance areas identified by management.[4] Once agreed on by the planning team, long-term objectives provide the basis for moving into integrated programs where accountability for specific results must be established."[5]

Integrated programs "identify and fix accountability for the specific actions and results required to accomplish long-term objectives."[5] They are still broad in nature but provide the basics for operational plans to be developed later. Below et al.[5] recommend seven steps to forming integrated programs: (1) identify the results needed to accomplish each long-term objective; (2) select the five to ten most critical results required to achieve the long-term objective; (3) Agree on approach; (4) For each integrated program, reach agreement on and document results concerning expected results, timetable, resources, accountability, and feedback mechanisms; (5) invite review and comment from the levels of management that will be implementing these programs; (6) Complete final documentation of the integrated programs; and (7) implement and evaluate the programs.

Financial projections, the last element of the strategic plan, pull together all the finance-related information into one place. They should include a forecast income statement, a forecast balance sheet, a capital expenditures forecast, key indicators of financial performance (forecast), and a financial summary.[5]

Stage 3: Strategic Implementation

Strategic implementation is the "process of translating the strategy of an organization into more specific functional-level strategies, programs, and budgets.[4] Operational plans serve the purpose. They are needed supplements to the strategic plan, because:

> Organizations are not what the organizational charts suggest: nice, neat, well-defined linkages with clear distinctions about who does what, when, where, and how. They are, instead, loosely knit confederations of individuals following dotted-line relationships, ad hoc alliances, and even their own whims. This is the reason for an action plan—some piece of writing that contains for all the protagonists to see (1) what is to be done; (2) why; (3) the names of who does what, when, where, and with what resources; and (4) no less important, how its accomplishment is to be gauged or measured.[2]

Components of an operational plan are the following[2]:

1. What you want to do
   - objectives
   - outcomes
2. Why you want to do it (the rationale)
   - information from environments
   - assumptions
3. Stakeholders
   - who has to be involved or informed
   - responsibility
4. Steps to be taken (the nitty-gritty)
   - what, when, where, how
5. Resources needed
   - people
   - money
   - information
   - facilities
   - technology
   - time
6. Measurement and control

Stage 4: Strategic Control

Strategic control is the "process of reviewing the goals of the organization, measuring the performance of the organization, comparing the goals with the performance, assessing the strategy, and taking corrective action if necessary."[4] Strategic control systems should (1) provide a means to coordinate the efforts of everyone in the organization, (2) motivate managers to achieve objectives, (3) provide an early detection system that indicates when strategic assumptions are wrong or when environmental conditions have changed, and (4) provide a method for management to intervene to correct an ineffective or inefficient strategy.[4]

For controls to be effective, they should be based on accurate, relevant, and timely information. They should be directed at controlling only the critical elements and should be flexible, cost-effective, simple, easy to understand, and timely. Finally, they should emphasize the exceptions.[4] The following steps frame a wise process for any new initiative: (1) setting objectives or standards, (2) measuring performance, (3) comparing objectives with performance, (4) determining the reasons for deviation, and (5) taking corrective action.[4]

DEPARTMENTAL STRATEGIC PLANNING

The organizational strategic plan with its mission should be the "hub of a great wheel," stimulating other specific plans for individual departments.[1] These departmental missions should be in line with the organizational mission but present values unique to the staff of different areas. Not unlike a marching band, the members should march to the beat of the same drum while they are playing different instruments. Going through a strategic planning process is an excellent learning experience for any department. Depending on the specificity of the organizational plan, departmental plans can be custom formatted to provide focused direction. In the emergency department, a planning effort would be especially useful to stimulate discussion among the multiple disciplines. Departmental plans do not have to be a full (seven section) plan:

> *Unit-plan development* could be implemented uniformly throughout the organization. However, a selective implementation plan based on the nature of the department's, or unit's, work and the readiness of the people within that unit for strategic planning is probably more realistic. There are certain functions, marketing or research and development, for example, that tend to be more future oriented, and for them a complete strategic plan, using the seven elements on a smaller scale, may be appropriate. In other areas, provision of unit roles and missions, long-term objectives, and integrated programs may be all that is needed. In still others, it may be sufficient simply to tie in their short-term operational plans with the organizational plan.[4]

BOX 5-4

EAST CAROLINA UNIVERSITY SCHOOL OF MEDICINE – DEPARTMENT OF EMERGENCY MEDICINE MISSION STATEMENT

The mission of the Department of Emergency Medicine is threefold: 1) to foster excellence in patient care for our community and serve as a tertiary care resource for the surrounding counties; 2) to provide the structure for, and support of, undergraduate and graduate medical education to develop motivated, industrious, enthusiastic and knowledgeable physicians; and 3) to continue to develop a faculty committed to exemplary patient care, leadership, teaching and expanding the knowledge base of Emergency Medicine through scholarly activities locally, state-wide, nationally and internationally.

During the planning period, the Department of Emergency Medicine will ensure competency-based education of student and resident physicians, expand and strengthen fellowship and research programs and continue to develop its national leadership role in Emergency Medicine education and the development of appropriate responses to national health care issues.

From ECU SOM, Department of Emergency Medicine: Faculty Retreat, Greenville, NC, 1986.

BOX 5-5

XXX EMERGENCY DEPARTMENT MISSION STATEMENT

The XXX Emergency Department is a team of skilled professionals. We are dedicated to compassion, sensitivity, efficiency and excellence in patient care. Our function is to advocate for the well-being and safety of the patient and family. Those in our care can expect to be treated with dignity, respect and courtesy. We will make every effort to meet the individual needs of our patients and their families in a positive, proactive manner.

We are committed to the education of medical, nursing, and allied healthcare workers. We will foster excellence in education and research that will contribute to the advancement of knowledge and medical care. We recognize the importance of community outreach and will develop and participate in programs that promote better health and safety to individuals and the communities we serve.

As a team, we are committed to treating each other with dignity, respect, and courtesy. We are all valued care givers, learners, and teachers, growing personally and professionally through collegial relationships. Our attitudes are positive, and our energies are goal and solution oriented. Our efforts are cooperative, in that we are expected to offer, as well as receive, support in our primary mission: PATIENT CARE.

Departmental plans are especially useful for communicating how different organizational projects can work together and interact. Too often an organization lets its many individual departments and initiatives spin in isolated orbit around different sets of goals, duplicating efforts. Specifying interdependent missions can lead to mutual understanding. The mission statement for the East Carolina University School of Medicine's Department of Emergency Medicine is shown in Box 5-4.

The mission statement from another emergency department has a slightly different tone. (Box 5-5.)

The ECU SOM Department of Emergency Medicine Unit Plan for 1990 to 1993 is provided in Appendix B.

PREPARING TO PLAN

For a planning process, whether organizational or departmental, to have the impact intended, careful preplanning preparation is necessary. Two essential ingredients to making strategic planning work are a viable planning process that all managers understand, and organizational commitment to both the plan and the planning process.[5] Once established, these factors set the stage for forming a planning team and choosing a team facilitator. The planning team needs to agree on terminology, approach, and separation of strategic from operational planning. The group may want to form an operating agreement that specifies appropriate group behavior and encourages participation. An operating agreement frees the team members to leave rank at the door and to communicate effectively without fear of offense or repercussions.

There are several techniques for getting group participation in the consolidation of the social, political, regulatory, economic, and competitive environmental issues. Ackoff[8] uses a question to stimulate the release of creative thought in planning: "If your hospital (or unit) were destroyed last night, what would you replace it with now—in the current environment?" His logic is that "Asking this question releases you from the burden of defending the status quo and justifying current behavior, practices, assumptions, and goals."[2] Listed below are three well-known, formalized methods for initiating group creativity:[4]

1. The Delphi technique is "the development, evaluation, and synthesis of individual points of view through the systematic solicitation and collation of individual judgments on a particular topic. Opinions are summarized and then sent back to the participating individuals for the development of new judgments concerning the topic. After several rounds of solicitation and summary, a synthesis of opinion is formed."[4]
2. The nominal group technique requires a group meeting to address a particular topic. Each member writes a list of ideas on the issue at hand. Then, members take turns sharing one idea at a time and recording them on a flip-chart. Members then build on each others ideas, adding more to the list. A vote is held, and discussion continues until consensus is reached.
3. In brainstorming, a group meets to discuss a particular issue. Members share ideas without constraints and explain them. The ideas are recorded but not evaluated.

As the planners discuss their environment and eventually make decisions that will bring more change to the organization, they must not forget that people will be affected. Communication strategies must be formed to manage the change process, keeping employees informed. As a suggestion, open employee forums are excellent feedback conduits.

SUMMARY

The importance of taking a strategic management perspective to planning should now be evident. Healthcare dynamics are always shifting while shaping people and organizations, and "planning is evergreen."[2] Continuous, intelligent planning does yield some sense of control. Whether the issue is personal success, departmental success, or organizational success, "If the ladder is not leaning against the right wall, every step we take just gets us to the wrong place faster."[1]

REFERENCES

1. Deleted in proofs.
2. Rovin S, Ginsberg L: *Managing hospitals,* San Francisco, 1991, Jossey-Bass.
3. Kotler P, Clarke RN: *Marketing for health care organizations,* New Jersey, 1987, Prentice-Hall.
4. Duncan WJ, Ginter PM, Swayne LE: *Strategic management of health care organizations,* Boston, 1992, PWS-KENT.
5. Below PJ, Morrisey GL, Acomb BL: *The executive guide to strategic planning,* San Francisco, 1987, Jossey-Bass.
6. American College of Emergency Physicians: *Policy summaries,* Dallas, 1994, ACEP.
7. East Carolina University School of Medicine: *Department of Emergency Medicine Unit Plan,* Greenville, NC, 1990-1993, East Carolina University Press.
8. Ackoff R: *Creating the corporate future,* New York, 1981, John Wiley & Sons.

APPENDIX

A ACEP Statement of Direction*

Approved Board of Directors November, 1995

Mission Statement

The American College of Emergency Physicians (ACEP) exists to support quality emergency medical care and to promote the interests of emergency physicians.

Preamble

Emergency Medicine encompasses the decision making and action necessary to prevent death or any further disability for patients in health crises, as well as health promotion and injury prevention efforts. Emergency Medicine is practiced as patient-demanded, broadly available, and continuously accessible care by physicians educated to engage in the recognition, stabilization, evaluation, treatment, and disposition of patients in response to acute illness and injury. The patient population is unrestricted and presents with a full spectrum of episodic, undifferentiated physical and behavioral conditions. Emergency medicine is an integral component of the health care system.

Value Statements

The Board of Directors has identified five value statements that serve as the guiding principles for the specialty of emergency medicine. These values, along with the goals and objectives that follow, are the foundation of ACEP's long-range planning process and through that process influence the annual budget, liaison relationships, committee objectives, and Council and Board actions.

The values of the American College of Emergency Physicians are:

- Quality emergency care is a fundamental individual right and should be available to all who seek it.
- There is a body of knowledge unique to emergency medicine that requires continuing refinement and development.
- Quality emergency medicine is best practiced by qualified, credentialed emergency physicians.
- The best interests of the patient are served when emergency physicians practice in a fair, equitable, and supportive environment.
- The emergency physician has the responsibility to play the lead role in the definition, evaluation, and improvement of quality emergency care.

Goals and Objectives

The board of directors has established six goals with corresponding objectives to provide direction for the operation of the College. The goals and objectives of the College are:

Advocacy

ACEP, as the voice of emergency physicians, is the key advocate for high-quality emergency care and public policy relating to emergency medicine.

Objectives

1. Managed care policies and procedures will protect the interests of emergency patients and emergency physicians and will recognize the role and responsibility of emergency physicians.
2. There will be sufficient emergency medicine training programs and emergency facilities to meet the needs of the public.
3. Mandated screening exams and other emergency services will be covered benefits for all patients.
4. Programs will be in place to assist emergency physicians in adapting to the changing emergency medicine practice environment.
5. Emergency medicine will be recognized as an essential element of the healthcare delivery system.
6. Based on research, ACEP will promote improvements in the emergency medicine practice environment.
7. ACEP will continue to support tort reform.
8. ACEP will work to ensure the continued high quality and availability of out-of-hospital emergency care.
9. ACEP will continue to support universal access to medical care.
10. ACEP will support programs and legislation to further injury prevention and control.

Education

ACEP will assure the availability of high-quality undergraduate, graduate, and continuing medical (CME) education in emergency medicine and will enhance the public understanding of emergency medicine.

Objectives

1. ACEP will continue providing high-quality CME products that address identified needs.
2. ACEP will continue to provide input into the standards of graduate medical education and assist new and existing residency programs in achieving them.
3. ACEP will foster and support public education about emergency medicine.
4. ACEP will continue to serve as a primary resource for career information and professional development in emergency medicine.
5. ACEP will enhance efforts to procure adequate CME funding for emergency medicine.
6. ACEP will ensure that ACEP's Undergraduate Medical Education Guidelines are implemented in all medical schools.
7. ACEP will make efforts to identify appropriate fellowship opportunities for emergency physicians.

Research

ACEP will support research that answers questions relevant to the practice and advancement of emergency medicine.

*From American College of Emergency Physicians, 1995.

Objectives

1. ACEP will identify and evaluate the most effective and efficient emergency medicine clinical technologies and patient care methodologies.
2. ACEP will acquire information and surveillance data on the emergency medicine practice environment, members and potential members.
3. ACEP will research and teach members what clinical practice data are needed, how to obtain it, and how to clearly present it in support of their own product.
4. ACEP will support the continued development and refinement of the scientific basis of emergency medicine.
5. ACEP will produce information concerning various levels of emergency department staff training and expertise required to practice high-quality emergency medicine.
6. ACEP will evaluate the effect of emergency medicine practice on emergency physician well-being.
7. ACEP will promote outcome research on clinical practice and out-of-hospital emergency medical services.

Professional Practice

ACEP will identify the elements of, and promote the effective and efficient practice of emergency medicine.

Objectives

1. ACEP will identify efficient and effective clinical practice models to assist members to adapt to changing healthcare environments.
2. ACEP will ensure that outcome measurement systems will be available as a tool to enable members to guide their emergency medicine practice.
3. ACEP will promote efficient and effective clinical practice models and they will be accepted by health system planners.
4. ACEP will work to assure appropriate value for the services provided.
5. ACEP will develop, validate and promote clinical guidelines.
6. ACEP will foster and promote the ethical practice of emergency medicine.

Communications

ACEP will have timely, effective communications with members and other constituencies.

Objectives

1. ACEP will be a recognized authority on emergency medicine and will serve as a clearinghouse on emergency medicine and related issues.
2. ACEP will effectively communicate the value of ACEP membership.
3. ACEP will foster greater interchange of information and discussion of issues with its members.
4. ACEP will enhance member satisfaction by increasing participatory opportunities and educating members on how to work effectively with College processes.
5. ACEP will serve as a forum for debate on issues relating to emergency medicine.
6. ACEP's key messages will be promoted uniformly in all College publications.
7. ACEP will expand its communication with other providers of emergency health care such as physician assistants, nurse practitioners and EMS personnel.

Organizational Viability

ACEP will ensure that sufficient resources (financial, human, and technological) and ongoing strategic planning systems are in place to effectively meet member needs.

Objectives

1. Total membership growth will meet or exceed the annual target set by the Board.
2. Sufficient numbers of members will be willing and prepared to assume positions of leadership in the College.
3. ACEP will ensure the availability of technological resources necessary to efficiently and effectively accomplish College objectives.
4. Non-dues revenue will meet or exceed annual targets set by the Board.
5. Growth of membership equity will meet or exceed the annual target set by the Board.
6. The Board will annually establish a benchmark by which to judge whether the number of staff is appropriate to meet the needs of the College, given the financial resources available.
7. The amount of non-dues revenue generated from nonmembers will meet or exceed targets annually set by the Board.
8. The annual staff turnover ratio will not exceed the target annually set by the Board.

APPENDIX

B Department of Emergency Medicine:

UNIT PLAN 1990-1993*

Vision Statement

The mission of the Department of Emergency Medicine is threefold: 1) to foster excellence in patient care for our community and serve as a tertiary care resource for the surrounding counties; 2) to provide the structure for, and support of, undergraduate and graduate medical education to develop motivated, industrious, enthusiastic and knowledgeable physicians; and 3) to continue to develop a faculty committed to exemplary patient care, leadership, teaching and expanding the knowledge base of Emergency Medicine through scholarly activities locally, state-wide, nationally and internationally.

During the planning period, the Department of Emergency Medicine will ensure competency-based education of student and resident physicians, expand and strengthen fellowship and research programs and continue to develop its national leadership role in Emergency Medicine education and the development of appropriate responses to national health care issues.

Priorities for Action

1. Achieve Distinction in Undergraduate Education
   a. Assist wherever appropriate with undergraduate programs in the Division of Health Sciences.
      Objective 1: Assign an interdisciplinary committee to evaluate the feasibility of developing a degree program in Emergency Medical Services.
      Evaluation: Arrange quarterly meetings to review the committee's progress and provide feedback to the department chairman.
      Results: Direct the degree program development based on analysis of committee findings and recommendations.
      Time Frame: Fall 1992, Fall 1993
2. Strengthen the Commitment of Excellence in Teaching
   a. Ensure that the curriculum committees will assume an active management role in the continuing evolution of the curricula.
      Objective 1: Ensure adequate rotational experiences for Emergency Medicine residents in other disciplines by reviewing and revising learning objectives/curricula for each off-service rotation.
      Evaluation: Meet with residents and directors of rotations in other departments to evaluate the success of each rotation in meeting its educational objectives.
      Results: Revise, delete or add new rotations.
      Time Frame: Spring 1992
   b. Prepare an adequate number of family and primary care physicians to meet the healthcare needs of eastern North Carolina with emphasis on rural practice.
      Objective 1: Provide medical students and resident rotators from other services an exemplary educational experience in the outpatient setting which will sharpen diagnostic and stabilization skills. Rotation opportunities for both rotating residents and medical students will be increased in order that all first year residents and fourth year medical students will complete a one-month rotation in the Emergency Department. Elective months will be available to senior residents.
      Evaluation: Monitor the yearly numbers and patterns of rotators.
      Results: Provide feedback to the Graduate Education Committee and the Student Affairs Office.
      Time Frame: Fall 1993
      Objective 2: Provide exemplary care, while reducing resident work hours and consequently resident work-related stress, in keeping with the revised ACGME regulations. This will be effected by increasing the total complement of Emergency Medicine residents, increasing the number of residents per shift throughout the day and decreasing the total weekly hours worked.
      Evaluation: Monitor the numbers of residents, positions filled and staff patterns maintained.
      Results: Provide feedback to the Graduate Education Committee.
      Time Frame: Fall 1993
      Objective 3: Provide close and continuous attending supervision to all in-training personnel in the clinical area by increasing the faculty complement.
      Evaluation: Evaluate faculty staffing based on patient peak flow patterns and feedback from rotators and quality assurance activities.
      Results: Adjust faculty staffing based on patient peak flow patterns and feedback from rotators and quality assurance activities.
      Time Frame: Fall 1991
      Objective 4: Ensure optimal learning opportunities for resident physicians by providing adequate patient volume, acuity and diversity, by: 1) working closely with private physicians and other services to provide emergency care for their patients in the department; 2) continuing outreach programs to regional community hospitals for patient referrals; and 3) continuing to develop the trauma team approach and incorporate the Emergency Medicine resident as a team leader.
      Evaluation: Audit patient flow identifying patient types, problems, acuity of illness and delays in the system. Identify resident involvement.
      Results: Provide data to the hospital administration and

*From East Carolina University School of Medicine: ECU-SOM Department of Emergency Medicine Unit Plan for 1990-1993.

devise alternative plans. Refine current trauma protocols.

Time Frame: Fall 1991

Objective 5: Increase direct Emergency Medicine participation with land and air medical prehospital care providers, by having an Emergency Medicine resident present with each Greenville scene-run and function as an active team member.

Evaluation: Monthly meetings will be held with the rotating residents to discuss feedback by the crew chief and review ambulance run sheets.

Results: Feedback will be provided to the Residency Director and the experience will be modified as needed to best utilize resident rotation time.

Time Frame: Summer 1991

Objective 6: Increase resident participation in scholarly activities by encouraging all Emergency Medicine residents to develop independent research projects or collaborate with the faculty in their ongoing projects.

Evaluation: Have the residents present their research at an annual departmental research conference.

Results: Feedback will be provided to the Residency Director and the experience will be modified to maximize the resident's exposure to research.

Time Frame: Fall 1992

Objective 7: Provide Advanced Trauma Life Support courses and Pediatric Advanced Life Support courses for eastern North Carolina.

Evaluation: Formal course evaluations by participants and informal discussions with instructors.

Results: Evaluations are incorporated into the planning of future courses.

Time Frame: Ongoing

c. Conduct ongoing research in the medical curriculum to introduce and evaluate innovations such as the role of information technology, use of standardized patient problem based learning and small group teaching.

Objective 1: Provide a state-of-the-art elective in air medical services for Emergency Medicine residents.

Evaluation: Monitor resident performance and feedback on the rotation.

Results: Modify the rotation curriculum based on resident performance and feedback.

Time Frame: Fall 1991

d. Develop and implement a competency-based clinical curriculum for all clinical courses.

Objective 1: Develop a fourth-year undergraduate Emergency Medicine curriculum which maximizes the student's exposure to areas of medical care uniquely provided by our specialty, while continuing to emphasize critical problem solving, prioritization of patient care and a compassionate, ethical approach to the patient.

Evaluation: Require each student to read assigned topics in a specified Emergency Medicine text, attend a didactic lecture series, and perform required clinical shifts in the Emergency Department, upon which he will be examined by a written and oral examination at the end of the rotation.

Results: Adjust the lecture series and teaching methods accordingly based on an analysis of knowledge and performance areas.

Time Frame: Fall 1991

Objective 2: Increase faculty commitment to, and excellence in, didactic undergraduate medical education.

Evaluation: Require students to evaluate faculty member's clinical and didactic teaching.

Results: Discuss evaluations with individual faculty members, including appropriate suggestions on improvements in lecturing and teaching style.

Time Frame: Spring 1992

Objective 3: Explore new venues by which Emergency Medicine faculty can increase the undergraduate medical student's early exposure to emergency care.

Evaluation: Review the current undergraduate medical curriculum and design electives and/or a lecture series that could be integrated into this curriculum.

Results: Revise or add new electives/lecture series in consultation with the Medical School curriculum committees.

Time Frame: Spring 1992

3. Develop a university culture based on respect for individual rights and human diversity

a. Evaluate and modify academic support services and counseling services.

Objective 1: Ensure the availability of academic support services, counseling services and remediation programs for residents in Emergency Medicine. Orient all new residents to these services.

Evaluation: Obtain resident and faculty feedback on the above programs.

Results: Modify the above programs based on appropriate concerns.

Time Frame: Ongoing

Objective 2: Explore an upper level resident/faculty member mentoring system for new residents.

Evaluation: Obtain resident feedback on the effectiveness and desirability of this program.

Results: Institute a mentoring program, if deemed desirable.

Time Frame: Spring 1992

4. Expand Doctoral Programs

a. Increase the number of fellows in the clinical sciences by one to two per year over the next five years.

Objective 1: Develop a structured curriculum for fellowship training in Emergency Medical Services, with a specific focus on rural care.

Evaluation: Fellows will be evaluated on their clinical performance, scholarly activity and teaching skills.

Results: The curriculum content will be adjusted according to an analysis of strengths and weaknesses of the fellow's performance.

Time Frame: Fall 1991

Objective 2: Develop and implement fellowship training in air medical services.

Evaluation: Fellows will be evaluated on their clinical performance and scholarly activity.

Results: The curriculum content will be modified based on an analysis of perceived strengths and weaknesses in performance and knowledge base.

Time Frame: Fall 1992

5. Strengthen the commitment to research, scholarship and creative activity.
   a. Support and encourage participation by all faculty in scholarly activity in its broadest sense.
      Objective 1: Increase the number and significance of faculty contributions to the medical literature.
      Evaluation: Monitor the publication of original research conducted by faculty in peer-reviewed journals.
      Results: Facilitate significant research through monthly research conferences and monitoring of funding sources.
      Time Frame: Ongoing
      Objective 2: Encourage faculty to present the results of their research and scholarly activity at scientific meetings.
      Evaluation: Monitor each faculty member's presentation record.
      Results: Discuss ways to facilitate presentations by individual faculty members.
      Time Frame: Ongoing
      Objective 3: Encourage faculty to develop areas of research interest that will provide a foundation permitting them to compete successfully for extramural research funds.
      Evaluation: Review individual faculty members' area of interest and attempt to match them to federal and private sources of research funding.
      Results: Match or modify each individual faculty member's research focus.
      Time Frame: Fall 1992
      Objective 4: Strengthen cooperative interdepartmental and extramural research efforts by maintaining up-to-date interest files on each faculty member or department division and eliciting similar information on other departments at East Carolina University and other Emergency Medicine programs nationally.
      Evaluation: Monitor the number and success of interdepartmental and extramural research efforts.
      Results: Modify individual faculty members' or divisions' approach to cooperative research to maximize their interactions.
      Time Frame: Fall 1992
6. Improve teacher education and stimulate improvement in public schooling.
   a. Become proponents of science education in grade school, junior high, and high school by establishing liaisons to these institutions and stimulating teachers of science.
      Objective 1: Encourage faculty and residents to provide their expertise to educate children on issues pertinent to Emergency Medicine, and encourage children to develop an interest in health and science.
      Evaluation: Monitor faculty and resident involvement with school and educational foundations involved in science and health education for children.
      Results: Encourage volunteer faculty and resident participation in this area as a means of public service.
      Time Frame: Ongoing
7. Advance the university effectively to external publics
   a. Encourage continued support for groups with critical healthcare problems including minorities, children, women, elderly, and the impoverished.
      Objective 1: Actively involve social services and protective services in the care and discharge planning of patients with critical health care problems.
      Evaluation: Obtain feedback from patients and social and protective services as to the effectiveness of these measures.
      Results: Use this feedback to continue to develop social and healthcare options for these patients.
      Time Frame: Ongoing
      Objective 2: Continue active faculty involvement in developing national policies and solutions for critical issues in health care.
      Evaluation: Monitor individual faculty involvement in national, educational, specialty and legislative key contact groups.
      Results: Discuss level of involvement and strategies to increase involvement with individual faculty members.
      Time Frame: Ongoing
   b. Cooperate within the School of Medicine to provide leadership for the continued development of primary, secondary and tertiary care for the region.
      Objective 1: Utilize clinicians from multiple departments to serve as faculty in advanced life support courses.
      Evaluation: Formal course evaluations by participants and informal discussions with instructors.
      Results: Feedback incorporated into the planning of future courses.
      Time Frame: Ongoing
      Objective 2: Develop an outreach program to Emergency Medical Services directors in eastern North Carolina to better integrate air medical transport in the local, regional and state EMS system.
      Evaluation: Survey EMS directors on the strengths and weaknesses of the program.
      Results: Incorporate survey results to modify programs as needed.
      Time Frame: Spring 1992
      Objective 3: Provide national education programs and become a recognized center of excellence and expertise for Air Medical Communications Specialists.
      Evaluation: Formal course evaluations by participants and faculty. Monitor faculty involvement in research and national air medical services advisory groups.
      Results: Feedback incorporated into center development.
      Time Frame: Fall 1993
      Objective 4: Improve public awareness of EMS through meetings, press releases and media education, cardiopulmonary resuscitation courses and talks at public schools and public service groups.
      Evaluation: Elicit feedback on effectiveness of education programs from the participants and public use of EMS system.
      Results: Modify educational efforts based on the above feedback.
      Time Frame: Summer 1992
      Objective 5: Develop a standardized curriculum for ini-

tial and continuing education training programs of various levels of EMS providers for eastern North Carolina.

Evaluation: Meet with EMS interest group and elicit feedback on the feasibility of implementing a standardized curriculum.

Results: If feasible, implement standardized curriculum in the different counties' training programs.

Time Frame: Fall 1992

Objective 6: Continue to work with the Trauma Service at East Carolina University School of Medicine to educate and provide rural healthcare providers and patients timely definitive trauma care.

Evaluation: Obtain feedback from outlying hospitals regarding their trauma care needs.

Results: Use this feedback to continue to develop and refine the system.

Time Frame: Ongoing

Objective 7: Increase the timeliness of high quality patient care in the Emergency Department.

Evaluation: Analyze the factors causing delays in patient care and mobilization from the department, and work with the hospital administration and other departments to modify or eliminate them.

Results: Improve patient flow in the Emergency Department.

Time Frame: Ongoing

8. Develop and Use Expanded Information Resources
   a. Develop programs for student and faculty training and continuing education in accessing, utilizing and evaluating information resources.

      Objective 1: Increase faculty computer literacy and use to prepare for increased use of on-line information resources in teaching and clinical practice.

      Evaluation: Monitor faculty continuing education and use of computers.

      Results: Improve faculty knowledge and use of computers.

      Time Frame: Spring 1992
   b. Develop with Pitt County Memorial Hospital a unified approach to computerized medical records, scheduling and resource management for inpatient and outpatient clinical settings.

      Objective 1: Provide faculty and resident education to ensure their ability to use new hospital systems as they are implemented.

      Evaluation: Monitor department use of computerized systems as available.

      Results: Use new computerized systems effectively.

      Time Frame: Ongoing
   c. Designate and establish population registries as a base for ongoing evaluation of healthcare issues.

      Objective 1: Increase the use of population registries such as the North Carolina Trauma Registry in ongoing research and quality assurance activities.

      Evaluation: Review use of and contributions to data banks in research protocols.

6 Conflict Management

Robert W. Strauss and Susan F. Strauss

"Meaning well and trying hard do not guarantee a good outcome."

Harles Cone

OUTLINE

Conflict is inevitable.

Whenever people work together, conflict will exist. This is especially true in a crisis-oriented environment such as the emergency department. Conflict is a natural consequence of incompatible behaviors and unmet expectations.

A prehospital care worker bringing an ill patient to the emergency department may expect a receptive, attentive, respectful staff who will stop what they are doing to attend to the new patient. Instead, he or she finds a busy, overwhelmed and somewhat rude staff member who expresses disappointment and anger on arrival of the emergency medical technician (EMT).

A patient with a perceived emergency wants to receive treatment **NOW** by a polite, respectful, competent and confident healthcare worker. The healthcare worker arrives in the patient's room one-half hour later to find a sarcastic and irritable patient claiming: "I thought you must have forgotten about me."

An emergency nurse in an understaffed department may not be able to keep up with the urgent patient care needs. A private attending leaves a busy office and arrives in the emergency department demanding that the nurse leave an acutely ill patient and attend to his or her (patient's) needs.

An emergency physician becomes increasingly frustrated as it seems that nothing is getting done and patients are languishing.

This chapter describes the origin of conflict in the emergency department and proposes effective techniques for managing conflict. Because most conflict is resolved at the personal (individual) level, the methods of resolution primarily address the individual.

BENEFITS OF CONFLICT

Conflict can be beneficial. High functioning organizations are not conflict free. Those who ignore the value of conflict may also overlook the conflicts that exist within their own organization and in so doing allow them to grow. Conflict seen as opportunity has many advantages including the following:[1]

- Improved solutions—A disagreement voiced and examined allows a deeper look into the problem, perhaps incorporating a perspective not yet considered. Attention to alternate views may integrate a broader solution responsive to several perspectives.
- Improved efficiency—Conflicts ignored or managed poorly lead to brooding and an unwillingness to participate in the solution. The organization will no longer function efficiently. Conflict addressed early diminishes anger and likely renders earlier success.
- Enhanced morale—Individuals recognize that they are respected and their ideas can contribute to the solutions of complex problems. Addressing the issues of people within the organization strengthens relationships and enhances competence.

When the conflict of an unhappy client, customer, or patient is acknowledged, the organization has an opportunity to change to meet the needs of those it attempts to serve (see Chapter 63). It is not enough to want to provide high quality. Quality can be sustained only in an organization that cares about the people who produce its products and deliver its services.

CONFLICT AND COMMUNICATION

When we learn, work, play, and worship, we are often participating in a group. Group interaction requires effective communication. Skillful communicators recognize the relative importance of words, tone, and body language when trying to persuade others of their belief.

Verbal content plays a relatively small role in the way we

communicate. Less than 10% of persuasion is a result of the actual words that are used. The majority of persuasion results from other forms of communication—the tone, posture, expression and movement of the communicator.

For example, we have all been to lectures where the lecturer was brilliant and the information important, but the presentation was in monotone; there was no movement and perhaps the presenter was reading from notes. In these situations, attention begins to wander, we become distracted and learning stops. Alternatively, those who speak with enthusiasm, expression, and movement are more engaging and, as a result, convincing.

Albert Mehrabian, one of the foremost experts in communication, performed experiments to demonstrate the importance of verbal and nonverbal communication (Box 6-1).[2] He looked at the contribution of verbal content, vocal expression, visual cues to persuasion, and believability. Morabian found that only a small percentage of what is communicated are the words that are actually used.

When speaking with people, we tend to overemphasize the content and try to convince them with the words. It is just as important to pay attention to expression and delivery.

Verbal Incongruence

On occasion, we encounter verbal incongruence. This occurs when there is disparity between the words and body kinetics, or the nonverbal expression such as tone and behavior. The following examples illustrate verbal incongruence:

- A parent yells at a child: "I'm not angry with you!" But the lips are tight, the body is tense, the posture is threatening and looming.
- An ataxic slurring patient in the emergency department with a strong scent of alcohol on his breath says: "I only had a coupla beers."
- On learning of his wife's sudden death, a grieving husband begins shaking uncontrollably and continues to say: "I'm fine! Really, I'm just fine!"

Our communication skills, both verbal and nonverbal, play a major role in the development or resolution of conflict in a nonstressed environment. Poorly developed skills often heighten discord and dissention in an emergency department—an environment intrinsically prone to chaos.

ORIGIN OF STRESS AND CONFLICT IN THE EMERGENCY DEPARTMENT

Stress is rampant in emergency departments. We confront situations daily for which we have little or no ability to find positive solutions. Many patients waiting to be seen believe that their problems are of an emergent nature and require immediate attention. Some of them are quite ill. Others may be in the hallway staring or even glaring at you while they wait. Meanwhile, the staff may be getting further behind and feeling overwhelmed, with raw nerves and "buttons" all ready to be pushed—a crisis in the making.

Patient Expectations—The 4 Cs

Patients arrive with certain expectations of the care and caring they will receive (Box 6-2). Their expectations in descending order of importance are as follows:

- Convenience (Rapid Care)—It is almost axiomatic that the most important aspects of emergency care from the patient's perspective are time and convenience. When patients have a choice about emergency care, they generally choose the place that will get them in and out most quickly. Patients place time pressure on us. We place time pressure on ourselves. After all "rapid assessment" is the *sine qua non* of emergency care.
- Caring—The next most important aspect of patient care is "caring." Rapid rapport and trust must be developed. Initially, the patient judges the staff not by the level of care but by the level of caring. Our responsibility is to take care of people's needs, both physical and emotional.

  Caring goes beyond providing a high standard of care. Patients have difficulty judging the level of care they receive. Most patients prefer a warm, friendly and concerned healthcare provider who delivers "good" care to a cold, unfriendly, and distant provider who practices on the cutting edge.
- Care—Because the actual quality of care is quite difficult for the patient to assess, this expectation generally is considered only when there is no improvement or "something goes wrong."
- Cost—Patients who are treated expeditiously, with caring and quality, tend to be less concerned about the cost of their care. Alternatively, cost may become an issue when a patient perceives that one or more of these aspects of care are glaringly absent.

The Healthcare Environment

An increasingly important factor in generating stress in the emergency department is the ever changing healthcare milieu. Healthcare reform brings with it pervasive pressures to contain costs while maintaining quality services. Managed care groups and hospitals carefully review and critique the use of resources in the emergency department and promote an increasingly limited battery of tests and procedures. Con-

BOX 6-1

PERSUASION: THE INFLUENCE OF VERBAL AND NONVERBAL COMMUNICATION

Mode	%
Verbal content	7
Vocal expression	38
Visual cues	55

BOX 6-2

PATIENT EXPECTATIONS: THE 4 Cs

Convenience
Caring
Care (Quality)
Cost

versely, specialty training, increasing malpractice fears, and quality review organizations at the national, state, and local levels create pressure to leave "no stone unturned."

Organizational Climate

The organizational climate in which we work places further stress on us. There is a significant inequality of status and pay. By these measures, physicians outrank the nursing staff; nurses outrank other nurses; and technicians and secretaries are often considered less significant team members. Intensifying this stress is the traditionally held belief that one person must be in charge of the patient care decisions. When the speaker has power over the listener and the situation is one of stress and crisis, the potential for conflict is far greater.

To some extent, we have created a downward customer service spiral. The increasingly limited financial resources of many institutions have resulted in substantial staff "downsizing", outdated equipment and facilities, and more prolonged "holding" of patients waiting for disposition. The result is poorer service. These and a multitude of other repercussions create further staff stress by frustrating our attempts to achieve goals of meeting the patients's needs and providing a quality service.

An Unhealthy Work Environment

We used to believe and promote that emergency healthcare workers were among the most psychologically stable workers. We thought that emergency personnel were a "special breed" who thrived on chaos and the high pressure and responsibility of the emergency department.

We now believe, however, that emergency healthcare workers are among the most psychologically unhealthy workers. Characteristics considered unhealthy in a work environment that are shared by emergency care givers include the following:

1. Intensive: The work is exhausting.
2. Dangerous: Emergency care is often a matter of life and death. The margin for error is slim and mistakes cannot be tolerated. Contagious diseases and increasing violence in our environment also carry personal risk to the healthcare provider.
3. Litigious: The fear of malpractice is pervasive among most emergency care practitioners.
4. Unpredictable: There is always a sense of the unknown pending. One moment the emergency department may be empty and 1 hour later full of multiply injured and severely ill patients.
5. Unmet expectations: When the patient or private attending arrives, only your total attention **now** will do.
6. Uncontrollable: There is often a sense of crisis and being out of control.

Shifts are often without break; sleep patterns are irregular. An increasing body of knowledge describes the biologic stress of changing sleep habits.

In describing stress and burnout among emergency care givers, Debra Slapper noted that:[3] "individuals prone to burnout are high achievers who have intense schedules, do more than their share on every project and don't admit their limitations . . . [And further] As we age, our bodies tolerate the physicial stresses less well. Twelve-hour shifts, eating on the run, no time for . . . breaks and sleep disturbances make us feel 70 when we are only 35." When combined with a lack of control over patient load, job insecurity, problems with professional and patient relations, and the emothional 'roller-coaster' of routine practice, it is understandable that many providers cannot cope with full time practice.[4]

MANAGING ORGANIZATIONAL STRESS AND CONFLICT

The institution of a continuous quality improvement (CQI) program is an excellent method of reducing departmental conflict. Unlike traditional quality assurance, with its emphasis on blame-fixing and outlier behavior, CQI emphasizes improvement in processes rather than in performance. CQI encourages staff input in process improvement, acknowledging their expertise in making systems work more efficiently. This arrangement philosophy diminishes departmental stress by sharing governance and placing value on staff input and function. Both elements are crucial in fashioning a team approach to problem solving and ultimately conflict resolution

In an organization committed to CQI, management will often meet one on one on a regular basis with employees to identify evolving problems or issues. Judgments about who is right or wrong are deemphasized; instead staff are empowered to work with management toward positive solutions. Issues are discussed in a timely manner and disagreement is acceptable. In short, creating a supportive and nurturing environment for staff and management alike will resolve many conflicts before they happen.

PERSONAL RESPONSE TO STRESS AND CONFLICT

On a personal level, how do we respond to stress and conflict? We respond by habit. Habits are simply learned patterns of behavior. Habits can be good. They allow us to perform without thinking. We perform thousands of minor activities during the day that have become habit and do not require conscious effort. When driving a car, habits allow one to watch the scenery, release a clutch, press a gas pedal, turn a steering wheel, and listen to the radio all at the same time.

The blending of our patterns of behavior comprise our individual personalities. We exhibit both routine (nonstressed) behavior patterns and "crisis patterns" when we are under stress. Although these behaviors may be effective in some environments, they are less productive in others. Some people confront stressful predicaments with maladaptive behavior patterns that exacerbate the situation, such as provocation, accusation, and/or disdain. We observe this repeatedly in people around us whom we describe as difficult.

CHANGING BEHAVIOR

The first step in changing behavior is recognizing that the only person over whom we have any significant control is ourselves. Why should we change our own behavior in response to a stressful situation?

Why Change

If you frequently become frustrated during times of stress and crisis, your conduct and communication skills may be part

of the problem and merit review. If you walk away upset, try to recall what happened and ask yourself, "What is my role in this?"

Think about one of the last difficult encounters you had at work. It is common to believe, "It sure seems like there are a lot of difficult people out there. And for the most part, I don't do anything to provoke them." Don't count on it. Often, the most difficult people don't realize that they are triggering stressful interactions.

Behavior patterns are difficult to change. They are fundamental components of our personalities. The adage that people learn from their mistakes is often untrue. Frequently, we repeat previous behaviors whether successful or not. Extrapolating from the experiments of the psychologist Guthrie, responses to stimuli tend to become habitual, or patterned behavior.[5] Thus it is likely that an inappropriate response to a stressful situation will occur again and again when confronted with similar circumstances. In fact, in times of crisis we tend to repeat a single individualized consistent personality style or behavior pattern learned in childhood as a response to stress.

How Does One Change: The Four Stages of Learning[6]

Most of our behavior patterns were learned as children and have become unconscious habits. To change behavior patterns as adults requires bringing the behaviors into consciousness and actively modifying them until they become unconscious again.

Stage I: Unconscious Incompetence. The first stage involves the recognition and determination that a new behavior is desirable. Generally, the processes necessary to accomplish the goal are poorly understood.

Child: wants to ride a bicycle, but doesn't know he or she can't.	Adult: wants to change a behavior but is unaware that his or her habits of interaction prevent success.

Stage II: Conscious Incompetence. The awareness of our inability can come in a variety of forms, many of them negative. Learning often occurs with falls and occasional psychologic injuries. It is key to recognize the feedback during change as an opportunity to improve.

Child: tries to ride the bicycle and falls off, becoming immediately aware of his or her inability.	Adult: receives input or criticism suggesting that the new behavior is ineffective.

Stage III: Conscious Competence. Trying to change what we do, to be different, is both a difficult and deliberate process.

Child: learns to ride by becoming attentive to balancing, turning the wheel, pedaling, speeding up, slowing, down, stopping, and more balancing.	Adult: with a conscious and determined effort, and occasional mishaps, behaves differently.

Stage IV: Unconscious Competence. Changing one's own behavior is difficult. It takes 18 months to 2 years of rigorous discipline for an adult to make a new behavior feel comfortable.[6] However, once a new habit successfully becomes a new pattern of behavior, "It's like riding a bike."

Child: rides easily without thinking about the process.	Adult: without conscious effort behaves differently.

CONFLICT RESOLUTION: GENERAL PRINCIPLES

Creating Trust

Effective communication occurs most easily in an environment of trust and respect. Supervisors and managers who reside in their offices except when criticizing or espousing memoranda create an environment of distrust and apprehension. It is the responsibility of the leadership to get close to the people providing the service or product so that they can understand the issues and conflicts first hand. Feedback or criticism of the night staff by emergency department leaders who never work nights or weekends may "fall on deaf ears." These comments may be resented and perceived as manipulating, self-serving, and condescending.

Alternatively, when a person identifies with you and believes you understand their issues, they are more likely to listen. It is necessary to both understand and be perceived as understanding the issue from the other's perspective before effective listening by the other side can occur.

Effective Listening

Effective emergency care often requires rapid problem identification. There is a tendency in some situations to move too quickly. Some healthcare providers interrogate patients with hurried, impatient questions and interrupted answers. Yet, success in obtaining information often depends on the trust and rapport we develop. If the person with the problem believes his or her issues are not being heard, he or she may well become frustrated, reserved, and vague, resulting in a breakdown in communication. Effective listening is a first step toward understanding the problem.

There is a tendency to believe we understand the problems of others because of our own past experiences. This is a projection of our own viewpoint, ignoring the speaker's. Without going through the process of listening, it is unlikely that we will understand.

Successful responses are neutral and without criticism. They simply accept the speaker's concerns and allow him or her to continue to explore and perhaps clarify feelings. Think of someone who "really listens" and the types of resources that person uses to make them effective listeners. There are several styles of listening including passive, reflective, and empathic.[10] Before reading the following responses, consider how you might respond to the comment:

"I just can't stop thinking about the child from the accident."

Impatient Response: "You're overreacting. You're getting too emotional about it. I would just put it out of my mind if I were you." Although perhaps well meaning, this advice attempts to substitute the perspective and experience of the listener for the feelings of the speaker. The speaker communicates criticism, dismissal, and lack of concern for the speaker's distress.

Passive Response: "Oh?" Passive listening simply requires the listener to be quietly attentive. This behavior generally will encourage the speaker to continue discussing the issue and often allow him or her to get to the crux of the problem. People problems take time to divulge and, like onions, may

require peeling away many layers before getting to the center. This type of response can also help defuse angry reactions. To feel comfortable when revealing a problem, one needs time and, at the very least, a neutral environment.

Reflective Response: "You can't stop thinking about him?" Reflective listening involves providing objective feedback to the person speaking. In its most rudimentary form, this simply involves parroting back the words. This technique encourages the speaker to clarify his or her feelings.

Empathic Response: "It sounds like you're worried about him." This listener has decided to try to understand the speaker, to get on the same side of the table. The listener has suspended his or her own frame of reference and attempted to rephrase content and reflect feeling. This type of nonjudgmental and concerned listening allows the speaker to open up most quickly and get to the core of the problem.

Eye Communication

Skilled communicators maintain good eye communication when listening to and speaking with others.[7] If you want people to listen to you or feel like you are listening to them, you must establish effective eye communication. Napoleon said: "To make oneself understandable to people, one must first speak to their eyes."

If you do not establish eye communication, the message is: "I don't want to be here or involved in this." Try the experiment of speaking with another using three different patterns of eye communication: minimal, intermittent, and continuous. Most others will unconsciously copy your lead. Turn sideways and rarely look into their eyes and they will do the same. Stand in front of them and look directly into their eyes when speaking and listening and they will, too. Note further, the discussion may get more conclusive.

Focusing on the Issue, not the Position

When dealing with conflict, it is necessary to focus on the issue, not the position.[8] This is true in complaint management, conflict resolution, or negotiation. Any difficult situation usually can be brought back to a level playing field by continuing to concentrate on the issue. Positions are always directed by underlying issues. Some of the most difficult people exhibit positional bargaining, such as shown in the following example:

Admitting Resident: "Why that's the third sick patient you've asked me to admit in the last hour. I won't do it."

The position is "NO!!"

Responding to the position is "taking the bait" and getting hooked into a win-lose situation. "Oh yeah! Well, you have to, and now! And if you don't, I'll call your attending." Positional bargaining may in fact get the desired result. However, it generally creates a winner and a resentful loser. And, if you are ever going to deal with the "loser" again, they will remember and may try to get you back.

The issue is "I'm tired, overwhelmed, and feeling out of control. I don't think I can handle another patient right now."

If one tries to understand the issue from the perspective of the admitting resident, the response might be: "Your night has been rough. I could hold the patient here for another 45 minutes while you catch up. I'll expect to see you at 3 AM, alright?" Trying to understand and then address the underlying issue may entail some minor compromise, but allows both sides to get their needs met.

Separating the People from the Problem[8]

We usually believe the people are the problem. After all, everyone has irritating behaviors. Although most of us have the potential to develop a mutually satisfactory and trusting relationship, we also may get angry and suspicious when offended. Our effectiveness in dealing with conflict in part depends on our ability to separate the person from the problem.

This process requires recognition that most people are not trying to create problems, but in fact, are trying to meet their own needs. However, in a stressful and hurried environment, they may communicate unskillfully and inadvertently aggravate a situation. The key to understanding the concept lies in the recognition that others have different perceptions of reality that are as valid as our own. To successfully resolve conflict, it is necessary to understand their underlying perceptions.

Note how differently the following scenario would conclude if the preexisting (underlying) perceptions were different:

Spoken Words	Underlying thought
A: Did you clean your car yet?	I have some free time, so if it isn't done yet, I can do it.
B: I told you I would do it when I get the chance and I will! Don't continue to bug me about it!	Nag! Nag! I've been busy doing more important things and now I'm being criticized for taking 5 minutes for myself to get a cup of coffee.
A: Well, never mind!	That's what I get for offering to help.

Avoiding the issue and concluding a negative motivation often create a self-fulfilling prophecy. When we perceive that the intentions of the other are dishonorable, we selectively interpret further actions in that same light. A poorly chosen word or a mishap may reinforce the negative perception and make a positive and supportive environment difficult to achieve. To resolve this conflict, the participants must examine the motivations of the other in a sincere and noncritical way. This may be accomplished by simply asking: "What was your reason for asking me if I had cleaned the car?" or "How did you feel when I asked if you had cleaned the car?" Eventually, by continuing to explore each other's motivations, both will see how they misinterpreted the other's intentions.

Responding to Emotion

It is tempting to respond emotionally to an obnoxious button pusher, to overpower them by getting angry. Responding emotionally to an emotional situation is loss of control. Yelling, crying, door slamming, and stomping away may provide temporary relief to the one who performs these behaviors. However, it will make resolution and subsequent interactions more difficult.

Emotional actions breed emotional reactions. Those who maintain composure and continue to focus on the issue enhance the resolution process.

Silence is an alternative response to hot emotional interpersonal conflicts. The more tension in a situation, the greater the desire for action. Action may lead to escalation, whereas silence may be neutral and encourage the parties to gain self-control. Silence is like the great Aikido master who allows

the opponent's own negative energy to move through space without affecting the master. It is difficult to maintain a steady stream of anger at someone who does not participate.

CONFLICT RESOLUTION: SPECIFIC SKILLS

We cannot change the personalities of others. However, if appropriate feedback is given, others may change their behavior toward us.

To encourage change, it is frequently necessary to provide feedback. In the heat of a stressful interaction, it is difficult for even the most composed to "put on the other person's shoes" and be open to criticism. Even with people we like, complaints ore often met with resistance.

Feedback and communication begin with listening. Properly used techniques can enhance conflict resolution, whereas imprudent feedback can exacerbate a poor interaction.

Avoid Negativism

First, eliminate the word *criticism* from your vocabulary. It connotes censure, condemnation, and disapproval. Using terms such as input or feedback will be more readily accepted as they connote a more objective observation. Second, when structuring feedback, focus on yourself, not the other person. This allows them to maintain self-esteem. Third, avoid labeling, personal attacks, and generalizations. For example, how would the following criticism be received: "You are always too argumentative!" This comment, while perhaps attempting to create positive behavior change, is more likely to lead to defensiveness and anger. It contains a labeling, generalized personal attack.

Well-formulated behavioral feedback includes a clear description of the behavior and how it affects you. This should include what you perceive and what you would like to see happen.

Gordon suggests structuring the feedback in the three parts:[9]

When . . . . ,
I feel. . . . ,
because. . .

For example:

When we argue,
I feel frustrated,
Because you don't give me respect for my ideas.

The "when" statement should be specific, concrete, and observable. Simply and objectively recount the occurrence, "When we argue." Be particularly careful to avoid attacks and labeling here. Avoid statements such as:

When: - you act the way you do (nonspecific)
- you behave like a jerk (labeling attack)

The "I feel" statement should contain a real and understandable emotion that is consistent with the situation. I feel angry, upset, embarrassed, or frustrated. Avoid nonfeelings phrases such as:

I feel: - like a child (how does a child feel?)
- like an idiot (not a feeling)

The "because" statement should be a specific result in the real world. You will discover and share your own motives. Avoid the temptation to blame. Focus on the way the behavior affects you and your perception.

Other common examples include a person who believes his or her opinion is overlooked:

When I'm ignored
I feel frustrated
Because I don't think that you trust my judgment

or the recipient of a degrading comment:

When comments like that are made,
I feel angry,
Because it's demeaning

Putting it into a three part complaint lets you and the other person know the problem, how it affects you, and why. If you can clarify it for yourself, you can clarify it for the other person. Adding, "What do you think?" or "How do you feel about it?" may help generate further discussion. The input of each party is required to effect change.

Avert Public Ridicule

We have all seen an angry person verbally abuse another person in a public venue. It makes everyone uncomfortable, and the unfortunate subject of the ridicule is likely to feel humiliated by this inconsiderate form of public exposure. The person expressing his or her discontent may not even recognize the inappropriateness of the behavior. You may be able to interrupt this dysfunctional communication and change behavior.

If a disruptive situation is occurring at the nursing station and you are uncomfortable with the expression of emotion in such a public arena, simply "move the melee." This could be a patient, a co-worker, a private physician, or an administrator. Do the following:

- Stand in front of the speaker, gain his or her attention, establish eye communication.
- Quietly and firmly say: "I want to talk with you about this over here" and move toward a more private space and then deal with the issue.

Few people will stand alone and continue to argue at nobody. Most will walk with you. The movement itself will begin to decompress the situation.

Responding to the Complainer

In our busy emergency departments, it is difficult to meet everybody's expectations. One of the results is complaints. Two of the most common are forms of: "It's taking too long!" or "You don't care!" People who are both waiting for a prolonged time and treated rudely may be particularly adamant in their expression of discontent.

When a person confronts us with his or her dissatisfaction, we are faced with an opportunity to provide immediate satisfaction in our response to the complainer. How we choose to respond may lead to immediate resolution or substantially exacerbate the problem.[10]

Blaming a Blamer. It is first necessary to recognize the person as a "blamer." Habitual blamers tend to be angry perfectionists who believe they should get their way and anything less is a catastrophe. They may believe that they have not gotten what they deserve because people are insensitive and purposefully obstinate. Blamers may use lots of personal pronouns, generalizations, and extremes of language to make their point. They tend to be dramatic, both in tone and gesture. Blamers may shake their finger, pound their fist, and

even be verbally threatening. The blamer, in essence, tries to place the responsibility for his or her problem on someone else. For example, a blaming patient who is tired of waiting might exclaim:

> "Why is it that every time I come here, I always have to sit around and wait for hours and hours! Don't any of you people care about anyone! Can't you see that I'm in agony!"
> Translation: "I want to be taken care of now!"

There are many ways to respond to this person. Before choosing, it is critical to recognize that this is *not* an attack directed at you. Although, it is tempting to take it personally, don't take the bait. Taking it personally, a blaming professional might respond by saying:

> "You know, we're very busy and we're getting to you as fast as we can. You are constantly interrupting the staff and delaying our getting to you. If you will just sit quietly and wait, we'll take care of you when it is your turn. There are people here who are really sick!"

Blaming a blamer rejects the placement of responsibility and places it back on the blamer. Joining this mud slinging contest only gets you dirty. There are no winners. Inevitably, it leads to escalation of the conflict. When the opportunity arises, the other person will get you back. It may be a letter to your chief executive officer or even the editorial section of the local newspaper.

Placating. Placating is in many ways similar to blaming.[10] The placater is self-blaming. The placater acts as if he or she is unworthy and personally responsible for the problem. The placater again uses many personal pronouns, generalizes, and places emphatic stresses on words. However, instead of being aggressive and placing the responsibility for the problem on others, a placater is apologetic and appears to assume the responsibility. A placater who is frustrated with waiting might say:

> "I don't know why it is that I always seem to come when it is so busy. I'm not a complainer, and I know that you doctors and nurses are so busy and my problem is so insignificant."
> Translation: "I want to be taken care of now!"

It is quite common for professionals in a service business such as healthcare to placate. The placating professional apologizes and seems to assume responsibility, such as:

> "I'm very sorry, I wish I could have been here sooner. You must be upset. Thanks for being so patient, I'm very sorry."

Placating in response to conflict works—to some degree. Generally, it avoids escalation and allows the other side to blame this obliging apologizer. This behavior however, causes the placater to feel inept and impotent. Further, it doesn't substantially improve the situation.

Being Objective and Then Giving Them What They Want. A more effective way of responding is to be objective and give them what they want.[10] This method eliminates all blame, deals directly with the issue of concern, and provides the complainer with what he or she really wants—attention and responsive behavior. The objective response avoids dealing with who is responsible. It is quite specific, limits the use of personal pronouns, and is even toned.

Objectively repeating the complaint back to the complainer from their perspective demonstrates that you understand the issue. Then, give them what they want—meet their need. In response to the complaint of taking too long, one might say: "Yes, it is frustrating to wait when ill. I am here to take care of you now. What is wrong?" If you are unable to provide the solution now, then let them know when you will, and do it.

To demonstrate all of these responses together, let's assume that a woman with severe chest pain is brought to the emergency department by ambulance. She is accompanied by her husband who is told to go out and provide registration information. He turns to you and says: "How can you think about paper work at a time like this!" You respond by . . .

Blaming: "You've got to do it or we can't do anything (e.g., radiographs) for your wife!" (You've just made him responsible for delays in his wife's care.)

Placating: "I know how you feel. I'm sorry, but we really need the paper work completed. Please do it. Sorry." (He'll probably do it, begrudgingly.)

Being Objective, Then Meeting the Need: "It is difficult to think about paperwork at a time like this. It is necessary. I will take care of your wife now." (You've listened to him, understood his underlying issue—his wife—and you are meeting his need.)

SUMMARY

The other person must be considered an equal who has real issues and real needs. The other person is not an adversary who must be overcome. Winning at another's expense does not work if future collaboration is necessary. Success requires a collaborative solutions in which both sides get their needs met. Each must be respected. It is important to work to satisfy their needs while attaining personal goals—to provide quality care for the patient in an environment of shared respect.

REFERENCES

1. Tjosvold D: *Learning to manage conflict: getting people to work together productively,* 1993, New York, Lexington Books.
2. Mehrabian A: *Non-verbal communication,* 1972, Chicago, Aldine-Atherton.
3. Slapper DR: Emergency medicine is here to stay. What about emergency physicians? In ACEP News 10:7, American College of Emergency Physicians, 1991.
4. Whitehead DC, Thomas H, Slapper DR: A rational approach to shift work in emergency medicine, *Ann Emerg Med* 21:10, 1992.
5. Hill WF: *Learning: a survey of psychological interpretations,* 1990, New York, Harper and Row.
6. Cone HE: *How to manage conflict, criticism, and anger,* 1988, Liberty, MO, Cone Resource Group Inc.
7. Argyle M: *Bodily communication,* 1988, New York, International Universities Press.
8. Fisher R, Ury W: *Getting to yes,* Boston, 1981, Houghton Mifflin.
9. Gordon T: *Leader effectiveness training,* New York, 1980, Bantam Books.
10. Elgin SH: *The gentle art of verbal self-defense,* New York, 1993, Barnes and Noble.

7 Time Management

John G. Keene

OUTLINE

Time is immutable. We cannot stretch, speed, slow, or save it. Despite all the books that have been written on time management, we cannot manage time. We can, however, manage ourselves and control how we use time.

Managing our time is no simple task given the demands of modern life. Our time can easily be consumed with the rush of responsibilities and obligations. Habit also plays a big part in how we use our time. To achieve greater success in life, we must manage ourselves. Therefore time management is life management.

Time management as the process of life management is a paradigm shift from the old concept of time management as a productivity and efficiency tool. The old model aimed at getting the most things done in the least amount of time. The new model is an effectiveness model based on the concept that to use time wisely, we must prioritize our desires, activities, and responsibilities so that we work on the things that are the most important to us first.

One could be efficient and generate a lot of work in a relatively short time while leading a meaningless and unfulfilled life. This occurs when we spend our time on activities that are not important or have little meaning for us. Benjamin Franklin said, "do not squander time, for that's the stuff that life is made of."[1] Our time is our life, and if we spend our lives involved in meaningless activities, activities that have limited personal value and provide us no satisfaction or reward, then we will find ourselves depressed and frustrated.

On the other hand, if we determine what is meaningful to us, develop the skills necessary to use our time wisely, and attend first to the activities that are most meaningful to us, we will lead satisfying, productive lives. Successful life management is achieved by (1) determining priorities and (2) establishing a system of organization, a framework within which we can accomplish our goals. The key elements of such a system are (1) staying focused, (2) obtaining feedback, and (3) ongoing evaluation/reevaluation.

This chapter provides practical tools to help you understand yourself better; to define your mission, roles, and goals; and to use this information effectively to manage your time and your life.

ESTABLISHING WHAT YOU WANT TO DO

The first step toward effective time management is to understand yourself well enough to define what is important to you and to prioritize your activities. An excellent exercise to begin this process is to make up a list of everything you would like to do in the next 20 years. The goal is to be exhaustive in composing your list. Try to put down as many things as you possibly can, stimulating your thinking about what you would really like to do. Most people think this will take hours to complete; however, most people have completely ex-

hausted their ideas in less than an hour. You can modify this process if you want to focus on one area such as running an emergency department by limiting your list to that area. Divide the list into five categories of activities: (1) family activities, (2) psychospiritual activities, (3) personal development activities, (4) health and fitness activities, and (5) professional/career activities.

Family activities include all of those items related to nuclear and extended families. These activities include time with spouse, children, and parents. Visiting relatives, family vacations, quality time together, and any other activity where the family is the key focus are be included.

Psycho spiritual activities include efforts to find spiritual meaning in our lives. This could include meditation, religious activities, contemplative walks, psychoanalysis, and other activities that focus on developing the spiritual sides of our lives.

Personal development includes all activities focused on us as individuals. This category could include reading great books, learning to play an instrument, learning a foreign language, taking classes, or other activities to broaden ourselves.

Health and fitness activities are those activities that care for our bodies. There is a growing body of evidence to support the fact that our mental processes improve as our physical condition improves. Physical conditioning can improve concentration, attention span, clarity of thinking, and the attitude with which we approach life. It makes sense therefore to devote a portion of our time to keeping ourselves physically fit. Fitness is important for time management; if by staying physically fit we are more effective, it is a wise investment of our time.

Professional and career activities are those activities related to our job or our work. It is not only the time we spend on the job, but also all those other activities surrounding our work such as continuing education, business trips, and reading.

It is vitally important to establish priorities in all of these categories to lead a balanced life. It is almost guaranteed that if we pick a single area, focus on it intensely, and pursue it single mindedly, we will be successful in that area; however, we may become seriously unbalanced by focusing all our energies and time on one thing. We need to balance our lives by paying attention to all five categories. In this way we will develop ourselves fully as human beings. This is critical to our effectiveness and ultimately our happiness.

The best time to make the list is now. An alternative, however, is to plan a weekend away from the chaos of normal life. This can be an exciting adventure, particularly if you go to an area that is emotionally stimulating such as the ocean, mountains, or desert. The environment becomes a tool to facilitate your thought process. It may be helpful to go with your spouse or someone who can be a sounding board for ideas as you begin to think about what you would really like to do for the next 20 years.

WHERE WE ARE VERSUS WHERE WE WOULD LIKE TO BE

The next step in becoming an effective time manager is to gain some insights into where you are now versus where you would like to be. Imagine that it is 5 years from now and you have been asked to write your own obituary. Write down how you would like to be remembered in relationship to the five main categories of human activity. This is an important exercise because it tells you what you would really like to achieve.

Once you have completed writing your obituary, read it aloud and then take a few minutes to jot down the areas in which there is a difference between what you are doing today and what you would like to achieve by the time you die. This can be a critical first step toward prioritizing what you are doing. If there are things in your obituary that you are not currently doing or have plans to begin, you should seriously reevaluate what you are doing. Goethe wrote, "the things that matter most must not be at the mercy of the things that matter least."[3]

PRIORITIZING AND GOAL SETTING

The next step in moving toward effective time management is to prioritize your activities through the process of goal setting. Brian Tracey, one of the masters of effective time management, aptly notes, "if you are not working toward your own goals then you are working toward someone else's."[4] At any point in your life, if you have not prioritized your activities, set goals, established plans for achieving those goals, and begun implementing those goals, then your life is drifting.

The "things I want to do" list has a variety of items ranging from important to "nice to do." In all likelihood it will be impossible to do everything on your list. To approach the task of using your time wisely and managing your list, you must modify the list so that it guides you. You can gain a sense of accomplishment by prioritizing the items on the list to help you focus on doing the most important things first.

Alan Lakein,[6] an early leader in time management, suggests prioritizing the items on your list by labeling them A, B, and C. A items are of utmost importance and provide the greatest success in leading the type of life you want. B items are important but are not *essential* to long-term success. C items consist of those nice things on the list that you would like to do some day, but that are not really important. Go through your lists, marking each item with an A, B, or C.

Once you have completed that process, make a new list consisting only of those items that you marked with an A, keeping them separated in the five categories. The A lists consist of things you consider critical to long-term success and your sense of well-being. Even those items considered to be most important must be prioritized. Rank the items in the A list in each of the five categories, with 1 being the most important. Start by asking the question, "If I can only do one thing in this category on my A list and I was assured of succeeding at it, what would it be?" Once you have chosen the first item, ask yourself the question, "If I could do just one more thing in this category on my list and was assured of succeeding at it, what would it be?" That will give you the second item. Go through each of the five categories to prioritize each list using that question. At the end of this exercise, you will have ranked the items most important to you in order of priority. You should now rewrite the lists in numerical order to create five lists, one for each of the five categories of human activities: family, psychospiritual, personal

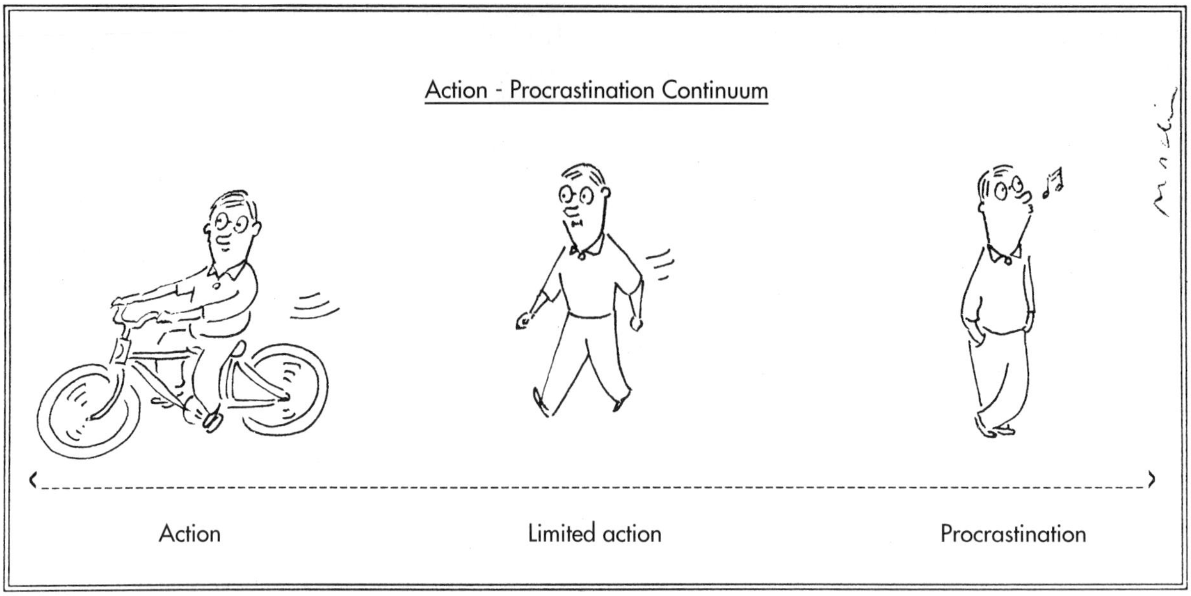

FIGURE 7-1 Action-Procrastination Continuum

BOX 7-1

ACTION PLAN FOR SUCCESS

1. Define your goal.
2. Specify the steps you will need to take to achieve that goal.
3. Identify the resources (human and otherwise) you will need to take these steps.
4. List the obstacles you must overcome to reach your goal.
5. Define the steps you will need to take to overcome these obstacles.
6. Set realistic deadlines for achieving each of these steps toward reaching your goal.
7. Program these steps into your daily activities in order that you can take action everyday toward meeting your most important goals.

development, health and fitness, and professional/career activities. These prioritized lists now become your list of goals.

Depending on the length of the lists, you may want to focus on the top four or five items in each of the five categories. This focuses your energies on the things most important in your life. By attending to all five categories, you will approach your life in a balanced way. You will attend to all of the parameters of your character, not just one.

MAKING IT HAPPEN

Up to this point you have been dealing with the things you would like to do as abstract ideas. To ensure success, those ideas must be converted into concrete plans with steps and deadlines. The key to success is not in having good ideas but in being able to turn those ideas into action. The following seven step process will help you convert your ideas into an action plan (Box 7-1).

Once you complete this process for each of the items you have determined are the most important in the five categories of human activities, you will have defined for yourself a master plan for living a balanced and successful life. At this point, take a moment to congratulate yourself for taking the first step in managing your life.

MOVING INTO ACTION

After developing a balanced set of goals and specific plans for reaching those goals you need to set them into action. Being able to initiate action is one of the key steps in effective time management. Many people get stuck at the wrong end of the action-procrastination continuum (Figure 7-1). This continuum describes the varying degrees of effectiveness observed in human beings in completing tasks and reaching goals. On one end of this continuum is effective action; on the other is total inaction. In the large middle zone is a range of limited action mixed with procrastination. This is where most people function.

Most people become frustrated in this middle zone of limited action. Action is spent achieving someone else's goals. Once you realize realistically where you are on the continuum you can begin to learn how to lead a life based on action.

Growing up we are socialized and we learn particular behavior patterns. These patterns become locked into habits. These habits guide our lives and form the barriers that keep us in the middle zone of limited action and procrastination.

To change our position on the action-procrastination continuum, we need to (1) develop new tools for overcoming

procrastination and inertia, (2) replace old habits with new effective, action oriented behavior patterns, and (3) adopt a daily prioritization model to guide our moment-to-moment choices.

NEW TOOLS TO OVERCOME PROCRASTINATION AND INERTIA

Work patterns are developed early in life, probably during the first 3 years as we learn to play. As we enter into school, these patterns are reinforced through our study habits. We generally carry those patterns throughout our lives. If you are plagued by ineffective action patterns and procrastination, three simple tools can be used to overcome these obstacles: (1) do it now, (2) schedule the time to do it, and (3) set deadlines.

Do It Now

W. Clement Stone,[7] an entrepreneur and author of numerous books on success, thought procrastination was one of the most insidious factors that blocked success. To counter this tendency, he would have his employees start each day by standing and shouting **"do it now"** 50 times. Numerous successful businessmen have credited their success to the training they received when they worked for W. Clement Stone.

This tool is simple. Every time you accept a new responsibility or task, remember to **"do it now."** The best time to tackle the project is when it is fresh in your mind and your energy is at its highest because you just accepted it. This tool is particularly helpful for those simple tasks that tend to pile up and get ignored.

If you get in the habit of doing things now, not only will you be much happier about the amount of things that you accomplish, but your reputation among your colleagues and superiors will grow as you become known as someone who can really get things done.

Schedule Time to Do It

If you cannot attend to something immediately, you can use the second tool: schedule time to work on it. Every task requires some time. The best way to ensure that you take that time to complete the task is to schedule it. This practice applies for tasks that take only a few minutes or many hours.

When you accept a new responsibility or task, if you immediately enter it into your schedule and define precisely when you will be accomplishing that task, you are going one step beyond accepting the new responsibility; you are committing time to complete it.

Set Deadlines

To ensure we complete our responsibilities, we frequently make lists. Lists can be helpful, but there are two inherent flaws in the list-making concept. The first is that there is no time line attached to a simple list. A simple list does not take advantage of time as a useful device for generating action. The second flaw is the inherent concept that when you complete the tasks on the list you will be "done." This stands in contrast to the way life works. Life is a never ending process. It is a never-ending and ever-changing list.

We fell into the list making trap. There were times when we had so many lists that we had to have a list to keep the lists straight. We became so obsessed with the lists that they became the end rather than the means. It was depressing because we never seemed to make headway on the mounting lists. Research into time management led to the understanding that we needed to get to the action step on each of the items. The best approach was to do things immediately and set deadlines. Doing things immediately would keep things off the lists and setting deadlines got them done. Part of this key to keeping the deadlines was to schedule time to do the jobs.

There is an effective way to modify a list to make it more effective. Simply add a column for a deadline beside each of the items. You can use the deadlines as effective incentives to move everything on the list into an action phase.

An adjunct to adding deadlines to your list is to write down the entry date. You could then make a rule to drop from the list anything that stays there longer than 1 month without any action. This clearly addresses your commitment to act on something that is on the list.

OVERCOMING HABITS: REPROGRAMING THE SUBCONSCIOUS

Concept

To overcome the habits that lock you into the ineffective part of the action-procrastination continuum, you must reprogram your subconscious. You must replace your old habits with effective new habits.

Included in the habits that may control your life are the habitual ways you perceive yourself. If you perceive yourself as inefficient or a poor time manager, these perceptions can be powerful obstacles to your growth and must be overcome. There are a number of highly effective techniques widely used by psychologists and a broad range of other groups to effectively change behavior. You probably know and practice many of these techniques. By using these techniques you change the way you perceive yourself and the way you react to situations.

Techniques

The following powerful techniques help reprogram and create new inner vision: (1) using positive affirmations, (2) acting the part, (3) teaching someone else, (4) sharing your commitment, and (5) Visualizing yourself in your new role.

Using Positive Affirmation. Positive affirmations are statements that you make to yourself about yourself. They are most effective in the present tense. By repeating a positive affirmation with conviction several times each day, it will soon become part of the fabric of your personality. For example, you would say "I am a nonsmoker" as opposed to "I will stop smoking." The former affirmation is both positive and in the present tense, whereas the latter example speaks about the future and has the negative connotation of quitting. For effective time management you may want to try a positive affirmation such as "I am an excellent time manager" or "I use my time well."

A good way to make positive affirmations more effective is to write them down on a card and put them on your mirror so that each morning when you go into the bathroom you will be reminded of your commitment to this affirmation. You could also put a card on the dash in your car and inside your briefcase. Each time you see one of the cards, repeat it, if possible, out loud with great conviction.

Acting the Part. Acting the part can be an excellent way to move yourself into a particular role. If you pretend that you are an excellent time manager you will gradually, over time, make this second nature and will no longer be acting.

Teaching Someone Else. Teaching is one of the best techniques for internalizing material. If you study the techniques of effective time management and then use them to teach someone else, you will be reinforcing this trait in yourself.

Share Your Commitment. When you tell someone about your plans, you create a public expectation that heightens your commitment to achieving that expectation. In short, you will always perform better when you think someone is watching. Your spouse or a close friend would be ideal for sharing such a commitment.

Visualize Yourself in Your New Role. The last technique for reprograming the subconscious is visualization. If you can see yourself functioning as an excellent time manager and can burn this image into your mind, you will become an excellent time manager. Visualize yourself in the present tense because the subconscious works in the present tense.

Athletes use this technique to enhance their performance. When a quarterback is stepping back to throw a pass, in the instant before he lets the ball go, he sees the trajectory of the ball and he can visualize his teammate catching it.

You can use the technique of visualization to assist yourself in reaching all your goals. The more clearly you can see yourself in a given role or achieving a certain goal, the easier it will be.

Harvey McKay, the author of *How to Swim With the Sharks Without Being Eaten Alive* and president of McKay Envelope Company, a very successful business, tells a story about how he used visualization.[8] Harvey is an avid baseball fan living in Minneapolis, Minnesota. Several years ago when Minneapolis was about to lose its baseball franchise, he organized a group of his friends and other businessmen to save the team by collecting money to build a new stadium. McKay became the chairman of the commission that was organized to build the stadium. His vision was that he would throw out the first ball in the new stadium. When he started he knew it would take about a year to raise the money for the stadium. At the end of 1 year he decided it would take 2 years. At the end of 2 years he reestimated 4 years. Finally after 7 years, McKay was able to realize his vision. He did throw out the first pitch in the Hubert Humphrey Metrodome. Harvey used his vision to inspire himself to work hard for 7 years to realize his goal. Visualization is one of the most powerful tools to influence your subconscious and your behavior.

TOOLS FOR DAILY DECISIONS

Learning to Stay Focused

By going through the goal setting exercises, you have prioritized the things you want to do in your life, identifying the top three or four goals within each of the five categories of human activity. To reach those goals, you need to stay focused on them. Here are three steps for staying focused: (1) review your goals daily, (2) use your goals in the daily decision-making process, and (3) review your progress daily.

Review Your Goals Daily. Begin each day by reviewing each of your goals in all five categories. Read them aloud to imprint them indelibly on your mind so that they become part of your moment-to-moment thought process. In addition, reading goals aloud provides an opportunity to ask "are these the right goals?"

Use Goals in the Daily Decision-Making Process. If you keep your goals in mind as you make your daily decisions about what you will and will not do, it will help in making your decisions. Ask yourself, "Will I be moving myself closer to reaching one or more of my goals by accepting this new responsibility or will it draw attention away from my efforts to reach these goals?" This question becomes a powerful framework for you to guide your choices.

Review Progress Daily. Review your goals every day and ask yourself the question, "What did I do today to help me achieve my goals?" It is important not to make this an exercise in self-recrimination. Rather it should provide an opportunity to either pat yourself on the back or take positive steps to renew your commitment to stay focused. It is a good idea to perform this review at roughly the same time each day so that it becomes a regular part of your life; just before you go to bed is an ideal time.

CONTINUOUS REVIEW

Continuous review of your goals and your plans on a daily basis is critical for success. It is important to give yourself positive feedback as you accomplish the steps you have defined. This will reinforce that you are working on the things that are most important to you. In addition, by reviewing your goals and plans on a daily basis, you will be able to recognize what you need to do to modify the goal or the plan to make them more achievable. You may need to break the steps into smaller and more tangible pieces.

A key element in achieving success is not only being able to visualize the goal, but to realize progress toward that goal on a daily basis. You need to reward yourself for taking those steps. Therefore if you have a well-thought-out plan with concrete steps that will lead toward your goal, you will know as you are taking those steps that you are moving closer to achieving your success. It is important that you give yourself credit for taking those steps and celebrate each of those steps as a piece of that long-term success.

You should plan to review and reassess your entire system of goals at regular intervals because things change. You need to keep your goals in tune with those changes. For some people this will mean reviewing and reassessing goals monthly, for others a yearly review is sufficient. The critical action is to take time to pull out your initial wish list and ask yourself whether your needs have changed and whether the plans you have laid out are the best for you.

Once you have decided what you want to do and how you are going to do it, you need to develop work habits and ways of doing business to maximize your effectiveness. Many different tools and techniques are presented. You will need to find those that work best for you (Box 7-2).

SCHEDULING SECRETS

Effective scheduling can be a tremendous asset in effective time management. The importance of getting things onto the schedule to ensure they are done has been presented; this section describes how to use your schedule; it is divided into five scheduling secrets (Box 7-3).

BOX 7-2

TIME MANAGEMENT TOOLS

Scheduling secrets
Telephone tips
Dealing with drop-in visitors
Procrastination
Inefficient meetings
Car time
Waiting in line
The coffee break
Processing paperwork
Delegating
Lack of focus

BOX 7-3

SCHEDULING SECRETS

Ending times
Accurate time allotment
Batching
"To do" files
Patterns

Ending Times

The use of "ending times" when scheduling is one of the most important tools at your disposal. Just as your budget tends to grow to match your revenue, a meeting or activity will grow to fill the time available. If no ending time is established, the meeting or activity will tend to drag on until it creates some form of conflict.

To avoid this time-wasting expansion of a meeting or activity, it is important to set the ending time when you schedule meetings. Most people find that if they only have an hour to deal with a certain number of issues they will pace themselves appropriately. You will find yourself being more effective by doing this, and your co-workers also will appreciate it.

Accurate Time Allotment

Accurate time allotment is a skill that must be learned. You must practice diligently to master it. It is tempting to optimistically plan to do two or three times more in a given time period than is reasonable. However, this practice leads to frustration over not completing those tasks and discord over being late if you squeeze in those last few minutes of work trying to complete them. It is not fair to the people with whom you will be meeting next. Try to learn to estimate time more accurately. For example, it probably takes 10 minutes to pack things, say goodbye to the staff, and then get to your car. If you think you can leave quickly, you will probably be late a lot. As soon as you realize it takes time to get out of the office and plan accordingly, you create appropriate expectations and can allot an accurate amount of time to leave.

Another example is planning a meeting. If you need to cover 10 items and you know each of them will take approximately 10 minutes to present and discuss, it is unfair to cram those 10 items into a 1-hour meeting. One of three things is going to happen: (1) you will not get through everything on the agenda, which may have certain consequences; (2) you may get through everything on the agenda, but some things may be dealt with ineffectively; or (3) the meeting will run over, which is unfair to other people who may have scheduled other meetings or activities to follow the meeting. It is probably better to schedule a little more time than you actually think you will need. If you finish early do not stick around squandering that extra time. Get on to the next meeting or to your next activity. Colleagues always like getting the gift of a little extra time.

Batching

Batching small tasks or similar tasks can be a useful way to let your schedule help you use your time more effectively. By scheduling a series of similar activities you take advantage of the phenomenon of "getting into an effective frame of mind."

Sometimes when you work on material in a particular area, you get deeply involved and your mind begins to engage the material in ways that allow for new insights and creativity. You can take advantage of this by scheduling similar topics in a series. As a result you may be far more effective in finding solutions and getting your tasks completed.

Batching also can be an advantage when you have a number of small tasks to accomplish such as brief letters and phone calls. To disperse these tasks throughout the day may work, but more often may be disruptive or tend to delay tasks.

"To-Do" Files

The fourth scheduling secret is to create "to-do" files. An excellent tool for this strategy is a chronologic file. You create one file for each day of the month, one file for each month of the year, and one file for each of the next 2 years. In all 31 files are labeled with the number for the days of the month, and 12 files are labeled with each of the 12 months and two additional files labeled for each of the next 2 years. Preferably, these files are kept in a desk file drawer for convenient retrieval.

This system provides a place to put things that inevitably are needed. In addition, it provides a way of scheduling more work. For example, if you are assigned the task of designing a quality assurance study, you would put the materials in the file for the day on which you intended to work on that task. Your commitment then is to accomplish everything that you have put into that file on that given day.

One method for coordinating this with your schedule would be to block time on your schedule to work on materials in your "to do file." Thus each day when you sit down to work if you are scheduled to process file items, you have the things that you need at your fingertips. Three potential pitfalls to avoid when using this system are the following:

- Be sure to schedule adequate time to accomplish the items you put in the file.
- If you place a critical item into one of these files, be sure to have a notation or tickler system to allow you to locate it if you need it before the scheduled work day.

- Do not put things in the files and then ignore the system, as you will lose files.

This system has numerous variations. You need to find the one that is most comfortable for you. The keys are to (1) find the system with which you are comfortable, (2) use it diligently, and (3) take control of your time by working with the system. A to-do filing system can: (1) help you schedule work, (2) make finding work materials vastly simpler, and (3) put the work materials at your fingertips. It cannot, however, make you do the work.

Patterns

The fifth scheduling secret is developing effective, consistent work patterns. Most humans are creatures of habit. Most people tend to develop routines for everything from eating, grooming, and family activities to job schedules and human interaction patterns. You can take advantage of this tendency and become more effective in managing your life and your time. Suggestions in this area would include scheduling work time for the same time slot each day and doing the same thing for returning phone calls.

TELEPHONE TIPS

Managing telephone calls effectively can be a tremendous asset in effective time management. Telephone interruptions are by far the most insidious time waster. We are programed to drop whatever we are doing to answer a ringing telephone. The perception is that if we do not answer the phone the caller might hang up. However, unless we are expecting an important telephone call, at least 80% of telephone calls have nothing to do with our goals. This means that if we interrupt what we are doing to answer the telephone and deal with the caller we are working on someone else's goals.

The following telephone tips are useful tools for controlling the disruption of the telephone call:

1. Take messages.
2. Give call back times.
3. Consider telephone calls as "mini meetings."
4. Set time limits.
5. Batch telephone calls.

The first line of defense we can use to protect ourselves from the interruption of telephone calls is to have our calls screened. One can either have a secretary or a telephone answering machine to perform this task. It is tempting to always be available to meet the needs of the callers by taking the phone call as it comes in. In some settings, this availability may be necessary to effectively carry out one's job. The price of providing this availability is the lost time that is required to regroup and continue what you were doing before the call arrived. The second cost is diminished effectiveness because you are unable to appropriately prepare for the phone call.

An important part of managing your calls is to give call-back times. By having your secretary give a call-back time or having this part of your answering machine message you will be more effective in managing your schedule and you will be helpful to others. This approach is critical in avoiding the frustration and time loss of "telephone tag."

An effective way to manage telephone calls is to consider each of them "a mini-meeting." Just as with any face-to-face meeting, the telephone call mini-meeting requires preparation to be maximally effective. At the least, this would involve setting an agenda and having all the appropriate materials available for the mini-meeting. Starting calls by reviewing your purpose and/or agenda helps focus everyone and identify other items to be discussed. If the person with whom you are having a conversation brings up agenda items that will exceed your time limit or about which you are not prepared, you are in an ideal position to schedule another mini-meeting.

Setting a time limit for the telephone call and sharing it with the person with whom you are speaking will prevent calls from dragging on. It is important to have a clock or a timer in front of you so that you can keep track of your time. The key is to stay focused on the purpose of the phone call and avoid distractions to stay within your time frame.

The last telephone tip has been touched on previously; batch your calls. If you schedule a specific time each day to make telephone calls, you can establish a rhythm that will allow you to be much more effective and not use up unnecessary time.

DEALING WITH DROP-IN VISITORS

Drop-in visitors interrupt your work plan by stopping in without an appointment to say "hello" or chat without a specific agenda. Sometimes they have a specific issue, but it is not directly related to your goals and priorities for that day. This can create a significant amount of frustration and may sabotage your schedule. The following strategies can help you with a drop-in visitor: (1) early redirection, (2) diversion/delegation, (3) scheduling a meeting, and (4) erecting barricades.

One of the best ways to handle the drop-in visitor is to redirect them based on your needs. After a cordial greeting, you could simply say, "I am really sorry but I have an important deadline to meet, can we get together at a different time?" Of course, you must be willing to set up a later meeting. An alternative is to offer someone else to help them. The difficulty of that technique is that the visitor needs to explain the issue so you are at least committed to hearing it. Another effective technique to keeping visits brief is to never let the person sit down. Greet the visitor at the door and simply do not let him or her pass or simply continue standing as the visitor enters the room. This sends the nonverbal message "I'm not in a position to meet now." If the person does not respond to this, you can use a redirecting statement.

If you are confronted with a drop-in visitor who falls into the category of "professional chatterer," you may want to use a diversion/delegation technique. This type of individual usually is gregarious and can be engaging. Unfortunately, when visitors drop in they tend to disrupt your day. An effective strategy is to engage them in a problem or issue, thereby diverting them from talking to you and then delegating that issue to them by suggesting that they become involved in finding a solution.

For example, we had the annoying problem of people waiting outside the front entrance of the hospital and dropping cigarette butts. After an appropriate greeting, the professional chatterer was shown the problem, and then delegated the problem by the question "Can you help out with this? Can you talk to the administrator?" This effectively diverted him. He got interested in the problem and it was easy to suggest that he take action immediately and exit.

This technique is particularly successful because it allows several positive things to occur. On one hand, you can give the professional chatterer some of the personal attention he needs. On the other hand, it allows you to handle the situation in a timely fashion so that your entire schedule is not disrupted. In addition, you can focus attention on issues that need to be dealt with.

The last method for dealing with drop-in visitors is to erect barricades. Many executives have their secretary's desk placed squarely in front of their door. No one can get in without going around the secretary. Your secretary becomes the gatekeeper and can protect you when you are working on things.

You will undoubtedly need to drop-in occasionally on someone. To avoid ambushing the person with whom you would like to meet, introduce your issue with a single sentence and then inquire if the timing is appropriate. For example, "I need to discuss the plans for the new emergency department. Is this a convenient time for you?" By extending this courtesy to others not only will they appreciate the courtesy you have extended, but they will frequently return the courtesy.

PROCRASTINATION

Procrastination is the antithesis of action. It is the habit of not doing something by putting it off. This insidious problem is extremely widespread and affects people in all aspects of life. This section describes several concrete methods for dealing with procrastination.

The following four common triggers precipitate procrastination: (1) the task seems too large, (2) you do not like the task, (3) you have a hidden fear of failure, and (4) you feel overwhelmed or too busy right now. Regardless of the trigger, the effect is the same. You enter a pattern of avoidance. Each time you put off a task, you reinforce the thought that triggered the initial avoidance. The more times you go through the process of putting off a given task, the harder it becomes to engage that activity. In essence, you are building a barrier between yourself and that task. Each time you put it off, you add to the barrier. This process becomes habitual, dominating key portions of your life.

To successfully overcome procrastination, you need to take the following steps: (1) recognize the triggers that put you into the cycle of procrastination, (2) develop techniques and strategies to move into action when you would normally procrastinate, and (3) reward yourself frequently for taking action. If you can identify the thought process that leads to your putting something off, you are taking the first step in uncovering the habitual behavior that constituted procrastination. The key is to break the cycle before it begins. Once you are in a patterned behavior cycle, it is difficult to function differently. The following nine procrastination preventing tools are useful in breaking the procrastination cycle.

Start Immediately

Anytime you are confronted with a task or an activity, begin working on it immediately. Even if you only finish a small amount, by taking action immediately, you have overcome inertia. Once you start something, it is much easier to continue.

Establish a Plan

A simple way to begin is to write out a plan. Use the same seven goal-setting steps:

1. Define successful completion for this activity.
2. Identify the necessary steps.
3. Identify the resources needed for completion.
4. Define the obstacles to a successful completion.
5. Identify the steps necessary to overcome obstacles.
6. Set up a timetable for each of the steps.
7. Reward yourself each time you take one of these steps.

This process should not be cumbersome. It should be simple, straightforward, and useful. It is a wonderful tool for moving you from inaction to action.

Do a Little Bit Each Day

By setting aside time each day, even as little as 15 minutes, to work on a large long-term project, you are more likely to complete the job. To wait for an opportunity where you have several hours or days to work on something is a set-up for procrastination. Invariably, some crisis will interrupt your plans and further delay work on the project. Doing a little bit each day is particularly effective when used in conjunction with developing a plan of breaking down a task into its component parts. Each part can be assigned to a particular day or series of days. The result is that you will effectively work your way through even huge projects, a piece at a time.

The technique of doing a little bit each day is also useful for ongoing responsibilities such as a quality assurance program. By setting aside 15 minutes each day to work on the quality assurance program, the task becomes surprisingly easy.

Schedule Your Impossible Tasks

If you block out time in your schedule to work on those "impossible tasks," you are more likely to complete them because you have made a commitment to that task. The key to successfully using this technique is to perceive your "appointment" to work on your task as important as any other appointment. In addition, a powerful psychologic step occurs when you publicly commit to do something.

Do the Hardest Part First

By doing the hardest part first, an important psychologic barrier is broken down. If you are able to eliminate the least appealing part of a difficult task by doing the hardest part first, you have changed your perception of the task. If you dive right in and complete the hard part, getting it out of the way, the easy parts become enjoyable. Completion of the hardest part is also an ideal opportunity to reward yourself.

Slice Up the Job

If you had to eat a whole pizza, contemplating the entire mass might be overwhelming. However, if you slice up the pizza, each individual piece is much more approachable. If you do the same to a job, it becomes much easier to accomplish.

Develop a System of Rewards

Part of the psychology of procrastination is that people get caught up in dreading the job to such a degree that they lose sight of any potential reward from completing the task. If you

set up a system of rewards, you can focus on the positive rewards rather than dreading doing the project. A successful system of rewards is established by creating steps that are easily achievable and providing rewards that are immediate.

For example, if you need to recruit a physician for your group and you dread making all of the telephone calls, a good reward system can be developed using your favorite foods. You can sit down with a glass of juice and a bunch of grapes (or whatever your favorite foods might be), and each time you complete a recruiting phone call you can reward yourself by taking a sip of juice and eating two or three grapes.

It really does not matter what the reward is or what the steps are. What does matter is that you are rewarding yourself immediately for achieving even a small part of your task. You can practice this with your children. For example, you can say to them, "when you clean up your room I have a surprise for you." You will be amazed at the results.

Time Trials

Time trials are an attempt to turn an onerous task into a game and have some fun rather than struggling. The object is to take each step in a project or a series of similar pieces and see how fast you can do them. You can combine this with a reward system and turn work into play. The idea of time trials may seem a little ridiculous; however, what you are doing is attempting to overcome the negative psychology of procrastination.

Procrastinators tend to spend all of their time dreading a job and never get around to spending any time working on it. If you change your perception of the job by making it a game, you no longer dread it and can actually enjoy it. Changing your perception of the task or responsibility is one of the keys of overcoming procrastination.

Avoid Pitfalls of Procrastinators

The five primary pitfalls of procrastinators are the following:

1. There is always more time tomorrow.
2. The best time to do something is always later.
3. Never start a project unless you can finish it.
4. It's best to get the little stuff out of the way first.
5. Don't do it if you can't do it perfectly.

Perhaps the most insidious pitfall for procrastinators is the idea that you will have more time to work on a project "tomorrow." The reality is that there are always new crises to interfere with your project, and it will keep getting delayed.

Similar to waiting until tomorrow, procrastinators are always looking for "the best time to do something." The ideal time never arrives and tasks are never completed. In reality the only time you have is the present; therefore the best time to begin anything is now.

The third pitfall is the tendency to resist beginning something until you can finish it. Some people can function with this concept; however, for most people it becomes an excuse, and jobs are delayed.

The fourth pitfall is the tendency to want to clear off the desk to get started on a major project. Instead you become occupied with the small stuff, consuming all of the time available for work. You have to resist the tendency to become occupied with anything other than what is scheduled.

The last pitfall is that procrastinators tend to think they have to be perfectionists. A huge barrier gets built thinking about how hard it will be to "get it right." As a general rule, it takes as much time to complete the last 10% of the job to make it perfect as it does to do the first 90%. Do not focus on perfection; focus on getting started.

INEFFICIENT MEETINGS

Meetings are important communication and action tools. They are indispensable in the business world. It has been estimated that half the time spent in meetings is wasted and a significant number of business people spend about half their time in meetings. You can lose up to 25% of your time through inefficient meetings. Therefore it is critical to take steps to ensure that your meetings are effective. The following seven rules can help in that process:

1. Define the purpose of the meeting.
2. Establish an agenda in advance.
3. Start on time.
4. Take careful minutes.
5. Keep focused.
6. Set deadlines.
7. Stop on time.

A valuable framework in which to consider the value of a meeting is to compare it to the meeting expense. The meeting expense is calculated by multiplying the time spent by the hourly compensation of each attendee and then adding those amounts. For example, if you have five administrators who meet for 3 hours once a month to discuss company policy, and each of the executives are paid $75 an hour, the meetings are costing the company $1125/month or $13,500/ year. The questions is, is the company receiving $13,500 worth of value by having those meetings. Viewed from this perspective, the importance of meetings may change. If you ask yourself before scheduling every meeting, "what will be the cost of this meeting?" you may decide to schedule fewer meetings. A brief telephone call or a memo may be all that is necessary.

Define the Purpose of a Meeting

Defining the purpose of a meeting is similar to establishing your goals. The purpose of the meeting is in essence the goal for that block of time. If the purpose of a meeting is established clearly and is shared in advance, the effectiveness of the meeting is increased by giving everyone the same expectation.

Establish the Agenda in Advance

Along with the purpose for a given meeting, you need to establish an agenda. This is analogous to defining the specific steps for a particular goal. The agenda also needs to be published in advance so that the people attending the meeting can be prepared. A useful technique is to list the people responsible for a each agenda item on the agenda. You also can highlight a given individual's tasks so that when the individual receives his or her copy of the agenda, the responsibilities will be obvious.

Start on Time

Always start meetings on time. It is not fair to those that have shown up on time to punish them by waiting for those who

are late. You are wasting the time of those who are punctual in deference to those who are disrespectful.

Some companies make a policy of locking the door when a meeting begins. This sends the powerful message that being on time is important. It also can have a dramatic impact on behavior.

Being on time is considered the sign of a true professional. Most people regard those who are on time as "class acts." It is considered to be a sign of respect and is great for business. People who are on time for meetings, assignments, reports, and in product or service delivery are perceived as providing a higher quality product. Many times being late simply means that you did not want to be there.

Take Careful Minutes

One of the great frustrations and inefficiencies of meetings is to have disagreements about the contents of the meeting, requiring yet another meeting. For example, you have negotiated with the hospital for the installation of a new monitoring system in the emergency department. Just before the shipment is ordered, you find the list of equipment for your department is far short of what you expected. To revisit this issue requires significant emotional investment and time.

The key to avoiding such problems is to take careful minutes and have everyone present sign off on them. In some situations, you may want to share copies of your minutes before the close of the meeting so that these things can actually be signed before the meeting breaks up. This technique can be extremely valuable in dealing with very sensitive issues.

This does not mean you have to take detailed minutes for every meeting that you attend; however, used appropriately, taking minutes, sharing them and having people sign off on them can be powerful tools for effectiveness and time efficiency.

Keep Focused

During meetings, always stay focused. Stick to the agenda and be sure to prioritize each item. Vilfredo Pareto, the Italian economist, pointed out that 80% of the goods and services come from 20% of the population. In other words, 80% of the wealth was owned by 20% of the population. This has become known as Pareto's 80/20 rule. It has been applied widely. It can be used in evaluating meeting agendas; 80% of the value of your meeting will be in 20% of the items. Put the important 20% at the beginning of the meeting so that if you run out of time, you will have gotten 80% of the value.

You will invariably encounter people who have their own agendas for meetings. If you have published your agenda in advance, you are in a position to deal effectively with their distractions by diverting the meeting back to the original agenda. It is important to acknowledge the importance of these individuals' issues. If you attempt to dismiss them, you will only heighten their resistance. If you acknowledge the importance of the individual's issues and make the commitment to deal with them at a future time, you can then refocus the agenda of the meeting.

Set Deadlines

Deadlines are extremely important to effective time use, especially for meetings. Within a meeting you can set deadlines for reading closure on an item. This will help you stay focused. In addition, whenever there is assignment of responsibility, it is critical to attach a deadline for completion of that item. Remember: An assignment or responsibility without a deadline is merely a conversation. Be sure to obtain the acceptance of each deadline by the individual(s) responsible and write them down.

Stop on Time

When you schedule a meeting always set the beginning and ending times. One of the most common time wasters are open ended meetings or meetings that do not end on time. Once you have passed the preset ending time, you have effectively converted to an open ended meeting. Always bring meetings to close on time. If agenda items require additional time you can choose to extend the meeting or schedule another meeting later. In either case, make this a conscious decision rather than relying on inertia.

CAR TIME

Lost time from a flat tire, a breakdown or a frustrating encounter with an auto mechanic aside, you are at the mercy of your car a significant part of your time. If this time is not used effectively, it will be lost to the task of transportation. The magnitude of the time loss is staggering. The average person driving 12,000 miles/year and living to an age of 72 years spends approximately 4 years in the car. With some creativity, this time can be used effectively.

Audiotapes are tremendous tools for enhancing the effectiveness of your car travel time. Meeting continuing medical education requirements is made much easier using audiotapes during car travel time. In addition, you can use this tool to explore new areas such as foreign languages, management skills, and negotiating skills. You should select tapes that provide information or help make decisions relative to your major goals.

A microcassette recorder also can be valuable in making your car time more effective. You can dictate letters, reports, and minutes of meetings.

A car phone can be an excellent way of conducting business during car time. The one disadvantage of making telephone calls in your car is that you cannot take notes or refer to materials. However, if you keep your calls brief, you can dictate your notes immediately after each call.

WAITING IN LINE

On the surface, waiting in line may appear to be an unavoidable time waster. This occurs in many forms each day, at the grocery store, in an airport, in a cafeteria, etc. You need to plan ahead to deal effectively with this problem. Virtually all your goals will require you to gain new information or stay current with literature. In setting up your plans for achieving your goals you will have identified at least some of this material. The key to successfully using the time that is usually lost waiting in line is to have some of this reading material available at all times. If you have a journal article or a book in your pocket, whenever you are waiting in line, you can pull it out.

To have this material readily available you can use the "flip and rip technique." Rather than reading a journal or maga-

zine from cover to cover, review the table of contents and identify articles of interest. "Flip" directly to that article, scan it to see if it meets your needs, and if it does "rip it out." Keep these articles in a "to-read" file and have several of them with you at all times. This technique is particularly helpful because it keeps you focused on the article about which you are interested. Also, you can avoid distracting advertisements. The marketing techniques used to create ads are designed to be distracting. Using the flip and rip technique you avoid them entirely.

You can use a similar technique with books. If you buy a paperback copy of a book, you can divide it into sections of about 50 pages, which are easier to keep in a pocket. You will be amazed at how many books this will allow you to read.

THE COFFEE BREAK

Every day presents numerous casual encounters that are opportunities for socializing. These encounters can consume significant time. In addition, they can be wonderful opportunities to spend time with people. The key is not to avoid these encounters, but rather to make a conscious decision about how much time you will devote to them.

The problem most people have with these encounters is lacking the discipline to limit their time or knowing how to disengage effectively. The best way to control the time spent in these casual encounters is to develop the habit of asking yourself at the beginning, "how much time do I want to spend socializing?" You then must learn to stick to that time commitment.

You can also practice bringing conversations to a close in a socially acceptable way. One powerful phrase suggested by Brian Tracy is, "well, I guess I've got to get back to work." This simple and powerful phrase will allow you to disengage. Keep in mind, the more abruptly you conclude a conversation, the more uncomfortable it may seem. It is important to look for a natural closure so that you make people feel comfortable.

PROCESSING PAPERWORK

Processing paperwork ranges from handling the mail to filing and writing reports. The amount of paper that you are required to handle or create can be quite large. At times you can be totally inundated and it can be an insidious time waster. The way you handle paper and the techniques you use to process it can make a difference in the amount of time processing paper consumes. It also has an important physiologic impact on our lives. The following suggestions can help maximize your efficiency in dealing with paperwork: (1) handle paperwork once, (2) file effectively, (3) manage your mail, and (4) procrastinate creatively.

Handle Paperwork Once

The first step in managing your paperwork is to learn to handle each piece the fewest times possible. Ideally, you would handle each piece a single time. Most people tend to lose a significant amount looking through large piles of paper. From the outset, you need to move things into the action mode. The first time you handle each piece of paper, you need to triage it into one of three locations: (1) the waste can, (2) process immediately pile, and (3) process in the future pile.

File Effectively

Papers that cannot be processed immediately should be kept in the action mode by scheduling a time to work on them and filing them systematically so that you do not lose time looking for them. The scheduling filing system previously discussed, which includes an action file for each day of month or some other form of a tickler system, is useful.

The main ideas in effective filing is to keep only those papers that will be useful in the future and in such way that they can be found. The logic you use in setting up your files must be readily identifiable, and it must be maintained consistently. Avoid the traps of "communications files" and "miscellaneous files." These files tend to become large and are difficult to retrieve items from. The tendency is to refer to them frequently when you cannot find something elsewhere. As a result a great deal of time is spent flipping through communications and miscellaneous. It is better to file things arranged to a specific plan so that you can find them easily and avoid the frustration of digging through large accumulations of paper.

Make a listing of your file headings and keep it handy to facilitate use of your system. It will also dramatically improve the consistency of your filing. Another key is to file things immediately rather than letting them pile up.

Manage Your Mail

Managing your mail is analogous to effective triage. Junk mail should be considered "DOA" and thrown away without even looking at it. Many times you can identify junk mail because the mailing label will be labeled "CAR-RT-SORT." This designation indicates that the piece mail is part of a bulk mailing. Unless the item is something that might be helpful to you, such as a catalog, throw it away. It helps to realize that all of the junk mail that you receive is someone's effort to "sell you something." This is an effort to meet their goals. The more time you spend handling junk mail, the more time you take away from your goals and work on someone else's goals.

Another tool to use in your mail triage is to look at the return address. If it is not someone you recognize, you are probably safe in assuming that it is someone else trying to sell you something and you can throw this piece of mail away. Another tool for effectively managing your mail is to have someone else prescreen it and remove all of the junk mail.

Procrastinate Creatively

Creative procrastination can be a valuable management strategy. You may be confronted with responsibilities generated out of someone else's need to deal with a problem. Sometimes if you "creatively procrastinate," the need for this item disappears or the problem solves itself.

DELEGATING

An important lesson in learning to be a good leader is to learn to delegate effectively. Effective delegation can empower those who report to you and increase the amount of work completed. Without effective delegation, you can get caught

up in mundane activities that consume your time and prevent you from working on your goals.

The following are five barriers to effective delegation: (1) fear of something going wrong, (2) feeling that others never get it right, (3) not wanting to give up the activity, (4) fear of dumping on others, and (5) not knowing how.

Many times delegation is hard because of a fear that something will go array, and there will be negative consequences such as job or business failure. An example is the salesperson who is so possessive of clients he or she becomes ineffective at sales. These individuals become involved in the operation and delivery of the product to the client, and their sales drop off. The key to overcoming this barrier is effective communication. If you let the person to whom you are delegating the task know your concerns, you are giving them the tools to complete the job properly. Asking for feedback and keeping communication open go a long way toward ensuring a positive outcome.

The corollary to the first barrier is the feeling that, "no one ever gets it right." Many times it is true that you can complete a task better because you know exactly how you would like it done. More often, however, if given a chance, other people will be able to do just as good a job as you would and sometimes even better. Frequently, the result of failure to delegate becomes overwhelming. Once you are seriously overcommitted, your effectiveness drops and your stress levels rise.

An imperfect decision made now is always superior to a perfect decision that is put off indefinitely.

Even if others will not do a job as well as you might have, it may be better to have them attempt the project because at least it will get done rather than be put off indefinitely.

Sometimes failure to delegate occurs because of simple enjoyment of doing the task. In making a decision about which things to delegate, you have to compare the task that you enjoy and the time it takes with goals and plans. Once you have made a conscious decision to delegate, you need to take steps to strengthen commitment to that delegation. One powerful tool is to make a public announcement. Another, is to commit it to writing. Both of these steps have a powerful impact on your mental image of your relationship to that task. Another step that can be useful is to turn over your files or reference material on that project. If you feel yourself being pulled back into a project that you have delegated, you need to pull out your list of goals and read through them reminding yourself that you have made an important decision not to work on that project in favor of using time to reach your goals.

The fourth barrier frequently encountered is this perception that others may believe that you are "dumping on them." This type of interpersonal pressure can be powerful; however, the perception is usually internal and would not be borne out by communicating with the individual to whom you would like to delegate the project.

The way you approach an individual to delegate something can also dramatically affect perception. For example, "I have this project, which is very important to the department because it should lead to dramatically improved patient care. I think you would be the ideal person to take charge of it because of your expertise in this area. Would you be willing?" You can always ask, "how do you think we should proceed?" By asking the individual you are giving that person options, thereby empowering them. By asking for input, you are involving the person in finding solutions. This is a powerful approach. By involving the individual in the process, you are conveying respect.

The alternative is to simply hand something to the individual and say, "do this." This authoritarian approach is sometimes quicker, but it will leave the person feeling dumped on. There is no sense of empowerment. The individual may feel dictated to. You also lose the opportunity to communicate respect to the individual.

The last barrier to effective delegation is the lack of understanding how to delegate. The most important component is effective communication. If you want to delegate something to someone, the person needs to understand why it is important to do it. That person also needs to have input into the process.

A part of the art of delegating is knowing how to respond to the person who resists taking on the project. For instance, the person may say, "I'm not sure I can do that, I have too many other projects right now." You could respond by telling the person to do it anyway, but this is likely to be met by anger and resentment. Suzette Haydon Elgin, an expert in communications, recommends that the first thing to do is acknowledge the concern. For example, you can say, "Yes, you are right, you do have a lot of things to do." When you acknowledge concerns, the individual is much more likely to work with you to find an answer. You can then follow your acknowledgment with a question saying, "Given your busy schedule and the importance of this project to the department, how can we move forward with this project?" This type of approach may take a little more time initially, but it dramatically increases the likelihood that the individual will approach the task with enthusiasm. In addition, you will be strengthening your relationship with that person rather than weakening it. You should practice this empowerment strategy whenever possible. You will ultimately save a tremendous amount of time as you strengthen relationships. By effectively delegating the things you need to delegate, you will be building relationships to make them more effective and ultimately gaining more time to work on your primary goals.

LACK OF FOCUS

Lack of focus takes many forms. It may be the reason not to work on a major project. For example, you become distracted by the articles on your desk and end up reading them instead of working on a major project. In another example, you open a drawer to get something and end up straightening the entire drawer. Another manifestation of lack of focus is feeling you must organize everything in your briefcase before you can get started. Generally, with lack of focus, you spend a great deal of time on minor tasks, making inefficient use of your time.

The solution to this problem is to gently refocus yourself every time you feel the urge to stray from a task you have scheduled. Sometimes you will need reminders to help you with this process, such as an index card with your goals listed on it that you can keep in front of you as a visual cue. It is important to be gentle with yourself when you need to refocus. If you berate yourself for having let your mind wander

or for getting distracted with a different task, you are framing the project in a negative message. This actually undermines the importance of the project. It is better to frame this refocusing in a positive thought such as, "it is good that I am getting back to work on my goal." If you pat yourself on the back for refocusing, you underscore the importance of your goals and that particular project. You can then enjoy the benefit of working on that project rather than thinking of the negative self-image of your inability to stay focused.

SUMMARY

Time management is life management. You manage your time by going through a process of setting goals and priorities. You then attempt to raise all of your decisions about time use to a conscious level and use your goals and priorities in making those decisions. In this way, you are attempting to work on the things that are most important to you. This will enhance your sense of accomplishment and self-worth.

In essence you need to change how you see the use of your time and the decision-making process. You can use the time management tools outlined in this chapter to facilitate this process. The result is that you will become more effective and accomplish more of the things that are really important to you.

REFERENCES

1. Franklin B: *Poor Richard's Almanac,* June 1746. In Beck EM, editor: *Bartlett's familiar quotations,* Boston, 1980, Little Brown.
2. Deleted in proofs.
3. Johann Wolfgang van Goethe cited in Covey SR: First things first, New York, 1994, Simon & Schuster.
4. Tracey B: *How to Master your time,* Chicago, 1988, Nightingale Conant.
5. Deleted in proofs.
6. Lakein A: *How to get control of your time and your life,* New York, 1974, Penguin Press.
7. Stone WC: *Success through a positive mental attitude,* New York, 1987, Simon & Schuster.
8. McKay H: *How to swim with the sharks without being eaten alive,* New York, 1989, Ivy Books.

8 Customer Relations in the Emergency Department

Daniel P. Walsh, Laura R. Seff, and Thom A. Mayer

OUTLINE

Although healthcare administrators have applied customer service strategies in hospitals for many years, a review of the healthcare literature yields little information about customer service in the emergency department environment. In recent years there has been a growing interest in customer service in the emergency department, fueled by new emphasis on benchmarking critical healthcare performance indicators and increasing competitive pressures.[1] Although much of the enthusiasm for patient relations programs comes from nurse managers and the immediate administrative directors of emergency departments, physicians are also beginning to recognize the need to develop customer service strategies.

Despite these changes, many healthcare providers continue to feel uncomfortable about calling patients customers and resist adopting customer-oriented behaviors and practices. Reasons for this resistance include the following: (1) emergency medicine personnel often see themselves as harried, overworked humanitarians with barely enough time to practice the essentials of emergency medicine and little time for anything else; (2) physicians in the emergency department are highly educated medical professionals with training in the direct delivery of healthcare, not classic business principles; (3) because they deal with life and death on an ongoing basis, physicians often resist issues perceived to be either "too touchy-feely" or "bottom-line money issues" and therefore nonsubstantive; and (4) emergency medicine residency programs do not incorporate education about customer service concepts and strategies in their curricula.

Every emergency department should have a patient relations program in place. The principles explored in this chapter provide a framework for developing such a program.

THE EMERGENCY MEDICINE CUSTOMER

The Customer Concept

Although many healthcare providers continue to resist the concept of "customers" in the healthcare setting, adaptation of business customer service philosophies and strategies is necessary. The increasingly competitive nature of all aspects of healthcare delivery is well documented.[2,3] As competition supersedes the underlying humanitarian motivations and becomes the determining force in which hospitals and physician practices survive, a business focus emerges as more common and, perhaps, more understandable than the traditional means of viewing the physician-patient relationship. Such an approach is extraordinarily popular at the present time, but requires careful understanding to avoid substantial pitfalls in its implementation.

An examination of the origin of the humanitarian motivations for medical and nursing practice is essential. The origins of medical ethics date 2500 years ago to the Hippocratic ethic, which comprises a complex body of knowledge that can simply be classified as the Hippocratic Oath. This oath identified the moral precepts of medical practice, and the less well-known deontological books, which describe the "etiquette" of medical practice or what is expected of an educated gentleman with medical knowledge.[4] These lesser-known deontological works included aspects of reputation, comportment, cleanliness, truth-telling, to which the Stoics later added concepts of duty and compassion. The Hippocratic ethic thus indicated that the physician was required to act with courage, temperance, justice, and most of all phronesis, the practical wisdom required to discern the right or good thing to do in a particular situation.[5,6] The basic Hippocratic texts, the Stoic notions of duty and compassion, congruent elements from Judeo-Christian traditions, and general concepts of noblesse oblige all combined to form an opinion about physician conduct that culminated in the 1847 Code of the American Medical Association.

For more than a century, this traditional, humanitarian approach to the ethics of medicine and the elements of the physician-patient relationship remained virtually unchanged. However, the confluence of several factors resulted in radical changes in both medical ethics and the foundings of the physician-patient relationship. First, in the middle decades of this century the technology of medicine exploded at an unprecedented rate, resulting in both essential understandings of cellular mechanisms of disease and a vast array of technologic, diagnostic, and therapeutic interventions. As a re-

sult, medicine expanded at a faster rate than did its ability to interpret such changes for the patient and public. This expansion of technology and therapeutic interventions did not necessarily come at the expense of medical ethics and virtues, but it is widely felt that this was in fact the case, at least as perceived by patients and the general community. For some, technical correctness became the primary goal in medicine, and the guiding principle of technical correctness is competence, not compassion. This is in no way meant to indict the entire medical profession, as there were many dedicated and compassionate physicians practicing diligently throughout this time. However, as medicine's technical competence and invasiveness grew, so did the trend toward specialization and subspecialization, which in many respects resulted in the perception by patients that physiologic and biologic needs were being met to a far greater degree than were their personal, emotional, and psychologic needs.

A major casualty of this transition was the nearly inexorable confusion between the virtue of beneficence, a core value of medical ethics in the Hippocratic formulation, and paternalism. Paternalism holds that the physician knows better than the patient what is in the patient's best interest, at least in the medical/technical sense, and perhaps in its moral, psychologic, and emotional overtones as well. Paternalism also connotes that the physician, as proprietor of medical knowledge, dispenses medications, advice, surgical procedures, and other interventions essentially without the patient's interference. The model of the physician as paternalist also strongly implies that the physician is the active, aggressive element of the physician-patient relationship, whereas the patient accedes to a defined role as the passive recipient of such "care."[7]

In sharp contradistinction, beneficence, in both its Hippocratic and modern senses, differs substantially from paternalism. In a beneficent model, the physician acts in the patient's interests, but with careful consideration from the patient of his or her respective needs. Most important, the physician as beneficent provider seeks three things. First, the physician seeks what is medically good for the patient, which is a blend between physiologic function and emotional and psychologic balance. Second, the physician seeks what is defined as good by the patient, particularly with regard to the context of the patient's way of life, family, and religious and emotional beliefs. Third, the physician should seek what is good for humanity and the human community overall, as it relates to the specific treatment of the individual. Finally, the beneficent model indicates that the physician seeks what is good for both individual patients and humanity overall in a spiritual sense, while considering both the physician's and the patient's spiritual/religious beliefs.

The increased capacity for technologic advances (often at the unintended expense of the virtue of compassion) and the confusion of beneficence and paternalism combined through several decades in this century with the general upheaval of moral changes, increased awareness of medical and technical knowledge on the part of patients and society as a whole, an increased trend toward consumerism, erosion of respect for traditional sources of moral suasion and authority, and a decline in agreement of a sense of community-shared values. All of these factors resulted in fundamental changes in the way in which the physician-patient relationship was viewed.

One of the results of this change was the application of concepts of consumerism and autonomy into virtually all aspects of medical relationships, including both physician-patient and nurse-patient relationships. (Similar parallels can be made for the nurse-physician relationship.) In addition to concepts of consumerism and autonomy, medicine became subject to increasing application of legal, economic, and business principles, all of which culminated in a change in the physician-patient relationship from essentially a medical, personal, and, optimally, ethical and moral encounter to one that can be typified as a commodity, albeit an extraordinarily complex one.

In the new healthcare environment, patients are no longer the lucky and grateful recipients of benevolent, autocratic caregivers. Patients today are better informed about many aspects of quality of care, and they often have choices in selecting where they receive medical care and from whom. Many patients consider themselves partners with the healthcare provider and expect to be included in the evaluation and decision-making processes. Whatever we choose to call them, patients have become customers because they make informed choices. As the transition from a physician-patient relationship has changed to a physician-customer relationship, at least in many respects, it becomes extraordinarily important to be able to define what a customer is. *A customer is anyone who is affected by either our processes or our products.* This definition is the simplest and most classic one derived from the continuous quality improvement literature, and it has been used in many healthcare settings.[8,9] When viewed in this way, the concept of the *healthcare customer* assumes a different and somewhat liberating dimension, particularly as it relates to understanding how our *processes* affect others. (Figure 8-1). Thus not only is the patient and family a customer, but so too are the myriad others who are affected by our processes: the medical staff, admissions personnel, the operating suite, intensive care units, payors, emergency medical services (EMS), and the community in general.

Patients are not the only customers in the emergency department. All participants in the emergency care delivery system are customers because they affect or are affected by the emergency care delivery process. In addition to the patient and their family, other customers include EMS personnel, managed care companies, insurance companies, local businesses, schools, and police agencies (Box 8-1).

There are also internal customers. Internal customers are those individuals who are part of the care delivery process in the hospital. The desired outcome of emergency medical care might be stated as a satisfied customer who achieves the best possible medical outcome. However, no individual provider has complete control over the care delivery process, and therefore no individual provider can ensure the desired result. Each provider in the emergency department and ancillary hospital departments is dependent on the skills and cooperation of other staff to reach the ultimate goal. This interreliance makes all emergency care providers and the other hospital staff who participate in the care delivery process internal customers (Box 8-2).

The debate about what to call those who have been traditionally referred to as "patients" detracts from the main issue—the need to accommodate internal and external participants in the emergency care delivery process to achieve the best results. This goal should form the foundation of any cus-

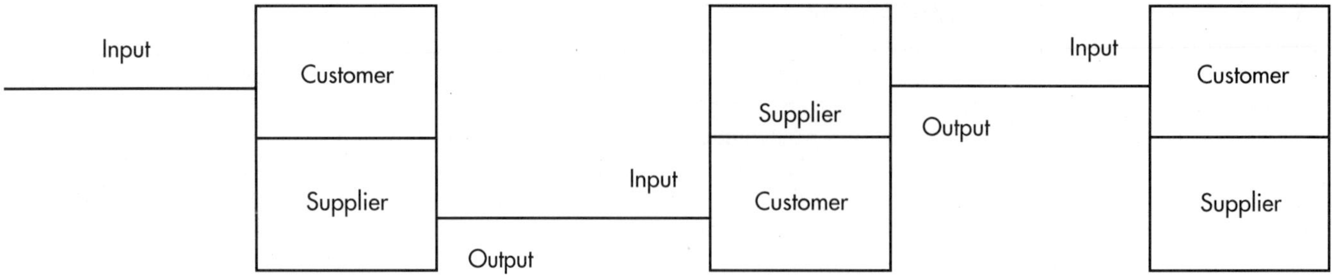

FIGURE 8-1 The Continuous Quality Improvement Supplier/Customer Continuum.

BOX 8-1

EXTERNAL CUSTOMERS

The Patient and family
EMT/Paramedics
Ambulance companies
HMOs and other directed care plans
Nursing homes
Occupational healthcare
Other referring hospitals
Funeral homes and the coroner
The media
Taxi cabs
Police
Schools
Athletic teams
Nursing and medical schools
Managed care programs gate keepers

BOX 8-2

INTERNAL CUSTOMERS

Fellow emergency department staff
Ancillary staff
Hospital administration
Hospital admitting staff physicians
Hospital admitting floor staff
Hospital volunteers
Chaplain service personnel
Nursing office and administration
Internal paramedic squads
Housekeeping
Dietary/nutritional services

tomer relations program. Further, the best way to understand customer needs is to survey them in an aggressive ongoing fashion because patient needs change over time.

How Customers Define Quality

It is important to understand what emergency department customers expect and recognize as acceptable service quality. Although patients may be sophisticated and highly educated in many fields, for the most part, they are not well educated in medicine. Because patients have limited ability to judge medical quality, their definition of quality is heavily based on other factors. Press, Gainey, and Associates[10] have performed patient satisfaction surveys in numerous emergency departments, collecting data on 28 areas of customer preference. Their results are included in Appendix A, but are summarized here.

"I was treated like a person." A person who discusses problems or has complaints of a private or personal nature, or a person who is extremely frightened about the possible outcome of an illness or injury expects to be dealt with on an individual basis. Individual attention and recognition put the patient at ease and lead the patient to believe that the physician is singularly concerned about his or her problem and looks at him or her as an individual.

"I got what I wanted." The patient and the patient's family have certain goals they wish to achieve during the emergency department visit. Sometimes these goals have little or nothing to do with the chief complaint. For example, a workers' compensation patient may present with a chief complaint of painful back secondary to a fall. The patient's goal in seeking emergency treatment may include narcotic medication on an ongoing basis or time off from work that has nothing to do with the healing process. It is important to acknowledge and discuss what patients and their families want, even if some or all of their goals cannot be met.

"I understood what was told to me." Almost universally, patients become intimidated when medical terminology is used, and they begin to nod in agreement even though they may not understand. However, if they do not understand the nature of their problem, how it was evaluated, why the recommended treatment was selected, and what to do with regard to follow-up care, there is a high likelihood they will feel at least some dissatisfaction.

"I was treated with respect." At the most basic level, patients want their privacy and dignity to be recognized and respected.

"I was kept informed." Patients want to mark the milestones of their progress in the emergency department. They do not mind waiting as much as they mind not knowing why they are waiting. The key is to keep people informed on a regular and frequent basis.

Patients also evaluate the quality of an emergency department based on small moments of truth throughout their visit. Was the patient greeted in a timely fashion by an individual who was friendly and concerned, who was identified by name tag, and who introduced him or herself? Was the treatment area clean and private? Was a concerned relative permitted to join the patient in the treatment area? Did the patient meet a physician who looked like a physician? Did the patient's visit run smoothly and in a reasonable time frame? These and

many similar aspects of the emergency department visit are totaled in a plus/minus fashion to form the patient's overall perception of quality.

Customer service is, in fact, one of the most understandable and easily gradable aspects of the patient's encounter. Customer service addresses those emotional and physical needs that are not necessarily part of the standard of care of emergency medicine, but are very important to the patient. Therefore customer service often equals quality care in the eyes of the patient.

How can we define *quality* as it relates to customer service? In traditional continuous quality improvement terms, quality exists to the extent that value is added to the encounter/service by the provider and/or the process. This concept of *value added* as the core definition of quality has the advantages of both utility and simplicity. The concept of value added is simple; anything that does not add value should be carefully examined with regard to its necessity for the process; value added is utilitarian in that it helps clarify the extent to which we in our processes do or do not meet the customer's needs.[11]

Further, when healthcare is conceived at least in part as a series of customer-supplier relationships in which value is added, it is also quite helpful in articulating that customer/patient satisfaction exists to the extent that the processes and providers are able to meet or exceed the customer's *prepurchase expectations.*[12] Next, to the extent that value is added and expectations are met and/or exceeded, quality and satisfaction exist; to the extent that they are not, dissatisfaction and disappointment result. For example, Inova Health System, a leader in healthcare quality improvement strategies, has defined quality as follows: "Quality consists of doing those things necessary to meet and exceed the needs and expectations of *those we serve* and doing those things right every time."

Although the specifics of the definition of customer service are important, equally important is that each institution carefully examines its own definition of customer service and how quality fits into that definition, as well as the specific elements of commitment behind it. For a customer service philosophy to be meaningful, managers and staff need to help coordinate as precisely as possible what is meant by terms such as quality, customers, patient satisfaction, and customer service.

BUILDING A CUSTOMER RELATIONS PROGRAM FOR THE EMERGENCY DEPARTMENT

Basic Elements of a Good Customer Relations Program

A successful customer relations program in the emergency department can result in increased patient satisfaction, a more positive experience for other external customers, and an improved work environment for internal customers. The foundation of such a program must be based on recognition of the inherent stresses and difficulties in the emergency department environment and a strong statement of values to which all staff can readily relate.

Although all aspects of healthcare delivery can be stressful and troublesome at times, the emergency department environment is particularly prone to difficulty. Virtually everyone who arrives as a patient begins the encounter from a negative perspective—they don't feel well, they don't want to be there, they're worried about the cost, they can't spare the time, etc. Even the most benevolent, kind-hearted care provider will be faced with hostile patients and family members. Customer relations programs for emergency departments must acknowledge this reality and incorporate strategies for coping with the environment.

Customer relations programs must be founded on values that are clearly stated and readily understood by the emergency department care providers. Furthermore, the values must reflect the patients' needs and concerns, as well as the needs and concerns of other external and internal customers. Without this foundation, staff will be unable to understand the appropriate focus or desired outcomes for their patient care activities.

Mission or value statements have been highly touted in recent years. Current literature recommends assembling all relevant staff and investing hours or even days in hammering out a written document identifying the entity's goals, mission, and values.[13,14] Another theory suggests that values must be stated from the top of the organization, with sufficient communication of those values to ensure staff understanding. In either of these scenarios, the behavior of the recognized leadership in practicing these values is critical to their recognition and acceptance by all staff. Chapter 5 details the process of generating and using mission statements.

Implementing a customer relations program should go beyond communicating the values. Emergency department staff must be educated in the principles of good customer relations and armed with the specific skills needed to convey a customer-oriented attitude in the stressful emergency department environment. Initiating effective training necessitates allocating appropriate resources including the financial resources needed to develop the program and materials and to hire a trainer, and the time for staff to participate in the educational activity. The recognized leaders of the emergency department (nurse manager, medical director) must participate in the training and demonstrate understanding and enthusiasm for the practice of good customer relations skills.

A single educational experience will not be sufficient to sustain positive behavior changes. Many emergency departments have gone down the path of initiating a substantial educational program, generating great enthusiasm and support, only to see the enthusiasm wane and the support fizzle from lack of remedial training and introduction of new techniques on an ongoing basis. Some people who have had this experience have erroneously concluded that customer relations training programs do not work. *To be successful, any training program must be designed to be ongoing with periodic introduction of new techniques, as well as planned activities, to remind staff about previously learned concepts and skills.* These activities may take the form of games or contests. Another effective approach is to incorporate reviews and introduction of new skills into monthly staff meetings. From time to time, it will be necessary to reassemble the staff for a more intensive program, again reviewing previously learned material, as well as introducing new concepts and skills. The combination of review and introduction of new ideas will sustain interest and enthusiasm for the customer relations program and will help staff maintain skill levels that will lead to posi-

tive outcomes (thus further reinforcing the desired behavior).

Another way to reinforce the desired behavior is to monitor and measure the results. Improved satisfaction for patients and staff is an obvious indicator of a successful patient relations program. Additional indicators include increased number of staff-generated improvement suggestions, fewer incidents of staff absence and tardiness, and a reduction in complaints from patients and other customers. Even process-oriented indicators such as turnaround times, patients leaving without being seen, and patients leaving against medical advice may improve. Indicators should be measured on a regular basis. Trended results should be widely reported among emergency department staff and other key emergency department customers. If results are not positive or are less significant than desired, it is important to identify what factors prevented attainment of expected results. The most dramatic improvements occur early on when there is the greatest opportunity and the greatest enthusiasm for the process. As time goes on, improvement tapers. If results flatten for a long time or begin to decline, a strategy must be developed for reenergizing the process, which may include some or all of the activities discussed previously.

Even when improvement programs are successful, leaders often overlook one of the most important opportunities to reinforce positive change. Accomplishments should be recognized and celebrated; perhaps by: (1) publishing notices in the hospital or local newspapers; (2) sending letters to administration, the hospital board of directors, and/or the medical staff touting individual and team accomplishments; (3) awarding prizes or trophies; (4) sending letters to individuals or groups who have performed well; and (5) organizing a special party or event.

Making the Care Delivery Process Customer-Friendly

Set the Tone When the Patient Checks In. In many respects the first encounter is the most critical in terms of forming a patient's opinion about the emergency department experience. Many emergency departments overlook the importance of training staff in the check-in area to be appropriately concerned, attentive, responsive, and informative. In fact, criteria for placing staff in this area should include a friendly personality, the ability to defuse anxiety, and a genuine sense of concern for people in distress. The check-in area should be easily identified. Protocols for the check-in staff should require that they explain to patients what to expect from the remainder of their visit, which should include triage, registration, evaluation by a physician or other appropriate clinical staff, testing as needed, treatment as needed, and either discharge or admission to the hospital. Patients' questions should be answered, or patients should be told to whom a question should best be directed.

Maximize Triage. At triage, patients are generally touched for the first time and have their first opportunity to explain the reason for their visit in detail. Triage is a second opportunity to help the patient relax by improving his or her understanding of what to expect from the rest of his or her emergency department visit. Good communication skills are extremely important. Triage must often be done swiftly and, fortunately, communication of concern, compassion, and professionalism is not a time-intensive activity.

Don't Lose Them at Registration. The process of registration is inherently distasteful because it involves dealing with information and money and in no way contributes to improving the patient's medical situation. It is extremely important not to ignore this process and the staff who administer it. In some emergency departments, the registration staff interview patients in the treatment rooms rather than requiring patients to sit in uncomfortable chairs in front of a desk and computer terminal. The availability of notebook and notepad computer formats makes this option feasible. Even if patients must pass through a registration area, every effort should be made to make this experience as brief, physically comfortable, private, and friendly as possible.

Keep Patients and Families Informed. In many emergency departments patients and family members sit for long periods of time without updates about the progress of their visit. It is important to have protocols that require physicians and other staff to see each patient at specified time intervals to assess any changes in his or her condition, ensure the patient's comfort, and answer any questions. At no time should a patient wait longer than 15 minutes without a visit from some member of the emergency department staff and a progress report. Some of these visits should be made by the physician and should offer patients an opportunity to ask new questions and obtain understandable information about their evaluation and treatment. Following this protocol will help overcome the common complaint, "I never saw the doctor."

Convey the Feeling That Time Spent with the Patient is Important. As part of patients' definition of quality care, healthcare providers are expected to spend sufficient time with patients to hear their concerns, answer their questions, and explain what they need to know. Physicians and other healthcare providers often feel there is not enough time to adequately meet these expectations. There are ways, however, to enhance the patient's perception about the duration and quality of physician encounters. First, it is important to express an awareness of the patient's time by acknowledging, explaining, and apologizing for any wait the patient experienced. Healthcare providers can also assure patients they are willing to take whatever time is needed to address all concerns and provide satisfactory care. Skilled communicators will be able to keep this promise without slowing the process. It is helpful to talk while examining the patient, particularly to explain what is being done and why. Whenever possible, spend a few moments sitting down. This often works well while taking the history. It is also important to touch the patient as frequently as appropriate. Premature movements toward the door before the patient is finished speaking should be avoided.

Address Nonmedical Needs. Attending to nonmedical needs can make a big difference in the patient's overall evaluation of the emergency department visit, particularly when a patient experiences a prolonged wait. Nonphysician care providers can offer patients and family members blankets, pillows, help to the bathroom, use of a telephone, and even a meal. When physicians have time it is helpful for them to assist with nonmedical patient needs as well. This conveys the message to all staff that these are not menial tasks, but rather an effective way to demonstrate caring behavior.

Be Proactive Versus Reactive. Proactivity is a powerful and necessary tool in a customer-oriented emergency department.

Proactivity arms staff with a positive sense that they can control what occurs in the emergency department. Reactive behavior stems from a feeling that the environment is not controllable. It is frequently accompanied by negative emotions such as anger, disappointment, and pessimism.

To establish a proactive emergency department, it is important to begin with an assessment of systems and processes that have predictably created problems for patients in the past. Likely cause(s) for the problems should be investigated. What aspect(s) of the system does not function correctly? Finally, systems and procedures should be modified to reflect needed improvements. In some cases problems may arise because a needed system does not exist. In that situation a system should be developed and monitored to ensure it accomplishes desired goals.

Use Patient Advocates. The most important patient advocates in the emergency department are the physicians, nurses, and other staff. At times, however, these individuals do not have sufficient time to provide the kind of support that patients and their families often require. Many emergency departments have begun to use staff or volunteers as designated patient advocates to serve as liaisons between patients and staff and who focus exclusively on identifying and meeting patient needs. Use of patient advocates does not absolve physicians, nurses, and other staff from the need to provide medical care from a patient-focused perspective. It does offer a safety net in a busy emergency department.

Include Customer Relations as Part of the Orientation/Expectations. One of the most often ignored problems with customer service programs or philosophies is that they are not clearly presented to the staff as expectations rather than optional programs that can be followed or not followed depending on the whims of the individual staff members. Customer service should be clearly identified in the orientation process and in the ongoing education of the physician, nursing, registration, and ancillary support staff. For those hospitals that use competency-based orientation, customer-relations should form an integral part of that process.

Customer-Friendly Communication Skills

Listening. Some people are intuitively able to listen well and others are not. People can improve their listening skills, however, with education and practice. Figure 8-2 depicts a self-test that will help assess a person's listening skills.

There are several barriers to effective listening. One is the environment. In a busy, fast-paced setting such as the emergency department, there are many distractions that make effective listening difficult. Speaker qualities such as irritating mannerisms or voice quality, or certain speech impediments may also create a barrier to effective listening and necessitate special concentration. The psychologist Carl Rodgers has stated that the greatest barrier to effective communication is our tendency to evaluate the speaker rather than the message.

Three types of listening are important in fully understanding a speaker's intent. The first is critical listening in which the listener attempts to determine the facts of a situation. This type of listening is most often practiced in the emergency department. A second type of listening is empathetic listening in which the listener tries to identify the underlying feelings as well as the factual content. This type of listening allows the listener the opportunity to understand and to offer appropriate comfort to the speaker. Finally, there is perceptive listening in which the listener seeks any hidden or unstated agenda or concern. Perceptive listening provides the listener with the greatest chance of fully satisfying the needs of the speaker.

Another important listening skill is active listening. In active listening the listener demonstrates both physical and verbal attention to the speaker by using attentive body postures and by effectively paraphrasing his or her understanding of the speaker's intended message. The key to active listening is accepting what the speaker says without deflecting or arguing with the message. This does not imply agreement but rather an implicit willingness to hear a message without evaluating it. Active listening combines both critical and empathetic listening. Active and perceptive listening are the keys to being an effective communicator and a customer-oriented listener.

Verbal Skills. Effective speaking is just as important as effective listening. One important verbal skill is use of free information in which recognition of cues provided by the speaker is acknowledged with direct language. For example, an elderly patient refusing admission to the hospital from the emergency department may mention a relative who is not present. The physician or nurse might use this free information by suggesting to the patient that the relative be contacted to assist the patient in making the decision. Use of free information makes the speaker aware that the listener is attentive to his or her needs and interests.

Another effective verbal skill is self-disclosure in which the listener uses the disclosure of certain personal facts about himself or herself to establish a feeling of commonality and intimacy with the speaker. Healthcare providers may use this technique to convey a personal experience with a similar medical situation to patients and their families. It is an effective way to support a medical decision when a patient is not comfortable. For example, a physician may tell the parent of a child with a head injury that she has a child of a similar age. The physician might go on to say that, considering the patient's present neurologic examination and normal activity, she would not order radiographs for her own child in the same situation.

In general it is important to use language carefully in the emergency department. Patients are sensitive to words that are too difficult or too simplistic. Patients may react to tone and pitch, as well as to the actual words used. The meaning of words can be dramatically changed depending on the inflection with which they are delivered. Speaking too quickly conveys a sense of being rushed or impatient and can often shut down effective two-way communication.

Body Language. Body language conveys much information about a person's thought processes and concerns. Eye contact, facial expression, hand positions and touching, arm positions, and stance signal positive, negative, or neutral feelings.

The signals from a patient's body language are important clues to his or her emotional state and may even assist the physician in arriving at a correct diagnosis. No one can mistake the message of a patient or family member standing half in and half out of the examination room, tapping a foot with arms folded, and looking intently at the nurses station. A patient's body language may telegraph distress intended to be

Instructions: Developing listening skills is an ongoing process. Discovering your attitude about listening is an important first step because attitudes determine your behaviors. Read each statement below. If a statement describes your listening attitude or behavior, mark yes; if not, mark no. Please be as candid and forthright with yourself as possible — the value of this assessment will depend on your sincerity in completing it honestly.

		YES	NO
1	I attempted to set aside my ego and focus on the speaker rather than on myself...		
2	I am not easily distracted...		
3	I value eye contact and maintain it most of the time...		
4	I wait for the speaker to finish before finally evaluating the message...		
5	I understand my biases and control them when I am listening...		
6	I listen for the speaker's emotional meaning, as well as subject matter content...		
7	I am a patient listener most of the time...		
8	I am interested in many subjects and do not tune out dry-sounding information...		
9	I refrain from constantly interrupting...		
10	I respond appropriately with a smile, a nod, or a word, as a speaker is talking...		
11	I listen carefully for a speaker's main ideas and supporting points...		
12	I ask questions for clarification...		
13	I am careful to judge the message rather than the speaker...		
14	I am aware of personal mannerisms that may distract a speaker...		
15	I restate or paraphrase what a speaker says to make sure I understand...		
16	I concentrate carefully and do not fake attention...		
17	I do not finish other people's sentences unless asked to do so...		
18	I take notes during meetings to record key points...		
19	When listening on the telephone, one hand is kept free to take notes...		
20	I keep my emotions under control...		

FIGURE 8-2 Listening attitude.

hidden. For example, a patient may be uncomfortable about a family member or friend who is in the room and thus may be reluctant to disclose all the necessary information about the medical situation. A patient's body language may also demonstrate impatience, frustration, or lack of understanding with the medical evaluation and care process. Emergency department care providers should be attentive to the patient's body language and, when tension or anger is detected, try to elicit the patient's concerns.

Emergency department care providers also need to be aware of the messages they send with their own body language. Customer relations training often incorporates an opportunity for trainees to be videotaped and to observe their own body language habits. This can be a powerful way to increase self-awareness about body language.

Box 8-3 shows the mnemonic GUEST, which can be used to remind emergency department staff about important aspects of listening, verbal, and body language skills.

Handling Patient Complaints

Most complaints are opportunities for improvement. Customers who give negative feedback about the quality of service provide a chance to solve problems. If the complaint comes while the patient is still in the emergency department, the physician or department manager should take the initiative to respond to the concern(s) quickly. If the complaint cannot be addressed during the patient's emergency department visit, the patient and/or family should be informed that the problem will be addressed, by whom, and within what time frame. It is helpful for the physician or manager to offer a business

BOX 8-3

VERBAL LISTENING AND BODY LANGUAGE SKILLS

G **GREET** the patient in a friendly manner.
U **USE** the patient's name. Make eye contact.
E Let the patient now what to **EXPECT.**
S Use active listening **SKILLS.**
T Close the interaction with instructions and a handshake **(TOUCH).**

BOX 8-4

POINT OF IMPACT INTERVENTION

1. Identify the problem and address it immediately.
2. Establish that you understand something has broken down in the communication process.
3. To the extent possible, wipe the slate clean.
4. Try to find out their expectations as precisely and in as much detail as possible.
5. Demonstrate that you are willing to negotiate and work with them to resolve issues.
6. To whatever extent possible, attempt to meet their expectations.
7. To the extent that you are not able to meet their expectations, offer reasonable alternatives.
8. When all efforts at Point of Impact Intervention have failed, always offer them the alternative of speaking to someone else in the emergency department or administrative chain-of-command to address their problems.

Courtesy Emergency Physicians of Northern Virginia, Ltd.

card or to write his or her name and contact phone number down so the patient will be able to follow up with any additional concerns or questions, or if the patient does not hear back with regard to the complaint. Use of the blameless apology as described previously, is often an effective way to take the sting out of patient concerns.

Sometimes patients' or family members' complaints escalate to a point where the patient and/or family member becomes agitated. When this occurs it is important for the healthcare provider to determine the cause of the distress quickly and to be proactive about calming down the situation. The care provider must become completely focused on the patient's concern. A patient or family member in an open area should be moved to a more isolated and private area as quickly as possible. This change will signal that the problem is being handled seriously while providing the physician or other care provider with the opportunity to take control of the situation. Changing the environment also has a calming effect on the person who is upset.

Clearly the focus of attention should remain on the patient. If family members are behaving inappropriately and reasonable intervention efforts do not calm them down, they should be asked to leave the treatment area, and in some cases, the hospital premises. Hospital security may need to assist with this process.

Once isolated, the patient must receive attention. He or she should not be moved and then left alone, even briefly. If the patient is already in a private area, the intervention process should be started immediately. The situation should be assessed to determine whether there is any imminent physical threat to healthcare providers, other patients, or the patient in question. Backup should be requested as needed. All the skills discussed earlier in this chapter should be used to determine the real problem. It is important to find out whether the patient is upset with something specific in the current emergency department visit or whether the patient is acting out a nonrelated frustration.

When the problem has been carefully assessed, the patient's options should be explained. The patient should be allowed to choose one or more options. This approach enables the patient to gain self-control and control of the situation. If the patient requires assistance in making the decision, resources available in the emergency department can be used. If the patient consents, family members can be asked to join the patient in the treatment room, or can be contacted by phone. Sometimes it is helpful to involve social services and/or clergy.

As the crisis winds down, it is important to summarize what has occurred and to make specific plans about how things should move forward. Proper follow-up should be arranged and the plan should be written, both for the patient's convenience and for documentation in the patient's record.

Patients who are intoxicated (alcohol or drugs), who have psychiatric disorders, or who have hostile or aggressive personality disorders are unlikely to respond to these techniques. Although it is important to handle these patients with kindness and compassion, it is also important to act quickly and decisively when their behavior escalates inappropriately. Every emergency department should have well-established and well-practiced protocols for dealing with this type of situation.

Point of Impact Intervention

At the Department of Emergency Medicine at Fairfax Hospital, a protocol called Point of Impact Intervention has been developed that uses these and other techniques (Box 8-4). Point of Impact Intervention reflects what most emergency departments have recognized: In the vast majority of patient complaints, the provider knew at the time of service that something was either "wrong" or, at least, distinctly different or unusual about the interaction with the patient and/or family. For most emergency departments, it is unusual to receive complaints from patients or families that involve situations in which the provider was completely unaware that a problem existed during the original interaction. The exception to this almost always relates to emergency department bills. Point of Impact Intervention reflects the policy that the provider should take immediate steps to help diffuse the situation and put the clinical encounter back on track, to the best extent possible. This goal applies whether the concern is with the emergency physician or with any other aspect of the emergency department experience. Because the emergency physician is the "Captain of the Ship," at least in the patient's and family's eyes, he or she should take the lead in helping to resolve concerns at the time that they occur, whether or not they have anything to do with the emergency physician. Simi-

larly, the emergency department nurse spends more time with the patient than any other healthcare provider in the system, so they should also be aware of the following concepts of Point of Impact Intervention:

1. *Identify the problem and address it immediately.* When problems occur, clarify questions and areas of difficulty with the patient or family. Give neutral responses as you establish clarity about the specifics of concerns and/or complaint. Don't interrupt; listen actively and empathetically. Acknowledge patient/family feelings, particularly feelings of anger, hostility, betrayal, etc. Remember that *acknowledging* the feelings does not imply that you either validate or accept responsibility, merely that you recognize the depth of the feelings and that you communicate this to them. Whenever possible, restate their concerns as you understand them, so that it can be clear where their concerns lie.
2. *Establish that you understand something has broken down in the communication process.* Use language such as, "I am not sure how we have gotten off track here, but I would like to address your concerns." Other helpful language includes the following: "I understand that you have some problems with what has happened here so far. I am sorry that happened, but I want to make sure that we can take care of you in the best way we can." It is difficult to overstate the value of two words at this stage in the conversation—*I'm sorry.* Even at times when it is unclear that there have actually been any genuine mistakes made by the emergency department staff or the processes involved, these two words can do a great deal to reestablish the communication necessary for ongoing care of the patient.
3. *To the extent possible, wipe the slate clean.* Although it is always better to start with a tabla rasa, that is not always possible. Certainly by starting the conversation with a clear understanding that you are sorry that this has occurred, you can begin to reestablish communication where it has broken down. The conversation should be polite but empathetic, stressing that you want to address the situation, but you also want to move the patient through the system unencumbered by whatever "baggage" has already been created. In some cases, this may mean that it is necessary to offer that a different staff member take care of the patient. For example, if a patient and family have had difficulty relating to a specific emergency department nurse, it is sometimes easier simply to offer transferred care to another nurse. Similarly, when double coverage is offered, it should be extended to certain patients who have problems with the emergency physician who began their care.
4. *Try to find out expectations as precisely and as detailed, as possible.* It is extraordinarily helpful to ask direct questions such as, "What are your expectations in this matter?" or "How could we have handled this differently?" In stating their expectations, the patient and family will realize that, in some cases, their expectations are unreasonable. In other cases, their expectations may be simply far different from what we have assumed them to be, particularly in regard to issues of being kept informed, being treated with courtesy, or having things explained in a timely fashion. For example, in a patient with chest pain, if the original electrocardiogram and history do not suggest a myocardial origin, explaining to the patient that the pain doesn't appear to be cardiac and that some other studies are necessary, rather than waiting until all studies are done before indicating the diagnostic possibilities, can help alleviate anxiety and concern.
5. *Demonstrate that you are willing to negotiate and work with them to resolve issues.* Often in cases of medication choices or diagnostic workup, the patient wants to have a voice and a choice. Offering patients with extremity trauma the option of pain medication early in the course of their care shows not only appropriate medical therapy but compassion for their pain. As Dr. Eugene Stead once said, "The physician who chooses not to listen to his patient does so at both his own risk and that of the patient."[15] Clear explanations of what will be done, why it will be done, and how long it is likely to take usually help ensure that the patient and family are satisfied with their experience.
6. *To whatever extent possible, attempt to meet their expectations.* The concept of previews in which the emergency physician tells the patient what he or she expects the results of the laboratory and radiographic findings to be, so that discharge planning can begin, even after the initial clinical encounter, can be quite helpful. For example, if a patient has costochondritis but radiograph is indicated to ensure there is no pulmonary pathologic conditions, explaining the likely etiology and that if the chest radiograph is negative the patient will be placed on antiinflammatory agents and a pain medication may help clarify issues before discharge. These issues may be as simple as an allergy to codeine that was not revealed by the triage nurse or that the patient prefers not to have any pain medication at all, which is somewhat less likely. Similarly, in a patient with back pain who is expected to have a negative radiograph but who will require bed rest, muscle relaxants, and antiinflammatory agents, telling the patient about this treatment before the radiograph is performed may help the patient discuss potential obstacles to such therapy with family, friends, or employer.

   When patients are asked to explain their expectations, not only are they often quite different from what we assumed, but they sometimes change in the course of the actual process of articulation. It is not uncommon for patients and/or families to realize the unreasonableness of their expectation if they are actually asked to articulate them. On the other hand, clinicians are often surprised by the simplicity and the ease in meeting certain patient requests. For example, some patients simply prefer to have an intramuscular injection of antibiotics because they know they are either too busy or too forgetful to complete the medication. Similarly, many parents prefer to discuss with the physician the antibiotic choices for a child with an acute infectious process such as otitis media.
7. *To the extent that you are not able to meet their expectations, offer reasonable alternatives.* There are times when patients have expectations that we cannot meet. If the patient wants 100 powerful narcotic pills, offer them a choice of other medications you are comfortable prescribing. If the patient is unwilling to discuss alternatives, it is unlikely the issue can be resolved, but at least you will be aware of the limitations. The patient, family, and oth-

ers who may observe the encounter in the emergency department will know that you are attempting to meet their expectations. One of the most difficult situations occurs when the patient and family want to be admitted to the hospital, but the clinical findings are not consistent with this request. The simplest way to handle this problem is to have the attending physician or the physician on-call for that specialty speak directly with the family. When disagreements cannot be resolved, be direct, clear, but unemotional in your language, such as "I'm sorry we disagree on this, but these are the alternatives that we have for treating you at this time. . ." At the end of the patient encounter, try to summarize for the patient and family what has occurred. If you will be referring areas for follow-up, explain how that will occur. Always try to refer patients to the emergency department if their symptoms do not improve in a specified time frame and if they are unable to contact their private or referral physician. If they have concerns about ancillary services such as registration, radiology, or laboratory, explain who you will be referring the problem to, in what time frame they could expect a response, and so on.

8. *When all efforts at Point of Impact Intervention have failed, always offer them the alternative of speaking to someone else in the emergency department or administrative chain-of-command to address their problems.* There are certainly some patients and/or families who "can't be pleased." If resolution cannot be reached even after all of the preceding points have been attempted, after it is still incumbent on the professional to offer follow-up in a different venue. For example, if the complaint is about the emergency department chair, offering the patient the chance to follow-up with either administration, the vice-chair of the department, or a representative from the medical staff helps assure that you are trying to be responsive to their needs and are happy to discuss what concerns they have with an independent, "outside" representative of the hospital.

Understanding and Overcoming Resistance

Healthcare providers hold several misconceptions that fuel their resistance to the concept of customers versus patients and the need to apply customer service strategies with emergency department patients. The ability to discredit the following arguments is essential to the successful implementation of a customer relations program.

"The customer is always right; therefore, if I disagree with a customer, I must be wrong." The customer is always right in the emergency department to the extent that the care provided should reflect the patient's concerns. Clearly, the patient's concerns do not always accurately reflect the real medical situation, and the physician who disagrees with a patient is not necessarily "wrong." However, addressing the medical situation while ignoring patient concerns generally does not lead to an acceptable outcome *in the patient's eyes.* Physicians and other healthcare providers in the emergency department must become skilled at assessing what is required to satisfy each patient's perceived needs while educating patients to modify unrealistic expectations for "satisfactory" care.

"Medicine is not business." In fact, healthcare is the largest business in the United States other than the federal government.

"I am a humanitarian. I don't want to be a used car salesman." The basic fallacy with this statement is the underlying assumption that being a humanitarian is somehow in direct opposition to being a salesman. Salesmanship is nothing more than the ability to negotiate successfully certain aspects of an encounter so that another individual understands and accepts your point of view. To provide medical care that meets patients' needs and expectation, healthcare workers must win patients' confidence and trust. Convincing a patient that a suggested method of therapy or diagnostic procedure will lead to the best outcome is a "sales" challenge. Healthcare providers must have good salesmanship skills to deliver the humanitarian services they are educated to provide.

"This isn't a restaurant and it certainly isn't McDonald's!" Emergency healthcare providers find analogies to fast food restaurants distasteful. Clearly the speed and impersonal aspects of a fast food operation are not analogous. However, fast food restaurants are also associated with consistent quality of service and product, and in this respect it may be useful to draw ideas from this highly successful service industry. One can compare the standard of quality of the food product to the standard of emergency medical care. However, expectations extend beyond product (or medical care) quality. Customers grade a restaurant on its ability to satisfy their emotional and physical needs, as well as on the quality of the food provided. Likewise in the emergency department, patients have certain emotional and physical needs that are not part of the standard of care for emergency medicine, but that significantly affect their sense of satisfaction with the care they receive.

"Some people are never satisfied and they don't deserve any extra consideration." Although the first part of this statement is undoubtedly true, the second half is self-defeating. Healthcare providers should understand that customer service does not necessitate accepting abuse from patients as a matter of course. It is reasonable to expect patients to adhere to reasonable standards of behavior if they are physically and emotionally capable. Nevertheless, everyone deserves consideration, including both the emergency department staff and even the most difficult emergency department patient. The best outcomes occur when staff are able to take the high road with difficult patients and use their communication skills and compassion to convey a consistent message of caring and concern.

"I'm too old to change my attitude." Everyone has certain "hot buttons" that trigger an immediate opinion about patients. These personal beliefs, which often strengthen with age, however, should not affect the delivery of appropriate patient care. Furthermore, the practice of customer service in no way indicates that one must change personal attitudes or beliefs, only that an individual must modify personal behavior to give each patient a feeling of genuine concern, as well as appropriate medical care.

"I'm tired of apologizing for things that are out of my control." The inference here is that apology is associated with blame. The practice of blameless apology, however, allows healthcare providers to show appropriate concern for a patient's complaint without accepting responsibility for causing the problem. Many times patients simply want to know

that someone is concerned about their complaints. When a physician, nurse, or other healthcare staff member demonstrates appropriate recognition of the concern and expresses regret for the patient's discomfort or inconvenience, the patient's hostility is usually diffused almost immediately.

"I am too busy with serious aspects of patient care to take time to practice customer service." It takes no extra time to shake hands with a patient and family members and express concern for the patient's problem. This behavior is easily integrated into the routine assessment process that is part of any emergency department patient visit. Techniques like active and attentive listening, sitting down while taking the history, and making sure to have hands-on contact with the patient also do not take extra time and convey the healthcare provider's interest in the patient's medical situation to patients and family members. After the physical examination, it takes only a few seconds before leaving the patient's bedside to explain what the patient can expect for the rest of the stay in the emergency department and approximately how long each step will take. A few invested moments at the beginning can save much time later by avoiding the need to deal with a frustrated patient or family member.

"We tried the "Customer Service" approach and we still got patient complaints." One of the misconceptions about the use of customer service strategies and having a customer-oriented attitude toward emergency medicine is that complaints will be eliminated. There will always be complaints and there will always be complainers. Complaints are volume and acuity dependent and occur at a normal frequency of approximately 3 to 5/1000 visits a year. No program should be developed and implemented for the purpose of eliminating complaints. The continuous quality improvement (CQI) approach for handling complaints, which centers on eliminating complaints that occur beyond the frequency of normal variability, is a more realistic and useful conceptualization. The real value of customer relations lies in the opportunity to minimize the number of dissatisfied patients. Studies have shown that 96% of customers who are dissatisfied with service do not actually complain. If there is a choice, these patients are likely to present to another healthcare facility when they need future emergency or in-patient care. More important, research indicates that patients who are dissatisfied with an outcome generally tell 20 other people about the perceived bad experience.

Motivating for Customer Relations

Although it could be argued that using a customer-focused approach to patients in the emergency department is simply practicing good medicine, some hospitals may choose to create incentives to motivate adoption of a customer relations program. Incentives may vary with different types of staff. For example, physicians may be motivated differently from registration staff.

When developing an incentive strategy, it is important to ensure that incentives will lead to desired outcomes. One of the most common mistakes with motivation plans is to intend to reward one outcome while structuring incentives that actually reward another. Techniques for avoiding this pitfall include involving the individuals targeted by the incentive. Incentive plans should be piloted and monitored carefully to ensure effectiveness.

Overall, external incentives for customer relations programs are of questionable value. The most effective strategy for gaining acceptance is to use patient satisfaction and complaint data to convince staff that a problem exists. Once staff believe there is a problem, they must be involved in developing solutions. A customer relations program is a natural outgrowth of this process. Recognition of successes, particularly those that result from group efforts, is perhaps the most effective way to reinforce good customer relations skills.

THE "IN-HOUSE VERSUS CONSULTANT" QUESTION

Once the decision has been made to implement an emergency department patient relations program, department and hospital administration must determine whether to develop the program in-house or to hire a consultant with skills and expertise in customer relations program development and implementation.

If the hospital has sufficient staff in the community relations and training departments, creating the customer relations program in-house is a viable option. One advantage of this scenario is the opportunity to include representatives of all of the emergency department units in planning and implementing the program. This maximizes the likelihood that the staff will be committed to the success of the program. Another advantage is the proximity of training staff who can ensure that training opportunities are ongoing, which is critical to the success of any customer relations program. In some cases, a hospital-wide program may be adapted for the emergency department. Obviously, one of greatest advantages of using in-house resources is the relatively low cost.

External consultants also offer advantages. Developing a comprehensive customer relations program is extremely time intensive. Many hospitals do not have the internal staff to devote to such a time consuming activity. External consultants also bring a certain expertise that may be more readily recognized by emergency department staff than the expertise of hospital employees. Consultants are able to stand back from a situation and objectively analyze what is needed. Finally, consultants are not invested in the politics of the hospital and therefore are in a position to offer advice and pinpoint problems that internal staff may be reluctant to address.

Whether a program is developed in-house or with a consultant, it will be important to establish a team of emergency department staff to participate in program development and implementation.

SUMMARY

The most important aspects of successful customer relations in the emergency department are commitment and leadership from the top. Everyone who works in the emergency department watches those in control to determine the appropriate customer service attitude. If physicians or charge nurses treat patients with a non-service-oriented attitude, other staff in the emergency department will treat patients accordingly. If the attitude from the chair of the department and nurse manager is one of customer service and compassion, the rest of the staff will act accordingly.

The next most important aspect of being successful in cus-

tomer relations is to have a proactive approach. There are no new problems or complaints in emergency medicine. Most individuals who are experienced in emergency medicine recognize that the same process problems recur. Proactivity offers a way out of that cycle.

Active and perceptive listening are also important aspects of customer service because they define the customer's perception of quality. These listening skills also give the healthcare provider clues to successfully resolve a complaint that may occur within the department. It is extremely important to understand that the customer's perception is his or her reality. Until that perception is changed, that reality will continue to exist.

The practice of customer service skills in the emergency department will help accomplish many goals of the emergency department manager. This approach will dramatically reduce stress within the department by minimizing the hostility and reactivity often associated with uncomfortable situations. When staff deal with each other as internal customers in a CQI format, not only will stress be reduced between departments, but morale will improve within the department and the hospital in general. The diligent practice of customer service will improve risk management because friends do not sue friends. The reputation of the emergency department as a customer-oriented facility will be enhanced. By providing staff with the skills to deal with the angry customer, overall complaints and liability will be reduced.

The practice of customer relations is a learned skill. Although some individuals are more intuitive and have a greater ability to adapt to the practice of customer relations, everyone can benefit from training in its techniques. To be successful, customer service training must be ongoing. An initial seminar may set the ground work and equalize techniques and skills among staff. This training and attitude, however, must be reinforced periodically.

An analogy can be drawn from early training in medical school. Every young clinical physician was told at one time to do for the patient what the physician would do or would have done for his or her own family member. The emergency department staff should be encouraged to do the same. With internal customers in ancillary services or with the patients and their families, staff should be as kind, respectful, and compassionate as they would be with their own family member. In this way, an excellent standard of customer service will always be maintained.

ACKNOWLEDGMENTS

The section on Physician-Patient Relationships is due almost exclusively to insights gained from the work of Edmund D. Pellegrino, MD, our nation's finest medical ethicist, whose influence is greatly appreciated.

REFERENCES

1. Mayer TA: Industrial models of continuous quality improvement: implications for emergency medicine, *Emerg Clin North Am* 10:523-547, 1992.
2. Montague J: The state of emergency, *Hosp Health Netw* 6:54-58, 1994.
3. Nelson EC, Wasson JH: Using patient-based information to rapidly redesign care, *Healthc Forum J* 6:25-29, 1994.
4. Hippocrates: *Hippocrates (I & II),* (Joans Whl-trans). Lobe Classical Library, Cambridge, Mass, 1981, Harvard University Press.
5. Aristotle: *Nicomachean Ethics,* 1106, A 22-24.
6. Pellegrino ED, Thomasma DC: *For the patient's good: the restoration of beneficence in healthcare,* New York, 1989, Oxford University Press.
7. Beauchamp TL, McCullough LP: *Medical ethics: the moral responsibilities of physicians,* Englewood Cliffs, NJ, 1984, Prentice Hall.
8. Pellegrino ED, Thomasma DC: *The virtues in medical practice,* New York, 1993, Oxford University Press.
9. Juran JM: *Juran on leadership for quality: an executive handbook,* New York, 1989, Free Press.
10. Press, Gainey, and Associates: *The Press Gainey emergency department report,* South Bend, Ind, 1992, Press, Gainey, and Associates.
11. Juran JM: *Juran on planning for quality,* New York, 1988, Free Press.
12. McMillian JR, Younger MS, Dewine LC: Satisfaction with hospital emergency departments as a function of patient triage, *Health Care Manage Rev* 11:21-27, 1986.
13. Bellow PJ, Morrisey GL, Acomb BL: *The executive guide to strategic planning,* San Francisco, 1987, Jossey-Bass.
14. Duncan WJ, Ginter PM, Swayne LE: *Strategic management of healthcare organizations,* Boston, 1992, Kent.
15. Wagner GS, Cebe B, Rozear MP, Stead EA Jr: *What this patient needs is a doctor,* Durham, NC, 1981, Duke University Press.

APPENDIX

A Emergency Department Patient Satisfaction

The Press, Ganey survey assesses emergency department attributes in 28 different areas. Analysis of thousands of patients indicate that 10 specific areas form the basis of emergency department patient satisfaction.

Press, Ganey Survey—Emergency Department Attributes

1. Waiting time to get to treatment area
2. Helpfulness of registration
3. Waiting time to see doctor
4. Doctor informative about homecare
5. Doctor informative about treatments
6. Comfort of waiting room
7. Privacy during registration
8. Staff cared about you as a person
9. Kept informed about delays
10. Medical care worth the money charged
11. Nurses informative about treatments
12. Let family/friends be with patient
13. Doctor took problem seriously
14. Courtesy of doctor
15. Courtesy of x-ray technician
16. Waiting time in x-ray
17. Courtesy of blood technician
18. Doctors concern for privacy
19. Skill in taking blood
20. Convenience of parking
21. Adequacy of information provided to family and friends
22. Nurses attention shown to you
23. Courtesy shown to family/friends
24. Nurses took problem seriously
25. Courtesy of nurses
26. Nurses concern for privacy
27. Technical skill of nurses
28. Waiting time to see doctor

Courtesy Press, Ganey Survey.

Factors Affecting Patient Satisfaction

1. Staff cared about you as a person
2. Kept informed about delays
3. Medical care worth the dollar
4. Nurses informed about treatments
5. Information to family/friends
6. Nurses' attention shown to you
7. Courtesy to family/friends
8. Nurses took the problem seriously
9. Courtesy of nurses
10. Concern for privacy

9 Managing Professionals in Organizations:

THE ROLE OF PHYSICIAN-MANAGERS

Thom A. Mayer

OUTLINE

The transition from physician to manager
Competencies for physician-leaders and managers

American medicine is in the midst of cataclysmic change. During the last decade, the development of integrated healthcare delivery systems has demanded an increased degree of cooperation among physicians, hospitals, and other healthcare organizations. One of the most significant transitions has been in the development of the role of physician-managers. Is the management of physicians different, and if so, why? A large body of knowledge indicates that there are significant differences between the management of physicians and other professionals. Not the least among these differences is the fact that physicians have received substantial education and clinical training, but in most cases have had little in the way of formal management training. The advent of combined MD/MBA programs, as well as the more widespread use of executive MBA programs, has changed the nature of physician competence in management. However, the majority of physician executives do not have advanced degrees in management.[1]

At the same time, physicians in leadership and management roles have a rich heritage in medicine, primarily in academic healthcare institutions, large hospital corporations, and physician practices such as the Cleveland, Mayo, Oschner, and Lahey clinics. However, the rate of acceleration of change in the healthcare industry, heralded by the development of widespread integrated healthcare delivery systems, physician-hospital organizations, and the advent of managed care, have all helped focus on the interdependency between physicians and hospitals, all of which requires a higher level of involvement of physician leaders and managers. Successful healthcare organizations share certain common characteristics, one of which is the capacity for physician and nonphysician management to work cooperatively, not competitively, in devising strategies, systems, processes, and structures that will allow effective delivery of quality healthcare in a fashion that addresses the needs of the clinical and nonclinical providers of that care, as well as the beneficiary of that care, the patient.

Unfortunately, inherent biases and the existing structures of many healthcare organizations have not positioned them for these changes. As Lord[2] noted, the strong history of relationships between medical staffs and their hospitals and administration reflect:

- *Separation* from administration (partially to preserve physician autonomy).
- *Representation* of physicians' interest as opposed to the organization's interest.
- *Focus* on quality of medical care (to the exclusion of nonmedical aspects of care and costs).
- *Assistance* in meeting accreditation requirements, often in a reluctant or grudging fashion.
- *Voluntarism* with brief leadership tenures and a "revolving door" aspect of physician leadership and management.

In contradistinction to this approach, new roles for physician-leaders and executives require new skills such as team building, collaborative decision making, strategic planning, and negotiation skills. Whereas physicians have been trained as individual decision makers, physician-managers are increasingly participating in multidisciplinary teams, in which collective skills are emphasized over individual skills. Detmer[3] makes the distinction between the "physician-manager," which he defines as a full-time executive without clinical responsibilities, and the "clinical executive," who acts in both administrative and clinical roles. Although such distinctions may have some meaning at the hospital or integrated healthcare system level, in most emergency departments the physician-manager is both a clinician and a manager. In fact, practical experience indicates that many of the most successful physician-managers and certainly the vast majority of emergency department chair obtain a substantial amount of their leadership *credibility* through their skills as clinicians. For that reason, only in unusual circumstances will physician-managers in the emergency department be totally immune from clinical duties and responsibilities. Nonetheless, in certain large organizations and in multihospital group settings, it may be necessary to have physicians in leadership roles without clinical responsibilities.[4]

Kurtz used behavior-oriented assessments to help delineate the differences between clinicians and managers.[7] These differences are listed in Box 9-1. In their clinical role, physicians have been trained as *doers,* inasmuch as they prefer hands-on involvement in patient care. However, in making the transition to a physician-manager, physicians must become planners or designers of clinical services and the manner in which those services interface with the healthcare organization. By nature of their training and philosophy, clinicians are used to one-on-one interactions and have based their decisions largely on their success in such interactions. However, management roles require interactions with multiple providers, often in diverse settings. Kurtz found that clinicians tended to be more detached, independent, and self-sufficient and were not "joiners" to the extent that managers are required to be.

BOX 9-1

MAJOR DIFFERENCES BETWEEN CLINICIANS AND MANAGERS

Clinicians	Managers
Doers	Planners, designers
One-on-one interactions	One to many interactions
Reactive personalities	Proactive personalities
Require immediate gratification	Accept delayed gratification
Deciders	Delegators
Value autonomy	Valued collaboration
Independent	Participative
Patient advocate	Organization advocate
Identify with profession	Identify with organization

Adapted from Kurtz ME: The dual role dilemma. In Curry W, editor: *The physician executive,* Tampa, Fla, 1988, American College of Physician Executives.

Provision of clinical services is reactive, inasmuch as the clinician waits for the patient and/or family to request medical care, as opposed to the proactive, anticipatory nature of management, in which initiation of change is required. One of the most impressive differences between clinicians and managers is that clinicians (particularly emergency physicians) require immediate gratification for satisfaction of their philosophic and personal needs, whereas managers must accept delayed gratification because the manifestations of their actions often take weeks, months, or sometimes years to fully develop. The clinical strategy in caring for a patient with heart failure or an arrhythmia is immediate; the strategy of pursuing practice diversification in occupational medicine is substantially delayed.

One reason that physicians are drawn to the practice of medicine is its sense of autonomy, inasmuch as the physician is the primary person responsible for deciding the principal courses of action in a patient's diagnostic workup and therapy. This role is in sharp contradistinction to the management role, in which delegation is a necessity. Leaders and managers often manage the process of problem solving and decision making, as opposed to making specific, isolated decisions themselves. This change from a paradigm of valuing autonomy to valuing collaboration is often difficult for the physician. Clinicians largely see themselves as patient advocates and identify with their chosen profession, whereas managers deal in more removed, detached frameworks and advocate the organization and its goals and objectives. Although those goals and objectives undoubtedly include the advocacy of quality care, this advocacy is several steps removed from bedside involvement.

THE TRANSITION FROM PHYSICIAN TO MANAGER

McCall and Claire[5] identified six critical transformations in the transition process from physician-clinician to physician-manager. The skills required and the psychologic demands are quite different for successful physician management than for successful clinician. Their work, based on interviews with physician-managers, helps delineate the importance of recognizing these factors during the transition process. They note that many of the skills of the physician adapt well to managerial roles, including the analytic skill of diagnosis, the self-confidence based on clinical skills, comfort with command, and the interpersonal sensitivity that comes with dealing with patients in difficult situations. However, it was quite clear from their study that these skills and abilities alone were not sufficient for the transition to a physician-manager. They identified six specific types of transitions critical to the overall shift, including three psychologic adjustments and three specific new skills or abilities.

The first psychologic adjustment is from hard-earned independence and autonomy as a clinician to much more dependent roles as a manager. As indicated previously, the clinical practice of emergency medicine allows a high degree of independent authority and discretion by the clinician. Despite the presence of protocols and increasing standards of care applied in the emergency department setting, the majority of the clinical practice of emergency medicine still includes an extremely high degree of autonomy. To adjust to the role of management, the physician must make the psychologic adjustment to being dependent on the actions of others. For example, as the chair of an emergency department, a physician in collaboration with his or her nursing colleagues adapts triage criteria to result in more efficient care. However, implementation of those criteria on a day-to-day basis requires dependence on multiple triage personnel. Because of the variability of response inherent in such a process, it is important for the physician-manager to be prepared to accept dependency on others.

Second, the physician-manager must make the transition from an identity as a physician-focused on individual patient care to an identity as a manager focused on the emergency department overall, as well as the overall institutional goals and objectives. McCall and Claire[5] noted that physicians are "fiercely independent, pursuing personal or professional agendas rather than department agendas." Although this is less often a problem in the emergency department because emergency department physicians are used to working in a team environment, it is nonetheless an important transition as a physician-manager attempts to integrate the emergency department into the institution overall and the healthcare system in general (see Chapter 10).

The third psychologic adjustment involves a transition from naivete about organizational dynamics to acceptance of organizational realities as a part of managerial life and recognition that specific skills and abilities are required for understanding organizational dynamics.

> The rationality of the clinic is based on fact, logic, and linearity. The rationality of the organization is very different—it rests in getting people to accept and act on a decision. Facts don't always triumph, people don't always rally around logic, and power, position, and different perspectives effect outcome. The politics of organizations can generate cynicism (among physician-managers).[5]

In addition to these psychologic adjustments affecting the transition from clinician to manager, the authors also noted that three new skills or abilities were necessary. These new skills and abilities can be quantified and taught, but are some-

what different from those assumed to be present in a clinical setting. The first involves a transition from demand and control in the clinical setting to persuasion, ambiguity, and communication skills in a managerial role. In fact, the expectations of patients and their families have changed substantially during the last several years, and it is far more common for successful clinicians to understand the need for communication skills with their patients in the clinical setting. When physicians take advantage of improved communication skills in the managerial setting, the transition from clinician to manager can be much easier.

The second of the new skills or abilities requires a transition from comfortable, established relationships with professional colleagues to authority-based, boss-subordinate relationships with former colleagues. This may help account for Shakespeare's dictum that "Uneasy rests the head that wears the crown." Emergency physicians in general have had a traditional lack of respect for authority based solely on hierarchy or bureaucracy. Although all emergency physicians practice in some form of group practice environment, their clinical roles have generally been independent, with clearly established communication lines with other emergency physicians and members of the medical staff. The transition to an environment where the physician-manager is actually in control of the destiny of other physicians can be extremely difficult, both for the manager and for the staff.

The third skill or ability requires changing from competence in medicine to competence in management. Regardless of how good a clinician is or how strong his or her interpersonal skills may be, it is important to recognize that organizational learning, negotiation skills, strategic planning, customer service, continuous quality improvement, and outcomes measurement are all distinct, quantifiable skills in which the physician usually has had little training. Taken together, these six areas involve a substantial change in issues concerned deeply with personal identity, from areas in which the physician has a strong sense of what Senge[6] refers to as *personal mastery* to new fields in which new competencies must be learned and new skills demonstrated.

In many cases, this transition may involve a profound sense of personal loss on the part of the physician, but it can also involve a great deal of excitement because it allows the physician to use additional competencies at a critical stage of his or her career. Indeed, in the Wisconsin Survey Research Laboratory study of more than 878 physician-managers, the reasons for switching to a career as a physician-manager were overwhelmingly proactive and positive, and involved a search for new opportunities and challenges.[7] The vast majority of such physicians clearly recognized the need for learning and demonstrating new talents and abilities in defined areas. In this sense, it appears that most physician-managers are moving toward a desired state, rather than moving away from a less desired or unpopular state. Although the duties and responsibilities as a clinical emergency physician can sometimes be onerous (and may help account for the "burnout" seen among emergency physicians), experience indicates that the majority of physicians pursuing management roles do so proactively rather than reactively. There is also a high recognition that medical management is, as Ellwood indicates, a "clinical science," that involves expertise in health management, medical management information systems, medical decision theory, psychology of organized medical care, and health promotion and disease prevention strategies.[11]

McCall and Claire[5] also noted that there were identifiable obstacles to the transition to the role of physician-manager, including three types of personal obstacles and one organizational obstacle. The personal obstacles that they identified were the physician-manager's own defense mechanisms (especially denial), errors in selecting physicians for management roles who were not suited or capable for them, and the physician-manager's inability to build new support systems to match the new competencies required in the physician-leader role. The organizational obstacle involves lack of design and poor preparation for the transition by the organization. This is an extremely important difficulty because the majority of hospitals and healthcare organizations have not put sufficient time and effort into thinking about how this transition should be made and how the physician should be prepared for it. For example, it is unusual to have physicians widely exposed to the simple human resources background necessary to take on a role as a physician-manager. They also noted that several problems were common as organizational obstacles (Box 9-2).

BOX 9-2

ORGANIZATIONAL OBSTACLES IN THE CLINICIAN TO PHYSICIAN-MANAGER ROLE

1. Failure to set clear objectives
2. Failure to delineate specific responsibilities
3. Failure to provide adequate and timely feedback
4. Failure to train/prepare the professional for the role
5. Neglecting to provide practical experience to develop managerial skills
6. Failure to mentor and/or guide physicians in this transition
7. Surrounding a physician with incompetent or inadequately trained staff
8. Failure to reward or recognize exceptional performance

Adapted from McCall MW Jr, Clair JA: In transit: from physician to manager (abstract), Philadelphia, 1990, Center for Applied Research.

COMPETENCIES FOR PHYSICIAN-LEADERS AND MANAGERS

Although the transition from clinician to physician-manager can be difficult, it is also important to recognize that there are (in addition to the specific body of knowledge that must be learned) specific competencies that can be identified as critical to roles of the physician-manager. The radical changes that American healthcare is undergoing point to the need for physician-managers to help guide such change. Many of the necessary competencies help initiate, develop, and sustain change for the organization. A level of complexity, intensity, and sophistication is required that differs in many important respects from those seen in the clinical environment, although

Table 9-1 New Physician Leadership Competencies

New competencies	New physician-leadership roles	Changes required in healthcare trends
Strategic business planning orientation	Strategic business partner	Increased governmental regulation through public-private partnerships
Empowering/developing others	Enabling/empowering manager	Accelerated development of organized physician career paths/practice options
Mission articulation	Cultural developer/mission implementor	Increase formation of physician-hospital economic and clinical alignments
Group leadership	Group/team effort leader; developer of vision	Focus on cost effectiveness, as well as revenue enhancement
Negotiation skills	Influence strategies user	Focus on vertically integrated healthcare organizations
Stakeholder relationship building	Consensus developer; stakeholder analysis	Continuous redefinition and documentation of standards and outcomes across stakeholder territory
Organizational awareness	Organizational systems alignment	Increased use of protocols, guidelines, standards and payment mechanisms

Adapted from Farrell JP, Robbins MM: *Healthc Forum J* 39-42, 1993.

there are certainly some similarities between the two. By the nature of their jobs, emergency department physician-managers are required to manage multiple constituencies, serve complex and often diverse organizational interests, and motivate and train highly skilled professionals to deliver high quality healthcare in a cost-efficient fashion.

Among the specific competencies required of physician-leaders-managers are strategic business planning, empowerment, staff development, mission articulation, group leadership, negotiation skills, change management, stakeholder relationship building, organizational awareness, and financial management skills[9] (Tables 9-1 and 9-2). Each of these competencies are addressed elsewhere, but it is important to recognize that these skills and abilities should not be viewed as denigrating the importance of quality medical care in emergency department environment. Rather, these competencies are required to help emergency medicine reach its fullest and most complete potential to help maintain its place as the "front line of American medicine." As other specialties develop these competencies, it is critical to ensure that emergency medicine managers are also highly trained, to best negotiate the resources and abilities necessary for the successful practice of emergency medicine in the future.

This approach makes the practice of emergency medicine more complete, in that it expands the specialty so that it is an art, a science, *and* a business. Dedicating oneself and one's organization to the transition to physician-leaders need not be at the expense of, and can be with the enhancement of, the clinical aspects of emergency medicine. In summary, it is important to recognize that the transition from a clinician to a physician-leader-manager is discrete and identifiable, with recognized obstacles to the transition. Nonetheless, when approached in a straightforward fashion and with a clear understanding that new competencies will need to be learned, the goal of managing professionals in organizations can be a satisfying, sustaining, and career enhancing. More importantly, it offers a substantial hope for further development of the clinical practice of emergency medicine, upon which all of our efforts depend.[10]

Table 9-2 Behavioral Indicators for Emergency Department Physician Leadership

Competency	Emergency department chair/president of group
Strategic business orientation	Effectively positions the group within the delivery system and the department within the hospital
Empowering/developing others	Empowers others to accomplish strategic goals; supervises and gives practical assistance
Mission articulation	Defines and promotes organization's mission within the system and assists group members in commitment to organization's values
Group leadership	Develops collaborative working relationships with parties to achieve departmental objectives
Negotiation skills	Forges strategic alliances, establishes key relationships, and develops agreements of tactical significance
Stakeholder relationship building	Develops strategic linkages focusing on achieving organizational goals; manages across stakeholder boundaries
Organizational awareness	Maintains understanding of system dynamics and organization's climate and culture

Adapted from Farrell JP, Robbins MM: *Healthc Forum J* 39-42, 1993.

REFERENCES

1. Kindig DA, Dunham N: How much administration is today's physician doing? *Physician Exec* 17:3-7, 1990.
2. Lord JT: The changing role of the organized medical staff: the challenge for medical staff leadership. In Lord JT, editor: *A guide for physician leaders,* Rockville, Md, 1992, Bader & Associates.
3. Detmer DE: *The physician as corporate practitioner and corporate leader,* Durham, NC, 1984, Duke University National Forum on Hospital and Health Affairs.
4. Dresnick S: The emergency department medical director. In Schwartz

G, Cayten G, Mayer T et al, editors: *The principles and practice of emergency medicine,* Philadelphia, 1993, Lea & Febiger.

5. McCall MW Jr, Claire JA: *In transit: from physician to manager,* Philadelphia, 1990, Wharton Center for Applied Research.
6. Senge P: *The fifth discipline: the art and practice of the learning organization,* New York, 1990, Doubleday.
7. Kurtz ME: The dual dilemma. In Curry W, editor: *The physician executive,* Tampa, Fla, 1988, American College of Physician Executives.
8. Kindig D, Dunham N, Man-Chun L: Career paths of physician executives, *Healthc Manage Rev* 16:11-20, 1991.
9. Farrell JP, Robins MM: Leadership competencies for physicians, *Health Forum J* 36:39-42, 1993.
10. Mayer T: The emergency department medical director, *Emerg Med Clin North Am* 5:1-29, 1987.
11. Ellwood PM: Shatluck lecture-outcomes management: a technology of patient experience, *N Engl J Med* 318:1549-1556, 1988.

10 Departmental Integration Strategies

Thom A. Mayer

The clinical practice of emergency medicine requires integration of the emergency department with multiple levels of the hospital, the Emergency Medical Service (EMS) system, and the community in general. On a given day in most communities across the country, the emergency department is called on to interact extensively with virtually all areas of the hospital at one point or another. Intensive care units, operating suites, imaging services, laboratory, medical/surgical floors, dietary, housekeeping, and medical records are all required to interact extensively with the emergency department during the care and the treatment of emergency department patients. Although the need for integration occurs on a de facto basis and is intuitive to those who practice emergency medicine, it is also important to recognize the prospective and strategic nature of approaching such areas of integration. It is precisely because of the interdependency between the emergency department and other areas of the hospital that those who are charged with management of the emergency department should ensure that a well-conceived and disciplined approach is taken to integrating the emergency department both within the hospital and throughout the community. The goals of this chapter are to identify those areas of both horizontal and vertical integration. Strategies that may be used to help smooth this integration process are also discussed.

HORIZONTAL AND VERTICAL INTEGRATION

The terms *horizontal* and *vertical integration* have been used in numerous settings to describe the need for organizations to take a broad and far-reaching approach to strategies that accentuate interdependencies between the organization and its related functions. Although these terms have been defined in various ways, horizontal integration of the emergency department refers here to integration within the boundaries of the hospital, medical staff, administration, and the governance function. In contrast, vertical integration of the emergency department refers to integration within the existing healthcare system, political structure, and surrounding community. Figure 10-1 illustrates the manner in which vertical and horizontal integration occur and the central role of the emergency department as the front line of American medicine.[1]

HORIZONTAL INTEGRATION STRATEGIES

Horizontal integration strategies are intended to ensure that the emergency department maximizes its potential for smooth and efficient relationships with other areas throughout the hospital. By far the most important of these horizontal integration strategies involves the *medical staff.* The objectives of each of the horizontal integration strategies should have clearly delineated goals, but the goals for integration of the medical staff should include the following:

- Establishment of a collegial, professional relationship.
- Education of medical staff with regard to emergency department operations and its complexity.
- Development of practical strategies to meet common needs.
- Development and implementation of mechanisms for dealing with problems, quality improvement concerns, etc.
- Establishment of mechanisms by which medical staff can evaluate their own patients in the emergency department.
- Providing a forum in which mutual areas of concern can be discussed (managed care, healthcare reform, gatekeeper concepts for prospective payment, etc.).

One of the most difficult aspects of integration with the medical staff involves the numbers of people involved. Regardless of the size of the emergency department group, members from various medical staff departments vastly outnumber the emergency physicians, so that emergency physicians must deal with the personalities and preferences of a large, diverse, and disparate group of people.

Several specific strategies can be helpful in dealing with this problem. First, when possible, surveys of the medical staff can be developed and kept in the emergency department (Figure 10-2). These surveys should reveal how the staff prefer to have their patients handled when they are in the emergency department, including when they would like to be called and subspecialty preference lists. However, given the increasing size of medical staffs and the changing nature of their practices, this strategy has become somewhat less practical than it had been in the past. Further, many medical staff members prefer not to state their preferences for subspecialty referrals in a written fashion.

Whenever possible, it is helpful to establish prospective guidelines with existing departments to help standardize the manner in which certain processes occur in the emergency department, as opposed to dealing with the whims of a large and changing medical staff. For example, should the attending primary care physician be called immediately after evaluation on patients who are probable admissions or only after

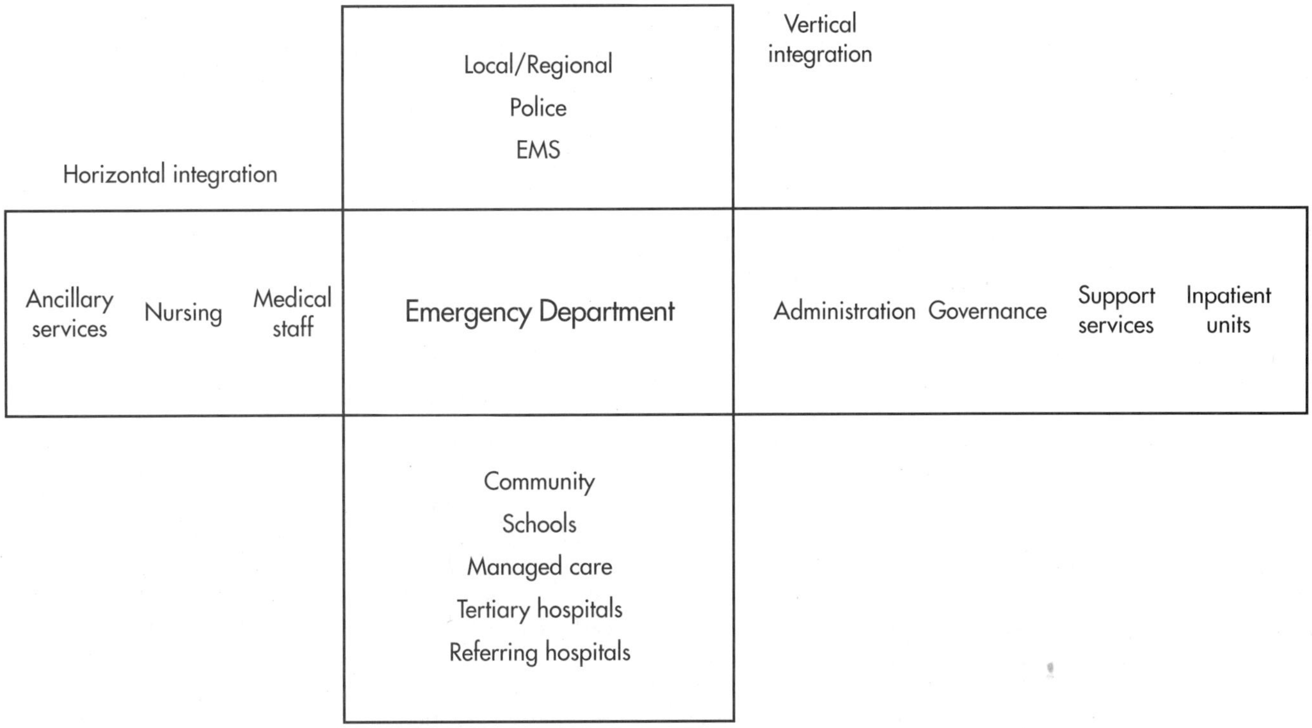

FIGURE 10-1 Vertical and horizontal integration of the emergency department.

diagnostic and therapeutic interventions have been completed? From a practical standpoint, most mature primary care physicians prefer to be called as soon as possible if it appears that a patient will need admission and/or substantial intervention, recognizing that the complete diagnostic and therapeutic workup have not been completed. Unless this question is handled in a standardized fashion, the emergency department is always open to the criticism by individual practitioners that they "didn't have all the data," "hadn't figured out what was wrong," or "were just acting as triage officers." From a strictly functional standpoint, calling the medical staff early has substantial advantages to flow patterns through the emergency department, but either style can be accommodated, although it is far more preferable to have a standardized, mutually agreed to approach to handling such aspects of care.

Establishing collegial and professional relationships with the staff is perhaps the most important issue in integrating the emergency department physician group with the medical staff. This includes aspects of both medical integration and social integration. From a medical standpoint, hospital-based physicians are often regarded as "contract groups" or "hospital employees." Although in some cases, employee relationships exist with emergency physicians and hospitals, the more the practice of emergency medicine is similar to that of the existing medical staff, the more chance there is for integration.[2] For that reason, fee-for-service or modified fee-for-service relationships are usually preferred, both because they make it clearer that the emergency physicians are similar to the existing medical staff and because it places some impetus on the practicing emergency physician for increasing flow through the department.

Prospective evaluations systems to ensure that quality improvement problems are addressed aggressively should be in place with all medical staff departments, through both usual medical staff mechanisms and other integration strategies. For example, it is important to ensure that each medical staff department have an identified liaison from the emergency department physician group. This liaison should act as a conduit for communication between the two departments. When possible, the liaison and/or chair of the department should attend medical staff department and section meetings to ensure that any problems or concerns about the emergency department can be addressed in an aggressive, straightforward, constructive, and proactive fashion. It is much easier to criticize a person or department that is not present. By attending department and section meetings, this problem can often be avoided.

The most consistent and important relationship between the emergency department and the medical staff of the hospital is through the patient care interactions that occur in the emergency department. By far the most common form of communication is by telephone about patients that are seen in the emergency department, whether they are to be admitted to the hospital or discharged. It is difficult to overestimate the importance of ensuring that such telephone communications are handled consistently, professionally, and succinctly. For example, when calling a surgeon in the middle of the night, it is far better to approach the need for consultation in a direct and straightforward fashion. "Jim, this is Thom Mayer in the emergency department, and I have a patient of Dr. Smith's, who asked that I call you. She has right-lower quadrant pain, a high white count, clean urine, and no other source for her pain; appendicitis needs to be ruled out. We have her set for admission or the operating room, depending on your clinical examination." Most medical staff

Medical Staff Emergency Department Preferences

Name ______________________________ Specialty ______________________________

_____ I wish to be called whenever my patients come to the emergency department.

_____ Call as soon as the patient arrives.

_____ Call when results are back and after treatment.

_____ Call when admission is necessary.

_____ I wish to be called only if admission to my service is necessary.

Specialty Referrals:

_____ Please call on each case.

_____ Please use the following:

Cardiology ______________________________

General Surgery ______________________________

Orthopedics ______________________________

Plastic Surgery ______________________________

Pulmonary ______________________________

Urology ______________________________

Others ______________________________

FIGURE 10-2 Medical staff preference form.

members prefer this sort of approach to a rambling, historical dissertation on the patient. Assuring that communicationsare clear-cut and straightforward, and that expectations are communicated clearly enhances the professional relationship between the emergency department physician and the medical staff. When orienting new physicians to the emergency department, it is important to ensure that they understand the importance of telephone communications with the medical staff. It is also important, whenever possible, to ensure that copies of the discharge summary on patients admitted through the emergency department are sent to the emergency physician. This approach helps assure that there is a quality improvement loop that is closed, but also helps give the emergency physician a better understanding of the long-term care provided to the patient in the hospital.[3]

Areas of professional disagreement must be handled in a

direct fashion. Although most emergency department chairs prefer to be informed about conflict between an emergency department physician and other medical staff members, in most cases the best way of handling the situation is to ensure that the parties involved speak directly to each other and work out their problems as professionals, at the same time keeping the emergency department leadership informed. It is of the utmost importance to ensure that all departments and sections of the hospital understand clearly that the leadership of the emergency department wants to be informed of *any* problems that relate to its function in a direct, real-time fashion. Nothing is worse than hearing second hand, through administration or the medical staff leadership, that there have been problems in the emergency department. It is imperative therefore to ensure that the emergency department chair communicate clearly to each department and section his or her desire to hear about problems immediately, so that they can be resolved in a professional and amicable fashion.

Most hospitals have some form of medical staff lounge, but it is relatively rare to see emergency department physicians in this area. Unfortunately, the lounge is an important area where discussions occur between medical staff members in both formal and informal fashions. For that reason, the emergency department chair and other emergency physicians should be encouraged to stop by the lounge on a regular basis, either while going on or off duty. This investment of time and effort is well worth the informal communication ties that can be developed in such a setting.

All emergency physicians should be active members of the local medical society and, to the extent possible, should seek leadership positions in that organization. The emergency physician group also should be aware of the need for social integration with other members of the medical staff, including athletic functions, social functions, and school and community service. All of these efforts help integrate the emergency physician group into the overall medical staff community.

Integration with the *nursing* functions of the emergency department is also a critical aspect of horizontal integration. The emergency department acts as a gateway to the hospital for virtually every floor and unit available, particularly the intensive care units, operating suites, medical/surgical floors, and pediatric floors. Strong working relationships between the emergency department and the nursing management are necessary in all of these areas. Although the majority of this interaction occurs at the level of emergency department nursing management, it is also critical to ensure that the emergency physician group be familiar with these sources and establish a close and collegial working relationship.

One of the more persistent and difficult problems facing emergency departments is scarcity of inpatient beds. This problem causes long delays in the emergency department after the patient has technically been "admitted" to the hospital. During times of such crises, close working relationships with nursing management on the floors and intensive care units can help diffuse this situation. Similarly, educational functions should be shared between the emergency department and the units and floors. Often these units and floors need inservice education or cardiopulmonary resuscitation training. The emergency department physician and nursing staff should help cooperate with the colleagues in the units and on the floors to help meet their educational needs whenever possible. When areas of disagreement or clinical care are raised, they should be handled in a prospectively defined and aggressive fashion. One of the biggest problems facing emergency departments is that many of the hospital staff truly do not understand the overall functions and complexity that occur in the emergency department. By relying on collegial relationships between the physician and nursing management in the emergency department and their colleagues on the floors and units, this situation can be alleviated over time.

Integration with *administration* is clearly one of the most important aspects of emergency department practice. The role of the hospital administrator is becoming increasingly difficult, complex, and confusing. Most emergency departments are well served when there is a climate of mutual respect between administration and emergency department management. Frequent and regular meetings should be held to help discuss goals and objectives and the progress being made toward attaining those goals and objectives. It is particularly important that emergency department management and its staff be seen as *problem solvers* as opposed to finger pointers. The multitude of problems that face American medicine in general, and emergency medicine in particular, can certainly create an environment where it is easy to assess blame, point out why progress cannot be made, or shift the focus and emphasis to other areas of the hospital or healthcare system. It is certainly the obligation of emergency department management to point out to the administration and medical staff the limitations of certain courses of action and lack of planning. Nonetheless, during any such interactions, it is extremely important to ensure that there is a constructive, positive, and reasoned solution to the problems. This transition to a problem solver from a problem identifier is an important aspect of the relationship between emergency department management and administration. To the extent possible, administration should be asked to identify their specific expectations, goals, objectives for the emergency department to ensure clarity with regard to how progress will be judged. Members of the administrative team usually have some form of ongoing human relations training and leadership development. Emergency department management should be integrated into those educational efforts so that the administrative and emergency department teams "speak the same language." This shared philosophic and educational background is a critical piece of the integration between administration and the emergency department.[4] Social interactions between the emergency department management team and administrative teams are usually rarer than those between emergency department physicians and medical staff members, but they can serve a useful function if kept on a professional basis.

One of the most neglected areas of horizontal integration relates to the *governance* function of the hospital. Hospital operating boards are the final authority to which administration and medical staff matters are referred. The leaders of the emergency department should be aware of the members comprising the hospital operating board and develop cooperative relationships with key members of the board. Care must be taken to ensure that this does not in any way circumvent the relationship of administration to the board, but rather serves to complement them. Members of the hospital operating board can be a rich source of advice and are most often happy to share experiences that they have had dealing with the com-

munity. This information can be of inestimable value to the emergency department management team. Chapter 14 lists the perspective of hospital operating boards when they interact with the medical staff in general and the emergency department in particular.

The emergency department has a strong interaction with other ancillary and support services in the hospital, including laboratory, radiology, anesthesiology, registration, and billing. The emergency department chair should have a strong relationship with his or her colleagues in pathology, radiology, and anesthesiology. These specialties share the hospital-based nature of emergency medicine, and it is wise to seek the counsel of such chairs, particularly if they have substantial and lengthy experience with the hospital. Combined skills of the physician and nurse managers of the emergency department should be used to establish good relationships with all of these areas of the hospital.

VERTICAL INTEGRATION

In addition to ensuring that the emergency department is integrated within the functions of the hospital, the emergency department management team should address the issue of vertical integration within the overall healthcare system. This involves relationships with the local and regional EMS agency, police, managed care providers, regional referral hospitals, and the political structure within which the hospital works. Part 10 addresses aspects of prehospital care in some detail, but it deserves reemphasizing that the EMS system is a major stakeholder in providing emergency department services. Both physician and nursing representation should be available to the EMS providers and, whenever possible, medical direction for the EMS system should be provided through the emergency department. Similarly, educational cooperation is essential with prehospital care providers because they form a critical part of the emergency department team. Police agencies have always had strong working relationships with the emergency department, and the increasing amount of violence in our communities indicates the need for ensuring that cooperation occurs at all levels. As with all other integration strategies, integration should be handled on a prospective basis and should include the top levels of management of the police force.

The emergency department is a substantial community resource, even though most community members hope they will never need it. The emergency department management team should have a plan for integration within the community, including public service activities, educational activities, injury prevention activities, and, whenever possible, speakers bureau or newspaper column information. At least one member of the emergency department physician group should be active with the local school authority, most of whom have some form of healthcare advisory board. As managed care becomes an increasingly substantial portion of the payor mix, the relationship with managed care providers will become even more critical than it currently is. Strategies for working with and negotiating with managed care are listed in Chapters 35 and 40, but it is important to recognize that integration with managed care can act as a strongly positive aspect of negotiations between the hospital and the managed care providers. Educating managed care agents with regard to the role that emergency medicine can play is crucial in this regard. Rather than railing at the reduced rates or capitation aspects that managed care may represent, it is important to negotiate from a position of strength and help educate the executives of managed care that emergency medicine can have relationships that are of mutual benefit and interest. When such relationships are in place, it reflects extremely well on the emergency department as it relates to overall negotiations between the hospital and the managed care provider.

Although many physicians avoid interaction with political elements of their profession, most emergency departments will be well served by ensuring that there is a strong and prospective relationship between the emergency department and whatever political entities are responsible for local and regional governance. This involvement must be handled cautiously and certainly in concert with administration and the governing boards of the hospital. Nonetheless, in most cases both administration and the board will welcome input and assistance in their interactions with the community political base, so long as it is carefully coordinated with their overall goals and objectives.

SUMMARY

Horizontal and vertical integration strategies form an important part of a successful emergency department. These strategies should be implemented after careful strategic planning and with the input of both physician and nursing management. All such strategies should be carefully coordinated with the administration and hospital operating board and should be monitored on an ongoing basis for their successful completion. As the healthcare environment faces an unprecedented level of change, these vertical and horizontal integration strategies must be able to respond rapidly with appropriate changes as well.

REFERENCES

1. Mayer T: The emergency department medical director, *Emerg Med Clin North Am* 5:1-29, 1987.
2. Mayer T, Cohen R: Entrepreneurism and benchmarks of emergency medical practice, *Ann Emerg Med* 13:129-131, 1984.
3. Dresnick S: The emergency department medical director. In Schwartz G, Cayten G, Mayer T et al, editors: *Principles and practice of emergency medicine*, Philadelphia, 1993, Lea & Febiger.
4. Johnson D: Administrative expectations of the emergency department, *Emerg Med Clin North Am* 5:149-154, 1987.

11 Conducting Effective Meetings

Robert W. Strauss

"90% of success is showing up!"

Woody Allen

OUTLINE

Meetings often seem like the bane of our existence. Most of us wonder how much easier our lives would be if we didn't have to participate in so many. The greater the success professionals achieve in an organization, the more time is spent in meetings. Managers spend more than 50% of the average work week in meetings,[1-3] in addition to the time spent preparing for and performing tasks assigned in a meeting. It sometimes seems as if an endless stream of meetings leaves us no time to catch up on the rest of our work.

This huge expenditure of time would be more acceptable if participants believed meetings were a valuable use of time. However, a poll of 471 management leaders conducted by Communispond reported that 70% of the participants found meetings "a waste of time."[2] A second survey performed by Accountemps found that the average executive spends 2 months each year in *unnecessary* meetings.[4] A third survey by Hofstra University and Harrison Consulting Services revealed that three fourths of business leaders spend more time in meetings now than they did a few years ago and expect to spend even more time in meetings a few years from now.[3]

The impact of a poor meeting is always detrimental. It steals time that could have been devoted to a more valuable effort. So why have meetings?

The fact is most groups and organizations can only function by having meetings. Major decisions affecting our lives are made daily in meetings. Congress approves budgets, an academic committee considers admissions, a jury decides innocence or guilt, a family decides vacation plans. Meetings can be successful.

WHY MEETINGS FAIL

What is the typical response to the question: "Why did this meeting fail?" Most respondents focus on three issues.[5-8]

The chair is disorganized. He or she has no control, establishes no order, is too talkative, unprepared, or does not communicate. The agenda was not followed. The chair's personality creates barriers to effective communication.

The committee members don't participate, are uninterested, unprepared, and don't pull their weight. They don't complete their assignments, show up late, talk during the meeting. There is too much arguing and conflict—one-upmanship by a dominant personality.

The meeting has no purpose. There was no preparation. Members don't know why they were gathered. It starts late and runs overtime. The room is too hot. Members couldn't see visual aids. The meeting was one digression after another.

Sound familiar?

THERE MUST BE A BETTER WAY

Whether you are running the meeting or just trying to survive it, it often seems like there must be a better way. There is. Effective meetings are purposeful, time efficient, focused, and well conducted. This chapter reviews the components of effective meetings with specific attention to:

- Why and why not to have a meeting
- How to prepare for a meeting in advance
- How to conduct a meeting
- Problem-solving techniques
- How to avoid common traps including the most difficult people
- What to do after everyone leaves

To transform a necessary and boring evil and make it into a creative center of communication, you must prepare, run the show without stealing it, and meet your objectives, as well as those of the group.

TO HAVE OR NOT TO HAVE A MEETING

The first issue to determine is whether the meeting is necessary.

Reasons to Avoid a Meeting

Meetings should be avoided (Box 11-1) or severely limited if they are only ritual. Unfortunately, rituals, like Linus' blanket, are not easily abandoned. Most meetings occur because there is always a meeting about the subject at this time of the day, week, or month.

If the person organizing the meeting is unable to develop a meaningful agenda, then this meeting should be carefully scrutinized for its value and purpose. Give consideration to looking for an alternative method for accomplishing the goal.

It may be unnecessary to have a meeting when there are no decisions to be made. This situation can occur when there is no question to be asked, no problem to be solved, or you already know the answer and don't need permission to accomplish the goal. It may also occur when greater involvement will only confuse the issue, as in "Too many cooks will spoil the broth."

Reasons to Have a Meeting

Meetings are the most efficient way to communicate some types of information and make some types of decisions.[1,2,5,9,10]

Information Transmission. This type of meeting provides a forum for the simultaneous dissemination of issues, not debate. It creates a pool of consistent knowledge. Typical examples include defining and promoting a group's mission, progress reports, educational seminars, and training sessions.

If a prolonged presentation is required, use visual aids to enhance interest. Multisensory communication is best. At the completion of this type of informational presentation, it is essential to check for understanding, reactions, confusion, or clarity.

Problem Solving. Problem-solving meetings are held to identify issues, develop solutions, make determinations, and implement the decision. The premise of a problem-solving meeting is that there is general agreement that a problem exists that members of the group can solve. A group is generally more creative and better at decision making than an equivalent number of individuals working alone.[2]

Group decision making creates commitment to the solution, which results in more effective implementation. If the problem is solvable by a single person, and commitment to the decision is unnecessary, the meeting is also unnecessary.

BOX 11-1

REASONS TO AVOID A MEETING

1. Ritual
2. No information to share
3. No decisions to be made
4. Sharing gossip
5. Showing off
6. Demonstrating power
7. Avoiding work
8. Can inform better by phone
9. Can inform better by email

ESSENTIAL COMMITTEES FOR EMERGENCY DEPARTMENTS[11,12] (Box 11-2)

The hospital's staff and administration carry out their business by committee. However, emergency care providers historically have been perceived as shift workers who put in their time and do little else to promote the mission of the institution. By working toward the common good of the institution, emergency physicians can be instrumental in implementing the institution's programs. Emergency physicians can have a voice and a presence that is crucial to recognition as peers. This participation will, over time, provide a broader perspective of the emergency department and its issues.

Members of the Department of Emergency Medicine should have representation on all key committees, including but not limited to those discussed in the following sections.

Executive Committee

Decisions affecting the entire medical staff are made here, and participation as an active voting member is critical. Participation allows you to present emergency department issues for definitive action. If you're not in, you're out.

Disaster Committee

An emergency care provider should chair this committee. Disaster management is composed of prehospital care, triage, rapid assessment, emergency intervention, referral, resource utilization, and communications, all of which are the foundations of modern emergency medicine. This arena is the perfect opportunity for emergency care providers to demonstrate their expertise to the staff and community.

Credentials Committee

This committee is pivotal and active participation may be crucial. This committee is charged with the responsibility of investigating and endorsing physicians for membership to the medical staff. Members of this committee delve into confidential matters. Presence on this committee avoids misunderstandings and promotes fair evaluation of emergency physician candidates.

Emergency Department Management Committee

Placing complete control of the emergency department in the hands of the physician or the nursing director is not always possible, or even desirable. Many directors want to share the

BOX 11-2

ESSENTIAL COMMITTEES

Executive Committee
Disaster Committee
Credentials Committee
Quality Improvement Committee
Emergency Department Management Committee

burden of responsibility with others who have strong interests in the success of the department. An emergency department management committee is an effective and politically expedient solution. The committee members should come from administration, emergency nursing, and the emergency physician group. This committee should provide a forum for consensus development, strategy, and team building.

Quality Management Committee

The emergency department plays a vital role in the provision of quality care in the hospital. Because of the importance and high visibility of the emergency department, the care rendered to emergency patients is scrutinized by the medical staff and administration. Institutional support for the emergency department quality improvement program will occur most easily when an emergency care provider is an active participant on the hospital-wide committee.

PREPARATION

Good meetings are well-orchestrated events (Box 11-3). The first critical element of successful meetings is planning.[11] Planning allows the group to accomplish its objectives smoothly and efficiently. Preparing for a meeting includes developing objectives, creating an agenda, inviting the appropriate people, and preparing the proper room logistics. Less time is spent in meeting when more time is spent preparing for them.

Determine the Purpose

Have you been to, or worse, run a meeting in which part way through you are uncertain about what you are trying to accomplish? Unfortunately, many meetings are poorly organized and seem to exist without purpose. Meetings without clear objectives waste time. When preparing for a meeting, simply ask yourself these questions:

- What do I want to accomplish as a result of this meeting?
- Will accomplishing this goal further the organization's mission?
- Could I effectively accomplish it without a meeting?
- What outcomes would demonstrate that I have successfully accomplished the objectives?

The more clearly the objectives can be stated, the more likely it is they will be accomplished. Establish priorities for the objectives so that the truly important issues receive appropriate attention. Once the objectives are clear, determine the type of meeting that will best accomplish these objectives.

Rule: "Write the minutes before the meeting." In other words, know what you want to accomplish, plan for it, and move things in the proper direction.

Develop an Action Agenda

The agenda is the single most important document required for a successful meeting.[2,5,9] An agenda is a road map, timetable, overview, advertisement, and goal-setter (Box 11-4). It cues the presiding officer, enlists attention of members, and keeps everyone moving in the same direction at the same time. More time spent preparing an agenda generally will require less time in the meeting. The agenda should be complete but accomplishable. If the time runs out before the meeting does, participants will be left with the impression of disorganization and poor prioritization. The agenda should be circulated in advance.

Write the Meeting's Objective. A statement of the meeting's objective will help the members mentally prepare for the discussion.

List Topics. Participants like to know in advance what will happen and what is expected of them. An agenda that is divided into its component parts will help organize and focus the discussion, allowing the chair to redirect a wandering group. It may be helpful to mark items for *information, discussion,* or *decision making* to cue members to the expectations.

Sequence Topics. Provide an orderly framework for the meeting's topics by placing them in a logical sequence. When subjects flow from one to another, it becomes easier to develop support for the issue, and the meeting becomes more manageable. A well-organized approach will facilitate work on key concepts. Some meeting leaders suggest beginning with topics that require more creativity, which also allows adequate time to be spent on the most complex issues. Others recommend an orderly progression of topics beginning with easier, less taxing topics, and proceeding to more difficult and complex issues. This method achieves group cohesiveness by establishing early success. Either approach can be successful, depending on the variables such as the chair's preference and the composition of the specific topic.

Circulate in Advance. Circulating the agenda in advance enables members to come to the meeting prepared. This practice also allows the group members to confirm the time of the meeting and review the topics for discussion. It compels the chair to consider each topic and be prepared. Advance circulation eliminates the most common cause of initial con-

BOX 11-3

MEETING PREPARATION

1. Determine purpose
2. Develop agenda
3. Select participants
4. Set setting
5. Seat for success

BOX 11-4

AGENDA ITEMS

1. Date, start time, end time
2. Location
3. List of individuals invited
4. Objective of meeting
5. List of topics including
   —brief summary
   —time allotted
6. Supporting documents

fusion seen at the beginning of a meeting. It is also a sign of courtesy to those attending the meeting.

Provide Supporting Documents. Supporting documents should be attached and sent early with the agenda so that members may become familiar with the information before the meeting. A requirement to protect confidential information is an exception to this practice.

Action Agenda.[13] Although some items require no further effort, others necessitate specific action by members of the group. Clarifying the steps, assigning specific responsibility, and gaining commitment will substantially increase the tasks that get accomplished.

Who Should Attend

The meeting planner must decide who should attend the meeting.[2,9,10,14,15] The basis of this decision is too often determined by considerations represented by the following statements: "They've always been at the meeting" (a ritual); Let's get a homogeneous group for quick and easy decisions (a rubber stamp); "Let's include everyone (a public relations event)." Inviting individuals who have no reason to be at the meeting is a waste of time and can be disruptive.

The appropriate list of attendees should be based on the need to be there. Relevant considerations for membership include knowledge and potential to contribute, power to make a decision, responsibility to implement a decision, and being affected by the decision (stakeholder analysis).[16]

Large groups (more than 12 to 15) often become ineffective at decision making. Homogeneity (choosing those with a similar perspective) leads to easy and quick decisions that have worked in the past. Few options will be considered and leadership challenges will be rare. A homogeneous group falls prey to "groupthink" and tends to exhibit stereotypic behavior and superfluous decisions.[17]

A more diverse or heterogeneous group will bring more information, alternatives, opinions, and creativity. This group will tend to make slower and more complex decisions. There will be less complacency and a greater drive for innovative solutions.

Set the Setting

Although the perfect meeting environment will not guarantee a successful meeting, an uncomfortable room that is hot, stuffy, noisy, and overly dark will guarantee failure. The following physical characteristics are important to consider.

Room Size. Choose a room that corresponds to the group's size. A small group in a very large room will create separation and distance between individuals.[1,9] Less communication will decrease the attention and focus on the issue, and the group will lose cohesiveness. A very small room with too few seats will quickly get hot, stuffy, and oppressive, squelching meaningful discussion.

Room Aesthetics. Dissention is more likely to occur when people are crowded into an unattractive room for a prolonged period. Poor aesthetics can produce monotony, irritability, fatigue, and hostility. A red room becomes unpleasant over a brief period of time. Lighter shades of blue and green are the most relaxing and conducive to successful group communication or "relaxed concentration."[1,14]

Consider the environment. The room should be attractive, clean, well ventilated, well lit, with an unobstructed view of the presenters and audiovisuals. Acoustics should be adequate and the temperature comfortable. The environment is rarely considered by meeting attendees unless there is a problem.

Refreshments may be appropriate. The meeting should make everybody feel nourished. "Breaking bread" creates a more cohesive group.

Seat for Success.[1,5,14] Seating configuration and room arrangement will dramatically influence the success of your meeting. The more formal classroom style limits interaction, whereas the more circular arrangements encourage it. You may wish to limit interaction in a meeting whose intent is to transmit information to a large group, such as a lecture or training seminar (Figure 11-1).

If your meeting involves fewer people (i.e., 7 to 15), and your goal is problem solving or decision making, consider a more decentralized seating arrangement (Figures 11-2 and 11-3). These groupings enhance group interaction. They are particularly suitable for meetings dealing with complex issues that require careful deliberation.

Maximum interaction occurs in circular arrangement. The leader loses the position of power, and the other members will feel equally powerful. Here, the risk is that there will be more frustrating disagreements. However, because satisfaction with decisions generally is based on participation, participants will tend to be more satisfied with and confident

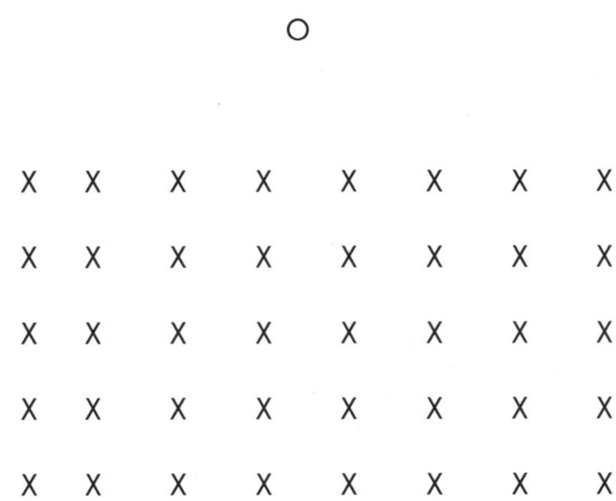

FIGURE 11-1 Formal classroom style seating used for information transmission. This style limits interaction.

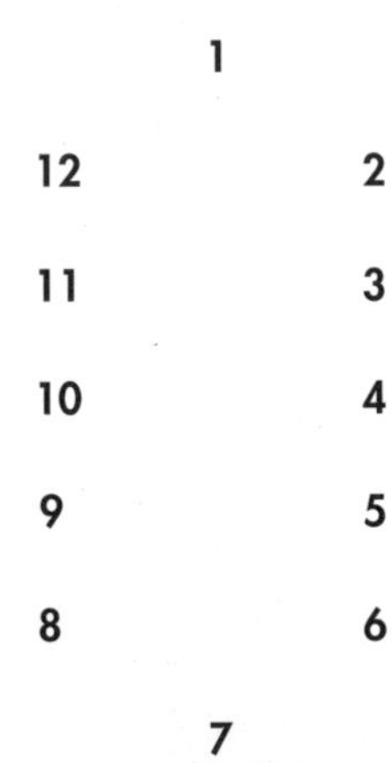

FIGURE 11-2 Rectangular table encourages limited interation and creates positions of dominance.

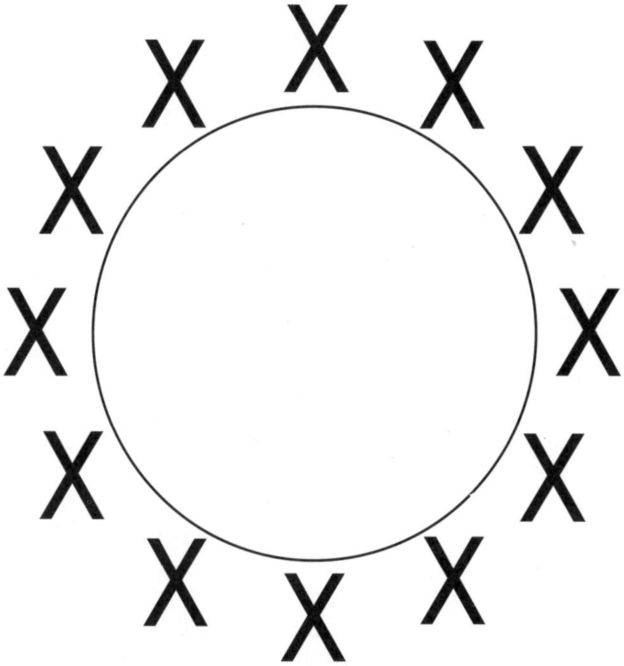

FIGURE 11-3 Circular table is decentralized style that creates maximum interaction and involvement, but limits control and eliminates positions of dominance.

about the solutions. The solutions will tend to be more detailed and contain fewer errors.

Positions of Power and Weakness. The positions of the group members in a noncircular seating arrangement will significantly influence their participation and control of the meeting (see Figure 11-2).

POSITIONS OF DOMINANCE. The head of the table[1,7] is the most dominant position. Leaders tend to sit at the head of the table (i.e., the short end of a rectangular table); therefore the people who sit at the head of the table tend to emerge as leaders. Sitting at the head of a table focuses attention on this visible position. It is easy to hear and be heard, to see and be seen.

POSITIONS OF NONDOMINANCE. Corner and Middle Seats[2-6,8-11] are the nondominant positions. Corner sitters tend to be inactive. Leaders who sit in a corner focus attention away from themselves and toward those sitting at the end. Tension may be evident when the leader sits in a position of nondominance. Sitting in the middle of the long side of a table will limit visibility and communication, particularly with those facing the same direction.

Strategic Placement of Group Members.[1,14] It may be possible to place members of the group to create the most favorable interaction. Any manipulation of seating must occur before the meeting actually begins. Methods include setting place cards, inviting a particular member to sit next to you, or having an ally invite someone to sit beside them. Specific placement strategies may include the following:

- Overly talkative members may be placed in a corner (i.e., position 2 or 8). This will minimize their interaction.
- Withdrawn members may be placed at the other end (head) of the table (i.e., position 7). This placement encourages participation, and the withdrawn member may emerge as more of a leader.
- Argumentative members should be placed apart but facing the same direction (i.e., positions 2 and 5). This limits conflict by limiting proximity and visual confrontation.
- A powerful opponent should be encouraged to sit next to the chair (i.e., position 2 or 12) and separated from his or her support system. Given the choice, adversaries tend to sit across from each other and surround themselves with their supporters. Note how frequently this occurs in a negotiation.

Inner Versus Outer Circle. A member who sits outside the inner circle will generally feel excluded; a member who sits in the inner circle will tend to participate more actively in the discussion. When attending lectures, many choose the front of the room because it encourages a sense of involvement and allows direct access to the speaker. The back of a room discourages involvement and allows the attendee to focus attention on other issues.

RUNNING THE MEETING

A poorly run meeting is like a poorly run resuscitation. No one is in charge and everyone present feels that things are out of control. Whether or not the desired outcome is achieved, everyone involved will believe the situation should have gone better.

Why are meetings so bad—why do they fall short? A study of business managers reveals that 78% have no formal training in running meetings.[2,18] This percentage is much higher for healthcare workers. As much as half of our nonclinical time is spent in meetings led by people who have no formal training. In what other field would professionals allow themselves to be consistently led or advised by someone with no formal training?

Setting the Tone

Take ownership of the meeting. The conduct of the chair determines the extent to which the committee will reach its potential.

As the leader, you must set the tone. Establish credibility. Arrive early and sit at the head of the table. Posture, confidence, and enthusiasm all influence the members of the group. If the chair is businesslike, committed, and task-oriented, the group members will actively participate. If the chair is lackadaisical and lacks focus, aimless discourse is the result. If the chair tells too many jokes, grandstands, or is confused, it will be contagious.

Skillful Guidance. Leadership is the ability to exert interpersonal influence. The chair should be seen as a type of stage director, bringing out the opinions and information, rallying the forces, channeling ideas into meaningful conclusions, and moving deliberately to the next issue.

Participation of the chair depends on the type of meeting. If the purpose of the meeting is to disseminate information, and the chair is the person with the greatest knowledge or expertise, the chair will do the most talking. However, if the meeting is intended as a problem-solving meeting, the participation of the chair should be limited. The chair should encourage the expression of all the opinions and generally refrain from advocating any particular viewpoint.

The rest of this discussion refers primarily to problem-solving meetings.

Chair's Opinion.[2] The chair's responsibility is to ascertain the group's resolve rather than imposing his or her own. Achieving this goal requires effective listening and keen attention.

RULE: The role of the chair is not to accomplish his or her goals, but to encourage the committee to recognize common goals and implement them. Accomplishing the goals should be the focus, not the leader.

The chair should advocate an opinion only after carefully listening to the opinions of others. This strategy allows other viewpoints to be heard and relevant concepts to be incorporated. The chair assumes a risk by advocating a particular solution. A chair who strongly feels one solution is best loses objectivity and is unable to be an effective facilitator.

On occasion, a particular decision of great importance may appear to have only one satisfactory solution. If this is the case, the method by which this issue should be resolved is by pre-meeting "jawboning." Do your homework. Solve the problem in advance. Take a stand only when the outcome is assured.

Managing Air Time

It is the charge of the chair to guide the discussion to a meaningful conclusion. This responsibility often requires active management of who speaks, as well as when and for how long they speak. There are many methods to control and limit the discussion on a topic.

Start and stop on time or even earlier. The chair should stress promptness. Late members shift the focus of the meeting from the topic being discussed and often require members to reexamine information or decisions that have already been addressed.

Limit time on the topic. Time limits, set in advance, will help govern the discussion. Within reason, adhere to those limits. This discourages rambling. When a topic requires more time than originally thought, seek group agreement to extend the time on this topic in exchange for decreasing time on another. Time limits for individual members may be necessary when there are a large number of people who would like to speak, the topic is controversial, or there are domineering members of the group.

Sequence discussants to provide order. It may be expedient for the chair to exercise control over who will speak next. Ask people to raise their hands, silently recognize them, and call them in order. Between discussants, state the sequence of speakers. This method lets members know that they will get their chance to speak. It allows them to attend to the discussion rather than focus their concentration on working their way into it.

Do not allow two members to maintain a back-and-forth debate when others would like to have their opinions heard. Simply state that others would like an opportunity to discuss the topic and describe the order of the next speakers. This process reminds the members that the chair will control the discussion.

Resolve issues in advance that do not require discussion in the meeting. Do not waste everybody's valuable time trying to determine information that may be obtained before the meeting. Assign a member in advance to provide materials or a list of possible solutions to a problem that does not require the group's deliberation.

Facilitating and Focusing the Discussion

The chair is a type of gatekeeper, encouraging pertinent discussion and curbing unnecessary input. The group must be guided to an end point, a decision. When the discussion is poorly focused, the chair must adhere to an orderly sequence of problem-solving steps (see Problem-Solving Techniques).

In a survey of 1000 business people from 3M and Unysis, the three most common problems cited in meetings were getting off the subject, not having clear goals or agenda, and meeting for too long.[19]

Wandering is considered the most common problem in meetings. The participants don't believe it is their responsibility to direct the discussion, and the group leader may not want to be overbearing. Participants become frustrated when they find the discussion is on the third tier of digression and someone is telling an anecdote.

It is the chair's responsibility to carefully monitor the discussion and focus the group's attention on the same issue. The chair must continue to silently pose the questions: "What are we talking about now?" "Is this relevant?" "Will this discussion move us toward resolution?" If not, "How can I refocus the discussion without stepping on the speaker?" This may be done by periodically summarizing the discussion and reflecting on its relationship to the agenda item.

Digressions may be dealt with by one of several methods. Subsequent agenda items should be noted as such with a commitment to deal with the issue later. Unrelated items should be recognized as important but not for the day's agenda. If this approach is unsatisfactory, the chair may offer to review the topic personally at another time or at the end of the agenda if time permits.

Drifting discussion requires refocusing by the chair. The better known or weaker the participants, the more easily refocusing is accomplished. The movement requires a balancing of discipline and sensitivity. It is crucial to maintain an awareness of the feelings of the participants.

Lack of clearly stated agenda/goals creates confusion. Establish a clear direction from the outset and adhere to it. Present a brief review of the agenda. Begin each topic with a concise presentation of the decision to be made (i.e., an orientation of the goals). Describe the method by which the goal will be reached. It may be helpful to provide an impartial review of the alternatives. Describing and following an intended order of discussion will help members stay on track while discouraging digression.

Closing the Discussion

Poor closure is a frequent problem of inexperienced group leaders. The discussion starts late, wanders without progress, and runs beyond the scheduled time. There are several common misconceptions regarding the closure of a discussion.

"The discussion must go on until everybody has said as much as they want to on the topic." Group input is critical. Yet it is not necessary for each member to participate in a limitless discussion. The chair is responsible for determining when the discussion has gone on long enough. This may occur when no new concepts are being presented or when the group appears to have reached consensus.

"Everyone must agree." Although it is preferable to reach unanimity of the group, it may not be possible. When the

chair recognizes that the sentiments of the individual members are established, it is time to conclude the discussion. The chair should then summarize the information and seek general consensus. Decisions made by consensus are preferable to those made by vote. It encourages the support of members who may be responsible for implementation.

"We must decide all of the details now." Determining the fine points may unnecessarily prolong a meeting. The specific components of a decision often are developed best in a subcommittee or by an individual who is responsible for the implementation.

When a stated goal of the agenda is met, conclude the segment with a summary of what has been decided. Describe the conclusion, assignments, and implementation method. Then move on to the next topic.

Bringing the Meeting to a Close (Box 11-5)

Ending the meeting well is as important as beginning it and running it. End the meeting when decisions are made, there is no new information, or the issues left can better be dealt with by subcommittee. Give everyone a brief opportunity to voice some final words. This technique allows members to voice an issue important to them when there may not have been a prior opportunity.

Summarize. Allot time on the agenda to summarize what has been accomplished. Review the meeting highlights. Compare the decisions to the goals. Praise the group and acknowledge their contributions. Always try to end on a positive note.

Clarify Responsibilities. Define what is to be done and by whom. Clarify actions that members have agreed to take and gain commitment for their completion. Set realistic deadlines for actions. It is often helpful to establish an agreed upon time frame for completion of each task. Each participant should leave with a clear understanding of his or her responsibilities.

Schedule Next Meeting. If a follow-up meeting is required, it may be appropriate to schedule it before adjourning, since all of the essential members may be together. This strategy will assist members to develop a commitment to the deadlines. An exception to this approach exists when the time frame for task completion cannot be determined in advance. Then, a general time frame and a mechanism for contacting members should be established.

Distribute the Minutes

The purposes of meeting minutes are to document what has occurred and remind participants of what is to be done. The minutes should enumerate the agreed upon actions, deadlines, and individuals responsible for completion of the actions. The chair is responsible for creating the minutes in a way that accurately reflects the essential elements of the meeting.

BOX 11-5

CLOSING THE MEETING

1. End on time
2. Summarize
3. Assign tasks
4. Schedule next meeting

Minutes should be distributed quickly. It is appropriate for the chair to communicate occasionally with the meeting members to check their progress on completing actions.

PROBLEM-SOLVING TECHNIQUES

Decisions involving a group are generally better and more satisfactory than decisions made by an individual. Group decisions also generate unity and cooperation, enhance communication, and develop commitment. A variety of problem-solving methods incorporate the advantages of the group participation in the decision-making process.

All of the problem-solving techniques have in common an orderly sequence of problem-solving steps:

- Identify problem
- Describe facts
- Determine alternatives
- Choose best solution
- Determine implementation method

This chapter reviews two problem-solving methods.

Brainstorming

Brainstorming is a simple, effective, easy-to-use method of problem solving that has broad application. Its value is derived from incorporating the creativity of groups and deferring to the judgment of individuals. Brainstorming encourages the group perspective and reduces personal bias. The steps of brainstorming are the following:

1. *State problem*—Determine the specific issue to be resolved by the group. Gain commitment from the group to focus on solving the problem. Describe the process and set time limits. Encourage a positive approach.
2. *Generate solutions*—Call for ideas, suggestions, and solutions from the committee members. Encourage each participant to say whatever comes to mind, no matter how well thought out. A nonthreatening environment in which each member feels free to express his or her ideas without fear of ridicule or criticism will engender the greatest creativity. There are no "bad ideas" or "wrong opinions." List each contribution. A structured exploration of ideas may follow.
3. *Develop criteria*—This important step provides a bridge between the generation and selection of solutions. It encourages the group to examine individual and group values. Agree on the standards against which the alternative solutions will be judged. This step may be difficult and may require thorough examination. Once the group agrees on acceptable criteria, selection of the solutions is easy.
4. *Compare alternatives to criteria*—Discuss each option in terms of the criteria developed by the group. Solutions that don't meet the most important criteria may be eliminated or receive a low ranking. Allow a consensus to emerge.
5. *Identify the agreed upon consensus*—When the group has reached consensus, the facilitator should review the group's decision. Test understanding and agreement, ask for commitment, and develop the implementation steps.

The Nominal Group Technique

The nominal group technique is an increasingly popular method of solving complex and controversial issues in a group format. This technique involves each participant and maintains confidentiality in decision making. The group gath-

ers in a room, and the facilitator poses the question and leads the group through the following six steps:

1. *Develop individual answers*—Each member of the nominal group develops solutions to the problem. These are written on paper for later reference and discussion.
2. *Compile group's solutions*—The facilitator asks each individual to contribute one idea at a time and then records each on a visible medium such as a flip chart or overhead projector. This process continues until all ideas are presented.
3. *Clarify each idea*—Each idea is reviewed. The facilitator and members of the group ask for explanations and clarifications.
4. *Take preliminary vote*—Each individual prioritizes and ranks the solutions. Then an anonymous vote of the group is taken to determine which alternatives are considered the best by the group.
5. *Discuss differences of opinion*—The initial ranking compiled by the group vote is discussed. Major discrepancies are examined to ensure each member clearly understands the information.
6. *Select preferred solution*—After the discussion is completed, members again prioritize their solutions. A final anonymous vote is taken and a solution chosen.

HANDLING AN IMPASSE

Problem-solving meetings depend simultaneously on active participation of the members and controlled flow of the discussion. However, some members may be too active and others may refuse to participate. It may be difficult to guide the discussion when members do not recognize their responsibility to participate in the decision-making process.

Although the leader is responsible for facilitating the discussion, he or she is not totally responsible for the success or failure of the meeting. This misconception places an unreasonable burden on the chair and sets up an antagonistic relationship between the chair and group members.

Dealing with Difficult People

Good group leaders have highly evolved interpersonal skills. They can balance the human need to participate with the group desire to control direction and input. It is necessary to withhold judgment so that potentially valuable participation and group creativity will not be stifled. Simultaneously, the leader must limit and guide the discussion to move it to conclusion.

Emotion. The expression of feeling may be discouraged by some group leaders because they fear the exposure of too much emotion. They may be concerned that emotional expressions will damage relationships and distract the problem-solving process. Alternatively, they may believe that the meeting can be a success only if everybody is affable and friendly. This approach creates a public relations event, not a decision-making meeting.

Exposure of true emotion may harm relationships, but is more likely to result in meaningful decisions. Emotional responses to issues should not lead the chair to panic but rather should be tolerated. In fact, the chair would be well advised to express gratitude for the display of concern about such an important issue.

Personalized emotional reactions directed toward an individual, on the other hand, should not be tolerated. Immediately, restore order by saying "This is not the forum for this particular discussion. Let's focus on the issue." This is an opportunity to refocus the discussion by providing an objective summary of the issue and the decisions that have been made.

Dominator. The person who does the most talking usually feels as though the most was accomplished. The dominator tends to monopolize the discussion at the exclusion of the other participants.[20] Dominators can appear in several forms. They may be very talkative, self-appointed experts, or an angry person with an ax to grind. The common characteristic is the desire to talk without listening; many want to run the meeting. Do not allow a member to inhibit group creativity by running the meeting into the ground.

The dominator is usually a valuable participant and should not be totally silenced. Doing nothing may allow the meeting to spiral out of control. Alternatively, a head-to-head confrontation may create an intolerable conflict. At best, the meeting becomes a spectacle; at worst, the chair will lose. In either case, many good ideas may be stifled and everyone present will be uncomfortable.

There are many more subtle and successful methods for dealing with the dominator. Arrange the seating to put the dominator in a less powerful position, such as a corner next to the chair. This positioning decreases the visibility and influence of the dominator on the rest of the group. Impose structure by obtaining group agreement to limit discussion by each individual to a certain length of time. Duly note what is said, and address the discussion to others by asking what they think. Maintain the focus of the discussion toward the chair; do not allow the dominator to be the focus.

Less subtle body language may be successful. Putting an open palm out, signaling "stop," will usually quiet the speaker. Standing will draw attention directly to the chair and away from the dominator.

If it is still difficult to control the dominator, take a break, and use the time to talk directly to this person. Explain the value of the group process and of allowing other, quieter participants to speak.

Silent Members. Even in the most participatory meetings, one or more members may not be actively engaged in the discussion. This may occur because the member(s) is shy or feels inhibited by more dominant members. To gain the greatest value of the group process, it is important for the leader to recognize the inactive members and encourage their input.

Avoid calling attention to silence as a means of changing it. Do not make a joke at the expense of a quieter member. Although perhaps well meaning, these techniques will discourage participation.

To encourage silent members, seat them in a power position such as the end of the table. Bring them out without a threat by asking a simple, direct question. Allow early and easy success by responding supportively and integrating their reply into discussion.

Handling Difficult Situations

Emotion, disagreement, and conflict in moderation may result in the most creative, well thought out decisions. However, when tempers rise and anger threatens the success of the meeting, the chair must take decisive action without be-

coming embroiled in the conflict. The only thing worse than watching a meeting deteriorate around you is participating in the destruction. The worst response is anger. It may relieve your tension, but it will add to everyone else's.

Focus on Issues. Frequently, the disagreeing members will have adopted different positions on the same issue. In an attempt to defend their position, the members may become contentious. This situation can usually be resolved simply by refocusing the discussion on the issue.

Process Checks. When the chair feels out of control of the process and recognizes that the discussion is wandering, several methods may be used to bring the meeting back into focus. The chair may ask a particularly rational member, "What do you think is happening?" This technique will usually bring the group's attention to the new speaker while the chair takes the opportunity to regain focus and control.

If the discussion is off track and both the chair and members seem confused, the chair might state, "We are clearly off track and moving in different directions. Does anybody have an idea of how to get back on track?" This usually works because the members all concentrate their attention toward reestablishing an orderly discussion.

Another successful technique is simply "taking a break." During the recess, the chair has an opportunity to gain composure, establish control over dominators, discuss methods of moving forward, and enlist support from group members.

SUMMARY

Meetings are conducted by, attended by, and intended for people. In the setting of a meeting, it is necessary to remember the basic needs of the participants. They need to participate in a meeting that:

- Is in a comfortable environment
- Values and appreciates its members
- Provides an orderly approach to issues (agenda)
- Uses time efficiently
- Accomplishes its tasks during and after the meeting

If you attend to the needs of the participants in a concerned and professional manner, your meetings can go far beyond the ordinary.

REFERENCES

1. Doyle M, Straus D: *How to make meetings work,* New York, 1982, Jove Publications/The Berkley Publishing Group.
2. Woods RH, Berger R: Making meetings work, *Cornell Hotel Restaur Adm Q* 29:100-106, 1988.
3. Tobia PM, Becker MC: Making the most of meeting time, *Train Dev J* 44:34-38, 1990.
4. Wakin E: Make meetings meaningful, *Today's Office* 25:68-69, 1991.
5. Ashenbrenner G: Planning effective meetings, *Business Credit* 90:43-46, 1988.
6. Bailey J: The fine art of leading a meeting, *Working Woman,* 12:68-70,103, 1987.
7. Blanchard K: Meetings that work, *Today's Office,* 22:9-11, 1987.
8. Zaremba A: Meetings and frustration, *Supervision* 49:7-9, 1988.
9. Michaels EA: Business meetings, *Small Business Reports* 14:82-88, 1989.
10. Clayton CK: A blueprint for productive meetings, *AGRI Marketing,* 29:70-76, 1991.
11. Strauss R, DeHart D: Medical staff interrelationships and clinical responsibilities. In Strauss R, editor: *In contracts: a practical guide to emergency physicians,* Dallas, 1990, ACEP.
12. Strauss R, DeHart D: Administrative responsibilities. In Strauss R, editor: *In contracts: a practical guide to emergency physicians,* Dallas, 1990, ACEP.
13. Cathcart J: How to plan a meeting, *Marketing Communications,* 12:82-83, 1987.
14. Linkemer B: *How to run a meeting,* New York, 1987, AMACOM.
15. Frank MO: *How to run a successful meeting in half the time,* New York, 1989, Pocket Books.
16. 3M: *How to run better business meetings: a referency guide for managers,* New York, 1987, McGraw-Hill.
17. Janis I: Victims of group think, Boston, 1972, Houghton-Mifflin.
18. Sigband N: Meeting with success, *Personnel Journal* 48-55, 1985.
19. Mosvick R, Nelson R: *We've got to start meeting like this!,* Glenview Ill, 1987, Scott Foresman.
20. Bean GJ: Don't let a dominator spoil the meeting for everyone, *Marketing Communications* 22:6, 1989.

SUGGESTED READINGS

Adler M: *How to speak, how to listen,* New York, 1985, MacMillan.

Bean GJ: Don't let a dominator spoil the meeting for everyone, *Marketing Communications* 22:6, 1989.

Blanchard K, Lorber R: *Putting the one minute manager to work,* New York, 1984, Berkley Publishing Group.

Brian LA: Toward more effective committee meetings, *Professional Safety* 36:28-31, 1991.

Crosby PB: *Running things: The art of making things happen,* New York, 1986, Plume Books/New American Library.

Drew J, *3M meeting management team: mastering meetings,* New York, 1994, McGraw-Hill.

Howard VA, Barton JH: *Thinking together: making meetings work,* New York, 1992, Quill/William Morrow.

Kieffer GD: Meetings of the mindless, *Across the Board,* 25:6-8, 1988.

Weiss DH: *How to deal with difficult people,* New York, 1987, AMACOM.

12 Emergency Department Interaction with Hospital Governance

William S. Tennant, Lloyd M. DeBoer, Stephen Cumbie, Richard M. Knapp, and Thom A. Mayer

OUTLINE

Governance of a hospital or healthcare system refers to the structure by which the multiple operating units of the present-day hospital and healthcare system are responsive to the entity or entities that retain the responsibility for quality, fiscal viability, and strategic direction of the organization and its ultimate role in the community. Although hospital administration and management are responsible for the day-to-day operations and implementation of the strategic direction of the institution, the board remains the entity to whom hospital management and the medical staff report on an ongoing basis. Although the specific structure of boards varies, virtually all healthcare institutions currently have a well-defined process by which all of the operations of the institution and its medical staff report their collective findings and recommendations to their parent board. This includes medical staff credentialing, quality improvement activities, promulgation of mission/vision statements, deployment of resources, and financial management. A careful reading of medical staff bylaws, rules and regulations, and administrative policies makes it clear that the ultimate source of governance for modern healthcare institutions is the healthcare system board.[1]

In this sense, the board acts as one of the four sides of successful emergency department practice (Figure 12-1), which also includes administration, the medical staff, and the patient/community. In many ways an understanding of the governance function of the board is the foundation on which the successful long-term practice of emergency medicine can be built. Yet many emergency physicians do not have a clear sense of the meaning of hospital governance and the critical role the board plays.

The chapter discusses the composition, purpose, and goals and objectives of typical healthcare boards; the changing nature of boards; the role of physician leaders in interacting with the governance structure; and the specific nature of the interrelation of emergency physicians with the board.

COMPOSITION, PURPOSE, GOALS, AND OBJECTIVES OF TYPICAL HEALTHCARE BOARDS

To begin to understand governance structures, it is necessary to ask the "Who, What, Why, and How" of such organizations. The "Who" describes the typical composition of a healthcare board. As recently as the last 10 years, boards often were composed of a group of self-perpetuating "pillars of the community," including community leaders and wealthy donors. Over time, potential new members of the board began to be nominated by organizations with substantial, and in some cases vested, interest in the operations of the institution. For example, it has recently become common for medical staff members to have either voting or ex officio seats on the board (often the president of the medical staff, members nominated by the county medical society, or, less commonly, members nominated from medical specialty groups). Similarly, community organizations, state or local governments, or citizen's groups have recently had a larger role in nominations to the board. However, as governance restructuring has attempted to streamline boards by consolidating functions, membership has been based much more commonly on qualifications tailored to the particular needs of the board in its deliberations.

In most cases, selection of board members is based on a combination of factors, including diversity of membership, community involvement, trust and expertise in healthcare, commitment, and ability to articulate the perspective of the organization, interest groups, or area of expertise that the board member represents. Because of the increasing consolidation of governance structures (see the following discussion), participating on boards represents a substantial time investment, particularly when board meetings, committees, and subcommittees are taken into account. It is unusual for boards to retain token membership from any groups that are not able to be represented on an ongoing basis by members who are able to bring continuity to the proceedings of the governance structure.

In its simplest terms, the "What" of boards is that they are responsible for overseeing the operations of the entire healthcare facility and are ultimately accountable for all of the assets that have been entrusted to that healthcare organization. *It is the job of the board to ask the extraordinarily difficult questions of how scarce resources will be deployed in an increasingly competitive environment, how relationships between hospitals and physicians will be structured, and where the organization should place its emphasis in helping to devise a reasonable healthcare structure that will serve both the organization and the community both now and in the fu-*

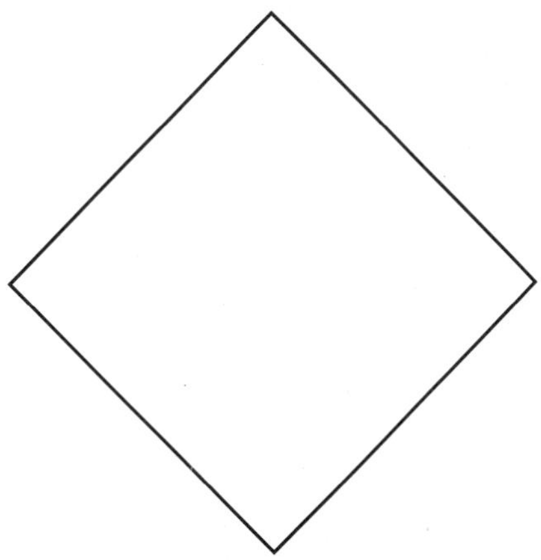

FIGURE 12-1 The healthcare system board is one of the four sides of a successful emergency department practice. All four sides must be addressed in an ongoing fashion.

ture. Box 12-1 lists typical specific functions for boards in healthcare institutions.

The "Why" of governance can be answered from the perspective of both the board itself and the healthcare system and the community. From the perspective of the community, it is necessary to have an oversight organization that is able to maintain accountability for the extraordinarily large amount of resources that any hospital requires to function. Even the smallest of hospitals accounts for millions of dollars in operating budgets and must maintain reasonable accountability to the public it serves. Even in proprietary hospital settings, in most cases the board has been structured to help ensure that such local accountability is addressed. From the perspective of the members of the boards themselves, most of them serve for a number of reasons including community service, a desire to give something back to the community, professional stimulation, and the enjoyment of participating in the growth of substantial local resources. The Greek word *koinonia,* which means a deep and abiding sense of community commitment, might best describe the primary reason that board members serve.

The typical board therefore usually consists of a combination of leaders of the community, including attorneys, physicians, elected officials, and representatives from business and education. Most healthcare boards are selected and maintained to ensure that there is application of broad areas of diversity of membership, which give both specific areas of expertise and substantial perspective to the deliberations of the board. As the source of ultimate accountability for the assets entrusted to it, the board's deliberations increasingly focus on the *wise use of assets*. The use of capital has received particular focus as that healthcare commodity has become increasingly scarce.

One of the most important functions of the board is to ask critical questions about operations, structure, and deployment of resources. As Elie Wiesel once observed, "The fundamental injustice of the human situation is that the most difficult questions are those that are least often asked."[2] It is precisely those difficult and fundamental questions that the board must have both the diversity and the commitment not only to ask, but also to ensure that appropriate answers are given. The ability to frame these fundamental questions in the right dimensions is essential to a well-functioning board.

BOX 12-1

PRIMARY FUNCTIONS FOR WHICH HEALTHCARE BOARDS ARE RESPONSIBLE (SPECIFIC FUNCTIONS WILL VARY FROM INSTITUTION TO INSTITUTION.)

- Strategic planning
- Strategic financial decision making
- Financial performance
- Governance
- Management compensation
- CEO selection and performance
- System operational performance
- Partnerships and affiliations
- Fundraising
- Quality improvement
- Compliance with accreditation/licensure requirements
- Community health improvement planning
- Prevention and health promotion planning
- Community relations interface
- Education and research policy/planning

CHANGING NATURE OF BOARDS

Few areas in society are changing as rapidly as healthcare. As what we do and how we do it changes, healthcare's structure evolves into new, challenging, but exciting directions. The structure of governance is also changing to meet the needs of the organization and the community it serves. A recent governance benchmarking study identified several trends among the systems studied, including changes toward the following areas:[3]

- Fewer governance layers
- Evolution of smaller boards and composition based on expertise and utility
- Redefined roles and priorities for greater clarity
- Greater use of councils, forums, and management assignments as integrating mechanisms
- Changing approaches to physician participation
- Consolidation of committees, clarification of charters
- Focus on strategy, strategic finance, and system oversight

An important trend has been the consolidation of boards to create "flatter" governance and organizational structures. This consolidation has had several benefits, including the following:

- Assurance of direct involvement in overall decisions, as opposed to fragmentation.
- Putting system boards closer to the direct action of healthcare delivery (and its problems).
- Ability to respond sooner to radical changes in the healthcare environment (e.g., from fee-for-service to capitation).
- More streamlined decision-making capacity.

As the healthcare environment has continued to change, many organizations have found that operating with multiple boards or levels of governance has become cumbersome, costly, difficult, and constraining. The problems facing healthcare organizations are many and include the need to focus on community health status, the requirement for streamlining and reducing costs (often involving downsizing), discovering new partnerships with physicians, moving to "covered lives" as a core business, increasing the role for primary care and preventive services, ensuring the ability to increase speed in product development, and a fundamental shift from operational to strategic knowledge and expertise as a core capacity.

All of these factors augur substantial and substantive changes in governance structure toward a flatter, more lean and efficient board structure that helps put trustees fundamentally closer to the organization's efforts to adapt rapidly, but intelligently to the changing healthcare market.

THE ROLE OF PHYSICIAN LEADERS IN INTERACTION WITH THE GOVERNANCE STRUCTURE

Not too long ago, common wisdom held that a physician need only practice good medicine to be successful. Although it is questionable whether that old saw was ever accurate, management skills are now considered to be essential to the successful practice of medicine, particularly emergency medicine. The application of sound business and management principles to the clinical practice of emergency medicine, as well as the business aspects of the specialty, has been essential to its success. Principles such as continuous quality improvement, change management, strategic planning, boundary management, and stakeholder analysis have all become a part of the day-to-day substance of the changing landscape of emergency medicine. Because hospital governance increasingly requires trustees who are articulate and expert in precisely these skills, it is important for physician leaders of the medical staff, including emergency physicians, to understand these principles and to practice them in the management of their specialty on a day-to-day basis.[4]

Healthcare boards have historically relied on articulate, experienced physician leadership to help guide the direction of the organization. Boards have often tended to put appropriate weight on the words and thoughts of physicians who could dispassionately discuss appropriate deployment of resources that best meet the needs of the institution and its patients. Unfortunately, some boards have also seen physician attitudes and behavior that could be described as narrow-minded at best and self-serving at worst. However, such physicians have tended to be in the minority, and their fellow physicians have often taken the responsibility for ensuring that a mature, balanced, and articulate perspective is given to the board from the physician community.

Members of the governance structure look to the medical staff and its physician leadership for assistance in several ways. First, and most important, board members look to some physicians to become *visionary leaders* of the medical staff, who are capable of understanding the need for change, communicating it to their fellow physicians, and helping play a substantial role in the development and implementation of change strategies. Second, physicians play an important role by virtue of their *medical expertise.* This expertise is critical in areas such as physician credentialing, acquisition and use of medical technology, and medical ethics. For example, some institutions have chosen to delegate decisions on capital budget requests to medical staff committees, which can help assess the relative need for certain technologies compared with others in the institution. Such an approach has the advantage that it allows substantial physician input, but also requires a great deal of leadership on the part of the physicians, who will be tasked with saying "No" to those budget requests that are not ranked highly enough.

A third important area is the ability to *present medical information objectively* and in a fashion that is concise, simple, yet comprehensive enough for nonphysician members of the board to understand. For example, the physician members or representatives to the board may be asked to explain why the substantial capital outlay may be necessary for three-dimensional magnetic resonance imaging equipment for tumor localization in radiation therapy in a hospital that has a substantial commitment as a cancer center. Similarly, it may be necessary to explain why substantial funding is essential for application of prehospital 12-lead electrocardiogram technology to help expand outreach and lower thrombolytic administration times in an institution with substantial commitment as a cardiac care center.

A fourth area needed from physician leaders is a sense of *organizational perspective.* Recognizing that the physician's primary duty is always to the patient, the governing board also recognizes that it is important for the physician leader to meet his or her duty to the organization and to the broader interests of all patients for which the organization cares. The financial pressure on healthcare institutions and the increasing presence of managed care represent two areas that may put substantial pressure on the physician to compromise either the interest of his practice, or that of the patients affiliated with that practice. However, a sense of organizational perspective is needed to help ensure that, whether in com-

mittees, at the executive level, or at the board level, physicians keep the best interests of the institution in mind. For example, in many states, the credentialing of podiatrists and nurse midwives is a matter of statutory compliance. If a physician is a member of the Credentials Committee, it is important that he or she responds appropriately to qualified individuals applying in these categories regardless of their personal preference or feelings about the role of such providers in the modern day healthcare institution.

A fifth area of importance for physician leaders is *consistency and constancy.* Foremost among issues of consistency is ensuring attendance at appropriate functions, particularly for physician members of the board. It is annoying for members of any committee or board to have "part-time members," particularly when other members of the committee have made the time and effort from their busy professional lives to ensure that they are available for the operations of the institution. Although most physicians are extraordinarily busy, it is important to ensure that appropriate time is budgeted for assigned meetings. When legitimate reasons arise for absences, it is important to extend the courtesy to the other members of the committee of informing them of your input on any issues to be addressed, as well as ensuring that the committee chair is aware of your absence and, where appropriate, the reasons for it.

An additional area of importance is ensuring that the physician debates issues vigorously and appropriately, but also in a fashion that allows for legitimate areas of difference. Once the discussion has been completed, however, an agreement has been reached or decisions have been made, and it is important for all members of the group to move forward as a team, supporting the collective decisions that have been reached. Physician leaders should identify areas in which real or perceived conflicts of interest arise and, where appropriate, recuse themselves from either debate or vote on the issue.

One of the most important roles of physician leaders is described by the literature on continuous quality improvement as the *Voice of the customer.* Continuous quality improvement defines a customer as anyone who is affected by the organization's processes or its products. In this regard, the physician is one of the most important internal customers of the healthcare process, and the hospital in particular. Moreover, the physician can offer an extraordinarily important perspective of one of the most important internal customers, particularly if the physician is able to dispassionately discuss the expectations of physician members from diverse backgrounds. Physicians can thus act as an important channel of communication to the board. Equally important, the physician can also ensure that appropriate information flows back to the physicians from the board level, establishing a means of ensuring that physicians are aware of the reasons for board decisions, deployment of resources, assignment of capital, etc.

Finally, as the role of the physician manager has developed, an expectation for *higher levels of management skills among physicians* has developed. Hospitals have always relied heavily on articulate and informed physician leadership to ensure that the institution continues to move forward in its goals and objectives. However, in the last several years, new talents, skills, and techniques have emerged at the physician level, which enables physicians to participate more meaningfully in management and in its interaction with the board. In many institutions, a new class of physician managers has developed at numerous operational levels, as well as at the top levels of management in some institutions. The use of many of the skills described in this book, including boundary management, negotiation techniques, strategic planning principles, continuous quality improvement, outcomes of management, and financial management, have all been important contributions to physicians' understanding of hospital operations.

RELATION OF EMERGENCY PHYSICIANS TO THE BOARD

One of the most essential features that both the board and administration look for from an emergency department group is the degree to which the emergency department physician group is able to identify the needs of the community and respond to them. The board also looks to the emergency department for substantial expertise not only in the clinical management of patients, but also in the operational management of the substantial resources required to meet those clinical needs. In all but the most rare circumstances, emergency physician groups have a captive audience, inasmuch as they are awarded exclusive contracts to evaluate and treat all patients in the emergency department (with the exception of those that the medical staff chooses to evaluate). With such exclusive contracts comes the need to offer an extremely high level of clinical service and management expertise.

Virtually all quality healthcare institutions have the *expectation* that quality of medical care is assumed. If the emergency physicians and nurses were not good practitioners, they would not be in the institution to begin with. In this regard, the board and management are looking for "Quality Plus," which simply means expertise above and beyond meeting the diverse clinical needs of the patients presenting to the emergency department. In addition, the management expertise to move the department forward toward its goals is also an essential expectation.

Other expectations from the board are a substantial capacity for change and adaptation. The modern healthcare system must anticipate the direction, magnitude, and pace of change in a multitude of different areas and requires that the emergency physician management team be able to respond in a similar fashion. Among the many skills required of the emergency physician group, one of the more important is *change management* (see Chapter 13).

A strong corollary to this capacity for change is a deep level of commitment to the institution. The board looks to all contract physicians including emergency physicians to have goals and objectives that are consonant with those of the organization overall. Although this statement is easy to make, its implications can be far reaching and yet quite subtle. For example, one of the goals of many healthcare institutions is to operate as a vertically integrated healthcare institution with substantial penetration in managed care, including control of specified numbers of covered lives within certain time frames. If the emergency department group operates on a historical fee-for-service basis and fails to participate in negotiated contracts with managed care providers,

the group may face serious questions with regard to its consistency with the overall objectives of the organization. This does not imply that emergency department physician groups should not expect reasonable compensation from managed care providers, and participate actively in negotiating such contracts; it simply recognizes the fact that it is important to do so in such a fashion that meets the institution's overall goals.

The interaction between the board and the emergency physician group should always be cooperative, collegial, and consonant with the objectives of the organization. It is extremely rare for hospital governance to want contract groups that are subservient, or less than full, active, and respected members of the medical staff. Instead, the board looks to its emergency physicians for guidance with regard to the role of the emergency department in achieving the organization's stated aims, caring appropriately for its patients, and participating in the dialogue about the strategic direction in which the organization will move.

Board members also have a fiduciary duty to the community at large to administer the assets with which they have been entrusted in the most effective, efficient, and responsible manner possible. At times, this may lead to economic tensions between the hospital entity or system on the one hand and individual physicians or groups on the other. From the perspective of governance, trustees and boards must make hard decisions in the ensuing months and years that may have adverse economic implications for physicians. Thus the existence of collegial relationships between board members and physicians should not be expected to prevent board members from making the hard decisions that relate to capitated care or other managed care initiatives. Simply stated, the board members' collective duty is to the community and institution it serves, and not specifically to physicians' economic interest.

Although it is unusual for the board to participate actively in the renegotiation of contracts with physicians, it is quite likely that the expectations of the board and management with regard to contract services will increase, particularly as managed care relationships become more common. As these changes occur, standardization of contracts, performance reviews, and contractual aspects with department chair are likely to become commonplace.

ADVICE FOR PHYSICIAN LEADERS

Physician leaders should address several specific aspects with the board. First, it is important to understand the role of the board and the institution in which the physician leader works. By contacting the administrator or the chair of the board, the physician can obtain written description of the role of the board within the institution and usually the overall strategic plan for the institution. Familiarity with how the board operates, its composition, and the strategic objectives of the organization is critical for all physicians to understand. Second, it is important to gain an understanding of how physician leaders can interact with the board and administration in enhancing the mission of the organization, accomplishing its stated purposes, and participating meaningfully in the organization's endeavors. Participation by members of the emergency department group in the hospital medical staff committee structure is an important first step in ensuring that all members of the group are commited to the institution.

Third, it is important for the leadership of the medical staff and the emergency department to get to know the members of the board. Although virtually all board members are extremely busy, most are willing to meet concerned members of the medical staff and discuss appropriate matters. Meetings should be scheduled to accommodate the board member's agenda, and most of them appreciate having some sense of what the substance of the meeting will be about. Most board members genuinely appreciate the opportunity to express their opinion about how the emergency department group can best fit the needs of the hospital, particularly as it relates to the overall strategic plan of the institution. Such meetings are an excellent opportunity for leaders of the emergency department to communicate to board members the philosophy of patient care commitment inherent in the emergency department physician group, as well as the substantial "safety net" that the department offers to the community at large.

During the course of meetings with members of the board, and in dealing with the board overall, it is imperative to establish a relationship of trust, cooperation, communication, and integrity. It is important to communicate an unwavering commitment to the institution and its strategic objectives to the board members and administration. In the past, some physician leaders have used their relationship with board members to help lobby either for commitments to areas that would result in financial gain for the physicians, or for development of individual physician's "pet projects" that are before the board for consideration. Although educating the board with regard to the unique perspective of emergency medicine is appropriate, caution should be undertaken whenever personal, professional, and financial objectives begin to coalesce to any substantial degree. If any potential conflict of interest develops, it is important to acknowledge such conflicts clearly and openly.

It is also important to use interaction with members of the board to understand how emergency department operations fit the overall strategic objectives of the institution. The board has a unique perspective with regard to the institution's resources, commitments, and its vision for the future. Interaction with board members and with the board as a whole can be invaluable in helping members of the emergency department team understand the direction in which the organization is headed and the emergency department's role within that plan.

Finally, it is important for emergency physicians to be clear to members of the management team and the board that the emergency physicians are committed to the organization and are willing to adapt, change, and facilitate the transition from our current state of healthcare delivery to the healthcare institution of the next century. This capacity to work as team members within the framework of a broader, more overarching goal occurs daily in the clinical delivery of care in the emergency department. Applying this principle to interactions with the board is a natural step toward the growth and development of the emergency department as a critical aspect of the institution's future.

Perhaps most important, interactions with members of the

board can be extraordinarily enriching to a physician, both personally and professionally. Board members' backgrounds represent a diverse and rich resource for any physician who takes the time and effort to engage them in constructive dialogue. The perspective they bring to an understanding of healthcare's role in the community is truly invaluable and is certainly worth the investment of time, energy, and effort to help ensure development of a strong and positive relationship between the emergency department and the board.

REFERENCES

1. Lord JT: The changing role of the organized medical staff: the challenge for medical staff leadership. In Lord JT, editor: *The physician leader's guide,* Rockville, Md, 1992, Bader & Associates.
2. Wiesel E: *Legends of our time,* New York, 1976, Paragon Press.
3. The Hay Group: *The Hay Report on governance benchmarking,* San Francisco, 1994, The Hay Group.
4. Bader BS: What the governing board expects from physician leaders. In Lord JT, editor: *The physician leader's guide,* Rockville, Md, 1992, Bader and Associates.

13 Transitional Leaders: MANAGING IN A CLIMATE OF CONSTANT CHANGE

Lloyd E. Greene

OUTLINE

Managing change has become a way of life for successful organizations. In commenting on the rate and consistency of change that organizations will experience, Jack Welch, Chairman of General Electric, has argued that "compared to the 1990s the 1980s will look like a walk in the park."[1] This is certainly a fact of life for healthcare organizations. The decade of the 1980s acquainted most healthcare managers with perpetual change. Managed care, externally imposed mandates, shifts in practice patterns, new technology, and emerging professional needs have all precipitated change. Tried and true practices, structures, and models, if not already discarded, soon will be. The turmoil, anxiety, and frustration that this change can bring to an organization are significant and are in part a function of our lack of coherence in responding to change. Some of us accept the need to change continuously and respond in a way that produces what Senge[2] calls generative versus reactive learning. Others are unwilling to accept or learn from change or find themselves deskilled in new environments.

For change to be both continuous and vital to organizational life, we must rethink how we arrange ourselves to benefit most from it. This is the essence of effectively managing change at the organizational or department level. Healthcare organizations are finding themselves much more in an open rather than a closed system model. Open systems are characterized by less control, less predictability, need for more resilience, and a need for a clearer sense of how they must interact with all of their constituencies, stakeholders, and a variety of environments, both external and internal. Organizations, particularly healthcare organizations, were viewed in the past as closed systems, in which the dynamics of an organization and locus of control were internally determined, chiefly on the basis of precisely defined roles and role relationships. In reality all systems are more or less open to direct or indirect influence from sources outside the system boundaries.[3] This chapter identifies kinds of change and some goals for effectively managing change and then discusses various approaches to effectively managing change.

KINDS OF CHANGE FOUND IN ORGANIZATIONS

Change can occur in a variety of organizational contexts. Don Berwick, MD, in a speech to the Quality Improvement Network on April 21, 1993, outlined two important kinds of organizational change.[4] The first, called *first order change,* is designed to "hold the course" and achieve stability. When you ride a bicycle to a specific destination, you make small adjustments as you ride. You turn the handle bars slightly back and forth in an effort to keep going straight. This is an example of first order change. These kinds of changes are familiar in your daily life at work and at home. At work it appears as the right hand column in your budget statement when we put parentheses around the deficit and not around a figure that is ahead of budget. The implication of the parentheses is that one wishes to make changes in the way expenses are being made so that "we can get back on budget." This kind of change is associated with course corrections.

The second type of change, *second order change,* is a change with a totally different intention, that is to break through to historic levels of performance of a system. First order changes are changes within a system. Second order changes are changes of a system. When you turn your bicycle to go north instead of east you are engaging in second order change. First order changes are addictive. They are reactive and pervasive. We are a culture interested in fixing problems and getting back on course. Improvement requires second order change. First order change helps, but breakthroughs in system performance require basic changes in the system as a whole—totally new ways to do things. Second order change usually presents most of the problems, anxieties, and difficulties associated with change and particularly draws on skills and vision of leaders to manage effectively. This chapter focuses on managing change in this context.

OUTCOMES FROM EFFECTIVELY MANAGING CHANGE

Change typically occurs as a means to an end. Organizations and departments embark on change efforts to respond to their environment, meet customer demands, and stay current in their market. Ray Stata, President of Analog Devices, argues that continual learning, and therefore change, is the only sustainable competitive advantage that organizations can have.[5] At the department or unit level, outcomes from change include getting staff and significant stakeholders to change behaviors, getting stakeholders to expect and look forward to change, getting stakeholders to ask for change, or have a grass roots interest in continuous learning and owning change. Demonstrating the value of change is important to effectively manage it. However, leaders must create fundamentally the culture for continuous change. This culture can be nurtured by creating a coherent system and foundation around which change can occur.

Approaches to managing change can be organized according to cognitive and psychodynamic models. Literature is replete with research, discussion, and case studies about cognitive models. The psychodynamic approach appears to be less documented in the literature, but nonetheless critical in effectively managing significant or second order change. Cognitive and psychodynamic models should be considered and used concurrently when managing change. Cognitive models take the approach that change can be dealt with as an intellectual exercise that involves certain skills, processes, and analysis. Psychodynamic models argue that in significant change, peoples' thoughts and feelings about the change must be considered to effectively manage it. The rest of this chapter reviews several cognitive and psychodynamic change models.

COGNITIVE MODELS FOR MANAGING CHANGE

Several cognitive approaches for planning and implementing change are responsive to the outcomes of achieving ownership, commitment, and creating a culture where change is endemic and actively sought in responding to environmental influences.

Programmatic Change Versus Task Alignment

Through a four-year study of organizational change at six large corporations, Beer et al.[6] found that the greatest obstacle to revitalization or change is the idea that it comes about through company-wide change programs known as programmatic change. They argue that programmatic change is at best problematic because it is guided by a theory of change that is fundamentally flawed. Programmatic change asserts that the place to begin is with the knowledge and attitudes of individuals. Changes in attitudes, this flawed theory goes, lead to changes in individual behavior. The thinking in this theory is that change in individual behavior repeated by many people will result in organizational change. Therefore change is like a conversion experience. Once people "get the religion" changes in their behavior will surely follow. According to the authors, this theory gets the change process exactly backward. They argue that individual behavior is powerfully shaped by the organizational roles that people play. Therefore they conclude, "The most effective way to change behavior is to put people into a new organizational context which imposes new roles, responsibilities, and relationships on them."[6] They advocate six steps to achieve task-aligned change.

1. Mobilize commitment to change through joint diagnosis of problems.
2. Develop a shared vision of how to organize and manage for competitiveness.
3. Foster consensus for the new vision, competence to enact it, and cohesion to move it along.
4. Spread this change revitalization to all stakeholders or departments without pushing it from the top.
5. Institutionalize the change through formal policies, systems, and structures including job descriptions and the way the work is to be done.
6. Continue to monitor and adjust strategies in response to problems in the revitalization process.

Force Field Analysis

Originally developed by Lewin[7] as a means for determining the energy in a social environment, force field analysis has become a useful tool for planning and analyzing the barriers to implementing change. Force field in its simplest form involves looking at the current state of a given situation to determine what forces keep it from improving or changing. Typically, this is diagramed with the current situation being at the center of driving and restraining forces. Figure 13-1 illustrates this model using employee communication as an example. Leaders or managers who are contemplating change can use this method to account effectively for the dynamics in a change effort. Those dynamics then are analyzed in terms of ways they can be changed. Lewin argues that the most effective way to get movement and therefore change is to remove restraining forces rather than adding driving forces. In the example depicted in Figure 13-1, this could involve removing some of the restraining forces preventing better employee communication.

Stakeholder Mapping

Gilmore et al.[8] at the Center for Applied Research have developed a tool known as stakeholder mapping that can be useful in change efforts. This tool has proved useful in looking at the individuals or key groups who will be important in accepting, owning, or implementing change (stakeholders). Gilmore et al. assert that people tend to focus on an issue or problem, but often fail to attend to how it is related to wider issues. In this context, for example, it is often helpful to identify the stakeholders who are most affected by or can affect the issue you are trying to address and change. They indicate that it is useful to list the major stakeholders who could be affected by a change, and for each note the following items:

- Actual evidence about the attitudes of the key stakeholders
- Each of these questions through the eyes of the stakeholder
- The nature of their stake; for example what do they care about with respect to the issue that is being contemplated to change?
- Values or interests
- Power to influence adoption and/or implementation of the approaches you favor, for example, central, influential or nonplayer?

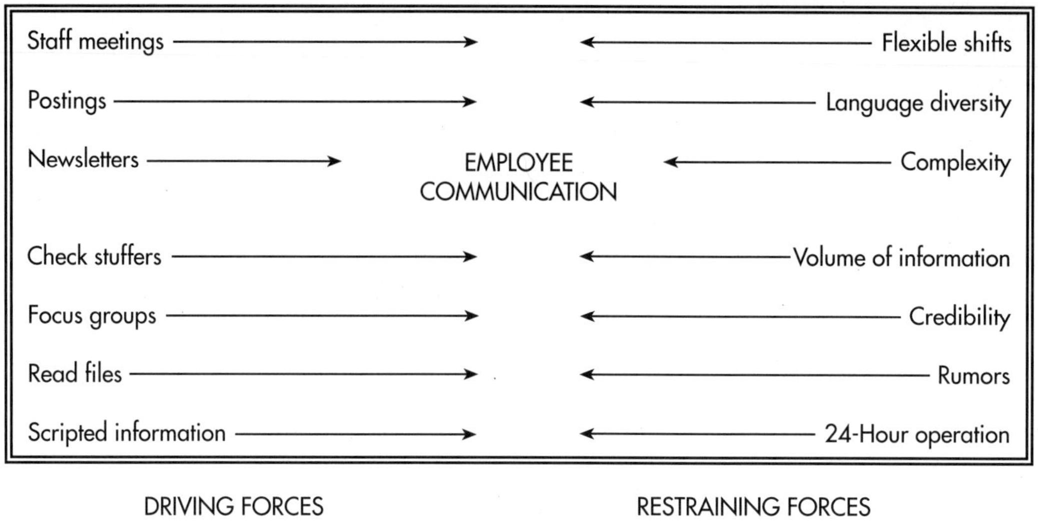

FIGURE 13-1 Force field analysis.

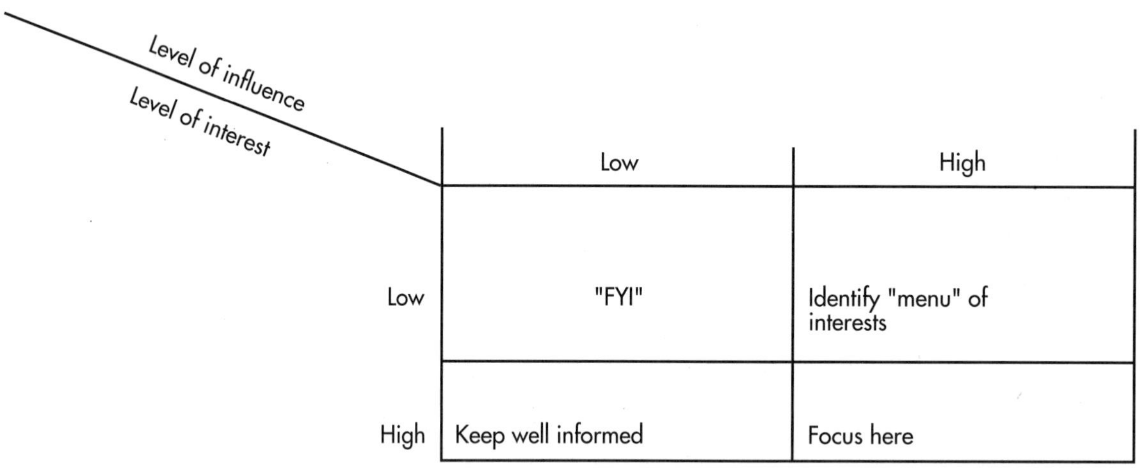

FIGURE 13-2 Stakeholder mapping.

- Who influences them and whom do they influence?
- What criteria they would use to evaluate and choose among alternative ways of dealing with issues?

Stakeholder mapping, then, involves creating a matrix characterized by level of influence on the horizontal axis and level of interest on the vertical axis. Figure 13-2 is an example of a generic stakeholder map. In creating this kind of matrix for key stakeholders, appropriate courses of action can be identified, which could be differentiated among stakeholders. All too often stakeholders are approached in undifferentiated ways with respect to contemplated change. This accounts for some of the difficulty that leaders or managers will encounter when trying to reach some of the change goals listed at the beginning of the chapter. It also accounts for missed opportunities and damaged relationships.

Vision

The term *vision* has achieved recent popularity as a method that leaders can use to develop a sense of purpose in an organization. Organizations continuously responding to change can be well served by having a sense of purpose that is shared by all stakeholders. Alignment of this kind is extremely helpful in containing the anxieties that change produces. Senge[2] has defined visioning as a way to paint a vivid picture of what you want your organization, department, or profession to look like in the future and make it real in the present. A vision in its simplest form is an expression of what you/we want to create. It answers the "what" question about organizations or departments. Senge argues that true dialogue and inquiry provide the basis for starting visioning work. As a technology, if applied in a thoughtful reflective way, it will uncover what is really important to a leader, manager, and his or her staff. The vision then becomes the stake in the ground around which change can be organized and become coherent and provides a sense of continuity and stability to staff.

Responsibility Charting

Gilmore et al.[9] have developed a method that can be applied in constantly changing environments in a way that addresses the ad hoc nature of roles that can and do exist.[9] Responsibility charting uses a matrix characterized by the specific task at hand. The horizontal axis lists the key stakeholders or actors in a change. The vertical axis lists the key tasks in a project or change. Role designations are then applied for each stakeholder for each task. Figure 13-3 illustrates a responsi-

Designing emergency departmet patient flow process	Nurses	Registrars	Physicians	Patients	Families	EMTs	Administration
1. Identify patient needs	R	C	R	C	C	C	A
2. Assess current process	A	C	R	I	I	I	I
3. Establish priorities	R	C	R	C	C	I	A
4. Design process	A	C	A	C	C	I	C

FIGURE 13-3 Responsibility chart. Standard symbols applied are *A,* approve; *R,* responsible; *C,* consult; and *I,* inform.

bility chart based on a patient flow project. The standard set of symbols applied are A, approve; R, responsible; C, consult; and I, inform.

Typically, responsibility charting is accomplished in a group setting. It can be used as a way for surfacing conflict about individual assignment of role for key stakeholders. It can provide specific, detailed information about key stakeholder roles and any product associated with change, whether it be the initialization, development, or implementation of change. Responsibility charting is best applied in situations in which defined roles, responsibilities, and dynamics of an organization are more networked, less bureaucratic or hierarchical, and thus more ad hoc.

General Cognitive Principles for Managing Change

People generally do not fear or dislike change; they fear or dislike the unknown. In rapidly changing environments, therefore, when outcomes are less predictable or are unknown, it is helpful for people to understand the processes being used to respond to change. For example, when cost reduction in an organization is an ongoing issue, and where position elimination or staff reduction is a by-product, it is helpful for people to know how this process will occur, and the timelines around which it should be accomplished. Similarly, when change engenders considerable rumor it is useful to disclose information about change sooner than later, and to disclose information about change to inside stakeholders rather than outside, if a choice needs to be made.

Although there are several other approaches to cognitive change, for example, the planned change models developed by Bennis et al.,[10] the models listed provide a useful framework to manage change on a cognitive level.

PSYCHODYNAMIC APPROACHES TO MANAGING CHANGE

Psychodynamic approaches to managing change involve techniques and processes intended to surface the feelings and thoughts people have about impending change or change that has recently been implemented. The goal of this approach is to help people move through various stages of response to change and ultimately to lead to a mind set that leaves people curious about, and open and committed to, change. It involves surfacing mental models, shaping those models, and helping people see the continuities and opportunities that can and do exist in change.

Psychodynamic approaches acknowledge the existence of at least two kinds of data that should be attended to when change is in progress. Those data are feelings that need to be given expression for constructive use of their energy, and second, the rationalizations and cognitive thought processes that will lead to constructive progress relative to change. The first section of this chapter referred to the cognitive processes. The next describes several approaches to managing the psychodynamic aspects of change.

Managing Boundaries

Organizations are typically depicted graphically by charts or boxes with names and titles and lines or arrows depicting hierarchical relationships. Organization charts of this type are meant to depict a neat and orderly flow of work and relationships. The reality, however, is that life in organizations is typically nonlinear, more dynamic, and more out of control than these charts, graphs, or models would indicate. Leaders and managers in organizations need to pay greater attention to the lines, arrows, or relationships between boxes than to the boxes themselves. More attention paid to the relationship boundaries that exist in an organization and the skills in attending to those relationships is more critical to getting work done in open system environments than in following traditional hierarchical or bureaucratic models. This shifts a leader's or manager's attention on a daily or episodic basis to the relationship issues.

Hirschhorn and Gilmore[11] have developed a useful model for managing relationship boundaries. They assert that boundaries are the differences that make a difference. Boundaries are identified as generic in all organizations and are characterized by four core relationships: *task, authority, identity,* and *political.* Table 13-1 indicates the framework around which boundaries can be characterized and used. In rapidly changing environments, Gilmore and Hirschhorn argue, it is critical to know what boundary you are in to effectively manage the issues at hand. Boundaries are defined based on the

Table 13-1 A Manager's Guide to the Boundaries That Matter

Key questions		Necessary tensions	Characteristic feelings
"Who is in charge of what?" →	AUTHORITY BOUNDARY	How to lead but remain open to criticism. How to follow but still challenge superiors.	Trustful Open Rigid Rebellious Passive
"Who does what?" →	TASK BOUNDARY	How to depend on others you don't control. How to specialize yet understand other people's jobs.	Confident Competent Proud Anxious Incompetent Ashamed
"What's in it for us?" →	POLITICAL BOUNDARY	How to defend one's interests without undermining the organization. How to differentiate between win-win and win-lose situations.	Empowered Treated fairly Powerless Exploited
"Who is—and isn't—'us'?" →	IDENTITY BOUNDARY	How to feel pride without devaluing others. How to remain loyal without undermining outsiders.	Proud Loyal Tolerant Distrusting Contemptuous

moment, not based on boxes or charts. It is critical for the right people at the right moment to be making decisions (the authority boundary), doing the right things (the task boundary), avoiding group-think and yet affirming group strength (the identity boundary), and finally knowing when negotiation is at play (the political boundary). The extent to which leaders and managers are aware of boundaries will help define their effectiveness organizationally. These boundaries are particularly at play in hospitals or departments in hospitals where professional identity can be a strength, or a liability; where authority frequently exists in the moment, for example, between a physician and a nurse in making decisions around patient care issues; and where the task boundary and political boundary play differentially, depending on the need at the moment. Hospital environments are becoming more and more negotiated environments in which no one person has the authority to make decisions, and where often the issues at hand can be effectively resolved with a collaborative model using principled negotiation.

Kurt Lewin's Three Stages of Organizational Change

Lewin[12] has characterized three phases of organizational change known as unfreezing, moving (changing), and refreezing. Lewin's use of these terms refers to the force field analysis model described previously. In any social situation, there is a field of social forces that maintains peoples' behavior within certain limits. This is a quasistationary equilibrium. To alter the behavior of persons in a situation, the equilibrium must be shifted to a new or different level, thus the term *unfreezing*. Unfreezing involves altering the limits of the equilibrium by creating the awareness of a need for and desire for change. In the popular jargon of paradigm shift, this is characterized by an initial stage of confusion during which the legitimacy of the dominant model or paradigm, or way of doing work, is literally under siege with few of the change questions answered. Normally, having people consider or reconsider how they think about doing their work requires establishing the need for the change and data that support the benefits or outcomes from the change.

Moving or changing involves actively manipulating certain of the social forces using force field analysis techniques, for example, decreasing those forces pressing toward a less desirable level of behavior and increasing those pressing toward a more desirable level of behavior. This process in a sense is a search for a new organizing logic that often arises from questioning some fundamental ways of getting work done. Thus the equilibrium level is shifted toward the more desirable level of behavior.

Finally, in refreezing, the equilibrium is stabilized at the desired level, ensuring that the social forces will remain stable and will not revert to the prior state. Lewin notes that "the unfreezing of the present level may involve quite different problems in different cases."[12]

One useful way to have people begin the unfreezing process is to have them talk about their thoughts and feelings about the impending change. Several useful methods can be used. One interesting exercise is to have people reverse roles in the "doer" and "planner" sense. This involves having those people who are planning the change take the role of the doer of the change, and having those who would be implementing the change take on the role of planner. Key questions in this exercise are: "What do you want from the other role in the environment of constant change?" "How would the planners want to implement the change?" "How would the doers want to be involved in the change?" Another version of this exercise is to have people take on the roles of various stakeholders in a change, for example, in a hospital environment, patients, board members, managers, nurses, technicians, and physicians. Another useful approach is to have people talk about how stakeholders would view the current environment they are in; how they might project their feelings about the

change raises important data. Data of this sort can be analyzed, trended, and used as a way to uncover significant feeling issues relative to change.

The Construction of Continuity

It is human nature to seek stability and predictability and to have anchors or continuity in one's life. The dynamics of change usually shake these foundations, or at the least, significantly challenge them. Bateson[13] has written about the issue of managing the paradoxes of stability and change. She argues that there is a continuum between continuity and discontinuity. In her view, the term *continuity* refers to a degree of sameness, primarily to sameness sustained through time. She argues that the leadership issue in any organization is to work with the relationship between continuity and discontinuity so that the benefits of both are available. Bateson has used exercises in which people focus on (1) the discontinuities in their life and (2) the continuities in their life. What she has been able to find through her research is that people can as easily make connections between various apparent discontinuities and therefore gain some sense of stability, direction, and coherence. The ability to find continuity in change is important for managing its psychodynamic aspects. It shows that there can be some stability and use of previous learning in change to create new ways of thinking, feeling, perceiving, and doing. Therefore continuity can provide for stability and discontinuity and can allow for paradigm shifts or second order change.

Mental Models

If change is fundamentally about learning, it is important to arrange ourselves so that we are continuously open to this learning. Senge[2] refers to one method for maintaining this openness as surfacing mental models.[2] Mental models are the fundamental ways we arrange and view the world. They are often characterized by conversations we have in our head about people, places, things, or events. For example, we may characterize a co-worker as ambitious, tenacious, impatient, or a great leader. This model or image of that person shapes the conversations we have with him or her. Argyris and Senge have developed an exercise called the left hand column, which is an effective way of surfacing mental models of this type.[2] The exercise asks people to think about a conversation they had recently that did not "go well," felt uncomfortable, or did not lead to the desired outcome. People are asked to record verbatim, if possible, the interchange in that conversation in the right hand column of a piece of paper. They then are asked to write, in the left hand column, phrases or thoughts that they would like to have said in the conversation. In examining themes in the left hand column, participants can usually identify those filters or mental models that impeded the conversation. This exercise opens up possibilities for use of that data to make these relationships or conversations more effective.

Closely aligned with maintaining an openness to change, and therefore learning, is what Senge[2] calls dialogue and inquiry skills. Dialogue is active and reflective conversation in which meaning is passed through a group. He contrasts dialogue with discussion in which people lob their opinions at each other. Dialogue literally means passing the meaning through in a conversation. Inquiry is contrasted with advocacy. We are probably all too aware of meetings or conversations in which people state their opinions as if they are axiomatic or true without doubt. Inquiry on the other hand allows people to be open to others' ideas, thoughts, or opinions and allows data to be used more productively to arrive at conclusions, decisions, or new learning. Dialogue and inquiry skills are critical in fast changing environments. Box 13-1 lists skills for dialogue and inquiry.

BOX 13-1

SKILLS FOR CREATING DIALOGUE/INQUIRY

1. Building on previous speaker
2. Paraphrasing previous speaker
3. Weaving together the views of two or more previous speakers
4. Being aware of your assumptions, biases
5. Being uncertain
6. Inquiry
7. Withholding judgment

The Stages of Death and Dying

Kubler-Ross[14] has researched the psychosocial stages associated with the death of a close friend or loved one. Those stages are denial, anger, depression, and acceptance. These stages can be coupled loosely with the feeling levels that people may experience in going through significant or second order change. Understanding that people may go through these stages helps in leading them through change. For example, when significant change is being asked for, people may be in denial: "The change is not right or may be unneeded." They may experience anger: "Why me or us?" They may experience a period of low energy before arriving at acceptance. Expecting these stages and engaging them are useful and can be accomplished through focus groups, conversations, structured exercises, or use of a skilled facilitator or outside consultant. To not acknowledge the possibility that people go through these stages will in many cases subvert the change process.

SUMMARY

This chapter provides a variety of cognitive and psychodynamic methods that can be useful tools in managing uncertainty. In a sense, according to Gilmore,[15] one can define the central challenge of leadership as uncertainty management. As we are increasingly facing second order change, that is, from a known current situation, to an emergent, yet to be discovered future state, we need a different kind of leadership that is comfortable with ambiguity and is able both to absorb some of the uncertainties and to allocate what remains in effective and fair ways to get others involved. The leader needs to contain some of the anxieties of his or her staff and at the same time know how and when to use skills to involve them.

REFERENCES

1. Welch J: Successful organizations—1992 and beyond, *The Westrend Letter* 2:13-17, 1992.

2. Senge P: *The fifth discipline: the art and practice of the learning organization,* New York, 1990, DoubleDay/Currency.
3. Sashkin M: A brief glossary of frequently used terms in organization development and planned change. In *1980 annual handbook for group facilitators,* New York, 1980, University Associates.
4. Berwick D: *Quality convictions: beyond the beginning,* A speech to the Quality Improvement Network Meeting April 21, 1993.
5. Stata R: Organizational learning—the key to management innovation, *Sloan Manage Rev* 30:15-31, 1989.
6. Beer M, Eisenstadt R, Spector B: Why change programs don't produce change, *Harvard Business Review* 68:158-166, 1990.
7. Lewin K: *Field theory in social science,* (D. Cartright, editor), New York, 1951, Harper.
8. Gilmore T et al: *Tools for systematic decision making,* Philadelphia, 1990, Center for Applied Research.
9. Gilmore T: *Responsibility charting,* Philadelphia, 1990, Center for Applied Research.
10. Bennis WG et al: *The planning of change,* ed 3, New York, 1976, Holt, Rhinehart Winston.
11. Hirschhorn L, Gilmore T: The new boundaries of the boundaryless company, *Harvard Business Review* 70:104-115, 1992.
12. Lewin K: Group decision and social change. In Maccoby EE, Newcomb TM, Hartley EL, editors: *Readings in social psychology,* ed 3, New York, 1958, Holt, Rhinehart & Winston.
13. Bateson MC: Managing the paradoxes of stability and change. In Srivastava S, Fry M, editors: *Executive and organizational continuity,* San Francisco, 1990, Jossey Bass.
14. Kubler-Ross E: *On death and dying,* New York, 1969, Collier, McMillan.
15. Gilmore T: Leadership and boundary management, *J Appli Behav Sci* 18:343-356, 1991.

PART TWO
Operations

14 Team Building: SOLVING PROBLEMS BY A MULTIDISCIPLINARY APPROACH

James Jay Hoelz

OUTLINE

Webster defines collaboration as "working together, cooperating".[1] Weiss and Davis[2] interpret collaboration as "interactions between nurse and physician that enable the knowledge and skills of both professionals to synergistically influence the patient care being provided." They also describe two key elements needed for a collaborative practice: cooperation and assertiveness. Cooperation is needed for individuals from different backgrounds and with different viewpoints to work together. Assertiveness is necessary for individuals to exchange knowledge and ideas.

The concept of nurse-physician collaboration has been discussed and studied since 1966. In 1967 Stein[3] wrote about the "doctor-nurse game." He accurately and humorously described the relationship between physicians and nurses during this era. His work can best be summarized by exploring the communication style between the two professions. "Nurses needed to communicate their recommendations without appearing to make them. Physicians requesting a recommendation needed to do so without appearing to be asking for it."[3]

Both physicians and nurses have expressed a desire to improve collaboration as evidenced by the formation of liaison groups such as those among the Emergency Nurses Association (ENA), the Society of Academic Emergency Medicine, and the American College of Emergency Physicians (ACEP). A representative from ACEP and from ENA are invited to attend the board meetings of each other's organization. The Emergency Nursing Foundation and the Emergency Medicine Foundation have collaborated on joint research grants to improve care for emergency patients.

Although the health care industry has made great strides since 1967, nurses, physicians, and other healthcare workers continue to struggle with collaborative efforts. Collaboration is imperative at this juncture of a problematic healthcare system and an unstable political environment. The questions are: How do we achieve this goal? And, why is this process so difficult?

OUTCOMES RELATED TO COLLABORATION

Several benefits result from collaboration. Knaus et al.,[4] in a study of 13 tertiary care institutions, demonstrated substantial differences in actual and predicted patient death rates. These differences could be linked to the interactions and communication style among nurses and physicians. Those institutions that encouraged and supported interaction and involvement by both the nursing and medical staff had the lower death rates.

Mitchell et al.[5] found similar results in the American Association of Critical Care Nurses (AACN) Demonstration Project at Overlake Hospital. The demonstration unit was organized to promote collaboration. Each unit coordinator made rounds twice a day with the charge nurse, reviewing questions about patient care, bed utilization, or other administrative issues. The medical coordinator was available to the nursing staff 24 hours a day. Mortality rates were significantly lower for patients who participated in this project, and results could be correlated with nurse-physician collaboration. Clearly, there is a benefit to the patient from effective collaboration between healthcare providers.

A second benefit from collaboration is improved job satisfaction. In 1982 and 1986, the American Academy for Nurses completed The Magnet Hospital Study. The following conditions promoted nurse recruitment and retention: high nurse/patient ratio, flexible staffing and scheduling, strong supportive nursing administration, participative management, and good nurse-physician relations.[6]

The third and perhaps most crucial benefit in today's healthcare environment is the ability to better serve the customer. As quality management, customer service, and patient focused care revolutionize healthcare, the institution that has established infrastructure and the commitment to working together will be successful. Organizations with collaborative practice models already functioning will be better equipped to adapt to changes in the regulatory, political, and social climate. Hospitals and departments without motivated, collaborative multidisciplinary teams will not be capable of meeting the challenges of the next decade, which will undoubtedly

include restructuring departments and services, reducing or redistributing resources, and redefining or redesigning roles.

BARRIERS TO COLLABORATION

The primary disadvantages in adopting a collaborative practice model is the time and energy necessary to change the current milieu, specifically, the historical adversarial relationship between nurses and physicians. Fagin[7] has identified the following barriers to collaboration: education, nurses' dissatisfaction, jurisdiction, sex-role stereotypes, hands-on versus intellectual activities, and social class.

Other studies have demonstrated distinct differences in perceptions and interests between nurses and physicians. Prescott and Bowen[8] found contrasting opinions when they asked physicians and nurses to describe the characteristics of a good relationship. Nurses stated that being mutually respected and trusted, being used as a resource in planning and decision making, and being supported by the physician in the presence of the patient were of primary importance. Physicians reported that the nurses' communication with them, the nurses' competence, and the nurses' willingness to help were important. Clearly, this difference in perception leads to increased potential for confusion, conflict, and constriction of a collaborative environment.

For any collaborative model to be successful, there must be overt administrative support. This support should be initiated by the Chief Executive Officer of the organization and disseminated by the Chief Nursing Officer and Chief Medical Officer of the organization. For the Emergency Department, this objective of collaboration should be embraced and actively supported by the medical and nursing directors of the department. A collaborative approach will surely fail without total support from all factions, from senior management to front line employees.

Collaboration and a team approach to problem solving must be a part of the mission of the department or organization. It must be one of the essential foundations on which improvements in patient care and operating processes are based.

It is also essential that both nursing and physician leaders recognize that there are historical, cultural, and societal barriers to collaboration. Identifying these barriers from the outset and realizing the potential effect on collaboration will help ensure the success of this effort.

SETTING THE STAGE FOR COLLABORATION

Four organizational elements are essential for a collaborative environment: flexible structure, horizontal communication, an environment for questioning, and a tolerance for failure.[9] The structure of the department must be adaptable so that hierarchical communication is not required to solve problems or to voice concerns. Problems and concerns should be solved through horizontal communication among various types of caregivers rather than through formal, vertical channels. Horizontal communication encourages and fosters multidisciplinary problem solving. An environment of questioning the status quo should be encouraged at all levels. Just because something has always been done a certain way does not mean it is the best way. Team members should be congratulated for initiating new ideas, not penalized for "bucking the system." Finally, the process of trying, failing, and trying again should be sanctioned, not punished. Failure should be viewed as one step closer to the best solution. When failure is tolerated as part of process improvement, creativity is fostered and team members are not fearful of the repercussions normally associated with failure.

For a team to be successful, it must have a mission or a reason for existence. Without a clearly defined mission, each team member will have his or her own agenda. There will be no methodology for improvement, no way to measure success, and in essence, no basis for collaboration. Members will be unsure of their purpose on the team and will grow disenchanted with the process. The mission should be determined by senior management, with clear parameters established through which change may be accomplished. Team members will decide how best to achieve and implement the mission outlined by management.

CHOOSING A MULTIDISCIPLINARY TEAM

The emergency department can have two types of multidisciplinary teams. The first is formed to solve a specific problem or concern, such as prolonged waiting time for triage (i.e., task force). This team would have a task to accomplish and would disband after the task has been completed. The second type of team may be formed to develop, plan, and monitor department progress toward a particular goal, such as quality (i.e., standing committee). This team will meet regularly and, although membership may change, the task is never complete.

The selection process for membership of each team should be consistent. It should include all parties that need to be involved in the problem's process and outcome. For example, if the problem to be addressed is laboratory turn-around time in the emergency department, the team should consist of a representative from each department or type of employee affected by this process. This team may include an emergency physician, an emergency nurse, an emergency technician, a unit secretary, a phlebotomist, a representative from specimen processing, a laboratory technologist, and the managers of the emergency department and the laboratory. Although managers may not have the in-depth knowledge of the process to recommend improvements, their presence is necessary to facilitate group problem solving and to provide visible support of collaborative decision making. The total number of members should be between 7 and 15 for optimal multidisciplinary problem solving. Less than seven may discourage adequate representation and diversity of opinion. More than fifteen creates an unwieldy group that inhibits problem solving.

SETTING OPERATING GUIDELINES

Many teams fail because they do not establish team operating guidelines before trying to problem solve. These operating guidelines include decision making, conflict management, ensuring team participation, ensuring task completion, the role of the leader and the note taker, and communicating

BOX 14-1

DECISION-MAKING GUIDELINES

We will attempt to make decisions by reaching consensus.
If we cannot reach consensus and a decision must be made, a majority of 75% will carry a decision.
If we do not have a 75% majority, we will table the decision, gather more information and discuss later.
Regardless of individual votes or opinions, the group decision will be supported by all members.
Members are expected to be active participants in discussion and decision making.
No decision is final—we will evaluate the effectiveness of our decision and alter if necessary.

information outside of the team. The team, with the assistance of a nonmember facilitator, should create these guidelines through group process. This approach will ensure ownership in the process and success of the team.

USING A FACILITATOR

As recommended previously, using a nonteam member facilitator is extremely helpful during the team-building phase and may continue to be useful in the process phase. A trained facilitator can assist the team in formulating operating guidelines and set a tone for cooperative, constructive participation. Being a nonmember of the group also provides value when the group begins to improve processes and to change practice. An outsider often provides an unbiased viewpoint, not steeped in the history and the politics of the situation and the institution.

DECISION MAKING

Each team should determine how decisions will be made. Most teams opt to use a consensus model. Decisions by consensus mean that although some members of the group may feel that a decision is not the best, they are willing to support and enact it. The decision then belongs to the team and not to particular individuals. This type of decision making facilitates cohesion. The team should also determine how to proceed if the members are unable to reach consensus. Does a majority of support constitute a decision and what comprises a majority: one half, two thirds? Box 14-1 is an example of one team's decision-making guidelines.

MANAGING CONFLICT

Multidisciplinary teams are formed because of the diversity of opinion and experience offered by individuals from different professions and/or departments. However, this diversity also leads to communication variances and the potential for conflict. In the initial phase of team development, it is helpful to use a tool to highlight differences in communication style and expectations. The Myers-Briggs Type Inventory is an excellent mechanism to examine individual communication styles and their effect on group dynamics. Scores reflect personality differences and their potential effect on communication. Use of the inventory encourages individuals to become familiar with personality differences and to use this familiarity to avoid conflict. Conflict usually arises when expectations are not met. Yet these expectations are often not clearly communicated. Defining a model for communication and managing conflict before its occurrence can help alleviate wasted time and energy. An example of a model for managing conflict is presented in Box 14-2.

BOX 14-2

MODEL FOR MANAGING CONFLICT

We will give each member time to voice his or her opinion without interruption.
We will value each other's opinion.
We will identify and admit conflict, confronting each other directly.
We will confront each other openly, honestly, gently, and professionally.
We will attempt not to personalize or internalize feedback.

BOX 14-3

PARTICIPATION GUIDELINES

Attendance is expected at all team meetings.
If a member misses a meeting, it is his or her responsibility to catch up on missed information.
We will respect the confidentiality of team discussions.
We will provide an atmosphere where team members feel free to express their opinions without fear of ridicule or recrimination.
We will ask the quieter members for input before making decisions.
We will attempt to schedule team meetings to facilitate maximum attendance.

ENSURING TEAM PARTICIPATION

Members will have different schedules and may have varying levels of commitment to the team. Members may miss meetings. It is essential to determine a model for ensuring participation at the start of the team process, such as the one listed in Box 14-3.

ENSURING TASK COMPLETION

It is essential to develop a model to ensure task completion. Team members will have varying work schedules and personal responsibilities that may interfere with the work of the team. If expectations are identified clearly at the start of the process, conflict may be avoided. Personal responsibilities are listed in Box 14-4.

BOX 14-4

PERSONAL RESPONSIBILITIES

Each individual is responsible for completing assigned tasks.
If an individual is having difficulty completing a task, it is his or her responsibility to seek assistance from other group members.
We will confront those who do not complete tasks and have not sought assistance.
We will ensure that tasks are reasonable in length and are assigned before the end of each meeting.
If a member is overwhelmed, it is his or her responsibility to seek assistance.

BOX 14-5

LEADER RESPONSIBILITIES

Keeps the group on track
Acts as liaison between senior management, external facilitator, and team
Arranges meeting logistics (time, date, place)
Calls special meetings as needed
Acts as focal point for communications for team members who are unable to attend meetings
Facilitates reassignment of tasks

ROLE OF THE LEADER

A leader, acting as team facilitator, is necessary to keep the team on focus and to keep the process in motion. The leader is not "the manager" of the team. They do not have more power over the process, they do not set agenda or direction for the team. They simply act to expedite change and improvement. Some role responsibilities of the leader are outlined in Box 14-5.

ROLE OF NOTE TAKER

Each team should have an identified note taker. Meeting minutes must be recorded and distributed to members. This role is intentionally not called the secretary, although the function is similar. Because each team may have a unit secretary or department secretary as a member, this role has been renamed so that it is not assumed that the unit or department secretary will play this role. The responsibilities of the note taker are outlined in Box 14-6.

CHANGING OPERATING GUIDELINES

The team should evaluate the effectiveness of the operating guidelines as they would any other decision. Evaluation should occur after the first or second meeting and every 1 to 3 months thereafter, depending on the frequency of team meetings. If the guidelines do not meet the needs of the group, they should be revised using the decision-making model adopted by the group.

BOX 14-6

NOTE TAKER RESPONSIBILITIES

Records minutes of team meetings, including discussion, decision, and responsibility for implementation
Ensures that minutes are legible and distributed to all team members
At the start of each meeting, identifies open issues and reviews minutes from last meeting
At the end of each meeting, gives overview of what took place and what will be in the minutes
Reviews unfinished business at the end of the meeting; reviews responsibilities and what will be discussed with small groups

COMMUNICATING INFORMATION TO OTHERS

Perhaps the most crucial activity for any team is communicating information, progress, and decisions to peers and coworkers who are not part of the team. Reaching successful decisions is it requires support from the group it will affect. Without adequate information, nonmembers will feel left out of the process, with decisions being made for them and not with them. The team members should develop a mechanism for communication so that nonmembers feel they have input into the process.

Some teams have found it helpful to divide nonmembers into equal groups and have a member of the team responsible for acting as a liaison to the team. Nonmembers should know who their liaison is, and the team should strive to develop an atmosphere that encourages questions and feedback from nonmembers. Success depends on the ability of team members to actively involve nonmembers in this process. To achieve this goal, members may need to actively seek out nonmembers, offer explanation, and solicit ideas and feedback.

Communication of team decisions is the key to either success or failure. Active and extensive communication with others will assure buy-in and support of changes. Poor or inadequate communication will allow nonmembers to harbor distrust of the group and therefore distrust of the process of change and the decisions made.

MEASURING SUCCESS

Each team needs to measure success in terms of two distinct parameters: the ability of the team to work collaboratively as a group, and the effectiveness of the team's initiated decisions. It is imperative to first evaluate the group's ability to work together. Are the appropriate individuals on the team and the appropriate departments represented? Do members on the team have equal say in the decision-making process, or do certain members exert more influence, either by their position or their status? Are individuals surfacing suppressed conflict? If so, is conflict being dealt with in an effective,

constructive manner, or is it being ignored and allowed to fester?

Teams should also examine their ability to successfully implement change. Has the mission been clearly defined and articulated to the team? Are individuals unsure of the goals of the group process? Has senior management clearly delineated parameters within which improvement can occur? Are efforts at change thwarted before implementation? Is management supporting the process? Has the team defined a specific methodology for investigating a process, examining options for change, choosing the best option, implementing the change, and evaluating the effect and potential success? Is the team communicating effectively with nonmembers to ensure trust, support, and feedback? These questions must be asked to evaluate the change process.

SUMMARY

The healthcare system is changing. Political, regulatory, and societal forces are exerting pressure for reform, restructuring, and reorganization. For healthcare professionals to achieve success in this environment, an environment that encourages and rewards collaboration for efficient and effective problem solving must be in place.

This chapter has defined collaboration, outlined the benefits and disadvantages to collaboration, identified how to choose a team, and how to prepare the team to work effectively. There are significant historical, societal, and cultural barriers to collaboration. Institutions, departments, and individuals must recognize the existence of the barriers and work to overcome them. Collaboration can succeed only if individuals are committed to cooperate and to be assertive, respecting each other's differences and celebrating these differences for the diversity they provide.

REFERENCES

1. *Webster's new ideal dictionary,* Springfield, Mass, 1978, G&C Merriam,
2. Weiss SJ, Davis HP: Validity and reliability of the Collaborative Practice Scales, *Nurs Res* 34:299-305, 1895.
3. Stein LI: The doctor-nurse game, *Arch Gen Psychiatry* 16:699-703, 1967.
4. Knaus W et al: An evaluation of outcomes from intensive care in major medical centers, *Ann Intern Med* 104:409-410, 1986.
5. Mitchell P et al: AACH demonstration project: Profile of excellence in critical care nursing, *Heart Lung* 18:219-235, 1989.
6. Kramer M: The magnet hospitals: excellence revisited, *J Nurs Adm* 17:354-379, 1990.
7. Fagin CM: Collaboration between nurses and physicians: no longer a choice, *Nurs Health Care* 13:354-363, 1992.
8. Prescott PA, Bowen SA: Physician-nurse relationships, *Ann Intern Med* 103:127-133, 1985.
9. Hoelz JJ: Shared governance: enhancing quality and satisfaction in nursing, *Med Surg Nurs Q,* 1:132-141, 1993.

15 The Role of the Emergency Department Medical Director

Thom A. Mayer

"Uneasy rests the head that wears the crown."

William Shakespeare, Henry IV

"In times of change, learners inherit the earth, while the learned find themselves beautifully equipped to deal with a world that no longer exists."

Eric Hoffer[1]

"Management is doing things right; leadership is doing the right things."

Warren Bennis[2]

"If management is doing things right and leadership is doing the right things, the emergency department medical director must do both consistently."

Thom A. Mayer, MD, FACEP

OUTLINE

The position of emergency department medical director is among the most sought-after and least understood in all of medicine. It is often assumed to be stimulating, rewarding, and gratifying. Nonetheless, many who have held the position have found it to be difficult, thankless, demanding, and even demeaning at times. In fact, all of these adjectives accurately describe the position of medical director of an emergency department. Because of the nature and complexity of emergency medicine, the job of coordinating the multidisciplinary services of a diverse group of providers under disparate circumstances is extraordinarily complex and difficult and requires tremendous talent, energy, and enthusiasm. However, guiding the development of an emergency department can result in gratifying improvements in patient care and staff development.

Regardless of the size, sophistication, or level of service provided in the emergency department, the necessary condition for success in emergency medicine is effective leadership and management.[3] It is impossible to deliver effective clinical care in the current healthcare environment without applying sound leadership and management skills. These skills allow clinicians the appropriate training, resources, facilities, and staff to deliver such care. The emergency department medical director must work collaboratively with other nursing and non-nursing managers to achieve two goals. The first goal is to develop systems and processes that consistently provide good outcomes for emergency department patients. These systems and processes must work in the absence of senior or middle management, functioning effectively 24 hours a day, 7 days a week. Second, the systems and processes must be designed so that the interests of both clinical patient care and the needs of the providers responsible for that care are considered. Much of the difficulty with the phenomena of stress and burnout (see Chapter 82) can be attributed to failure to take the needs of the provider into account in designing emergency department processes. In the past, emergency department medical directors were often viewed as being in a position of power, control, and authority. Nothing could be farther from reality. The job is a critical one, but the key competencies for success in our rapidly changing healthcare environment are collaboration, cooperation, empowerment, aligning incentives, and "stewardship," to use Peter Block's concise term.[4]

Previous emergency medicine textbooks have relegated a single chapter or small section on management of the emergency department and the roles and responsibilities of the emergency department medical director.[5-7] The central goal of this textbook is to present the entirety of the body of knowledge on emergency department management, including the application of business principles to the practice of emergency medicine. Therefore in some respects, the textbook itself is a description of the roles necessary for effective emergency department management. This chapter focuses specifically on the medical director's role in the development, implementation, and ongoing monitoring of the emergency department's journey toward using sound scientific management principles. The major sections of this textbook are instructive in helping frame a discussion of the

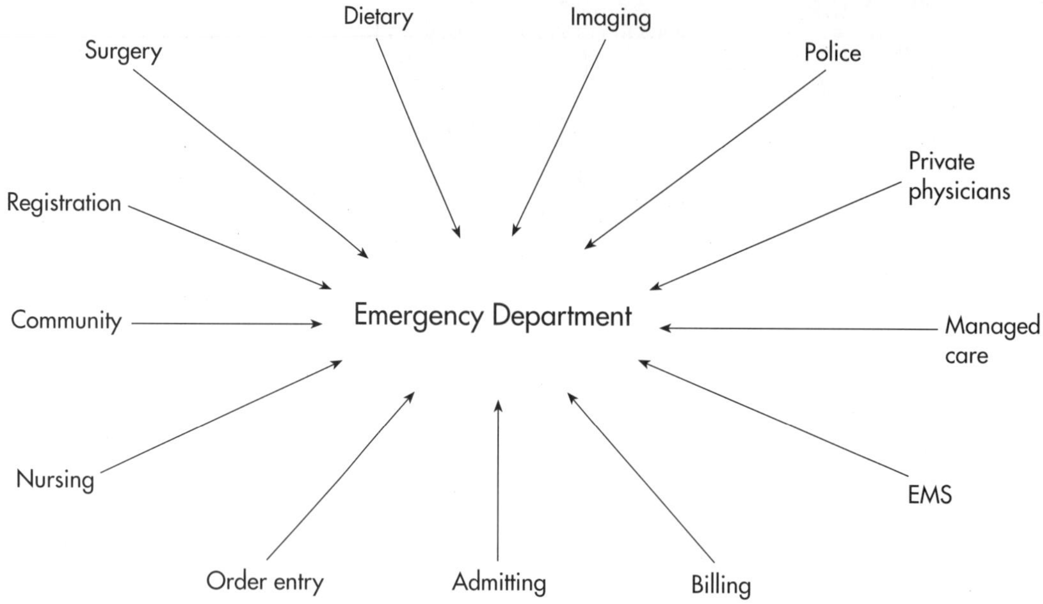

FIGURE 15-1 The emergency department is a process-rich environment. Regardless of size or volume, all emergency departments have multiple, cross-functional processes at work on each patient. Success requires careful, sequential coordination of these processes.

emergency department medical director's roles and responsibilities. Those sections include:

- Management principles
- Operations
- Contract management
- Financial management/reimbursement
- Quality
- Risk management/legal
- Human resources management
- Practice diversification
- Professional relationships
- Prehospital care

The role of the medical director is to integrate all of the skills represented in these sections into the planning, implementation, and evaluation of all emergency department operations. However, rather than simply reiterating these functions in this chapter, the focus is on broader strategies that enable the emergency department medical director to perform his or her job most effectively. Of necessity, the chapter overlaps in some areas with others. Readers are referred to other chapters for more in-depth treatment of specific topics of interest.

THE TRANSITION FROM PHYSICIAN TO PHYSICIAN-MANAGER

The difficult and daunting job of the emergency department medical director can be successfully undertaken only when there is an effective transition from being strictly a clinical care provider to a physician-manager. Chapters 1 and 9 discuss this transition in some detail, but it is important to recognize that a physician-manager requires talents, skills, and techniques that allow him or her to operate both as a clinician and as a manager of services. Coordination of clinical and administrative issues is an essential, fundamental core proficiency for the medical director. Nonetheless, this is an extraordinarily difficult and complex transition, primarily because the provision of patient care itself comprises extraordinarily diverse and complex processes that must function smoothly and efficiently. The emergency department is the locus of multiple, cross-functional processes that are active in even the simplest of patient encounters.[8] These interdependent encounters include triage, registration, resource allocation, diagnostic evaluation (including ancillary services), therapeutic interventions, patient and family education, discharge processing, consultation, and, in some cases, admission to the hospital. Figure 15-1 illustrates the complexity of the processes involved in emergency department evaluation and therapy. Further, if any step in this multitude of processes is performed incompletely or inaccurately, it will matter little to the patient or family that the other functions were performed correctly. In the emergency department environment, designing a system that allows for 999 of 1000 processes to function correctly is a recipe for failure, not success. It is instructive in this regard that the concept of process management, which is an essential part of quality improvement activities, is taught in a game known as "Friday Night at the ER."[9] This game is structured to teach process management through a practical example of the interrelationship of cross-functional processes. It is entirely appropriate that business consultants have viewed the emergency department as *the* quintessential example of the complex interaction of cross-functional processes.

As Figure 15-2 illustrates, most emergency departments are organized in at least four distinct, separate, yet interrelated functions, which usually report through different vertical structures:

- Emergency department physicians: Provide clinical care and coordination of medical resources

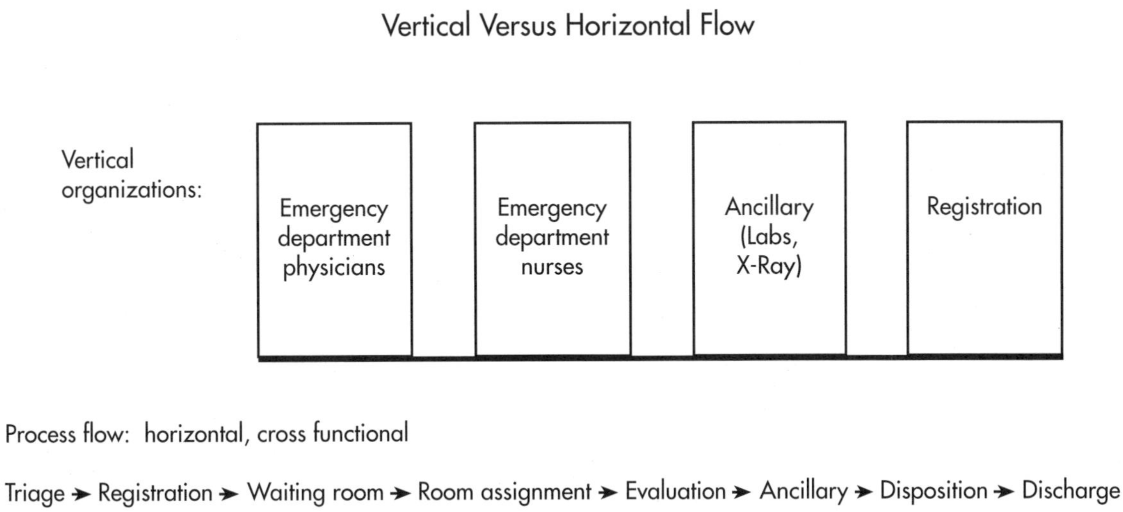

FIGURE 15-2 Vertical versus horizontal flow.

- Emergency department nurses: Perform triage, primary nursing functions, and coordination of nursing resources
- Emergency department ancillary services: Provide laboratory and radiologic and other services
- Emergency department registration: Handles financial functions, including hospital admissions

Intertwined in these core functions are other essential providers including unit secretaries, emergency department technicians, housekeeping, security, volunteers, and social work. Despite the multiple vertical silos present in emergency department operations, the patient moves through the clinical encounter in a horizontal, process-oriented fashion. *Managing the clinical encounter across these cross-functional processes is at the heart of the role of emergency department medical directors and their nursing colleagues.*

An additional essential competency of an emergency department medical director is the ability to work in a collegial and cooperative fashion with the other managers of emergency department functions, including nursing, ancillary services, and financial services. The importance of physician-nurse relationships is discussed in detail. It should be said at the outset that the relationship between the emergency department medical director and nursing director is among the most important in the entire emergency department. This relationship requires a substantial commitment of time, effort, and energy to ensure that it is managed cooperatively and prospectively. These two healthcare professionals should strive to ensure that they have a common vision for the emergency department, as well as, to the best extent possible, a common philosophy of management and a clear understanding of the working relationship. They should meet frequently, usually at least twice a month, to discuss departmental operations, problems, and future directions. There should be a clear understanding that each will inform the other of any issues or problems that may affect them, using telephone, voice mail, e-mail, memos, or face-to-face meetings so that each can be informed of departmental operational problems on a timely basis. The relationship should be highly supportive both in emergency department operations and the meetings that affect them. Similarly, the emergency department medical director must work cooperatively with the managers of other departments so that services and processes can be coordinated smoothly and prospectively.

BOX 15-1

QUALIFICATIONS OF EMERGENCY DEPARTMENT MEDICAL DIRECTOR

Clinical Qualifications
- Demonstrated clinical excellence
- ABEM certification or preparation
- "Merit badges" optional
- Commitment to education

Management skills and experience

Communication skills
- Written
- Verbal
- Listening

Integrity and intellectual honesty

QUALIFICATIONS

The qualifications necessary to function as an emergency department medical director vary. For example, the specific qualifications required to run an academic emergency department in a 700-bed academic teaching institution with 80,000 emergency department visits may be somewhat different from those required for an emergency department in a 250-bed community hospital with 25,000 emergency department visits. However, several essential characteristics should be sought in any emergency department medical director (Box 15-1).

Clinical Qualifications

The emergency department medical director should, at a minimum, have board certification or board preparation in emergency medicine. Although the supply of board certified emergency physicians is still somewhat lower than the demand, even small hospitals in rural settings should make it their goal to ensure that the physician charged with oversee-

ing clinical care responsibilities in the emergency department is board certified. For children's hospitals, the director should be board certified or board prepared in pediatric emergency medicine, the examination for which is jointly administered by the American Board of Pediatrics and the American Board of Emergency Medicine (ABEM). Board certification in emergency medicine or pediatric emergency medicine provides some relative assurance of clinical competence, but also indicates that the director has completed a process of stringent peer review that will serve well in dealing with the multiple problems that he or she will face as a director. Although the emergency department medical director should be a trusted and experienced clinician in emergency medicine, he or she may not be the *best* clinician among the emergency physicians serving the hospital. Indeed, one of the marks of a mature physician-manager is to surround himself or herself with highly qualified clinicians, any one of whom may be able to outshine the director in a given clinical category. Nonetheless, demonstrated clinical competence and the respect of one's colleagues is essential for all emergency department medical directors.

Successful completion of various protocol-oriented courses are a common issue facing emergency physicians. Certification in Advanced Trauma Life Support, Advanced Cardiac Life Support, and Advanced Pediatric Life Support courses has often been thought essential for emergency physicians. However, if a candidate has successfully completed the ABEM certification examination, the attainment of such certifications are largely superfluous. Certification in such courses therefore should be guided by hospital policy, regulatory requirements (e.g., level I trauma center verification), and the dictates of the emergency department physician group. Regardless of certification status in such courses, knowledge of the precepts and protocols used in these courses may be of assistance to the medical director with regard to the educational functions of the department. In most cases, maintaining at least some emergency department physicians with instructor level status in such courses can be of significant benefit to the department's long-term patient care, public relations, and educational functions.

Management Skills and Experience

Chapters 1 and 9 describe management skills in detail, particularly with regard to the transition from being a physician to a physician-manager. Nonetheless, the medical director must have the ability to recognize potential problems, describe accurately the components constituting them, communicate clearly and effectively with others both the nature of the problem and the reasons for it, recommend appropriate solutions, and successfully follow through on such recommendations. Although previous experience as a medical director can be helpful, attention to the particular mind set of a physician-manager (see Chapters 1, 9, 10, and 11) is in many respects more important. This mind set largely consists of the elements of collaboration, empowerment, and stewardship mentioned previously. Management training itself can be attained through masters programs, readings in the management literature, and courses offered by the American College of Physician Executives, the American College of Emergency Physicians, and business schools with programs designed for physician executives.

Communications Skills

The medical director must have excellent written, verbal, and listening communication skills. Written communications form an important part of the medical director's job. The director should be an effective, terse writer, capable of reducing problems or issues to a single page that outlines the issues, addresses its components, and suggests solutions. In other words, the director must have good editing skills. Physician-managers should also be aware of the "power of the carbon copy." Issues that cross boundaries with other areas of the hospital should be copied to representatives from affected departments. The medical director also should ensure that a written record of any important verbal conversations is available. Whether the conversation has been in person or via telephone, a brief letter summarizing the issue and its resolution should be generated to create a "paper trail," documenting the manner in which issues are to be addressed. All written correspondence should be edited carefully to ensure that there are no personal attacks, injurious comments, or other language that might be construed as being harmful. When addressing areas of performance deficiency, failed service, or other deeply felt issues, the facts can nearly always be presented in a way that speaks to the depth of feeling of the moment.

Verbal communications are also an essential skill for the medical director. The director must have the ability to communicate effectively in bedside clinical care. The emergency department staff should have a healthy respect for the verbal abilities of the medical director, which always starts with their assessment of the manner in which the physician handles bedside communication with the patient and their family. Such verbal communication should always be deeply imbued with a deep sense of respect for the value of the person. For example, referring to "Mrs. Smith in bed 3 with abdominal pain" is a completely different verbal communication than "the belly pain in 3." To some, this level of communication may seem unimportant; however, the patients, their families, and the emergency department staff readily notice such detail in verbal communication. The medical director therefore should have an extremely high degree of professionalism in all verbal communications, whether in the clinical or management settings.

A critical component of communication skills is the ability to listen effectively. At times it seems that we expect managers to have all of the answers; in fact most people would prefer to have someone who is capable of listening intently and in an open fashion to their communication. In many cases, it is helpful to repeat what has been heard to ensure that effective communication of the issues has occurred. All physician-managers should be familiar with the literature on improving written, verbal, and listening skills.

Integrity

Although these qualifications are fairly specific and quantifiable, perhaps the most important criteria for a medical director is integrity and intellectual honesty. By the very nature of the job, the medical director must often make difficult judgments, astutely assess complex interpersonal relationships, and acknowledge existing deficiencies of the emergency department staff and the processes under which

they function. Confidentiality, trust, and maturity are the attributes that emergency department personnel respect most. The medical director should have a strong sense of personal worth, decency, and integrity to deal successfully with the problems indigenous to the job. These are not areas in which specific requirements can be set, and yet they are among the most important for successful completion of the job as medical director. Intellectual honesty in particular is an extremely important attribute. Because of the multiple vertical reporting structures in an emergency department, there is often an attempt to find fault or lay blame on someone else's doorstep. At times, the blame truly does belong either with the physician group, an individual physician, or the medical director. Under such circumstances, having the intellectual honesty to address the issue is critically important for long-term success.

ORGANIZATIONAL STRUCTURE

Chapters 3 and 4 address the issue of organizational structure in the emergency department in some detail. As we have indicated, however, most emergency departments have at least four vertical structures through which operations report, despite the fact that the patient moves in a horizontal, cross-functional fashion across these somewhat artificial separations. The keys to organizing a structure in the emergency department are to ensure that the following are created:

- An integrated emergency department, capable of delivering a seamless service
- Appropriate access to the decision-making levels within the organizational structure
- Internal fairness and parity in the structure
- A foundation of excellent patient care

Many hospitals have addressed the issue of organizational structure by ensuring that there is a multidisciplinary committee or council in which information with regard to emergency department operations is discussed, disseminated, and decided on a routine basis. At a minimum, such committees should include representatives from all of the operational areas of the emergency department, including physicians, nurses, unit secretaries, registration, laboratory, imaging services, respiratory services, social services, and emergency department technicians. Figure 15-3 describes a typical committee and its functions with regard to ensuring that an ongoing organizational structure is in place that addresses the needs of the patients and the providers who care for them. The specific organizational structure is in some respects less important than is assurance that there is an effective ongoing

INOVA HEALTH SYSTEM
FAIRFAX HOSPITAL
DEPARTMENT OF EMERGENCY MEDICINE
1995
Emergency Department Operations & Quality Council Members

1. The purposes of the Emergency Department Operations and Quality Improvement Council are:

    1. To Allow for Exchange of Information on Emergency Department Operations
    2. To Assist Emergency Department Leaders on Management Issues
    3. To Guide and Assist the Department's Quality Improvement Teams
    4. To serve as an Forum for Management and Leadership Development

2. Membership:

    ☐ Chairman, Emergency Medicine
    ☐ Chief, Pediatric Section, Emergency Medicine
    ☐ Operations Manager, Registration, WCC, ED, CTAII
    ☐ Supervisor, Emergency Department Registration
    ☐ Director Quality Improvement
    ☐ Emergency Department Staff Nurse
    ☐ Vice Chairman, Emergency Medicine
    ☐ Quality Management
    ☐ Supervisor, Immediate Response Lab
    ☐ Assistant Director, Radiology Department
    Administrative Manager, Radiology Department
    ☐ Clinical Specialist for the Emergency Department
    ☐ Emergency Department Social Work
    ☐ Patient Care Director, Emergency Department
    ☐ QI Facilitator

FIGURE 15-3 Emergency department operations and quality improvement council.
(Courtesy Fairfax Hospital Department of Emergency Medicine, Falls Church, Va.)

3. Agenda

- Fixed Agenda Items
  1. Overall Department Operation
  2. Emergency Nursing
  3. Emergency Physicians
  4. Radiology
  5. Registration
  6. Laboratory
  7. Access of Reston
  8. Quality Improvement
  9. Pediatric Emergency Medicine
  10. Social Services

- Reports
  1. JCAHO Update
  2. Nursing Council

- Additional Agenda Items
  1. Open Forum
  2. Adjournment

FIGURE 15-3, CONT'D. For legend see opposite page.

means of communications between the multiple providers of care in the emergency department.

SPECIFIC ROLES

One of the most important roles of an emergency department medical director is to coordinate with nursing and non-nursing managers to ensure that the emergency department is committed to excellence, is fair and reasonable in its management structure, undergoes constant improvement, and continues to be responsive to the needs of its patients and the providers who provide their clinical care. In that regard, the emergency department's leadership must define three primary roles: establishing the boundaries of the organization, providing a constant commitment to excellence and quality, and developing the emergency department providers. Each of these is addressed in some detail.

Boundaries of the Organization

In addressing the boundaries of the organization, the emergency department medical director must begin by assessing the core functions and processes of the emergency department. Is the emergency department a community hospital resource for convenience care? A level I trauma center? A pediatric emergency medicine center? A gatekeeper for primary care physicians and managed care organizations for after hours care? A regional tertiary care resource? All of the above? All of these questions must be asked from a macromanagement standpoint to ensure that the managers and providers of clinical care have a clear understanding of the boundaries of the emergency department. These boundaries must be discussed in some detail with administration, the medical staff, and the hospital governance structure to ensure that there is consonance in the vision of the emergency department's function. In addressing these questions, the department will begin to address issues of strategic planning and mission statements, which are discussed in detail in Chapter 5. Regardless of the current strategic plan or mission statement, virtually all emergency departments are undergoing constant change, and therefore the boundaries of the organization are subject to revision.

In addition to establishing the boundaries of the organiza-

tion itself, the emergency department medical director also must have a clear sense of the boundaries of his or her specific job. These boundaries are largely defined by two important sources: hospital administration and the emergency department physician group. These two sources largely define the specific contractual roles and responsibilities in the job description for an emergency department physician. Appendix A lists several such job descriptions, which tend to focus on areas such as medical affairs, administrative responsibilities, and nursing interactions. Although such delineations are important, rather than focus on these specific areas, this chapter speaks to the broader issues of establishing the boundaries of the organization, ensuring the commitment to excellence for the department, and developing its providers.

Current Assessment. The first step in establishing the boundaries of either the organization or the role of the emergency department medical director is to ensure there is an accurate, concise assessment of the current status of the department and its leadership. Box 15-2 lists the primary questions of the initial assessment. The first step in that assessment is determining the core businesses of the emergency department including aspects of primary, secondary, and tertiary care. In determining the core business, statistical analysis of acuity of care, percentage of patients admitted to the hospital, financial payor mix, impact of managed care will be helpful in ensuring there is a clear understanding of the primary function of emergency department and how revenue is generated. The second aspect that must be addressed is the current status of resources available, including physical plant, nursing resources, technicians, emergency department physicians, core secretaries, registration personnel, and ancillary services such as radiology and the laboratory. These resources should be detailed at some length, so that there is a clear understanding for all parties involved. A third aspect that needs to be addressed is assessing whether the current resources match the previously identified core business for the boundaries of the organization that have been established by administration, the medical staff, and the emergency department leadership. If prompt emergency department care is a stated goal, but there are insufficient space and staff to deliver this goal, this problem must be discussed honestly and openly.

The leader should then assist in establishing the initial goals of the emergency department. Succinctly stated, "What needs to be done *now?*" Assessing these goals involves determining the internal and external stakeholders of the emergency department (see the following discussion) who should help participate in establishing a clear understanding of the current situation, as well as offering insight on future direction. Once short-term goals are determined, the emergency department medical director must ask the difficult question, "What magnitude of change is required to complete these goals?" In some cases, the magnitude of change will be relatively small and can be dealt with somewhat easily. Far more commonly, the degree of change requires a clear understanding of change management and its principles. The topic of change management is addressed in Chapter 13, as well as in the following paragraphs.

In continuing the current assessment, the emergency department medical director determines whether the appropriate tools and structure will be made available to complete the magnitude of change required. In addition, it must be made clear how success will be measured, when it will be measured, and by whom. A further area of importance is assessment of the current culture of the organization. What are the primary mind sets and decision-making processes of the leaders of the organization? Are the organization's imperatives derived from quality improvement, management by objective, concepts of learning organizations, reengineering, etc? Finally, in completing a current assessment of the emergency department and predicting changes that need to be made on both a short- and long-term basis, it is important to be conservative and judicious in establishing goals and strategies. As in many organizations, the progress of change is far less dependent on the energy and skills of the leader than on his or her ability to empower and steward the staff to effect change.

BOX 15-2

BOUNDARIES OF THE ORGANIZATION: INITIAL ASSESSMENT

1. What are the core businesses of the emergency department?
   - Statistical analysis of acuity of care
   - Percentage of patients admitted to the hospital
   - Financial payor mix
   - Impact of managed care
   - Specialty services (trauma care, pediatric, cardiac, etc)
2. What resources are available to deliver such care?
   - Physician resources
   - Nursing resources
   - Technicians
   - Ancillary services
   - Physical plant
   - Additional support and services
3. Do the current resources match identified needs to reduce the core business?
4. What are the initial goals of the emergency department? What needs to be done *now?*
5. What magnitude of change is required to complete these goals?
6. What is the current culture of the organization?
7. Have I been conservative and judicious in establishing goals and strategies?

Stakeholder Analysis and Boundary Management. Stakeholder analysis and boundary management are two separate but closely related tools of benefit to the emergency department medical director in defining the boundaries of the organization.[10] Stakeholder analysis simply identifies key stakeholders within any given process or product, delineates their "stake" or position on a given issue, and attempts to seek input and enlist support for necessary changes in the process. Using this tool requires a clear understanding of the process, its component parts, and sufficient recognition of organizational dynamics (including resistance to change).

In the 1990 General Electric Corporation Annual Report, Chief Executive Officer Jack Welch described his vision of "A boundaryless company where we knock down the walls that separate us from each other on the inside and from our key constituencies on the outside."[11] Welch recognized the

need for an organization in which vertical hierarchies are replaced with horizontal, functional networks and in which cross-functional teams participated with suppliers and customers to improve services. In the past the traditional boundaries of organizations were structured along areas of function, hierarchy, and geography. Boundaries were "hard wired" into the very structure of organizations in a rigid fashion. This organization approach had at least one advantage. Managers and employees within the structure usually had roles that were simple, clear, and relatively stable, even if they were not particularly functional.

As the importance of developing "seamless" and "boundaryless" operations emerged, traditional boundaries began to be replaced in a functional fashion by new boundaries. Hirshhorn and Gilmore[10] have defined these as task, authority, identity, and political boundaries (Figure 15-4).

The *authority boundary* seeks to determine "Who is in charge of what? What am I authorized to do?" In traditional organizations, those in authority were easy to identify; they were the bosses who issued the orders the workers followed. However, as organizations have become more flexible, the individual with formal authority is not necessarily the one with the most up-to-date information about a given patient or customer need. This boundary can be seen in the emergency department where the nurse spends substantially more time with the patient than the physician and therefore usually has more access to information about how the patient feels, what the response has been to therapy, and interaction with the family. The authority boundary has in many respects been a major determinant of the interaction between emergency department physicians and nurses (see Physician-Nurse Relationships). In addressing issues on the authority boundary, several questions must be asked. Where does the individual, process, or organization get its authority to do its work? How does each of the providers within the process or organization hold others accountable, particularly in areas of cross-functional dependency? Who is responsible for what aspects of patient care? Are these responsibilities cross-trained, or are they solely delineated to specific individuals or job descriptions? The last two questions have significant overlap with the task boundary.

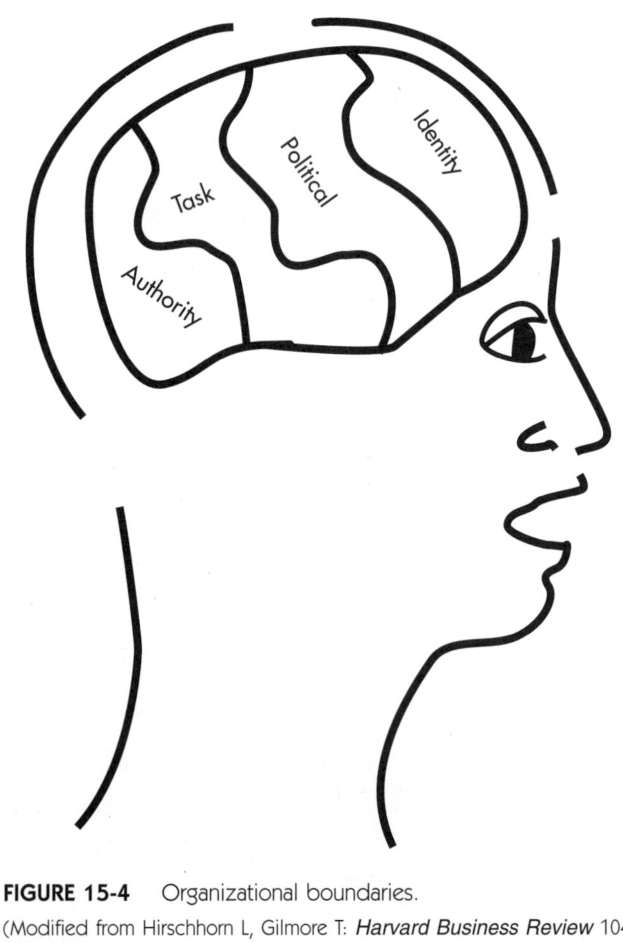

FIGURE 15-4 Organizational boundaries.

(Modified from Hirschhorn L, Gilmore T: *Harvard Business Review* 104-115, 1992.)

The fundamental question of the *task boundary* is "Who does what?" In the complex setting of the emergency department, every patient encounter requires multiple providers who complete multiple tasks under highly differing conditions. In traditional emergency department structures, there has been a contradiction between the specialized tasks performed by the emergency department personnel and the need for shared purposes, which is at the heart of a well-functioning emergency department. Ideally, emergency department providers should address the task boundary in such a way that the work can be divided up so that their separate efforts can be coordinated to provide good clinical care and customer care in a process that promotes teamwork. In traditional organizations, managing the task boundary is largely a matter of overseeing formal interactions among different personnel. As emergency departments have adopted cross-training, quality improvement, and reengineering methods, however, individuals have increasingly had to depend on others who would, in a traditional environment, be considered outside their realm of control or in such specialized jobs that there was no shared understanding of purpose.

The *identity boundary* is an essential component of defining the organization because it primarily asks the question "Who is and isn't 'us'?" Who are the members of the emergency department team and what are the criteria for membership? What loyalties do the emergency department team members feel toward each other, and what are the extent of those loyalties? How clearly are the identities of the team members aligned with the purposes they provide? Initially, people acting at the identity boundary trust insiders, but are wary of outsiders. As the focus on identity boundaries increases, staff tend to become more energized and motivated because the "team spirit" involved in identity boundary management is usually infectious in nature. However, relationships at the identity boundary can also run the risk of disrupting the interrelationship between the emergency department and other areas of the hospital if the boundary is drawn so sharply that emergency department team members do not collaborate with their colleagues in other areas.

For emergency department providers, the *political boundary* is important because it speaks to the power of the emergency department as it relates to the larger context of the hospital and healthcare system. The fundamental question of the political boundary is "What is in it for us?" It seeks to understand the context in which the emergency department fits with other stakeholders in the healthcare system and also addresses issues such as how power is negotiated among the different stakeholder groups. Properly framed, the political

boundary for an emergency department is powerful, founded as it is on the essentials of patient care, interaction with the community, and interrelationship with other aspects of the healthcare organization. Although in many hospitals, *politics* is a term of pure derision, it is a necessary outgrowth of the interaction of the multiple stakeholders involved both in and with the emergency department. When operating at the political boundary, staff face the challenge of defending their interests and those of their department without undermining the effectiveness and coherence of the organization as a whole.

Table 15-1 summarizes skills required to manage effectively across the authority, task, political, and identity boundaries. Using these skills in boundary management and stakeholder analysis can assist emergency department managers in identifying specific strategies to address needed change within an emergency department setting. In addition, it can be helpful in identifying common areas in which dysfunctional relationships both within and outside departments can exist. Because of the highly cross-functional nature of emergency department operations, "managing across the seams" forms an important part of the leader's task. Being aware of boundary management and stakeholder analysis issues therefore is important to a properly functioning emergency department.

Change Management. Chapter 13 addresses change management in detail. Being able to manage change effectively forms an essential core competency for the emergency department medical director and his or her colleagues. The changing landscape of healthcare is one reason why an understanding of the science of change management is essential. Further, as more focus is placed on redesigning or reengineering processes, understanding the obstacles to change assumes increased importance. There are numerous formulations of the theory of change management, but the ideas of several seminal thinkers can be helpful to emergency department managers.

Schein has delineated the theory of change as transition from the comfortable present to the uncertain future, in which he describes the concepts of anxiety one and anxiety two. Anxiety one is the inability or unwillingness to learn something new because it appears to be too difficult or too disruptive. The present state of affairs, regardless of its difficulties, is in almost all cases easier to accept *prima facie* because of the uncertainty and difficulty of the alternatives. The most common response to anxiety one is similar in many respects to the formulations of the stages of denial of death as described by Kubler-Ross:[13] denial, anger, depression, and acceptance. Denial is at the essence of anxiety one in that it simply refuses to accept either the necessity for change or the inevitability that change will occur. Denial as a response may range from apathy to anger, which constitutes the second stage in the process. Common responses at this stage include the insistence that the change will never work, that the individual is withdrawing from the organization, that management will be sorry, or, in the clinical setting, that the change could affect patient care. Anger often gives way quickly to depression, which is commonly manifested as dwelling on the past, sulking, associating with others who share the fear of change, and resisting other new changes, procedures, or tasks. Finally, as an understanding of anxiety one increases, there are early signs of acceptance, often manifested by probing questions about the nature of the change, the reasons for it, and the details of the new process. In addition, anxiety one often provokes the most basic of defense mechanisms, including projection of anger or depression on others, which in the emergency department most often manifests itself as physician-nurse discord.

The essential problems in dealing with anxiety one are the obstacles to understanding, which include an inability to grasp a problem, limited skills to reinvent or reenvision the problem, and limitations of learning new processes within the organization. Anxiety one is in contrast to anxiety two, the downside associated with *not* learning, changing, or adapting. Whereas anxiety one is readily apparent in change management process, anxiety two must often be developed by managers and providers alike to make sure that it is apparent to all of those affected by the change management process. This requires disconfirmation, or demonstration that the current system *is* broken, including highly visible demonstrations, intense communication, and economic education of the consequences of failure to change. *Schein astutely observes that significant change cannot occur until anxiety two exceeds anxiety one.* One of the roles of the leader in assur-

Table 15-1 Key Boundaries and Their Implications

Boundary	Key issues	Shaping factors	Skills
Authority	Control, accountability	Number of levels Culture of "direct talk" Delegation practices	Setting/accepting limits Letting go Challenging upward Absorbing risk/uncertainty
Task	Productivity, effectiveness	Division of labor Work design Organization design Customer requirements	Linking data to performance Balancing integration and specialization
Sentient	Loyalty, identity	Professional groupings Cultural identities Regional ties Group identifications	Promoting identification, avoid groupthink Understanding stereotyping
Political	Rewards, equity, security	Differing interests Power distribution	Negotiating differences Linking conflict to collaboration Understanding the dynamics of bargaining, gaming

Adapted from the Center for Applied Research, Courtesy of Mal O'Connor.

ing that the staff understand that anxiety two exceeds anxiety one is the creation of so-called *safe pathways,* which help providers understand that there is psychologic, economic, and clinical safety in moving from the current process to the new process. Perhaps the most appropriate metaphor is seeing someone cross a narrow bridge over a high chasm, but negotiating the bridge successfully to the other side. Once it has been demonstrated that the bridge is safe, others are more likely to follow this safe pathway to the other side.

An illuminating and entertaining example of the principles of change management is drawn from the Bible and is given by Hammer,[14,15] the originator of the concept of reengineering. Hammer uses the story of Exodus, as recounted in the Books of Exodus in Numbers and refers to it as "The Case of the Road to the Promised Land." It covers the journey of the Israelites from slavery in Egypt to the Promised Land in Israel, which by any standard is a drastic improvement. However, between the old (slavery) and the new (promised land) lies something very bad—40 years in the desert. Hammer notes six lessons in the biblical story (Box 15-3). The first lesson concerns what it takes to get started in any change management effort because the process of change itself is extremely difficult. Although people may agree as to the unpleasantness of the current situation, they almost universally are terrified of what resides outside the boundaries of their familiar, day-to-day lives. Why then did the Israelites agree to follow Moses? Hammer offers two answers, which he refers to as the wedge and the magnet. The wedge is simply something that causes you to let go of the past (in Schein's formulation, anxiety two), which in the case of the Israelites was Pharaoh's Army, a formidable and particularly ill-tempered force. Hammer points out, however, that although fear of destruction is a powerful incentive to change, it is rarely enough because it does not provide a direction toward which one can move. Therefore in addition to a wedge, there must be a magnet, which draws you toward a specific goal: the wedge repels; the magnet attracts. In many cases, the magnet is a vision, just as it was in Moses' time. However, the vision must not only be that of the leader, it must also be translated in a meaningful fashion to the followers.

The second lesson of the Exodus story is the need for the leader to clearly demonstrate willingness to take risks in the change process. This willingness is illustrated by the events at the Red Sea, in which Moses tells his followers that the sea will part and they will walk safely to the other side. According to Hammer, the children of Israel said, "You first." Moses' willingness to step into the sea demonstrated to his followers his own personal courage. Hammer's third lesson derives from the battle of the Israelites and the Amalekites, in which Moses directs the battle from the top of the mountainside, during which the battle always turned in favor of the Israelites when Moses' arms were raised to the sky, but in which the Amalekites prevailed whenever his arms fell to his side. Moses enlisted his brother Aaron and his nephew Hur to hold his arms up when he grew too tired, thereby ensuring victory for the Israelites. This illustrates the critical importance of support and alignment among those who are charged with the effort of change management. Conversely, dissension and discord in this group must be resolved before successful change management can occur. In some situations, consensus may require changes in staff.

The fourth lesson from the Exodus story illustrates the need for constant vigilance and visibility, the need to see and be seen. When Moses left his people to climb to the top of Mt. Sinai and receive the Ten Commandments, the people quickly slipped back into debauchery and idol worship. Change requires leaders who are constantly vigilant and constantly visible to those they are leading; otherwise the organization tends to revert to previous patterns of behavior. The fifth lesson from the Exodus story illustrates the role of exaggeration, romanticism, and loss. As the Israelites traveled through the desert, they were provided with the proverbial "manna from heaven," which sustained them through their journey. However, after a time they complained to Moses about this miracle food, preferring to remember, the "flesh pots of Egypt, the fish, the melons, the onions." What they were remembering is what they perceived as the good old days, even as they conveniently forgot that they were in slavery at the time. Clearly, the lesson here is that all change is loss, which is amplified and exaggerated routinely. No matter how bad the old situation, it always has some redeeming qualities. A substantial amount of change management is assisting people in dealing with this loss, particularly before the new process is fully in place.

Finally, the last lesson from the Exodus story arises when the Israelites approach the perimeter of the Promised Land, only to learn from their scouts that, although it is indeed a land flowing with milk and honey, that it is also inhabited by giants, who made them feel as if "we were as grasshoppers in *our* eyes."[16] Hammer points out that this illustrates the fear, inadequacy, and need for personal transformation in any change management effort. Simply stated, if you believe you can't change, you won't. In the case of the Israelites, the Lord decreed that that generation would die in the desert and that only the next generation, who presumably did believe in their future, could enter the Promised Land.

Hammer further delineates five principles for overcoming resistance to change. The first of these principles is that resistance is natural, inevitable, and should be expected. The

BOX 15-3

CHANGE MANAGEMENT: THE CASE OF THE ROAD TO THE PROMISED LAND

The Exodus from Egypt: the wedge and the magnet

The Parting of the Red Sea: Leading by Personal Example————→The Battle Against the Amalekites: The Importance of Support and Alignment The Episode of the Golden Calf: The Need for Constant Vigilance and Visibility: The Need to See and Be Seen————→ The Complaints About Manna: Exaggeration, Romanticization, and Loss————→The Report of the Scouts: Fear, Inadequacy, and the Need for Personal Transformation

Hammer uses the parable of the Exodus from Egypt and the journey to the Promised Land as an example of difficulties that must be overcome and decisions that must be made in any change management initiative.

Adapted from Hammer M, Stanton SA: *The reengineering revolution: a handbook,* New York, 1995, Harper Collins.

essential cause of failure in many change management efforts is not the resistance itself, but the failure of leadership to anticipate, recognize, and deal with it.

The second principle is that resistance can often be disguised, "under the surface" and is seemingly subterranean in nature. As Hammer indicates, "The naive expectation is that resistance will be manifested as sabotage. Would that it were so! Explicit resistance has the virtue of being on the surface, open to view and response."[15] Instead, resistance is nearly always subtle and hidden in nature and therefore must be sought out. As John Kenneth Galbraith observed, "Faced with the alternative between changing one's mind and proving it is unnecessary, just about everybody gets busy on the proof."[17]

The third principle is that resistance has many motivations, and the astute leader will anticipate and understand these motivations. Not only will there be resistance among people who clearly "lose" because of the change, but even presumed "winners" can often turn out to be enemies of change. At its essence, this lesson recognizes that fear constitutes a major part of change, the reaction to which is as varied as the personalities and interests of the people involved in the change effort.

The fourth principle for overcoming resistance to change is to deal directly with people's concerns about change rather than their arguments against it. The effective leader should anticipate the depth of emotion that change engenders and confront it directly, preferably by finding ways to contain rampant anxieties.

Finally, the fifth principle is recognizing that there is no single, prescribed way to deal with such resistance, but rather that leaders must individualize their approach in applying incentives, information, interventions, indoctrination, and involvement to deal with the issue at hand. Hammer's work discusses these issues in more detail.[14,15,18]

An additional formulation of practical importance in change management is that of Kotter.[19] Drawing on his experience with more than 100 companies, Kotter delineates eight principal steps in successfully transforming an organization through the change management process (Box 15-4). The first of these is establishing a clear sense of urgency, demonstrating the necessity of dealing with change in a timely fashion. This first step is far from easy and requires a clear understanding of the difficulty in driving people out of their comfort zones. The leader must clearly, concisely, and compellingly demonstrate the cost of failing to act on the issue (anxiety two, in Schein's formulation). According to Kotter, approximately 75% of the managers of an organization must be convinced that change is necessary for successful change management to occur.

The second step is to form a powerful guiding coalition that is of single mind with regard to the need for change, along with at least a general outline of the process through which the change will occur. The key players within the organization must be prospectively dealt with in this regard, so that the message sent to the rest of the organization is clear and unwavering. In many cases, forming this coalition may require replacement of some people at the management level, if they are unable or unwilling to recognize both the need for change and the necessity of a unified approach.

The third step in transforming the organization is creating a vision of the future that can be easily communicated to those faced with the change. The vision should not only be clear, but also should have supporting strategies for achieving that vision, so that the change is seen as something desirable, not nebulous. Kotter indicates that the vision should be able to be communicated in 5 minutes or less, generating a reaction that signifies both interest and clear understanding.

BOX 15-4

EIGHT STEPS TO TRANSFORMING YOUR ORGANIZATION

1. **Establishing a sense of urgency**
   Examining market and competitive realities
   Identifying and discussing crises, potential crises, or major opportunities
2. **Forming a powerful guiding coalition**
   Assembling a group with enough power to lead the change effort
   Encouraging the group to work together as a team
3. **Creating a vision**
   Creating a vision to help direct the change effort
   Developing strategies for achieving that vision
4. **Communicating the vision**
   Using every vehicle possible to communicate the new vision and strategies
   Teaching new behaviors by the example of the guiding coalition
5. **Empowering others to act on the vision**
   Getting rid of obstacles to change
   Changing systems or structures that seriously undermine the vision
   Encouraging risk taking and nontraditional ideas, activities, and actions
6. **Planning for and creating short-term wins**
   Planning for visible performance improvements
   Creating those improvements
   Recognizing and rewarding employees involved in the improvements
7. **Consolidating improvements and producing still more change**
   Using increased credibility to change systems, structures, and policies that don't fit the vision
   Hiring, promoting, and developing employees who can implement the vision
   Reinvigorating the process with new projects, themes, and change agents
8. **Institutionalizing new approaches**
   Articulating the connections between the new behavior and corporate success
   Developing the means to ensure leadership development and succession

Adapted from Kotter JP: *Harvard Business Review,* 1:59-67, 1995.

The fourth phase of the process is communicating that vision in a repetitive and consistent fashion. Too often, leadership assumes that communicating the vision once, twice, or even ten times is sufficient to drive the change management effort. Instead, communication of the vision should virtually permeate the organization during the initial phases of the change management initiative.

The fifth step is to empower others to act on the vision by eliminating obstacles to change, changing systems or structures that undermine the vision, and encouraging risk taking, nontraditional ideas, and creative methods of achieving the vision. If the change initiative is present only to the extent that management is present to act on it, it is virtually sure to fail. Instead, all levels of the organization must be empowered to act on the vision in creative ways.

The sixth step in the change management process is planning for and creating short-term wins. At the outset, visible performance improvements should be designed and demonstrated to help sustain the change management effort. Further, the employees involved in these improvements should be clearly recognized and rewarded for their successes.

Once the change initiative has begun to show progress, the seventh step is to consolidate improvements and accelerate the pace of change. As the change management initiative gains credibility, systems, structures, and processes previously thought to be "untouchable" in a change process will become accessible as change accelerates. This seventh step is essential for developing the critical mass necessary to drive the pace of change.

Finally, the eighth step in the process is to institutionalize the new approaches that have been generated, emphasizing cross-functional connections between new behaviors and the success of the organization.

The final tool can be of benefit to emergency department managers during change management initiatives derived from the work of Block.[20] He points out that those who need to be influenced during the change process should be evaluated on two essential dimensions, agreement and trust. People either agree or disagree about where the effort is headed, and we either trust or distrust each other concerning the way we operate in pursuit of that future. Using the two dimensions of agreement and trust, the manager can create a matrix (Figure 15-5) to help assist in evaluating appropriate strategies for influencing them during the course of the change process. Using stakeholder analysis, a political strategy can be developed to help identify who among the stakeholders in the process needs to be influenced to bring about change. Each of these people can then be placed on an appropriate part of the matrix, based on evaluation of his or her agreement or disagreement with the change, as well as the level of trust in which the manager holds them. This tool helps realign incentives of key stakeholders during change efforts.

The first category in the matrix is *allies,* in whom there is high agreement with the change process and high trust. With allies, the key to success is firming an agreement on the process or vision, reaffirming the quality of the relationship that generated the trust, acknowledging any substantial doubts or vulnerabilities of the change effort, and asking for their advice and support in the course of the effort. In addition, it can be helpful to help ensure that allies have a chance to interact with each other, to help build even further support for the change effort.

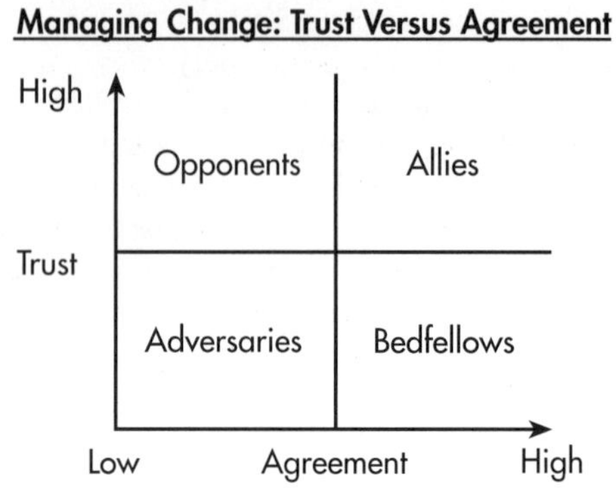

FIGURE 15-5 Managing change: trust agreement: Block's model of change management suggests placing stakeholders on a grid assessing both trust and agreement. Stakeholders can then be classified as opponents, allies, adversaries, or bedfellows, with appropriate strategies for change management assigned to each group. (Adapted from Block P: *The empowered manager: positive political skills,* San Francisco, 1987, Jossey-Bass.

The second category is *opponents,* in whom we have a high degree of trust, but who have a low level of agreement with the change management effort. The task of the opponent is to bring out the best in us, because we trust their motivations and can rely on them to state their objections to the change in a straightforward and highly visible fashion. By challenging the change management effort openly, we become visibly involved in a productive dialogue that allows reasonable debate. In dealing with opponents, it is important to reaffirm the quality of the relationship and the fact that it is based on trust while stating differences in positions. Those differences should be stated in a neutral way and should include a reasonable effort at articulating the position of the opponent to change. At this stage, the opponent should be engaged in useful dialogue to problem-solve how objections to the change effort can be resolved.

The third category in the matrix is *bedfellows,* people who agree with us about how to proceed, but in whom there is a low to moderate amount of trust. Typically these are people who are aligned with the vision of the change effort, but in whom there is distrust with regard to past behavior, mechanisms of dealing with change and/or the people involved in it, or the sense that the bedfellow does not give us the whole story when issues are discussed. In dealing with bedfellows, it is important to reaffirm the agreement while acknowledging that caution exists. It is important to be clear about what is desired from bedfellows in terms of the change management effort and the continued working relationship. They should be kept well informed, and the manager should expect to be well informed in turn. Bedfellows should be encouraged to be clear, concise, and straightforward in their understanding of and objections to the change effort. Most important, ground rules of the relationship must be established with regard to how the change effort will be managed because the relationship is not primarily based on trust.

The fourth category in the matrix is *adversaries,* in whom there is both low agreement and low trust. As Block astutely

notes, calling someone an adversary is "a position of last resort. . . People become adversaries only when our attempts at negotiating agreement and negotiating trust have failed."[20] The essential connection to adversaries is that they can become the object of our envy because they act (and get away with it) in a way that we do not permit ourselves to act. Specific strategies for dealing with adversaries are to state the vision again clearly in a neutral way that indicates our best understanding of the adversary's position, to identify any of our own contributions to the problem, and to conclude the summary of the plans with no specific demand because both trust and agreement are low.

Two additional categories deserve some comment. Although they do not appear on the matrix, some stakeholders are those in whom there is low trust and unknown agreement: We don't trust them but we don't know where they stand with regard to the effort, often because they do not know themselves. Block identifies these people as *fence-sitters* who are usually people with strong interpersonal skills, good communications skills, and a knack for framing issues so that apparent conflicts disappear by their constantly stating alternate points of view. The cardinal virtues of a fence-sitter are caution and patience. In many ways, fence-sitters are a bureaucratic prototype and therefore the strategy is to try to flush them out, find out where they stand, and encourage them to take a position (any position) with respect to the change management project. In most cases, fence-sitters are not worth excessive effort in the midst of a change management process. Finally, there is a similar group of people in whom we have a high level of trust but who are also undecided with regard to the project. These people might be called the *undecideds*. In most cases, it is useful to treat undecideds with a high degree of respect in a similar fashion to the strategy outline for opponents.

For most change management efforts, efforts should be focused on those in whom there is a reasonable degree of trust, which suggests that opponents, undecideds, and allies should receive the most focused effort. Regardless of the specific formulation used in the change management effort, attention to this science and the tools and techniques it offers is important to the emergency department medical director and his or her colleagues. Dealing with change in an effective way is a fundamental challenge for all emergency department leaders.

Commitment to Excellence and Quality

One of the most fundamental roles of a leader in the emergency department is to demonstrate a consistent, passionate, and nonwavering commitment to excellence in the clinical care of patients in the emergency department setting. Although the term *quality* is perhaps overused, its essential meaning is to describe products or services that add value. Quality exists to the extent that value is added to that product or service by the provider.[21] The more value added, the higher the quality of the service. Perhaps a better standard to which to commit is that of excellence, which communicates clearly that the product or service has been carefully constructed and appropriately revised to meet the highest possible standards. In examining this commitment to excellence, the emergency department medical director should make a current assessment of the department, similar to that outlined in the section Boundaries of the Organization. However, assessment of clinical excellence and quality requires substantially more effort and diversity, particularly given the large number of clinical functions performed within the emergency department. For example, an emergency department may be excellent at providing general medical care for undifferentiated emergencies, but may not have the same level of capability for major trauma patients or pediatric emergencies. For that reason, any assessment of the existing state of clinical excellence requires more detailed and comprehensive clinical review of charts, outcomes, and patient and medical staff satisfaction.

Managing Resources. One of the most important roles of an emergency department medical director is managing the financial and nonfinancial resources necessary for the provision of excellent clinical care. As indicated previously, the various sections and chapters of this textbook are designed to delineate the specific tools and techniques available for managing these various resources. Similarly, the job descriptions listed in Appendix A delineate specific functions for the medical director. However, these competencies must be unified by a leadership and management approach capable of taking a global view of the *overall* resources available to the emergency department. For example, an emergency department is charged with developing a "fast track" alternative to normal operations. Careful consideration must be given to what, if any, additional resources will be required to implement this change. To begin with, the emergency department medical director (along with his or her management colleagues) needs to ensure that there is a clear understanding of the goals for the service. More rapid care? More cost-competitive care? To function as an after hours gatekeeper for minor illnesses? As a competitive alternative to urgent care centers? As a means of "decompressing" the main emergency department? Consideration must be given to whether additional staff and space will be provided to the emergency department to develop such a program. If not, it is likely that using existing resources (both staff and space) could result in actually *lengthening* the turnaround times for patients who are neither acutely ill nor well enough to fall under the fast track system. Further, is the system designed with the patient's input, to ensure that it has the customer's needs in mind before designing the space and policies for the service? Finally, what information systems will be put into place to track progress of the product line, and under what time frames will reassessment and evaluation occur?

These parameters and more form a part of the overarching management of resources required to determine the success or failure of the program over time. To an increasing degree, aligning incentives, managing relationships, establishing the milieu for collaboration, and empowering employees form the basis of managing resources, as opposed to more traditional concepts of counseling or terminating employees, controlling resources, and micromanaging. The other chapters in Part 2 provide more detail about managing emergency department resources.

Customer Service. Emergency medicine is by nature a personal service business, in which emergency department team members cooperate to deliver excellent medical care in an environment that meets or exceeds the patient's expectations. Customer satisfaction exists to the extent that the prepurchase

expectations of a product or a service are met[22]; to the extent that these expectations are not met, customer dissatisfaction occurs. One of the most attractive concepts from the quality improvement literature is the definition of a customer as anyone who is affected by our processes or our products. This definition conveniently allows for clarification of customers as either internal customers (those within the organization, primarily involved in the processes used in developing the product or service) or external customers (those outside the organization, who are more focused on the product or service itself). In the emergency department environment, there are several essential internal customers to the process, including our emergency department colleagues, the medical staff, and administration. The most important external customers to emergency department services are patients and their families, although payors are becoming an increasingly important class of external customer.

SERVICE TO THE PATIENT AND FAMILY. Chapters 8 and 52 delineate essential components of customer service in the emergency department. However, our *raison d'être* is the patient. When designing our commitment to excellence and quality, it should always be undertaken with the input of the patient and in a way in which, to the best degree possible, we are able to meet his or her expectations. Although we are not always able to meet these expectations, it is incumbent on emergency service providers to help narrow this gap whenever possible, and, in all circumstances, to help educate the patient with regard to the capability of the department to deliver on certain expectations. Service to the patient should thus imbue all levels of the organization from the emergency department physician and nurse to the housekeepers and security guards. Customer satisfaction leads to employee satisfaction, and aggressive customer service programs can be of benefit to both the patient and the provider.[19-22] Whenever possible, emergency physicians should visit patients they have admitted to the hospital. Not only is this good customer service, it is also an opportunity to obtain follow-up on the patient's progress and often leads to positive, collegial discussions with medical staff members on rounds. Emergency physicians should also have business cards printed, which should be shared appropriately with patients.

SERVICE TO ADMINISTRATION. It is imperative for all emergency department medical directors to understand the concept of service to the hospital administration. As financial and nonfinancial incentives become more aligned between hospitals and physicians, hospital administrators look to all hospital-based or contract management physicians to work closely and cooperatively with the needs of the institution. (Box 15-5.) Most hospital administrators view the emergency department medical director as primarily responsible for ensuring that operations and clinical competence in the emergency department are provided in a seamless fashion. The emergency department medical director should meet frequently with the appropriate administrator to ensure a common vision for the emergency department and a clear understanding of day-to-day operations. These meetings should form a regularly scheduled part of the relationship. The emergency department medical director should use this time carefully, giving prospective thought to the issues to be discussed. In many cases, it may be preferable to provide a written agenda in advance of the meeting to ensure that the administrator is aware of the relevant issues. Stakeholder analysis and boundary management skills should be used to keep appropriate administrators informed of issues that affect their departments. For example in many hospitals, the administrator responsible for ancillary services is not responsible for emergency services. If the emergency department has issues with either the laboratory or radiology departments, copying the appropriate administrator, as well as the administrator responsible for the emergency department, should be considered.

BOX 15-5

SERVICE TO HOSPITAL ADMINISTRATION

1. Align strategic incentives
2. Meet frequently with appropriate administrator
3. Use meeting time judiciously
4. Use stakeholder analysis and boundary management
5. Ensure the administrator is part of the emergency department team
6. Establish management credentials
7. Use the guidance and advice of the administrator
8. Understand the organization's philosophy, common language, and accounting principles
9. Inform administrators prospectively of potential problems
10. Be responsive

The emergency department medical director must ensure that the administrator to whom he or she reports feels a part of the emergency department team. Anything less than a feeling of being one of "us" is counterproductive. The administrator responsible for the emergency department should be invited to selected emergency department staff meetings, emergency department physician group meetings, and social functions. In developing the relationship with the administrator, it is important both to establish your management credentials (to the extent that they exist) and to let him or her know you value management skills as the application of sound business principles to clinical practice. Whenever possible, enlisting the administrator's guidance to access management information, courses, or advice, can help further develop a personal and professional relationship. The medical director should emphasize his or her willingness to learn additional management/administrative skills and techniques. In particular, the medical director should spend a great deal of time learning the organization's philosophy, common language, and accounting principles.[24] Is the organization driven by total quality improvement or more traditional management approaches? Is there an imperative to reengineer, redesign, or develop patient-focused care initiatives in the hospital? Does the financial office develop profitability reports by service line based on partially allocated or fully allocated costs? What is the impact of indirect costs on the profitability of service lines? Whenever possible, the medical director should attend appropriate management team meetings to ensure they are carefully integrated into the overall operations of the hospital and to gain exposure to the organization's philosophy and operational structure.

The medical director should keep the administrator informed prospectively with regard to any serious problems

that are developing in the emergency department. In pointing out these problems, he or she should be a problem-solver, not a finger pointer. The medical director should be capable of concisely and dispassionately stating the elements of a problem, offering alternatives, and recommending a course of action. In this regard, responsiveness is a key quality characteristic for any emergency department medical director. When issues are identified that require action, a timely, thoughtful, and responsive nature is essential for the successful discharge of his or her duties. When disagreements occur, they should be calmly discussed in private, never in a public setting. If issues with which the administrator does not agree will be raised at the meeting, these differences should be discussed in detail before any public discussion of them. A close, collegial relationship between the emergency department medical director and administrative colleagues can form a powerful partnership that benefits the patient, medical staff, hospital, and emergency physician group.

SERVICE TO THE MEDICAL STAFF. An additional customer to whom the medical director should be responsive is the medical staff, including both the formal structure of the medical staff and the individual physicians comprising it (Box 15-6). Many physicians in private practice view the emergency department (as well as other hospital-based/contact management groups) as practicing in a fundamentally different situation. The emergency department medical director and physician colleagues should make every effort to close this gap, emphasizing common ground as opposed to differences. For example, for those emergency departments practicing fee-for-service emergency medicine, it is essential for the medical director to stress to the medical staff that they are compensated in highly similar ways, based on volume of patients and quality of service.

Emergency medicine is not only a personal service business between the physician and the patient, but also a personal service business between the emergency physician and the attending medical staff. The medical director should assist his or her physician colleagues in establishing a climate of mutual respect and appreciation between the emergency department physicians and attending physicians in the hospital.

BOX 15-6

SERVICE TO THE MEDICAL STAFF

1. Align strategic incentives
2. Establish a climate of mutual respect and appreciation
3. Provide succinct, focused clinical summaries
4. Assist medical staff members in the emergency department
5. Attend department/section meetings
6. Visit the physician's lounge
7. Copy attending medical staff on emergency department record
8. Obtain discharge summaries on admitted patients
9. Use stakeholder analysis and boundary management
10. Solve problems in private
11. Inform appropriate medical staff leaders of potential conflicts

Clearly, the primary basis of this positive climate is delivering excellent clinical care that is responsive to the needs of the attending physician. For example, in addition to providing excellent evaluation and therapy for a patient with a myocardial infarction, it is also helpful to ensure that the emergency physician provides a succinct, focused summary to the medical staff on the telephone, allowing them to ask pertinent questions when necessary. Emergency physicians should make clear to the patient that their care is going to be discussed and coordinated with their private physician, particularly in an era when the role of the primary care physician and managed care is of increased importance. When medical staff members come to the emergency department, every effort should be made to assist them in delivering care to their patients as promptly as possible. (This does not mean that the emergency department should be used for elective procedures.)

The emergency department medical director should regularly attend meetings of departments and sections of the medical staff (with the approval and consent of the respective chair and section chiefs). This practice helps ensure that any issues with the emergency department can be discussed in an open and professional fashion. In many cases, small problems can be dealt with immediately, instead of being allowed to grow into larger issues. Similarly, the medical director and other emergency physicians should be encouraged to spend time in the physician lounge, discussing issues and/or problems with medical staff members. A great deal of discussion occurs in the physician's lounge, and it is important for emergency department physicians to be available to address any questions about their department. Whenever possible, a legible copy of the emergency department medical record should be forwarded to the patient's private physician, which helps inform the physician of the care delivered in the emergency department and often increases the respect for the diagnostic and therapeutic interventions that occur. Similarly, the emergency physician should routinely review discharge summaries on admitted patients and copies of office notes from attending physicians.

When complaints or concerns arise from the medical staff, they should be handled *immediately* by the medical director. Whenever possible, the attending physician and emergency physician should meet to resolve any issues, questions, or concerns about clinical care. When conflicts do arise between individual physicians and/or departments, it is important to prospectively assess stakeholder issues relating to the problem, including speaking to all parties involved and ensuring that the facts are known in advance. Whenever possible, such problems should be resolved in private, as opposed to during a meeting. The medical director should have sufficient moral character to apologize freely for mistakes made in the emergency department, while at the same time defending staff who may have been criticized unfairly.

The tools of stakeholder analysis and boundary management are essential in dealing with the medical staff. The medical director should ensure that boundaries between and within departments are respected and addressed appropriately. The medical director should be aware of potent allies within the medical staff who can be of assistance in negotiating solutions to difficult problems. In particular, when important issues will be subject to close votes in committee,

informing appropriate medical staff members in advance of the issues, potential solutions, and suggested resolution is a critical aspect of boundary management. In this regard, the emergency department medical director should have a reputation for honesty, fairness, and common sense that is earned through previous interactions with the medical staff.

Despite attention to all of these issues, conflict can still arise. When this condition occurs, it is important to remember that many medical staff members retain the dated concept of emergency physicians as hospital-based physicians who are pawns of administration. Such physicians routinely expect emergency department medical directors to side with the hospital in all matters. Although the emergency department medical director and the physician group should be aligned strategically with the objectives of the hospital, the medical director must be willing to honestly express his or her opinion, even when it may conflict with that of the administration. Most hospital administrators understand this concept, but concept should be discussed (in advance if possible) with the administrator. The emergency department medical director should seek to resolve disputes in private, as opposed to public, forums, particularly when the emergency department is going to win on a given issue, because it is better to handle such victories in a private setting as opposed to subjecting the "loser" to what might be perceived as the humiliation of defeat. Areas of known conflict with the medical staff, should be addressed preemptively and solved in face-to-face negotiations whenever possible. Hospital administrators should be kept informed about any substantial differences between the emergency department physician group and other members of the medical staff. Their advice and/or perspective can be extremely helpful in resolving difficult issues.

The emergency department medical director must help manage the relationship between the emergency department physician group and the medical staff to the best extent possible. Identifying the needs of the attending physician prospectively, attending department and section meetings, and socializing with the attending physicians are ways to establish a common dialogue. Similarly, emergency physicians should participate actively in both the medical staff structure and in the county/state medical society, demonstrating their commitment to the needs of the medical community.

Physician-Nurse Relationships. The interaction between physicians and nurses is among the most complicated, confusing, and compelling in all of medicine. Nowhere do physicians and nurses work more closely for long periods of time under varied conditions than in the emergency department. For 8 to 12 hours at a time, teams of doctors and nurses work side-by-side to meet the needs of patients, their families, and the other customers of emergency department processes. To a significant extent, the growth and success of an emergency department can be gauged by the quality of the relationship between the emergency physicians and emergency nurses. Despite these working conditions, little explicit thought and effort usually have addressed how physicians and nurses are educated, trained, motivated, and rewarded to do emergency department operations. The emergency department medical director must work extremely closely with his or her nursing colleagues to ensure deep understanding of this important relationship and must commit substantial time and effort to learning how such relationships can be further developed.

The origins of physician and nursing education can be instructive. American medical education has been based for decades on an authoritarian, hierarchical educational model, with relatively strict progression of the student, resident, and junior physician through the stages of education and development. Medical schools and residencies in particular have reinforced classic concepts of doling out information, procedures, and prestige based on the level of training of the student or physician. The titles themselves reflect this authoritarian structure: junior student, senior student, intern, junior resident, senior resident, chief resident, fellow. Such hierarchic structures are also maintained during the initial phases of clinical practice, with the use of titles such as independent contractor, junior partner, and senior partner.

Similarly, physician education is highly "ends-driven;" The primary, driving goal is to make a specific diagnosis and offer appropriate treatment. In an increasingly technologic environment, physicians have developed a near obsession with ensuring that all available technology is brought to bear to make the most accurate diagnosis, resulting in the best available treatment. Although the means of attaining the diagnosis and treatment are important, the primary focus is on the end result in American medical training and practice.

Nursing education, on the other hand, is far less authoritarian and hierarchical in nature, beginning in nursing school and continuing through nursing practice, which is in many respects more collaborative in nature than medical education and practice. Further, nursing practice itself is highly process-driven, as opposed to ends-driven, with the primary focus on the manner in which interventions are undertaken. One need look no further than the policies and procedures manuals of most emergency departments to see evidence of this contrast. Nursing policies and procedures tend to be highly process-driven, which is reflected in the delineation of purposes and objectives. Physician protocols are more algorithmic, reflecting some process orientation, but driven, seemingly inexorably, toward specific ends.

One of the most fundamental differences between emergency physicians and emergency nurses is the increased amount of time that the nurse is able to spend with the patient. Emergency physicians are usually limited to discrete, though repeated, interactions with patients and their families, that tend to be quite end-focused. The questions a physician asks involve time, intensity, duration, and quality of symptoms. This staccato litany of questions includes review of systems, past medical history, family history, and social history, often read off of a specific form recorded both for medical and billing purposes. Nursing interactions are more long term in nature and reflect a deeper understanding of the underlying nature of the patient's clinical presentation, social problems, and family interaction. In the best of emergency departments, mechanisms are in place to ensure that communication between emergency physicians and nurses routinely reflect these interactions so that the nurse is able to collaborate openly with the emergency physician in transmitting information about the patient. In this way a common understanding is reached with regard to the nature of the problem, and the most appropriate treatment.

How can the emergency department medical director and nursing director best cooperate to ensure optimal emergency department operations? The seminal work of Katzenbach and Smith in defining teams is instructive, terse, and accurate:

> A team is a small number of people with complementary skills who are committed to a common purpose, performance goals, and approach for which they hold themselves mutually accountable.[24a]

In addressing the concept of teams in the emergency department, the focus here is on the operational teams that work clinically in the emergency department at any given time. For that reason, the definition's focus on a *small number of people* is helpful, particularly because larger groups face difficult logistical issues, often fail to interact constructively as a group, and have difficulty in agreeing to a shared, common purpose. In fact, even in the busiest of emergency departments, a small team of approximately 20 to 30 people work at any given time to see that the patient receives maximal benefit. That fairly small group of people operates with *complementary skills,* including technical functional expertise, problem-solving and decision-making skills, and interpersonal skills. In the emergency department environment, it is important to recognize the complementary nature of the skills and training of physicians and nurses. For example, the time and depth that a nurse is able to give to a patient could potentially paralyze an emergency department if that same amount of time and depth were exercised by the emergency physician, who is expected to play a central role in maintaining patient flow through the emergency department. In developing or selecting teams, it is essential to consider these complementary skills. The operational processes of an emergency department should reflect the wisdom of the emergency department leadership in considering such skills. Conversely, it would be an error of equal significance to overemphasize skills alone because teams often serve as vehicles for personal learning and development, helping hone and develop skills in a way that medical school, residency training, and nursing school cannot.

This small group of people with complementary skills must then commit to a *shared common purpose and performance goals,* which they should have a voice in formulating. All members of the team should be able to articulate clearly and concisely this shared common purpose and ways in which the individuals will interact to meet these goals. One area in which emergency departments often perform well is ensuring a commitment to a *common approach,* particularly given the protocol-oriented nature of many emergency department operations. All members of the team should have a common understanding of how certain problems will be addressed, whether those problems are clinical, social, or interpersonal. Only when such a common approach is widely known do professionals have the confidence to approach the diverse problems present in the emergency department, assured that their colleagues have a clear understanding of their roles and those of others. Finally, teams should be structured to provide *mutual accountability,* which stands as a litmus test of the quality of the team's purpose, approach, and success. When mutual accountability is not present, the team has rarely formed a common purpose and approach that can sustain them during difficult periods.

Two relationships help form a team paradigm in the emergency department: the charge nurse-charge physician relationship and the medical director-nursing director relationship. The charge nurse and charge physician must have clearly delineated roles and responsibilities (Boxes 15-7 and 15-8), in which they cooperate closely to ensure that the department is effectively managed on a shift-to-shift basis. Equally important is a strong, supportive, and cooperative relationship between the medical and nursing directors. Not only must these two professionals be role models for the staff, but their collaboration should itself provide a model for the rest of the staff to follow. Their relationship of trust and mutual respect is *the* essential building block for a strong emergency department.

What can the emergency department medical director and nursing director do from a practical standpoint to ensure a team approach to the physician-nurse interaction? First, it is necessary to be proactive in considering the team concept. There should be a clear understanding of the boundaries of the relationship, boundary management issues, and the perimeters of practice in which physicians and nurses interact. The approach must always be collaborative, both at the management level and at the bedside. Substantial efforts should be invested in ensuring that fragmentation of emergency department operations and processes does not occur. For decades, emergency departments have heard the nonproductive language that "that's a nursing problem" or "it's a doctor problem." Such a "zero sum mentality" is common, but it should be recognized as an essentially destructive form of communication. Instead, the department should proactively establish the concept of a team of professionals working collaboratively to address the needs of both the patient and the providers. When service failures occur, instead of creating divisiveness, they should act to strengthen the bonds between team members, as well as the processes in which they function.

Second, the medical director and nursing director should clearly and concisely communicate the desired results of the team. These goals often include not only patient care, but also the working relationship and interdependency of team members. Emergency department leaders should seek "small victories," such as letters of compliment from patients, and celebrate them publicly. Cooperative and collaborative behaviors should be encouraged, and those who exhibit them should be developed as role models for the department.

Third, it is essential to keep the communication line open, particularly at the bedside. Emergency nurses spend substantially more time with patients; and the emergency physician should listen carefully to their insights, judgments, and evaluations. Further, mature emergency physicians have always actively sought the opinions of emergency department nurses with regard to the patient's clinical presentation, progress, and response to therapy. From a theoretic standpoint, modern learning theory emphasizes the concept of *double loop learning,* as presented by Argyris,[24] which is typified by continual feedback loops of information during the course of the learning process. The concept of double loop learning lends itself to the interaction between nurses and physicians in the emergency department, in which multiple providers obtain information from diverse sources that must be assimilated to help establish a learning environment in which the patient's diagnosis and therapy can be effectively understood (Figure

BOX 15-7

CHARGE NURSE RESPONSIBILITIES

Emergency Department

Charge Nurse Responsibilities

Effective: Revised:

Patient Care Administrator
Emergency Department

I. Description

A more senior clinician who has knowledge of intradepartmental and interhospital policies and procedures. This nurse monitors the quality of patient care in the department by matching patient needs with departmental resources.

II. Responsibilities

1. Has the authority to make management decisions in the absence of the Patient Care Director or Assistant Patient Care Director.
2. Coordinates interactions between RN staff, EDP, PMDs, secretaries, ancillary staff, incoming ambulance and helicopter personnel, and communications nurse.
3. Maintains communication with senior EDP and/or Pediatric EDP regarding critical patient needs in the department.
4. Communicates with Patient Care Director, Patient Care Administrator, or Administrative Director, as needed.
5. Makes decisions with regard to use of on-call nurse and relays information to Administrative Director when appropriate.
6. Assigns CODE BLUE, CODE YELLOW, and M-SET response nurses when appropriate.
7. Ensures that assigned department tasks are completed by designated staff and signed off on daily checklist.
8. Facilitates rapid patient flow through department by making frequent rounds.
9. Assists with patient care as needed and coordinates help for nurses who need assistance.
10. Coordinates crisis intervention for family with social workers and clergy.
11. Documents significant occurrences or interventions on 24-hour shift report.
12. Ensures appropriate completion of Medicus cards.
13. Becomes main source of communication for nursing in the emergency department in a disaster situation.
14. Assists Northern Virginia Community College and George Washington preceptors with assigning students to appropriate emergency department staff.
15. Assigns primary nurses for acutely ill patients based on nurses' workload and availability when necessary.
16. At beginning of each shift, sees that narcotics are counted accurately and that *all* sets of keys are in the department before previous shift leaves.
17. Assigns staff mealtimes and facilitates breaks.
18. Checks staffing numbers on graphic sheet to facilitate department coverage for 24 hours and make appropriate calls to cover staff call-ins.
19. Receives report from on-going charge nurse and makes walking rounds.
20. Carries M-SET beeper at all times.
21. See that all personal property is returned to owner or that it is sent to Lost Property Department according to hospital policy (see Emergency Department Valuables Standard).
22. Responsible for supervision of nurse technicians on each shift.
23. Responsible for leaving and routing appropriate documentation of incidents, employee accidents, quality committee reports and transfer forms.

III. Expected Outcomes

1. Patient flow through department is improved.
2. Patient needs are better matched to departmental needs.
3. Nurses with excessive workload are assisted.
4. There is improved organization and communication in the treatment area.
5. Acutely ill patients are appropriately assigned to a primary nurse.
6. Assignments are completed.
7. Ensure communication.

BOX 15-8

CHARGE PHYSICIAN DESCRIPTION

Emergency Department

Charge Physician Description

Effective Date: **Revised:**

Chair, Emergency Medicine **Vice Chair, Emergency Medicine**

Objective:

To describe the roles and responsibilities of the emergency department Charge Physician.

Policy:

1. The Charge Physician has overall responsibility for the delivery of quality medical care in the emergency department, including clinical and nonclinical aspects of care. The Charge Physician should work closely with the Charge Nurse to ensure that the clinical and administrative needs of the emergency department are met on a timely basis.
2. The Charge Physician has responsibility for ensuring professional and timely communication between the emergency department physicians and:
   - Nursing
   - Private Medical Staff
   - Administration
   - Emergency Medical Services
   - Patients and Families
   - Community
   - Media

   The Charge Physician and Charge Nurse should be notified of any significant problems with regard to potential problems in any of these areas.
3. The Charge Physician should work closely with the Charge Nurse on assessment of mobilization of resources for patient flow including:
   - Remaining up-to-date with numbers of patients presenting to the triage desk and waiting for rooms.
   - Assisting the Charge Nurse in determining flow patterns and use of resources within the emergency department to meet patient care needs.
   - Working cooperatively with the Charge Nurse to ensure that appropriate actions are taken when potential delays in patient treatment occur, whether they are a result of numbers of patients, numbers of physicians or nurses, backups in the laboratory, availability of rooms, or other.
4. The Charge Physician's responsibility for making the decision to call in back up physicians and add additional coverage. In general, backup physician coverage from the call list should be used when charts accumulate on the physician deck (greater than six charts) for 1 hour or longer. However, the Charge Physician should use backup coverage at any time when adding additional physician resources could be expected to improve patient care or the timeliness thereof.
5. Ensuring that private medical staff are able to communicate with emergency department physicians whenever such physicians call in about patients. The Charge Physician need not take every call, but simply help ensure that the Communications Nurse is able to forward calls to available emergency physicians by Spectra-Link telephone.
6. Overall communication with EMS should be handled by the Charge Physician as it relates to medical control issues. Code Blues and Code Yellows should be alternated between physicians seeing acute side patients, except for pediatric trauma cases, which should be referred to the pediatric emergency physician.
7. Charge Physician will act as a resource to emergency physicians and nurses with regard to patient complaints or dissatisfaction within the emergency department. In coordination with the Charge Nurse, the Charge Physician will be available to use Point of Impact Intervention strategies to help resolve patient complaints at the time they occur. If necessary, the Administrative Physician on-call or Chair also can be called to assist in these matters.
8. The Charge Physician will be assigned prospectively according to the emergency physician schedule. Rotation of the Charge Physician will not be subject to specific shifts, but according to a preset schedule that attempts to facilitate the preceding functions. Changes in the emergency physician schedule should consider the assignment of the Charge Physician and should be communicated to the Chair's office, Communications, and Charge Nurse.

15-6). For example, in the course of the care of a patient with congestive heart failure, the emergency physician and nurse cooperate collaboratively with multiple inputs of information from diverse sources, including EMS providers, the patient, the family, past medical history, medical records, and attending physicians. This information is assimilated into the patient's entry level status at the time of treatment in the emergency department, to which are added technologic pieces of information such as the electrocardiogram, chest radiograph, pulse oximetry, and laboratory studies. During the course of evaluation and therapy in the emergency department, these data points are constantly reassessed by both the physician and nurse, who participate in the patient's care from similar yet different vantage points. Without double loop learning, it is impossible to ensure that such a complex learning environment can result in effective patient care.

Fourth, medical and nursing directors need to recognize authority, task, political, and identity boundaries addressed previously, and at the same time focus on outcomes, not on "who's the boss here?" The interaction between emergency nurses and physicians should allow boundary management issues to be handled aggressively, but professionally. The nature of the protocol-oriented approach in emergency medicine, including concepts such as advanced triage and advanced interventions, attests to the degree to which most emergency departments cooperate in managing such boundaries on an ongoing basis.

Fifth, the emergency department leadership should seek input from team members when redesigning processes that affect them. Effective emergency departments have a long history of enlisting input from the providers to assist in process management and quality improvement issues (Part 5).

Finally, the medical and nursing directors should cooperate closely to ensure a sense of empowerment and stewardship within the emergency department. Although the leadership can help define the collaborative nature of the desired approach, it is incumbent on the providers themselves to accept responsibility for managing such relationships in the midst of a sometimes confusing emergency department. When areas of objection or concern occur, they should be dealt with at the time they occur, but not at the bedside or within earshot or view of patients or family. When necessary, team members should meet with their respective nursing and physician colleagues to help resolve areas of substance.

DEVELOPMENT OF THE PROVIDERS

The emergency department medical director must provide an environment in which the emergency department staff can continue to grow and develop both as individuals and as professionals. This role requires a clear understanding of a combination of disciplines, including management principles (Part 1), understanding of emergency department operations (Part 2), and familiarity with principles of human resource

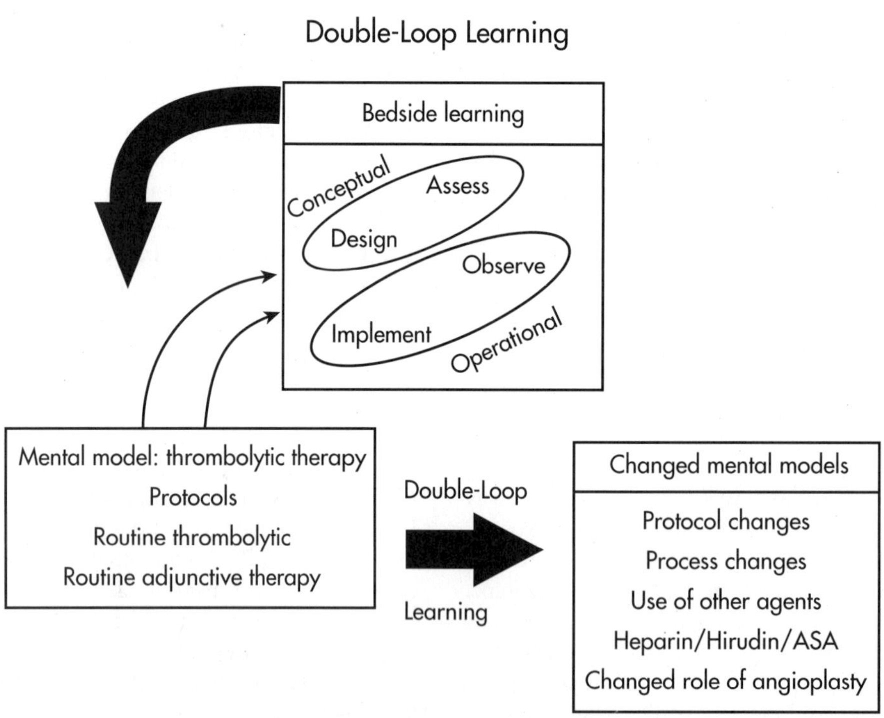

FIGURE 15-6 Single-loop and double-loop learning: thrombolytic therapy example. Argyris and Kim have indicated that single-loop learning occurs when single-dimensional questions elicit single-dimensional answers, without fundamental questioning or changing of the mental model governing the issue. In the example of thrombolytic therapy, single-loop learning asks, "Is the patient a candidate for thrombolytic therapy?" and applies appropriate protocols and therapies. In double-loop learning, the feedback from bedside learning questions the mental model itself and forces it to adapt to fundamental changes of the system and/or process.

(Modified from Kim DH: The link between individual and organizational learning, *Sloan Management Review* 37-50, 1993.

management (Part 7). The medical director must understand that developing the providers of emergency department care is in many respects his or her most difficult role. It requires a clear understanding of a fundamental, basic truth: Development of the providers requires a spirit of continuous improvement, which can arise only out of developing an organization that continues to learn. Development of the emergency department providers requires an understanding of the principles of the learning organization, selecting the right staff, orienting that staff appropriately, developing appropriate performance reviews, ensuring that retention and development programs are in place, and providing appropriate team-building activities.

Learning Organizations

The concept of learning organizations was first developed by Senge.[25] He defines learning organizations as "places where people continually expand their capacity to create the results they truly desire, where new and expansive patterns of thinking are nurtured, where collective aspiration is set free, and where people are continually learning how to learn together." Senge draws heavily on multiple sources of organizational learning theory[26,27] and suggests the use of five component technologies within the organization to develop this commitment to learning:

- Systems thinking
- Personal mastery
- Mental models
- Shared vision
- Team learning

Organizational theorists have studied the learning process in detail, but a universally accepted, practically applicable definition has been somewhat elusive. Nonetheless, the literature suggests that organizational learning is a process that occurs over time and is linked with tying knowledge acquisition to improved performance. In learning organizations the acquisition of knowledge allows modification of behavior to reflect new knowledge and insights that benefit both the providers and the customer (e.g., patient, family members, EMS, medical staff, administration). This definition emphasizes that knowledge acquisition alone is not enough. The processes that result in patient care must be changed as a result of the knowledge acquisition for true organizational learning to occur. As Garvin[28] noted in his commentary on learning organizations, "Without accompanying changes in the way work gets done, only the *potential* for improvement exists." For example, the advent of thrombolytic therapy represents a knowledge base of importance to emergency medicine. However, that knowledge must be applied to the processes in the emergency department to result in better patient care, because the technology itself is of little value unless it can be applied in as rapid a fashion as possible, which requires changing existing processes and the ways of thinking.

Senge's five component technologies are described in more detail in Chapter 1. It is important for the emergency department medical director to understand the concepts of the learning organization to ensure that the providers of emergency department care can be developed in an environment that encourages organizational learning. The medical and nursing directors should work collectively at ensuring that the system is able to move from a superficial knowledge to a deep understanding of the system. It is not enough to know *how* things are done; one must also know *why* things occur and *how they can be changed* to bring about improvement. Finally, building learning organizations is not an individual task, but demands the participation of the entire emergency department team because it involves a shift that goes to the core of our culture. In the past, managers were expected to know how the process worked and design changes in that process in relative isolation. The new culture of learning organizations and continuous improvement requires a substantial shift of culture to learning by individuals and the organization itself, which results in better care for the patient.

Selecting Emergency Department Staff

The emergency department is always a process-rich environment and is often confusing. Working there requires tremendous skill and ability by a diverse group of team members to result in effective patient care. In past decades, many hospitals viewed the emergency room as a place to send staff with bad attitudes or who couldn't "cut it" on the floors, intensive care units, operating suites, or other areas of the hospital. As the modern concept of the emergency department has developed, it has become increasingly apparent that providing emergency department care requires many skills, including clinical, interpersonal, and management skills. For that reason, a careful and prospective approach to selecting the emergency department staff is essential for success. Several steps are required.

First, the medical director and nursing director should have clearly articulated expectations of the staff. These expectations should include a straightforward understanding of the vision, mission, and goals and objectives of the emergency department. Before hiring any staff, these expectations should be made clear, as should elements of clinical, interpersonal, personal, and professional commitment. Concepts such as effective problem resolution and methods for handling patient complaints should be addressed in a straightforward fashion. All potential emergency department staff should have a clear understanding of what the organization does, how it does it, and how it reacts and adapts to changes, improvements, complaints, and adversity.

Second, group investment in the hiring process itself is necessary. The decision to hire a specific staff member from a pool of applicants needs to be made carefully, and "buy in" from stakeholder groups should be carefully considered. Depending on the level of the position, colleagues from nursing, medical staff, and administration may be included in the course of the interview and decision-making process. In general, any physician hired for a supervisory position should be interviewed by appropriate stakeholder groups. Once a candidate is chosen, this strategy also can help ensure that key stakeholders from other areas are invested in the success of the individual. The level of the person involved in the interview process is often interpreted by the candidate as a symbol of commitment to and importance of the position. For example, if an emergency department medical director candidate is not interviewed by the president of the medical staff, chief executive officer of the hospital, or appropriate community members, a clear message is being communicated that the emergency department is not a high priority for the institution.

The interview process itself should be highly substantive, exploring important issues of approaches to problems, philosophy of care, and cultural fit with the institution. For example, if a candidate applies to a position in which management is highly participative, but the candidate has a high degree of authoritarian, hierarchical need for control, it is unlikely that the person can be successful. In most cases, the interview process should be summarized, preferably in writing, so that those responsible for selecting the emergency department staff members can communicate clearly their reasons for favoring one candidate over another.

Finally, the potential for growth within the emergency department environment should be a strong consideration in selecting emergency department staff. In most cases, the original interview process can help medical and nursing directors identify areas in which growth and development of the individual can occur. One question has been particularly helpful in selecting emergency department staff and should usually be asked after an initial bond of trust has been developed in the interview: "What is the worst thing I am going to hear about you, and from whom will I hear it?" The thoughtfulness and reflection inherent in the answer can be helpful in selecting emergency department staff.

The orientation process is addressed in Chapters 73 and 74, but should be handled with a great deal of prospective thought and should be guided by clearly established policy. In most cases, it is important for emergency physicians to work one to two shifts with another physician to learn the specific vagaries of the emergency department, its flow patterns, relationship to the medical staff, and other characteristics. After the initial integration of new staff into the department, it is usually a good idea to review progress and assess questions at 1-, 3- and 6-month intervals and 1 year into the new staff's tenure.

Performance Review

The concept of performance review has undergone considerable revision over the last several years. Traditional performance reviews assess the conformance and/or capability of an individual according to preestablished standards laid out by the organization. These reviews have fairly clearly defined categories by which the individual is evaluated and therefore yield reasonably clear expectations with regard to performance criteria and their assessment. Block,[4] Kohn,[29] and others,[30-31] however, have questioned the role of such traditional performance reviews and their outcome on organizations and the individuals who comprise them. A central concern is that such performance reviews are essentially controlling, confining, and ineffective. Block in particular suggests that "We need a reward system that gives preference to service over self-interest.[4] He suggests three essential elements to help develop a performance review system that emphasizes stewardship over power and control. First, the performance review should *affirm the purposes of the organization,* including its commitment to excellence, the boundaries of the organization, and the development of the providers with whom the individual works. Second, the performance review should help *"share the wealth" of the organization.* In many cases, pay increases themselves depend on the results of the performance review. However, such reviews are increasingly structured to help individuals expand their personal and professional horizons, as well as maintain or increase financial compensation. In addition, some organizations have developed concepts such as gain sharing, cross-training compensation, and even development of equity options. Finally, performance reviews should drop the cloak of secrecy. Secrecy about performance review is often a symbol that there are inequities within the structure that cannot be justified, even perhaps to those who benefit most from them. Performance reviews should be shared with other staff members, but the process of daily feedback to the staff should help reaffirm the overall purposes of the organization. Performance reviews therefore should not come as a surprise to individual staff members, but simply confirm or summarize the period under review, with specific attention given to prospective goals and objectives for the individual and group.

Physician Retention and Development

Effectively managed emergency departments seek physicians who are responsible, innovative, and motivated by commitment to and satisfaction from daily emergency department practice. The cost of turnover is extremely high among professionals and is estimated to be at least 1.5 to 2 times the actual salary in replacement costs. It is to the emergency physician group's advantage to ensure that not only are the right staff selected, but that a specific physician retention and development program is in place. The physician group should help establish long-range goals that facilitate interchange among individuals in several different areas, including the following:

- Daily work demands and stresses
- Job security
- Wages
- Benefits
- Provision of adequate leadership
- Equity and parity in participation
- Professional status
- Support for the professional and his or her family
- Personal and professional development

A formal physician retention and development structure should be in place for every emergency department medical director. It is also important to recognize the need to individualize specific programs within these areas to help meet the needs of the diverse group of physicians who comprise the emergency department team. For example, in many cases physicians have less interest in short-term earnings than in developing job security and planning for retirement, their children's education, and a more long-term strategy to creating wealth. Most important, the physician retention and development program must be adapted over time to meet the changing needs of the group members.

Counseling, Discipline, Dismissal

Although in most cases creating a learning organization, selecting the right staff, orienting them appropriately, and helping them coalesce as a team results in good outcomes, counseling, discipline, and even dismissal of staff are sometimes necessary. The most important aspect of counseling and discipline among emergency department providers is to ensure that it is handled in a professional, fair, and equitable fashion. Any such sessions should be held in private, to ensure confidentiality and lack of intrusion on the patient care pro-

cess. The staff should be encouraged to settle minor differences among themselves when they occur. For example, if specific practice habits cause annoyance or dismay to specific doctors or nurses, those professionals should be encouraged to help resolve those issues at the time, rather than dealing with it later. "Keeping small problems small" is an important strategy in the emergency department environment. It is also critical to ensure that the enforcement of any counseling or disciplinary procedures is handled impartially. If the staff believe that discipline is being used in a punitive fashion only against specific members of the staff, it can have a substantially deleterious effect on emergency department operations and morale. Specifically, if "favorites" of the medical or nursing director are perceived to "get away with" behaviors that others are disciplined for, this is a serious problem.

Similarly, complaints or concerns should be dealt with quickly, usually within the same business day and always within a few days of being informed of them. Each complaint should be addressed with the individual at or near the time that it occurs. In some cases, managers have not informed individuals of complaints about them until they have reached a certain number or intensity, only to be informed by the staff member, "You never told me about this." Whenever possible, written documentation about the nature and type of complaint or concern that has been raised needs to be provided to the professional. Staff members should be regularly informed about the frequency of complaints and how they compared to those for other staff members. Considerable thought must be given to the counseling and disciplinary procedures among both nursing and physician staff. In most hospitals, a clearly defined Human Resources policy governs the disciplinary process. Such policies typically progress along specified steps:

- Verbal warning
- Written warning
- Decision-making leave day
- Termination

Although it may not be necessary for the physician group to have a similar structure to that of the hospital, it is important to have some sense of parity between the physician and nursing structures, particularly with regard to process and severity.

In some cases, contract termination or reassignment of staff is necessary. When this is the case, several steps should be followed closely. First, it is essential to obtain appropriate legal advice whenever contract termination is being considered. Attorneys can help ensure that the appropriate process is followed, documentation is in place, and appropriate thought has been given to other alternatives. Second, written documentation of the events leading up to the termination must be in place. Contract law in the appropriate jurisdiction should be researched to ensure substantial compliance. Third, it is important to think the issue through carefully, yet expeditiously. Questions the medical director should ask himself or herself include the following:

- Am I being fair?
- Is this in the best interest of
  - Patient care?
  - The physician group?
  - The hospital?
  - The individual physician?
- Are there any other alternatives to contract termination that would *definitively* resolve the issue?

When contract termination is necessary, it is critical to ensure that key stakeholders are alerted in advance, but with absolute maintenance of confidence. Any time an emergency physician is relieved of his or her duties, the administrator, chief of staff, and other important stakeholders must be informed, but the information must not reach the physician before the medical director informs him or her. Once the decision is made, it is usually best to move quickly yet judiciously. The medical director should give considerable prospective thought to how the information will be communicated, what is going to occur, what alternatives are available, and what the effect of the contract termination will mean to both the corporation and individual. In most cases, it is preferable to deliver such news in person, although, depending on the inflammatory nature of the contract termination, it may be preferable to have witnesses and/or attorneys present. If attorneys will be present, it is usually best for the physician also to have counsel present.

When the actual meeting occurs, it is best to briefly lay appropriate groundwork, but move to the termination itself in a rapid fashion. In explaining reasons for the termination, address the behavior or the problem, not the person. The medical director should be firm in his or her decision, unless the individual presents serious reasons for reconsideration. However, in most cases, contract termination would not have been decided unless all other alternatives had been exhausted. For that reason, it is generally unwise to reconsider the termination, even briefly. Similarly, the medical director should outline the plan for completion of duties or activities with the emergency department and assist, to the best extent possible, in the transition to a new position. A written letter should summarize the meeting, including all pertinent points raised. That letter should be direct and straightforward in describing how the contractual relationship will end, including the transition period.

After contract termination has occurred, the medical director must be cautious with other staff members. Other members of the physician group should be dealt with individually in a frank and straightforward manner, while protecting the confidentiality of the individual physician terminated. Contract terminations of emergency physicians generally cause substantial concern and/or turmoil among other emergency department staff, who may be rallied to support the individual. When possible, these issues should be dealt with prospectively, but should always be handled in a straightforward and intellectually honest fashion. The medical and nursing director should work carefully on any staff termination to help address such boundary management issues.

Personal Development

The medical director and his or her colleagues should work carefully to help establish a program for the personal development of individuals involved in the emergency department. At the department of emergency medicine at Fairfax Hospital, management has developed the Emergency Department Survival Skills Course to meet this need. This course

reflects the philosophy that emergency medicine is a specialty that requires a specific set of skills and abilities, beyond clinical competence, to be able to provide high quality clinical care, high quality customer care, and ensure the long-term viability of the providers of such care. The course involves training in areas such as customer service, stress recognition and management, conflict resolution, time management, communication skills, and team building. Many of these skills relate not only to the professional environment in the emergency department, but also to the development of the individual on a personal basis. Experience with such an approach indicates that it reduces patient complaints, increases customer satisfaction, and increases employee satisfaction. In addition, long-term stability of emergency department providers has improved with this approach.

Regardless of whether a formal professional and personal training approach is in effect, the emergency department medical director should make every effort to help in the personal development of the members of the emergency department team. Appropriate guidance, leadership, and support should be given to team members whenever they ask. Clearly, these conversations should be handled in a private, professional fashion, strictly respecting the boundaries established by each individual.

The Manager Under Fire

Regardless of the time and attention placed in ensuring that leadership and management issues are addressed, emergency department medical directors occasionally come under substantial criticism for the manner in which the department is functioning. When such circumstances arise, several steps are important (Box 15-9). First, remove the "I" from the issue. This simply means that, although the criticism seems (and in some cases, is) personal, the medical director should not react directly to it. This approach requires substantial integrity and self-control, but is an essential component of dealing with criticism.

Second, focus on the substance of the criticism, and define areas of required improvement. It is important at the outset of the process to listen carefully, rather than defending either the director or the emergency department. There is always a strong temptation to immediately generate answers to the criticisms involved, but it is best at this stage to listen carefully to what is being said, reserving comments or rebuttals for a more appropriate time. After listening to the substance of the criticisms, restate the issue so that it is clear that the area of concern is understood. At this stage, it may be appropriate to begin to state potential qualifications and/or inaccuracies in the original statement of the problem. However, a detailed response to the criticism should usually be reserved for a later time.

Third, set specific priorities and action plans to address the areas of criticism. This approach should involve a collaborative approach among team members involved in the area under criticism, using appropriate elements of boundary management.

Fourth, set specific time frames under which the problem will be analyzed and solutions presented. Such time frames help ensure a brief "breathing period" during which the problem can be analyzed, while also establishing an appropriate sense of urgency among team members to address the issue within a specific time frame.

Fifth, use all available resources to address the problem, including consultants if necessary. Too often solutions to problems are somewhat "patch work" or Band-aid in nature. To develop a thoughtful, reasoned, and successful solution, all appropriate resources, including data gathering, should be brought to bear on the issue.

Sixth, arrange for follow-up mechanisms with appropriate time frames in which interval successes or failures are evaluated.

Seventh, document improvement on a frequent basis. Make sure that information is fed back to those who have criticized either the individual or the department on a regular basis. Make it clear that improvement is occurring and emphasize the leadership role that the emergency department and the medical director have played in this improvement.

Finally, whenever the medical director or the emergency department are "under fire," these problems should be approached with tenacity and ferocity. The solutions to the criticisms raised should be aggressive and decisive, but responsive in nature. When the emergency department and its leadership are criticized, the medical director should understand that his or her practice, standing in the community, livelihood, and professional career are on the line. Just as desperately ill patients can be resuscitated and revived to live long and productive lives, so too can emergency department operations and those who lead them be infused with an aggressive spirit of enthusiasm to help improve areas of perceived lack of performance.

BOX 15-9

THE MANAGER "UNDER FIRE"

Remove the "I" from the issue.
Focus on substance; minimize the emotion.
Set specific priorities and action plans.
Set specific time frames.
Use all available resources.
Arrange follow-up mechanisms.
Document improvement; celebrate success.
Be aggressive, tenacious, and when necessary, ferocious.

SUMMARY

Although the roles of the emergency department medical director are diverse and difficult, the position can help create satisfying improvements in patient care, develop the emergency department, and expand the horizons of the team members who comprise that department. By focusing on a commitment to excellence, establishing the boundaries of the organization, and developing the providers, emergency department medical directors can help ensure the viability of their emergency department and the patients who rely on it.

ACKNOWLEDGMENT

Dr. Lorna Facteau and Deborah Royalty, MEd reviewed the manuscript and added greatly to its clarity and content.

REFERENCES

1. Hoffer E: *The passionate state of mind,* New York, 1955, Doubleday.
2. Bennis W: *On becoming a leader,* Reading, Mass, 1989, Addison-Wesley.
3. Mayer TA: The emergency department medical director, *Emerg Med Clin North Am* 5:1-28, 1987.
4. Block P: *Stewardship: choosing service over self-interest,* San Fransisco, 1993, Barrett-Koehler.
5. Schwartz GR, Cayten CG, Mayer TA et al, editors: *Principles and practice of emergency medicine,* ed 3, Philadelphia, 1992, Lea & Febiger.
6. Rosen P, Barkin RM: *Emergency medicine: concepts in clinical practice,* St Louis, 1992, Mosby.
7. Tintinalli JE, Chrome RL, Ruiz E, editors: *Emergency medicine: a comprehensive study guide,* ed 4, New York, 1995, McGraw-Hill.
8. Mayer TA: Quality improvement in emergency medicine. In Schwartz GR, Cayten CG, Mayer TA et al, editors: *Principles and practice of emergency medicine,* ed 3, Philadelphia, 1992, Lea & Febiger.
9. Golden K: *Learning systems thinking with Friday night at the ER,* Chicago, 1995, Breakthrough Learning.
10. Hirschhorn L, Gilmore T: The new boundaries of the "boundaryless" company, *Harvard Business Review,* 70:104-115, 1992.
11. Welch J: *1990 Annual Report,* General Electric.
12. Schein EH: How can organizations learn faster? The challenge of entering the green room, *Sloan Manage Rev* 34:85-92, 1993.
13. Kubler-Ross E: *On death and dying,* New York, 1969, Macmillan.
14. Hammer M, Champy J: *Reengineering the corporation: a manifesto for business revolution,* New York, 1993, Harper Collins.
15. Hammer M, Stanton SA: *The reengineering revolution: a handbook,* New York, 1995, Harper Collins.
16. *The Holy Bible,* Revised Standard, Numbers 13:33.
17. Galbraith JK: *The affluent society,* New York, 1958, Doubleday.
18. Hammer M: Reengineering work: don't automate, obliterate, *Harvard Business Review* 68:104-112, 1990.
19. Kotter JP: Leading change: why transformation efforts fail, *Harvard Business Review* 73:59-67, 1995.
20. Block P: *The empowered manager: positive political skills at work,* San Francisco, 1987, Jossey-Bass.
21. Juran J: *Juran on planning for quality,* New York, 1988, The Free Press.
22. McMillan JR, Younger MS, DeWine LC: Satisfaction with hospital emergency department as a function of patient triage, *Healthc Manage Rev* 11:21-27, 1986.
23. Johnson DV: An administrative perspective on emergency medicine, *Emerg Med Clin North Am* 5:149-154, 1987.
24. Argyris C: Education for leading—learning. In *The learning organization in action,* New York, 1994, American Management Association.

24a. Katzenbach JR, Smith DK: *The wisdom of teams: creating the high-performance organization,* Boston, 1993, Harvard Business School Press.

25. Senge PM: *The fifth discipline: the art and science of the learning organization,* New York, 1990, Doubleday.
26. Ackoff RL: *Creating the corporate future,* New York, 1981, John Wiley & Sons.
27. Stata R: Organizational learning: The key to management innovation, *Sloan Manage Rev* 30:63-64, 1989.
28. Garvin DA: Building a learning organization, *Harvard Business Review* 71:78-91, 1993.
29. Kohn A: Why incentive plans cannot work, *Harvard Business Review* 71:68-73, 1993.
30. Ridge JT, Larsen JA: Why some long-term incentives fail. In Nalbantian HR, editor: *Incentives, corporation, and risk-sharing,* Totowa, NJ, 1987, Rowman & Littlefield.
31. Deci EL, Ryan RM: *Intrinsic motivation in self-determination in human behavior,* New York, 1985, Plenum Press.

APPENDIX A Fairfax Hospital Position Description

Position Title: Chairman & Medical Director
Department: Emergency Medicine

POSITION SUMMARY

Under the direction of the Vice President/Chief Operating Officer (COO) or his designee the Assistant Administrator for Emergency, Trauma & Ambulatory Services (Assistant Administrator), provides operational administrative/clinical medical direction and leadership for the Fairfax Hospital Emergency Department (Department). Develops, implements, and administers policies and procedures as they apply to the provision of emergency services. Supervises, in conjunction with the Assistant Administrator, the administrative and clinical personnel assigned to the Department. Identifies, in conjunction with the Assistant Administrator, strategies, plans, and budgets for the Department. Consults with the Emergency Department Physician Advisory Committee and the Emergency Department Management Group as appropriate in carrying out duties and responsibilities including setting priorities and time lines.

Key Duties and Responsibilities

1. Medical Affairs

1.1 *Patient Care, Policies, Procedures, and Admission Criteria:* Develops patient care policies and procedures for the Department and secures the approval of these policies and procedures from either committees of the medical staff and/or administration. Implements and ensures compliance with all approved policies and procedures.

1.2 *Patient Care Management:* Responsible for the overall supervision of nursing and ancillary support staff employed in the Department, including the Patient Care Administrator (PCA) and the Patient Care Director (PCD).

1.3 *Quality Improvement/Assurance:* In conjunction with the Associate Administrator for Patient Care Services, develops the Department Quality Improvement (QI) and Quality Assurance (QA) Program including the total scope of care that is consistent with those of the JCAHO, the American College of Emergency Physicians, and the system-wide QI program of Inova Health System. Provides guidance and assistance to the Chairperson of the Department QI/QA Committee, PCA and the PCD in implementing the QI/QA program. Ensures implementation of resultant recommendations.

1.4 *Continuing Medical Education and Research:* Plans and implements the ongoing continuing medical education (CME) and research programs related to emergency medicine for the appropriate Department clinical staff.

1.5 *Medical Staff Bylaws Rules and Regulations:* Ensures that the Department conforms with the bylaws, rules, and regulations of the Fairfax Hospital Medical Staff and all appropriate Federal, State, or Local laws and regulations. Serves as the medical representative to the Medical Executive Committee, Planning & Programming, Emergency Department Physician Advisory Committee, and Trauma Committee. Abides by the bylaws, rules and regulations of the Fairfax Hospital Medical Staff.

1.6 *Physician Credentialing and Privileging:* Develops and implements a process for the evaluation of physician criteria and the granting of privileges to provide emergency medicine services in accordance with hospital and Medical Staff bylaws, rules, and regulations. Develops and implements emergency medicine medical staff evaluations.

1.7 *Medical/Administrative Staff Liaison:* Acts as formal liaison between the Department staff and Fairfax Hospital administrative, medical, and ancillary staff. Includes formal and informal action with elected and appointed representatives of the medical staff.

2. Administrative Responsibilities

2.1 *Department Service Management:* Provides administrative direction and leadership for the Department and emergency medicine physicians.

2.2 *Administrative Policies and Procedures:* Develops, reviews and approves all operating policies and procedures for the Department in conjunction with the Assistant Administrator.

2.3 *Planning and Department Development:* In conjunction with the Assistant Administrator identifies and recommends objectives for the Department consistent with Fairfax Hospital goals. Implements programs necessary to accomplish approved objectives and plans. Serves as the Fairfax Hospital medical and administrative representative in the development of Emergency Medicine Services within Inova Health System.

2.4 *Personnel Management:* In conjunction with the Assistant Administrator, recruits, hires, evaluates and develops all supervisory, support and nursing personnel for the Department.

2.5 *Staff In-Service Education:* Ensures that an effective program of in-service education is implemented for nursing and support personnel in the Department.

2.6 *Capital Expenditures:* Reviews and recommends all capital equipment and facility renovation orders for the Department.

2.7 *Supply Procurement:* Reviews and recommends all supply and vendor specifications for the Department.

2.8 *Licensure and Accreditation:* Assures the compliance of the Department with JCAHO standards and Virginia Public Health regulations, as well as with other Federal, State and Local regulations and other professional accreditation standards applicable to the Department.

2.9 *External Representation:* Represents Fairfax Hospital interests to external organizations concerned with emergency medicine patient care and management.

3. Knowledge, Skills, and Abilities

3.1 Licensed as a physician in the State of Virginia.
3.2 Board Certified by the American Board of Emergency Medicine and Board Eligible in Medical Management by the American Board of Medical Management.
3.3 Special training and certification in Advanced Trauma Life Support and cardiac resuscitation.
3.4 A high level of interpersonal skills to allow effective communications with a wide variety of hospital personnel, physicians, and the general public.
3.5 Significant hospital-based emergency medicine care experience and expertise.
3.6 Documented interest and experience in emergency medicine education and research, including lecturing, publishing and participation in clinical and administrative peer review literature.

4. Reporting Relationships

4.1 Reports to the COO or his designee for administrative and contractual matters and to the Medical Staff Executive Committee for clinical quality of care matters.
4.2 In conjunction with the Assistant Administrator has supervisory responsibility for all nursing and ancillary support staff employed in the department, including the PCA and PCD.

DEPARTMENT
Job: Medical Director of Emergency Center
Reports to: *Professionally* As Related
Administratively Administrative Director, Medical Staff

Basic Purpose

Plans, organizes, controls, and directs the Emergency Department. Assumes full medical and management responsibilities for the quality and quantity of work performed at the main hospital building and as otherwise required.

Supervision Received

The Medical Director of the Emergency Center is governed by hospital bylaws, policies and procedures, rules and regulations of the Medical Staff and shall be accountable medically to the Executive Committee and administratively to the hospital Assistant Vice President.

Supervision Exercised

The Medical Director of the Emergency Center shall provide medical and administrative supervision to all staff assigned to the stated department.

Typical Duties

1. Develops departmental policies to achieve objectives of the department and The Toledo Hospital.
2. Analyzes and interprets various records, reports, and other data for the purpose of giving recommendations to the Medical Staff and to the hospital Administration in such matters as operations, budgets, staffing, technology, and quality of care.
3. Prepares, submits, and monitors financial budgets to justify continued funding for ongoing and new departmental operations.
4. Participates in educational programs for a reasonable period of time providing teaching and clinical services for medical students, physicians, nursing personnel, and others to develop and promote improved patient care skills and treatment programs.
5. Advises and consults with other physicians as requested.
6. Provides guidance and advice to solve problems that surface from time to time in the course of daily departmental operations.
7. Monitors the performance of personnel in the department.
8. Keeps abreast of stated discipline knowledge and trends and assures quality of patient care.
9. Provides medical direction for the Emergency Department.
10. Develops policies and procedures, as well as protocols, equipment, and staffing needs.
11. Promotes clinical research as deemed necessary.
12. Advises on medical and administrative problems and on questions of policy and public relations as they relate to medical practices.
13. Initiates and directs staff conferences for instructional purposes and discusses administrative and medical problems.
14. Investigates and studies new developments in medical practices and techniques, adapting them to specific hospital needs.
15. Represents hospital in meetings of professional groups when appropriate.
16. Performs other duties as might be reasonable and related.

GENERAL INFORMATION

Must be a Doctor of Medicine, Board Certified in Emergency Medicine with experience, not including residency, and be a member of The Hospital Executive Committee.

Chain of Command. Recognizing that the Medical Director will not always be available, an Assistant Medical Director should be named. This person will be responsible to act on behalf of the Department Director when the Department Director is not available.

THE EMERGENCY DEPARTMENT MEDICAL DIRECTOR

Duties and Responsibilities of the Emergency Department Director

Patient/Family

1. Ensure overall quality of patient care:
   a. Clinical
   b. Interpersonal
   c. Patient/family expectations.
2. Maximize ability to deliver timely care.
3. Integration with medical staff practices.
4. Address concerns and questions of family members.
5. Ensure appropriate patient discharge instructions.
6. Address patient education.

Medical Staff

1. Coordinate overall patient care.
   a. Individual patients
   b. Treatment protocols
   c. Patient transfer agreements
   d. Individual physician practice patterns
   e. Credentialing of ED physicians
2. Expedite patient flow from ED to physician practices.
   a. Admitted patients
   b. Discharge patients
3. Respect medical staff's right to see patients.
4. Attendance and participation at Medical Executive Committee.
5. Attend department meetings (medicine, surgery, pediatrics, etc).
6. Handle all patient complaints and document follow up.
7. Medical Staff committees
8. Social interaction
9. Aggressively respond to medical staff complaints/concerns
10. Coordinate involvement with related physician services.
    a. Pathology/Laboratory
    b. Radiology
    c. Intensive Care Units

Administration

1. On call, immediate availability to respond to problems
2. Assess overall status of the ED.
   a. Anticipate problems
   b. Respond to identified problems in a timely fashion
   c. Monthly volume trends
   d. Payer mix
   e. Number of admissions
   f. Medical staff concerns
   g. Nursing needs
   h. Community and board concerns
3. Meet regularly (at least monthly) with administration.
4. Respect table of organization and reporting structure.
5. Document response to problems ("paper trail").
6. Develop and monitor Quality Assurance/JCAH issues.
7. Participate in hospital risk management efforts.
8. Develop appropriate ED pricing strategies.
9. Personnel management
   a. Physician
   b. Nonphysician
10. Develop marketing and public relations programs for the ED.
11. Ensure appropriate quality care.
12. Participate in community and hospital disaster planning.
13. Provide long-range planning input for ED.
14. Advise on drug, equipment, and staffing needs.

Emergency Physicians

1. Provide a stimulating professional environment.
   a. Clinical
   b. Interpersonal
   c. Physical facility
   d. Financial
2. Physician recruitment
   a. Expectations = reality
   b. Interaction with staff
3. Ensure appropriate physician staffing.
4. Coordinate clinical care of the ED.
   a. Procedures
   b. Protocols
   c. Medical staff interface
5. Educate with regard to the broad perspectives of the ED (Cheerleading)
6. Scheduling
7. Continuing Medical Education
8. Assess clinical status.
9. Consideration of career development concerns
10. Social interaction
11. Coordinate monthly meetings.
12. Coordinate interface with nursing, ancillary services.
13. Coordinate interface with administration.
14. Encourage medical staff and community involvement.

Nursing

1. Foster *appropriate* communication between ED nurses and physicians.
2. Ensure appropriate patient care.
3. Develop policies and procedures.
4. Participate in nursing quality assurance.
5. Promote nursing in-service education.
6. Address nursing complaints.
7. Advise appropriate personnel on nursing problems.
8. Advise on triage (function, education, monitoring, etc).

Emergency Medical Services

1. Medical Direction (where appropriate)
2. Educate ED physician and nurses.
   a. Protocols
   b. Standing orders
   c. Telecommunications
3. Education
   a. Training
   b. In-service programs
4. Ensure participation in EMS quality assurance.
5. Handle complaints from EMS regarding ED operations.
6. Attend EMS meetings.

Community

1. Public service lectures
2. Education

Courtesy Fairfax Hospital, Falls Church, Vir; The Toledo Hospital, Toledo, Oh; Bruce Janiak, MD; and Thom A. Mayer, MD.

16 The Role of the Nursing Director

Celia H. Dover

OUTLINE

The roles and responsibilities of today's emergency department nursing director are more complex than they were a decade ago. Because of the rapid and drastic changes that have occurred in healthcare, the emergency department has become increasingly important to the hospital's financial viability, service, identity, and delivery.

Titles of emergency department nursing directors are numerous: head nurse, supervisor, manager, emergency department coordinator, and division director. Although the titles vary, the roles are the same. The emergency department nursing director must effectively direct, integrate, and coordinate diverse fiscal, socioeconomic, and operational components of the emergency department. Medical, administrative, and other groups may concern themselves with discrete aspects of the department, but the nursing director must integrate all efforts to ensure total quality management and fiscal viability. In some departments, nursing and medicine assume a central role in integration.

QUALIFICATIONS AND RESPONSIBILITIES

Ideally, the emergency department nursing director will possess a background in emergency nursing with a broad knowledge and skill base of emergency care practice. Diverse management abilities and leadership skills are essential to this role and facilitate the development of an effective, quality-oriented staff.

The Joint Commission on Accreditation of Healthcare Organizations (JCAHO) has recently defined a set of standards that identify the characteristics and processes of leadership (Leadership L.D.2.1-L.D.2.10).[1] These standards stress the need for an organization's leaders to define a strategic plan that is consistent with the organization's mission and vision; to clearly communicate the mission, vision, and plan throughout the organization; and to fulfill the organization's vision by providing the framework to accomplish the goals of the strategic plan. The four processes of planning, directing, implementing and coordinating, and improving are essential for the organization's service leadership (Box 16-1). Standard Emergency Services 2.3 defines a general standard for emergency department nursing management that requires relevant training, experience, and current competence.[1]

The Emergency Nurses Association's Standards of Emergency Nursing Practice are recognized as guidelines for providing the highest level of emergency nursing care.[2] These standards define four components that apply to the emergency department nursing director's performance: practice, research, education, and professionalism. These components are integrated into emergency nursing practice and help define the scope of responsibility. Although these standards provide an excellent framework for practice, each individual institution will determine the more refined qualifications and position descriptions for the position of emergency department nursing director.

Box 16-2 illustrates a common listing of basic requirements for the emergency department nursing director position.

The duties delegated to the emergency department nursing director far exceed the parameters of clinical nursing practice. The clinical practice and management functions must be separated and defined so that the nursing director has the time and resources for addressing all system components. The emergency department nursing director must have the authority to manage each area of responsibility. The role responsibilities are extensive and present a challenge in our current fragmented healthcare system.

Nursing Care Practice and Personnel

Clinical direction involves all activities that address the clinical performance of personnel in the department: nurses, aides, technicians, emergency medical technicians (EMTs), paramedics, nurse practitioners, nurse clinicians, and others who perform clinical duties in the department. In some emergency departments, nurse practitioners may be considered medical staff and report directly to the medical director.

The emergency department nursing director is vested with independent decision-making authority to implement strategies, programs, and patient care consistent with the institution's policies, goals, and objectives. Appropriate structural and practice strategies can be undertaken within any emergency departments that preserve and promote high standards of practice. With an understanding of all constraints, the highest level of practice effectiveness must be demanded by the emergency department nursing director and all practitioners themselves.

To attain and retain credibility in the department, the nurs-

BOX 16-1

JCAHO LEADERSHIP STANDARDS

Standard

LD.2 Each hospital department has effective leadership.

Intent of LD.2

Department-level leadership is as important as the hospital's senior leadership. Department leaders embrace common qualities of effective leadership shared by all hospital leaders. Specifically, department leaders help create an environment or culture that enables a hospital to fulfill its mission and meet or exceed its goals.

Department leaders clearly convey the hospital's mission to all staff. They support staff and encourage in them a sense of ownership of their work processes. They also hold staff accountable for their performance. Department leaders motivate staff to improve their performance continuously, thereby improving the hospital's performance.

Ultimately, department directors are responsible for the operation of their department, and for the measurement, assessment, and continuous improvement of the department's performance. The best evidence of effective leadership is a department that operates effectively and efficiently.

Patient care services are organized, directed, and staffed in keeping with the scope of services offered.

Standards

LD.2.1 Directors integrate their department's services with the hospital's primary functions.

LD.2.2 Directors coordinate and integrate services within their department and with other departments.

LD.2.3 Directors develop and implement policies and procedures that guide and support the provision of services.

LD.2.4 Directors recommend a sufficient number of qualified and competent persons to provide care.

LD.2.5 Directors determine the qualifications and competence of department personnel who provide patient care services and who are not licensed independent practitioners.

LD.2.6 Directors continuously assess and improve their department's performance.

LD.2.7 Directors maintain appropriate quality control programs.

LD.2.8 Directors provide for orientation, in-service training, and continuing education of all persons in the department.

LD.2.9 Directors recommend space and other resources needed by the department.

LD.2.10 Directors participate in selecting outside sources for needed services.

From Joint Commision on Accreditation of Healthcare Organizations: *The 1996 Joint Commision accreditation manual for hospitals,* vol I, Oakbrook Terrace, ILL, 1995, JCAHO.

BOX 16-2

BASIC REQUIREMENTS FOR ED NURSING DIRECTOR

- Graduate of a National League of Nursing accredited school of nursing.
- Valid state RN license.
- BSN required, MSN preferred.
- Minimum of 4 years emergency nursing experience.
- Minimum of 2 years management experience.
- Management, leadership, and clinical skills.
- Effective communication skills.
- Certified Emergency Nursing (CEN) preferred.
- Advanced Cardiac Life Support (ACLS) preferred.

ing director must possess clinical competence. Remaining clinically active in the department not only supports clinical performance and role modeling, but also allows the director to experience the morale and functional stability of the human resource component of the department.

The emergency department nursing director's respect and regard for the human resources component of the department affects the performance, productivity, and efficiency of the overall operations. If staffing turnover rates are low, replacement, recruitment, and training costs are low. People management is a fundamental skill for the emergency department nursing director. Characteristics of the workplace must be considered to improve the quality of the environment. Staff morale and job satisfaction frequently outweigh other benefits of employment.

The emergency department nursing director can convey respect and a belief that staff members are responsible for their actions and are capable of using their own resources to solve problems. Care and concern for the individual are expressed by communicating that the person's ideas, feelings, and opinions are valued.

With the stress and demands of work in the emergency department, the emergency department nursing director's empathetic understanding can contribute to a staff member's growth and learning and promote an ability to act effectively. Communicating interest about how the staff is responding to work experiences and seeing and understanding from their point of view facilitate an effective cooperative relationship.

Administrative Leadership

Administration of the department involves much more than answering complaints or conducting staff meetings. Budget considerations, planning strategies, efficiency factors, patient satisfaction, and liaison with other departments are all important components. The emergency department nursing director must be an innovator, catalyst, goal setter, planner, and visionary.

The emergency department interfaces with more facilities and services than any other hospital department. Although it is central to operations and generates its own patient load, it is dependent on many other internal and external entities for achieving efficient care delivery. Internal services involve laboratory, radiology, materials management, admitting/registration, security, and social services. External services in-

clude emergency medical systems, police, media, coroner, and visitors. The nursing director plays a vital role in promoting and enhancing affiliations with each service provider. The nursing director must understand the function and value of each service. Open communication and regular meetings with both internal and external services promote emergency department operational efficiency.[3]

The many decisions that must be made by the emergency department nursing director may be reached by delegation to committees. The productivity of the emergency department is greatly enhanced if committees are used efficiently. The nursing director needs to know how to select and structure groups for projects and how to effectively run the meetings.

In determining the need for a committee, the nursing director must consider issues such as the number of people involved, the degree of power given to the group, and the goals and objectives of the committee. The jobs of the committee need to be clearly assigned, a leader should be elected or appointed, written records should be kept, and the expected results should be identified.

Committees are not designed to handle day-to-day decisions, but are the best available technique for arriving at joint conclusions and determining actions. Using a committee structure to handle the larger issues such as policy changes or long-term plans precipitates an honest, open, participative leadership style.

Quality Assurance/Risk Management

The nursing director must ensure that patient care and satisfaction are at a maximum level and there is proof of improvement as a result of the quality assurance efforts.[4] Quality and risk monitoring criteria in the emergency department must include practice-related indicators, as well as the patient's perception of quality. Because patients generally cannot judge the quality or appropriateness of the emergency care, their perceptions are based on individual staff members and how the patient's emergency was managed. A patient encounter with negative outcomes often causes the kindness and caring of the staff to be overlooked. A dissatisfied patient usually relates his or her negative experience to anyone who will listen.[5]

The patient satisfaction survey is the most effective measure for identifying problems related to a patient's perception of quality of care. Regular monitoring of staff courtesy, timeliness, and ancillary services provides valuable information for addressing quality and patient satisfaction in the emergency department.

Risk management activities must include chart review to identify problems, educate staff, and avert legal problems. Litigation is a particularly sensitive area in the emergency department and a primary impetus for quality and risk monitoring. Positioning all staff to function with an awareness of quality and risk issues involves strategic planning and the implementation of a broad-based program.

Receiving pertinent, significant information on patient care is crucial to the success of both risk management and quality assurance. Incident reports have become associated with threats and other negative connotations and have been replaced with occurrence, situation, or event reports. The reporting of an event or happening that is not consistent with the routine operation of the emergency department or the routine care of a particular patient should be reported and reviewed by the emergency department director.

Risk management and quality assurance often combine educational efforts. Education may be directed to a specific employee or physician who has been identified by the system as having a particular problem. More frequently education efforts reach a larger audience. Teaching new residents and nurses about malpractice claims, risk management, and quality assurance should be a high priority. Departmental orientation programs should introduce all new employees to the principles of risk management and quality assurance and instruct them regarding particular reporting obligations should an occurence happen.

Building an Effective Team

The team concept is essential in the practice and administration of emergency care (see Chapter 14). The nursing director plays a primary role in promoting the integration and collaboration of physicians, nurses, support/clinical staff, and other ancillary staff. Effective emergency department operation requires diverse staff to merge their respective resources and skills to deliver timely, efficient, and high quality emergency care. The emergency department nursing director must promote a team atmosphere in which goals and objectives are shared. The shared goals and objectives enhance productivity and allow for shared accountability in patient outcomes. A unified nursing director and emergency department physician management team is also essential to overall team building. The combined knowledge base, skills, and consistency of purpose of this leadership exemplifies practice commitment.

Emergency care offers unique opportunities and challenges in the practice of teamwork. The emergency department nursing director and the physician director should be the role model for teamwork. Planning for a department's growth and progress should be a joint effort between nursing and physician leadership to ensure that goals are agreed on and supported by all. When the top leadership works together effectively, departmental teamwork is a natural result.

Managing Change

The emergency department nursing director must possess innovative solutions to change and be prepared to manage an environment of rapid technologic, socioeconomic, and financial change. In response to these changes, the emergency department nursing director must be prepared to manage the varying levels and training requirements of the staff. Staff education is a continuing process that encompasses every level of personnel, from the clerical staff to the physicians.

The differentiation of educational duties within the emergency department is the prerogative of the nursing director. The most efficient and economic means for achieving the educational requirements of the department vary among institutions. The educational functions of some institutions are included in the functions of the staff development department. These departments are responsible for both orientation and in-service and continuing education of all departments. However, because emergency departments are very specialized, it is increasingly difficult for the staff development department to provide specific educational programs that meet departmental needs. A sharing of staff development activi-

ties between the emergency department nursing director and the staff development department facilitates a joint assessment of educational needs. This arrangement allows the nursing director to identify which in-service and education programs are needed by the staff, whereas the staff development department assists with material and personnel to help with planning, conducting, and evaluating the programs.

Clinical nurse specialists (CNS) are particularly beneficial in an emergency department in planning and implementing educational programs for the staff. Because of their greater depth of knowledge and skill, CNS can be a tremendous assistance in the education and development of emergency department personnel.

Participation in emergency department staff development can be shared by the staff. Participation in the needs assessment, planning, and presentation of programs by the emergency department nursing and physician staff assists in the provision of an education program that is of value to all emergency care providers.

The fragmented healthcare system, industry, and socioeconomic factors such as violence, substance abuse, overcrowding, and funding deficits further complicate the change agent role.

To facilitate change in this difficult and complicated emergency care environment, the emergency department nursing director must be knowledgeable about information unique to the department. Information about patient acuity, source of payment, and peak volume times should be used by the nursing director when initiating change at any level. An understanding of and ability to articulate the problems unique to emergency care are powerful tools when initiating change at the departmental, hospital, community, state, or federal level. Objective presentation of factual, scientific data along with receiving of input and ideas from all identified participants facilitates effective change in the emergency department.

Change is a complex, continuous process that can rarely be rushed or imposed on unwilling participants. Before the onset of any change process, the readiness to participate and support for the project by those who will be involved must be assessed. Each situation and emergency department have unique features that influence the response to innovation. The nursing director should plan and evaluate carefully all aspects of the identified change and direct the project toward its goal. Change that is presented positively by the nursing director can be implemented in a manner that builds morale, improves attitude, increases productivity, and promotes innovation.

Communication

Two-way communication between management and staff enhances the leadership capabilities of the nursing director and is fundamental to change management, emergency department survival, and success. The staff have reasonable solutions to problems because of their understanding and involvement with the issues. Allowing staff input conveys that the nursing director wants feedback about how to improve effectiveness. Management-staff communication decreases the time spent on nonproductive dialogue and increases the time directed toward problem identification and resolution.

Effective communication is often facilitated through staff surveys, which encourage employee input without fear of reprisal. Departmental newsletters are an effective method of communicating administrative directives. Staff empowerment occurs through the effective dissemination of important organizational information.

The challenge to any emergency department nursing director is to ensure that the predominant communication networks increase the effectiveness of the group and avoid communication patterns that undermine, interrupt, or otherwise impede effective functioning. The emergency department nursing director must be especially astute at assessing the communication mechanism to identify the communication channels and the accuracy or inaccuracy of the messages, and promoting efficient communication or alleviating the causes for disruptive communication.

It is important to recognize how people communicate to detect incomplete and inaccurate information before its transmission causes havoc. Every department should provide for communication in three directions: upward, downward, and horizontal.

Upward communication is essential to make decisions based on valid and accurate information. Upward communication also gives employees a feeling of belonging and being part of the department when they know that what they think is important to the effective functioning of the team. Communication modes such as group meetings, conferences with individuals or small groups, suggestion boxes, and responses to memoranda tend to encourage upward communication.

The most frequent forms of downward communication are instructions, policies, and procedures. The effectiveness of downward channels of communication can be determined by the frequency with which employees complain that they never know what is going on.

Horizontal communication is necessary for the organization and coordination of activities. Time and energy are saved when co-workers readily discuss projects, make plans together, and provide each other with evaluation of ideas or plans.

Considerable peer support and a team spirit atmosphere can be generated through active, open, and honest communication. For horizontal communication to be effective, participants must trust one another and respect each other's opinions.

Deliberately creating and unifying a group of emergency department personnel into a group of people who function as an effective and efficient team and thereby accomplish specific goals is one of the most important roles of the emergency department nursing director.

Ensuring Compliance with Policies, Regulations, and Standards

The emergency department is affected by federal, state, and local requirements: JCAHO standards for accreditation; fire, safety and building codes; Environmental Protection Agency (EPA) requirements; hospital policies and procedures; departmental policies and procedures; Centers for Disease Control and Prevention (CDC) guidelines; Occupational Safety and Health Administration (OSHA) guidelines; Medical Staff bylaws, rules, and regulations; and regulations resulting from the Consolidated Omnibus Budget Reconciliation Acts

(COBRA) of 1985 and 1989. This multitude of regulations is used as the basis for practice directives in the emergency department.

The emergency department must have a policy and procedure manual that includes written procedures for activities that occur or are related to emergency department operations. Everything stipulated by a regulatory agency should be covered in this manual.

Administrative approval is required for additions or modifications of policies and procedures, and all require an annual review. The nursing director must communicate all general hospital policies to the staff because many of these policies apply to all staff.

Clear and concise presentation of policies and procedures that affect the staff in a meeting that encourages interaction and input assists in the communication of this information. Direct involvement in the policy-making process, whenever possible, enhances the "buy-in" of information by the staff.

The development of a committee that involves professional nurses from the emergency department in decision making is an effective way to give nurses a voice in the decisions that affect their clinical practice. It is important to provide guidelines for the function of this type of committee. The emergency department nursing director should attend as a consultant; all shifts and levels of personnel should be represented. Participation must be voluntary, and specific goals should be identified.

Marketing/Public Relations

Marketing strategies are used to create the image desired by the institution and the emergency department. The emergency department's role in public relations as the "front door to the hospital" has become more and more crucial as hospitals compete for in-patient admissions.

Considering these factors, the nursing director must apply consumer-oriented strategies in the emergency department. Emergency department consumers include patients/visitors, hospital employees, staff physicians, third party payors, Emergency Medical Services providers, police, and media. Each consumer group listed has the potential to control services or revenues, as well as the ability to contribute to the success or failure of the emergency department.

Marketing the emergency department has potential for improving the market share of consumers and achieving a better payor mix from the community. Consumers able to shop for healthcare will look for ease of access, atmosphere and ambiance, comfort, timeliness of service, courtesy, and cost of care relative to service.

The effective emergency department nursing director will communicate and involve all levels of staff in marketing efforts. The rationale behind marketing efforts fosters understanding and cooperation from staff. As the front-line providers of patient care, these personnel must buy into and assist with the development of marketing strategies for the emergency department.

Staffing the Emergency Department and Improving Productivity

Productivity challenges in the emergency department are unique in that fluctuating patient volumes and acuity alter the accurate assignment of staff to the workload. The unique nature of the practice setting may prohibit the sharing of staff from other nursing units. These factors contribute to the emergency department's reputation as being the most difficult department to staff.

Regardless of these circumstances, the most efficient use of human resources is in the appropriate assignment of staffing patterns to the relative workload. Staffing patterns should reflect the mix that best assesses and treats the various patient types, volumes, and levels of acuity.

The introduction of patient classification systems (PCS) has substantially altered the scheduling function, providing a work measurement standard by which to assign professional staff. The system identifies several patient categories based on the level of resources used. Each category denotes an incremental time–work-load measure, based on the average number of minutes of nursing time per encounter. Newer models are addressing cognitive complexity (the degree of analysis needed to care for the patient) and work environment complexity (the number and type of patients needing nursing care simultaneously).[6] The complement of the PCS-based staffing and peak workload periods achieves the optimal professional staffing configuration based on a measurable workload.[7]

Managing Finances and Budgeting

The financial management of the emergency department is primarily the responsibility of the nursing director. A solid grasp of the operational objectives, emergency department charges, revenues, collection rates, and expenditures is essential to the budgeting process.

Capital, program, and operational budgets processes begin with the development of departmental goals and objectives. Once departmental goals have been clarified, the process must be reconciled with the hospital's pressing goals and objectives and approved by administration.

Information about volume and patient mix, supplies, equipment, and pharmaceutical costs must be collected and analyzed. Capital equipment requests must be thoughtfully planned and evaluated to best meet the needs of the patient population and the emergency department.

The emergency department nursing director must involve the physician director and medical staff, as well as other emergency department staff, in budget preparation. Front line caregivers possess an understanding of supply and equipment utilization that can help save revenues and improve use of the purchased product.[3]

A discussion of the financial status of the department and the cost of all aspects of emergency care with each level of emergency care provider clarifies accountability and responsibility. Efforts to control the budget and practice within its limits will be more successful if all levels of staff are aware of and participate in the budget preparation process.

SUMMARY

The role of the emergency department nursing director is primarily to define new roles for emergency care facilities and providers and position both for the changing healthcare en-

vironment. This role combines a broad emergency care skill and knowledge base with diverse management skill and authority to direct one of the most important resources of the hospital and healthcare.

The responsibilities of the nursing director are varied and range from managing clinical nursing practice to managing finances and budgeting. Socioeconomic trends present challenges to the nursing director role, as the impact is seen in emergency departments. The nursing director's understanding of the relationship between outside influences and the operational intricacies of the emergency department enhances the financial viability of the institution and positively affects quality of care.

REFERENCES

1. Joint Commission on Accreditation of Healthcare Organizations: *The 1994 Joint Commission Accreditation manual for hospitals,* Oak Terrace, Ill, 1996, JCAHO.
2. Emergency Nurses Association: *Standards of emergency nursing practice,* ed 2, St Louis, 1991, Mosby.
3. Buschiazzo L: *The handbook of emergency nursing management,* Rockville, Md, 1987, Aspen.
4. Rowland HS, Rowland BL: *Nursing administration handbook,* ed 3, Gaithersburg, Md, 1992, Aspen.
5. American College of Emergency Physicians: *Emergency medicine risk management: a comprehensive review,* Dallas, 1991, ACEP.
6. Prescott P: Nursing intensity: needed today for more than staffing, *Nursing Economics* 9:409-414, 1991.
7. Frank I: *Managing emergency nursing services,* Rockville, Md, 1989, Aspen.

17 Emergency Department Facility Design

Stephan G. Lynn and Norman Rosenfeld

OUTLINE

Although emergency physicians, nurses, and their colleagues daily enter their hospital's emergency department and may focus on the signage on the street, may remember the paint color in the reception area and know that the cardiac room is next to the ambulance entrance, they rarely reflect on the impact that features of that department's design may have on our daily lives. The way in which the elements of the emergency department are integrated into a whole, the relationship of ancillary services and equipment to patient care areas, the location and physical relationship of triage to entry and treatment areas, and even the color scheme may affect professional performance. The way in which an emergency department is designed may determine the following:

- The ability to provide high quality patient care
- The speed and efficiency at which care is provided
- The number of staff necessary to provide that care
- A substantial part of the patient's perception of care
- The satisfaction derived from the roles as emergency care providers

Few have the opportunity and responsibility to design a new emergency department "from scratch"; many have or will have the opportunity to participate in the renovation of an existing emergency department. This chapter underscores the important role that facility design plays in delivery of quality of care.

NECESSARY FIRST STEPS IN THE DESIGN OF AN EMERGENCY DEPARTMENT

The move from concept to a functioning facility requires several important steps, which are described in Box 17-1.

GOALS AND OBJECTIVES FOR THE NEW FACILITY

It is critical to define goals and objectives and to establish expectations of the new or renovated facility before planning for its design. An emergency department may be built as an integral element of a newly constructed hospital facility, either contained within the hospital facility or as a separate wing integrated with the hospital. Facilities may be renovated for a number of reasons; to improve community access to hospital facilities, to accommodate new patient care services, or most importantly, to enhance patient care. Renovation may be dictated by increased patient volumes or the community perception of unmet need in the community. Frequently, emergency departments are reconstructed to accommodate new product lines: fast tracks, pediatric or psychiatric facilities, observation units/holding areas, chest pain facilities, occupational medicine, women's health, trauma or other designated specialty care, Emergency Medical Services (EMS) base station facilities, or other specialized functions to better serve the present patient population or to attract new patients. In this way, the emergency department and its design play a major role in the hospital's effort to change the quality of care delivered, improve its image, enhance its market, or compete with the strategies of other providers.

Planning for renovation should begin with a formal review of the hospital and the emergency department mission statement; if either is not current, the initiation of an emergency department project should provide the impetus to review the hospital's goals and mission. Because the emergency department is so critical to the function of the entire hospital and the health of its community, this process is important and should be broad based.

SELECTING AN ARCHITECT

The architect's role in developing the program and plans for an emergency department and in working constructively with a large number of emergency department and hospital staff is crucial; selecting this architect requires a careful and structured process. It is important to remember that designing and supervising the building of an emergency department is a highly specialized skill; not every architect will have the experience and knowledge to accomplish an appropriate end result; even an architect well known to the hospital or one having designed many previous hospital projects may not be the ideal candidate for the design of the emergency department.

The architect selection process should begin by establishing an emergency department project team and defining its responsibilities. The appropriate emergency physician, nurse, and emergency department administrator are important members of this team. The emergency department team must de-

BOX 17-1

FIRST STEPS IN THE DESIGN OF AN EMERGENCY DEPARTMENT

1. Establishing goals and objectives for the new facility
2. Seeking an architect
3. Preparing a functional and detailed space program
4. Defining regulatory constraints and the "certificate of need" process
5. Creating a diagramatic plan
6. Determining a project budget

BOX 17-2

CONSIDERATIONS FOR SELECTING AN ARCHITECT

- Size and longevity of the firm and its key staff. Request their professional credentials and areas of expertise along with resumes of those individuals who would be assigned to your project
- Description, geography, and construction cost of past, present, and future projects with special emphasis on emergency department design
- Client references
- Historical performance on cost projections and adherence to budgets and schedules
- Information gathering, processing, and disseminating techniques. How will the architect's team work with the emergency department project team to program and plan the new emergency department? What are their methods for providing space, function, and budget solutions?
- Personality of the principals responsible for the project and their ability to communicate with the emergency department design team

BOX 17-3

CONSIDERATIONS FOR THE FUNCTIONAL PROGRAM

Services provided

- Emergency care
    - Trauma
    - Burn
    - Hyperbaric
    - Spinal immobilization
    - EMS base station
- Separate chest pain/cardiac facility
- Admitting/holding units
- Urgent care
    - Fast track
    - Scheduled revisits
    - Women's health
    - Occupational medicine
    - Observation units

Patient volume

- Patient type
- Patient acuity
- Average versus peak
- Trends and projections of volume and acuity

fine the clinical needs that result in the design of the new department. Although many other clinical specialties will have interest in the design, they should not be members of the primary design team; their needs and the competing requirements for limited space and construction dollars must be balanced by the clinical priorities of emergency medicine. Functional relationships and space allocation must be integrated to create a functioning whole according to the emergency medicine–based principle of architectural triage (see the following discussion). Members of the hospital's planning, design, and engineering departments should join with representatives of finance and operations to complete the emergency department project team.

In considering an architectural firm, the design team should inquire about the criteria shown in Box 17-2.

In the process of selection of and communication with the architect, the administrators will be responsible for the hospital interests such as legal, public relations, and finance. The emergency department director will coordinate input from all of the clinical areas within and without the department and will assume all of the familiar roles of the triage officer. The architect will direct this information gathering and will coordinate the work of a wide range of consultants including engineers, interior designers, and equipment and cost consultants.

PREPARING A DRAFT PROGRAM AND A BUDGET

Planning should begin with a functional program, which includes the elements of service that a Department of Emergency Medicine wishes to or is required to provide to its patients. Next a space program will be developed to reflect areas needed to provide the services identified for patient profiles and projected volume of service. The functional and space programs will be converted into a project budget for construction and equipment and will be the basis for projected staffing and operating costs.

The functional program includes the services to be provided in the facility and the patient volume served by category. The functional program should consider the many current and emerging areas of service (Box 17-3).

All of these services are reflected in the final design plan but require validation by management systems within the emergency department (triage options available, relationship of registration to chart generation, dictation/transcription systems, storage of supplies and medications), as well as by functional relationships (see Creating a Functional Design Plan).

Accurate estimates of projected emergency department patient volume are critical in designing an effective emergency department. Chi Systems, Inc. created a series of numerical projection methods for emergency department patient volume (Box 17-4).

Using all of these rough rules of thumb, one can project a peak shift workload and a nonurgent peak shift workload.

BOX 17-4

PROJECTION METHODS FOR EMERGENCY DEPARTMENT PATIENT VOLUME

- Peak month workload (PMW) = 10% of annual visits
- Average daily workload peak month (ADWPM) = PMW/ 30.5 days
- Peak daily workload (PDW) = ADWPM + 2.33 × the square root of ADWPM
- Peak shift workload (PSW) = 50% PDW
- Nonurgent volume = 40% PDW
- Nonurgent peak shift workload = 75% of nonurgent PDW

(Adapted from Hayward C: Functional and space programming. *Emergency department design,* Dallas, 1993, ACEP.)

Next, one needs to know the time patients spend in each room; remember that this does not equate to time from emergency department registration to discharge. Departments may vary because the time depends on the time from registration to physician evaluation and laboratory and radiography turnaround time. In many emergency departments, patients usually spend about 120 minutes in a room, and nonurgent patients spend about 45 to 60 minutes.

By integrating these estimating methodologies, the number of treatment spaces required can be estimated. Assuming the plan is for 30,000 annual emergency department visits (planning for a 10% annual increase in a department that presently sees 27,000 visits). The peak monthly work load (PMW) would be 10% of the annual visit volume or 3000 visits. To calculate the average daily workload peak month (ADWPM) 3,000 is divided by 30.5 to get 98 visits. The peak daily workload is then calculated: PDW = ADWPM + 2.33 × the square root of ADWPM (98 + 2.33 × square root of 98 = 98 + 2.33 × 9.9 = 98 + 23 = 121 visits on the peak day). The peak shift workload (PSW) is 50% or 61 visits per peak shift.

The nonurgent peak daily workload is about 40% of the peak daily workload (121 × 0.40) = 48 and 75% of the nonurgent peak daily workload is 36 patients, the nonurgent peak shift workload.

To convert these figures into a number of patient care rooms, each emergency patient requires about 2 hours and each nonurgent visit requires about 1 hour (61 emergency visits × 2 hours = 122 visit-hours / 8 hours per shift = 15 emergency care rooms and 36 nonurgent visits × 1 hour = 36 visit-hours / 8 hours per shift = about 5 nonurgent care rooms). This technique of rough estimate is a reliable starting point for the functional plan—the number of acute and nonurgent rooms needed to accommodate predicted peak volumes.

To convert these room numbers into space, we need to know that American Institutes of Architects (AIA) standards and common practice provide at least 120 square feet per emergency treatment room and at least 80 square feet per nonurgent cubicle. Furthermore, it is important to understand that these room sizes reflect "net square feet," the space between the walls that is actually available for patient care use; to convert to "gross square feet" (the space including the thickness of the walls and the corridors and entry vestibules necessary to pass between typical rooms) net square feet is multiplied by 1.5.

BOX 17-5

MINIMUM REQUIREMENTS FOR FULL-SERVICE EMERGENCY DEPARTMENTS

Marked entrance, at grade level, protected from the weather
Treatment room—120 square feet (11.15 m^2) contains examination light, work counter, hand washing facilities, medical equipment, cabinets, medication storage, adequate electrical outlets, counter space
Multiple bed treatment rooms—80 square feet (7.43 m^2) hand washing facilities provided for each four beds or a major fraction thereof
Pelvic examination rooms shall allow for the foot of the examination table to face away from the door
Trauma/cardiac rooms—250 square feet (23.23 m^2) additionally including radiography illuminators, monitors, immediate access for attire used for universal precautions, doorways shall be a minimum of 5 feet (1.52 m)
Provisions for orthopedic and cast work; may be in trauma room
Scrub stations adjacent to trauma and/or orthopedic room
Patient toilets (two, where there are more than eight treatment rooms)
Nurses station—preferably permitting visual observation of all traffic into the unit
Securable closets or cabinet compartments for staff
Access to staff toilets, lounge, and lockers
Security station
Infectious isolation room
Bereavement room
Secured holding room

(From *Guidelines for construction and equipment of hospital and medical facilities,* Washington, DC, 1990, American Institute of Architects Committee on Architecture for Health and U.S. Department of Health and Human Services.)

To quickly convert the number and size of treatment rooms to the total size of the emergency department (to quickly add in an estimated space allocation for the waiting/reception room, the clean and dirty utility rooms, the office space and all of those other necessary functions that have not been considered, the number of the treatment rooms required is multiplied by 600 (15 emergency care rooms × 600 conversion factor = 9000 square feet for the total emergency department size). To arrive at the same number in a more precise manner, all of the support services required to support complete emergency care can be added to this estimate.

The *Guidelines for Construction and Equipment of Hospital and Medical Facilities* published by the American Institute of Architects Committee on Architecture for Health with assistance from the US Department of Health and Human Services (1990) lists the **minimum** requirements for full-service emergency departments (Box 17-5).

Construction budgets require in-depth consultation with the architect and construction manager. The cost will vary substantially depending on whether the construction is part of a more major construction project, new construction, or

renovation. It may depend on the exact location within the construction site or the status of the soil and bedrock and varies dramatically in different parts of the country. Rarely can any project be completed for less than $150/square foot.

DEFINING REGULATORY CONSTRAINTS AND THE "CERTIFICATE OF NEED" PROCESS

Regulatory constraints defining the process of approval and necessary elements in the design of hospitals and emergency departments vary in each locality. In some areas, it is necessary to file a certificate of need (CON) that will be evaluated by the state or local department of health or another governmental agency; in these locales, approval of the CON is necessary before building can begin. Such minimum acceptable standards and the formal process of filing and approval of the CON are designed to establish a consistent level of quality in the emergency departments construction projects designed to serve the community. The architect plays a key role in ensuring that the functional and spatial program, as well as the budgets for equipment, staff, and construction, meet the local requirements. The architect assists in preparing the documents necessary to achieve approval.

At a minimum, design and building codes, shown in Box 17-6, will need to be incorporated into the building plans. It will probably be necessary to meet these standards to achieve regulatory or CON approval.

Usual requirements for completing the certificate of need request for proposal are shown in Box 17-7.

It is important to plan in advance for these review processes; they require substantial collaborative efforts between the architect and the emergency department design team and substantial time in the planning and design process. Delay in gaining regulatory approval not only may result in delay or deferral of a construction project, but also may significantly increase its cost.

CREATING A FUNCTIONAL DESIGN PLAN

Emergency Department facility planning is guided by principles that are specific to emergency department design. Understanding these basic elements of emergency department design will allow the creation of a functional environment that will facilitate patient care, improve both staff and patient satisfaction, and enhance perceptions.

The Integrity of Emergency Medicine

The emergency physician should assume a lead role in the project team. Just as emergency medicine is recognized as a clinical specialty, independent and distinguishable from all others, so must the emergency physician determine the best options for clinical space allocations and resource deployment. Design cannot be completed without the participation and advice of other clinical specialties such as radiology in which the technical knowledge is beyond the scope of most emergency physicians. The contributions of other specialties must be synthesized by the emergency department design team before it can be functionally integrated into a coherent whole. In addition, emergency department staff input is critical to design the optimally efficient emergency department, and representation on the design team by several staff members is highly desirable. Because there is usually competition for limited space, equipment, and budget, the final clinical priorities should be mediated, determined, or established by the emergency physician to ensure that the most basic principles of our specialty are appropriately translated into a form of architectural triage—the most basic element of emergency department design.

Architectural Triage

Just as in clinical management, the facility design of the emergency department should follow basic principles of triage. Architectural triage results in space conforming to function in the same way that the triage officer organizes treatment priorities. One should be able to enter the emergency

BOX 17-6

DESIGN AND BUILDING CODES NECESSARY FOR CERTIFICATE OF NEED APPROVAL

- *Guidelines for construction and equipment of hospital and medical facilities*, Washington, DC, American Institutes of Architects
- *Accreditation manual for hospitals*, Chicago, Joint Commission on Accreditation of Healthcare Organizations
- State and local building codes
- State and local health agency codes and licensing requirements
- National, state, and local fire codes
- Federal, state, and local access standards for those with disability

BOX 17-7

CERTIFICATE OF NEED REQUIREMENTS

- Statistical data
  - Annual emergency department visits in the recent past, present, and future
  - Clinical Case Mix
    - Ambulance arrivals
    - Admissions
    - "True" emergencies
    - "Nonurgent" patients
    - Major trauma
    - Ob-gyn patients
    - Psychiatric emergency patients
    - Pediatric emergency patients
  - Demographic origin by Zip Code or region of patients
  - Demographic projections
  - Payor case mix
- Functional and spatial plans
- Construction budgets
  - Construction cost
  - Equipment cost
  - Financing cost
  - Agency review and legal costs
- Time frames for project

department at the point of maximal acuity, usually the ambulance entrance, and walk past adjacent treatment areas, moving in a continuous pattern of patient acuity to the waiting room, the lowest point on the triage scale. This carefully organized flow pattern is realized in the smooth structural integration of clinical activity in the emergency department as a result of a responsive architectural design. The plan provides the appropriate segregation of clinical populations (the separation of the trauma patient from the pediatric patient and the separation of the waiting room from the ambulance entrance); moreover, it locates the trauma and cardiac rooms close to the ambulance entrance and integrates the trauma room, cast room, and imaging facilities. It manifests itself in function-specific design characteristics to parallel treatment requirements (high ceilings, high intensity illumination, and a neutral color palette in the acute areas; lower ceilings, lower lighting levels, sound-absorbent materials, and brighter colors in the less acute areas).

Adjacency Relationships

The relationship of the emergency department to the hospital's community outside the hospital and to other hospital clinical areas is critical not only to ideal function but also to the quality of total patient care within the hospital-based healthcare system. The emergency department should be located within the hospital so that it is strategically accessible to the major traffic corridors that bring patients to the department. This location results in easy pedestrian, vehicular, or public transit access and visibility to the neighboring community. In most design plans, the relationship of the emergency department to its neighboring community is more important than its relationship to in-hospital clinical areas. Because the emergency department is the true "front door" of the hospital and the most common entry for patients and their families, its location on the hospital site is as important as its relationship to other hospital areas. Current trends indicate that patient entry to the hospital system through the emergency department approaches 50% in many areas, and as such more patients will define their perception of the hospital through its emergency department than through all other areas.

The relationship of the emergency department to other in-hospital clinical facilities is of great importance. Easy access to imaging (particularly complex imaging), the operating room, and the critical care complex is necessary to ensure quality patient care. In hospitals where these facilities are not horizontally contiguous, they will share the same elevator bank with the emergency department to ensure rapid access. The elevator should be key-controlled, with constant availability for the emergency department; it should be accessible without crossing hospital traffic patterns to protect the privacy of patients and not expose visitors and families to patients being transported. The ideal plan might contain a double-sized elevator accessible only from the acute area of the emergency department adjacent to the ambulance entrance and the cardiac/trauma rooms. This elevator would provide patients transport to the operating room and intensive care units above without crossing other hospital traffic. Ideally, it would provide roof level access to the heliport for receiving or transferring patients from the emergency department, trauma, or other critical care/operating room areas.

The emergency department waiting/reception room should have direct access to the hospital and its outpatient facilities so that patients can access both areas without traversing the acute clinical areas of the department. In many hospitals, the emergency department and the main entrance to the hospital are the only two areas staffed with security guards on a 24-hour basis; consequently, the main security office should be located near the department. A secondary security outpost located within the emergency department may become the primary security location for the hospital on the night, weekend, and holiday shifts. An ideal design would provide a single security station within the department to allow security staff visual access of the waiting room, entrances, psychiatric component, and the acute care area. A glass-enclosed structure located at the junction of these several functional areas would achieve that end.

The emergency department is an important user of both the imaging services and the hospital laboratory; the proximity and turnaround time of these diagnostic services is important to efficient clinical care in the department. An adjacent location is preferred in facilities that see less than about 50,000 patients/year. Because emergency department patients must travel to the imaging suite, the radiology area should ideally share a corridor (with exclusive use by patients) and be adjacent to the trauma and cardiac acute areas of the emergency department. The same radiology facilities could be accessed from the opposite direction for general hospital use (See Figure 22-5). Emergency department and hospital populations should have equal access to diagnostic radiology, but with separate traffic patterns. When emergency department volumes exceed 50,000 annual visits, fixed radiologic equipment for routine chest, abdomen, and bone films and a computed tomography scanner can often be staffed and cost-justified within the emergency department proper. Here, too, they should be adjacent to the areas of highest acuity within the department. Some hospitals will use emergency department-based radiology equipment and technicians to provide off-hours imaging services for the entire hospital. An area for emergency department patient radiography waiting should be designed so that stretcher, wheel chair, and ambulatory patients can be observed by the emergency department nurses and physicians.

Because pneumatic tube or other automated systems can transport specimens to the laboratory, and computers can return the results in a time-efficient manner, the location of the laboratory in relation to the emergency department is no longer as important as in the past. Emergency departments that see 50,000 annual visits will find it cost effective to provide on-site laboratories to perform routine "stat" tests (e.g., complete blood count with differential; electrolytes, blood urea nitrogen, and glucose; urinalysis, urine and/or serum pregnancy; creatine phosphokinase with isoenzymes; blood gases) and to store at least two units of O negative blood. Analysis of the use of the central hospital laboratory will usually indicate that the emergency department is the only 24 hour/day user, and in most hospitals will use almost 25% of the laboratory's services. If the emergency department "stat" laboratory is located at a corner of the facility and accessed by pass-throughs, one from the core of the emergency department and one from the corridor of the hospital, the traffic patterns of the emergency department patients' specimens and those of the other hospital patients can be kept separate,

ensuring confidentiality and integrity of the department, with minimal disruption by the inflow of specimens from other areas of the hospital.

Attention should be given to the location of the emergency department in relation to the medical records, pharmacy, and the central supply areas of the hospital to ensure convenient access to these important support functions. If the emergency department can be located proximate to the respiratory therapy department, social work services, and the admitting office, it will become more convenient and efficient for those services' staff when they come to the emergency department. Most hospital emergency departments admit on average 40% of the patients and the majority of patients in the evening, on holidays, and on weekends.

Separation of the Ambulatory from Ambulance Entrance

A well-designed emergency department will visually and functionally separate its ambulance and ambulatory entrances. This separation of these different patient groups is appropriate to maintain the visual privacy and confidentiality of each group and to allow the safe and secure entrance into the same emergency department of patients arriving by different means and types of vehicles. Critically ill or injured patients arriving in rapidly moving ambulances do not easily mix with and should not be viewed by relatively healthy ambulatory patients or friends or relatives visiting the department. This separation will occur naturally in a department that is architecturally triaged.

Separation of walk-in from ambulance entry may be more difficult in emergency departments with smaller volumes because of the limited amount of area and frontage. Such separation may also require duplication of triage staff. In these facilities, the placement of the ambulance and ambulatory entrances around the corner from each other may allow physical separation, but permit the same staff person to assess both groups at entry. Ambulatory entrances require the most public visibility through location and signage; EMS services will usually know how to find the ambulance entrance.

Acuity Requires Visibility; Privacy is a Luxury and is Limited

The area within the emergency department designed and equipped to accommodate acutely ill patients should allow physician and nurse staff constant visibility of each acute patient; likewise, each patient must have the security of knowing that emergency practitioners are within constant sight. This design should be accomplished without allowing patient-to-patient visibility.

In most cases, it is best accomplished by locating patient treatment positions radially around a central core of physician's and nurse's work stations. The privacy divider that separates the patients from staff could be either a cubicle curtain or break-away sliding glass doors with a privacy curtain on the inside. Consideration should be given to ensure that no object within the central core is higher than 40 inches (the standard height for a stand-up writing desk) and low enough so that a patient lying on a standard (36 inches high) stretcher can maintain visual contact with the staff (Figure 17-1). Sliding glass door dividers (foot walls) with a 5 foot opening will allow a standard 30-inch stretcher with a staff person alongside to pass while a patient car is in progress and will pro-

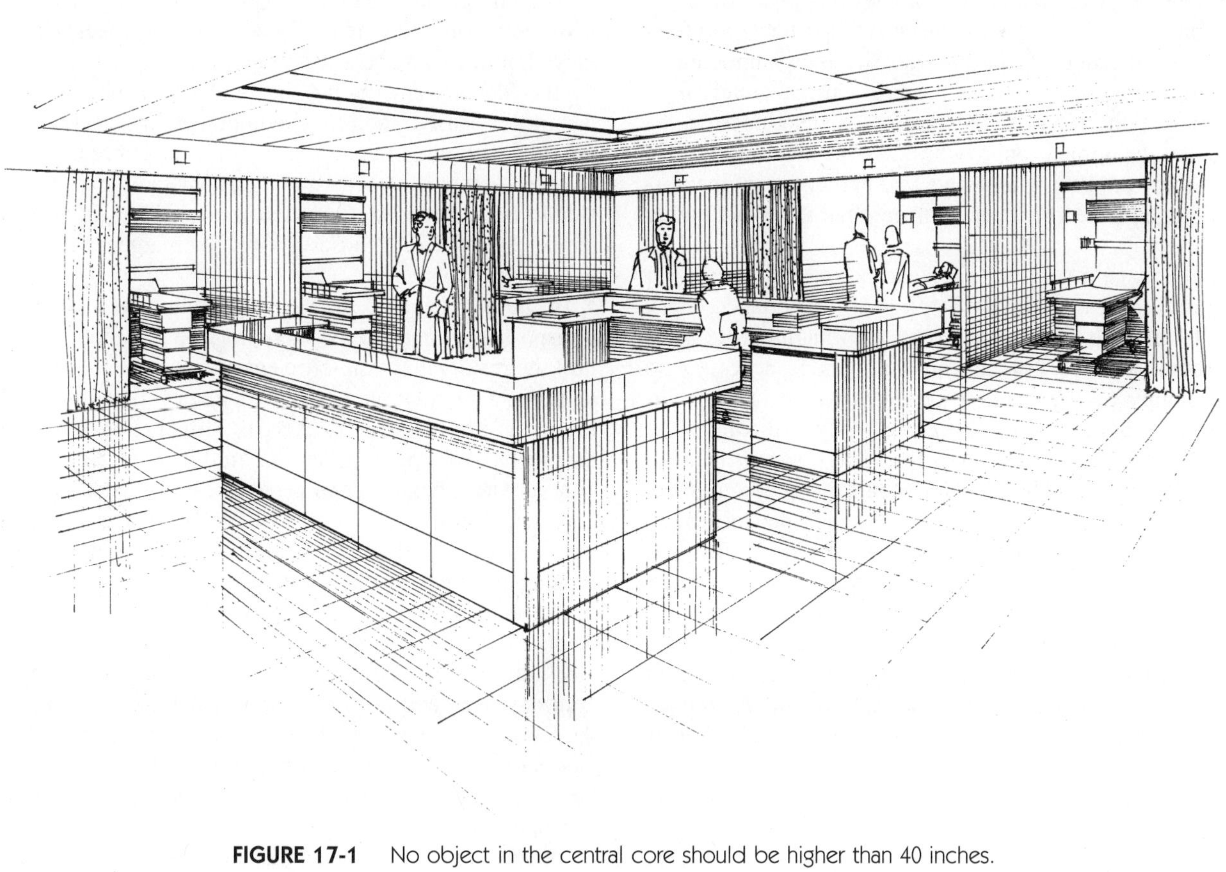

FIGURE 17-1 No object in the central core should be higher than 40 inches.

(Copyright Norman Rosenfeld Architects, New York, NY.)

vide auditory and olfactory privacy and isolation from infectious disease.

Greater flexibility can be achieved in the function of the emergency department acute care patient room by placing flexible folding ceiling-to-floor wooden partitions between the rooms. These partitions will allow visual privacy and a high degree of auditory privacy between the rooms, while providing the opportunity to open the divider and create a double-sized room (Figure 17-2). This would be useful for the management of a cardiac arrest, which might occur in a standard room; for the management of five or six seated patients observed for mild smoke inhalation; or for the treatment of a family unit of two within one space. When it is decided that the privacy of the patient within a room and the peace and quiet of those adjacent is best protected by a totally enclosed room with walls and doors (e.g., the cardiac or trauma rooms), policy should require such rooms to be staffed continuously while occupied.

Privacy is a luxury that cannot often be provided in the acute care setting of the emergency department; nonetheless, certain areas (e.g., ob-gyn rooms, quiet consultation rooms, and nonacute pediatric rooms) require less visibility and a higher degree of privacy. In considering the issues of patient privacy, it is important to satisfy visual, auditory, and olfactory privacy. Nevertheless, it is the design team's responsibility to preserve the patient's dignity, even at the expense of some elements of patient privacy. Those rooms designated for patient privacy may require visual assessment at the discretion of the staff. This can be accomplished by incorporating curtained or venetian blind glass vision panels in the walls adjacent to the doctor's/nurse's station or to the corridor. Staff-controlled privacy in a psychiatric room is maintained by placing a curtain or blinds outside the vision panel to be controlled by the staff without entering the room. Locating toilet facilities near these "private" rooms (e.g., ob-gyn) will provide an even greater degree of privacy for these special patients.

Many emergency departments are adding a quiet/consultation room to their facilities; these rooms provide a comfortable private environment for staff and family to spend a greater than normal amount of time discussing sensitive issues. They may be used to inform and provide privacy for the family that is grieving, dealing with the acute loss of a spontaneous abortion, supporting a family member of a patient that is acutely ill or injured, or in some settings providing a setting for complicated discharge instructions. The area should be located so that it can be directly accessed from the waiting/reception area and from the acute care area of the emergency department and is usually furnished as a typical practitioner's office with a desk, chairs, sofa, and table. In many emergency departments, this area serves the additional function of accommodating the press, fire services, or police officers when the need arises. This use would be facilitated by providing four to six telephone jacks with either emergency department or hospital phone lines and by providing portable telephones of the same numbers.

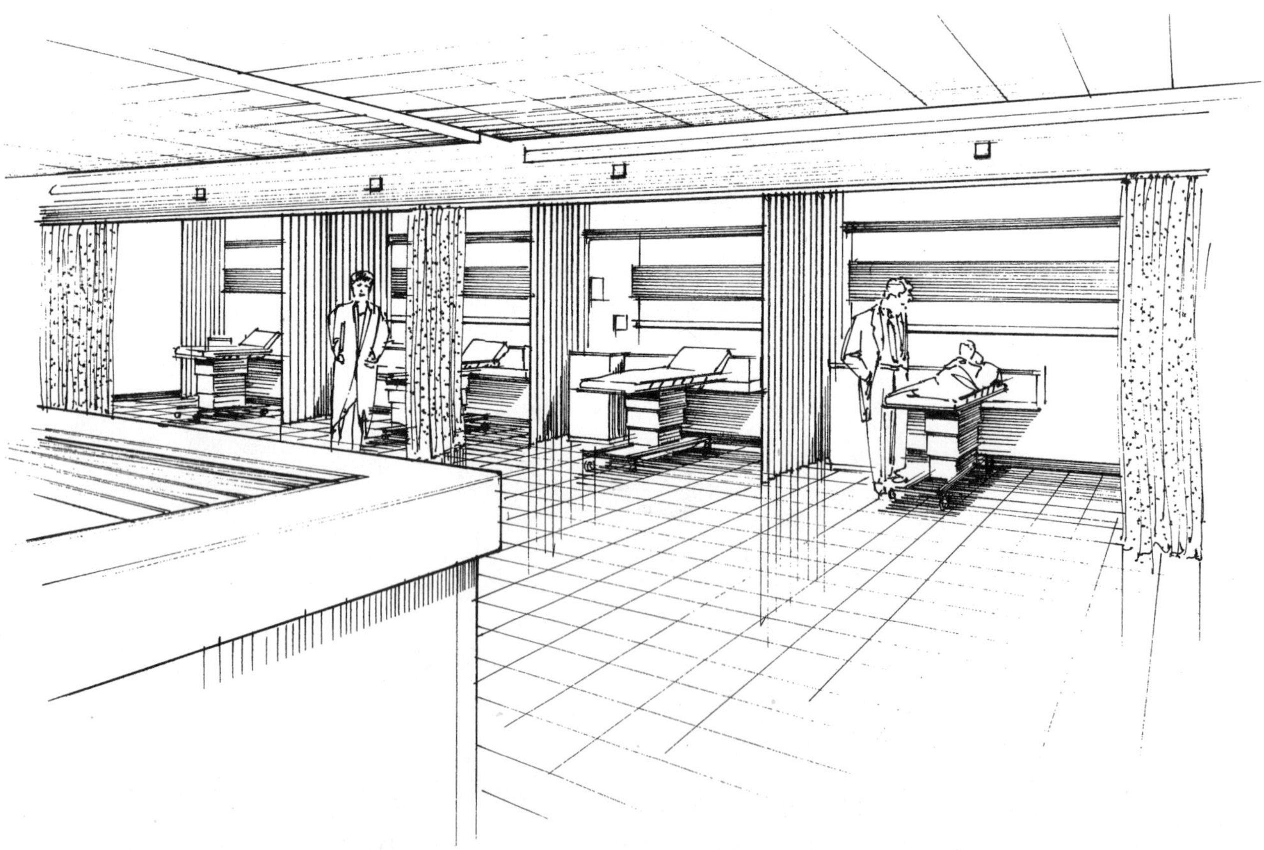

FIGURE 17-2 Wooden flexible folding partitions should be provided between acute care patient rooms for greater flexibility and to provide visual and auditory privacy when needed.

(Copyright Norman Rosenfeld Architects, New York, NY.)

Ambulatory Care Cubicles

All emergency departments regularly see patients who require attention but need neither privacy nor recumbency during most or all of their care; patients with apparent sprained ankles, minor injuries, rashes, ocular foreign body sensation, mild asthma, and many other similar problems would fit into this category. In planning emergency departments in which there are either spatial or financial limitations (almost all that are built), it is appropriate to consider designing space that will allow patients to be treated either in a remote area of the acute emergency department or in a designated fast track area within cubicles that require less space than standard stretcher areas. An "ambulatory care cubicle" (of at least 3 by 5 feet, but usually no more than 25 square feet) with partition sidewalls and cubicle curtain front walls can easily accommodate a single seated patient (Figure 17-3). The area can be outfitted with a "school desk" (stationary chair with a tablet arm and a storage shelf underneath) that will provide seating and patient storage and a flexible bracket arm wall-mounted lamp. These cubicles will accommodate a single practitioner treating one patient at a time. One or two larger cubicles with dental/ENT chairs, a sink, wall-mounted suction and oxygen, and portable or wall-mounted slit lamps will allow the evaluation and treatment of more complicated patients, with special eye/ENT/oral surgical needs in the same treatment area. These cubicle treatment areas may be located in the fast track or in the acute emergency department and should ideally bridge the two when both exist in the same emergency department. They should be accessible to both patient populations without traversing the space of the other area. Providing storage space for the equipment frequently used in such areas and allowing easy access to these areas without traversing the emergency department proper will accommodate these ambulatory patients, and will allow them to be treated and released without entering the acute emergency department. In many settings this planning/service concept has allowed the treatment of 30% of patient volume in as little as 10% of floor space.

In Search of the Ideal Emergency Department

The principles of emergency department design discussed earlier have been used as the basis for diagraming the ideal department (Figure 17-4). The plan is not meant to be nor

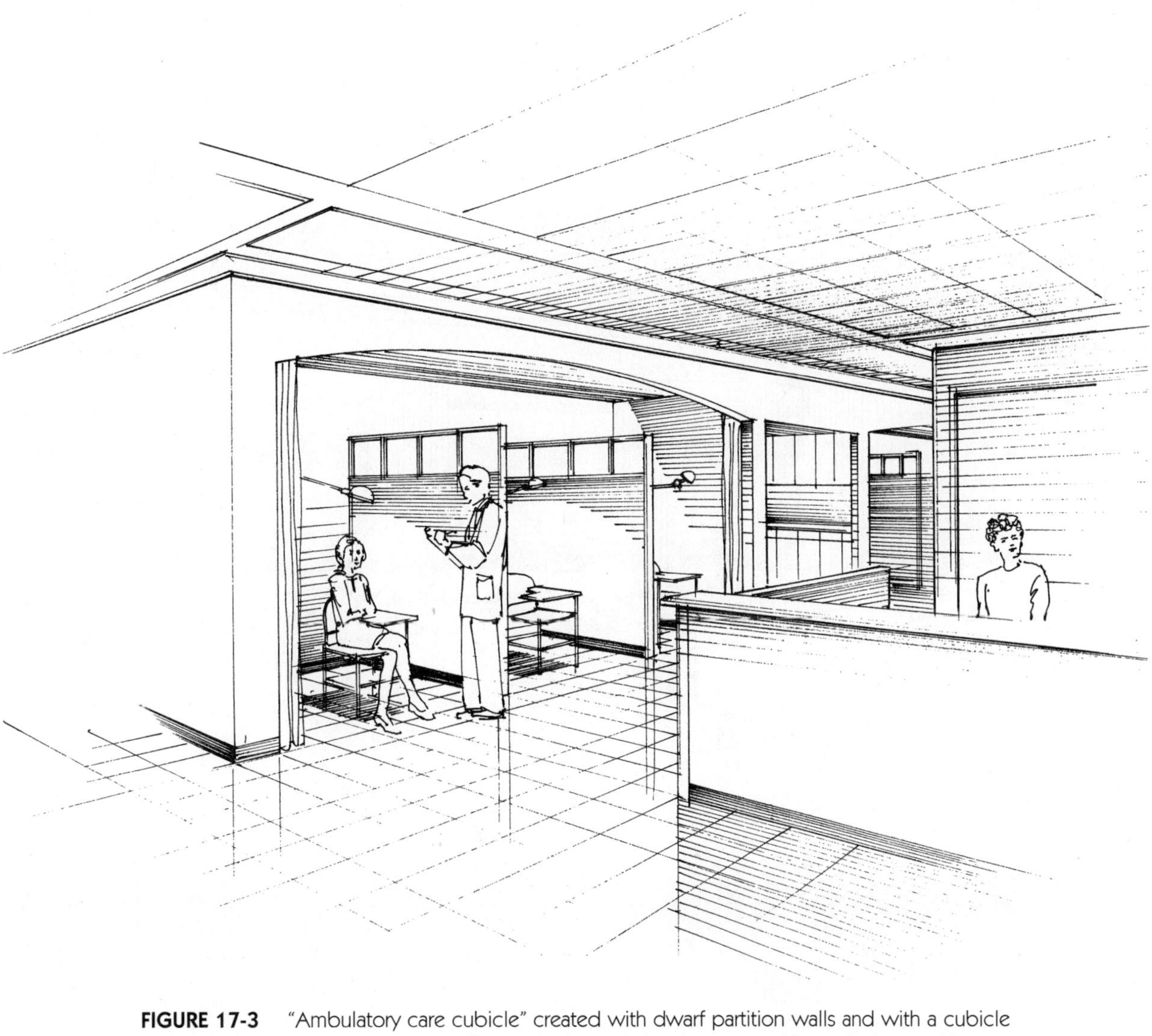

FIGURE 17-3 "Ambulatory care cubicle" created with dwarf partition walls and with a cubicle curtain for visual privacy accommodates a single seated patient treated by a single practitioner. (Copyright Norman Rosenfeld Architects, New York, NY.)

could it easily be used for any specific facility. Rather it represents the component elements of a plan functionally organized so that it can be expanded or contracted, can have modules removed or added, and can continue to provide the appropriate functional relationships needed for high quality patient care in a cost-efficient environment that is satisfying to both patient and staff. The plan illustrates all of the elements of structure and function that would exist in a large multispecialty emergency department that provides service to a diverse patient population.

In this plan, the ambulance and ambulatory entrances are widely separated, providing easy access to each and privacy and security for both patient populations. An optional internally controlled vestibule entrance leads to the psychiatric area so that police and EMS may bring patients who need immediate psychiatric screening directly to the psychiatric emergency department. This concept requires dedicated nurse staffing of the psychiatric emergency department and may result in the retriage of some patients back to the acute emergency department after delivery to the psychiatric emergency department. For control and security reasons, there are only two other entrances to the hospital—one allowing direct access of triaged patients from the waiting/reception area to the hospital outpatient area and one from the acute emergency department to the hospital. A limited number of entrances and exits provides greater security and enhances control of patient flow. Glass vestibules at both entrances provide necessary visibility of entering patients and weather protection.

Triage should be located in the direct visual and physical path of the patient entering the ambulatory vestibule. Wayfinding, if necessary, can be enhanced by creating a floor design (e.g., "checkerboard tiles") or by directive ceiling lighting (a lowered or raised ceiling area with indirect lighting) to emphasize or define the path to triage. The triage area should be designed to accommodate two nurses in parallel. Even in low-volume emergency departments, the normal but often unpredictable influx of patients may require double-teaming in this most critical entry area. The triage nurse should have clear visual access of the entrance and the entire reception area so that he or she can observe pretriage and posttriage patients and assess or reevaluate all patients (and friends and relatives) for triage options. Maximal visibility of triage must be complemented by a separate area adjacent to or behind the triage area that affords the triage nurse and patient privacy for brief physical assessment or for the communication of confidential information. This dual design feature integrates the often conflicting roles of triage—access and visibility along with privacy. Ideally, the design of triage should allow high priority patients to enter the central core of the emergency department through the rear of triage without reentering the reception area.

Registration is usually parallel in design and function to triage. Both are high visibility because of their function and both are vulnerable to angry or destructive patients or their relatives. Consequently, security in the reception area and for triage/registration takes on particular importance. A security

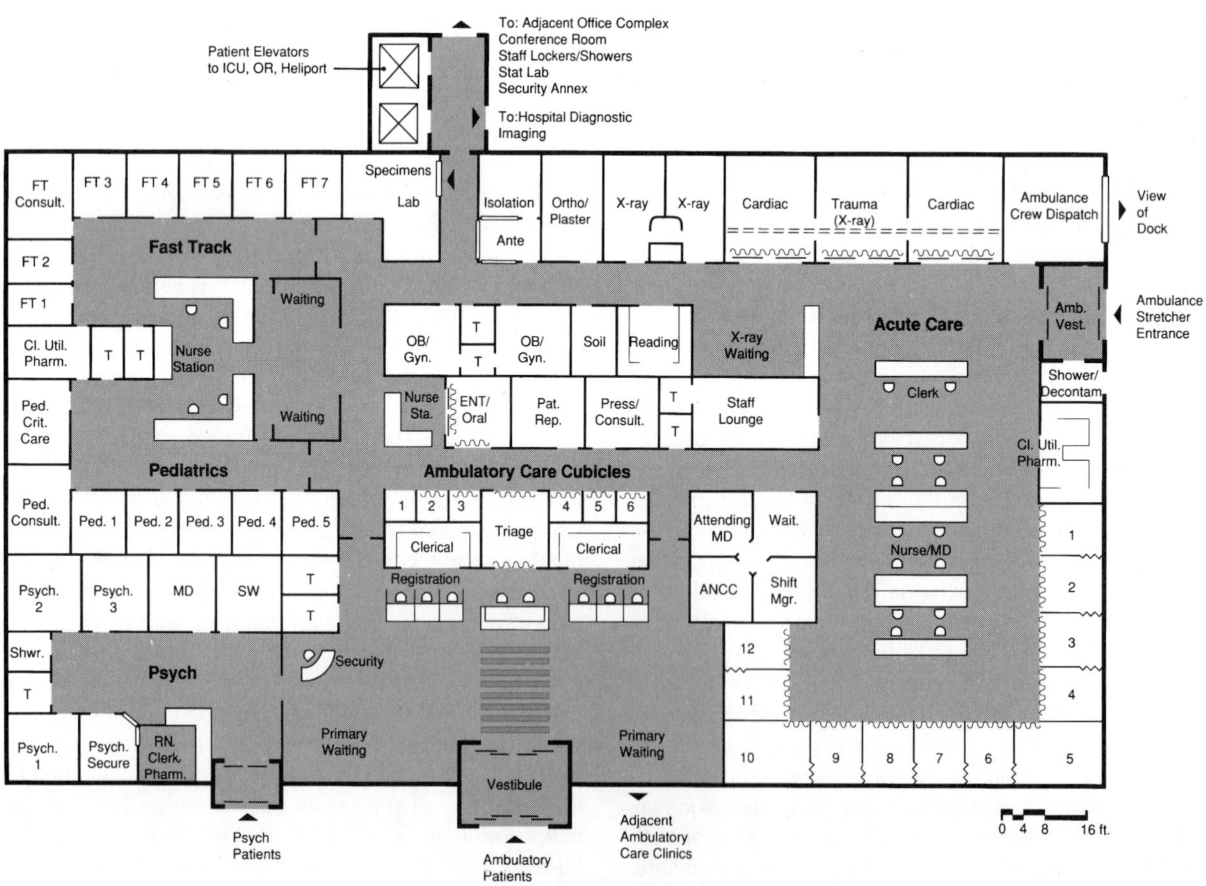

FIGURE 17-4 Idealized emergency department.

(Copyright Norman Rosenfeld Architects, New York, NY.)

officer located in the emergency department should have a fixed desk location adjacent to the psychiatry area, with full view of the main waiting area and external and internal entrances of the reception area, triage, registration, and the rest of the reception area. This 24-hour security desk should receive the "panic alarms" and video camera transmissions from other areas in the emergency department and should be continually staffed. Often the security desk will share responsibility with the telephone operator as the hospital's off-hours command post, receiving all building system alarms, medical crisis alerts, and community disaster alerts. Depending on patient population, triage and registration may need to be secured by Lexan or shatterproof glass. Specific security design solutions should consider the need to pass papers, take vital signs, and talk to patients. The level of security must be weighed against the message of separation and lack of trust (lack of security) that may be transmitted to patients and their families. Other design elements in the reception area include a drinking fountain, separate male and female bathrooms, public telephones, and magazine racks for pleasure reading and emergency department-supplied medical information. Because the first impression of many patients and their families will occur in the waiting/reception area of the hospital's emergency department, interior design elements—plants, artwork, color palette, wall coverings, and lighting—will be particularly important. Chairs and furniture in the reception area should be constructed of durable, nonabsorbent materials. This is important not only for cost efficiency and appearance, but also for hygiene and infection control.

There are three connectors from the reception area to other areas of the emergency department: one to the psychiatric emergency department, one to the pediatric emergency department and fast track, and one to the acute care emergency department. All of these doors should be controlled by staff on the inside inviting patients and relatives in or by the security guard electronically opening the door from the security desk (the doors visible directly or by mirrors). The route from the reception area to the main hospital should be direct with minimal disruption to the emergency department, either by patients or families.

The psychiatric emergency department should be located adjacent to the main ambulatory entrance, with the security guard positioned at its entrance. A second vestibuled entrance from the exterior would be desirable. This second entrance would be most valuable if a larger percentage of the psychiatric emergency patients arrive by ambulance or by police because it offers both an opportunity for a second exit for staff and a potential security hazard as an entrance. Access must be carefully controlled by the psychiatric nurse(s) from within the psychiatric nurse's station. This station should provide secured visibility to the entrances, waiting area, and all of the psychiatric patient rooms, with a one-way see-through glass to the secure room. A separate physician interview room and the emergency department social worker's office are necessary components of this patient care complex. Separate toilet and shower facilities allow this area to be fully independent. All doors should open out (so that they cannot be barricaded from the inside) and are lockable from the outside only; all light fixtures are flush with the wall, nonbreakable, and controlled from outside the room; all sinks and fixtures are specially designed for psychiatric use; door closers should not protrude (so as to prevent opportunities for hanging). All rooms should have vision panels with curtains or blinds on the outside. The secure room should have a one-way vision panel to the nurse's station or a recessed video camera with screen in the nurse's station. A separate waiting area for this component is important to both the psychiatric and nonpsychiatric patients.

The ambulatory care cubicles and the eye/ENT/oral surgery cubicle are immediately adjacent to both entrances to the emergency department. These areas act as a bridge between the acute and less acute areas and are accessible from and usable by both areas. Most important, patients can be treated and released from this area, never having to enter the central core of the emergency department. With a separate nurse/physician work station in the area and with storage of most of the equipment and supplies necessary to provide care within the area, a physician/nurse team can provide most of the needed care without having to leave the area.

The patient representative's office and the quiet consult/press/police room is located in the area that bridges the reception area and both the acute and urgent areas of the emergency department. This arrangement allows staff to meet with patients, families, friends, and police and press in a quiet area of the department, with easy access to the reception area that neither interferes with nor is affected by the patient care in the acute emergency department.

The pediatric emergency department and the fast track share an entrance, nurse's station, waiting area, and a clean supply/pharmacy area. This plan offers operational economies and spatial efficiency for the fast track, which is likely to be open for a limited portion of the day. The least desirable feature is the shared pediatric and adult waiting/reception area. These can be designed as more separate areas at some expense in space and staffing. Each area has a consult room where nurses and/or physicians may spend a longer period of time discussing patient care plans or issues of treatment or diagnosis with patients and their families. The pediatric emergency department has its own critical care area.

The acute care emergency department is entered from the ambulance entrance or through the reception area. An ambulance room/EMS dispatch center is immediately adjacent to the ambulance entrance with a large window overlooking the ambulance bay. It contains the communications systems, secondary supply depot for EMS staff, and work area/lounge for prehospital personnel. For security reasons, it is entered only from within the emergency department.

Adjacent to the ambulance entrance is the shower/decontamination room; it has a separate secured exterior entrance to allow access without contaminating the primary ambulance area. It has a secondary entry through the ambulance vestibule to permit patients who require a shower or decontamination to enter without leaving the confines of the department and to provide access to the department for decontaminated patients. Guidelines for the control of radioactive wastes require that the drainage of fluids from the floor and the exhaust of air and gases from this area be handled by systems that are separate from the rest of the hospital and that collection systems not enter the common waste flow of the hospital's effluents. Alternative stretcher-mounted tray systems are available to capture fluid drainage into a single secure barrel that may be safely and appropriately disposed of.

The ability to close down the ventilation systems in this area separately from the rest of the hospital may provide cost-efficient and effective means of controlling and safely handling the wastes from this area.

On entering the central core of the acute care emergency department, the nurse/physician/clerk area is outfitted with work surfaces, storage space, and charting desks all below eye level (below 40 inches), with no visual obstruction from supporting columns, supply carts, or furniture in the center of the work space. All staff standing in any part of the central core should have maximum visibility of all patient areas; similarly, patients looking in from their stretchers/treatment areas can see the staff in the work areas.

A complex of critical care/trauma/cardiac rooms is immediately adjacent to the ambulance entrance. The divider between these areas and the work area is a sliding break-away glass door system that accommodates a 60-inch passage. Inside is a curtain that adds visual privacy to the auditory and olfactory privacy provided by the glass wall divider. The adjacent critical care rooms can be separated by standard floor to ceiling walls or as illustrated in the diagram by 5 to 7 foot high lead-lined dividers over which passes a single ceiling-mounted radiographic unit. This arrangement eliminates the need for portable equipment and provides for in-room radiography, with a single unit providing superior resolution films in all of the critical care rooms. The arrangement is ideal in maintaining the ability to continue critical patient management while obtaining critically needed radiographs promptly.

A double-sized dedicated elevator is adjacent to the ambulance entrance and the critical care rooms directly connecting the emergency department to other hospital floors that may contain the critical care unit, operating room, complex imaging, and a roof-top heliport. This elevator is the primary connection between all of the critical care services of the hospital and must deliver its patients on each appropriate floor only into privacy-protected patient-only areas without cross traffic of hospital visitors.

All of the acute care rooms have curtain dividers at the foot of the stretcher, which separate them from the central nurse/doctor work area. Separation between treatment positions is by folding wall dividers that provide visual and auditory privacy between rooms and allow the flexibility, on opening, of creating double-sized rooms. Wood-slotted dividers add a warmer feel to the area and pose no special asepsis problem. All of these rooms are fully and equally equipped with medical gases, services, and supplies so as to be used completely interchangeably.

The ED imaging area is contiguous to the critical care rooms and adjacent to the corner of the central core. It contains standard fixed table radiography rooms, a compact "daylight" developing area, a radiologist's reading room, and a patient waiting area. The reading room, by design, has no door and allows easy access for the radiologist to the staff and provides the opportunity for the radiologist to venture into the department. This plan encourages emergency department/radiology bedside consultation to determine the most appropriate imaging mode. An added benefit is the sharing of the knowledge that "clinical correlation is needed" with the emergency physician before dictating the radiograph reading. The radiographic patient waiting area allows the staff to maintain visual observation with them as they wait. Radiographic equipment in the trauma/cardiac rooms is adjacent and conveniently accessible to the radiography staff (Figure 17-5).

Two obstetrics/gynecology rooms are situated in a quiet corner to allow use and access by both the acute care emergency department and the fast track. They share a toilet facility. The entrance vestibule creates privacy within the rooms, and the room is designed for maximum privacy with the patient facing away from the door.

An isolation room with an anteroom for staff to gown, glove, mask, and scrub is located off the central core. As the number of persons with AIDS, tuberculosis, and other infectious diseases continues to increase, these patient rooms will be required. The use of glass sliding doors for both the room and the anteroom will provide isolation and maintain the ability to observe the patient.

The orthopedic/plaster room is located adjacent to the radiography suite but off the central core. It contains the sink with the plaster trap and all of the equipment (e.g., plaster, fiberglass, crutches, canes, knee immobilizers) frequently used in the management of orthopedic patients.

The staff lounge is located immediately off the central core of the emergency department so as to allow easy access by the staff and, with the door open, afford some visual and auditory connection with the acute care area, even while in the lounge. The lounge has a dedicated toilet. Depending on hospital and emergency department policy, a staff food refrigerator, sink, and a microwave oven may be provided. The easy accessibility of the staff lounge will discourage and signal the undesirability of eating, drinking, or newspaper reading in patient care areas. A staff locker and shower area is designed outside and adjacent to the emergency department so that the staff may enter and exit the hospital passing through this area and enter the department only through the hospital entrance in uniform/without coats and parcels and ready to provide patient care.

The clean supply and pharmacy area is open and visible to the central core. This arrangement provides easy access and high visibility and provides far more security than enclosed units. A nourishment center should be part of this area, including storage space for refrigerated foods and a rewarming area. A single soiled holding area is used by all of the modules of the emergency department.

An optional office complex within the department is provided for those staff with primary clinical responsibility (e.g., the attending physician, the assistant nursing care coordinator, and the emergency department junior administrator/clerical supervisor). It shares a waiting area and allows a convenient location to perform administrative functions while maintaining responsibility for patient care. This on-site management complex facilitates the location of the major emergency department administrative suite at a location either adjacent to or remote from the department. In some designs, the primary office complex may be located on the floor immediately above the emergency department, with easy stairway/elevator access to the department. (First floor hospital space is usually limited and consequently quite valuable.)

The emergency department stat laboratory is located in an area accessible by all modules of the department from within.

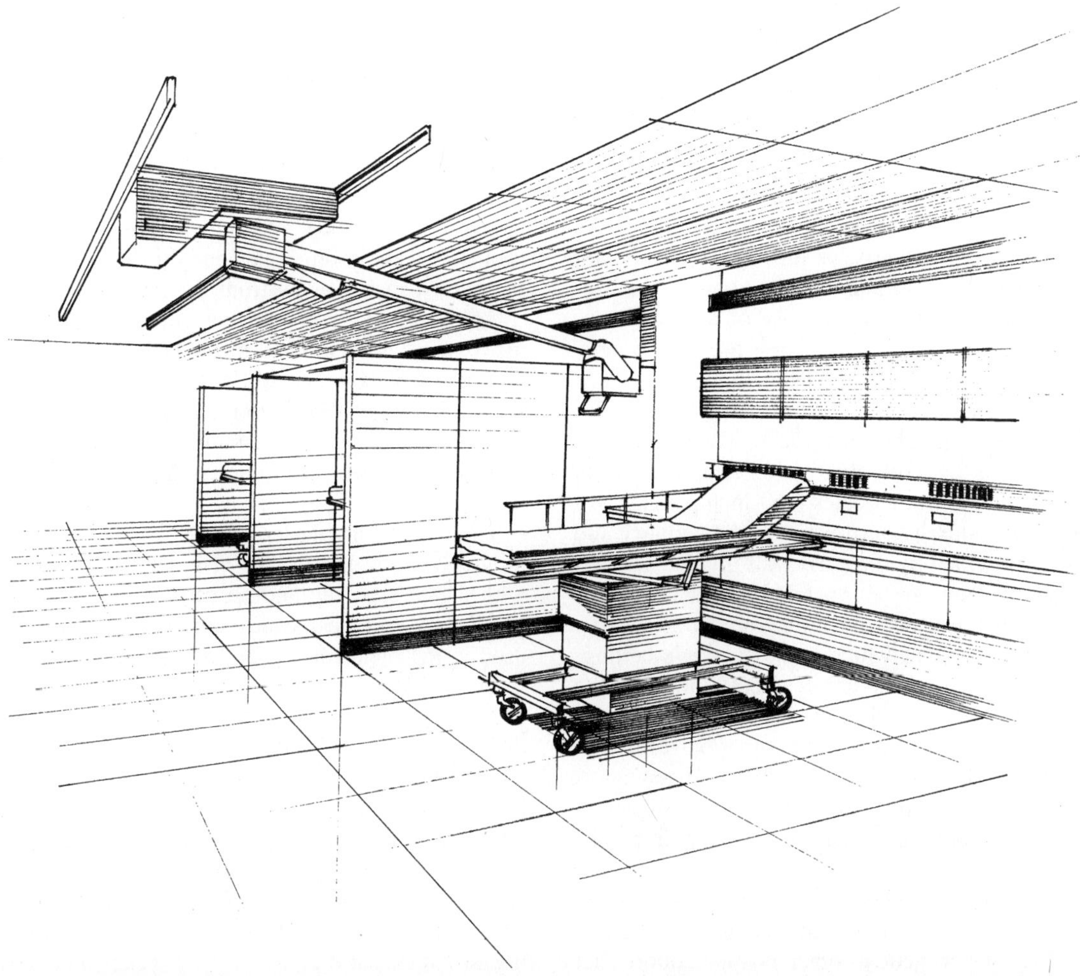

FIGURE 17-5 Adjacent critical care treatment positions separated by lead-lined partitions, at a height of 5 feet, can be commonly served by one track-mounted radiography unit.
(Copyright Norman Rosenfeld Architects, New York, NY.)

It has a pass-through entrance from the hospital corridor so that it may serve as the stat laboratory for the entire hospital and can be accessed without traversing the emergency department.

This ideal emergency department plan represents a conceptual model that can and will be modified, expanded, or diminished in a number of different ways to make it hospital-specific. These changes must always recognize the needs of the patients, staff, and hospital.

A well-designed emergency department can enhance both the management and delivery of emergency medicine. Emergency department design concepts can affect policies and procedures of patient care. Often the design of an emergency department can have an impact on a hospital's scope of services and range of populations served. Although good design does not deliver good patient care, an appropriately designed facility can be of great assistance to both physicians and nurses in providing timely and effective emergency care.

18 Managing the Overcrowded Emergency Department

Stephan G. Lynn

OUTLINE

The emergency department is frequently thought of as a microcosm of the hospital as a whole; almost everything that happens every day in the hospital, happens in the emergency department. The emergency department is also the "front door" of the hospital—the portal of entry in the hospital that sees the highest volume of patients and that is closest to "the pulse of its community." For these reasons, the emergency department is the only department in the hospital to experience overcrowding, a problem that represents the convergence of local hospital policy and national healthcare policy.

Overcrowding in the emergency department is a significant problem that has several manifestations and many causes. In its classic form, it occurs when admitted patients cannot leave the department because all staffed inpatient and intensive care unit (ICU) beds in the hospital are occupied and no beds are available in neighboring facilities for transfer.[1] This is clearly a hospital problem, an inability to accommodate admissions from the emergency department, which is manifested in the emergency department. The solutions are within the hospital; only coping mechanisms are available within the emergency department. Overcrowding of another type occurs when large numbers of patients come to the triage desk and seek care in the emergency department, overwhelming the ability of the staff and the facility to expeditiously accommodate additional patients; here, overcrowding occurs largely in the waiting room of the emergency department. This problem is related more to the nature of the emergency department's community, state and federal health policy systems, and systems of reimbursement for healthcare. It has little to do with local hospital policy.

Both of these conditions are problems of access: the first, access of patients to in-hospital resources and beds manifested by admitted patients waiting in the emergency department; the second, access of patients in the community to healthcare manifested by seeking that care in the emergency department. The department staff may seem to be "innocent bystanders" with respect to both of these problems (the first, an afterload problem, the second, a preload problem); however, as caregivers who feel significantly responsible for their actions and who assume a role as patient advocates, emergency physicians and nurses have a critical role to play in the resolution of both problems.

TOO MANY PATIENTS, TOO FEW AVAILABLE BEDS

The essence of classic overcrowding is simple: There are too many patients who require acute inpatient care and too few hospital beds or too few hospitals available to care for these patients. Patients who are admitted must be held in the emergency department until a bed becomes available or the patient is transferred to another institution. When a large percentage of a community's emergency departments become overcrowded simultaneously and adopt ambulance diversion or some other limited availability status, the problem rapidly escalates to "emergency department gridlock," a particularly difficult problem in which no emergency department in the community can safely accommodate additional patients.[2]

Scope of the Problem

In 1989 the American College of Emergency Physicians (ACEP) conducted a survey of its chapters to assess the extent of overcrowding; 41 state chapters reported overcrowding.[1] In 1991 the National Public Health and Hospital Institute published its survey (based on results from fall 1988); 239 emergency department directors from hospitals that were member institutions of the National Association of Public Hospitals and/or the Council of Teaching Hospitals reported the following:

- Private hospitals reported hospital mean occupancy rates as high as those in public hospitals.
- Three of four institutions studied reported increased rates of emergency department utilization.
- During one reference month (August 1988), 40% of reporting hospitals diverted ambulances at least part of the time.
- Emergency department directors at 65% of the institutions reported that overcrowding was having moderate to severe negative impact on their quality of care.[3]

In January 1993 the Government Accounting Office (GAO) reported the responses of 689 valid surveys of 1073 questionnaires selected as representative of the nation's 5298 hospitals that had emergency departments. In 1990 (the GAO study year), one in three hospital emergency departments nationwide reported a delay of 4 hours or more in transferring admitted patients to inpatient beds, affecting 18% of admit-

ted patients nationwide. Admission delays were reported by half of urban hospitals and three fourths of large hospitals (more than 300 beds). In the study year, 61% of urban area hospitals requested diversion of ambulances at least once during the year, 13% of urban hospitals requested diversion more than 100 times, 23% reported that diversion lasted 8 hours or more, and more than half of those that requested ambulance diversion reported that the frequency of these requests increased from 1985 to 1990.[4] All of these studies document that many emergency departments nationwide experience difficulty finding inpatient beds for patients admitted through the department; many hospitals—public and private, urban and rural, large and small—experience overcrowding.

Contributing Factors

There are many causes of emergency department and hospital overcrowding; most are the result of inadequate or reduced funding for emergency healthcare during a period of increasing demand. The GAO reports that hospitals that experience delays of more than 4 hours in obtaining beds for patients had several conditions in common (Box 18-1).[4]

Lack of availability of ICU and emergency department beds was the cause of ambulance diversion in 45% of hospitals nationwide surveyed by the GAO.[4] ACEP's survey[1] identified the major contributors to the problem of overcrowding as a growing shortage of healthcare professionals (e.g., nurses, especially critical care nurses, and emergency physicians), increased use of emergency departments as a route of admissions (the American Hospital Association reports an increase from 30% in 1980 to 40% in 1990), high inpatient average daily census, hospital bed reductions or conversions to special uses not affected by diagnosis-related groups (DRGs) (e.g., alcohol or drug detoxification, psychiatry, or rehabilitation), closure of hospitals or emergency departments, prolonged use of acute care beds by patients who could otherwise be accommodated in nursing homes or at home if resources were available, increasing numbers of poor or uninsured patients,[5] increasing numbers of patients with AIDS, and increasing numbers of drug-related admissions (e.g., trauma, overdose, and infectious complications).[6]

Management of Hospital Overcrowding

Emergency departments exist primarily to provide comprehensive emergency care and stabilization; once stabilized, patients requiring admission should be expeditiously transported to an appropriate inpatient unit. When this cannot occur, hospital overcrowding results. In this setting, major changes in department management may be necessary to maintain the standards of adequate basic emergency care under increasingly adverse circumstances. Overcrowding causes diversion of resources (e.g., space, staff, time) to support prolonged inpatient care within the emergency department; this usually results in fewer resources available to support emergency care, the primary purpose of the department. Initial management measures should focus on recognition of the impending overcrowding crisis so that procedures can be initiated to enhance the efficiency and capacity of the hospital's inpatient units to admit and accommodate patients before they back up in the emergency department. Initial management should be aimed at preventing overcrowding before it occurs and has a negative impact on the care of all patients in the department. Changes in emergency department management should be initiated only if the hospital management changes fail; if the problem is particularly severe, changes in the Emergency Medical Services (EMS) may be necessary.

Documentation of the scope of the problem at the hospital is necessary to convince administrators to lend their efforts to make the changes in inpatient management necessary to improve the quality of emergency department patient care when the hospital becomes overcrowded. Department admission logs and change-of-shift reports provide a valuable data source. To collect documentation of the nature of hospital and overcrowding, the log should include criteria such as those shown in Box 18-2. A change of shift report may be maintained to document the number and status of patients at fixed

BOX 18-1

PERCENT OF HOSPITALS WITH DELAYED EMERGENCY DEPARTMENT ADMISSION

Hospital occupancy rate greater than 60%	84%
Increased visits because of:	
Illegal drugs	78%
Violence	78%
AIDS	74%
Alcohol abuse	74%
Inability to staff emergency department with nurses	54%

From *Emergency Departments: unevenly affected by growth and change in patient use,* United States General Accounting Office, GAO/HRD-93-4:1-72, 1993.

BOX 18-2

CRITERIA FOR EMERGENCY DEPARTMENT ADMISSION LOGS

Patient name and medical record number
Emergency department admission diagnosis
Bed type required
- (medical, surgical, etc., isolation, ICU, private or service, etc.)

Times
- Registration
- Initiation of physician treatment
- Admission decision
- Bed assigned
- Bed available
- Patient to floor

Comments
Summary data by day
- Total emergency department admissions
- Total admissions for each bed category
- Total patient hours from admission decision to transport ("boarder hours")
- Total hospital admissions from all sources (from admission's office)
- Percentage of all hospital admissions through the emergency department

times during the day. Box 18-3 shows the information to be recorded.

From this information, trends per shift, per day, per month, and average times from registration to physician evaluation, from evaluation to admission decision, and from admission to floor can be extracted. Using other data sources (emergency department statistics and hospital census data), correlations can be made between inpatient census and waiting times and department walkouts, between ICU and emergency department census, and between bed type and waiting times. All of these will be valuable in defining strategies to alleviate the problem of department overcrowding.

Inpatient measures to deal with overcrowding need to be activated expeditiously so that the hospital can accommodate patients and ideally avoid overcrowding. The ultimate goal is to reverse hospital overcrowding and to prevent emergency department backup. To choose when to activate these contingency plans, many hospitals have established the following trigger points: overall inpatient census of 85%,[7] a medical-surgical census of 90%, and only one or no available critical care beds.[2] All concerned must agree on these trigger points and the activation of contingency plans and/or the meeting of a special bed management committee to define crisis management policy during times of overcrowding. This committee should have broad and definitive decision-making authority, should meet before emergency department and hospital overcrowding occurs, and should establish contingency plans that will allow the admissions office and the on-call administrator to take definitive, independent, and preapproved action at the time of a crisis, even if the committee is not able to reconvene. These management strategies include all of the following management practices designed to improve the quality of care and/or the hospital's fiscal bottom line.

Inpatient Length of Stay. Individual physician and departmental average length of stay should be evaluated. Corrective action should be taken to reduce length of stay that is at variance with accepted norms. This approach is clearly the most effective and cost-efficient way to alleviate overcrowding in the DRG era of prospective payments.

Intent to Discharge Policy. A system needs to be established to allow physicians to notify the admissions office of a patient discharge the evening before it occurs; this protocol will allow efficient early discharge and rapid bed turnover.

Discharge Notification by Inpatient Units. Inpatient staff, unit clerks, and head nurses must learn that an important part of the hospital's mission is its financial viability, and the reason for their employment depends on their ability to accommodate the next admission on their inpatient floor. Prompt notification of the admissions office of expected discharges and efficient management of bed turnover is mandatory. Because this action will result in a positive work increment for the inpatient staff involved with the arrival of the next admission, positive incentives and effective monitoring of bed turnover may be necessary to accomplish the efficient transition from the last discharge to the next admission in the same inpatient bed.

Discharge Lounges. To facilitate early and efficient discharge of patients in inpatient units, an area on each patient floor (patient lounge) or a central area within the hospital may need to be equipped and staffed to care for discharged patients who are not yet ready to leave the hospital (ride home has not yet arrived, escort not available until after the work day).

Elective/Emergency Admission Priority. There should be a preestablished and agreed upon policy that defines a priority for different categories of hospital admissions; this policy will allow the admissions office to assign beds to urgent elective and emergency department admissions and nonurgent elective admissions scheduled for invasive procedures. All must agree on a policy that will determine when elective admissions should be deferred because of high hospital census or emergency department overcrowding.

Admissions Coordinator. The hospital needs to assign an Associate Director of the Admissions Office whose primary function is to visit the floors of the hospital regularly, find beds that are or are about to become available, facilitate the turnover of these beds, and be vested with the authority to discipline inpatient staff who do not meet the hospital's expectations with respect to bed turnover.

Physician/Admissions Office Liaison. In a crisis such that occurs with severe hospital overcrowding, a physician may need to be assigned to work closely with the admissions office to ensure that access to inpatient beds is based completely on medical need. This physician will serve as an arbitrator for the best interest of all of the hospital's patients in determining whether the admitted emergency department "boarder" patient or the semiurgent elective patient at home gets the last available inpatient bed.

Flexible Bed Designation. At times of hospital overcrowding and high inpatient census, policy must guarantee maximal bed flexibility. Beds that might otherwise be reserved and staffed and equipped to provide limited roles (e.g., medical, surgical, private, research, metabolic, female) must become interchangeable at times of crisis.

Alternate Level of Care (ALC) Patients. At some hospitals, ALC patients may continue to occupy acute inpatient beds when their medical and social needs would be better met by home healthcare or in a nursing home, but no such resources are available. This inefficient bed use may block emergency department admitted patients (and elective admissions) from access to inpatient beds. Social workers, discharge planners, and legal advocates must work in tandem to guarantee rapid

BOX 18-3

CHANGE OF SHIFT REPORT CRITERIA

Diversion status and times
Patient name
Emergency department location
Working diagnosis
Admission status
Time of emergency department registration
Summary data
Total admitted patients in emergency department
Total patients in emergency department
Total patients in and awaiting triage
Total patients triaged and in waiting room

and appropriate placement of ALC patients to provide more hospital beds available for acute inpatient care.

In-house Transfers. Transfers between different inpatient beds to facilitate patient comfort or physician convenience must be limited during times of overcrowding; each transfer requires the time and staff work equal to both the discharge and admission of an inpatient.

Over Census Beds. Within the limitations of applicable laws and regulations, additional locations on the inpatient units not normally used to care for patients should be identified. In times of emergency department overcrowding, these nontraditional patient care locations (hallways, lounges, a second bed location in a single patient room, reopened inpatient units that were temporarily closed) need to be used in place of equally nontraditional locations for patient care in the emergency department. Most of these nontraditional inpatient bed locations will provide more privacy, quiet, access to telephones and TV, ability to turn out the lights at night, and ability to accommodate visitors than any location in the emergency department. From the perspective of patient care, almost any nontraditional inpatient bed location is preferable to the hallway in the emergency department.

If 10 admitted patients waiting for inpatient beds in the emergency department can be located in nontraditional locations on 10 floors, each with 20 beds, the incremental workload for inpatient nurses would be 5% per floor; if those patients remain in the department, the emergency nurses may need to exceed their normal patient care capacity by 30% to 100%. If the hospital can create flexible staffing and facilities to care for monitored inpatient needs (available critical care space), there will be a greater pay-off in relieving department overcrowding.

"Thirty-Minute Rule". Some hospitals seem to have a disincentive for inpatient clerical, nursing, and housekeeping staffs to recognize and to report available beds for patients waiting in the emergency department. There is a substantial work increment for these staff if there is a new admission that cannot be delayed beyond the end of their shift. Some hospitals have initiated a policy that 30 minutes after the admissions office has assigned an inpatient bed for a patent, the emergency department will send the patient to the inpatient unit on a stretcher. The patient will be cared for on that unit (even if the last patient has not yet left the bed, the housekeeper has not cleaned the room, or the inpatient nurse is not available to accept report). Only a nursing supervisor can intervene and allow the patient to remain in the emergency department. This policy creates a powerful incentive for inpatient staff to turn over beds efficiently.

Holding Unit. In hospitals in which the "boarding" of admitted patients in the emergency department has become a regular phenomenon, separate staff, facilities, and equipment have been allocated to provide interim inpatient care for patients for whom an inpatient bed is not available. Additional space and staff allocations are needed to create a unit that improves patient care; neither should occur at the expense of emergency department staff or space.

Inpatient Billing. Most third party payors allow inpatient billing for patients maintained in the emergency department who have an order written for admission to the hospital, a complete history and physical examination recorded, and an inpatient attending physician's signature. This rule usually applies to patients who begin their hospital stay in the emergency department and are subsequently accommodated in inpatient units, but is also applicable to patients admitted in the department and subsequently discharged, never having left the department. (This situation most commonly applies to patients with diagnosis of chest pain/rule out myocardial infarction after an appropriate number of negative electrocardiograms and creatine phosphokinase results have been returned while the patient remains in the department.) In some institutions, there may be a substantial income stream from patients admitted and discharged from the emergency department.

Inpatient Physician Responsibility. Inpatient physicians (private attending physicians, critical care physicians, inpatient housestaff) should assume clinical responsibility for ongoing inpatient care of patients detained in the emergency department (routine orders for medications, history and physical examination documentation). As long as the patient remains in the department, it should be the responsibility of staff to continue to provide emergency care (e.g., arrhythmia management, emergency management for hyperkalemia). The well-documented order of the appropriate inpatient attending physician should be necessary to discharge a patient from the emergency department who has been admitted to the hospital.

Direct Admission Policies. Patients admitted (or transferred) to the hospital with an inpatient bed available at the time of arrival should be assessed in the emergency department for stability (remaining on the ambulance gurney) and sent promptly to the inpatient floor bed, if the patient is deemed stable. It is presumed that all such admitted patients are sick, and only instability should be a criterion for remaining in the emergency department.

Initiating Overcrowding Measures

Emergency department measures to deal with overcrowding should be initiated only when hospital policy changes do not result in the expeditious availability of appropriate inpatient beds for admitted patients. Substantive modifications in the process of and patient care plans for emergency department management will be necessary to preserve acceptable standards of patient care. Most of these changes will facilitate the provision of inpatient and critical care management in the department long beyond the time frames usually expected. Overcrowding cannot be managed by "working harder;" basic changes will be necessary to meet inpatient care standards within the department for those "boarder" admissions who dwell there, while maintaining the usual standards of emergency care for those patients requiring it.

Supplemental Staffing Contingency Plans. The hospital and emergency department staff should agree in advance on criteria that define when additional patient care providers (both physicians and nurses) need to be called on to reinforce the emergency department staff. In planning staff allocations for the department, appropriate staff need to be added to the inpatient units and ICUs so that they may accommodate admitted emergency department patient boarders before adding staff to the department. It is presumed that it is better for inpatient staff to provide inpatient care in inpatient facil-

ities than to make our best effort to provide inpatient care in the emergency department.

Furthermore, inpatient staffing ratios need to be made flexible at times of overcrowding. Adherence to inpatient staff/patient ratios (e.g., critical care nurse/patient ratios of 1:2) should not interfere with the transfer of department patients to the ICU when additional beds are available, but adequate staff to achieve the usual ratios are not available. This strict adherence to inpatient standards of care cannot be tolerated when the same staff/patient ratios cannot be maintained in the emergency department to care for the same patients.

Inpatient Charts. Complete inpatient charts (binders, order sheets, progress notes, and ancillary reports) must be generated in the emergency department to document inpatient care provided there.

Inpatient Staffing Models. To provide inpatient services in the emergency department, allocated staff should be cross-trained or new staff provided to perform routine morning phlebotomy and ECGs, to support dietary needs, to schedule and arrange complicated procedures (exercise tolerance tests, radionuclide cardiac scans), and to administer medications on a scheduled basis (e.g., intravenous penicillin every 4 hours).

Expand Emergency Department Formulary. Pharmaceuticals not regularly used in the emergency department (chemotherapeutic agents) must be made easily available.

Revised Floor Plans. Nontraditional patient care spaces (e.g., hallway spaces, in front of the view box, next to the linen closet) need to be formally designated so that staff can locate patients quickly; such locations should be chosen carefully to provide maximal access to care while maintaining the potential for privacy when appropriate.

Emergency Department Cost Accounting Systems. To differentiate standard department expenses from those of admitted inpatient boarding in the emergency department, hospital cost allocation for the department needs to be revised so that the medical record number of admitted patients attributes the high cost of inpatient ancillary services and pharmaceuticals to a separate "Emergency department admitted" account or to the patient's inpatient account.

Fast Track. The establishment or expansion of a fast track parallel to the emergency department with appropriate staff and space will allow patients with less urgent problems to be seen more quickly and in a way that does not compete with the department for staff, space, or time. Persistent overcrowding will sometimes cost-justify a fast track patient care area at a lower total emergency department patient volume than would otherwise be the case.

Emergency Medical Services System Changes

Overcrowding will necessitate changes in the EMS System when it occurs regularly in several emergency departments in the same community at the same time. These EMS management systems require substantial interhospital cooperation, well-defined EMS authority, and an integrated system of ambulance dispatch. EMS policies will need to define the following:

- Consistent, agreed on, easily defined and verified criteria for diversion
- Regular communication of EMS diversion status by each hospital to EMS; regular communication from EMS to all ambulances
- Protocol to reevaluate or cancel diversion status when simultaneously requested by several nearby emergency departments
- Criteria to override diversion status (with a safeguard to allow dispute resolution only after patient care in the department is guaranteed)

Federal legislation requires that the circumstances, indications, stability, and interhospital transfer of patient care responsibility be clearly documented. Hospital or EMS systems need to expedite interhospital systems of transfer at times of overcrowding. In shared and mutually produced manuals (or computer databases), each hospital should define its total bed capacity, special bed capacity (e.g., medical-surgical, ICU, ob-gyn, psychiatry, burn), and person or title of individual (with telephone numbers) to contact for administrative and medical approval for transfer (specific, as appropriate for type of bed, time of day, or day of week). Such information will facilitate the interhospital transfer of patients when necessitated by hospital overcrowding or for any other reason.

TOO MANY PATIENTS, NOWHERE ELSE TO GO

Since the end of the 1980s, much attention has been directed at the overcrowding of the classic type (described previously). At the same time, it has become increasingly clear that there is another trend in the use of the nation's emergency departments: overcrowding in the waiting room with too many patients who have nowhere else to go. Total patient volume seen in the emergency department nationwide is rising; the department is a major point of access to healthcare and, for many, the only source available. This "safety net" role for the nation's emergency departments at one time allowed emergency physicians to "travel first class" on the "moral and ethical high road" for many years, but recently it has made the department the target in healthcare policy planning to contain cost and to reduce "inappropriate utilization," a major area of interest of a GAO document, released in 1993.[4] This second form of emergency department overcrowding is less well defined and less well studied, but no less important.

The GAO reports that 86% of the emergency departments studied reported seeing more patients in 1990 than in 1985, with the largest increase seen in rural (27% increase), in small urban hospitals (30% increase), and in small hospitals (30% increase). Between 1985 and 1990, volume rose from about 84 million to 99 million, an 18% increase; at the same time hospital admissions decreased by 7% and visits to physician's offices increased by only 11%. Factors driving up emergency department utilization most often cited in the GAO survey included the number of people without health insurance, a rise in the number of elderly using emergency department services, and an increase in people with more serious illnesses. The GAO reports that of the nearly 100 million emergency department visits in 1990, about 43% were considered nonurgent (a retrospective determination that the discharge diagnosis is not life- or limb-threatening or does not require immediate care). Rural and small hospitals were more likely to report high proportions of nonurgent visits than were

other hospitals. The most frequent reason given for nonurgent use was that the patient did not have a primary care provider. In 1990, of the almost 40 million nonurgent visits, 15 million were made by people who did not have a primary care provider; another 6 million were unable to find their primary care providers. At the same time, 82% of the hospitals reported that sources of primary care were available in their communities. Thirty-six percent of patients with nonurgent conditions in the emergency department sought care there because their primary care provider had closed his or her office or because of "convenience."

Growth in visits to the emergency department was highest in patient populations insured by public programs. From 1985 to 1990, while volume of visits grew nationwide by 19%, Medicaid patient visits increased 34%, Medicare by 29%, and uninsured volume by 15%. In 1990 37% of all Americans were insured by Medicare, Medicaid, or were uninsured (13% of Americans had their healthcare coverage provided by Medicare, 10% through Medicaid, and 14% were uninsured). At the same time, 56% of emergency department care was in these categories (Medicare was 20% of volume; Medicaid was 17% of volume, and the uninsured was 19% of volume).

The emergency department is the only portal of entry into the healthcare system that is mandated by federal legislation (Consolidated Omnibus Budget Reconciliation Act [COBRA] legislation of 1986 and following) to provide care to all who seek it. Furthermore, the emergency department provides all of the convenience features (open 24 hours and on weekends and holidays) no longer available in the primary care system. The increase in patient volume causes problems because it has occurred among a disproportionate number of uninsured and poorly compensated (Medicare and Medicaid) patients. As a result, a concurrent flow of financial resources, allowing expanded staffs and facilities, has not occurred to accommodate patient care needs. Until major changes occur in the way in which emergency care is compensated and healthcare, in general, is reimbursed for those with no insurance and for those with government insurance, it is likely that there will continue to be too many patients with nowhere else (or nowhere better) to go than the emergency department.

With both types of overcrowding occurring concomitantly in many emergency departments throughout the country, it is not surprising that it is becoming increasingly difficult to provide adequate emergency care. Emergency departments will continue to provide a major part of the critically important safety net of our nation's healthcare system. Unfortunately, our current capacity to meet the needs of our patients is being stretched to the limit. Long-term solutions require a substantial reallocation of societal resources. A major overhaul of the way in which emergency and indigent health care is financed, a substantial increase in the number of available well-qualified emergency physicians and nurses, an increase in available primary care providers and an expansion of their times of availability, and nationwide effective programs of injury and disease prevention are needed. Successful resolution of hospital and emergency department overcrowding represents a significant challenge, perhaps the greatest challenge facing our profession today.

REFERENCES

1. Lynn SG, Hockberger RS, Kellermann A et al: *A report from the American College of Emergency Physicians task force on hospital overcrowding and emergency department overload,* Dallas, 1989, ACEP.
2. Lynn SG, Kellermann AL: Critical decision making: Managing the emergency department in an overcrowded hospital, *Ann Emerg Med* 20:287-292, 1991.
3. Andrulis DP, Kellermann A et al: Emergency departments and crowding in United States teaching hospitals, *Ann Emerg Med* 20:980-987, 1991.
4. *Emergency Departments: unevenly affected by growth and change in patient use,* United States General Accounting Office, GAO/HRD-93-4:1-72, 1993.
5. Gallagher JE, Lynn SG: The etiology of medical gridlock: causes of emergency department overcrowding in New York City, *J Emerg Med* 8:785-790, 1990.
6. Kotelchuk R: Down and out in the "new Calcutta": New York City's health care crisis, *Health PAC Bull* 19:4-10, 1989.
7. Storer RH, Hancock WM: *A simulation study of parameters affecting hospital unit occupancy and implication for unit sizing,* Ann Arbor, 1976, University of Michigan Press.

19 Development of the Triage System

Susan W. Somerson and Vincent J. Markovchick

OUTLINE

The concept of triage or sorting was originally developed for mass casualty, disaster, or battlefield situations in which decisions had to be made about the allocation of resources and medical care. This concept has been expanded to urgent care centers and emergency departments in which unscheduled patients arrive by ambulance or other means seeking emergency or urgent care.

In recent decades, fewer primary care providers and limited hours led to limited office availability for nonurgent complaints. Emergency departments, traditionally viewed as the site for care of acute and urgent conditions became identified by the public as accessible sources for care of nonurgent conditions. The net effect for the department was a slow but steady increase in the percentage of patients presenting with nonurgent complaints, with subsequent congestion of the overall department. Other factors contributing to increased patient census are the following:

1. Patients fearful of losing a much needed job who use the emergency department because it is the only source of care available after "normal business hours"
2. Reintegration of chronically mentally ill patients into the community, without systems to support them in a noncloister environment
3. Private physician referral of patients to the hospital with an order for routine radiographs or laboratory workup
4. Uninsured patients who are unable to obtain evaluation in a community-based setting in a timely manner

Emergency department leadership recognized the need for a strategy that could quickly identify and separate emergently ill and injured patients from those with nonurgent or chronic complaints. Application of triage principles was the response. Because it is estimated that currently there are more than 90 million visits annually to emergency departments in the United States, it has become imperative for the emergency department to use a system for rapid identification and sequestering of the acutely ill/injured patient from those with nonurgent conditions.

TRIAGE ENVIRONMENTS

Within the hospital and prehospital settings, four major environments for triage have been identified: disaster triage in the field, disaster triage in the emergency department, field triage through communication with base command, and routine emergency department triage.

The first, disaster triage in the field, is generally a functional responsibility of the Emergency Medical Services (EMS) personnel. Depending on regional practice and the established plan, representatives from local hospitals may be involved in on-site management. Ensuring a smooth transition from field to hospital requires collaborative planning among representatives from medical facilities in the community, EMS, and other municipal services in the development of a community-wide disaster management plan. Medical facilities within the community must ensure active participation by all involved in developing the plan to effect a smooth transition from the field to facility.

On-site triage at a disaster scene is generally performed by the most senior practitioner on site. The role is similar to triage concepts applied on the battlefield—rapid assessment and rank ordering of victims for transport to hospitals for definitive care. On-site interventions are limited to those that can rapidly and effectively reverse death, overall, increasing the likelihood that the greatest number will survive. Some municipalities may incorporate a second level of triage at the disaster site to oversee patient distribution among a number of facilities within the community. The goal of this second level of triage is to match the capabilities of facilities within the community with injuries sustained by victims and to ensure that no emergency department is overwhelmed with casualties.

Operationalization of the second triage environment, disaster triage in the emergency department, varies among facilities, dictated by the respective hospital and departmental

plans. Disaster triage may be supervised by a physician/nurse team, physician, or nurse alone. This individual should be supported by a number of ancillary staff to facilitate victim movement once disposition has been determined. As with field disaster triage, the priority function of the individual performing disaster triage is to evaluate rapidly each arriving victim and assign a priority for care. Some institutional plans also may call on this individual to assign a specific destination for care; in other plans, the assigned priority dictates disposition. The same philosophy with regard to treatment of victims as that seen with on-site disaster triage is applied to ED disaster triage. Interventions are limited to those that are life saving and can quickly reverse an otherwise moribund situation. Triage during a disaster has different goals and processes than routine triage; therefore all staff must be familiar with both processes and knowledgeable with regard to when to use each one.

In the third environment, field triage through communication with base command, decisions relate to whether a patient should be transported to a hospital, the modality of transport (air versus ground, lights and siren), and appropriate hospital destination. When multiple patients are involved, the patients who must receive priority for transport must be identified. Protocols can be developed to cover triage decisions made by prehospital providers, backed up by on-line direct communication with base station personnel.

The final triage environment, routine emergency department triage, is the most frequently used and highly developed of the four environments. It is the topic of the rest of this chapter.

THE TRIAGE PROCESS AND TRIAGE SYSTEMS

Triage is a hierarchic decision making process with regard to the acuity of a given patient relative to overall acuity and activity within the department. The goal of this thought process is to answer the question, "Where does this patient fit at this time into the hierarchy of the department?" Thus the triage process is performed frequently and at times, subliminally by all levels of emergency department practitioners on a daily basis.

A triage system, however, is much more complex and complicated, relying on the support and collaboration of staff in the emergency department, other departments within the hospital, community providers and facilities, and the EMS system to achieve desired effects. Although the triage process is used in a triage system, the intricacies of a true system are much greater.

Generally, there are three classic triage system models, each defined by its characteristics within seven functions/parameters (Table 19-1). Rarely, however, is any one model found in its purist form. More often, there is a hybridization, a blending of different attributes from the three classic models. For example, a given triage system may resemble the spot check model in which a registered nurse (RN) serves as the triage staff, gathering subjective and objective data that are documented in a consistent manner. However, that same emergency department may elect to operate in a manner more consistent with comprehensive triage, using four triage categories and having an operational requirement to discuss cases with a physician before referral to community resources. Similarly, institutional limitations may prohibit the ability to initiate laboratory or radiology studies before evaluation in the treatment area, such as one might find in a comprehensive triage model.

Developing an efficient and effective triage system depends on matching attributes of the different models with the resources of the hospital to produce the highest level triage system possible for the greatest number of hours possible. A smaller emergency department may not have the patient vol-

Table 19-1 Classic Triage Models

Title	Staff	Assessment	Categories	Disposition	Documentation	Reassessment	Diagnostics, treatments initiated
Traffic cop	Nonprofessional; clerk, security	Chief complaint	2—sick/not sick	Waiting room or treatment area	Little or none	None	None
Spot check	Healthcare provider: RN, MD, LPN, paramedic	Chief complaint, subjective and objective data	3—nonurgent, urgent, emergent	Waiting room, treatment room, refer out, or treat and discharge	Done; quality and quantity are inconsistent	None	Simple treatments; e.g., ice to ankle, sling applied
Comprehensive	RN, Nurse practitioner, Physician's assistant, or MD	Chief complaint, subjective and objective findings; limited physical examination	4-5—Life-threatening, urgent, semi-urgent, non-urgent, referral; each category has specific time parameters for reassessment	Waiting room, treatment room, refer out, or treat and discharge	Always present; may include completing designated data fields on each patient to ensure critical aspects evaluated and recorded	Done while awaiting treatment room; as per specified times for assigned category	Simple treatments and diagnostics in triage area, e.g., glucometer, pulse oximetry, may request laboratory or radiology studies

Adapted from Thompson J, Dains J: *Comprehensive triage,* Reston, Va, 1982, Reston Press.

ume to mandate dedicated triage staff on each shift. In such a setting, it may be acceptable to have the charge nurse called to the department entrance to triage patients as they arrive; alternatively, a rotation of staff may be called to triage. Perhaps there may be enough traffic to warrant dedicated triage staff between certain hours only. In busier departments, a dedicated triage staff may be responsible for obtaining subjective and objective patient data while a float ancillary staff is assigned to obtain laboratory workup, vital signs, or requesting/obtaining other diagnostic procedures. In those departments with high volume, a system that requires two professional staff for triage may be required.

As any triage system is designed, certain legal and quality tenants must be upheld and incorporated into final strategies. The Consolidated Omnibus Budget Reconciliation Act of 1985 (COBRA) and the Omnibus Budget Reconciliation Act of 1989 (OBRA) mandate that all patients presenting to an emergency department must have a medical evaluation before inquiry is made about the patient's financial status. Another aspect of the OBRA regulation requires that emergency conditions be stabilized to the highest level achievable by the sending facility. Although this requirement rarely affects the triage staff, a troublesome situation may develop if triage staff are empowered (either formally or informally) to independently determine patient stability and initiate transfer without physician consultation. As protocols and procedures for triage operation are standardized, aspects of this regulation must be clearly addressed and strategies to ensure compliance incorporated.[1]

In addition to federal regulations, state or local regulations may impact triage system design. Physician, nursing, and administrative leadership should investigate these topics and ensure that triage system design incorporates strategies for complying with any relevant state or local regulations.

The second mandate of triage system design should have delivery of quality care as one of the desired outcomes. This facet can be facilitated by development and implementation of collaborative operational agreements among nursing, physician, and hospital administrative leaders. Operations can be formalized by the establishment of care guidelines, prerequisites for triage staff, and patient classification/urgency ratings. Consensus among nursing, physician staff, and hospital administration will foster a united front in terms of performance expectations of physician, nursing, and support departments.

An important aspect of quality care is the patient's satisfaction with the visit. The emergency department is the point of entry for many patients and may represent a patient's only experience with the hospital; thus, a positive impression is most important. Any individual who arrives with a health complaint should be met by a professional who is concerned about the health problem before the patient is screened for financial and insurance information to: identify and rectify life/limb threatening emergencies; foster the impression of patient care as a priority; and to enhance the image of the institution. If patients perceive their healthcare needs are considered first and foremost over the financial well-being of the institution, complaints should be minimized. Once the patient has been deemed stable and in no need of immediate treatment, demographic and financial information can be obtained. Triage staff have the unique opportunity to set the tone for the patient's interpretation of the entire hospital experience.

Finally, the operating triage system must comply with medicolegal mandates. Triage system operations must ensure that triage staff function within their respective scope of practice and that physician staff respond to triage staff requests as required by their scope of practice. Expanded activities, such as the authority to request diagnostic studies from triage or ability to refer to another care provider, should be clearly and specifically delineated, including under what conditions the triage staff may perform these activities and any prerequisites (such as physician consultation or medical screening) that must exist before implementation.

COMPONENTS OF A TRIAGE SYSTEM

When contemplating the initiation or modification of an existing triage system, several pragmatic/structural aspects must be considered:

1. Who will staff the triage area? How many are needed? What is the level of practice? What prerequisite educational programs are required?
2. What space and equipment should be dedicated to triage?
3. What documentation formats should be used?
4. What departments and systems are available in the emergency department, hospital, and community to make the triage system most effective and efficient?
5. What method of communication is available between the triage setting, treatment area, and other areas in the hospital and the community?
6. How will evaluation of treatment protocols and patient classification ratings be achieved?
7. What security issues are important to address?

Personnel

Several desirable attributes should be considered when deciding which category of practitioners should be designated to function as triage staff. Intuitively, it should be assumed that individuals working in this area are clinically knowledgeable, with demonstrated capacity for critical thinking. The ability to rapidly elicit pertinent history and display expertise in physical assessment skills will enhance accuracy of conclusions. Individuals functioning in the triage office must be organized and possess the ability to remain poised under pressure. Triage staff should demonstrate exemplary interpersonal skills. To be most effective in the triage role, staff must be capable of establishing rapport and a trusting relationship within a few minutes of meeting the patient. Doing so increases the likelihood that the patient will be totally truthful in relating the problem. The importance of a caring, concerned attitude cannot be overemphasized. A staff member may be an expert clinician, but the display of nonverbal behaviors suggesting boredom or preoccupation with other concerns will negate the ability of that individual to function effectively in a triage setting. Conversely, a less than expert but caring practitioner may find that a patient volunteers information that would otherwise be withheld; the practitioner thus obtains additional information to more accurately triage the patient.

Except in unusual circumstances or extremely high volume emergency departments, physicians are rarely involved in

triage. However, a physician must be immediately available and accessible to the triage personnel to assist in decision making when questions arise. Most often, the RN is used for triage; some institutions have had success with advanced practice nurses in the form of nurse practitioner or clinical nurse specialist.[2] The number of personnel assigned to triage should reflect department needs. Often, one RN is sufficient; in some institutions, the RN may be assisted by ancillary staff or another RN. Hours of operation will also reflect department demands. There may be a need for a dedicated triage nurse around the clock; or only during specified peak flow hours. Coverage for the triage position may be filled by personnel designated exclusively for that role or may be shared by members of the department on a rotating basis.

Prerequisites in terms of training or experience are set by each institution, again guided by the demands and resources available to each department. Some institutions mandate a minimum amount of experience in the emergency department, either in total or within that department, before assignment in triage. Other departments may require triage staff to maintain nationally recognized credentials such as advanced cardiac life support (ACLS), pediatric advanced life support (PALS), emergency nursing pediatric course (ENPC), or certified emergency nurse (CEN). Existing staff development resources may be available to support the design and offering of specific triage courses or preceptorships that must be completed before functioning independently as triage staff. The exact requirements ultimately determined as prerequisites must be weighed against the attributes and needs of the department.

Because OBRA regulations require that all patients presenting to the emergency department receive a medical screening evaluation, each institution should describe the process by which an individual is credentialed to provide this evaluation and to be revalidated periodically.

Ancillary personnel such as nursing assistants, technicians, EMTs, and paramedics can be invaluable members of the triage team, particularly in high volume departments. These staff can assist in decision making by collecting and reporting data such as vital signs, obtaining and performing spot urine human chorionic gonadotropic (HCG) hormone assays, and blood glucose measurement. Alternatively, they can speed patient care after disposition by facilitating completion of laboratory studies, radiographic examinations, or other diagnostics requested by triage staff. As with so many other facets of a triage system, specific duties will be reflective of institutional needs and abilities. In some emergency departments, ancillary staff may merely transport patients to treatment areas; in others, they may draw blood and send specimens to the laboratory or initiate the process to request radiographs.

In busy institutions or during high volume hours, consideration should be given to having some type of support personnel available to relieve triage staff of nonmedical issues. A receptionist, volunteer, or security staff can provide direction to patient rooms or parking or information about other nonclinical topics. Although triage staff is generally sought out by family and friends of patients as an information source, busier departments may be able to identify a volunteer to function as a liaison between the patient's primary caregivers and family, thus freeing triage staff to concentrate on their triage duties.

Space Requirements

The space available for the triage area will be dictated somewhat by the current configuration of the emergency department. In some instances, minor remodeling in the department can achieve the desired effect. Major remodeling or new department construction plans are ideal opportunities to optimally configure a triage area. The ideal triage area has several characteristics; configuring one area to meet all of them can be challenging.

First, the triage area should be adjacent to the emergency department entrance for patients and positioned to allow triage staff to observe patients as they walk toward and into the department. Departments using a semienclosed office as a triage area may wish to consider a one-way mirror in the office to permit visibility while maintaining the privacy of patients in the triage office. If there are doorways into the triage area, they must be wide enough to accommodate wheelchairs and stretchers. The area should be large enough to hold a sufficient amount of frequently used supplies and equipment and have enough space to permit initial patient resuscitation if needed. To facilitate transfer to definitive treatment if an emergent situation arises, the route from triage to treatment areas should be clear and unobstructed. Finally, there must be a sink within or adjacent to the triage area for compliance with infection control practices.

Institutions with a single entry for ambulatory and ambulance patients must decide whether triage staff will be responsible for evaluation of all patients or only those patients who do not arrive by stretcher. Department flow may be enhanced if patients arriving by ambulance proceed directly to the treatment area where staff perform triage. In some instances, the triage decision may be to send the patient back to the initial triage area. This type of triage system requires constant communication between triage and treatment area personnel.

Institutions with widely separated entrances for ambulatory and ambulance patients may find it necessary for treatment area staff to triage patients arriving by stretcher. If the two separate entrances are physically close and department volume is manageable, triage staff may be able to evaluate both categories of patients. Field evaluation performed by prehospital providers will often speed the decision-making process for triage staff.

Ideally, the physical configuration of the triage area should allow staff to expand or minimize the level of privacy. Privacy encourages patient disclosure and allows for a limited physical examination by triage staff if needed. Triage can be performed in a private nook or office equipped with curtains or doors to enhance privacy as needed; alternatively, some departments may have space for an adjacent examination room that can be used if needed. The need for privacy and the degree attainable are mediated by issues of security, which are discussed later.

Regardless of exactly where triage is performed, there should be sufficient space to accommodate a desk and two chairs. When determining space requirements, the institution's patient population profile should be considered. Departments that care for large numbers of elderly patients re-

quire a larger triage area that can easily accommodate wheelchairs. Similarly, a high volume of pediatric patients will necessitate a table or crib for assessment of infants. An area large enough to accommodate a stretcher is invaluable, should a patient have a syncopal episode.

In addition to spatial requirements for furniture and stretchers, space should be allotted for equipment needed to obtain vital signs and other diagnostic adjuncts in triage. The amount of space required is dictated by the extent of assessment and diagnostic tests performed at triage. At a minimum, space should be allocated for a blood pressure machine and thermometer system. If more sophisticated testing is performed such as obtaining blood glucose, pulse oximetry, or urine HCG measurements, additional space is needed not only to hold the supplies, but also to provide a means for acceptable handling and disposal of blood and body fluids. Busier departments that plan to have ancillary staff gather vital signs or other diagnostic samples may find that a separate space that is adjacent to triage (capable of containing the staff and supplies) will ease congestion within the formal triage area.

In some department systems, a computer terminal and keyboard are essential components in the triage area. Software may act as a decision tree for the staff, a vehicle for documenting triage findings, or communication to treatment area staff. If software is a component of your triage system, additional desk space (and therefore possibly a larger desk) must be dedicated for the terminal and keyboard.

Equipment and Supplies

As with all other aspects of triage system development, the extent of equipment and supplies stored in the triage area will parallel the expectations of triage staff as delineated in the specific department plan. Consideration should be given first to supplies needed to support airway, breathing, and circulation. The exact amount and type of equipment for a given department should be guided by the physical proximity of the treatment or resuscitation areas to the triage area. The closer the proximity of the triage area to the resuscitation area, the less need for resuscitation equipment at triage. A dedicated stretcher should be immediately available for rapid transfer of critically ill or injured patients to the resuscitation area.

Other supplies needed in triage should be tailored specifically to the existing triage and treatment protocols. Suggested items used for patient assessment are listed in Box 19-1. Although the automated blood pressure cuff is a useful tool to obtain pulse and blood pressure reading and increases triage staff's efficiency, staff should not become so dependent on it that they cannot obtain this information "the old fashioned way." Automated devices do not obtain respiratory rates or evaluate the pulse for irregularities, two "basic" assessment data points that may become minimized or lost in the shuffle of automation.

Equipment needed for temporary or ameliorating treatments are considered next. Suggested supplies are listed in Box 19-2. The extent of patient treatments initiated in triage is determined by patient condition, lag time to treatment area, and procedures permitted by departmental protocols. The longer the anticipated delay to definitive treatment, the more need to have and use extensive supplies for first-aid interventions in triage. Other than those instances in which the patient is taken directly to the treatment area, some sort of intervention such as minor hemorrhage control, wound dressings, and ice packs, should be initiated if possible. The patient with an ankle injury will not suffer any long-term poor outcomes if ice application is initially deferred during a 5-minute registration process. However, the institution stands to gain far more, in terms of positive reactions and perceptions generated, when ice is applied immediately.

In some departments, a collection of resource material may be useful in the triage area. Resources include emergency nursing, triage, and drug references. Some departments may have detailed decision trees or treatment protocols available for staff unfamiliar with a given patient presentation. A listing of resources for nonemergency issues and needs such as

BOX 19-1

TRIAGE SUPPLIES/EQUIPMENT FOR ASSESSMENT

Pulse oximeter
Snellen chart
Glucometer
Flashlight
Otoscope
Thermometer
Automatic blood pressure device
Tongue blades
Nonsterile gloves
Spot urine HCG supplies
4×4 gauze
Supplies for occult blood detection
Masks, eye protection
Clean catch urine cups
Cotton-tipped applicators
Sink

BOX 19-2

TRIAGE SUPPLIES/EQUIPMENT FOR TREATMENT

Oxygen administration devices
Suction
Needle disposal unit
Dressings/Kling
Cervical collar
Suture removal kits
Sling
Splinting material
Emesis basin
Saline solution
Betadine solution
Hydrogen peroxide
Tissues
Rigid eye shields
Born on Arrival (BOA) kits
IV and intermittent infusion device start kits
Ice bags/ice chest

social services, support groups, clinics, abusive situations, and shelters can be compiled and categorized. Once identified, such resources within the facility and community will expand the options triage staff can offer patients.

As mentioned earlier, a sufficient number of stretchers and wheelchairs must be available adjacent to both the triage office and the ambulatory entrance to the emergency department. A dedicated stretcher or wheelchair for transport of critically ill patients is essential. Nothing is more disconcerting and tension producing than waiting with the family of a patient having crushing chest pain while someone attempts to find a wheelchair to take them to the treatment area. Similarly, there is an expectation that when a family member is driven to the emergency department with an ankle injury, a wheelchair will be available so that the patient does not have to walk on the injured ankle. The patient and family will form negative impressions of the department if these vehicles are not available.

Finally, each member of the staff should consider how the triage area will function in case there is a need to convert from conventional triage to disaster triage. Plans for this conversion should be clearly outlined in the institution's disaster plan. Details of the structure and function of such an area are beyond the scope of this discussion. The reader is referred to resources discussed in Emergency Department Disaster Management (Chapter 96) when developing this aspect of a triage system.

Documentation Systems

As with every other aspect of triage system development, the documentation system should be guided by the needs and capabilities of the department and institution. The one constant is that the triage process must be permanently documented in some manner; how that end is achieved can be accomplished in a variety of ways.

In some institutions, staff make handwritten notes of their findings. These may be recorded in a designated area on the patient's emergency department record, on a separate triage form, or on a nursing documentation record. Alternatively, triage findings and interventions may be entered into a computer system capable of replicating triage information on the emergency department medical record or nursing record. Regardless of where the information is recorded, several formats can be used. Most triage documentation allows some space for a freehand note related to the patient's presenting complaint. Additional space may be available for triage staff to document essential subjective and objective information based on experience and expertise. Alternatively, some models include detailed checklists for patient systems evaluation. In some documentation systems, all sections must be completed; in others, the triage nurse is free to select and complete applicable sections. Often, the finalized documentation system is a blending of the two, with space for a narrative note, as well as data points that must be evaluated and recorded. Triage specific software is also available and may be useful if the department has a management information system that is compatible with a given program.

Although all triage documentation systems have the option to record a great deal of information, a minimal data set contains four points in the triage note: (1) the patient's presenting complaint, (2) some degree of objective assessment, (3) acuity rating, and (4) disposition. Using this system, a patient in extremis might be described as "patient brought by family who report he's 'sick'; presents pulseless and apneic." Coded notations would also indicate emergent classification with disposition to the Code Room.

The preceding example represents minimal documentation; in less emergent presentations, additional data points should be elicited and recorded. These data points should be consistent with the Uniform Emergency Department Data Set currently being developed through the Center for Disease Control. These points may include a history of the presenting complaint, a focused physical examination, medication history, allergies, and significant medical history. In addition, subsets of the population such as female, pediatric, and trauma patients may have additional data points that should be collected such as weight, menstrual history, and mechanism of injury. Time of initial contact with triage staff should be recorded either automatically or by hand. Many of the data fields that an emergency department determines to be mandatory can be incorporated into a check system within the triage documentation space to enhance completion by staff. Required data fields can be shaded on a handwritten triage document; if a computer model is used, the program can be configured to require completion in designated fields before movement to the next screen can be achieved.

Communication Systems

In most departments, the goals of triage will be best achieved when staff are physically stationed in the triage area during most of their work shift. To best achieve this state, a communication system is needed that allows triage staff to rapidly communicate with a variety of contact points without leaving the triage area. Within the emergency department, staff first need some communication system between the triage and treatment areas. Of particular note is the need for a mechanism to contact the charge nurse and an attending physician. Some departments may have communications systems by computer links or Management Information System (MIS) that enhances communications and requests for services.

To ensure that each patient presenting to the emergency department is triaged to the most appropriate treatment area for his or her respective needs, the triage nurse needs access to services and resources outside the department, but within the institution. Examples include obstetric units, pediatric and adult specialty clinics, admissions office, and paging services. To facilitate contact, there should be at a minimum a posted list of frequently called extensions; more useful is a phone capable of accepting speed dial numbers in the triage office.

Similarly, triage staff may need to access or be available to resources and referrals outside the institution. Again, a list of frequently called numbers or phone equipped with programmed speed dial is invaluable. Establishment of a dedicated phone line for physician offices or managed care providers to use when referring patients for emergency department evaluation will project a "user-friendly" format and facilitate care of those patients. Equipping this line with voice mail or a recorder allows the referring provider to leave vital information and eliminates phone interruptions for triage staff. Some institutions may have designated phone lines for

Table 19-2 Chest Pain Resulting from Trauma

Category	Disposition	Findings
1—Critical	Immediate emergency department treatment area; notify attending physician and charge nurse	Penetrating chest trauma Blunt chest trauma with hypotension Blunt chest trauma with unstable vital signs
2—Serious	Immediate emergency department treatment area; notify charge nurse	History of blunt trauma <24 hours Severe pain Poor general appearance, for example, pale, diaphoretic Hypoxia (O_2 saturation <90%) Unilateral decreased breath sounds
3—Urgent, stable	Registration; for treatment in emergency department	None of the above signs or symptoms are present Vital signs are stable Trauma >24 hours and <1 week
4—Routine	Registration; for treatment in fast track	None of the above signs or symptoms are present Vital signs are stable Minimal pain

field EMS units with incoming ambulance patients that triage staff can monitor or answer.

To enhance communication between patients and triage staff, a system must be developed to ensure that triage staff are aware of new patients in a timely manner. Departments with a high volume and a corresponding wait to see the triage nurse may find it necessary to use a two-tiered system. One triage staff member assumes responsibility for brief contact with all patients entering the department. This staff member essentially performs a primary survey with identification of presenting complaint. Patients determined to be emergent are immediately escorted to treatment areas; others are directed to the secondary triage staff for further evaluation. Even those departments that are not continually subjected to high traffic will often have bursts of activity, where triage staff may be confronted by several patients presenting at once. A number of plans ensure that no one is lost in the shuffle. Some departments have found it useful to have patients record name, presenting complaint, and sign-in time on slips of paper or cards. Once the cards are delivered to triage staff, they can be perused to determine who needs evaluation first. Other departments may use a log book in which patients record name and arrival time; confidentiality issues preclude notations of chief complaint, which is an obvious downfall of such a system. Still other departments have no sign-in system; rather patients ensure they will be seen by taking a number or waiting near the triage area. The latter systems have the greatest potential for disaster, such as the inability to recognize an acutely ill patient who enters into cardiac arrest in the waiting room. This deficiency can be partially overcome if triage staff are observant for some of the subtle physical cues ill patients may display, and if triage staff recognize the need to suspend the triage of one patient to perform a brief inquiry of other patients awaiting evaluation.

PATIENT CLASSIFICATION/URGENCY RATINGS AND TREATMENT GUIDELINES

Within any emergency department, consensual and collaborative development of patient classification systems and guidelines for treatment is critical for successful operation of a triage system.

Patient Classification/Urgency Ratings

Group members charged with development of urgency ratings should first reach consensus on patient classification systems. The true challenge in establishing classification systems is to make it simple, easy to use, and comprehensive.

As described earlier, classification systems may have from two to five categories. Once the group has agreed on the number of categories to be used, discussion should begin about the attributes or patient characteristics that can be found within each category. Characteristics may be based on patient presenting complaint and history, physical findings, vital signs, or a combination of all three. Group members need to try to create operational definitions or philosophies of each classification. Often, examples of presenting situations applicable to each category can help to convey a sense of perspective for each category; however, these examples should not be used blindly. It is advisable to devise protocols that are complaint specific and address acuity levels because patients present in this manner. Departmental need can best be served by first evaluating and categorizing the high-volume or high-risk complaints seen in a particular department. The triage classification/urgency rating assigned will then dictate the patient's disposition from triage. Guidelines for classifications may be formulated in a narrative, outline, or algorithmic format. Tables 19-2 and 19-3 represent classification guidelines for patients presenting with chest pain.

In this system, those patients described as emergent are transferred directly to the treatment area, and the attending physician and charge nurse are notified. A patient classified as urgent would be brought to the treatment area and the charge nurse notified. A patient meeting criteria for the non-urgent classification would be sent to the waiting room or registration area. When formulating guidelines for classification, it is important to make them specific for the personnel and facility in which they will be used. For example, if an emergency department has a fast track area, guidelines should be written that account for this area.

Table 19-3 Chest Pain Resulting from Medical Condition

Category	Disposition	Findings
1—Critical	Immediate ED treatment area; notify attending physician and charge nurse	CPR being performed Patient with chest pain or altered level of consciousness and: • Arrhythmias • Malfunctioning pacemaker • Dyspnea/apnea • Hypotension
2—Serious	Immediate ED treatment area; notify charge nurse	Chest pain with one or more of the following: • History of cardiac problems • Pain with exertion • Severe, crushing pain • Substernal location • Poor general appearance, for example, pale, ashen • Dyspnea • Radiation of pain to arms, jaw • Diaphoresis • Nausea • Hypertensive (SBP >180, DBP >110) • Hypotensive (SBP <90) • Tachycardic (HR >100) • Bradycardic (HR <60) • Hypoxic (O_2 saturation <90%) • Irregular pulse without previous history Unilateral decreased breath sounds
3—Urgent, stable	Registration; for treatment in ED	None of the above signs or symptoms are present Vital signs are stable Presence of fever (T >100.6° F) See appropriate protocols for wheezing, cough, chest trauma, etc
4—Routine	Registration; for treatment in fast track	None of the above signs or symptoms are present Vital signs are stable

ED, Emergency department; *CPR*, cardiopulmonary resuscitation; *SBP*, systolic blood pressure; *DBP*, diastolic blood pressure; *HR*, heart rate; *T*, temperature.

Some institutions using a triage classification/urgency rating of *nonurgent* or *routine* may authorize triage staff to refer these patients to another source of care, either on campus or outside the hospital following a medical screening examination. If staff are permitted to refer, the agreed on guidelines will require an additional step of a medical screening examination by qualified medical personnel before finalizing the referral.

While formulating patient classifications with corresponding disposition options from triage, the work group should also address management of patients who subscribe to an Health Maintenance Organization (HMO) or other managed care provider. Often the provider will not authorize treatment without prior approval, except in the case of an emergency condition. Patients presenting with overt emergency conditions should be treated immediately. Those patients with nonurgent or nonurgent-*appearing* complaints are troublesome to the triage staff and the emergency department. Every patient arriving in the emergency department should have an evaluation by triage staff with registration and triage findings recorded. This evaluation should be made before inquiry about financial capabilities to ensure compliance with OBRA regulations. After initial triage, phone contact with the provider with regard to patient treatment and disposition should be initiated.

The most troublesome question arises when a managed care provider denies the visit and asks that the patient be sent to the primary care provider. The emergency department staff and the hospital need to discuss how these situations will be handled. A medical screening examination must be performed by qualified medical personnel (as defined by the institution's rules and regulations) before referral. Often, an adequate determination cannot be made about the safety and wisdom of allowing the patient to leave for the managed care site *without* performing a physical examination or diagnostic workup in the emergency department. Inviting representation from the managed care providers as the triage disposition protocols are developed may help create a working relationship that will resolve specific cases as they arise. In the final analysis, the prudent emergency department should hold and evaluate those patients where there is a reasonable suspicion that an emergency condition exists, even if the managed care provider has denied the visit.

Treatment Guidelines/Protocols

Once a classification system has been developed, the next task is to define broad actions for patients falling into each classification. This process represents rudimentary steps toward standing orders to begin treatment. Although nursing staff are capable of identifying patient problems and initiating nursing measures toward resolution, they cannot independently assign medical diagnoses or initiate diagnostic tests or treatments. When staff other than physicians function in the triage role, their practice must be limited to the legally

defined scope of care. Through collaborative agreements, triage staff may be authorized in certain situations and under physician-approved standing orders to independently take actions falling outside the strict interpretation of nursing scope of practice. Such actions may include initiating treatment and requesting laboratory or radiology studies. Because under these circumstances, the nurse may initiate such actions *before the patient is seen by a physician,* staff must be extremely vigilant in not overstepping their authority. The key lies in collaboratively identifying the extent of expanded authority that the physician group staffing the department collectively can accept and are willing to grant. Although attending physician and nursing staff are the primary participants in creating these guidelines, there should be representation and support of hospital administration, most notably through risk management participation.

Guidelines may range from simple directions to exhaustive listings of actions to be taken and under what conditions. The written guidelines should be an available reference to the staff in the triage area, either as a manual or by computer access. Optimally, they should not be so cumbersome as to mire triage staff and slow the flow through triage. If physicians are present in the emergency department, broad guidelines may be developed with an admonition to verify questionable situations or troublesome patients with physician consultation. The less on-site medical consultation available, the more specific and detailed the directions.

These collaboratively developed guidelines may include not only authority to initiate diagnostic procedures, but also therapeutic interventions that can be implemented in triage. Often, many of these interventions are simple nursing maneuvers such as application of a splint, dressing, or ice. In some instances, there may be an opportunity to initiate treatments that exceed nursing measures and enter the realm of standing orders. Examples of the latter include the option to administer tetanus immunization at triage or insert an intermittent infusion device for serial glucose measurements while the patient is in the waiting room.

SUPPORT SYSTEMS

Optimal functioning of a triage system depends on the collaboration and buy-in of a number of support systems within the emergency department, the facility, and the community. Some support systems may need to be available 24 hours/ a day, 365 days a year. In other instances, the department may have to limit hours of operation for some support services to best allocate available resources.

One example of a support system within the emergency department is the fast track area. Operation of a designated area within the department allows triage staff to segregate patients with minor, nonurgent complaints from those with more serious or comprehensive problems that require the resources of an emergent care area. Emergency departments accustomed to treating a high volume of patients with nonurgent complaints or with limited access to primary care providers are often forced to relegate these patients to a low treatment priority. Sitting in the waiting room, these patients watch the more acutely ill called for treatment first while they continue to wait. Triage staff often bear the brunt of anger expressed by these patients for the delay, and the staff may expend extensive time and energy trying to provide explanations and diffuse anger. Furthermore, patrons who frequent the emergency department quickly learn what constellation of symptoms will guarantee a quick trip to the acute area. Thus emergency departments that have a high volume of nonurgent patients may wish to consider operating a fast track area, at least on a limited basis. This area can result in more effective patient care and efficient department operations and can enhance public relations.

Another source for divergence of triage staff attention is the need to respond to a variety of requests not related to patient evaluation. Such requests include parking facilities or directions to an inpatient room, hospital cafeteria, or another department within the institution. Some of these requests may be decreased by ensuring that the emergency entrance is used exclusively for patients, family, and staff in the emergency department; however, family and discharged emergency department patients may need answers to some of these questions. Family and friends of patients often approach the triage nurse for follow-up information or a status report on a specific patient. Although part of the role of triage staff is to act as a resource, such activities can draw staff away from the more critical role of evaluating new arrivals. It may be useful to have clerical or volunteer staff assist families in securing this information. For critically ill patients, it is more appropriate for a professional to speak with and be the information source to the family; this duty may fall, at least initially, to the triage nurse. More often, however, a family member's simple request, such as an opportunity to visit with the patient, can be managed by a volunteer acting as a liaison with the patient's primary nurse. Sources for volunteers may be the traditional hospital volunteer corps; alternatively, students in any of the healthcare disciplines may be willing to act as ombudsman.

Each institution needs to identify support systems within the hospital that can be useful to the emergency department in assisting to ensure that patients are cared for in an area that matches need and acuity. Often, another department within the hospital can deliver care in a more cost-effective and expert manner than the emergency department and its staff. Examples of such entities include outpatient registration areas to initiate laboratory or radiology requests of private physicians, pastoral counseling, and social service offices. Patient care areas more appropriate for a given presentation may exist; examples include the labor and delivery unit for women beyond a given gestation or clinics or private physician offices that are agreeable to seeing specific categories of patients such as pediatric, psychiatric, dermatologic, and dental. Referral to such specialty areas should be included in triage classification/urgency ratings. In most instances, triage staff should make every effort to contact staff in the specialty site and discuss the patient with them before referral.

Triage staff also should have available to them a listing of support agencies in the community to whom individuals can be referred. In some instances, referral alone may be all that is required; in other cases, referrals can supplement care delivered in the emergency department. Examples of such agencies include a listings of clinics or other public health resource for routine and on-going care, support groups for specific concerns such as human immunodeficiency virus (HIV) and sudden infant death syndrome (SIDS), or groups

addressing abusive situations. Some requests of triage staff may be directed at meeting social rather than physical needs. A listing of agencies in the community available to meet needs such as free meals, housing, transportation, or indigent medical care will greatly increase the triage staff's effectiveness and efficiency.

SECURITY ISSUES

The incidence of violence directed against emergency department staff and patients warrants incorporation of security personnel and protocols in the emergency department team. Triage staff are particularly vulnerable to the threat of violence for two reasons. First, by virtue of its function of evaluation of incoming patients, the triage area is located near the entrance. Second, the triage process is generally the individual's first contact with staff. Triage staff often have no advance notice about emotionally labile, angry, or potentially violent patients and therefore may quickly and unexpectedly find themselves in a violently escalating situation. Several physical, operational, and interpersonal strategies can be incorporated into a triage system to minimize and deal with the issue of violence.

The first strategy is to ensure the presence of security personnel. Hospital entrances that are open 24 hours a day should be monitored by hospital security. The entrance is of course one of these accesses, and, more so than routine employee entrances, needs to have the *presence* of security staff at all times. Patients and families arriving in a fearful, anxious, or intoxicated state may react in an unconventional manner, and trained security officers are invaluable in deescalating such situations. The immediate availability of security personnel is required to ensure the safety of all patients, visitors, and staff. Personal safety demands that staff should not proceed outside to retrieve patients unless escorted, preferably by a member of the security staff. Public relations perceptions will be diminished as emergency staff and family members wait for a member of security staff to respond so that staff can go outside to bring in a patient from the family's car. It is far more practical, both from a public relations perspective and a staff safety perspective, to have security personnel immediately available 24 hours a day in the emergency department.

In institutions with a high emergency department volume, consideration should be given to creating a satellite security station near the department. This satellite could be the command post for a given cadre of security staff assigned within the hospital. A similar strategy could prove useful in smaller institutions that cannot justify assigning a security staff member to the emergency department. Creation of a satellite unit permits the addition of other tasks (such as watching television monitors), therein making the position more efficient. In addition, several systems of "panic buttons" can be installed in the triage office or worn by the triage nurse.

Placing security staff or a security satellite in overt view near the emergency department notifies patients and visitors that security staff are immediately available. This subtle show of force may be sufficient to dissuade potential disrupters. Patients or staff may be unable to control threatening or violent behavior. A quick response by a force of security may terminate such behaviors.

Other strategies to ensure safety of triage staff affect the physical design and furnishing of the triage area. Configuration of the desk and chairs can act as a barrier to a patient or family who demonstrates unexpected violent behavior. Most people will accept two chairs separated by a desk as a normal configuration for interaction between strangers. Those institutions that have a separate room for triage will need to incorporate an escape mechanism for triage staff. Optimally, an unlocked and outward opening door should be installed in the wall opposite the door used by the patient to enter the triage office. A belligerent patient would need to overcome the barrier of the desk; such a barrier would allow triage staff time to exit through the escape door.

Finally, didactic and practical instruction in identifying and managing situations with a potential for violence is becoming increasingly available. Interventions include verbal and nonverbal messages to deescalate events, as well as physical approaches to limit injury to patients or staff. Exposure to this sort of instruction can be invaluable to triage and all emergency department staff.

IMPLEMENTING OR MODIFYING AN EMERGENCY DEPARTMENT TRIAGE SYSTEM

Preliminary planning for initiation or modification of a triage system should be undertaken by a task force of emergency department staff. Planning steps will include identification of desired goals, as well as an analysis of departmental demands and resources available to achieve the desired goals. Membership on this task force should include not only leadership representation from nursing, medicine, and administrative branches in the emergency department, but from clinicians practicing on a daily basis who can provide insight into "front line" operational issues.

The group should first identify needs or problems that may be resolved through initiation or modification of a triage system. In some instances, needs may have already been identified and quantified through ongoing data collection and analysis. For example, quality monitoring studies such as patient satisfaction surveys, emergency department length of stay studies, or an analysis of discharge diagnoses to elicit the percentage of the population having a nonurgent problem have the potential to highlight problems. In other instances, needs and problems are initially perceived by staff members. Box 19-3 lists some commonly identified needs that can be mitigated in part by triage system development. The listings in this box are not comprehensive; rather, they provide a basis to promote discussion within individual departments. When faced with global complaints, such as "the wait is too long," the group will need to examine this issue to identify all the reasons for these waits. This step is critical to the process. If a problem cannot be stated specifically, it will be impossible to solve it.

Quantification of a staff-perceived problem through data collection and analysis will provide objective evidence to confirm or deny the existence of problems. Such data may already reside in performance improvement (P&I) studies, or a study can be created to capture the data. Regardless of how they are gathered, these data will not only reveal the magnitude of the problem, but also will provide a baseline measurement for evaluation of the effectiveness of any interven-

BOX 19-3

RATIONALE TO INITIATE OR MODIFY A TRIAGE SYSTEM

Speed patient through the system

Enable early request and processing of laboratory, radiology so results available when patient seen by physician
Identify nonurgent patient and direct to fast track area
Refer patient to area where services needed can be provided at less cost and by staff more skilled in that aspect of care; for example outpatient lab, labor and delivery, social service, community resources

Make patient visit more cost effective

Refer patient to provider where needs can be managed at a lower cost; for example labor and delivery, HMO, public health facility/clinic
Verify managed care agreements before initiation of in-depth evaluation/treatment

Identify patient with actual/potential emergent conditions

Identify overtly emergent; for example gun shot wound
Identify subtle presentations with potential for serious outcome; suicidal, myocardial infarction presenting as jaw pain
Desire to match triage acuity with patient's urgency as per diagnosis at disposition from emergency department

Initiate infection control procedures

Identify and isolate suspected active tuberculosis, childhood diseases at triage

Enhance communications between triage area/receiving area and treatment area

Contact point for physicians outside hospital to refer in patients

Enhance public relations, perception of emergency department

Initial contact to be a healthcare provider
Healthcare worker initiates treatment to make patient/family feel better, less anxious
Healthcare worker is a contact person for family/friend to obtain ongoing information about patient status
Healthcare worker is able to give immediate feedback to anxious patient at triage; for example "no fever", "this is not the pain pattern typically seen with heart attacks", etc

Comply with federal/local regulations

COBRA/OBRA; initial evaluation by qualified personnel before questions regarding financial status

Cost effective operation of the hospital

Match patient needs with low overhead departments, or departments skilled in care of particular problem; clinics, outpatient laboratory, employee health

tions initiated. For example, the staff of an emergency department without any triage system may have intuitive feelings that sick patients have an unacceptably long wait before being placed in a treatment room. Data could be collected with regard to the time from arrival to the emergency department to the treatment room of those patients sick enough to ultimately be admitted as inpatients. Findings can be benchmarked with national or regional norms to determine whether a problem exists. It may be helpful to identify two acceptable timeframes: one for patients admitted to critical care units and another for patients admitted to routine beds. Once a functioning triage system has been established or modified, repeating the original time study will provide objective evidence about the effectiveness of the triage system.

After defining discrete goals and obtaining baseline data, the task force can begin to identify strategies to address needs and evaluate the feasibility of the proposed remedies. Task force representatives should contact emergency departments with similar attributes in terms of patient volume and acuity to learn what strategies other hospitals have found helpful. These strategies can be adopted or modified to meet the requirements of the emergency department. Other members of the task force can be assigned to perform a literature review. Some emergency-oriented journals offer monthly columns that describe how different departments have remodeled their facility or set up triage systems. In short, group members should be encouraged to explore available resources to find out what other institutions are doing.

Analysis of your own departmental demands and resources before the development of the triage system increases the viability of proposals. Box 19-4 offers some variables that will impose limitations on department operations; such variables need to be addressed in proposed strategies. As an example, consider the variable of literacy level within the population of a given emergency department. A department that serves a population that can read and write might use a scheme of asking patients to write name, time of arrival, and nature of complaint on index cards. Triage staff then have the capability to establish priorities for individual patient evaluation. This scheme would be ineffective in an emergency department that serves a population with poor literacy skills, and an alternative strategy for patient "sign-in" would need to be developed.

Once a given strategy for change has been proposed, the task force will next need to evaluate the degree of cooperation required from other departments and services. Logically, proposals that primarily affect aspects directly under emergency department administrative control of the department are more likely to succeed than plans that cross department boundaries. Thus a proposal that expands ancillary staff duties to include obtaining vital signs at triage is more likely to succeed than a proposal to initiate radiography requests at

BOX 19-4

ASSESSING DEPARTMENTAL NEEDS, RESOURCES, AND DEMANDS

Staff	How many staff are available? On each shift? What is the breakdown of professional/technical/ancillary staff?
	What is their level of training?
	What is the current expertise specific to the triage process and triage system operation?
	How many staff hold national credentials such as certified emergency nurse? Other credentials?
	What other responsibilities might triage staff have?
	What other tasks could be assigned to a permanent triage staff?
	What are the staffing levels of support departments (e.g., radiology, laboratory) on each shift?
	How many physicians are available on each shift?
	Residents versus attending? What is the level of training?
Patients	How many patients are seen in a day? A week?
	What are the distribution patterns within the day or the week?
	What is the predominant nature of presenting complaints? (urgent? nonurgent?)
	What primary care providers are available to patients, and what are their hours of operation?
	What is the predominant language within the patient population? What are alternative languages? What is the literacy level?
	What is the predominant profile of patients within the department? Elderly? Pediatric? Walk-in? Referrals from smaller institutions? Referrals from other institutions such as nursing homes?
	Are there specialty physicians on staff at the hospital who regularly refer patients to the emergency department for evaluation? (e.g., oncologists, HIV care providers, sickle cell patient providers)
	What is the usual mode of patient arrival?
Institution/ facility	What departments are capable and willing to assist the emergency department, for example, Security, labor and delivery, Outpatient laboratory, Radiology, Clinic system?

triage. To achieve the most effective triage system, interdepartmental collaboration will be required as the system evolves; however, interdepartmental proposals can be deferred until the system is well established.

The proposed strategies should be analyzed with regard to potential impact on the emergency department, identification of colleague and system supports, and documentation avenues that will need to be developed or modified. Examples of colleague support includes consensus on policies defining triage classifications, guidelines for referring patients to other departments, and creation of curriculum for a triage workshop. Another example of an impact on an existing department is the identified need for physical renovation to create a triage area or make an existing area safer or more efficient.

SUPPORTIVE FORCES

When campaigning for the creation or modification of a triage system, key personnel will find a greater likelihood of success if forces that obstruct or support the planned change are identified early.

Supportive forces for development of a triage system can be summarized into five major areas:

1. Identification of emergently ill and injured patients
2. Compliance with federal and local regulatory agencies
3. Enhanced flow through the department
4. Financial incentives for the department and facility
5. Enhanced public relations and patient satisfaction

Rapid Identification of Acutely Ill or Injured Patients

The rapid identification of patients needing immediate treatment is a commonly identified rationale for implementation of a triage system. This need will likely be the driving force for acceptance by the emergency department staff. Although even a lay person can recognize a gunshot wound or crushing chest pain as an emergent situation, educated triage staff should be able to identify and act on patients who present with subtle manifestations that underlie life-threatening conditions.

Triage decision making is an organized process based on essential data obtained from the history and physical assessment of the patient. If this decision-making process occurs in an organized manner, with appropriate guidelines that stress in the differential diagnosis the most serious condition possible given the presenting complaint, vital signs, and assessment data, the vast majority of unstable or potentially unstable patients should be identified within minutes of arrival to the emergency department.

Federal and Local Regulatory Agencies

Perhaps the most obvious and compelling rationale for initiation or modification of a triage system relates to federal and local regulatory agencies. OBRA regulations clearly mandate patient evaluation before inquiry about financial status. The same regulation imposes significant fines and possible loss of Medicare reimbursements to institutions that fail to comply with this order. Thus the most simplistic of triage systems, one where the patient is first evaluated by a healthcare provider, has essentially been mandated by federal law. The Joint Commission on the Accreditation of Healthcare Organizations (JCAHO) is another regulatory agency that imposes a clear mandate for patient evaluation by qualified personnel at triage.[3]

Enhanced Flow Through the Department

Use of a comprehensive triage system will enhance patient flow through the department in several ways. First, patients

can be referred to another resource, effectively reducing the number of patients a department will need to manage. Within larger departments or those with specialty subareas, patients can be triaged to the area most closely matched to their needs. Thus, nonurgent patients can be funneled to a fast track area; patients with complaints of a surgical, medical, gynecologic, or psychiatric nature can be referred to these specialty subareas within the emergency department. Comprehensive triage permits staff to request certain studies from the triage area. Rather than send a patient with an injured wrist to the waiting room, the patient is sent to radiology for films. In this scheme, radiographs are completed and ready for review at the time the patient is first seen by a physician, resulting in a shorter stay in the emergency department and fostering patient satisfaction.

Financial Incentive for the Department and Hospital

Use of a triage system can facilitate assurances of reimbursements for patients covered by managed care organizations. In those instances where the managed care provider refuses authorization, the patient is identified as at risk for nonpayment before extensive hospital resources are utilized, including admission. Facilities offering inhouse specialty departments (such as labor and delivery [L&D], outpatient laboratory and radiology) can be assured that triage staff will match patients to services needed by directing patients to the most cost-effective department in the hospital capable of caring for their specific problem. Examples of this are the triage of third trimester pregnant women to L&D where the staff with expertise and equipment necessary to evaluate them is available. Female patients with minor gynecologic complaints could be referred to a female health center or gynecologic clinic where the staff may have more expertise and experience in meeting some of the educational needs.

As noted previously, when triage staff are authorized to initiate diagnostic studies at triage, the emergency department length of stay for a given patient can often be significantly shorter. Shorter length of stay allows a greater number of patient evaluations within a given time frame and ultimately more cost-effective use of personnel and resources.

Patient Satisfaction and Public Relations

An often overlooked benefit of a triage system is the enhanced public relations and corresponding patient satisfaction. To capitalize on this aspect, criteria applied in selection of triage staff should demand excellent interpersonal skills as well as clinical expertise. As the point of initial contact between patient and the institution, triage staff will set the tone for the patient/family perception of the visit. If the initial impression is poor, the ensuing staff and events will likely also be viewed as poor. Admittedly, initially negative perceptions developed at triage can be modified by subsequent staff behaviors throughout the rest of the visit. However, to effect this change, staff will need to exert a great deal of energy to overcome initial perceptions. It is far more efficient to create a positive initial impression than work to overcome a poor initial impression.

Another aspect of triage that enhances patient perception is the fact that the initial contact in the emergency department is with a healthcare provider. Simple treatments such as application of a dressing or ice will facilitate patient comfort and foster a sense of concern for the patient. In those instances where the presenting complaint is not amenable to a bandage or splint, triage staff can offer a psychologic bandage such as commentary on a good blood pressure or lack of a fever. Patients may still be sent to the waiting area, but they take with them a positive thought to hold during the wait—either the ankle feels better because of the ice, or although they do not know what is wrong with them, their blood pressure is good. Overall the patient feels less anxious from the triage contact and somewhat more positive about the wait for treatment. Finally, when the initial contact in the emergency department is with a healthcare provider concerned about the patient's problem rather than the registration clerk asking about insurance and financial concerns, it sends a strong message to the patient about the priorities of the emergency department and the institution.

FORCES THAT OBSTRUCT TRIAGE SYSTEM DEVELOPMENT

Early identification of forces that will obstruct development of a successful triage system permits the creation of strategies to deal with these forces before implementation.

When attempting to initiate the most basic triage system, the first resistance felt is likely to originate in the emergency department staff. Physician, nursing, and clerical staff may not believe there is a problem with the present system. Strategies should focus on uncovering objective data that reflect the rationale for implementation of a triage system or modification in the current triage system.

Review of incidents within the department in which there was a bad patient outcome may be useful, particularly if it can be shown that early evaluation by triage staff could have changed the outcome. Similarly, time studies of a patient visit may provide objective data to heighten staff awareness about the length of time required for a patient to move through the department. Staff can then begin to initiate strategies that might decrease overall length of stay through the development of a triage system.

Surveys can be designed to focus on those particular points regarding patient satisfaction and public relations that implementation of a triage system could remedy. Questions should specifically focus on initial contact with hospital personnel, patient's belief about staff competency, perceived caring and concern about the patient, and satisfaction with the speed of service.

An argument against implementation of a triage system could be the need for additional personnel to staff the area. The position of triage staff might be viewed as an "easy" assignment, requiring limited physical exertion. Depending on patient flow for a given shift, the nurse may be perceived to have "down" time. Creativity can overcome some of these charges. Triage staff can be expected to occupy "down" time with activities to support the department. Examples of such activities include reviewing records from the prior day for performance improvement activities, being responsible for patient follow-up and call backs, or drafting the next nursing staff schedule. Department management should identify a list of tasks that can be performed by triage staff to mitigate this argument.

The most basic triage system will require services from departments outside the emergency department, such as security, for effective and safe operations. As a given triage system increases in sophistication, the support of other departments such as radiology, laboratory, and specialized care settings becomes imperative. Convincing these departments of the merit of a triage system may require buy-in from hospital administration through clear savings in terms of dollars, decrease in poor patient outcomes, or improved patient satisfaction data.

EVALUATION OF EFFECTIVENESS

Perhaps the most frequently used studies to evaluate triage system effectiveness are time studies. Specific parameters to be measured include arrival time to treatment area time, time from arrival in the treatment area to physician evaluation, overall emergency department length of stay, and wait time for diagnostic study results.

Another frequently used study evaluates patient satisfaction. Honest responses are more likely if patients have the opportunity to complete the survey after discharge, but within a few days of the emergency department visit. To ensure collection of a representative sample, the survey tool should be mailed to a random sample of visits, perhaps every tenth patient registered. Use of such an instrument permits the collection of other data related to the visit and patient perceptions in addition to those of the triage experience. Staff responsible for designing the survey should ensure that two to three questions specifically address aspects related to triage (e.g., length of time to being seen by triage staff, behavior of triage staff, importance of first being seen by a nurse).

Once a triage system has been developed, a variety of studies can be performed to evaluate the functioning of the triage system and personnel. One example is a random sampling of emergency department records to compare the triage impression and disposition with the final diagnosis and management. Specifically, there is a search for the degree of undertriage and overtriage performed retrospectively. Undertriage (that is, failing to recognize and respond to a patient who is subsequently found to be critically ill/injured) should be minimal, with each case reviewed with the respective staff. Overtriage (that is, assigning a falsely high priority to a patient) is the more desirable end of the spectrum, creating a "safety net" for patients. However, excessive overtriage can be problematic because it negates two goals of triage: identification of emergently ill/injured and minimizing congestion within the department.

Individual triage staff can benefit immensely by reviewing the records of patients they triaged the previous day. Contrasting triage impressions against the final diagnosis and disposition allows each staff member to gain a sense of respective "batting average." Feedback is quick and private and permits staff to learn from their experiences in a private manner. Designating 15 to 20 minutes each day for triage staff from the prior day to complete this activity will enhance compliance.

SUMMARY

Triage is a team effort. It begins in the prehospital arena and continues on arrival in the emergency department and beyond, with the reassessment and reevaluation of patients while they await treatment. Development of triage guidelines also is a team effort. Guidelines should be flexible and amenable to timely revision based on continuous quality improvement evaluation. Triage personnel must be properly trained in use of the triage guidelines and in public relations. Emergency physicians must be immediately available to support triage personnel. If the triage system is successful, there will be an overall improvement in emergency department patient care and public relations for the entire institution.

REFERENCES

1. COBRA/OBRA, 42 United States Code Sec. 1395dd.
2. Burgess K: A dynamic role that improves the service: combining triage and nurse practitioner roles in A&E, *Prof Nurse* 7:301-303, 1992.
3. Joint Commission for Accreditation of Healthcare Organizations: *1994 accreditation manual,* Emergency Services 2.2.4, Oak Terrace, Ill.

SUGGESTED READINGS

Lyle N, Abel C, Faircloth K et al: *Triage: meeting the challenge,* Chicago, 1992, ENA.

Pardee D: Decreasing the wait for emergency department patients: an expanded triage nurse role, *J Emerg Nurs* 18:311-315, 1992.

Purnell LD: A survey of emergency department triage in 185 hospitals: physical facilities, fast-track systems, patient-classification systems, waiting times, and qualifications, training and skills of triage personnel, *J Emerg Nurs* 17:402-407, 1991.

20 Patient Classification Systems

Paula Tanabe

OUTLINE

Rationale for developing a patient classification system
Factors to consider when developing a patient classification system
- Blend of nursing services
- Skill performance of RN and Non-RN staff
- Performance of outpatient procedures
- Indirect nursing care
- Nonproductive and unavailable time
- Emergency department patient population characteristics (patient care mix)

Types of patient classification systems
- Prototype system
- Medical- and nursing-diagnosis–based systems
- Factor analysis

Planning phase
- Soliciting support
- Resources
- Patient log analysis
- Determination of nursing care time
- Determining categories
- Validity
- Time-in-motion studies

Implementation of the system
- Pilot study
- Classification of the patient
- Data entry systems

Patient acuity and nursing resources
Revenue-generating capability
Currently available systems
Summary
Glossary of terms

A patient classification system (PCS) can be an invaluable tool for the nurse manager. It allows the manager to quantify nursing care and help predict staffing needs, and it provides nursing with a mechanism to charge for their services.

A PCS also provides valuable information for the emergency department physician and administrator. Many mission statements for emergency departments contain the goal of delivering high-quality care in a timely manner. A PCS can provide documentation of acuity of care, which can lead to evidence for the need for increasing nursing care hours to deliver care in the desired high-quality, timely manner.

A PCS "groups patients according to some observable quality or characteristic that enables users to estimate the amount of nursing time that the groups of patients require".[1] The decision to implement a PCS requires extensive planning and information and a commitment to the project. A major factor to consider is whether to develop your own system or purchase a commercially developed system already in existence. Regardless of the choice, the planning and implementation phases require the involvement of many departments and personnel. These areas will be discussed throughout the chapter.

RATIONALE FOR DEVELOPING A PATIENT CLASSIFICATION SYSTEM

Before PCSs, staffing patterns in the emergency department were based on the department's census. As patient acuity increased over the years, census-based staffing was inadequate for nursing care delivery because it did not reflect the complexity of patients' needs. An alternative staffing method was needed that considered both acuity and volume. Patient classification systems were developed to solve this problem. Nursing care hours per day can be calculated retrospectively.[2]

Patient classification systems provide the nurse manager with a wealth of information in the following areas, which will be discussed in greater detail in this chapter[1]:
- Emergency department patient population characteristics
- Blend of nursing services required
- Calculation of revenue generated by nursing

FACTORS TO CONSIDER WHEN DEVELOPING A PATIENT CLASSIFICATION SYSTEM

The decision to implement a PCS represents a significant challenge to the emergency department nurse manager. Many factors must be considered before examining available systems or collecting preliminary data. The following factors should be considered:
- Blend of nursing services provided (mix of Registered Nurse [RN] and non-RN services)
- Skill performance of RN/non-RN staff
- Performance of outpatient procedures
- Indirect nursing care
- Emergency department patient population characteristics (patient care mix)

Blend of Nursing Services

One of the most important factors to analyze is the RN/non-RN ratio of patient care providers. Does the emergency department utilize non-RN patient care providers that are a part of the nursing budget? This will eventually become important when determining staffing needs. It is also important to determine the times when an RN and non-RN staff perform the same skill. Do RNs always delegate venipuncture to a technician, or only when one is available? This will need to be closely examined during the time-in-motion studies.

Skill Performance of RN and Non-RN Staff

The roles of the following patient care providers who are not part of the nursing budget must also be analyzed, as well as the frequency in which they provide the activity (always, usually, or occasionally): electrocardiography, respiratory, and laboratory technicians. When these technicians are unable to perform the skill, do RNs complete the function? If they do, these skills must be evaluated via a time-in-motion study and included as a part of direct nursing care. All direct patient care activities (hands-on care), including initial and continued patient assessments provided by the RN and RN assistive worker, must be considered and included in the time study.

The role of the medical staff should also be considered. Is the emergency department in a small community hospital where the RNs may provide more technical skills, or is the department in a large teaching hospital where residents assist more with technical skills? Greater complexity of skill performance may require greater nursing resources.

Performance of Outpatient Procedures

Many emergency departments provide outpatient procedures. If RNs participate in any of these procedures, time-in-motion studies should be performed for these procedures, since these activities will affect nursing resources that are necessary for these procedures. For example, the emergency RN may assist with the following procedures:

Endoscopy
Bronchoscopy
Employee health needs (e.g. administering vaccines)
Dialysis
Outpatient blood administration

Indirect Nursing Care

All indirect patient care (non–hands-on care) activities in which the RN engages must also be evaluated, and time studies must be performed. The following is an incomplete list of indirect nursing care activities to consider[3]:

Answering the telemetry radio
Stocking
Response to in-house cardiac arrests
Narcotics count
Calling the laboratory and radiology department for test results
Calling reports to the units
Preparing laboratory slips
Patient teaching
Transporting patients
Equipment checks
Triage nursing
Continuing and mandatory education

A list developed by Buschiazzo[3] provides examples of direct and indirect nursing care activities (Box 20-1). Triage has been traditionally included as part of indirect nursing care. Regardless of patient acuity, a triage nurse must be present. This time should be calculated as part of the fixed, indirect patient care activities, which will be discussed later.

The time it takes to complete indirect care must be closely studied, and an average time calculated. This time will eventually be added into the 24-hour total of nursing care hours needed to provided adequate staffing.

BOX 20-1

PATIENT CLASSIFICATION

Direct nursing care time

1. Assessment
2. Physical care
3. Planning care with physician
4. Time spent on obtaining laboratory results
5. Documentation on patient's record
6. Teaching of patient or significant other
7. Psychologic support of patient or significant other
8. Social support of patient or significant other
9. Time spent on transfer to receiving area
10. Giving report to receiving nurse
11. Discharge planning

Indirect care or responsibilities

1. Charge nurse: administrative responsibilities
2. Counting narcotics
3. Taking or giving report at change of shift, between breaks
4. Checking equipment
5. Stocking of supplies
6. Return from transfers
7. Transfers to and from another facility
8. Code response outside of the emergency department
9. Nursing time spent on errands to laboratories, central supply, etc.
10. Calling to determine if a bed is ready for transfer
11. Repeat calls for test results
12. Triage

From Buschiazzo L: Adapting PCS to emergency services, *Nurs Manag* 16(5):34 B, 34 D-E, 34 H, 1985

Nonproductive and Unavailable Time

In addition to direct and indirect patient care activities, nonproductive RN time must also be evaluated. Nonproductive time includes break and meal times. An average amount of nonproductive time is determined and eventually subtracted from the total hours worked in a shift. For example, a nurse working 8 hours may actually be available for only 7.25 hours, and this amount of time, not 8 hours, would be used in eventually determining how many nurses are needed in a 24-hour period. Unavailable time consists of sick and vacation days. This amount of time is also used later in determining staffing needs. Figure 20-1 illustrates the differences between nonproductive, direct, indirect, and unavailable time.

The role of all advanced practice nurses in the emergency department must be evaluated. Do these nurses provide direct patient care? If they do, the decision must be made to either include or exclude their time providing patient care as part of the PCS. Their salaries are usually not built into the PCS but are figured into a department budget.

Emergency Department Patient Population Characteristics (Patient Care Mix)

The emergency department's patient care mix must be closely examined. What are the characteristics of the population that your department serves on a daily basis? Does your depart-

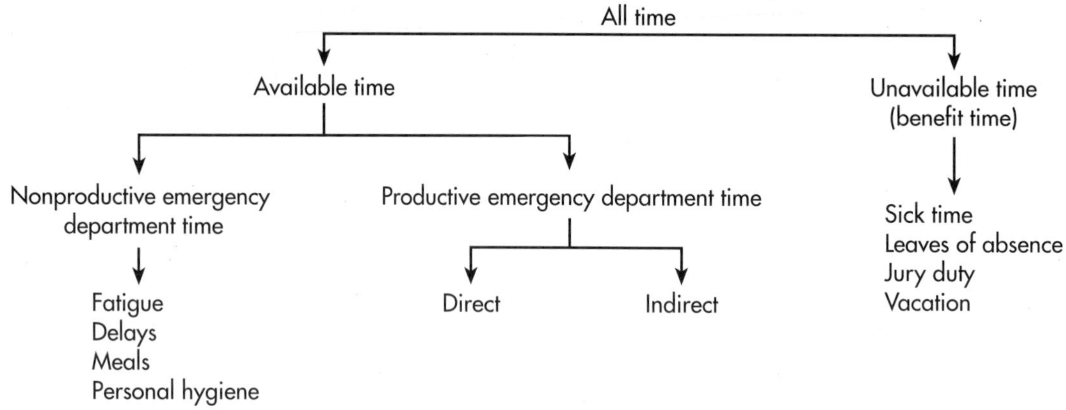

FIGURE 20-1 Nonproductive, direct, indirect, and unavailable time.
(From Emergency Nurses Association: *Emergency department patient classification systems,* 2 ed, Chicago, 1995, The Association.)

ment see a large percentage of patients who are acutely ill, or is your department used by the majority of patients for primary healthcare? A greater number of acutely ill patients increases the acuity of the population, whereas a greater volume of non–acutely ill patients will be reflected in a greater census. Both acuity and volume are important factors that influence nursing resources. The census should be evaluated for past and current trends. Admission rates must be evaluated. An increase in admission rate will probably have a greater effect on patient acuity and nursing care time delivered than will an increase in census. A nurse spends more time providing care to one patient being admitted with a small-bowel obstruction than to 10 patients with flulike symptoms.

Admissions should be further analyzed for type of admission. Critical care admissions will greatly increase nursing care needed. The availability of critical care and general inhouse beds is another factor to consider. Are emergency department patients being held in the department for hours after beds are requested because open patient beds are unavailable? Does the emergency department have a holding area for these patients, and does the department staff the area? If emergency RNs are monitoring these patients, perhaps an observation charge should be built into the PCS. Time studies could estimate the average time spent monitoring these patients, and this time could be built into the PCS as an indicator in the factor analysis system or placed as a criterion under the prototype system. Both systems will be discussed in detail in the next section of this chapter.

TYPES OF PATIENT CLASSIFICATION SYSTEMS

Two main categories of PCSs exist: a prototype or factor analysis system. An inherent weakness of all systems is the provision of retrospective data. Inpatient classification systems provide the user with current nursing needs of the unit. Only retrospective data are provided by emergency department PCSs because of the short length of stay of the patient population. However, these data can be analyzed in time segments (e.g., 1-hour time blocks) to help determine the usefulness of variable staffing throughout a 24-hour period. It is the task of the nurse manager to analyze the data and identify trends over time that can be accurately interpreted to predict future nursing staff needs.

Prototype System

The prototype PCS places the patient in a specified broad category that describes his or her nursing care needs. Categories are developed according to selected criteria.[4] Criteria should be based on the nursing process (Table 20-1). For each category an average amount of nursing time is determined. A panel of experts (experienced emergency nurses) can provide this information, as well as a retrospective chart review.

Compared with a factor analysis system, a prototype system, once established, requires less work on the part of the nursing staff to maintain. Nurses determine which category the patient should be placed in versus tallying every procedure and nursing skill used for the patient, as is needed in a

Table 20-1 Prototype System Based on the Nursing Process

Nursing process/action	Category 1	Category 2	Category 3
Assessment	Triage and discharge only	Every 30 minutes	More frequently than every 30 minutes
Patient teaching	Simple (e.g., infection precautions, discharge changes)	Moderate (e.g., crutch walking)	Complex (e.g., new diabetic teaching)
Interventions	Simple (e.g., wound irrigation, suture setup)	Moderate (e.g., nasogastric tube or urinary catheter insertion)	Complex (e.g., arterial line monitoring)

factor analysis system. However, the prototype system is very subjective, is difficult to monitor, has poor interrater reliability, and can be easily manipulated by staff, which compromises the accuracy of the data collected.[2] For example, staff nurses may believe that the care required was really greater than the category in which the patient fits. The nurses may then place the patient in the higher category, and reliability of the data is compromised. Another example would be the nurse who does not completely understand the categories and places patients in inappropriate categories.

Medical- and Nursing-Diagnosis–Based Systems. Two prototype methods of categorization have been used less frequently: medical diagnosis and nursing diagnosis. When medical diagnosis is used, the discharge medical diagnosis categorizes the patient. Certain medical diagnoses fall into specific categories. A patient who had a cardiac or traumatic arrest would be placed in the highest category, and a patient with flulike symptoms would be placed in the lowest or least acute category. A panel of experts determines which medical diagnoses should be placed in each category. This is a very simple method to use, and data are easily retrievable from old charts. However, caution must be used, since this method alone does not accurately capture nursing care provided, which is the major reason for making use of a PCS.[2]

A nursing-diagnosis–based system promotes professionalism, is in accordance with the Emergency Nurses Association Standards of Practice,[5] and promotes the utilization of nursing diagnoses. However, nursing diagnosis is not widely implemented in emergency departments throughout the country and may not accurately reflect the time or acuity of nursing care delivered.[2] For example, the diagnosis of ineffective breathing pattern may apply in a patient whose trachea is intubated or in a patient having a mild asthma attack. Nursing care delivered would vary greatly depending on the condition of the patient. Further specification of acuity levels within each diagnosis is necessary before widespread use of a PCS using nursing diagnosis is possible.

Factor Analysis. The factor analysis method places patients in categories based on previously identified, weighted critical indicators. These indicators are identified after careful analysis of all nursing activities that are performed. Varying degrees of intensity are determined, for example, frequency of nursing assessment (initial, frequent, or continuous). Other examples of indicators include the initiation of an intravenous line, medication administration, patient teaching, and levels of psychosocial support provided. All pertinent indicators that apply to the patient are checked and totaled. This total determines the patient classification category, or acuity, of the patient.[4]

Factor analysis provides objective information, is associated with high interrater reliability, and can easily be replicated. Difficulties with this system include its complexity; in addition, it is more time-consuming to implement and maintain, and it may not include all descriptors of nursing care.[2] Table 20-2 compares the prototype and factor analysis systems.

Table 20-2 Prototype System Versus Factor Analysis

Descriptor	Prototype	Factor analysis
Reliability	Variable, moderate to low	High
Implementation time	High	High
Implementation cost	Low	High
Maintenance work	Low	High
Category base	General classification	Individual indicators
Complexity	Moderate	High

PLANNING PHASE

Planning is the most important phase in implementing a PCS. It is important to identify the institution's primary goal for implementing the system. Is it to provide a revenue-generating mechanism for the department, or merely to document nursing time and defend staffing ratios? What is the desired change to be effected?[1]

Soliciting Support

All departments and personnel affected by implementation of a PCS must be approached, and the impact of the PCS on the emergency department's relationship with the departments clarified. Support of the emergency medical director is desirable. Hospital administration, information systems support, billing, and various other departments that may be affected by the implementation of the system must be consulted and informed of the project. There is a greater chance of successfully implementing a change when those affected by the change are supporting it. This is best accomplished by soliciting their input from the start versus advising them of the change after it has been made.

The emergency nursing staff is probably the most critical group from which to gather support. Nursing staff will be responsible for collecting additional data or completing additional forms as a part of the PCS implementation. Without the support of the nursing staff the system will never be successfully implemented. Compliance with completing patient classification cards will be poor and data will be inaccurate. The nursing staff can be instrumental in all phases of the project's planning and implementation.

The support of emergency nursing staff can be sought in many ways: via staff meetings, in-service training, or other self-governance committees. If the emergency department uses clinical ladders, this would be an excellent project to be involved with to promote clinical advancement. Participation in the project should be reflected in evaluations and merit reviews.

Resources

At this time, it is advisable to analyze the department's resources that are available for the project. The implementation of a PCS requires computer hardware and software, significant financial resources, and information systems personnel who are available for consultation. Do you have the resources to develop your own system, or can you purchase an already developed system? If developing your own, and resources are very limited, you may choose to develop a prototype model, since this system requires fewer financial, computer, and personnel resources to institute and maintain.

Patient Log Analysis

Once a core group of those involved has been formed, planning begins. The emergency department's patient registration log should be closely analyzed to collect information as follows. Length of stay should be determined and broken down into time-based categories.[2] This information can be used later to help determine times for the categories once they are selected. All the other factors related to the emergency patient census and characteristics should be analyzed. Some of these factors include percentage of admissions, pediatric census, population characteristics (cardiac, medical, trauma, etc.), and peak periods of emergency department visits. This information provides the manager with trends that are unique to the department, which reflect consumption of nursing resources.

Determination of Nursing Care Time

All nursing care that is performed by RNs and non-RNs is determined and classified according to direct, indirect, nonproductive time (meals, breaks, etc.), and unavailable time (vacations, sick days, etc.)[2] (Figure 20-1). Estimated times for each direct activity should be determined, and a total indirect, nonproductive, and unavailable time per 24-hour period is estimated.

Determining Categories

In developing a prototype model, the next step is to analyze the average length of patient stay and break this into the number of categories you choose for your system. Natural breaks in time can frequently be determined. Once the number of categories has been selected, patient descriptors for each category must be determined. Descriptors for each category should clarify nursing care delivered.[2] The following are potential descriptors that could be used for each category: patient status (stable, unstable, or emergent), frequency of RN assessment, and complexity of nursing care delivered. In a four-category patient status system using frequency of RN assessment; a category 1 patient may require only initial triage, whereas a category 2 patient may require only one reassessment during the emergency department stay; a category 3 patient may require reassessments every 30 minutes, whereas a category 4 patient may require reassessment at least every 15 minutes. Thus it is apparent that the prototype system is general and places patients in broad categories. After evaluating the descriptor criteria developed for each category, an estimated nursing care time is developed for each category.

The procedure for developing a factor analysis category is slightly different. Again, all direct and indirect activities must be timed and weighted. The importance of weighing activities is illustrated by the following example. The administration of an intravenous medication would be weighted more heavily than the administration of an oral medication. Intravenous medications require more preparation time and monitoring of the patient's response. This should be reflected accordingly in an acuity system. Indicators of direct patient care are selected. Broad categories are developed with more specific indicators. For example, medications may be a category with the following indicators to be checked when appropriate: oral medication, intravenous piggy-back, and continuous vasoactive intravenous drip. The continuous vasoactive drip would carry a higher weighted score. These scores can be acuity or time based. All the appropriate indicators are then checked for each patient, and a patient acuity score is determined. Value ranges for each category are determined and based on the patient's acuity score, and the patient is automatically and objectively placed in the proper category.

Validity

Once the patient categories have been developed, they must be analyzed for content validity. Content validity is defined as "the degree to which items adequately represent the universe of the content"[6]. Applied to a PCS, content validity determines whether the PCS is, indeed, measuring nursing services that are delivered. This can be determined by having a group of experts or staff nurses review the categories and match indicators with category definition (e.g., by time, frequency of assessment, etc.). Content validity should be established for both prototype and factor analysis systems.

Validity must be further established via time-in-motion studies. Actual performance times are compared with projected performance times for a procedure (e.g., factor analytic) or a patient type (prototype). If you are purchasing a system, you should still perform these studies to compare your actual time with the time defined in the system. If the times do not correlate, you may choose to revise the system if allowed by the company, select another system, or develop your own system. This is a crucial step. If a selected system does not adequately represent the emergency department nursing times, the data will not be adequate to determine staffing needs or generation of revenue.

Time-in-Motion Studies

Time-in-motion studies measure the actual time necessary to provide all direct and indirect nursing care activities that were previously estimated. There are various ways to collect these data. If financial resources are limited, devising a data collection tool that is user friendly allows the staff nurses to time their activities as they are being performed. The tool must be easy to use and adequately explained to all personnel. Advantages of involving staff nurse personnel include initiation into the change process and increasing their familiarity with the system. A disadvantage of using staff nurses to collect these data is collection of potentially unreliable data; in addition, the staff nurses' workload is increased.[2,6]

Using nonparticipant observers for data collection, if possible, provides more reliable data but in some cases the data may be less valid. Nurse researchers use stopwatches, observe nursing care time, and record each activity and cognitive complexity of the activity. One disadvantage of using nonparticipant observers is the difficulty in estimating the cognitive process behind the observed patient care activities. The observer may not be aware of what the RN is doing or thinking.[2] However, for objectivity purposes it is much better to use nonparticipant observers for data collection.

Measurement of nursing activities should be collected on all shifts, on all days of the week, and for a sufficient period of time, perhaps for 2 or 3 weeks.

Interrater reliability is another important criterion to evaluate during data collection. Interrater reliability determines the degree to which two different observers measure the same variable or task consistently.[7] It is important that each person measuring the performance of a task measures it in the same manner and same time period. It is important that if

two different observers watch a nurse perform venipuncture, each records the same time and if measured, cognitive complexity. Each descriptor in each category should have at least 10 observations rated by different staff at the same time. Interrater reliability of 90% is desirable.[2] Each observation is recorded, and the values must correlate with 90% accuracy. If one nurse timed the duration of an activity as 5 minutes and another timed it as 10 minutes, interrater reliability would be low. If interrater reliability is found to be low, then either the categories or the descriptors or both must be reviewed and revised. Reliability is also assessed by having nurses match hypothetical patients or actual cases with their appropriate classification and calculate the percentages of agreement. Again, 90% agreement for each case is desirable.

Once time-in-motion studies are complete, the indirect, nonproductive, and unavailable times must be determined. These times will eventually become a part of determining the number of full-time equivalents (FTEs) needed per 24-hour period.

The times for each patient classification category are totaled. The actual total is compared with the estimated time previously developed during initial work on category development. If this difference is poorly correlated (using Pearson's product-moment correlation coefficient), the category times must be reevaluated. There are various statistical procedures that can examine the degree of fit between actual and projected nursing time involved in patient care activities, including analysis of variance.[2] When the data categories, descriptors, and times have been adequately validated, the system is ready for implementation.

IMPLEMENTATION OF THE SYSTEM

Several factors should be considered when implementing the PCS, including the following: performing a pilot study, deciding who will classify patients, and data entry systems.

Pilot Study

Once the system is ready for implementation, a pilot study should be performed. The purpose of the pilot study is to compare the actual staffing that is used with the predicted staffing based on the information collected. The pilot determines whether the selected PCS is feasible and provides data necessary to examine staffing and revenue generation. The length of the pilot study should be determined, as well as who will actually record the category and where. Pilot studies can be as long or short as the nurse manager believes is necessary to obtain adequate data to properly evaluate its initial effectiveness.

Classification of the Patients

Will the staff nurses or secretarial personnel be required to complete an indicator sheet or determine the patient classification category? In a prototype or diagnosis-based system the nurse should probably determine the category. These systems require judgment as to the complexity of the nursing process performed. More analysis than simply checking off tasks is required.

Data Entry Systems

Is the emergency department log computerized, and will the category be recorded on the log? To obtain optimal use of the PCS, the category should become a part of the permanent record. This also assists in the billing process if the system will be used to generate nursing revenue. The PCS provides objective data (particularly if a factor analytic system is used) to justify nursing care charges. For example, a set charge could be determined for each category.[2]

At the end of the pilot study the nurse manager should compare the predicted staffing needs with the actual staff used. Large variances between predicted versus actual staffing should be closely examined, and categories or descriptors revised before actual implementation.[2] For example, perhaps the time estimated for a specific category is actually underestimated by 30 minutes. This category should be revised to reflect this, or the PCS will grossly underestimate the necessary amount of nursing resources. Any difficulties experienced with the system by the nursing staff or other departments involved with the system should be resolved at this point.

Once established, the PCS should be monitored over time. Reliability checks should be conducted frequently to ensure staff compliance and accuracy in filling out the cards or entering data and in determining the correct category. Any major changes in the emergency department will affect the nursing care that is delivered and necessitate system alterations. For example, the addition of new skills, a change in the RN/non-RN staffing mix, and a change in the patient population are variables that may require adaptation of the system. The development and implementation of a PCS is a task that is never complete.

PATIENT ACUITY AND NURSING RESOURCES

Although the PCS provides many advantages for the emergency department manager, the most important is the provision of objective, accurate documentation of nursing care delivered. These data can be used to defend current staffing needs and will identify trends and the need for increased staff, both RN and non-RN.

The utilization of a PCS provides the nurse manager with the information to predict the minimum number of nurses needed to provide nursing care based on acuity versus volume. The actual determination of nursing care hours needed is a relatively simple step in the overall task of designing and implementing a PCS. Several references are available for additional, more specific examples of calculating nursing care hours.[3,7-11]

The following example illustrates the process of determining the average daily nursing care hours required after examining 1 month's worth of data (Table 20-3). Initially the number of patients for each category and day is tallied for a 1-month period. The total number of patients per day per category is then multiplied by the average time determined for a patient in that category. This example illustrates an RN-only staff. For example, in Table 20-3 a category 1 patient uses an average of 14 minutes of nursing care. On September 1, 27 patients were in category 1, resulting in 378 minutes of nursing care time for category 1 patients on 1 day. This process is applied to all categories of patients, and a final tally of nursing care *hours* is determined. A total of 9593 minutes, or 160 hours of *direct* nursing care was required for that particular day. At this point the figure that was determined to represent average *indirect* nursing care is added to this value. The triage and charge nurse are included as a por-

Table 20-3 Emergency Department Patient Classification Worksheet

Category 1 = 14 min. × 1 hr. = 14 min.
Category 2 = 24 min. × 2.2 = 53 min.
Category 3 = 53 min. × 4.3 = 228 min.
Category 4 = 85 min. × 4.5 = 383 min.

Month Nov. 1985
Average daily hours required 227
Required FTEs 46.9

Date	Cat. 1	Total min.	Cat. 2	Total min.	Cat. 3	Total min.	Cat. 4	Total min.	Total hrs. direct	Average indir.	Total req. hrs.	Req. staff
9/1	27	378	56	2968	19	4332	5	1915	160	62	221	29.3
9/2	51	714	43	2279	18	4104	12	4596	195	62	257	33.2
9/3	33	462	30	1590	10	2280	6	2298	111	62	173	22.3
9/4	74	1036	32	1696	12	2736	12	4596	166	62	228	29.4
9/5	25	350	52	2756	18	4104	5	1915	152	62	214	27.6
9/6	29	406	52	2756	29	6612	3	1149	182	62	244	31.5
9/7	33	462	44	2332	12	2736	12	4596	169	62	231	29.8
9/8	28	392	41	2173	11	2508	9	3447	142	62	204	26.3
9/9	21	294	40	2120	17	3876	13	4979	188	62	250	32.3

Month required average hours	6810
	÷
Days in month	30
Average daily hrs.	227

Adapted from Buschiazzo L: *Nursing management,* 16(5):34B-34H, 1985.

tion of the indirect time. As shown in Table 20-3, 62 hours of indirect nursing care was determined to be the average amount of indirect nursing care provided per day. It has been estimated that as much as 50% of nursing care time can be spent performing indirect nursing care.[2] The total nursing care hours necessary for September 1 was 222 hours.

Calculations vary according to the type of shift worked (i.e., 8, 10, or 12 hours). Meal and break times must be subtracted from the base hour. In the example in Table 20-3, nurses worked 8-hour shifts; 7.75 hours was the time used as actual work time. This time appears to represent only 15 minutes of nonproductive time and may actually be too high. Other examples[2] calculate 7.0 hours of actual hours worked for an 8-hour shift.

On September 2, 257 hours of nursing care hours were required. This total is divided by 7.75 (actual work time per shift). The number of nurses who were needed to provide nursing care for that day was 33.2. At the end of the month, staffing requirements were totaled (227 hours per day), divided by 7.75 (29.29), and multiplied by 1.6 (46.86), the conversion factor for 1.0 FTE required to cover vacation, sick time, and the like (unavailable time). This calculation results in an average requirement of 46.86 FTEs for September. Similar calculations can be performed at the end of a year. The example in Table 20-3 accounts for all direct, indirect, and nonproductive nursing care time. The addition of nurse assistive personnel, managers, and educator positions must be added into a final budget.

It must be remembered that a number of staff must always be present to provide for minimum safety. The manager should calculate enough nursing resources to provide care for trauma patients, cardiac arrest patients, or the sudden influx of acutely ill patients that occurs daily in most emergency departments. Staffing numbers must be determined after a careful analysis of the department's particular patient care mix and trends.

If large variances exist between what the PCS predicts as staffing needs and what you have previously been operating with, the PCS may demonstrate the need for more or less staff. If the need for less staff is demonstrated, a further evaluation of your categories, descriptors, and times is necessary. If the system demonstrates the need for more staff, data are available for use in negotiating new positions.

REVENUE-GENERATING CAPABILITY

A PCS provides an objective method of determining a nursing charge. Nursing remains one of the few groups of professionals in the hospital who provide direct patient care and do *not* charge for services.

Careful thought and cooperation from the emergency medical director and hospital administrators must be attained when developing nursing charges. It must be clear that the emergency department will receive a portion of the reimbursements obtained.

The PCS provides a database that clearly differentiates nursing care and could be used in determining charges. It has been recommended that acuity data and pricing be evaluated separately.[21] For example, many emergency departments throughout the country provide wound checks at no charge. This patient still uses nursing time but has a low acuity category; however, if the department does not charge for the visit, it would not be appropriate for the nurse to charge for services. Using the PCS to help generate revenue is another advantage of the PCS.

CURRENTLY AVAILABLE SYSTEMS

Many systems are currently developed and available for purchase.[2] If financially feasible, purchasing a system significantly reduces the time required for implementation of the system and provides many advantages. A thorough evaluation of the system is necessary before purchase. Systems for purchase frequently have other features, including automated registration, charting functions, order entry, and quality improvement capabilities. These provide significant advantages

and allow for maximum utilization of a computerized system. A careful analysis of cost, hardware required, computer support, and the capability of the system to merge with the hospital's currently existing computer system is important.

SUMMARY

Instituting a PCS in the emergency department represents a significant challenge to the emergency nurse manager, whether the decision is to purchase a currently existing system or to develop a department-specific system. The reasons for choosing to institute the system must be clear. In the planning stages many factors must be considered that will significantly impact the design and selection of the appropriate system. Patient data and department resources must be analyzed to decide which type of system to implement. The planning and implementation stages require a significant time commitment, and time-in-motion studies should be conducted. The reliability and validity of categories selected must be examined. Once the system has been implemented, the advantages to the nurse manager are endless. An objective method of predicting nursing staffing needs has been developed. The opportunity to generate revenue from nursing care delivered is now possible.

Glossary of Terms

Descriptor: Characteristics used to describe something.

Direct nursing care: Nursing care provided that requires hands-on or direct verbal communication with the patient or family.

Indirect nursing care: Activities of nursing care that are affecting patient care but are not provided in the presence of the patient.

Interrater reliability: The ability of several observers to watch the same task and measure it consistently with each other.

Nonproductive time: Nursing time that is not spent in providing care, for example, meals and breaks.

Panel of experts: Individuals who are considered experts and are consulted for their opinions.

Patient classification system: A system utilized to describe patients and the amount of nursing care that they require. This system has many other advantages.

Productive time: A combination of direct and indirect nursing time.

Time-in-motion studies: Studies that measure and record the actual time it takes to perform various activities. The activity is measured numerous times, and an average of these times is used to determine the actual time.

REFERENCES

1. Krizek MB, Chernow PM: Implementing a patient classification system in the emergency department, *Emerg Nurs Reports* 1:9, 1986.
2. Emergency Nurses Association: *Emergency department patient classification systems manual,* Chicago, 1990, The Association.
3. Buschiazzo L: *The handbook of emergency nursing management,* Rockville, Md, 1987, Aspen.
4. Stolley J, Hachmann D: Establishing reliability and validity of an ED patient classification system, *J Emerg Nurs* 15:6, 1989.
5. Emergency Nurses Association, editor: *Standards of emergency nursing practice,* St Louis, 1994, Mosby.
6. Buschiazzo L: Adapting PCS to emergency services, *Nurs Manage Crit Care Manage Ed* 16:5, 1984.
7. Polit D, Hungler B: *Nursing research principles and methods,* ed 2, Philadelphia, 1983, JB Lippincott.
8. Bulter W: ED patient classification matrix: development and testing of one tool, *J Emerg Nurs* 12:5, 1986.
9. Schulmerich S: Developing a patient classification system for the emergency department, *J Emerg Nurs* 10:6, 1984.
10. Schulmerich S: Converting patient classification data into staffing requirements for the emergency department, *J Emerg Nurs* 12:5, 1986.
11. Kromash E: Patient classification and required nursing time in a pediatric ED, *J Emerg Nurs* 10:2, 1984.

21 Patient Throughput

Richard F. Salluzzo, George Terranova, and Vincent Verdile

OUTLINE

No aspect of emergency care is more scrutinized than the ability of a given emergency department to evaluate, treat, and make a disposition for a patient in a reasonable amount of time. The patient throughput process consists of an enormous number of individual steps, all of which can be quite complex, making the overall process (particularly in a high-volume emergency department) difficult to manage. Without question, patient satisfaction is to a large extent dependent on how well the flow through the emergency department is managed. Equally important, optimal use of resources will not occur without certain core efficiencies in the throughput process.

The purpose of this chapter is to describe the most important steps in patient throughput and define strategies that might be effective in making throughput more efficient. In addition, we will review some of the management pitfalls that occur when trying to improve patient throughput, and we will examine newer informational technologies that can lend valuable assistance in improving this process.

The format of the chapter consists of a step-by-step evaluation of the throughput process with an emphasis on ways to identify and resolve problems in process.

TRIAGE

The triage process is a critical step in patient throughput from the standpoint of both quality and resource utilization. Decisions made at triage that affect throughput include the decision about which patients are appropriate for a fast track if one exists, which patients can go directly to radiography if such triage guidelines are in place, and which patients are high priority and require immediate medical attention. In addition, triage is an important interface point in terms of patient satisfaction.[1]

For triage to work well there has to be departmental consensus on the model of triage to be employed. For instance, in a very-low-volume emergency department, triage may essentially perform a pass-through function with the triage nurse spending only a brief time with the patient. In a high-volume, complex emergency department, the model may be that of comprehensive triage in which initial vital signs are obtained, x-ray triage occurs, and, in general, thorough nursing assessments are performed on the patients. Whichever model is used for your department, parameters of timeliness and quality must be measured on a regular basis.

The complete triage-to-registration process should not take longer than 10 to 12 minutes, even if a comprehensive triage model is in place. As with any process in the emergency department, the mean time and the spread around the mean are equally important. For instance, if the mean time for the triage process is 6 minutes but half the patients require 10 minutes and the rest only 2 minutes, there may be an acceptable delay at the triage desk for half the patients. The importance of consistency in all key processes of patient throughput cannot be overemphasized.

The best way to evaluate and improve the triage process is to have a multidisciplinary team consisting of nurses, physicians, and senior emergency department clerks evaluate and modify the existing process so that it is more consistent, effective, and timely. Although the management team is capable of designing an effective process change, its acceptance by a disenfranchised staff may be limited. For this reason, reliance on teams is essential to operationalize good ideas about fundamentally important processes in the department (Fig. 21-1).

REGISTRATION

The registration process should not take more than 5 to 8 minutes on average, if there is an appropriately trained staff. In general, one registration clerk is needed for every 7000 to 10,000 annual emergency department visits to maintain effective flow.[2] The use of a training manual and trainers among the staff and an effective orientation period are important tools if ward clerk performance is to be optimized.

To ensure outstanding registration clerk performance, several parameters ought to be measured, such as registration time, numbers of errors, patient satisfaction, and courtesy of phone answering. An important issue in terms of registration clerk management concerns reporting lines for the clerks. The emergency department physician manager must be ultimately responsible for the clerk management term.

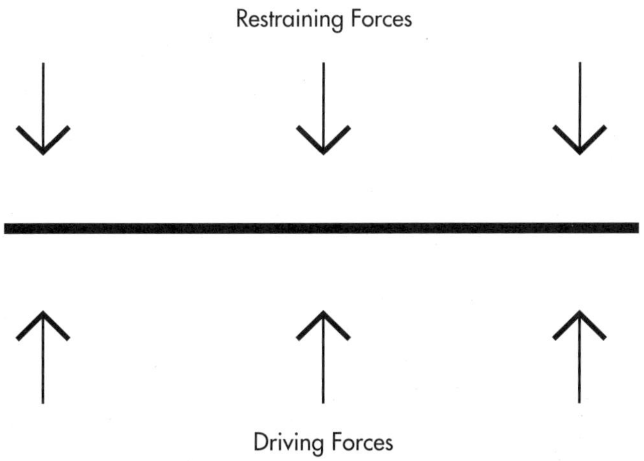

FIGURE 21-1 Lewen force field.

NURSING EVALUATION

Once a patient has been effectively triaged and registered, a staff nurse should see that patient within a reasonable time, which can vary based on patient acuity. In general, a patient should not have to wait more than 15 minutes for this nursing contact. There should be at least one Registered Nurse (RN) for every 5000 annual emergency department visits, although this number may vary depending on case mix, time spent in the emergency department, number of admitted patients, facility design, and other factors.

Primary nursing has proven quite effective in facilitating optimal patient throughput and enhancing patient satisfaction.[3] In this nursing model, one nurse is primarily responsible for a given emergency department patient and that nurse should be intimately familiar with the status of that patient's healthcare plan. The primary nurse should provide the patient with regular updates concerning anticipated testing or consultation, inform the physician of the patient's clinical status, and interface with family concerning patient care issues. For effective throughput to occur, there should be optimal interface between the physician and nurse in terms of communication and work sharing. It may be worthwhile to charter a Quality Improvement team in the emergency department to carefully review how physicians, nurses, and patients interface so that improvements in this process can be made.

PHYSICIAN EVALUATION

In some instances (i.e., patients who are critically ill) a nurse and a physician evaluation occurs simultaneously. For nonacute condition a physician should provide an evaluation within 20 minutes of the patient's arrival in the room. For effective physician evaluation of patients, there must be adequate physician staffing, and most studies indicate that emergency physicians can evaluate between two and three patients per hour of an average emergency department patient mix.[4] Physician staffing should reflect this average productivity level. Approximately 70% of emergency department visits occur between 10 AM and 10 PM. For example, if an emergency department has 30,000 annual patient visits, approximately 20,000 of those visits will occur between 10 AM and 10 PM. This means approximately five patients per hour will be seen during this period. Clearly, an emergency department of this volume would need at least two physicians during peak hours or approximately 36 hours per day of physician coverage.

Since emergency department physicians are often managing several patients simultaneously, they tend to do a hurried initial evaluation, order a broad spectrum of tests, and then reevaluate the patient sequentially. There are times when this approach is the only one that can be adopted, given the status of the department. On the other hand, a well-thought-out strategy after the initial patient evaluation with appropriate test ordering prevents delays in waiting for unnecessary test results and diminishes the number of false-positive test results that occur. These two issues often cause untimely delays in patient throughput. In addition to ordering only those tests that are necessary, the physician must be aware of when test results become available so that he or she can act quickly on these results. Ideally there should be some form of a notification mechanism to let the physician know when these test results are ready for interpretation.

If time allows, it is also helpful to sit down and spend a few minutes with the patients early in their emergency department course to assure the patient and family that they are not being rushed through the system.[5] In addition, the physician can give patients realistic parameters for the timeliness of their diagnostic and treatment regimens to prevent unrealistic expectations concerning how long they will be in the emergency department. These two strategies significantly enhance the patients' perception of both the quantitative and qualitative aspects of the emergency department visit.

LABORATORY ORDERING

To improve laboratory throughput times in the emergency department, it is essential that an effective database be created to evaluate laboratory performance. It is important that the laboratory provide a daily tracking of throughput times on tests performed in the department. The emergency department management team can then get a sense of when delays occur and which tests tend to be more slowly performed. There are many steps from venipuncture to the posting of test results, any of which may cause significant delays in obtaining those results. An audit of this process, preferably with a flow diagram, should be conducted to understand where the delays occur. Once armed with this information, the emergency management team can create a rational strategy about how to improve the process. For instance, many emergency department managers assume that a STAT laboratory (see Chapter 25) on site in the emergency department will automatically improve patient throughput times. In certain emergency departments, however, with high patient volume and acuity several other processes provide bottlenecks to patient throughput, in addition to the laboratory process. In those situations, improving one process (i.e., the laboratory process) may not have any impact on overall throughput. Depending on the complexity of your emergency department, you may find it useful to create a multidisciplinary Quality Improvement team to review the laboratory ordering process.

BOX 21-1

POINT-OF-SERVICE LABORATORY TESTS

Streptococcus sp. throat culture
Urinalysis
Urine pregnancy test
Spun hematocrit
Pulse oximetry
Diagnostic peritoneal lavage (DPL)
Finger-stick glucose test
I-STAT electrolyte levels
Electrocardiogram
Cardiac enzyme test
Ultrasound

There are a number of strategies that should help improve laboratory throughput times. For instance, certain tests might best be performed by the emergency staff to prevent untimely delays (Box 21-1) (e.g., urine pregnancy tests, urinalysis, spun hematocrit, and finger-stick glucose). In addition, the emergency department physician director should carefully review utilization of laboratory tests to ensure that unnecessary test ordering is not occurring. Most important, the laboratory and emergency department should meet and agree on certain performance standards that are reasonable for the various laboratory tests. As already mentioned a Quality Improvement team should review the laboratory ordering process to determine where inefficiencies are occurring.

RADIOLOGY

Many of the issues related to the laboratory process also apply to ordering x-rays. To effectively manage this process, it is critical that the emergency department management team have a reliable database that specifies laboratory performance by time of the day, day of the week, and specific tests ordered. In addition, evaluation of this process by a Quality Improvement team that is multidisciplinary should also occur. Once a clear understanding of the process as it exists is obtained, modifications of that process can be suggested and implemented. As with laboratory performance, it is important that certain preestablished standards that are mutually acceptable to the department of radiology and the department of emergency medicine be created and tracked. For example, the two departments might agree that 40 minutes is a reasonable time to complete a computed tomography scan. Usually, plain films should be completed in 30 minutes or less. Once such performance standards are created, they should be monitored on a regular basis, preferably as part of a daily management report but at least on a weekly basis. Although mean performance from the radiology department is important, consistency in that performance is just as critical. For instance, if the mean performance time for a given test is 45 minutes but half the patients require 20 minutes for their studies and the other half, 70 minutes, there will be unacceptable delays for a significant proportion of the patients, despite a reasonable mean performance time for the test.

USE OF CONSULTANTS

Consultants play a key role in the practice of emergency medicine and have significant impact on patient throughput times. To effectively manage consultant performance, a database must be created quantifying the performance of consultants. As with laboratory and radiology performance, mutually acceptable performance standards should be created between the emergency department and the various consulting services and this performance should be regularly monitored. Certain practice protocols and guidelines can be set in motion to facilitate the use of consultants and in some cases to obviate the need for initial consultation in the emergency department. In general, consultation should occur within 45 minutes of speaking to the consultant so that unnecessary patient delays in disposition do not occur. Keeping the patient and family aware of the need for consultation helps them understand the need for a longer emergency department stay.

DISCHARGE PROCESS

Discharge is another important step in the throughput process that should be evaluated for its effectiveness. For instance, if the nurses, exclusively, discharge patients and the nurses are busy with other tasks, it may be that one or more of your patients wait a considerable time before discharge. A review of this process by appropriate staff members may result in significant modifications that improve the overall efficiency of this process. In general, patients should be routinely discharged within 10 minutes from the time the discharge decision is made. As with other process change, the modified discharge process ought to be monitored to ensure consistency and adherence to performance standards. Computerized discharge information, which eliminates the need for handwritten or preprinted disease or treatment specific instructions, is one method to reduce the time needed to discharge a patient.

INFORMATION SYSTEMS

Several software packages that are available to emergency departments allow access to the main hospital data banks, tracking of emergency department patients, order entry, and other important functions.[6] It is unclear whether such systems will have dramatic impact on throughput time, but they certainly should be of some benefit in this regard. Chapter 29 discusses in detail various information systems for the emergency department of the future. It is clear, however, that the use of these software packages makes data collection and retrieval much easier, and information tracking remains one of the key ingredients in monitoring and improving performance in the department. The emergency manager should consult with hospital administrators on plans for information system upgrade and, clearly, should be part of the hospital team that reviews various information systems options.

FAST TRACKS

The use of a fast track or a minor care area in the emergency department can certainly improve patient throughput times[7]

(see Chapter 31). Fast tracks offer several advantages in terms of cost-effective care delivery. First, physician extenders can be used at a definite cost savings. Second, minor cases can be segregated in this area so that nursing and physician staff are not attempting to take care of the very sick and minor cases simultaneously. This creates a much more effective division of labor. An example of the impact a fast track can have is a 60,000-visit emergency department that had average throughput times of 180 minutes and reduced the average throughput time to 115 minutes within 3 months of staffing a fast track area. Of the 60,000 visits, the fast track treated 17,000 with an average throughput time of 60 minutes. The area used physicians' assistants exclusively. Incremental resource allocation was minimal except for the renovation of additional space for six stretchers. As this example shows, not only can fast tracks improve overall throughput times, they can do so in a cost-effective manner.

MONITORING PATIENT THROUGHPUT

In this chapter we have discussed several steps in the throughput process, as well as how to set reasonable standards for a given process. In addition, we have discussed ways to evaluate and improve that process through the use of Quality Improvement teams. Given the importance of throughput times on patient satisfaction, daily tracking of individual patient throughput is desirable.

Most registration systems can be modified to include fields that monitor the patient's course through the emergency department. Times of triage, registration, and discharge can be easily retrieved. The chart can also be designed to capture initial nurse and physician patient encounter times once the patient is in a room. The chart design should also include consultants' response times. When an advanced information system with order entry capabilities is in place, it is quite easy to retrieve laboratory, radiology, and other ancillary data as well. If such a system is not in place, it is important to create a manual or semimanual system that provides this information.

As we have emphasized in this chapter, throughput consists of many discrete processes, all of which require reasonable efficiency and consistency if the overall process is to be effective. According to the time lines we created in this chapter, a non–fast-track patient not requiring the use of laboratory or radiology services should be processed through the ideal emergency department in approximately 60 to 70 minutes. A patient receiving laboratory and radiology services requires approximately 90 to 110 minutes. Actual throughput times in your department may be less if individual steps require less time than in our model.

One of the problems in managing patient throughput is developing consistency. For instance, your emergency department might have a mean throughput time of 110 minutes for a given week, month, or year. However, there will be many individual shifts and days when throughput times are two or three standard deviations from the mean. Not only are mean throughput times important, but so is the spread around the mean (i.e., the amount of variability). Great unreliability in this process is unacceptable, even if the mean times are reasonable. When an emergency manager tries to assess the causes for this variability, he or she generally considers several important factors, including census, staffing, laboratory and radiology throughput times, number of admissions, and number of ambulances (Box 21-2). Analyzing the data by univariate analysis and multiple regression demonstrates an inability to account for a large part of the variability in throughput times. For instance, Reilly and others[8] looked at approximately 25 factors affecting emergency department throughput and found that only 4 factors—the number of admissions, the number of traumas, the number of pediatric cases, and nurse staffing—impacted throughput times. Even more surprising, these factors accounted for only 30% of the variability in throughput time. The daily census had little impact on throughput time. Whether the emergency department saw 100 patients or 140 on a given day did not correlate with throughput times for that day.

There is no question that an emergency department manager can make substantial improvements in patient throughput by means of the strategies discussed in this chapter, such as creation of a fast track, ensuring that admissions leave the emergency department promptly, improving laboratory and radiology throughput times, and ensuring adequate staffing. On the other hand, even when these and other processes are thought to be optimal, there is still quite a bit of variability in mean throughput times. There are now several software packages that allow a more accurate evaluation of the fac-

BOX 21-2

FACTORS AFFECTING PATIENT THROUGHPUT

- Facility size and design
- Case mix
- Number of admissions
- Average time spent in emergency department by admissions
- Number of ambulances
- Number of traumas
- Census
- Nurse, physician, and ward clerk staffing
- Radiology throughput
- Laboratory throughput
- Pediatric cases
- Pediatric admissions
- Number of x-rays ordered
- Number of laboratory tests ordered
- Fast-track census
- Fast-track throughput
- Time of day
- Day of week
- Month
- Consultant throughput times
- Type of consultants
- Patient flow per hour
- Specific physician performance
- Specific nurse performance
- Number of unit admissions
- Number of patients older than 65 years
- Number of patients less than 3 months of age

tors affecting patient throughput (unpublished data, Sun-Health, Charlotte, N.C.). These programs allow the emergency manager to create a model that duplicates performance in his or her department. With these models any given factor can be changed while holding all other factors constant so that the impact of that factor on throughput times can be evaluated. For example, if the average laboratory turnaround time in your department is 70 minutes, the impact of halving this time to 35 minutes can be ascertained with a simulation program. This type of analysis is important because when evaluating the emergency department in real time, it is impossible to change just one factor and hold all others constant: hence the true impact of changing one process can never really be measured. By this kind of analysis, the emergency manager can quickly assess which factors are having the most impact on throughput time and, consequently, where the resources of the department ought to be directed to have maximal impact.

SUMMARY

In this chapter we have discussed a step-by-step approach to improving patient throughput in the emergency department. We have emphasized the most important processes and factors associated with this process and how they may be modified. In addition, we briefly mentioned the newest technology by which this process can be analyzed.

REFERENCES

1. Macleod AJ, Freeland P: Should nurses be allowed to request x-rays in an accident and emergency department? *Arch Emerg Med* 9:19-22, 1992.
2. Schulmerich SC: Converting patient classification data into staffing requirements for the emergency department, *J Emerg Nurs* 12:286-290, 1986.
3. Bursch B, Beezy J: Emergency department satisfaction: what matters most? *Ann Emerg Med* 22(3):586-591, 1993.
4. Graff L, Radford M: Formula for emergency physician staffing, *Am J Emerg Med* 8(3):194-199, 1990.
5. Bjorvell H, Stieg J: Patients' perceptions of the health care received in an emergency department, *Ann Emerg Med* 20(7):734-738, 1991.
6. Chuan Hu S: Computerized monitoring of emergency department patient flow, *Am J Emerg Med* 11(1):8-11, 1993.
7. Wright S, Erwin T, Blanton DM et al: Fast track in the emergency department: a 1-year experience with nurse practitioners, *J Emerg Med* 10:367-373, 1992.
8. Reilly K, Salluzzo RF, Mulholland D, et al: Factors affecting patient throughput times in an academic emergency department, *Acad Emerg Med* 2(5):440, 1995.

22 Developing Policies and Procedures

Kathleen M. Richmond

OUTLINE

Management role in policy development
Policies and procedures for the emergency department
Policy and procedure requirements
Development of policies and procedures
Policy and procedure format
Liability issues
The emergency department policy and procedure manual
Use of the policy and procedure manual
Summary

Policies and procedures are formal, written communications within an organization. A policy is the basic governing principle that outlines the structure and course of action for patient care; a procedure is the outline of steps used in the process of performing that patient care. The Joint Commission for Accreditation of Healthcare Organizations (JCAHO) has set standards by which a healthcare institution is judged. The use of policies and procedures is one of the ways that accrediting bodies/organizations measure and evaluate healthcare institutions' compliance with established national standards of care. Productivity and efficiency in healthcare organizations correlate with policies and procedures based on high standards and professional norms of excellence.

A high degree of coordination is needed in healthcare institutions because of the complexity of their structure. One method organizations use to promote internal coordination is through formulation of rules, manuals, job descriptions, policies, and procedures. Specialty units/departments, such as the emergency department, must provide specific policies and procedures to guide staff in definitive care of their distinct patient populations.

MANAGEMENT ROLE IN POLICY DEVELOPMENT

In a traditional model of organizational theory, management's role includes planning methods and procedures to accomplish goals of the organization and establishing standards by which actual results can be compared. Managers in healthcare institutions have relative control over patient care policies and practices and must be able to determine, translate, and implement relevant implications for the department's scope of responsibility. Management is accountable for ensuring institutional/departmental compliance with professional, regulatory, and government standards of care for provision of effective, high-quality patient care. Emergency department policies and procedures should be developed in accordance with current standards for emergency and trauma care recommended by professional organizations such as the American College of Emergency Physicians, the American College of Surgeons, the American Heart Association, and the Emergency Nurses Association. Patient care decisions should be consistent with professional standards, rules, and regulations of governmental authorities and policies of the facility.

Management should involve various healthcare professionals in the development, implementation, and monitoring of departmental policies and procedures. Physicians traditionally have authority to formulate standards, supervise, and control most healthcare services. According to JCAHO recommendations, there should be provisions for nursing department/services to participate in policy decisions affecting patient care services in the hospital. Therefore it is essential that policy decisions involve both medical and nursing professionals.

POLICIES AND PROCEDURES FOR THE EMERGENCY DEPARTMENT

Policies and procedures provide the framework within which emergency department healthcare workers operate. They provide order and guides to situations to ensure safe patient care. Policies and procedures function as a map for emergency healthcare workers who may lack practical experience and expertise in a specific patient care situation. By breaking down activities into elements and providing pertinent rules, policies and procedures permit emergency staff to act with relative safety in providing patient care. Policies and procedures provide rules of order and control as a basis for safe care in the emergency department.

Substituting written rules for medical and nursing judgment may not be necessary or medically appropriate in all emergency situations. Written policies and procedures standardize activities and demand conformity. Detailed policies and procedures may lead to a sense of more complexity than is necessary in a given patient care situation without regard for individual patient differences. It is a medicolegal liability to have emergency department policies and procedures that cannot be adhered to as written. Therefore emergency department policies and procedures should be written in an outline format to guide rather than confine the healthcare professional.

POLICY AND PROCEDURE REQUIREMENTS

Emergency department services are directly and indirectly affected by federal and state legislation and regulatory agencies, including requirements for trauma center designations, disaster planning, and emergency medical services (EMS). Historically, there has been mandated reporting of various types of emergency cases (e.g., abuse and neglect situations, injuries related to use of motorized vehicles or weapons, and illnesses resulting from specific infectious diseases). More recently, the Consolidated Omnibus Reconciliation Act of 1985 (COBRA) mandated triage and transfer policies for emergency departments of hospitals that participate in the federally funded Medicare program. Many of these requirements and mandates are among those included in the JCAHO standards for emergency services.

The JCAHO standards require patient care in the emergency department to be guided by written policies and procedures. There must be a well-defined plan of emergency care provided by qualified individuals and appropriate services based on community need. Organization, direction, and staffing of the emergency department must be appropriate to the scope of services offered. The emergency department must be appropriately integrated with other departments and services of the hospital. The emergency department must be designed and equipped for safe and effective patient care. Documentation of emergency care must be incorporated into the patient's permanent medical record, and appropriate quality control mechanisms must be established. Emergency department policies and procedures should incorporate these standards, as well as those requirements related to emergency services in other hospital department/services standards. JCAHO-required policies are listed in Box 22-1. These policies vary from year to year based on current JCAHO requirements. The reader is referred to the most recent JCAHO publication for the current information.

Emergency department manuals should include all JCAHO-required policies and procedures as outlined in the standards and may include others that the individual department finds helpful or necessary.

BOX 22-1

POLICIES REQUIRED BY JCAHO

- Location, storage, and procurement of medications, blood, supplies, and equipment
- Care to minors and unconscious patients
- Notification of the patient's personal physician
- Confidentiality of patient information
- Authorizing release of information and materials to police or health authorities
- Patient transfer and discharge
- Emergency medical record and consent for treatment
- Infection control measures, including prevention of cross-infection and contamination
- Equipment failure
- Safety practices
- Traffic control, including visitors
- Dispensing of medications
- Handling and safekeeping of patients' valuables
- Disaster preparedness
- Scope of treatment allowed in the emergency department, including general and specific procedures that may not be performed by medical staff
- Other than physicians, who may perform special procedures
- Use of standing orders
- Property exchange necessitated by the transportation and transfer of patients
- Circumstances that require the patient to return to the emergency department for treatment
- Management of radiation exposure or contamination
- Alleged sexual assault or molestation protocols
- Alleged or suspected child abuse protocols
- Management of pediatric emergencies
- Reporting of individuals dead on arrival (DOA) to the proper authorities
- Evidence collection and preservation in DOA cases.
- Management of substance abuse patients or emotionally ill patients who become difficult to handle
- Initial management of patients with burns, fractures, hand injuries, head injuries, multiple injuries, poisonings, animal bites, gunshot or stab wounds, or other acute problems
- Guarding unconscious or irrational patients from harm
- Tetanus and rabies immunization
- Private attending physicians' patients in the emergency department
- Telephone orders from private physicians
- Telephone advice to patients
- Emergency staff caring for delayed admission inpatients in the emergency department

JCAHO, Joint Commission for Accreditation of Healthcare Organizations.

DEVELOPMENT OF POLICIES AND PROCEDURES

Guidelines for the proper development, review, and distribution of policies and procedures vary among institutions. Each individual emergency department must operate within the larger structure of the hospital organization, which will have its own guidelines for policy and procedure development. Ideally, the emergency department will form a committee for developing departmental policies and procedures.

The emergency department policies and procedures committee, consisting of representative emergency staff physicians, nurses, and assistive personnel, serves as a review board for all policies and procedures. Individual committee members or small subcommittees rework initial policy drafts according to their areas of interest or expertise. Final drafts are submitted to hospital administration for approval according to institutional protocol.

The committee also reviews and revises current policies and procedures on a routine basis to ensure compliance with current standards and regulations. An annual review process of all policies and procedures is mandated by the JCAHO; however, reviews/revisions may need to be done more frequently, if indicated. As technology changes, standards change. Policies and procedures must be regularly reviewed and updated to reflect the most current practice standards.

POLICY AND PROCEDURE FORMAT

The administration of the institution generally dictates the format to be used by individual departments for its policies and procedures. Polices and procedures that apply to all areas of the institution are part of the administrative manual. Specific department policies and procedures are included in

BOX 22-2

FORMAT FOR POLICY/PROCEDURE

HEADING: Department name
Policy/procedure number/code
Effective date
Date of original/previous policy/procedure
Page number of total pages
SUBJECT: Title of the policy/procedure
PURPOSE: General overview statement of need for policy procedure
POLICY: Broadly stated governing principles (organized in outline form)
A.
1.
2.
a.
b.
B.
C.
PROCEDURE: Responsible person(s) and specific methods or steps required to accomplish desired outcome (organized in outline form)
RESPONSIBLE PERSON *PROCEDURE*
1.
a.
b.
(1)
(2)
(a)
(b)
i.
ii.
2.
3.
APPROVAL SIGNATURES AND DATES:
1. Manager (of issuing department)
2. Medical director
3. Administrative vice-president

the individual department manuals. The administrative manual includes those shared policies and procedures in each department's manual. Where multiple departments share the same policy and/or procedure, the policy and procedure will appear in each department's manual. For example, the policies and procedures for patient restraint in the emergency department are included in both the Emergency Department Manual and the Security/Safety Department Manual.

Policies and procedures may be written as a combined format, eliminating the need for individual numbering of policies and procedures. The combined format generally includes the subject, purpose, policies, and procedures (Box 22-2).

Policies and procedures for an entire institution are numerous and are usually categorized within an organized identification system according to administrative protocol. Individual department manuals may be alphabetized or segmented into groups of policies/procedures for easy reference.

BOX 22-3

POLICIES WITH HIGH-RISK POTENTIAL

Use of restraints
Obtaining consents
Patients who leave the emergency department against medical advice
Treatment of alcoholic/substance abuse patients
Telephone advice given by emergency staff
Triage protocols
Patient transfers

LIABILITY ISSUES

Hospital and department policies and procedures establish standards that the institution requires employees to meet. Deviation from the guidelines contained in the policy and procedure manual may indicate that an employee has failed to meet the accepted standard. Policies and procedures should define what can and cannot be done in the emergency department and identify who may perform specific procedures. Institutional and departmental policies and procedures do not relieve professional accountability for actions taken and judgments made, including delegation of patient care activities. Emergency department policies and procedures must correlate with professional standards of emergency care and institutional quality assurance protocols.

The hospital's legal resources generally define areas of high liability for the particular facility and its emergency department. The geographic location and demographics of the service area of the hospital, level of care required and expected by the predominant clientele versus the level of care that can be provided, and lack of alternate local healthcare resources may be contributing factors to the liability risk of any emergency department. Generally, areas of high-risk potential exist in all emergency departments. Special medicolegal consideration should be given to policy and procedure development for these areas. A policy or procedure with high-risk potential should be routed through the institution's risk management department and/or legal counsel for final review and approval before implementation (Box 22-3).

A policy does not need to be in writing to be considered legally valid. Unwritten directives that are common knowledge and practice in the department carry the weight of written policy with regard to liability for the staff and the institution. Therefore all policies should be written to address common knowledge and practice of the department.

Written policies and procedures are necessary for consistency in patient care. Policies are considered minimal standards for medicolegal purposes and should be followed as such. Failure of staff to conform to an existing policy creates a potential liability for the emergency department, as well as the hospital.

THE EMERGENCY DEPARTMENT POLICY AND PROCEDURE MANUAL

A comprehensive policies and procedures manual contains all policies and procedures that relate to the functioning of the

BOX 22-4

EXAMPLE OF TABLE OF CONTENTS FOR A COMPREHENSIVE MANUAL OF EMERGENCY DEPARTMENT POLICIES AND PROCEDURES

Section 1:
Emergency Department Structure and Administration
- Communications—intradepartmental
- Community-based emergency services
- Contact of family physician
- Use of nonlicensed assitive personnel in the emergency department
- Individual and/or shift responsibilities
- Location and description of the emergency/trauma department
- Medical staff call roster and alternates
- Nursing personnel
- On-call policy
- Physician direction and staffing
- Physician privileges
- Qualification of practice for registered nurses
- Quiet room
- Responsibility and accountability to the medical staff and hospital administration
- Role of department in relation to prehospital care/EMS
- Scope of care
- Service charges
- Trauma center concept
- Unit meetings

Section 2:
Patient Care Protocols
- Abdomen—blunt and penetrating trauma
- Admission into the emergency department
- Admission of a patient from the emergency department
- Animal bites
- Assessment of patients before registration
- Autologous blood transfusion
- Births in the emergency department
- Burn management
- Cardiopulmonary resuscitation
- Cast removal
- Chemotherapy administration
- Chest—blunt and penetrating trauma
- Code blue
- Communicable disease
- Drug abuse patients
- Ear irrigation
- Emergency department nursing before physician arrival
- Eye irrigation
- Follow-up care
- Fracture and orthopedic injury management
- Head injury management
- Inpatient observation
- Intravenous drug administration
- Medications in the emergency department
- Multiple trauma patient management
- Noninvasive blood pressure monitoring
- Noninvasive pacemaker
- Pediatric emergencies
- Pelvic examinations
- Peripheral vascular injury management
- Physician evaluation of all patients
- Poison ingestion management
- Rapid transfusion protocol
- Respiratory care
- Sexual assault examination
- Standards of emergency nursing care
- Tetanus prophylaxis
- Treatment in the emergency department
- Unconscious patients
- Psychiatric/emotionally ill or disturbed patients
- Venereal disease
- Wound preparation

Section 3:
Patient Care Record
- Confidentiality of patient information and record
- Discharge instructions
- Emergency department record—protocol for use and completion
- Medical records department
- Use of standing orders
- Use and documentation of transfer form

Section 4:
Quality Assurance
- Antibiotic review
- Competency assessment and documentation—unit specific
- Culture report follow-up
- ECG reading follow-up
- MICN certification requirements (as applicable)
- Nursing staff performance/assessment
- Orientation policy
- Patient classification system
- Patient and family/caregiver education
- Quality assessment and improvement monitoring

Section 5:
Safety/Risk Management
- Abused child/elder
- Against medical advice patients
- Bullet removal
- Call backs in the emergency department
- Consent for emergency treatment
- Coroner's cases
- Disaster plan
- DUI blood sampling kit
- Expired patients
- Infection control
- Information released
- Insect control in the department
- Interhospital patient transfer
- Left without being seen patients
- Maintenance of equipment in the emergency department
- Narcotics/narcotic counting
- News media
- Nonsterile equipment cleaning
- Notification of police
- Procedures not performed in the emergency department
- Refusal of treatment
- Reporting of HIV testing
- Restraints in the emergency department
- Safety
- Traffic control
- Triage personnel
- Valuables

EMS, Emergency medical services; *ECG,* electrocardiogram; *MICN,* mobile intensive care nurse; *DUI,* driving under the influence.
NOTE: Some policies/procedures listed in the patient care protocol section may be placed in the safety/risk management section or vice versa (e.g., sexual assault examination, abused child/elder).

emergency department and provision of patient care. Inclusion of administrative and other hospital departments' policies and procedures that relate to emergency department operations is essential. The manual may include the emergency department's services and scope of practice, goals and objectives, job descriptions, community and referral resources, floor plan, staffing patterns, and organizational chart.

The manual should contain a table of contents in the order dictated by the institution but cross-indexed alphabetically for easy reference. External disaster plans and EMS standard operating procedures may also be included or cross-referenced as part of the emergency department's policies and procedures manual. Box 22-4 is an example of a comprehensive table of contents for an emergency department manual.

USE OF THE POLICY AND PROCEDURE MANUAL

The contents of the policies and procedures manual must be relevant and useful to the emergency department staff. The staff need to be aware of the existence of the manual, and refer to it for guidance in matters of high-risk and/or infrequently performed procedures. Policies and procedures must be appropriate and meaningful to the staff who are expected to use them.

New employee orientation should include use of the emergency department policies and procedures manual. Updates of the manual's content must be communicated to current staff to ensure compliance to the policies and procedures. Policies cross-referenced from administrative or other hospital department manuals must be easily accessible to the emergency staff for review, as needed.

SUMMARY

Development of policies and procedures for the emergency department is an integral part of management's scope of responsibility. Policies and procedures should be complete without being complex in content. Policies and procedures provide guidelines to safe and effective patient care that comply with accepted standards of emergency care and regulatory agency requirements. There should be multidisciplinary involvement in the formulation of emergency department policies and medicolegal input for high-risk areas. Annual review and update by department professionals is the minimal requirement to ensure current practice and technology in all policies and procedures.

The emergency department policies and procedures manual must be easy to access and use, and employees should be knowledgeable about its content. Well-defined policies and procedures, when properly used, increase the quality of patient care and decrease medicolegal liability for the emergency department, its staff, and the healthcare institution in which they operate.

ADDITIONAL READINGS

American Nurses Association: *Code for nurses with interpretive statements,* Kansas City, Mo, 1985, ANA.

Benner P: *From novice to expert: excellence and power in clinical nursing practice,* Menlo Park, Calif, 1984, Addison-Wesley.

Bethel P: Nursing care procedures: an operational focus, *Nurs Manage* 22:47-49, 1991.

Emergency Department Nurses Association: *Standards of emergency nursing practice,* St Louis, 1995, Mosby.

Fiesta J: Legal aspects: standards of care, *Nurs Manage* 24:30, 32, 1993.

Hamilton G, editor: *Presenting signs and symptoms in the emergency department: evaluation and treatment,* Baltimore, 1993, Williams & Wilkins.

Joint Commission on Accreditation for Health Care Organization: *Accreditation manual for hospitals, 1993,* Oakbrook, Ill, 1992, JCAHO.

May H, et al, editor: *Emergency medicine,* ed 2, Boston, 1992, Little, Brown.

Rosen P et al, editor: *Emergency medicine: concepts and clinical practice,* ed 3, St Louis, 1992, Mosby.

Shortell S, Kaluzny A, editors: *Health care management: a text in organization theory and behavior,* ed 2, Albany, NY, 1988, Delmar.

Van de Leuv J, editor: *Management of emergency services,* Rockville, Md, 1987, Aspen.

23 Nurse Practitioners in the Emergency Department

Suzanne M. Wall and Maureen Scahill

OUTLINE

In the 1960s the roles of both Nurse Practitioners (NPs) and Physician's Assistants (PAs) were developed to address a perceived shortage of primary care physicians. Over the years, these roles have expanded beyond primary care to a vast array of other areas and needs such as occupational medicine and orthopedics. During these past three decades physicians, patients, and institutions across the United States have come to depend on these practitioners. Larger numbers of people are seeking help with their healthcare needs in the emergency department annually, and as this provision of healthcare becomes more competitive and costly, new strategies to optimize patient care and maximize reimbursement are being used. The use of NPs and PAs in emergency care is one answer to optimize the provision of services in the emergency department.

On completion of this chapter the reader will be able to:

1. Describe the educational preparation of the NP.
2. Describe the scope of practice of the NP in the emergency setting.
3. Illustrate how an NP may be used in emergency services.
4. Discuss issues associated with the NP role, such as reimbursement, collaborative and independent practice, and prescriptive authority.

EDUCATION, CERTIFICATION, AND LICENSURE

Nurse practitioners are educated in graduate programs or certificate programs in community hospitals. These programs run for 9 to 24 months and offer a master's degree or certificate of completion. Some programs may also be structured as a post-master's certificate program. Specialization in areas other than primary care may occur through postgraduate education programs or on-the-job training. Completion of these programs prepares NPs to provide healthcare to a wide variety of patients, including emergency department patients. The estimated cost of this NP education is approximately one fifth that for medical school education.[1]

Certification of NPs, by the American Nurses Association (ANA), or American Academy of Nurse Practitioners (AANP), recognizes individuals who have met a national standard of practice and education. Beginning in 1992, NPs seeking certification must show evidence of advanced nursing education at the master's level or higher.[2] Certification demonstrates commitment to the profession and renewal requires continuing education and ongoing clinical practice by the individual. Certification is a voluntary process but in some states is a prerequisite for NP licensure.

Licensure varies by state, usually falls within the scope of the Board of Nursing, and entitles the nurse to practice (using the "Nurse Practitioner" title). Several states have joint regulation of practice by the Board of Nursing and Board of Medicine. As of 1996, nurse practitioners in 48 states have some degree of prescriptive authority.[3] However, there is wide interpretation of prescriptive authority. Of these 48 states with prescriptive authority, 15 identify independent prescribing. Independent prescribing is defined when the following criteria are met: (1) there are no physician cosignature requirements, (2) the Board of Nursing is the authorizing body for NP prescriptive authority, and (3) prescribing is not statutorily defined as a medical act.[3] The regulatory agency governing NPs in an individual state should be contacted regarding the specifics of that state.

EMPLOYMENT COSTS

The NP is regarded by many researchers, physicians, and nurses to be both complementary and substitutive to physicians in primary care because of the significant overlap of nursing and medicine functions in primary care. This substitutive role has been used to assist in determination of employment costs for NPs.

Substitution ratios have been determined by several different researchers for office visits in primary care practices.[4] These substitution principles rely heavily on appropriate delegation of responsibilities and on matching productivity between the two provider groups. In general it was found that with appropriate delegation of duties, four nonphysician healthcare providers could replace two to three physicians, with substitution ratios ranging from 0.50 to 0.75. That is, one NP could replace 0.50 to 0.75 of a physician's duties. Record and Schweitzer[5] applied these substitution ratios to an economic model simulating different practice and patient characteristics and found an overall substitution ratio of 0.63.

Salaries for NPs in 1995 averaged $50,000. Average salaries for NPs in 1992 were $45,000 and for physicians,

$130,000,[6,7,8] making the salary differential $85,000. This salary differential gives an employment cost ratio of 0.35 (45,000:130,000).

Federal law mandates direct reimbursement rates for Medicaid-funded pediatric and family services within the scope of individual state laws. Medicare reimbursement is also mandated; however, this is limited to specific situations, which are addressed later in this chapter. Using the values identified previously, one NP could substitute for 0.63 of a physician at 0.35 the physician cost. Even with the lower reimbursement rates, considerable savings can be realized. Thus in general, with proper delegation by a physician, an NP can perform approximately two thirds of the physician's duties at approximately one third the cost.

In the emergency department, delegation of patient care responsibilities to NPs for nonurgent complaints frees physicians to care for the more acutely ill. Careful review of patient logs should reveal specific patient populations that may be managed by NPs in a given setting. Review of patients who have left without being seen may reveal additional numbers of patients who could be managed by an NP, thereby capturing revenue that may otherwise be lost. These numbers determine a given volume of patients appropriate for management by the NP. Making use of the NP to care solely for patients with these nonurgent complaints, even at the lower Medicare reimbursement rate of 75% that of physicians, may help capture increased revenue by decreasing the numbers of patients who have left without being seen.

BOX 23-1

SAMPLE PRACTICE AGREEMENT

The Emergency Medical Associates of Strong Memorial Hospital or designees, agree to work in a collaborative practice with ______________.

Consultation with collaborative emergency physicians will be initiated by the nurse practitioner in situations that are outside of the scope of nurse practitioner practice. A note that the collaboration has occurred will be entered into the patient record by the collaborating emergency physician.

Should an emergency absence of a nurse practitioner occur, coverage will be provided within the department in accordance with current practice.

Referrals to other care providers, including but not limited to, physicians and social workers may be initiated by the nurse practitioner. Such referrals, with rationale for referral, will be entered into the patient record by the nurse practitioner. Written reports from consultants to whom patients have been referred will be discussed between the emergency physician and nurse practitioner.

Resolution of disagreements between the nurse practitioner and collaborating physician regarding matters of diagnosis and treatment are discussed and negotiated. If the issue is clearly a nursing problem, the collaborating physician will defer to the nurse practitioner; if the issue is a medical problem, the nurse practitioner will defer to the collaborating physician.

Nurse practitioners and physicians will participate in collaborative chart review. A random assignment of charts will be audited on a daily basis. A record of audited charts will be kept in the Director's Office.

Courtesy Strong Memorial Hospital of the University of Rochester, New York.

SCOPE OF PRACTICE

Clinical Responsibilities

Nurse practitioners, like physicians, are educated to use independent, professional judgment in the evaluation and treatment of patients.[9] As professionals, NPs recognize the limitations of their competence and know when to refer to other providers in terms of their ethic and legal obligation to the patient.

Practice Agreements. Independent practice of NPs is currently legislated in a handful of states. Oregon, one of the states that authorize the greatest independence, states that the NP is "independently responsible" for the provision of patient care and that the Board of Nursing is responsible for defining the NP scope of practice.[3] Collaborative practice is defined by the ANA as "a collegial working relationship with another healthcare provider in the provision of patient care. Collaborative practice requires the discussion of patient diagnosis and cooperation in the management of care."[10] In states that mandate collaborative practice, the use of a practice agreement and patient care protocols helps protect the patient, NP, physician, and institution. Practice agreements in collaborative practice (Box 23-1) should include provisions for unit coverage, responsibilities of care, and provisions for dispute resolution.

Protocols. Practice protocols assist NPs and their collaborating physicians in providing high-quality care and in some states are required for NP practice. A nurse practitioner can not legally "practice" medicine, but in collaboration with the physician can carry out medical acts.[11] Guidelines for the assessment, diagnosis, and treatment of a given illness (e.g., pharyngitis) set the standard for care. These standards may be developed along a site-specific framework or adapted from among the many different protocols available commercially. Commonly performed emergency care skills and procedures should be identified and the validation of knowledge assessed through a competency-based orientation period. Many of these procedures and skills, such as suturing and splinting, are not readily obtained through sources other than on-the-job training. Nurse practitioners, physicians, or PAs who possess these skills should be used to assist the new NP to become proficient in these commonly performed procedures. These validated skills and procedures should be included in the practice protocols (Box 23-2). Whatever source is used, both physician and NP should agree on the protocol and sign and date the defined protocol. These protocols should be reviewed and updated annually, at least, and should remain available on the unit for quick reference.

Collaborative practice with physicians is common for both NPs and PAs. Nurse practitioners, however, are able to conduct nursing practice without specific physician supervision. The PA is employed to assist in specific physician practices and is limited to carrying out medical tasks. The independent nursing practice of the NP may be a distinct benefit in the emergency department. The Joint Commission on Accreditation of Healthcare Organizations (JCAHO) requires specific nursing and medical documentation in the patient

BOX 23-2

SAMPLE EMERGENCY DEPARTMENT NURSE PRACTITIONER SKILLS INVENTORY

General Skills
- Obtain and document a detailed medical history focusing on the patient's presenting chief complaint
- Obtain and document an appropriate physical examination focusing on the presenting condition
- Order appropriate radiographic studies for the initial assessment of patients
- Order appropriate laboratory studies for the initial assessment of patients
- Write orders for medications and treatments
- Write prescriptions

Life Support
- Advanced Cardiac Life Support (ACLS)
- Pediatric Advanced Life Support (PALS)
- Advanced Burn Life Support (ABLS)
- Trauma Nurse Core Course (TNCC)

Orthopedic Procedures
- Assess and splint simple fractures of the long bones
- Apply skeletal traction
- Assess and manage sprains and strains

Minor Surgical Procedures
- Administration of anesthesia by local infiltration
- Perform digital block
- Irrigate, debride, and suture simple lacerations
- Incise and drain uncomplicated superficial abscesses
- Minor burn care
- Foreign body removal from superficial cutaneous sites
- Nail trephination
- Arthrocentesis

Other Procedures
- Insertion of nasogastric tubes, gastric lavage
- Performing arterial puncture for obtaining blood gas levels
- Anterior nasal cautery and packing
- Slit lamp ocular examination
- Ocular tonometry
- Foreign body removal from superficial cornea and sclera

record.[12] The NP is uniquely qualified to fulfill both documentation requirements. This ability to document both nursing and medical care may free the staff nurse from documentation time that may be better spent in direct care.

The ability to practice independently as well as collaboratively with physicians in the care of emergency patients makes the NP a versatile care provider. Determining patients who may be evaluated and treated independently by the NP in the emergency care setting enhances effective treatment of patients with minor or primary care needs. Fast-track or "quick-care" areas may be implemented (Box 23-3). Care for emergency patients after discharge is an appropriate advanced practice nursing function. Follow-up care for patients is often difficult to access, and many emergency treatments depend on reliable follow-up. Nurse Practitioners are cost-effective and appropriate healthcare providers to reassess wounds and lacerations, evaluate response to treatments, and reevaluate therapies. For example, the patient with community-acquired pneumonia could easily be reassessed by an NP in a follow-up, aftercare clinic affiliated with the emergency department or institution.

BOX 23-3

CONDITIONS APPROPRIATE FOR INDEPENDENT CARE BY THE NURSE PRACTIONER IN THE EMERGENCY DEPARTMENT*

Pharyngitis
Upper respiratory infections
Otitis
Asthma
Back pain
Extremity injuries
Urinary tract infections
Sexually transmitted diseases
Minor lacerations
Prescription refills
Headache
Rash
Foreign body removal
Minor burns
Localized allergic reactions
Minor ophthalmic complaints
Incision and drainage of abscesses

*Not inclusive: these are suggestions only.

Collaborative practice with physicians in the emergency department expands the breadth and depth of the patient population that may be seen by both providers. Care of more acutely ill patients may be accomplished by using the NP in the front line of care, either in an expanded triage role or to primarily assess patients seeking acute care. The NP is able to gather history and physical assessment data, order appropriate diagnostic studies, and begin the process of treatment or admission. Discussion and collaboration with the emergency physician validates or expands on measures taken by the NP. For example, the febrile patient with abdominal pain can have the history taken, laboratory studies ordered, pelvic examination performed, and diagnosis and treatment of pelvic inflammatory disease begun by the NP.

Nonclinical Responsibilities

The NP fulfills not only clinical, patient-care related activities, but also the roles of administrator, educator, and researcher. Both the Emergency Nurses Association[11] and the ANA[10] outline the importance of these facets of the NP role.

Administrator. As an administrator the NP may function as a coordinator for group practice, administer an NP-managed fast track,[13] organize schedules, and monitor budgets. Thus NPs are uniquely qualified to address legislative issues and health systems management issues at the institutional, local, state, and national levels. A unique perspective of patient care from both a nursing and medical viewpoint and knowledge of the societal problems of those seeking primary care within the emergency care system make the NP a strong patient advocate.

Educator. As an educator the NP provides both formal and informal programs of staff education and nursing, medical, and dental student education. This educator role helps model the professionalism of the NP to other disciplines and fosters awareness of collegiality between professions.

Researcher. As a researcher the NP with an advanced degree is qualified to assist or direct clinical research in the emergency care setting. The emergency department is an area of great potential for nursing and medical research, and the NP is uniquely positioned to participate in both arenas. The collaboration of NPs and emergency care physicians is an area with little objective data to validate the benefits of such an association and could present fertile territory for research.

Quality of Care. Professional responsibilities of the NP include maintaining standards set by the institution, state and federal government, and professional associations. Self and peer evaluations assist the NP in monitoring the quality of care provided. Peer review is a process by which NPs monitor, assess, and judge the quality of care. In a collaborative practice the physician and NP may review each other's care as a means to improve the overall quality of care. This peer review may be mandated in some states but should be a vital component of any NP practice.

Numerous studies focusing on the provision of NP services and their quality of care have been evaluated by the Office of Technology Assessment (OTA).[1] The OTA metaanalysis concluded that "within their areas of competence, NPs . . . provide care whose quality is equivalent to that of care provided by physicians." Not only are patients satisfied with the care they receive from NPs, but physicians who work with NPs are satisfied with their performance—more so than physicians who have little contact with NPs. In the arena of problems requiring technical solutions patients were more satisfied with the care provided by physicians, which reflects more extensive technical training on the part of physicians. In the effectiveness of interpersonal management, number of diagnostic tests ordered, thoroughness of diagnosis, and outcome measures, however, care given by NPs was superior to that of physicians as measured in both process and outcome measures in 12 different studies.

REIMBURSEMENT STRATEGIES

Federal law currently mandates direct Medicaid reimbursement for pediatric and family NPs for services that the NP is legally authorized to perform under state law, whether or not under the supervision of a physician.[8] The Health Care Financing Administration (HCFA) does allow the states to tailor the definition of NP to suit their individual needs by requiring only that the NPs be licensed and engaged in pediatric or family practice within the scope of the state law. HCFA's broad definition of services could be logically assumed to cover adult-care NPs performing patient care within the zone of overlap between adult and family scopes of NP practice.[9]

Medicare reimbursement for NPs is directed through Medicare Part B. Each state has specifics of availabilitv of a separate provider number and special coding for reimbursement. If a physician is present, services the NP provides will be "incident to" the physician's. The physician is not required to interact with every patient but is available on-site for consultation as needed. These incident to reimbursement rates will be the same as those of the physician. When the physician is not on-site, the reimbursement rates will vary. The setting, rural, urban, or contract Health Maintenance Organization (HMO), will determine the reimbursement schedule.[11]

With the arrival of capitation of care, Nurse Practitioners are in the forefront of providing cost-efficient services. Under capitation contracts, a fixed-dollar amount is allotted to HMOs and hospitals for care provided to patients. Since NPs are cost-efficient providers of services and have lower fixed costs (i.e., salaries), they may provide cost-competitive services. Negotiation of contracts for capitated care should include language for reimbursement of services provided by nurse practitioners.[3,11]

CLINICAL PRIVILEGES

It is necessary to acquire clinical privileges within the framework of the employment setting. In an institution the corporate board is responsible for granting clinical privileges. The board may give this authority to the hospital director or chief executive officer. Other institutions may require the entire board to grant privileges. An important step in this process is to determine the applicant's competence.

The professional disciplines of nursing and medicine are responsible to review the qualifications of the NP. For a physician the medical director would be responsible for this duty. For an NP this role may be filled solely by the nursing director or by a joint practice committee comprising nurses and physicians. The professional discipline groups have the responsibility to verify the applicant's credentials and competence.

The professional discipline(s) bases judgments on national and/or state standards, certification board examinations, and continuing education requirements. The individual practitioner's scope of practice should also be reviewed in this context. This is particularly important when the practitioner may be functioning in a role outside the realm of traditional practice (e.g., the NP in the emergency department setting).[14] In addition to reviewing certification credentials and scope of practice, the professional discipline may require verification of advanced training specific to the practice setting. For example, in the emergency department practice Advanced Cardiac Life Support, Pediatric Advanced Life Support, Advanced Trauma Nursing Course, or Emergency Nurse Pediatric Course certification may be required.[14] There are published guidelines available that can be used to develop a formal policy for granting the NP clinical privileges.[15]

Gaining clinical privileges has been a long-standing practice for physicians; however, it is a somewhat recent practice for nonphysician providers. Nonetheless, this process has become well established in many institutions and is a growing practice in many other settings.[15] Nurse Practitioners employed by institutions or hospitals are generally credentialed by the employing institution. In private physician practices such as emergency medicine contract groups clinical privileges are granted by the physicians' organization. In some of these organizations there are joint practice committees as well.[14]

The institution or private practice committee establishes a regularly timed interval (frequently annually or biannually) for reviewing credentials, practice scope, and treatment guidelines. This process is to ensure continued competence and accommodate any changes in practice. The practice committee may want to alter the NP's scope and duties. For example, the NP may plan to add joint aspiration or chest tube insertion to clinical practice and treatment guidelines for specific situations. The NP would submit evidence of advanced education and training in this procedure. Regular review and renewal of clinical privileges would include assessment of proposed changes.

In summary, the chief executive officer and institution's board have the sole authority to grant clinical privileges. They are ultimately responsible for the practitioner's activities within the scope of that particular practice. The professional discipline(s) is the advisor and validator. The individual practitioner has professional and personal accountability to fulfill the requirements set by the practice setting.

SUMMARY

Collaborative practice, with nurse practitioners and emergency care physicians working together to optimize patient care, will benefit *all* parties in the healthcare arena. Evidence supports the facts that NPs can provide services to patients with primary care needs who arrive at the emergency department and that NPs can collaborate with physicians to provide care to the more acutely ill population. The use of NPs fulfills both nursing and physician requirements for JCAHO documentation, as well as clinical, administration, research, and education roles in the emergency department.

Limitations on prescriptive authority in some states and third-party reimbursement limitations make it difficult for some patients to be adequately availed of the comprehensive services that can be provided by collaborative practice in the emergency department. Continued lobbying by physician, nursing, and consumer groups should assist in making these care choices more readily available.

REFERENCES

1. United States Office of Technology Assessment: Nurse practitioners, physicians assistants, and certified nurse midwives. *Policy analysis,* Washington, DC, 1986, United States Government Printing Office.
2. Price MJ, Martin AC, Newberry YG et al: Developing national guidelines for nurse practitioner education: an overview of the product and the process, *J Nurs Educ* 31(1):10–15, 1992.
3. Pearson LJ: 1992-93 Update: How each state stands on legislative issues affecting advanced nursing practice, *Nurse Practitioner* 18(1):23-38, 1993.
4. Poirer-Elliott E: Cost-effectiveness of non-physician health care professionals, *Nurse Practitioner* 9(10):54-56, 1984.
5. Record JC, Schweitzer S: Potential effects on staffing and costs: estimates from the model. In Record JC, editor: *Staffing primary care in 1990: physician replacement and cost savings,* New York, 1982, Springer.
6. Smithing R, Wiley M: Nurse practitioner salary survey results, *Nurse Practitioner* 20:78, 1996.
7. Brider P: Where did the jobs go? *Am J Nurs* 93(4):31-40, 1993.
8. Burda D: Physician pay, perks vary by employer, *Mod Healthc* 23:16, 1993, p 58.
9. Safriet B: Health care dollars and regulatory sense: the role of advanced practice nursing, *Yale J Regulation* 9(2):419-488, 1992.
10. American Nurses Association: *The scope of practice of the primary health care nurse practitioner,* Kansas City, Mo, 1985, The Association.
11. Emergency Nurses Association: Position statement: advanced practice in emergency nursing, *J Emerg Nurs* 17(6):33A, 1991.
12. Joint Commission on Accreditation of Healthcare Organizations: *Accreditation manual for hospitals,* Oakbrook Terrace, Ill, 1992, Joint Commission on Accreditation of Healthcare Organizations.
13. Covington C, Erwin T, Sellers F: Implementation of a nurse practitioner–staffed fast track, *J Emerg Nurs* 18(2):124-131, 1992.
14. Sherwood TA: A word about clinical privileging, *Nurs Manage* 22(2):52-52, 1991.
15. Melvin N: Developing guidelines for clinical privileges for nurse practitioners. In Steel, JE, editor: *Issues in collaborative practice,* New York, 1986, Grune & Stratton.

ADDITIONAL READINGS

American College of Emergency Physicians: *Guidelines for the role of nurse practitioners in emergency department (policy statement),* Dallas, 1995, American College of Emergency Physicians.

Cohen MM, Lanigan A: *Nurse practitioner protocols,* Tallahassee FL, 1989, Sunbelt Medical Publishers.

Emergency Nurses Association: *Advanced practice in emergency nursing: position statement,* Park Ridge, IL, 1994, Emergency Nurses Association.

Greensher A, Roemer H, Siemering K: *Ambulatory protocols for emergency care,* Bowie, MD, 1984, Prentice-Hall.

Hoole AJ, Greenberg RA, Pickard CG: *Patient care guidelines for nurse practitioners,* ed 3, Boston, 1988, Little Brown.

24 Nursing Methodologies: TEAM, PRIMARY, AND MODULAR

Regina M. Heiser

OUTLINE

Team nursing
Primary nursing
Modular nursing
Resources in emergency care
- Emergency medical technicians and paramedics
- Physician extender roles
- Unlicensed assistive personnel: nursing assistants, aides, patient care technicians

Nursing care model decision-making
Trends affecting nursing care model utilization
- Evaluation of nursing care models

Although emergency departments may vary in shape, size, and technology use, several similarities exist between rural and urban emergency departments. First, there is a diversity of patient and family needs that range in acuity from the most severe trauma to the nonurgent condition. Second, there is an unpredictable patient volume and, third, health services are expected to be provided on a 24-hour a day, year-round basis. Although the similarities between emergency departments are easily identified, it is the differences in patient population, nursing philosophy, size, location, and nursing activity that determine which nursing care model delivery system will be used.

The responsibility for providing adequate staffing of qualified professional nurses to ensure the delivery of safe care in the emergency department rests with the emergency nurse manager.[1] However, because of changing acuity levels, patient volume and mix, and nursing responsibilities, one universal staffing pattern or system cannot be effective for all emergency departments.

There are several nursing care delivery models functioning in hospitals and emergency departments. Some of these are primary nursing, team nursing, and modular (or zone) nursing. Each model has its advantages and disadvantages, and more than one model may be used within organizations. A trend in the future may be differentiated nursing practice. Differentiated nursing practice is a philosophy that recognizes role differentiation among nurses based on individual knowledge, skill, education, competence, and independent judgment. Any model or nursing care delivery system can be enhanced by the implementation of differentiated nursing practice.[2] Differentiated practice improves the delivery of patient care by providing a structure that efficiently utilizes scarce nursing resources while enabling nurses to optimize their practice and obtain compensation for their expertise.[3]

TEAM NURSING

Team nursing arose in the immediate post-World War II era as an attempt to organize a stratified nursing work force composed of professional, licensed practical, and ancillary support staff.[4] Team nursing is a hierarchic labor pattern in which specific nursing tasks and functions are performed based on rank. Patient care is supervised by the Registered Nurse (RN), or team leader, while care is delegated to various nursing support staff based on skill level and patient needs. Team nursing promotes differentiation between nurses (RN and Licensed Practical Nurse [LPN]); however, differentiation is based on educational levels or degree. Competency, skill, and clinical decision-making are additional abilities that differentiate nurses as they progress through stages of growth from novice to expert.[5] These abilities are not recognized in a team nursing model. The advantages of team nursing include a lowered cost for care because lower-skilled workers are utilized for lower-skilled work, combined access to knowledge and team expertise when working with difficult patients or patient situations, and the opportunity to foster leadership.[6] Critics of team nursing state that it fails to provide continuity of care because tasks are stratified based on nursing skill mix and work is task-oriented, not patient-centered. Delegating care to others increases nursing time spent in nonnursing functions. It is also a task and skill some nurses have difficulty doing. Subsequently, job satisfaction suffers as a result of a diminished nurse-patient relationship. Problems with accountability for care provided by other staff are identified by nurses as another dissatisfier. The disadvantages of team nursing promoted changes in patient care delivery that would evolve into primary nursing.

PRIMARY NURSING

In the early 1970s, the replacement of ancillary nursing personnel (LPNs and aides) by professional RNs began to impact and restructure team nursing. By the mid-1980s, primary nursing was the major nursing model.[4] Primary nursing can be described as both a philosophy of nursing and a method of organizing care.[7] The advantages of primary nursing are imbedded in its philosophy of accountability to the patient for patient care, nursing autonomy, the advancement of nursing as a profession, and the individualization of care based on the nurse-patient relationship. In team nursing the team is accountable for the delivery of patient care. In primary nursing the primary nurse is accountable for the patient's plan of care 24 hours a day for the duration of the nurse-patient contact.

Philosophically, primary nursing is a form of managed care. Primary nursing is a means to promote staff and patient satisfaction, enhance the quality of care, reduce hospital costs for care, and increase retention of nurses by increasing job satisfaction.[7,8]

The disadvantages of primary care include high recruitment and retention costs for an all-RN labor force, the mismatch between high-level nursing staff and low-skill tasks, the lack of team identity causing diminished nursing collaboration, and the lack of opportunity to develop leadership skills.[6]

The cost-effectiveness of primary nursing is controversial: some studies have reported this model to be more cost-effective,[9-12] and other studies found no difference between the cost of team and primary nursing.[13-15] Data from these studies cannot be subject to meta-analysis as a result of the variety of data collected and the time period analyzed.

A five-year cost comparison study by Gardner[8] of primary and team nursing showed that primary nursing provided higher-quality care than team nursing. Quality of care was measured by the Quality Patient Care Scale (Qualpacs) designed by Wandelt and Ager.[33] Patient stress was reduced on primary care units as measured by the Hospital Stress Rating Scale.[16] Infection and postoperative complications were monitored through quality assurance data, which showed no difference between primary and team nursing models. On primary care units nurses with higher educational levels were retained longer, resulting in cost savings. Costs were reduced in primary care areas because: 1) fewer supervisors and nursing administrators were needed, 2) fewer agency nurses were utilized, and 3) primary nurses were able to manage a higher and more complex patient: staff ratio than team nurses.[8]

MODULAR NURSING

Modular nursing has been described as a variation on team and primary nursing combining attributes of both systems.[6] Modular nursing, also called "district" or "zone" nursing, is a means to provide care for patients of varying acuity with a mixed nursing skill level. Modules are based on a geographic location of a group of patients. Staffing patterns for a module may consist of an RN and LPN team, an all-RN team, or an all-LPN team with an RN as charge nurse over several modules. The assigned nurse team is responsible for all patient care within its module. Advantages of modular nursing include increased continuity and quality of care when nurses are assigned to the same group of patients, collaboration among group members, increased efficiency and time savings, and decreased sense of isolation.[17] A disadvantage of modular nursing is increased planning time to coordinate care. No data on cost analysis of modular nursing are available. Shukla's[13] analysis of all three models, concluded that quality of care was not affected by the nursing care delivery system used. However, quality of care was affected by nurse competency in the delivery of care. Competency was rated by nonparticipant observers on units with similar patient needs. Cost analysis data show team nursing was the least expensive delivery care model.

RESOURCES IN EMERGENCY CARE

How can high-quality, cost-effective care be provided in emergency departments? This question is debated not only in emergency departments but throughout the healthcare system. Factors that impact the healthcare environment such as increased patient acuity, budgetary constraints, diminished ancillary support in radiology, materials management, social services, technologic advancements, healthcare reform, and the trend for outcomes management and evaluation also influence how staff and resources are used in emergency departments.

Emergency nursing is a specialized practice. The use of non-RN caregivers such as emergency medical technicians (EMTs), Paramedics (EMT-Ps), LPNs, Licensed Vocational nurses (LVNs), unlicensed assistive technicians (UAPs), nurse aides, nursing assistants, orderlies, emergency department technicians, and physician assistants (PAs) has created role confusion in the delivery of patient care in many emergency departments. The Emergency Nurses Association (ENA) states that all personnel in non-RN caregiver roles should be supervised by registered nurses.[1] However, state Nurse Practice acts mandate which personnel the Registered Nurse can supervise and, in many states, non-RN caregivers cannot be supervised by registered nurses. Problems that identified when non-RN caregivers are not supervised by nurses include inconsistent delivery of quality care, quality assurance, and collaborative practice.[1]

Since the 1950s, the numbers, titles, and job descriptions of non-RN caregivers have increased in an attempt to meet the need for emergency services and relieve nurses of non-nursing tasks.[18] In 1991 the American Hospital Association reported a 60% savings in nursing salaries when non-RN caregivers were employed. Using non-RN caregivers is a means to control rising hospital costs. However, the dissemination and utilization of technology accounts for the major portion of all healthcare costs. "Of the estimated sevenfold real increase in healthcare spending since 1950, new technologies and practice patterns account for up to 90% of the growth."[19] Variables such as length of stay, morbidity, and mortality are directly related to nursing resources in the provision of care and must be evaluated objectively before budgetary constraints are placed on nursing personnel.

Emergency Medical Technicians and Paramedics

The use of EMTs and EMT-Ps in the emergency department setting is cause for concern for several reasons: (1) variability in prehospital education, training, and preparation; (2) lack of role differentiation and responsibilities for care among RN staff, EMTs, and EMT-Ps; and (3) professional and personal liability for care provided in the emergency department by prehospital care experts.[18] A significant concern is the use of on-duty prehospital personnel to assist in emergency department care. Questions arise regarding patient abandonment and continuity and quality of care when on-duty personnel are activated to respond to a prehospital call for services.[20]

The National Association of Emergency Medical Technicians supports the use of EMTs and EMT-Ps in the emergency department to the fullest extent of their licensure and certification but not as a replacement for emergency care nurses.[21] Legislation proposed by the Alabama State Committee of Public Health (1991) introduced the utilization of EMT-Ps in emergency departments under the supervision of a physician or an RN. This proposal was in direct violation of the Nurse Practice Act of Alabama. In 1992 results of an ENA survey showed more than half of all states reported past or present experiences with the use of non-RN caregivers in the emergency department. The ENA position statement regarding non-RN caregivers in emergency care states that "all non-RN care givers involved in providing nursing care within the emergency care setting shall be directly supervised by and responsible to professional emergency registered nurses. In no case does ENA advocate the use of non-RN caregivers to provide nursing care in place of emergency nurses."[22]

Physician Extender Roles

Physician Assistants (PAs) trained in emergency care are another care-extender alternative. Physician Assistants are academically and clinically trained professionals who work under the supervision of a licensed physician.[23] Advantages of emergency-trained PAs include (1) less supervision time than medical residents from rotating specialties; (2) expertise in emergency medicine; (3) reduced waiting times resulting in increased patient satisfaction, reduction of malpractice liability, increased patient volume resulting in increased revenue; and (4) money saved in salaries.[23] These same advantages apply to nurses functioning in emergency departments as Family Nurse Practitioners (FNPs) or Case Managers. The concept of Nurse Practitioners (NPs) as physician extenders developed from the educational format of NP programs. Physicians and nurses were jointly responsible for directing NP programs. With the advent of increasing recognition of the NP as a nursing specialist, this perception has changed and continues to change.[24] Advanced practice nursing roles offer a unique service that extends beyond basic nursing care.

Unlicensed Assistive Personnel: Nursing Assistants, Aides, Patient Care Technicians

The use of UAPs as care-extenders was widely accepted during World War II with the creation of team nursing and the need for increased nursing care. With the advent of primary nursing, many hospitals released their UAPs for an all RN staff and then found themselves unable to provide adequate nursing when faced with a severe nursing shortage. Nursing assistants were recruited, again, into acute and non-acute care areas. UAPs are employed by 97% of hospitals and have a role in both direct and indirect patient care.[25-28]

The advent of healthcare reform has resulted in reengineering and restructuring of many processes within the hospital and healthcare system. Reengineering or "down-sizing" has resulted in the replacement of RNs with technicians and other care-extenders. This has been applauded as a money-saving effort and criticized for its impact on patient care.[29,30] The Magnet Hospital's study evaluated the relationship between staffing and quality care. Adequate staffing and high-quality care were highly correlated to job satisfaction and RN retention.[31]

The role of UAPs in the emergency department is longstanding. UAPs provide many non-nursing functions such as patient transport, housekeeping duties, inventory management, messenger services, or phlebotomy services. This allows nurses to focus on patient care, education, and manage patient flow within the department. Additional advantage to nursing assistant utilization in emergency departments involves lines of supervision, accountability, and responsibility. UAPs and nursing assistants are supervised by RN personnel. The roles and responsibilities of UAPs and nursing assistants are developed and overseen by emergency department nurse managers. Issues of delegation, consistency of performance, and training are critical to the successful use of UAPs in emergency departments.

Few, if any, emergency departments function without using non-RN caregiver personnel. Emergency nursing is unique in its reliance on triage, rapid assessment, decision-making skills, and proficiency in organizing and performing tasks. The role of non-RN caregivers can be a valuable adjunct to nursing care.

NURSING CARE MODEL DECISION-MAKING

How does a manager know which nursing care model is best suited for the emergency department? Traditionally, emergency department models were based on history—the "we have always staffed this way" model—or on the model used within the hospital (primary, team, or modular).

Whatever nursing care model is used in the emergency department, it must be the system that provides the best quality of care with maximum efficiency. For large, busy emergency departments, the model may include triage and/or fast-track patient services. Small emergency departments may use primary or team nursing in a zone or territory format. Patient acuity, volume, services provided (level I trauma care, in-house endoscopy performed in the emergency department, outpatient services, tertiary care vs. primary care), and patient mix are factors that influence the utilization of nursing care models. No longer should patient care census be the only variable used to determine staffing patterns. The ENA supports the continuing development, implementation, and evaluation of patient classification systems.[32]

Patient classification systems, while still not completely accurate in predicting staffing needs, are currently the best measure of patient acuity and volume. Patients are classified into a basic three-tier system that determines the need for care, such as emergent, urgent, and nonurgent. Some systems are based on a five- to seven-tier system that attempts to classify patients into a broader scale (see Chapter 20 for further information).

Some emergency departments classify patients at triage and at discharge in an attempt to capture the acuity of patients who have acute changes in status while in the department. Many classification systems are not only useful in ensuring that the most acutely ill patients obtain treatment in a timely manner, but are also being linked to financial reimbursement for nursing care services provided in the emergency department.

TRENDS AFFECTING NURSING CARE MODEL UTILIZATION

Several trends in emergency care have the potential to impact nursing care delivery systems in the emergency department.

With the increasing use of triage as an effective, efficient means to identify patients needing acute care, staffing needs and patterns are affected. Increased staff is necessary to provide triage personnel. Research demonstrates that expert nurses are more accurate at predicting admissions and patient needs than are novice triage personnel.[34] The use of non-RN caregivers as triage personnel may continue to pose problems for emergency departments.

The advent and implementation of fast-track systems will impact nursing care delivery models. Fast-track systems provide a means to quickly give care to patients with nonurgent conditions during hours when emergency departments are traditionally at peak operation. Fast-track systems can be staffed by PAs, a physician, and an RN, or NPs. This variety of staffing allows for flexibility but has the potential to create additional role confusion in emergency care.

Trends that have the potential to decrease staffing needs, promote cost containment in healthcare, and expedite patient care involve the use of critical pathways; advanced patient classification systems; case management through implementation of clinical guidelines; use of computerized patient tracking systems, emergency nurse practitioners; work redesign, such as flexible staffing, float or stat pools; and salaried nursing staff.

Evaluation of Nursing Care Models

Evaluating staffing patterns and nursing care provided in the emergency department can be a manager's nightmare. Although several computerized systems work effectively for the in-house patient population, these systems, when applied to emergency patients, cannot capture the unpredictable volume and acuity of the emergency department. It is essential that models be evaluated in relation to cost, efficiency, and patient outcomes, and any information system implemented in the emergency department must be able to provide these data.

Nursing care delivery systems should agree with departmental goals. Many emergency nursing departments have a philosophy of care that the nursing care delivery system should support. For example, if the emergency department philosophy is individualized patient care, primary nursing within a zone format may be the best choice for that department.

A manager must have a working knowledge of patient census, acuity, and patient needs and outcomes (desired and actual) to determine which nursing care delivery system will provide the most benefit. Staffing patterns are also impacted by length of patient stay, amount and type of patient teaching (preoperative, discharge, admission, or transfer), numbers and types of procedures performed in the emergency department requiring nursing assistance, and the types of nursing duties performed (triage, nonnursing responsibilities performed by nursing, on-duty management staff, patient follow-up activities, or referrals).

Staffing patterns and nursing care delivery models are affected by nurse retention, recruitment, and turnover. For example, team nursing utilizes a team leader. If an emergency department is a mix of novice staff with few proficient or expert staff members, team nursing may be an effective care delivery model while novice staff is maturing and gaining skills.

Cost containment is a challenging issue to all managers (see Chapter 46 for more information). Collaborative practice between nursing and emergency physicians is essential for quality, cost-effective patient care. Standards of care, clinical guidelines, and critical pathways are a means to affect both quality and cost of care. These should be developed collaboratively and impact nursing care delivery models in the decision as to who, when, and how care will be differentiated.

Evaluation of nursing care delivery systems is conducted using classification and quality assessment data. For example, the acute myocardial infarction patient should not only be treated emergently in terms of nursing and physician care, but also must receive the same quality of care in terms of pharmacologic support or electrocardiogram response time as a patient in the cardiac intensive care unit. According to Sovie,[29] "we must critically examine what needs to be done, what difference it makes in patient outcomes, and the best way to do it to produce the desired results."[35] Ultimately, each emergency department has the opportunity to become an autonomous unit where creative approaches to patient care are a continual challenge.

REFERENCES

1. Emergency Nurses Association: *Position statement: nurse staffing in the emergency care setting,* Chicago, 1991, The Association.
2. Ehrat KS: The value of differentiated practice, *J Nurse Adm* 21(4):9-10, 1991.
3. McClure ML: Differentiated nursing practice: concepts and considerations, *Nurs Outlook,* 39(3):106-110, 1991.
4. Brannon RL: The reorganization of the nursing labor process: from team to primary nursing, *Int J Health Services* 20(3):511-523, 1990.
5. Benner P: *From novice to expert,* Menlo Park, Calif, 1984, Addison-Wesley.
6. Curran CR: There is no pure air, there is no pure water, and there are no pure nursing care delivery models! *Nurs Econ* 10(2):157-158, 1992.
7. Higgins M, Dixon P: Skill mix and the effectiveness of nursing care, *Nurs Standards* 7(4):19-21, 1992.
8. Gardner K: A summary of findings of a five-year comparison study of primary and team nursing, *Nurs Res* 40(2):113-117, 1991.
9. Wolf GA, Lesik LK, Leak AT: Primary nursing: the impact on nursing costs, *J Nurs Adm* 16(3):9-11, 1986.
10. Jones K: Study documents effect of primary nursing on renal transplant patients, *Hospitals* 49(24):1975.
11. Marram G: The comparative costs of operating a team and primary nursing unit, *J Nurs Adm* 6:21-24, 1976.
12. Betz M: Some hidden costs of primary nursing, *Nurs Health Care* 2:150-154, 1981.
13. Shukla AK: All-RN model of nursing care delivery: a cost-benefit evaluation, *Inquiry* 20:173-184, 1983.
14. Schultz MA, Bender MA: The change to primary nursing: a high-quality endeavor, *Health Matrix* 4(3):25-28, 1986.
15. Chavigny K, Lewis A: Team or primary nursing care? *Nurs Outlook* 32:322-327. 1984.
16. Volicer BJ, Burns M: Preexisting correlations of hospital stress, *Nurs Res* 24:408-417, 1977.
17. Bennett MK, Hylton JP: Modular nursing: partners in professional practice, *Nurs Manage* 21(3):20-24, 1990.
18. Curry JL: Oil on troubled waters: unlicensed assistive personnel in the emergency department, *J Emerg Nurs* 18(5):428-431, 1992.
19. Manning WG, Newhouse JP, Duan N et al: Health insurance and the demand for medical care, *Am Econ Rev* 77(3):251, 1987.
20. Wisecup JW: Paramedics in the emergency department, *J Emerg Nurs* 18(5):372, 1992.
21. National Association of Emergency Medical Technicians: *Position statement: role of the emergency medical technician in the emergency department,* Kansas City, MO, 1992, The Association.
22. Emergency Nurses Association: *Position statement: the use of non–registered-nurse (non-RN) care givers in emergency care,* Chicago, 1993, The Association.

23. Sturman KM, Ehrenber K, Salzberg, MR: Physician assistants in emergency medicine, *Ann Emerg Med* 19(3):304-308, 1990.
24. Kitzman H: The CNS and nurse practitioner. In Hamric AB, Spross JA, editors: *Clinical nurse specialist in theory and practice,* Philadelphia, 1989, WB Saunders.
25. Huber DG, Blegen M, McCloskey JC: Use of nursing assistants: staff nurse opinions, *Nurs Manag* 25:64-68, 1994.
26. Mills ME, Tilbury MS: Restructuring safety, quality, and cost: nursing administration's perspective, *Nurs Policy Forum* 1:17-19, 1995.
27. Manuel P, Alster K: Unlicensed personnel: no cure for an ailing healthcare system, *Nurs Health Care* 15:18-21, 1994.
28. Boston C, Vestal K: Work transformation, *Hosp Health Netw* 12:50-55, 1994.
29. American Nurses Association: How hospitals are saving: work redesign tops cost-cutting efforts, *Am J Nurs* 95:70, 1995.
30. Anders G: Hospitals RX for high costs: fewer nurses, more aides, *Wall Street Journal,* Feb 10: section B1,B4, 1995.
31. Kramer M, Schmalenberg C: Job satisfaction and retention: insights for the '90s, *Nursing* March/April 50-55, 1991.
32. Emergency Nurses's Association: Position statement, nurse staffing in the emergency care setting, Chicago, 1991, Emergency Nurse's Association.
33. Wandelt MA, Ager JW: *Quality patient care scale,* New York, 1974, Appleton-Century-Crofts.
34. Hawk M: Triage nursing expertise: the difference between novices and experts, *J Emerg Nurs* 17:6, 429, 1991.
35. Sovie MD: Clinical nursing practices and patient outcomes: evaluation, evolution, and revolution, *Nurs Economics* 7(2):79-85, 1989.

25 Patient Disposition

Thomas A. Scaletta and Ellen Taliaferro

OUTLINE

The practice of emergency medicine generally focuses on short-term problem solving, but many outpatient management plans require attention to long-term issues. Therefore, to provide quality patient care and to minimize medicolegal risk, every patient who is registered into the emergency department but not admitted to the hospital requires an appropriate, individualized aftercare plan. In most emergency departments this applies to 80% to 90% of all patients seen. Thus busy emergency departments are constantly challenged to provide appropriate dispositions.

Certain Emergency Department patients (i.e., those with multiple medical problems) are in need of *comprehensive* aftercare plans.[1] For instance, a victim of domestic violence arriving at the emergency department with a facial fracture has two serious problems. The fracture must be treated appropriately, specific aftercare instructions given, and a follow-up referral arranged. In addition, a safe environment and ongoing counseling should be offered.

Clinical standards for the practice of emergency medicine must be complaint specific and focus on difficult disposition decisions.[2] When discharging patients, the following issues should be addressed:

- It must be determined, to the extent possible, that the patient will be able to perform self-care in a competent and rational manner, or suitable supervision must be arranged.
- Complications or worsening/recurrence of the disease process must be anticipated, and the patient must be instructed on how to recognize and respond to these possibilities.
- Arrangements must be made for the patient to receive follow-up care from a competent physician who is prepared to care for the patient's problem.[3]
- The patient or family needs to understand the nature of the care provided, as well as the discharge arrangements.

EFFECTIVE PATIENT DISPOSITION

Process of Disposition Determination

The disposition decision process is extremely challenging and complex; once the diagnosis has been made, there are many uncertainties associated with this process. It is often difficult to anticipate the likelihood of worsening of a disease state (e.g., an oral antibiotic failure) or to foresee an abrupt recurrence of a chronic problem (e.g., an asthma exacerbation). The degree of divergence from a patient's baseline level of function weighs heavily in the disposition decision. However, when this is determined indirectly either from the medical record or through recollections from the private physician, it may be imprecise and result in overly optimistic assumptions. The disposition decision is further muddied because, although objective hospital admission criteria for certain medical problems have been developed and reported in the literature, in many cases such criteria remain vague and subjective.[1]

Compounding social factors must be incorporated into the disposition decision. These include level of literacy, amount of familial support, homelessness, lack of healthcare insurance, chemical dependency, and involvement in abusive relationships. There should be a strong liaison between the emergency department and the hospital social services department, since many patients will need temporary housing, counseling referrals, cab vouchers, medications, and visiting nurses. Knowledge of the local demographics of an emergency department population, including prevalent languages spoken, enhances communications and makes the disposition process more effective. Emergency physicians should base all disposition decisions on the projected likelihood of a favorable outcome and should practice within a wide margin of safety.

Difficult Disposition Decisions

The emergency physician should speak with the assigned continuing care provider about every difficult disposition decision. It is not enough to discuss only cases requiring admission.[3,4] Speaking with private physicians allows communication of important medical information, ensures close follow-up, and maintains good public relations. The emergency physician remains the most appropriate and responsible physician to render a disposition decision, since he or she has performed the most recent interview and examination.[4,5] In light of this, no bargaining should occur with an off-site physician when the emergency physician believes a hospital admission is absolutely necessary. However, when dealing with borderline disposition decisions, the emergency physician may appropriately agree to discharge a patient if early follow-up is ensured by the continuing care provider. Such patients should be given detailed instructions and discrete parameters for their immediate return to the emergency department. Meticulous documentation becomes a medicolegal necessity: including all conversations with the continuing care provider.

Conflict Resolution

Disagreement concerning the proper disposition of a patient is common among physicians (especially among those with differing specialties), since criteria for hospital admission for many medical problems are relatively subjective. In addition, emergency physicians generally have a lower threshold for admitting patients than continuing care providers, since the patient's medical baseline or ability to follow aftercare instructions cannot be established without the benefit of a long-term patient-physician relationship. Unresolved disagreement with the emergency physician over an admission decision mandates that the admitting physician evaluate the patient in the emergency department and write a note of intent to assume care of the patient. Emergency physicians must always remain staunch patient advocates and never succumb to the pressures of merely wanting to accommodate the continuing care provider in making a particular disposition. Patients and their families should be kept informed of irreconcilable differences in medical opinion so they can contribute to the final decision.

Economic pressures may lead many private physicians and hospital administrators to discourage the admission of medically indigent patients. "Pre-established guidelines for interfacility transfer or treatment of private health plan patients in emergency situations will avert patient anger and frustration as well as adverse outcomes that compromise care."[1]

To solve disagreements, "principled negotiation," as described in *Getting to Yes*,[6] should be used over traditional positional bargaining. Positional bargaining can be illustrated by the following hypothetic conversation at a garage sale:

Mr. Smith: I'll give you $10 for that old lawn mower.
Ms. Jones: Old? Why it's only been used a couple of times! I want $100.
Mr. Smith: For that piece of junk? How about $30?

Positional bargaining may be effective but strays from honesty and fairness. As an alternative, principled negotiation uses objective facts to focus on relevant issues, not on the individuals with differing views. For instance:

Mr. Smith: I'm interested in that lawn mower.
Ms. Jones: I've had it for over 10 years and have had no problems. The blade needs to be sharpened though.
Mr. Smith: I saw a similar model for sale in last week's newspaper for $50, but it was sold when I called.

Paraphrasing the issues demonstrates full understanding of the other party's concerns. There are no longer opponents, only proponents inventing creative ideas for mutual satisfaction.

When negotiation fails, an "expert" should resolve disputes. Preapproved hospital executive committee policies and procedures should be in place and used to settle disagreements between physicians. When this method fails, an appropriate and responsible arbitrator with extensive clinical experience should "break the tie."[1] The departmental chairman or the chief of medical staff is generally the most appropriate arbitrator. When others are involved in the decision-making process, the emergency physician's medicolegal risk is reduced but never eliminated. If admission disputes for certain medical problems continually recur, then interdepartmental policies should be agreed on to provide long-term solutions.

Use principled negotiation to settle admission disputes as follows:

1. *By avoiding positional bargaining.* Remove emotions, blame, and confrontation from the negotiation process. Maintain composure and be diplomatically persistent.
2. *By presenting only relevant objective facts.* Reference prior studies, textbooks, or policies. The goal is always optimal patient care and advocacy.
3. *By creating options for mutual gain.* For instance, when possible, seek a more sympathetic admitting physician.
4. *By using a suitable arbitrator to settle unresolved disagreements.*

For further information concerning principles of negotiation see Chapter 6.

Emergency Physician–Patient Communication

Physician approachability improves patient satisfaction and compliance and may correct any misunderstandings about the seriousness of a diagnosis and the importance of the aftercare plan.[6,7] Not all malpractice claims are filed because of a suboptimal outcome: the patient may simply feel he or she was treated poorly. The attitude of the entire emergency department staff is critical. Simply keeping families and significant others updated on a patient's progress greatly improves relations. The main reasons for breakdown in emergency physician–patient communication are poor rapport and lack of explanation of the diagnostic plan.[8] Emergency physicians must show respect and compassion for patients and continually educate them about their illnesses. When the potential for bad outcomes is emphasized, those who fare well are generally pleased with their emergency department care.

So as not to undermine the patients' confidence in his or her medical care, it is recommended that discussions regarding disagreement between physicians not occur in the presence of patients, families, or significant others unless a resolution cannot be reached between physicians.

DISCHARGE TEACHING

Role of the Emergency Physician

Emergency physicians are ultimately responsible for disposition decisions and should guide nurses and house staff in the disposition process.[1] To create the best aftercare plan, the emergency physician should inquire about the patient's living arrangement, occupation, alternatives for continuing medical care, and ease of transportation to follow-up appointments.

The emergency physician should fully explain the diagnosis, treatment, and optimal aftercare plan to the patient. Outlining the pertinent risks of noncompliance with the aftercare plan allows the patient to make an informed decision of whether to follow the instructions.[1] In the interest of efficient time management, the emergency physician should begin patient education regarding self-care once it is likely that the patient will be discharged. When contemplating several possible diagnoses, the emergency physician's degree of certainty or uncertainty for each should be explained to the patient. This practice is seldom perceived as incompetence.[9]

Role of the Emergency Nurse

Emergency nurses play a vital role in patient disposition and should allocate adequate time for teaching and reinforcing aftercare instructions to patients, families, and significant others. Many nurses are more sensitive to relevant psychosocial issues and less intimidating than physicians, allowing patients, family members, and significant others to ask more questions. Some emergency departments use audiovisual materials to emphasize important instructions.[1] Nurses must be sure a patient acknowledges full understanding of the problem and plan and before obtaining his or her signature.

A designated nurse with special education and interest in delivering aftercare instructions often does the best job but can "burn out" because of the repetitious nature of this task.[1] Also, a single nurse delivering aftercare instructions for all the emergency department patients creates yet another queue that increases patient waiting time if backlogs occur.

Ancillary Services

Certain specially trained individuals can be used for certain aspects of discharge teaching of emergency department patients. Examples include involving physical therapists for crutch training, respiratory therapists to demonstrate correct use of inhalers, or specialized nurses for diabetic patient teaching or burn care.

Non–English-speaking patients should be provided with appropriate aftercare instructions that they can understand. The 1993 Joint Commission on Accreditation of Hospital Organizations (JCAHO) standard (ES.1.5) states the following: "When required frequently in the emergency care area, there is a means of communicating in the languages of the predominant population groups served by the hospital's emergency department." When available, in-house language translators should be present at discharge to address any questions the patient, family members, or significant others might have of the nurse of physician and must record the aftercare instructions in the patient's native language. When an in-house translator is unavailable, the emergency department staff can use the AT&T Language Line Services, which provide translation of virtually any language by telephone for subscribers.*

Socioeconomically deprived patients present special problems. Medical social workers are trained to solve some of these problems by arranging necessary shelter, transportation, and access to appropriate resources (i.e., visiting nurses, delivered meals, or support groups). Psychiatrists or crisis workers help greatly in determining the appropriate disposition of patients with mental illnesses and can provide information on resources for ongoing treatment or counseling.

Patients identified as *chronic* emergency department users can be categorized by their primary underlying problem (i.e., chemical dependency, psychiatric disorder, or chronic medical problems), and an appropriate case manager assigned to each. Emergency department recidivists usually represent a small proportion of total patients but per individual use a great deal of emergency department resources. Case managers can oversee the medical care of these patients and ensure that their continuing care occurs outside the emergency department whenever possible.

CONTENT OF AFTERCARE INSTRUCTIONS

Description of the Diagnosis

It is important to provide the patient with a concise description of his or her diagnosis. Avoidance of medical terminology allows clearer understanding by patients. Patient education materials can be purchased or adopted from medical texts that are geared toward the general public. Special attention should be made to address the following facts: 40% of adult patients in the emergency department read at or below an eighth-grade level, and 20% are functionally illiterate. This is important because most of the current patient reference materials are written at a high school or college level.[9-11] To improve comprehension use simple sentence structure, vocabulary devoid of medical "jargon," and plenty of diagrams as ways to ensure that the discharge instructions are below an eighth-grade level of comprehension.[11,12] Repetition and highlighting of important points are extremely helpful.

Problem-Specific Aftercare Instructions

The development of standardized protocols for follow-up care is beneficial in the care of common, specific problems. For example, consider the results of a study of 197 parents of children with otitis media who were seen at the Children's Hospital of Wisconsin in Milwaukee. Those who were given *standardized* instructions, either verbal or written, had significantly increased knowledge of their children's illnesses within 3 days of the emergency department visit, were more satisfied, and had a significantly lower revisit rate than those with *nonstandardized* instructions.[12]

In addition to instructing the patient in what *to do* for self-care, it is essential to explain what *not to do*. Set objective limits to guide the patient as to which activities are appropriate and which are inappropriate.[3] Recommendations should be specific to the patient's occupation, hobbies, personal priorities, social situation, and education level. "If . . . then" statements should dominate the instructions.

---

*411 Pacific St., Suite 301, Monterey, CA 93940 (1-800-752-6096).

Warning Symptoms

Discharge instructions should explicitly list symptoms that may be associated with a worsening medical course and would necessitate an immediate return visit to the emergency department. A generic statement (e.g., "If your illness worsens or any concerning symptoms develop, return to the emergency department immediately. Do not wait until your follow-up appointment.") is helpful, but the absence of specificity makes interpreting "concerning symptoms" difficult for patients. Emergency department aftercare instructions should include the names of the healthcare providers and the telephone number of the emergency department to allow easy recontact should questions arise or problems occur at home.

Prescription Information

Written information should be given to patients for all medications prescribed or dispensed from the emergency department. Generic and trade names should be included, as well as reason for the drug's use, time and route of administration, proper dosage, frequency, and duration—all in plain language.[13] Patients are more compliant when they understand the seriousness of their disease and how therapy will lead to improvement.[14] It is important to list only common or serious side effects and adverse reactions and to indicate when patients should discontinue a medication. An all-inclusive list of side effects and adverse reactions may prove more problematic than helpful.

In some emergency departments drugs are dispensed directly to the patient. Although this practice guarantees that patients obtain their medications, it must comply with federal and state regulations. In some states only physicians or pharmacists can complete drug labels and dispense medications. Dispensing schedule-2 medications, which requires triplicate prescription forms, should be an unusual event for emergency physicians, and specific reasons for using these drugs must be carefully documented.

Disclaimers

Disclaimers are important components of aftercare instructions. Standard disclaimers explain the hospital's system for informing patients of culture results or discrepancies in electrocardiogram or radiograph interpretation. It is important that patients are informed of the dangers in *not* complying with the aftercare instructions. This practice will minimize the medicolegal risk when problems occur as a result of noncompliance.

Referral Information

All emergency department patients need a designated referral for follow-up care within a specified time interval. Referral information should include the name of the continuing care provider or clinic, address and phone number, and business hours. Emergency departments able to assign "on-the-spot" referral appointments may well increase patient compliance with follow-up.

Medical Work and School Excuses

All work or school excuses should remain part of the medical record. The date of return and any activity restrictions should be expressly stated. When duration of activity restriction is unclear, the emergency physician should defer to the referral physician, who may discontinue or extend the restrictions at the time of the follow-up appointment. Patients visiting from out of town may require documentation of the need to alter travel plans.

Injury and Illness Prevention Information

During discharge teaching, emergency physicians and nurses play a key role in the area of injury and illness prevention. Standard injury prevention warnings can be given either routinely or when particularly applicable. Examples include the following:

- Always wear a seatbelt when driving a car and a helmet when riding any cycle.
- Never drive while under the influence of alcohol or drugs.
- Smoking is a serious health risk and should be discontinued at once.
- See your doctor for regular checkups and to arrange tests that screen for cancer.

In one study the issues most important to patients at an urban, public hospital were firearm homicide prevention and safe sex.[15] These highly relevant, preventive healthcare topics are only recently being routinely incorporated into emergency department aftercare instructions.

Signature and Documentation

Signatures acknowledging the patient's understanding of their aftercare instructions may shield the emergency physician from some degree of medicolegal liability when patients are noncompliant.[3] Preceding the patient's signature should be a statement like the following: "I completely understand and will follow all the above instructions." Getting the patient's signature, or that of a responsible third party, in legal terms, "puts them on notice." Documentation must reflect that the aftercare instructions were given and that the risks of noncompliance are fully understood.[16] A copy of aftercare instructions should become part of every patient's permanent medical record: it becomes critical evidence if a lawsuit is filed. During discharge teaching the potential for problems, such as complications, treatment failures, disease recurrence, or other maloccurrences, should be emphasized. Patients must be informed of the risk of noncompliance.

COMPUTERIZED AFTERCARE INSTRUCTIONS

Computer programs that generate individualized aftercare instructions strengthen the multidisciplinary discharge process by increasing patient satisfaction, improving staff efficiency and effectiveness, adding information to existing databases, and satisfying the JCAHO standards for discharge planning.[17] Currently at least 10 software programs are available for creating aftercare instructions. Before choosing any one of these programs, the emergency department clinical directors should review several programs, since there is a great deal of diversity in the systems and in the user's expectations.

The most basic system is a stand-alone microcomputer with a monitor and printer. There is a fundamental dichotomy between MS-DOS and Macintosh operating systems and software. When purchasing hardware, there are many cost-benefit considerations: faster processors, larger hard disk space, increased RAM, and laser printers "speed up" the process but increase expense. Choosing one system over another depends on available resources and prior experience specific to the emergency department and staff.

One sophisticated, important feature of the more advanced programs is the ability to interface with the hospital's mainframe computers. This avoids the need to reenter information, such as patient demographics, while simultaneously providing computer storage of discharge information that can be used for documentation and periodic reporting purposes.

The software should be well documented, and ongoing technical support is crucial. There is always an initial learning curve before an end-user can easily navigate any program. Many systems are mouse driven and may be modified to incorporate touch screens or light pens. Nearly all programs use menus to choose among various diagnoses, medications, follow-up plans, and other parameters. Excellent measures of user friendliness include the time it takes a new user to generate discharge instructions and the ease by which any mistakes can be corrected.

It is important to critique the end product—the medical content and accuracy of the aftercare instructions. Ideally the reading level should be below eighth grade.[11,12] Most programs provide conversion to Spanish, and some allow increased text size for visually impaired patients. The system should allow the user to choose multiple diagnoses and medications for a single patient when necessary. Some programs incorporate medication interactions and allergy cross-checking. Standard disclaimers and injury prevention warnings are universal.

Most programs contain a database of all possible follow-up physicians or clinics, which can be regularly updated. Some allow information about the daily on-call physicians to be printed automatically when a certain medical or surgical specialty is selected, to facilitate appointment making.

Customizability allows discharge instructions to be permanently modified to accommodate institutional or physician biases or unique patient populations. In addition, outdated information can be continually updated by the emergency department staff responsible for maintaining the program. Immediate, on-line editing allows instructions to be personalized for individual patients whenever necessary.

Most programs can produce school or work excuses when applicable. Some programs can automatically create prescriptions using a second printer. The most advanced systems integrate registration information on a real-time basis into a database that can be used to write periodic reports, identify high-risk patients, perform time-study analyses, or simply keep a log of the instructions that specific patients received.

Cost of hardware ranges from $2000 for a single basic workstation (i.e., hard disk, monitor, and printer) to $20,000 for a network of three high-quality workstations. Software prices for simple systems start at about $1000. Advanced systems capable of interfacing with hospital mainframe computers cost over $10,000. Voice-activated dictation systems designed for "paperless charting" and aftercare instruction generation can exceed $50,000.

FOLLOW-UP CARE AND COMPLIANCE

Studies have shown a 30% to 50% follow-up rate in both urban and suburban hospitals. Researchers at the Oregon Health Sciences University discovered seven predictors of good compliance with follow-up. These predictors were found to include older age, referral back to an established clinic, evaluation by a consultant in the emergency department, and the use of "mandated" clinic appointments assigned in the emergency department.[18]

Some patients, when discharged from the emergency department, design their own self-care and may completely ignore the emergency department aftercare instructions.[3,19] Interestingly, one study found that 10% of patients sought additional medical care within 72 hours after leaving the emergency department, *independent* of their scheduled follow-up appointment.[10]

One axiom of emergency medicine is that every patient, by definition, had an "emergency" and ought to be followed up.[3] There are several options for arranging follow-up care after an emergency department visit. A specified appointment with a continuing care provider or clinic can be made from the emergency department. As an alternative, the patient may be instructed to arrange his or her own appointment with a certain provider or clinic.

Some facilities arrange for patients to be scheduled for return to the emergency department on a particular date and time. This practice may enhance department revenue, but it may contribute to emergency department overcrowding and patient dissatisfaction when unexpected waits occur.

In some circumstances it may be appropriate for patients to simply receive a list of warning signs and be instructed to seek medical care should concerns arise. However, "as needed" follow-up requires that the patient make a judgment regarding disease severity, and this practice increases medicolegal risk. "Mandated" follow-up, on the other hand, leaves no room for misinterpretation.

Patients requiring reevaluation should be referred to an appropriate continuing care provider within a *predefined* time interval. In reality, follow-up appointments are often made at a time mutually convenient for the patient and the continuing care provider, rather than within the time interval specified by the emergency physician. This practice is not acceptable if the emergency physician believes that it will compromise the care of the patient. To arrange timely follow-up, cases should be discussed with the continuing care provider and a copy of the emergency department chart forwarded to that provider.[1] The 1993 JCAHO standard (ES.7.1.1)[20] recommends as a quality improvement measure that "a copy of the record of emergency services provided be available to the practitioner or medical organization responsible for follow-up care." Many private physicians routinely investigate the well-being of their patient upon receiving a copy of the department record.

For underprivileged patients at teaching hospital clinics, waits of weeks or months may occur before follow-up appointments can be scheduled. "Overbookings" may be arranged for more urgent cases by obtaining special approval from consultants.[18] Whenever waits for follow-up care impose a significant risk to the well-being of patients, clinical directors and hospital administrators should intervene. Medical social workers may be able to arrange community agency referrals (e.g., visiting nurses or "free" clinic visits) for interim evaluations.

Patients visiting from other cities or countries must be advised on how the aftercare instructions can be blended into their travel plans and should be given a copy of their emergency department records and test results.

QUALITY IMPROVEMENT IN THE DISPOSITION PROCESS

Indicators

Standard Quality Improvement (QI) indicators to evaluate discharge instructions include routine chart audits, review of unscheduled revisits (especially those requiring admission), and measurement of compliance with JCAHO standards. Focused studies of problem areas can be designed whenever necessary.

A review of revisits within 72 hours to one emergency department found that about half were attributable either to deficiencies in patient education or to noncompliance with discharge instructions.[21] It is important to define emergency staff roles for discharge planning and development of materials targeted for the representative patient population.[1] Discharge planning can be taught to emergency staff by nurse educators, clinical nurse specialists, QI personnel, or risk managers. Such training is seldom implemented.[1]

Patient Recontact

Calling patients after emergency department visits reinforces aftercare instructions, confirms follow-up appointments, and identifies patient complaints or questions. In addition, telephone contact promotes patient satisfaction and improves public relations for the department.[1,22]

A prospective study was conducted to evaluate the effect of telephone follow-up on patient care and satisfaction when predetermined high-risk criteria were met. All charts were reviewed during the study period, and 15% of patients were selected for recontact. Calls were assigned to an emergency nurse, social worker, or emergency physician on the basis of preestablished criteria that corresponded to the staff's expertise and training. Of those patients selected, 81% were contacted after an average of 1.6 attempts with calls averaging 70 seconds in duration. Forty-two percent of the patients contacted required clarification of their discharge instructions. Of seven patients stating that their condition had worsened, six required direct medical intervention. Ninety-five percent of all patients questioned were positively influenced by telephone follow-up.[23]

Another study of patient understanding and compliance with discharge instructions involved patients arriving at the emergency department with asthma.[24] Patients were contacted by telephone, and an average of 1.7 attempts was necessary to reach patients with calls lasting an average of 6 minutes. Of the studied population, 82% reported an improvement in their medical condition, 16% were unchanged, and 2% were worse. In 17%, follow-up was urged; in 9%, instructions were reinforced; and in 8%, the follow-up appointment was made for the patient.[10]

In urban, public emergency departments, where about 40% of patients are unable to be reached by telephone, reminder cards with appointment information can be mailed.

MEDICOLEGAL ISSUES

Transfer Laws

Discharge of patients relates to the patient transfer requirements outlined in the Consolidated Omnibus Budget Reconciliation Act (COBRA) of 1985. Legally the definition of "transfer" includes any movement of a patient "outside a hospital's facilities by any person employed or affiliated with the hospital."[25-28] Thus a patient discharged home is technically transferred. Emergency physicians must be aware of the regulations governing the COBRA legislation (see Chapter 61).

Discharges Against Medical Advice

Adult patients of sound mind desiring to leave against medical advice (AMA) have the right to do so. The emergency physician must show concern, not frustration, for these patients while informing the patient of all risks and providing the most appropriate aftercare plan possible given the discharge circumstances.

It must be stressed that only competent patients can leave AMA, and the objective criteria by which functional competence is determined (outlined in the Emergency Doctrine[26]) must be documented. Functional competency is a continuum and should be correlated with the degree to which a medical problem represents a threat to a patient's life or quality of life. Alert, appropriately acting adults, to be deemed fully competent, must pass the mini-mental status examination and the Shiller test. This test considers the following question: "Does the patient have sufficient mind to reasonably understand the condition, the nature and effect of the proposed treatment, and the attendant risk in pursuing the treatment and in not pursuing the treatment?"[27] Patients determined to be functionally incompetent must be safely and respectfully detained until potentially life-threatening problems are addressed and the patient is able to care for himself or herself.

Documentation must include objective clinical parameters defining competence and a statement that the patient fully understands the risks in leaving AMA. A standard AMA form should be used to facilitate proper documentation. Obtaining the patient's signature on the AMA form demonstrates acknowledgment of personal responsibility for leaving AMA. When the patient refuses to sign the AMA form, a witness should sign and attest that the risks were explained. Documentation (devoid of euphemisms) should reflect that the patient was fully informed of all health risks, no matter how improbable or morbid.

A retrospective chart review of 52 consecutive patients leaving AMA from a suburban moderate-volume emergency department revealed that the level of functional competence of these patients was not recorded in one third and a follow-up referral was not made in more than one third. Documenting that patients understood their diagnoses occurred 36% of the time; that they understood their treatment, 44%; and that they understood the consequences of refusing care, 57%. Eighty-two percent of patients left AMA because they disagreed with the management plan, yet only 30% were dissatisfied with their interaction with the emergency physician.[28]

The emergency physician should never allow the patient's decision to leave AMA to adversely affect the quality of care delivered, including discharge instructions, medication prescriptions, and follow-up appointments. Such patients should be informed of alternate forms of treatment that could solve the medical problem, and these treatments should be made available whenever possible.[29] The patients must be assured they will be welcomed back into the emergency department should they reverse their decision to leave AMA. Patients that leave AMA must be treated with respect and concern by every member of the emergency staff. Only then are they likely to heed medical advice and, perhaps, reverse their decision. Careful documentation of aftercare instructions, including comments regarding alternate forms of treatment, must be a part of all AMA discharges.

Physicians in Training

In many teaching hospitals, supervising attending physicians review all admissions before the patients leave the emergency department. If inadequate staffing levels prevent attending physicians from seeing every patient, then predefined *high-risk* patients and problems should mandate supervision. Standardized approaches for managing various medical problems through written protocols reduce medicolegal risk.[9] This practice prevents rotating house staff from omitting a key component of the physical examination or a necessary study. This practice also addresses differences in attending styles. Certain supervising attending physicians adopt a "surveillance strategy" and actively seek out concerning cases, while others passively become aware of problems only when brought to their attention.[2]

In teaching hospitals, admitting residents must not be allowed to refuse admission for any patient without attending physician approval. Management alternatives can be discussed, but the ultimate decision must be made by the most senior physician present—usually the attending emergency physician. When disputes cannot be resolved, the attending admitting physician should evaluate the patient in the emergency department and assume his or her care. Such situations will inconvenience the patient and are risky in medicolegal terms for the admitting attending physician.

Some attending physicians on medicine and surgery services believe it is appropriate for their residents to function autonomously "as their agents" and act independent of the emergency physician. This practice is ethically, medically, and legally wrong. The most senior physician is usually the emergency department attending physician, who therefore must approve of all plans that affect patient care. The emergency physician remains primarily responsible for a patient until proper transfer to another attending physician occurs. Patients, families, and significant others must understand who are the house staff, who are the attending physicians, and what this difference means.[29]

Alcohol- or Drug-Impaired Patients

A study of 163 emergency department patients at a university hospital and a Veterans Affairs Medical Center who were under the influence of alcohol had blood alcohol levels (BALs) drawn that averaged 235 MG/DL. Of those thought to be impaired at discharge, only 6% were advised not to drive home and 25% were placed in the care of a responsible person.[30] Failure to diagnose or to arrange proper treatment for drug or alcohol abusers represents incomplete patient care and may expose others to the risk of injury.[31]

To confirm clinical sobriety, the emergency physician should document a normal neurologic examination (specifically mental status, speech, and gait) and ensure that the patient has a plan for food and shelter. If a BAL is drawn, the emergency physician is legally justified in holding the patient until the level is at or below the "legal limit." Although many emergency physicians are reluctant to allow the law to impact their practice, holding a patient until the BAL is predicted or measured below the "legal limit" is the only way to minimize the inherent medicolegal risk. If the BAL is not drawn, the patient may be safely discharged when functional competence and clinical sobriety can be documented.

Alcohol- or drug-impaired patients must be advised not to drive or operate machinery and should be referred for substance abuse treatment. Whenever possible, a designated driver should be assigned or an alternate method of transport arranged. When a third party assumes responsibility for a patient, the name of that person and relationship to the patient should be recorded on the emergency department chart.

Reportable Conditions

It is important for the emergency physician to become familiar with state regulations regarding child, spousal, or elder abuse reporting. Patients who are victims of violent crimes should be encouraged to file a police report and given appropriate counseling. The emergency physician has a duty to warn a third party of potential harm when, for instance, a hostile patient leaves the department with the intent to harm another. Many states are moving toward mandatory reporting of family violence. Therefore it is important that consideration of local and state laws be incorporated into the discharge planning process.

Most states require reporting to the Department of Motor Vehicles medical problems that could potentially cause sudden loss of consciousness. Such patients must be told that a report has been filed and not to drive, operate machinery, climb ladders, swim alone, or become involved in any other situation that, if consciousness were lost, could threaten their lives. While such reporting commonly occurs after a seizure disorder is diagnosed, it must be contemplated for chemical dependency, recurrent hypoglycemia, and any other mind-altering condition.

Minimizing Medicolegal Risk

Particularly distressing situations occur when a patient or third party refuses necessary treatment, demands unnecessary treatment or admission, or insists on an unnecessary or hazardous transfer to another institution. When such circumstances pose a significant medicolegal risk, advice should be immediately sought from the hospital attorney or risk manager. Patients should be encouraged to speak directly with their private physician or a consultant about management disagreements so that the emergency physician does not appear obstructive.[3]

Emergency physicians are legally responsible for patients after discharge. Tort laws state that the person who could have best prevented a problem is the one most responsible for its occurrence. "Proximate cause" defines how directly an event is related to the bad outcome and is somewhat arbitrary.

An imperfect emergency department visit resulting from problematic medical care, scant documentation, misinformation, or poor patient relations, when combined with a maloccurrence, may invoke a lawsuit. In the Harlow case of 1982 a misdiagnosis of muscle spasm resulted in a $6 million lawsuit after a herniated disk at the vertebral level C4-5 caused quadriplegia. The defense attorneys "urged better documentation of the discharge instructions" to include warning symptoms necessitating follow-up care and obtaining the patient's signature.[32] Plaintiffs have excellent recollections of their emergency department visit—they have been contemplating the events since the problem occurred—and juries are swayed by such detailed testimony. Because considerable time passes before cases are tried, the emergency physician often has difficulty recalling the particular emergency department visit. For this reason, when any potential medicolegal problem is identified, the emergency physician should immediately record a statement and submit it to the hospital's risk manager.

Programs to minimize medicolegal risks in the emergency department can lower insurance premiums. The Commissioner of Insurance for Massachusetts in July 1990 granted a 20% discount for organizations in compliance with the Massachusetts-ACEP Risk Management program, which includes specific discharge instruction sheets for certain "high-risk" diagnoses.[33]

SUMMARY

This chapter emphasizes the importance and complexity of the patient disposition process and discharge teaching in achieving successful outpatient management. Communication skills between the emergency physician and both the patient and his or her primary care provider are essential in determining the most appropriate disposition. Emergency physicians and nurses must realize that delivering excellent aftercare instructions is an integral part of a winning risk management program and greatly improves patient satisfaction. The use of available computerized programs improves staff efficiency and provides personalized, well-understood aftercare instructions.

REFERENCES

1. Hellstern RA, editor: *Managing the emergency department: a team approach,* Dallas, 1992, ACEP.
2. Overton DT, guest editor: Quality in emergency medicine, *Emerg Clin North Am* 1992. 10(3):477-648, 1992.
3. Henry GL, editor-in-chief: *ED risk management,* Dallas, 1991, ACEP.
4. McMillan JR, Younger MS, DeWine LC: Satisfaction with hospital emergency departments as a function of triage, *Health Care Manage* 11(3):21, 1986.
5. Verdile VP: The telephone in emergency practice, *Foresight* 27:1-6, 1993.
6. Ury W, Fisher R: *Getting to yes: negotiating agreement without giving in,* New York, 1983, Penguin.
7. Peck CL, King NJ: Increasing patient compliance with prescriptions, *JAMA* 248(21):2874, 1982.
8. Chande VT, Bhende MS, Davis HW: Pediatric emergency department complaints: a three-year analysis of sources and trends, *Ann Emerg Med* 20(9):1014, 1991.
9. American Health Consultants Inc., editors: *Reducing risk in the emergency department,* Atlanta, 1989, American Health Consultants Inc.
10. Powers RD: ED patient literacy and the readability of patient directed materials, *Ann Emerg Med* 17:124, 1988.
11. Jolly BT, Scott JL, Feied CF et al: Functional illiteracy among ED patients: a preliminary study, *Ann Emerg Med* 22(3):573, 1993.
12. Isaacman DJ, Purvis K, Gyuro J et al: Standardized instructions: do they improve communication of discharge information from the ED? *Pediatrics* 89(6.2):1204, 1992.
13. Sbarbaro JA: Strategies to improve compliance with therapy, *Am J Med* 79(6A):34, 1985.
14. Monane M, Gurwitz JH, Monane S et al: Compliance issues in medical practice, *Hosp Physician* April (29) 1993, pp. 35-39.
15. May JP, Martin KL: A role for the primary care physician in counseling young African-American men about homicide prevention, *J General Intern Med* 8:380, 1993.
16. Horty J, editor: Home instructions must be clear and documented, *Patient Care Law* December 1985–January 1986, pp. 1,4.
17. Siders AM, Peterson M: *Increasing patient satisfaction and nursing productivity through implementation of an automated nursing discharge summary.* Proceedings of the Annual Symposium on Computer Applications in Medical Care, 1991, pp. 136-140.
18. Magnusson AR, Hedges JR, Vanko M et al: Follow-up compliance after emergency department evaluation, *Ann Emerg Med* 22(3):560, 1993.
19. Kerr EA, Siu AL: Following after hospital discharge: does insurance make a difference? *J Health Care for the Poor and Underserved* 4(2):133, 1993.
20. *JCAHO manual for hospitals,* Emergency services, Oakbrook Terrace, Il, 1993, JCHO.
21. Keith KD, Bocka JJ, Kobernick MS et al: Emergency department revisits, *Ann Emerg Med* 18(9):964-968, 1989.
22. Levy R, Goldstein B, Trott A: Approach to quality assurance in an ED: a one-year review, *Ann Emerg Med* 13(3):166-169, 1984.
23. Jones J, Clark W, Bradford J et al: Efficacy of a telephone follow-up system in the emergency department, *J Emerg Med* 6(3):249, 1988.
24. Murphy JG, Jacobson S: Assessing the quality of emergency care: the medical record versus patient outcome, *Ann Emerg Med* 13(3):158, 1984.
25. Frew SA, Roush WR, La Greca K: COBRA: implications for emergency medicine, *Ann Emerg Med* 17(8):835, 1988.
26. Lewis SM, McCutchen JR: Emergency exceptions to informed consent. In: *Emergency medicine malpractice,* New York, 1987, John Wiley & Sons.
27. Schwartz M: The patient who refuses medical treatment: a dilemma for hospital and physician, *Am J Law Med* 11:147-194, 1985.
28. Dubow D, Propp D, Narasimhank K et al: ED discharges against medical advice, *J Emerg Med* 10(4):513, 1992.
29. Henry GL: Risk management and high risk issues in emergency medicine, *Emerg Med Clin NA* 11(4):905-922, 1993.
30. Simel DL, Feussner JR: Driving-impaired patients leaving the ED: the problem of inadequate instructions, *Ann Intern Med* 112(5):365, 1990.
31. Lowenstein SR Weissberg MP, Terry D: Alcohol intoxication, injuries and dangerous behaviors and the revolving ED door, *J Trauma* 30(10): 1252, 1990.
32. Hill HE: $6 million discharge instruction: *Emerg Depart Law* 21:1, 1989.
33. Blau ML: Emergency physician's gain malpractice discount. *Physician's News Digest* 3(6):8-9, 15, 1990.

26 Emergency Department STAT Laboratory

Joel M. Bartfield

OUTLINE

Decreasing the time spent waiting for laboratory results in the emergency department has the potential to positively affect patient care. In some circumstances, time to administration of therapy can be shortened and overall patient throughput time may also be shortened. This can lead to improved patient and healthcare worker satisfaction and help to diminish emergency department overcrowding.

Establishing a STAT laboratory in the emergency department is a potential way to decrease the time delay for laboratory results, although such a project may involve a significant amount of personnel and expense. Therefore before considering an ED STAT laboratory for an individual department, the allotment of resources should be justified. This chapter discusses this issue and the logistics involved in setting up an ED STAT laboratory. The potential impact of an ED STAT laboratory on the rest of the hospital is also discussed.

STEP 1: GATHERING DATA

Before spending the time and energy required to establish an ED STAT laboratory, its impact on patient care should be evaluated. Information should be gathered concerning the present system so that interventions will be data driven rather than based on a manager's intuition regarding "what should work to improve patient care."

If the goal is to decrease patient throughput time, two principal questions must be answered: What is the turn-around time for individual laboratory tests? and How often is patient disposition or treatment delayed because of these turn-around times? The process for obtaining a laboratory test result should be broken down into individual segments, including the time required to obtain specimen, label specimen and requisitions, transport specimen, perform laboratory test, and communicate result to the emergency department (Box 26-1). Audits should be performed to obtain data for each of these components. For instance, during a given week, clerks can be instructed to record the times they receive, send, and obtain results on emergency department laboratory specimens. By using a "flow diagram" approach in examining this process, bottlenecks can be identified. This evaluation of the laboratory process should be performed by a team of experts (i.e., laboratory technicians, doctors, nurses, ward clerks, and nurse assistants).

Determining the impact of laboratory turn-around time on overall patient turn-around time is more challenging. Specific questions must be addressed, such as the following: Is patient disposition often delayed pending laboratory evaluation? Are there significant delays in treatment as a result of laboratory delays? Devising strategies to answer these questions may well require prospectively gathering data on consecutive emergency department patients by using an unbiased, well-trained observer. Although this requires a great deal of time and effort, it is an important step in determining the possible impact an ED STAT laboratory might have on patient turn-around time. For example, it is entirely possible that an audit examining time delays will reveal that times can be considerably shortened by having a laboratory in the emergency department. However, if other factors (x-ray or consultation) are the rate-limiting steps in patient throughput, improving laboratory performance is unlikely to have much impact.

WORKING WITH DATA TO IMPROVE PERFORMANCE

The review process should be conducted in a completely unbiased manner, and the changes made should be data driven rather than based on preconceived ideas about "what should work best for the emergency department." After carefully analyzing the data, potential schemes to improve overall patient care by decreasing laboratory turn-around time should be formulated. Establishing an ED STAT laboratory may correct certain problems but have virtually no impact on others.

Before assuming that an ED STAT laboratory will significantly shorten the time required to run certain tests, the audit data must be scrutinized carefully. Are there significant delays in running all laboratory tests or only certain tests? Will an ED STAT laboratory be able to perform the tests that currently have long delays? Can an ED STAT laboratory perform tests significantly faster than the hospital laboratory? Are there ways to work with the director of the hospital laboratory to minimize the time required to perform particular laboratory tests? Before establishing an ED STAT laboratory, it is obviously appropriate to carefully explore the latter question. Working closely with the hospital laboratory is not only cost-effective but is likely to meet with much more support than attempting to establish a new system such as an ED STAT laboratory.

BOX 26-1

INDIVIDUAL SEGMENTS AFFECTING LABORATORY TURN-AROUND TIME

Obtain specimen
Label specimen
Fill out requisition
Transport specimen
Perform test
Report result

MECHANICS OF SETTING UP AN ED STAT LABORATORY

Previous studies have demonstrated that certain limited tests can be made in the emergency department with a reasonable degree of accuracy as compared with the hospital laboratory.[1-3] However, there are many issues that must be considered before setting up a formal ED STAT laboratory. It would certainly not be cost-effective to attempt to perform every test currently offered by the hospital laboratory. Laboratory tests that should be considered for inclusion are high-volume tests, tests that are easy to perform, and tests for which results have historically taken a long time to obtain from the hospital laboratory. Obviously, adequate and appropriate space must be allocated. A room dedicated as the ED STAT laboratory must be available. The size of the room will be predicated on the amount of equipment required to perform the laboratory tests that have been chosen to be included. In addition to the startup costs to purchase and/or lease equipment and materials, other ongoing costs include equipment maintenance and upgrading and salary lines for ED STAT laboratory personnel.

A decision must be made regarding who is ultimately responsible for the ED STAT laboratory. Will the operation be managed by the emergency department or the hospital laboratory, or as a joint venture? The person who oversees the ED STAT laboratory will be responsible to ensure that the laboratory is in compliance with all state and local regulations. The laboratory also must meet requirements for accreditation by the College of American Pathologists and the Joint Commission on the Accreditation of Healthcare Organizations. In addition, issues regarding quality management must be addressed.

IMPACT ON HOSPITAL

Establishing an ED STAT laboratory may significantly affect the overall workings of the hospital laboratory. If a substantial volume of testing is decentralized from the hospital to the ED STAT laboratory, it is possible that the main laboratory would be forced to restructure in certain areas.

SUMMARY

Setting up an ED STAT laboratory has the potential benefit of improving patient care by decreasing patient turn-around time. Other positive aspects include a source of potential revenue. The feasibility of setting up an ED STAT laboratory must be carefully explored. This chapter explores some of the pros and cons of establishing an ED STAT laboratory in an individual department.

REFERENCES

1. Howanitz PJ, Steindel SJ, Cembrowski GS et al: Emergency department stat test turnaround times: a college of American pathologists' Q-Probes study for potassium and hemoglobin, *Arch Pathol Lab Med* 116(2):122-128, 1992.
2. Spivey WH, Unger HD, McNamara RM et al: A clinical evaluation of the QBCII® centrifugal hematology analyzer in the emergency department, *J Emerg Med* 7:329-333, 1991.
3. Bartfield JM, Robinson D, Lekas J: Accuracy of microcentrifuged hematocrits in the emergency department, *J Emerg Med* 11:673-676, 1993.

27 Materials Management in the Emergency Department

Marilyn P. Swinford

OUTLINE

Nursing administrators and managers have a vital role in the purchase of equipment and supplies required for the provision of emergency services. Nurses across the nation participate in the design, acquisition, utilization, and evaluation of state-of-the-art emergency care products. Collaboration among emergency department managers, materials managers, physicians, nurses, and company representatives is critical to meet the emergency department's supply and demand needs.

Materials management is described as the management (handling) and control of supplies and equipment and related activities from acquisition to disposition. This continuum includes the functions of supply specification, purchasing, receiving, supply processing, distribution, inventory control, supply utilization, standardization, value analysis, and forecasting.[1] The emergency department manager must understand the various methodologies used to provide supplies and how those methodologies can optimize materials management for the emergency department.

BUILDING A MATERIALS MANAGEMENT PHILOSOPHY

Organizational structure, size and location of the institution, existing and potential departmental resources, and scope of emergency services influence the development of a materials management philosophy. Issues to consider include the institution's and the department's organizational structure, product evaluation and purchasing methods, capital purchases, service contracts, charging methods, supply, and inventory. Several departments may collectively purchase items.

CENTRALIZED VERSUS DECENTRALIZED MATERIALS MANAGEMENT PHILOSOPHY

Supply acquisition and disposition may involve a structure that is centralized, decentralized, or a combination of both.

Centralized

A centralized materials management department often includes the purchasing department, stock area, and receiving dock personnel, but generally not members of nursing service. The centralized method usually applies to hospital-wide usage items, including common patient care supplies (intravenous [IV] fluids and tubing), office supplies (paper goods and forms), and dietary and pharmaceutical items. The purchasing agent is charged with getting the best buy. The greatest benefit of centralized management to the institution and ultimately to the emergency department is cost containment. The centralized team buys in large numbers, standardizes supplies used within the institution, uses a review process to monitor purchases, reduces shipping and freight charges, and endorses protection through the use of large service contracts.

Decentralized

Decentralized purchasing moves the purchasing decisions away from the materials management department to the individual department. Decentralized purchasing may be appropriate for specialty unit items. These include emergency department specialty orthopedic appliances (e.g., cervical stabilization devices and custom suture trays). Similar nursing units may use group purchasing for specialty items resulting in dollar savings and the ability to purchase state-of-the-art products. This type of purchasing is still considered decentralized because the nurse manager is actively involved in purchase decisions.

Combination

Purchasing using a combined centralized and decentralized approach is the most widely practiced method. Materials managers have expertise in purchasing that most nurses do not possess. They have specific information of manufacturers and vendors who carry product lines, a working knowledge of contract negotiation, historical knowledge of the institution's previous buying practices, and familiarity with other departments' existing stock. The emergency department manager may be unaware that an item is in current use and available in another area. Nurses have clinical information, such as the ability to identify the need for a product and the direct application of a product, that the nonmedical person does not possess. Combined purchasing involves a collaborative approach. It blends the centralized buying power of the purchasing department with custom or specialty purchases chosen by the end user.

COLLABORATION BETWEEN EMERGENCY DEPARTMENT MANAGERS AND MATERIALS MANAGERS

The emergency department manager is responsible for creating a strictly controlled materials and supply budget. The technical expertise and financial skills necessary for department operations is enhanced by open communication between the emergency department manager and materials manager. A product evaluation process may be the best venue for these individuals to discuss common concerns related to supply selection, cost, and product performance.

Product Evaluation

Product evaluation can be a time-consuming responsibility for the emergency department manager, who must be aware of changes in technology and availability of equipment while fulfilling other managerial roles. Working with suppliers, vendors, and company representatives can be facilitated by the manager's specifying what information is needed and what products are to be reviewed. Unit-based product evaluation committees with the aim of cost containment can help streamline and standardize operations.

A product evaluation committee commonly consists of multidisciplinary membership, including hospital purchasing director or purchasing staff representative, nursing clinical specialist, nursing educational service representative, nurse manager, staff nurse, pharmacy and laboratory personnel, and physician. This collaboration provides the committee with individuals whose everyday practice is affected by which products are purchased, reviewed, or deleted. The chair is usually the director of the materials management department. The chair directs the committee toward products developed by companies with which the institution has existing contracts, when possible. The committee chooses the best product from an already narrowed field.

The methodology adopted by a products committee varies among institutions. The committee members may appoint a representative for each item reviewed. The representative obtains information from the vendor and presents it to the committee. The product should be evaluated for safety, quality, price, serviceability, and standardization. Other factors influencing purchase decisions include storability, availability, delivery time, educational support, service and repair records, other hospital user experience, competitive product comparison, and independent company studies of the product's effectiveness.[2]

Committees may review certain items on a scheduled basis. This eliminates vendors from presenting similar items at each visit; for example, IV infusion devices and IV supplies may be reviewed annually. Other items (catheters, monitor electrodes, dressings) are scheduled for review during a particular month. This system helps the group prioritize and systematically review all necessary equipment. Product evaluation ends with a written report to administration giving recommendations on product purchases.

Staff Input

Emergency department staff nurses work in an environment that demands functional design and adequate supply availability. They are key individuals in the success of materials management as it affects the daily operations of the emergency department. Emergency department team members have a significant role in achieving success with charge mechanisms and in product evaluation. Emergency department nurses can recognize misuse by using a continuous quality control program. Beginning with in-hospital services, staff awareness of issues involved in efficient control of supplies can be heightened. Direct observation of emergency department staff practice assists with developing supply storage systems and establishing par levels necessary to support practice. Examination of product usage reports and monthly charges may encourage the nurse who has a poor attitude or a lack of motivation to identify issues pertaining to cost-effectiveness and to develop measures to improve compliance in charge processes.

PURCHASING METHODS

Emergency managers must educate themselves to understand, choose, and direct the purchase of healthcare products. Purchasing groups, distributors, medical suppliers, and manufacturers provide purchasing information. Company representatives are a primary source for product information. Exhibitors at local, state, and national conventions provide nurses, educators, and researchers the opportunity to preview many items. For example, The Emergency Nurses Association (ENA) Annual Scientific Assembly presents an opportunity for an outstanding group of vendors to display state-of-the-art equipment and technology.

Purchasing personnel are important resources for locating suppliers and contractors, developing contract language, and obtaining vendor references. They provide price quotations for budget projections, identify realistic lead times for acquiring technical information, and expedite contract performance.[3]

Purchasing Contracts

Purchasing contracts should be based on actual usage and accurate usage projections. Projections may be based on historical data such as patient census. By examining census patterns, the emergency department manager can propose month-to-month delivery schedules. Examination of monthly usage reports, generated by accounting or data audit departments, may be a more accurate means to project supply needs. By examining a 3-month trend for usage, an annual projection can be made.

Automatic shipment is one type of purchasing contract and constitutes an arrangement between the supplier and the department to routinely send items in predetermined amounts. When considering automatic shipments, the emergency department manager should be certain the contract allows for adjustment of the shipment to allow for variations in demand for the item.

Purchasing Groups

Purchasing groups or consortiums represent a collection of hospitals. Purchasing departments should have a directory listing of these groups. Purchasing groups negotiate with manufacturers and distributors to obtain the best prices for their members based on volume buying. This concept is good for smaller institutions with lower usage volumes or larger institutions with purchases of smaller quantities. Hospitals with few personnel resources benefit from contracting with purchasing groups. For many institutions, purchasing groups handle the bulk of the workload. Purchasing groups usually have a "sole source" mandatory contract by which the institution must abide or incur a penalty. For example, the purchasing group has a contract with Manufacturer A and Manufacturer B for urologic supplies. The hospital wishes to buy a urologic item from Manufacturer C. Under terms of the purchasing group/hospital contract, purchasing from Manufacturer C will result in a financial penalty to the hospital.

Distributors

Distributors working alone or with groups can obtain noncontract items. Because there is no affiliation with a particular supplier, the distributor is allowed to do individual buying. The advantages a hospital can realize from use of distributors are as follows: distributors sell in small units of measure (e.g., box versus case); distributors sell direct to hospitals, whereas many manufacturers do not; distributors' delivery times are more frequent than manufacturers; and there is no charge for freight. Hospitals can expect to pay distributors a markup for their service; however, this may be offset if the distributor offers a discount or promotional programs. Distributors may be the sole resource for smaller hospitals or any institution that embraces the philosophy of independent bargaining.

Medical Supply Houses

If the hospital has limited or no on-site storage capacity, a medical supply house may be used to obtain supplies on an as-needed basis. To be of greatest benefit to the hospital, the medical supply house should be geographically located to readily provide items when needed. The emergency department manager with limited or absent storage capability will probably use the supply house out of necessity. If the supply house cannot provide supplies in a timely fashion, the emergency department manager may need to confront the hospital administration to determine other options. This may include creating a storage area in the emergency department for frequently used items. If administration views storage as unnecessary use of space, the manager may want to present a cost comparison of frequent low-volume buying versus bulk buying and storage. Tracking frequency of item unavailability may be helpful in documenting effect of low supply as it relates to patient care.

Direct Purchasing

Direct purchasing from the manufacturer may be appropriate for special orders. However, it is an expensive means of acquiring supplies because of small numbers and long-distance shipping rates. Most capital purchase items, such as stretchers and monitoring equipment, are obtained from the manufacturer via direct purchase. Noncapital items include all other items whose cost falls below the amount determined as capital by the hospital. These may include orthopedic splints, surgical instruments, and suture.

Supplier Changes

Despite the purchase method chosen, hospitals may be faced with or may choose supplier changes during the year. Supplier changes can occur for the following reasons:

1. Financial savings can be achieved for the department.
2. Purchasing group or vendor contract states that the hospital must change because the original company subcontracts or changes to another for the supply item.
3. The quality of the existing product may not be acceptable to the hospital.
4. The supplier deletes the existing items and the manager is forced to change.

Because of a change in the institution's supplier, product inservices and training may be necessary for the staff. By shopping among vendors, dealing with supply houses, or buying from purchasing groups, the manager may find new sources of inventory and establish new ties with vendors.

EQUIPMENT AND SUPPLIES SUGGESTED FOR EMERGENCY FACILITIES

Each emergency department must determine the need for supplies based on patient population and scope of services. Many hospitals spend 40% or more of their total budget on supplies alone.[4] *Emergency Care Guidelines* includes recommendations for resources necessary for the operation of an emergency department.[5] The Joint Commission on Accreditation of Healthcare Organizations has established general guidelines for facility design and equipment necessary for safe patient care in the emergency department. Specific guidelines are further delineated based on the level of service of the department—level I, II, III, or IV.[6]

Hospital-Wide Items

Items used by several departments are often kept in central storage areas and are accessible to all patient care areas. Items may be obtained via delivery carts or elevators that service the patient care area, by sending emergency department personnel to the central storage areas for pickup, or by having the supplies delivered by personnel from the central storage area. Supplies used throughout the hospital include patient care items, pharmaceuticals, linens, and dietary items. Items for office supply (pens, certain forms) may be ordered on a weekly or biweekly basis. These items are expensed to the department by the stock room or purchasing department.

Hospital-Wide Services

Hospital-wide services used by many areas include laboratory, dietary, and radiology services. For example, the laboratory provides phlebotomy services to all patient care areas. The phlebotomist brings all supplies (syringes, needles, vacutainers) to the patient care area. The cost for the service and associated equipment is passed on to the patient, not to the emergency department.

Patient Care Items

Certain patient care supplies are bulk items used in all patient care areas. Items used to provide routine care are usually standardized within the institution. An example is bedpans. Bulk purchasing and standardization of the item assists in maintaining emergency department supply.

Department-Specific Items (Specialty Items)

Surgical services, obstetric/gynecologic services, and critical care areas need many specialty items. In the emergency department these items may be determined by physician practice, staff preference, patient preference, and prehospital compatibility (for example, a cervical spine immobilization collar). The emergency nursing manager may assume the purchaser role when specialty items are needed. Selecting the item, determining the quantity of item to have available on the unit (par level), and evaluating the item may become the tasks for employees within the department, similar to the process assumed by members of the product evaluation committee.

Pharmaceuticals

The quantity and variety of drugs for the emergency department stock should be based on analysis of routine usage. Quotas can be set and are appropriate when using automated drug dispensing systems. Infrequently used drugs should be kept in the smallest quantities possible or dispensed directly to the patient, preventing an inventory buildup. This practice should reduce the emergency department's liability for storage of outdated drugs.

CAPITAL PURCHASES

Capital purchases include major purchases (radiology equipment), improvements (remodeling), or projects (implementation of a fast track) acquired during the budget period. Capital expenditures for equipment are defined by each institution on the basis of cost and expected life span of the equipment. There are several options available to the emergency department manager for purchasing capital equipment.

1. Purchases expensed entirely at the time the purchase is signed. It is hoped that the revenue generated by the capital item will equal the expense of the item in a relatively short time.
2. Purchases based on payment after installment and implementation in the department.
3. Lease versus purchase options.
4. Cost-per-use options. For example, if an item will be used for several years, a purchase agreement may include spreading out the cost of the equipment over several years. This allows the manager to equate or balance the cost with revenue generated.

Hospitals may use consulting services such as MD Byline (Dallas, Texas), MedEcon (Louisville, Kentucky) and ECRI (Plymouth Meeting, Pennsylvania) when considering capital purchases.[3] Hospitals pay a fee for such services. In return for the fee, the hospital receives information concerning reasonable price ranges, equipment performance levels, and service capabilities. Vendors may be recommended for possible negotiations. The consulting service provides any information obtained while assisting the hospital with the capital purchase to update its own database.

Capital equipment acquisition involving a substantial cash cost should be considered separately from routine supply purchases. The hospital or department will want a list of specifications to be agreed to by the company selling a piece of capital equipment. These specifications may include purchase price, installation cost, trade-in, or salvage. The manager should plan for capital expenditures by projecting a 3- to 5-year budget for equipment upkeep and replacement.

SERVICE CONTRACTS

Service contracts are offered on capital equipment purchase items and many specialty items used in the emergency department. A working knowledge of the hospital's philosophy and the maintenance or repair services available within the institution influences the decision to obtain a service contract. The institution's philosophy may be that it is better to have service contracts on all items to cover repair in case of supply interruption, malfunction, or failure. Other institutions may manage repairs internally at a rate lower than the service contract rate. An exceptional biomedical service department within the facility may influence the decision not to have service contracts because in-house personnel can accomplish maintenance and repair. If the item is near the end of expected service or if the equipment becomes outdated, the contract may be dropped because it would be wiser to purchase new equipment than to repair the original item. Service contracts are estimated to represent 30% to 40% of a manufacturer's profits.[3] Most service contracts can be modified and should be examined to be sure the hospital is getting adequate service for justifiable cost. In cases where only one company produces an item, hospitals can contain costs by negotiating service specifications.

Items to negotiate in a service contract include hours or days of service availability, response times, process of acquiring service, upgrades, software enhancements, staff training, and impact on operating budget (often 10% of purchase cost).[3] Many department managers budget for service contracts monthly. It is therefore necessary to consider the added cost of a service contract above the original purchase cost. The emergency department manager can negotiate service contracts item by item. For example, payment for labor may be included but not for travel expenses of repair personnel. Usually a 12-month warranty for parts and services is obtained for major purchases. Terms and length of warranty are negotiable. The manager may try to obtain an extended warranty in lieu of a sizable price discount, or try for both.

CHARGING MECHANISMS

Charge structures are influenced by many factors, including Medicare reimbursement, national and regional practices, and third party payer requirements. Private insurance companies, commonly referred to as third party payers, reimburse the hospital for certain supply items. If the items are believed to be nonessential to the healing process the company may choose not to reimburse for billing of that item. Charging mechanisms are usually developed by the institution and adapted to the emergency department. The price increase for supplies and equipment use for the upcoming year is generally determined at the time the annual budget is prepared. General pricing information can be obtained from the federal General Accounting Office. Additionally, the Consumer Price Index for Hospitals is an indicator for costs of paper goods and plastics. The index, reflected as a percentage point, may help the manager with budget projections based on proposed or anticipated cost increases.

Nursing staff should be encouraged to explore efficient methods for patient charging, which may directly increase time for patient care. Charging mechanisms may involve use of ticketing and sticker systems, custom charge forms, computer entry at central stations, bedside computers, and bar coding.

Managers must identify items charged to the department and nonchargeable patient supplies (e.g., pens, cups, forms, syringes). Programs and services that can be charged to the patient are established by Medicare, Medicaid, and third party payers. Neither the hospital nor the emergency department can bill patients for items not allowed by third party payers. An administrative representative, usually a billing specialist or the materials manager, serves as a valuable resource to the emergency department manager in identifying which items can be charged to the patient. The hospital-allowed markup of the item (cost posted to the patient's account) is set according to third party payer standards and may not exceed a certain percentage.

The emergency department manager must determine whether supplies are to be charged individually or clustered in a procedure charge. Charging supplies individually may result in greater revenue to the emergency department. However, in the hectic emergency department environment this practice may be impractical. For example, personnel must charge for each item used in suturing a wound, including instruments, antiseptic, anesthetic, dressings, and suture. The emergency department pace may make it impossible for the personnel to track charges accurately on all patients for all procedures. An alternative is to establish a procedure charge, which reflects the combined cost of all supplies for suturing a laceration (e.g., establishing a sterile setup charge or basic tray charge). This charging mechanism may be more convenient for personnel and ultimately results in better compliance with charges. Nonchargeable supplies (e.g., syringes, Band-Aids, cotton swabs) are often expensed to the unit at the time of delivery. The manager must include cost of the supply delivery into the routine operational expenses for the department. These may be posted daily, weekly, or biweekly based on the delivery schedule.

Ticketing and Stickers

The use of tickets or stickers involves placing a sticker or leaving a ticket on all chargeable supplies. As the item is removed from stock for patient usage, the sticker is filed (usually on patient charge cards) for later entry on the patient's bill. The system has considerable human error in that stickers are often lost in the hurried patient care environment or are not matched to the individual patient for whom the item was used. The system involves all the emergency department personnel in applying, removing, and collecting stickers. File cards placed at the bedside may increase compliance versus placing stickers on charts located away from the patient care area. Cards are attached to the patient chart at time of discharge to allow entry of ticket or sticker information into the computer.

Custom Charge Forms

Supply order forms and custom charge forms specific to the department have been used by nursing departments for years. Charge forms are ideally a single page, listing the most frequently charged items, and may be kept with the patient chart or in the patient care area. Quantities of items are marked as used. These data are either directly entered into a computer by emergency department personnel or sent to the billing specialist. Custom charge forms should decrease the need for ticketing and stickers.

Computer Systems

The use of computer systems permits entry of charges directly to the data audit department or business office for patient billing. Charge order entry screens with alphabetic or frequency listing are created, and patient charges are entered for supplies and services at the conclusion of the emergency department visit. This system helps eliminate the many steps often required to track the item from the time it is removed from stock to the time it is charged to the patient. Order entry may be done by clerical staff within the department, billing specialists, or the clinician. This system requires excellent charting of patient care services and items for order entry. A system of tickets or stickers may help the nurse recall supplies used. A custom charge form (a hard copy of the emergency department computer screen) is useful in times of computer downtime or failure.

Bedside Computers

Institutions with bedside computers may allow the clinician to enter charges at the time of use. In some systems, the charge may be related to the procedure. For example, the nurse documents "IV access" on the bedside terminal. Charges for fluids, tubing, needle, and infusion devices are then automatically entered.

Bar Coding

Computer entry via bar coding is a widely used charge process by retail and grocery stores that has finally made its way to healthcare institutions. By scanning the bar code for the supply or service, the charge is entered. Quantity of items may be selected by rescanning the bar code for the number of items used or by bar coding a quantity value.

Staff education about hospital services and supply charges is necessary to maintain compliance with any charge system. Hospital personnel may be unaware of the impact of patient care costs, especially with usage items that are not directly charged to the patient. Additional considerations affecting the development of a successful charge program include the following:

1. Third party payers are demanding documentation for items for which the patient is billed.
2. The operations budget of the department will be affected as much by the waste of less expensive miscellaneous items as by the loss of specialized equipment and supplies.
3. Theft among hospital employees must be addressed to review the impact it has on department costs.

SUPPLY INVENTORY

Supply inventory guidelines may be set by hospital administration, the materials management department, or the unit manager. This large-scale inventory may include items stored in central stock areas and pharmacy. Hospital-wide inventories may be conducted monthly or annually to assess supply volumes. Specific problems can be associated with low or surplus inventory (Box 27-1). Inventories are scheduled to meet the manager's need. Annual inventories may alert the manager of duplicated or obsolete items. Based on inventory findings, the manager may consult the product evaluation committee to recommend alternative supplies. A monthly inventory of stock allows the manager to check for expiration dates and assess the amount of storage space available. Routine inventory of stock is conducted by day or by shift, comparing actual stock to established par levels. This maintains necessary quantity of stock for routine operation. An inventory schedule for selected items may be necessary to fulfill terms of a contract. For example, a supplier who provides a specialty suture tray may request quarterly inventory to determine the volume to be shipped.

Infrequently used items or items needed for disaster preparedness should be inventoried periodically. This will ensure that items are present and can be located quickly. Special inventories may be conducted in times of national or international disaster or events. Recently, institutions conducted a special inventory during Operation Desert Storm to determine current supplies in anticipation of medical supply shortages stateside.

BOX 27-1

INVENTORY PROBLEMS

Low inventory

1. Misuse of valuable nursing time spent looking for or obtaining patient care items.
2. Possible misuse of supplies substituted for missing items.
3. Increased level of frustration and stress resulting in low job satisfaction.
4. Potentially serious and in some cases even life-threatening patient care consequences.

Surplus inventory

1. Hospital funds are tied up in excessive product inventory and are not available for other purchases.
2. Extra space is required to store the additional inventory.
3. Improper rotations and use of dated supplies may occur.

STORAGE SYSTEMS

Supply storage involves the process of supply inventory combined with a procedure for ensuring that supplies are available to nurses when needed. "Supply availability and orderliness are considerations in designing or selecting devices or systems for storage. The selection process for shelves, bins, carts, cabinets is an important one."[3]

Several resources are available for the emergency department manager to review storage system recommendations. The American College of Emergency Physicians, in *Emergency Department Design,* discusses facility design for the emergency department.[7] The ENA Monograph Series, *Leadership in Management in Emergency Nursing,* has two modules discussing patient flow and facility design.[8] The ENA Trauma Coalition has published a resource document for nursing of the trauma patient focusing on special needs for trauma care.[9] Each of these documents addresses supply availability, and some provide stocking guidelines.

Exchange Carts

An exchange cart system uses an exchange of a full bin of products for a used bin as indicated. Industrial principles for exchange carts can be applied to nursing units. Keeping twice the amount of supplies on hand than that needed enhances productivity. Exchange cart systems have historically been used in surgical services because of the predictability of number and type of cases to be performed on a daily basis. Such systems are well adapted for emergency department use. A usage trend can be plotted by the manager to establish par levels. Depending on the available space for storage and patient census, exchanges may need to occur by shift or by day.

Fixed and Mobile Shelving

Alternatives to exchange cart systems include fixed and mobile shelving. Fixed and mobile shelving with par levels requires restocking at some point by someone who may be a nursing or materials management employee. Wheel-mounted mobile shelving units shuttle across tracks, compact together, and require only one "transposable" access aisle per bay or movable carriage.

ACQUISITION SYSTEMS

Acquisition systems for stock inventory include central stores, bulk stores, just-in-time (JIT) systems, and stockless systems.

Central Stores

Central stores refers to an area that houses backup supplies used in every department. Departments replenish the supplies kept on the unit from the central store. Although commonly used, some institutions may elect not to have this warehouse surplus storage because it requires mass duplication of supplies.

Bulk Stores

Whereas central stores provide a warehouse for virtually all supplies, bulk stores involve large storage areas in the institution for quantities of routine high-volume items. Operating on a first in, first out (FIFO) philosophy, the inventory should ideally turn over monthly; however, 14 or 15 "turns" annually is acceptable. Some supplies will turn 30 or so times per year, such as intravenous supplies. Considerations for using bulk stores must include the physical space available to store items and the attention to expiration dates.

Just-In-Time System

The JIT system is a concept developed by Japanese industries to have stock delivered as needed. Stock items spend minimal time on loading docks or in stockrooms, but instead go quickly to the unit. Under this system, required materials are delivered by the original supplier to the location where they are used at the precise time they are needed. For example, in industry the parts are placed on the assembly line where and when they are needed. The success of the system relies on the manager's ability to predict the need for supplies. In JIT systems, contingency planning must occur in the event the stock runs out. Advantages of the JIT system:

1. Supplies are delivered in a timely manner to the point at which they will be used.
2. The department does not house any materials and inventory, thus avoiding overhead costs.[10]

Stockless Systems

Stockless systems eliminate a stockroom or central service area. Stockless purchasing represents buying supplies for direct utilization by the respective departments without a duplication or accumulation in the central stores.[1] Items are kept in the emergency department, and timely delivery of goods from the manufacturer is essential. This system is best suited to institutions in urban areas where supplies can be obtained with quick notice and delivery. The institution is paying the vendor to do what the materials manager does. The vendor must package and ship the items in units ordered by the department and in quantities specified by the department. This process is more customized, usually at a higher cost. The cost of eliminating the materials manager may be matched by vendor charges for the customized service. Fluctuations in patient census, coupled with not having close suppliers, may make it difficult to use a stockless system. Under the philosophy of stockless purchasing, central stores should provide a minimum supply of an item to adequately handle a maximum number of customer units or departments as opposed to a maximum amount of an item being used to supply only one or two units.

The average amount of inventory to be kept in the stockless area should approximate a 2-week supply. Setting quotas for the stockless system is the key. To establish quotas, the manager determines the quantity of the items used during the previous year. When divided by 26 this amount should be fairly indicative of a 2-week supply.[11]

Advantages of a stockless system are as follows:

1. It eliminates at least one and perhaps two levels of costly supply duplication, at a cost savings.
2. It allows for better and more efficient utilization of central stores by freeing space.
3. There is less handling, which means fewer worker hours for the receiving and supply function.
4. It provides for more control over "unofficial" inventories, those supplies that have been expensed and dispensed.[11]

One disadvantage of a stockless system is that the manager may fail to plan for seasonal influences on frequently needed items. A 2-week supply in one season may be inadequate in another season (e.g., pulse oximetry digit sensors during asthma season and suture sets during summer season).

Pharmaceutical Dispensing Systems

Pharmaceutical dispensing systems have been developed and enhanced to provide the emergency department with a wide variety of medications. Many systems also incorporate charges when the system is accessed. PIXSIS and Documed are examples of medication delivery systems. These and similar systems use par levels for pharmaceuticals and incorporate a user-friendly charge process, which may greatly increase time for patient care.

SUMMARY

Clear understanding of fiscal and inventory issues allows the manager to choose a materials management philosophy that results in well-planned supply acquisition, resource allocation, and charging mechanisms.

REFERENCES

1. Housley C: *Hospital material management,* Germantown, Md, 1978, Aspen Systems Corporation.
2. Eusebio E, Horger-Scheuber M, Jorlett J: Product selection in the hospital: controlling cost, *Nurse Manage* 16(3):44-46, 1985.
3. Guerin T: Materials management considerations in critical care areas, *Crit Care Nurs Q* 15(3):56-62, 1992.
4. Smith T: Materials management: a model for product review, *Nurs Manage* 16(3):51-54, 1985.
5. American College of Emergency Physicians: *Emergency care guidelines,* Dallas, 1991, ACEP.
6. Joint Commission on Accreditation of Healthcare Organizations: *Accreditation manual for hospitals,* vol 1, Chicago, 1992, JCAHO.
7. Riggs LM, editor: *Emergency department design,* Dallas, 1993, American College of Emergency Physicians.
8. Emergency Nurses Association, Monograph series: *Leadership in management in emergency nursing: enhancing patient flow and facility design,* Park Ridge, Ill, 1993, ENA.
9. Emergency Nurses Association, Trauma Coalition: *Resource document for nursing of trauma patients,* Denver, 1992, ENA.
10. Blaney DR, Hobson CJ: *Cost-effective nursing practice guidelines for nurse managers,* Philadelphia, 1988, Lippincott.
11. Housley C: Stockless purchasing makes dollars and sense, *Dimens Health Serv* 54(5):24-26, 1977.

28 Patient Interview

Howard A. Freed

"He cures most successfully in whom the people have the greatest confidence."

Galen, as quoted by Osler

OUTLINE

It is traditionally taught in American medical schools that of all the steps in a patient's workup (history, physical examination, laboratory testing, x-rays, etc), the history is the most important step. Specifically, most physicians have been taught that the diagnosis is apparent in the large majority of cases after the history alone, and it is true that either the diagnosis or important hints about the diagnosis virtually always come from the patient's history.

It is ironic, therefore, that such a minuscule proportion of a physician's training involves interviewing skills.[1] For example, in one recent textbook of medicine, only 2 of the book's 1500 pages addressed patient-physician communications. Systematic training and continuing medical education in interviewing skills is almost nonexistent. Much of what is written on the subject is filled with vague generalizations of little practical value to the practicing emergency physician. For example, consider the following advice offered in Cecil and Loeb's *Textbook of Medicine:*

> *Communication on a Cultural Level is enriching to the patient-doctor relationship. This can be based on a mutual interest in the arts, literature, history or even politics. . . . The patient profits as he is exposed to the disinterested comments of a wise and cultured scientist.*[2]

It is hard to see how advice on this level will be of much value to the practicing emergency physician and his or her patient. For the interview to be of value, the goals of the encounter must be made explicit.[3]

PHYSICIAN'S GOALS

The typical emergency physician desires a brief, friendly, efficient conversation with the patient. A minimal amount of extraneous conversation is generally desired, unless invited by the often busy physician. The physician wants to be treated with respect and have the interaction lead to the correct diagnosis.

PATIENT'S GOALS

The patient has been driven to go to the emergency department by a relatively strong need and wants that need satisfied even when it is totally unspoken. The patient desires comforting and reassurance. The patient wants to be treated with respect and wants the correct diagnosis to be made.[4]

COMMON NEEDS/DIFFERENT NEEDS

The preceding analysis reveals that the patient's goals and the physician's goals have elements that are shared and elements that are divergent. The common ground is that both parties want to be treated with respect and both desire that the correct diagnosis be made (Box 28-1). The patient wants the need that brought him or her to the emergency department to be addressed, wants to be comforted, and wants quick and effective treatment. The doctor is under pressure to be correct in the evaluation of the patient's problem and to prescribe appropriate and quick treatment.

Each party's goals may or may not be met during the physician-patient interaction. Although there are many ways to analyze this situation, the interaction can be looked at as a "win or lose" situation.

Win-Win

In the win-win situation the physician and patient "hit it off well" and seem to be fast friends. The conversation is cheerful and friendly, and even if the interaction is not completely efficient and directed, each side is trying to cooperate with the other. The patient and physician spend a small amount of "quality time" together.

Win-Lose

In the win-lose interaction the patient more or less wins, but the physician loses. The interaction is inefficient because the physician is dealing with a rambling, tangential, inconsistent, or otherwise frustrating patient. The physician "does his job,"

BOX 28-1

GOALS OF PHYSICIAN/PATIENT INTERVIEW

Physician goals

Brief and efficient interaction
Minimal extraneous conversation unless invited by the physician
Be treated with respect
Make a correct diagnosis

Patient goals

Meet need that caused the patient to go to the emergency department
Be comforted and reassured
Be treated with respect
Get a correct diagnosis

and may even offer the patient the appropriate comforting and reassurance due in a professional interaction. The diagnosis and standard medical care may be correct, but the physician is frustrated even to the point of rage over the patient's talkative and tangential conversation while the physician is trying to move along to other pressing needs.

Lose-Win

In the lose-win interaction the physician wins, but the patient loses. The physician is able to get in and out efficiently with a minimal amount of extraneous conversation. The diagnosis is quickly reached, and basic, standard medical care is prescribed and documented on the chart. Unfortunately, only some of the patient's needs are met. The driving need that pushed the patient to come to the emergency department may never have been addressed or even spoken. The patient and his or her family are frustrated and are likely to be angered at the size of the physician's bill.

Lose-Lose

In the lose-lose interaction both the patient and the physician walk away angry. There may be hostile or antagonistic behavior and remarks. The physician may be brusk and disrespectful, and the patient may be overtly insulting or vulgar. Patients in this type of interaction often leave against medical advice and often refuse to sign the paperwork. Even when a diagnosis is made and the standard care prescribed, both the patient and physician come away from the interaction angry and thinking poorly of each other.

OBSTACLES TO IMPROVING PATIENT-PHYSICIAN INTERACTIONS

Sweeping improvements in interactions with patients and improving one's interviewing techniques are difficult. A number of significant barriers to improvement exist.

Lack of Time Spent on the Problem

Most practicing emergency physicians spend either no or little time actively improving patient interviewing skills. In the barrage of ongoing continuing medical education (CME) activities and offerings available to the emergency physician, improving interviewing skills is almost unheard of.[5] Similarly, most physicians do not spend a great deal of their private educational time working on these skills. This is surprising because there is a remarkable consistency in the kinds of encounters physicians find frustrating.[6]

BOX 28-2

TIPS FOR SUCCESSFUL INTERVIEWING

- Adult-to-adult amenities—introduce yourself; be polite.
- Be supportive.
- Pay attention to subtle and nonverbal communications.
- Pause and offer to answer questions.

Lack of Proven Effectiveness of Teaching Tools

One of the reasons that there is not much CME activity regarding interviewing skills is that little is known for certain on how to teach these skills effectively. It is much easier to measure the effectiveness of teaching scientific facts and concepts. Although information on effective teaching of interviewing skills exists,[7-13] it is not widely disseminated.

Lack of Motivation

Peer pressure to improve interviewing skills and techniques is rare among emergency physicians. Tangible evidence of individual motivation to improve in these areas is uncommon. Evaluation of emergency physicians is increasingly common by superiors, government officials, and a variety of others concerned with the quality of care. Although physicians are evaluated by many different criteria, skill in interviewing techniques is rarely assessed except indirectly (e.g., patient unhappy and complaining about care, causing some type of case review to be done).

Need for Personal Change

A physician's response to information found on a physical examination and laboratory workup is relatively devoid of emotional content and relatively easy to change. On the other hand, the physician's patterns of conversation, demeanor, and interpersonal skills are more difficult to change. Improvements and interview techniques require a change in long-established, personal work habits and traits of the physician. This is rarely easy, particularly given the previously mentioned factors (relatively little time spent on the problem, lack of effective tools, and lack of motivation).

TIPS FOR SUCCESSFUL INTERVIEWING (Box 28-2)

Adult-to-Adult Amenities

Introduce yourself.[3] Be polite. Ask the patient's permission occasionally during the physician-patient interaction ("May I listen to your heart?"). Say goodbye when the interview is completed.

Be Supportive

Avoid interactions such as the following transcribed, real patient interview:[1]

Doctor: "Exactly where is the pain?"

Patient: "It's so hard for me to explain, I am trying to do as well as I can." *(turning to husband)* "Aren't I doing as well as I can?"

Doctor: "Well, is the pain high up in your belly or down low."

Patient: "I kept getting weaker and weaker. I didn't want to come to the hospital. I was so frightened." *(weeping)*

Doctor: "Did the pain come before the weakness or afterward?"

Ignoring the emotional content of the patient's speech is rarely a successful strategy.

Pay Attention to Subtle Communications

Verbal clues (tone of voice, inflection, etc.) and nonverbal communication should be heeded and responded to with empathy. "Between-the-lines" messages are as real as the spoken words, and the interview should not proceed as if nothing were happening when the patient is obviously becoming angry or tearful.

Pause and Offer to Answer Questions

One of the patient's goals is always to obtain information.[3] Even the busy emergency department physician needs to take a moment, without rushed words or body language, and be available for questioning by the patient. An interview is rarely successful overall if the patient walks away with major unanswered questions. Emergency physicians always provide information, but it does not always answer the patient's major questions.

METHODS TO TRACK PHYSICIAN PERFORMANCE

The emergency department manager has a variety of tools available to assess and track physician performance and patient interactions. Verbal and written complaints about the emergency department physicians expressed by patients, families, and other attending physicians can be tracked. The average or typical number of patients leaving against medical advice (AMA) can be measured, and each physician's performance can be monitored and compared with his or her peers looking for outlier activity. Patient satisfaction surveys, both written and by telephone, may reveal a pattern of behavior that is problematic. Direct observation of physician interviewing skills on the job is relatively easy to do, although objective assessment of performance is not possible.

REFERENCES

1. Platt FW, McMath JC: Clinical hypocompetence: the interview, *Ann Int Med* 91:898-902, 1979.
2. Beeson PB, McDermott W: *Cecil-Loeb textbook of medicine,* Philadelphia, 1967, Saunders.
3. Rosenzweig S: Emergency rapport, *J Emerg Med* 11:775-778, 1993.
4. Cassel EJ: The nature of suffering and the goals of medicine, *N Engl J Med* 306:639-645, 1982.
5. Rosenzweig S: Humanism in emergency medicine, *J Emerg Med* 11(5):556-559, 1993.
6. Platt FW, Carroll JG, Keller V, Gordon GH: Three strategies for improving communication with your patients. ACP Observers: ACP, January 1993.
7. Suchman AL, Mathews DA: What makes the patient-doctor relationship therapeutic? Exploring the connexional dimension of medical care, *Ann Int Med* 108:125-130, 1988.
8. Platt FW: *Conversation failure: case studies in doctor-patient communication,* Tacoma, Wa, 1992, Life Sciences Press.
9. Bertakis KD, Roter D, Putnam SM: The relationship of physician medical interview style to patient satisfaction, *J Fam Prac* 32:175-181, 1991.
10. Cohen-Cole SA: *The medical interview: the three function approach,* St Louis, 1991, Mosby.
11. Lipp MR: *Respectful treatment: a practical handbook of patient care,* ed 2, New York, 1986, Elsevier.
12. Collenda CC: Training in empathy, *Am J Psych* 146:125-126, 1989.
13. Levy R, Gale MS: Interactional approach to the difficult emergency department patient, *JACEP* 6(1):7-9, 1977.

ADDITIONAL READINGS

Dailey RH: Approach to the patient in the emergency department. In Rosen P (editor): *Emergency medicine: concepts and clinical practice,* ed 3, St Louis, 1992, Mosby.

Lipkin M, Putman SM, Lazare A: *The medical interview,* New York, 1995, Springer-Verlag.

Platt FW: *Conversation repair: case studies in doctor-patient communication,* Boston, 1995, Little Brown.

29 Application of Computers in the Emergency Department

Karen Sue Hoyt

OUTLINE

HEALTHCARE DELIVERY SYSTEMS IN THE NEXT DECADE

Healthcare Integration

The healthcare industry has faced change before, but this time these new directions are more dramatic and with greater consequences than at any other time in healthcare history. Healthcare delivery systems will begin to explore new strategies for the integration of the range of primary to tertiary care services offered in the emergency department. Hospitals and healthcare organizations will continue to face competition for urgent care services.[1] This approach will foster closer analysis of cost reduction measures, such as more automation and computerization. As a part of healthcare integration, managed care competition has brought forth an even greater need for the transfer of information across computer networks that link hospital emergency departments with affiliate hospitals, urgent care centers, and even remote clinic sites within the system.

Restructuring Workflow and Patient-Centered Care

In recent years there has been increasing emphasis on restructuring workflow to achieve the most cost-effective outcomes. Simultaneously, there has been an emphasis on patient-centered care. This means making systems that are "seamless" from the patient's perspective and moving the delivery services to the patient whenever possible. This workflow restructuring necessitates the need for providing timely, accurate, and integrated clinical, management, and financial information systems, which also ensure patient confidentiality.[2] The transfer of information by computers has eliminated the need for asking the patient the same information more than once. Automated discharge instructions, for example, also provide patients with simple-to-read forms that are thorough and complete.[3] This is in addition to the time savings for emergency department physicians and personnel.

Clinical Resource Management

Clinical resource management (CRM) departments within institutions have now been established nationwide. The goal of CRM is to reduce hospital costs by managing the use of ancillary services while continuing to provide quality patient care. This means appropriate use of laboratory tests, radiologic procedures performed, and the number and type of pharmaceuticals ordered for the patient. Studies indicate that physicians accessing resources by computer show lower resource utilization.[4] Another important CRM principle is to lessen variation in practice patterns and to produce more refined outcome measures. Emergency department algorithms and clinical policies allow emergency physicians and nurses to provide standardized care and to decrease practitioner variation.[5] Clinical diagnostic and decision-making software also can assist with these efforts. Additionally, although the need for determining outcomes over the long term continues, access to longitudinal patient data is also needed.[6] This information will have to be entered, stored, and retrieved from computer systems.

Information System Mandates

The Joint Commission on Accreditation of Healthcare Organizations (JCAHO) has already set standards on information systems management. In 1994 the JCAHO collected data from hospitals on clinical indicators to measure the quality of a hospital's care. This data collection is now mandatory.[7]

The Computer-Based Patient Record Institute, Inc, (CPRI), a nonprofit organization founded in 1992 in response to a 1991 Institute of Medicine study, stated that,

> in keeping within the context of computer applications . . . this committee recommends that an independent, national organization be created to accelerate the development, deployment, and use of computer-based patient records in the United States.[8]

The application of computers in the emergency department, therefore, is a technical imperative.

This chapter focuses on the use of computers in the delivery of patient-centered care. This care is provided by physicians, nurses, and support staff working in the emergency department setting. It is critical to keep in mind the changes occurring in healthcare and the overall information system requirements as computers are introduced into the emergency department environment.

INFORMATION SYSTEMS FOR THE EMERGENCY DEPARTMENT

Central File Server

Graphic operating systems (i.e., Windows) with high-level security that interface with hospital information systems are available today. These systems contain primarily patient admission, discharge, and transfer (ADT) information, along with the patient's financial data. They have an order entry function that gives the emergency department the ability to order laboratory and radiologic procedures on-line, as well as receive results. The retrieval of the these results then appears on these systems.

The trend seems to be personal computer (PC) systems connected to servers with less reliance on the mainframe. The systems are networked to hospital information systems for easy access to mainframe information. Many emergency departments with information systems capability usually have both mainframe and stand-alone terminals that may or may not communicate with each other.

Point-of-Care Terminals

At registration there will be mobile, preregistration, or self-registration options. At the bedside there will be wall-mounted units or rolling, wireless units. Point-of-care terminals in the emergency department are usually part of a stand-alone emergency department system. These terminals are used for patient charting at the bedside. The nurse validates data captured from monitored interfaces. These sources provide timely and accurate clinical information about patients. Desk-mounted units will have touch screen or keyboards for clinical information input. Check off lists will be used primarily for ease of charting.

Other Computer Software

Voice-Controlled Computer Software. In the last decade, communications technology for the emergency care setting has become more advanced. For instance, voice-activated systems have been introduced. This technology is potentially useful, but it has limitations that must be understood to be used effectively.[9] Database transcription services, however, are still the preferred method of generating a quality electronic record.

Hand-Held Devices. Several hand-held devices are available for recording patient information. Light-weight, palmtop devices are used at various points of care for easy data entry into computer systems.[10]

Other Emergency Department Software. Medical management information offers software on history taking, patient interviews, differential diagnoses, and patient management. Computer-aided diagnostic and decision-making and expert systems software are also available for the emergency clinician. Patient acuity and classification systems for billing along with scheduling (staffing) systems for the department have been used.

COMPUTERIZATION IN THE EMERGENCY DEPARTMENT

This section explores emergency department computer acquisition and data requirements, with an emphasis on obtaining clinical database information. The information needed to care for an emergency patient is best appreciated if it is based on patient flow through the department. Integration into an electronic medical record will be underscored during this process.

Data Elements

Integrating emergency department systems with hospital information systems (HIS) begins by creating an integrated emergency department electronic information infrastructure. To understand this integration, the emergency department must recognize the data elements it is attempting to capture in the system. These data elements should be based on the seven principal functions of the emergency department chart: (1) medical management/care, (2) quality improvement/management, (3) risk management, (4) reimbursement/billing, (5) clinical resource management, (6) regulatory/legal, and (7) research.[11] The categories essential for the development of a computerized emergency department medical record are outlined in box 29-1.

Electronic Registration

An important part of choosing a computerized emergency department system begins with method of patient registration. General patient information is obtained at the time of registration, which prepares for later possible hospital admission. Alternative methods of registration include preregistration from another database within the system, mobile registration via hand-held units, or self-registration on site by the emergency department patient. Because patients enter the system in a variety of ways (e.g., ambulatory, ambulance, helicopter), several options should be contemplated. Preauthorization information can now be obtained by electronic photograph identification.

BOX 29-1

AMERICAN COLLEGE OF EMERGENCY PHYSICIANS EMERGENCY DEPARTMENT MEDICAL RECORD ELEMENTS

Essential emergency department medical record elements categories include the following:

1. Prearrival information
2. Hospital record numbers
3. Initial encounter data
4. Patient demographics
5. Responsible parties
6. Emergency notification
7. Signature authorizations (legal agreement)
8. Clinical evaluation (history and physical)
9. Diagnostic interventions
10. Treatment interventions
11. Clinical course summary (progress notes and evidence of medical decision making)
12. Communications (private physicians, consultants, required reporting to agencies)
13. Final diagnostic/clinical impressions
14. Disposition

With the advent of healthcare reform, the medical identification card is used. This card contains information about the patient from demographics to an entire medical history. Information is updated with each clinic, office, or emergency department visit.[10]

Patient Tracking/Status Screen

The bar coded/electronic bracelet is used for emergency department patient tracking. This process begins the tracking process of the patient both within the department and to other departments (e.g., laboratory and radiology). A status board screen then displays the tracking information not only to personnel, but also to significant others in the emergency department waiting area.

Triage Information

Triage information is acquired from many sources. For patients admitted by ground or air transport, prehospital or transfer information is downloaded at the time the patient enters triage from electronic ambulance record systems. This includes clinical information from portable monitors (such as electrocardiogram [ECG] readings), which are transferred onto emergency department monitors by cartridge or disk.

Other triage needs include basic clinical information such as chief complaint, medical history, allergies, current medications, vital signs, and patient assessment data, which are entered electronically into a clinical information system at the bedside. Standardized treatment protocols, driven by the patient's chief complaint, prompt order entry of laboratory results and radiographs into the system.

Bedside Charting

Clinical information systems are used for bedside charting.[12] These systems have the capability to copy forward information or cross-chart information onto other flowsheets or forms for entry into the system only once. An example might be allergies, which need to appear on the emergency department admission sheet and at the bedside nursing documentation flowsheet.

Medication administration can be ordered immediately with approved computerized care algorithms at the point of care. Drug dosage software, already in use in emergency departments, calculates accurate drug doses and intravenous drip rates for the patient. These calculations are based on information obtained at triage in which the patient's age, height, weight, preexisting conditions, and chief complaint were entered.[13]

Electronic Discharge/Patient Teaching

At a minimum, discharge information must include patient diagnosis, interventions, medications given or prescribed, and referral information. Discharge and teaching instructions should be available in multiple languages. Prescribed medications should be cross-referenced for allergies and adverse drug reactions if the patient is on multiple medications. Electronic discharge should also prompt the system to provide appropriate medication administration information at the time of discharge.

Patient/family education is a key component to patient continuity of care. Computerized touch screen videos, for example, could be used to educate families using written diagnosis-specific aftercare instruction. These videos could be played while families are in the waiting area.

BOX 29-2

COMPUTER SELECTION COMMITTEE COMPOSITION

- Emergency department director
- Emergency department nurse manager
- Emergency department advanced practice nurse
- Representative from administration
- Medical records representative
- Data processing/information systems representative
- "Super/end user" (medical and nursing staff representatives)
- Support service representative (e.g., registration clerks, laboratory personnel, and respiratory therapist)

FROM SELECTION TO DIRECTION: PREIMPLEMENTATION

Selecting an Information Systems Committee

Choosing a particular computer system for the emergency department begins with the creation of a computer selection committee. The computer selection committee must consist of key stakeholders; not only those who will benefit from the use of the system, but also those who will use the system on a daily basis. Some of the members who should be selected for this committee are listed in Box 29-2.

The information systems selection committee serves another purpose. It can be used during and after system selec-

BOX 29-3

QUESTIONS TO ASK BEFORE PURCHASING AN EMERGENCY DEPARTMENT COMPUTER SYSTEM

I. What is the cost of the system?
   A. Hardware (including maintenance and upgrades)
   B. Software (including upgrades and new releases)
   C. Connectivity (e.g., wide area network)
   D. Client support (on-line support, repairs)
   E. Additional resources to support system (e.g., human)
   F. Customization costs (by vendor or hospital)
   G. Training costs
   H. Technical consultant fees if applicable
II. What is the reliability of the system?
   A. System architecture (e.g., distributed architecture, relational database)
   B. System performance (and ease of movement between screens)
   C. Frequency of downtime
III. Can the system (screens) be customized?
   A. By the hospital
   B. By the vendor
IV. Can the system interface/integrate to other systems and monitors?
   A. Interface capability to hospital information system and satellite clinics
   B. Ancillary services interfaces (laboratory, radiography, pharmacy) for order entry and resulting reporting
   C. Admissions, discharge, and transfer interface
   D. Does the system have the ability to download data from portable monitors/devices (e.g., electrocardiogram monitors, intravenous pumps, pulse oximeters)?
   E. Integration to a computerized patient record
   F. Order entry and results reporting to and from mainframe system/server
V. What is included in the software package?
   A. Patient registration
   B. Triage
   C. Patient tracking
   D. History and physical
   E. Physician order entry
   F. Nursing documentation at the bedside
   G. Results reporting
   H. Discharge instructions
   I. Prescriptions
   J. Phone directory with autodialing for physician referral
   K. Show reference (on-line protocols/algorithms)
   L. Medication administration dosage calculations
   M. Coding/billing features
   N. Query capability to produce ad hoc reports for the following:
      1. Patient acuity
      2. Patient flow
      3. Staffing requirements
      4. Waiting times
      5. Patient diagnoses
      6. Text processing
      7. Quality improvement
VI. What standard reports are included with this system?
VII. What are the security features?
   A. Passwords
   B. Levels of security
VIII. Satisfaction
   A. Patients
   B. End user (nursing and other ancillary services)
   C. Physician

tion to assist in the preparation of the emergency department specifications workbook that outlines the customers' (in this case the emergency department) configuration requests. It describes in minute detail the attributes of each flowsheet, the stipulations for printed reports, and other vital specification requirements including monitored interfaces.

Finally, and most important, this committee can be used as the coordinating body for customization changes after installation. The emergency department information systems committee should be given the authority to approve all flowsheet and configuration changes. The hospital medical records and information systems departments and the forms committee of the institution should also review the printed reports if they are not represented on this committee.

Selection Criteria

Questions to be asked when selecting a computer system for the emergency department are listed in Box 29-3. Other hospital end users, systems administrators, managers, and physicians should be interviewed.[14]

The Justification Proposal

All emergency department computer systems must have some cost/benefit justification if they are to be approved by hospital administration.[15] Systems should improve department productivity. The standard of care for emergency patients should be enhanced while realizing appropriate use of clinical resources.

Once there is significant interest in and support for a computerized emergency department system, the next step in the process is to prepare a justification proposal. Box 29-4 lists the components to include when writing the justification proposal.

Selling the Proposal

The proposal is next presented to key administrators for determination of purchasing. The "sell" to administration may consist of not only the written justification proposal, but also a more formalized presentation including a slide presentation or computer demonstration. Many hospitals use an information systems prioritization process that lists criteria for proposal completion. This process may require background information in the proposal document from the finance or data processing department or may require a key administrator to

BOX 29-4

PREPARING A JUSTIFICATION PROPOSAL FOR AN EMERGENCY DEPARTMENT SYSTEM

I. Introduction to a clinical information management system (CIMS)
II. Why a CIMS?
III. Comparative analysis of a patient care information system and a CIMS
  A. Differences
  B. Interface
IV. Preparation of the quotation
  A. Hardware
  B. Software
  C. Additional features costs
  D. Service and support agreement
  E. Other costs (wiring, cabling, local area network connections)
V. Benefits of a CIMS system
  A. User benefits
    1. Physicians
    2. Nurses
    3. Managers
  B. Benefits for the medical center
    1. Quality
      a. Accuracy
      b. Timely data capture
      c. Improved operations
      d. Legibility
      e. Completeness of emergency department record
      f. Standardized format
      g. Improved access to information
      h. Enhanced communication
      i. Easy auditability
      j. Validity (includes monitor interfaces)
      k. Quality assurance/quality improvement
      l. Risk management/clinical resource management/research
    2. Quality of care: detailed discharge instructions to patients
    3. Costs
      a. Reductions/revenue enhancement
      b. Nursing time/productivity
      c. Staff turnover/recruitment/marketing
      d. Reimbursement
      e. Supplies/resource use/resource management
      f. Regulatory compliance
      g. Changing practice style/procedure standardization
VI. Costs/benefits analysis
  A. Cost of a CIMS
  B. Savings
    1. Elimination of transcription costs
    2. Reduction of coding/billing errors
    3. Enhancement of reimbursement through accurate documentation of level of service provided
    4. Overtime reduction
    5. Eliminates missing emergency department record
    6. Forms usage reduction
    7. Supply and expense reduction
    8. Cost avoidance of additional personnel
    9. Revenue enhancement
    10. Break-even analysis
    11. Determining return on investment
VII. Additional considerations
  A. Password capability and levels of security
  B. System interface issues
  C. User orientation
  D. User acceptance of the system
  E. Competition
  F. System review
  G. System expansion

champion the proposal. It is important to solicit input and support for the system by other departments. Securing buy-in from others who will ultimately use the system is also wise. Evidence of support might be in the form of letters of support from physicians who will use the system or from managers from other departments who will benefit from computerization of the emergency department. Staff and even patient surveys are helpful in determining the value of the system. At some institutions pilot projects are negotiated through joint ventures with the vendor.

Contract Negotiations

After the selection process has occurred through the request for proposal (RFP) process or occasionally through sole source justification if only one vendor meets system requirements, contract negotiations begin. Signing of the contract with the vendor may take days to months. In some cases the purchasing department will assist the emergency department in the contract signing to be sure that the hardware and software purchases are agreeable and that the appropriate service and support agreements are in place.

Additional Support

At this point added human or other resources may be needed to prepare for system installation and ongoing support. These items should have been secured in the justification proposal. In some cases a nursing informatics person or a systems administrator may be hired or shared with another department. In many institutions the advanced practice nurse works with the vendor to write the system specifications and to train the staff. Support is usually provided by the information systems/data processing department. See Box 29-5 for a sample job description of a systems administrator.

FROM SELECTION TO DIRECTION: IMPLEMENTATION

Kick-off Meeting: Introduction of the System

After the contract is signed, it is important to schedule a kick-off meeting that includes the selection committee and all related parties. The vendor can also be present to demonstrate the system to staff and others who will be using the system.

BOX 29-5

SAMPLE JOB DESCRIPTION FOR A SYSTEMS ADMINISTRATOR AT UCSD MEDICAL CENTER SAN DIEGO, CA

Function/ task no.	Major functions and tasks
A.	**GENERAL SYSTEM RESPONSIBILITIES**
1.	Maintain system integrity; troubleshoot and resolve problems.
2.	Monitor system activity; check system logs in a proactive manner.
3.	Maintain system network; configure system set-up and changes; troubleshoot networking issues and maintain modem communication link.
4.	Establish and maintain communication with customer service and support; report system problems in a timely manner.
5.	Establish and maintain in-house user support policy, including after hours support.
6.	Provide first line support for end users; provide education as appropriate.
7.	Establish and maintain a contingency plan and backup procedures in the event of system failure.
8.	Maintain system components and history in the Medical Center problem management system.
9.	Maintain system problem log/resolution in Medical Center problem management system.
10.	Develop written documentation of system configuration, implementation, and operation, copy filed on UCSD Medical Center's Help Desk for emergency support.
11.	Participates in on-call rotation for troubleshooting computer problems in various departments.
B.	**HARDWARE/EQUIPMENT SUPPORT**
1.	Install new or replacement equipment on the local area network in accordance with Medical Center standards.
2.	Establish and maintain hardware support policies; return defective equipment for replacement; maintain accurate shipping records (date out, serial number, how shipped).
3.	Maintain records of all installed equipment, serial numbers, and placement location.
C.	**SOFTWARE SUPPORT**
1.	Install supplied software "Patches" and "Updates" in a timely manner.
2.	Test software upgrade/replacement in a "nonproduction" mode before implementation.
3.	Schedule system downtime as required by software updates.
4.	Implement security procedures as defined by the policies of the facility; maintain the password database accordingly.
5.	Maintain all customer-owned files and databases.
6.	Develop tools (e.g., shell scripts) to support operations and maintenance activities.
7.	Liaison between vendors, both hardware and software, that interact with the system.
8.	Maintain software upgrade/replacement history in Medical Center change management system.

Skills and knowledge	Selection importance
In-depth working knowledge of standard personal computer operating systems, network, and applications software.	Required
Strong technical knowledge of personal computer and mainframe computer components, various types of communication devices, and computer related equipment and supplies.	Required
Knowledge of computer programming languages, library editors, computerized file structures, data elements, and applications program structures.	Required
Familiar with system design process, including needs assessment and cost/benefit analysis.	Required
Ability to use advanced problem determination programs and equipment in problem analysis.	Required
Skill in implementing environment or software changes to effect problem resolution situations.	Required
Ability to organize and write procedures and documentation for Help Desk to resolve problems.	Required
Ability to conduct training sessions for end users in the effective use of their systems.	Required
In-depth working knowledge of programs and functions. Must be able to work in the component, problem, financial, and change management subsystems.	Required
Excellent verbal communication skills. Must be effective across a broad base of users and user experience.	Required
Excellent problem-solving skills; ability to communicate system needs to various groups clearly and concisely.	Required
Experience with server, local area networks, and modem communications.	Required
Skill in microcomputer hardware troubleshooting and replacement.	Required
Ability to write shell and C language programs.	Required
Familiarity with hospital/medical environments.	Preferred
Have a thorough understanding of the organization, functions, and goals of the data processing department, especially the end user support concepts.	Preferred

BOX 29-6

Approved by____________________
Date____________________

Subject: *Accountability/Passwords/Security*

Purpose: This policy explains the accountability policy, use of passwords, and security for the system.

Policy: All data entries **must be signed** (legal signature) using the individual's assigned password. Passwords are considered **strictly** confidential.

Scope: Registered Nurses (RNs) and Respiratory Therapists (RTs), clinical nutrition, pharmacy, unit secretaries, and technicians.

General Information:

1. A password has been issued to all employees. Passwords are **strictly confidential** and should not be revealed to others. Computer functions will **always** be linked to that user's password **regardless of who enters it.**
2. All data entries must be signed with this password; the password assigned to each user is equivalent to a **personal computer signature.**
3. After the password is entered into the system the user's initials will be linked to the data that have been entered. These initials will appear on the **printed report** (chart copy) and in the full signature of the **show detail** (popups) section on the screen.
4. Charting on the system using another employee's password is **strictly forbidden,** and use of any other user's password is considered misrepresentation.

Registry Personnel:

5. All registry personnel will be issued a password at the beginning of the shift by the Relief Charge Nurse or Assistant Nurse Manager.
6. The password issued for registry personnel is considered valid and operational each time the individual is assigned to the patient care area.
7. Registry personnel are required to adhere to the policies and procedures set forth by the department and the hospital.

Site Preparation

Site preparation is an important component of system implementation, or "going live." For example, if a large system with many bedside workstations has been approved, a staging area may be required to check all the computer hardware when it arrives. The system is then delivered to the emergency area, and the software is loaded onto the system. This is called *burning in,* or testing the system. Other installation considerations include connectivity to both system and device interfaces.

Screen Design

As mentioned, a specifications workbook outlining specific configuration requests and documentation requirements assists in delineating the design of each emergency department screen. For example, the configuration workbook defines the elements for a status screen. This document is composed in conjunction with the vendor because there may be questions about the feasibility and functionality of the configuration request.

When creating emergency department screens or flowsheets for computerization, necessary data elements should be incorporated into an emergency department medical record. The Centers for Disease Control (CDC) has developed a uniform emergency department data set based on specialty organization input. It is due to be released in 1997.

The Emergency Nursing Uniform Data Set (ENUDS) represents emergency nursing's effort to standardize the collection, storage, and retrieval of essential, comparable, core nursing data. ENUDS is part of the CDC uniform emergency department data set. ENUDS is an expansion of the Nursing Minimum Data Set (NMDS), including first assessment initial patient acuity (triage classification), nursing diagnoses, interventions, outcomes, and intensity of nursing care. The NMDS includes 16 elements that have been categorized into three groups: (1) nursing care, (2) client demographics, and (3) service.[16] These items of information are used on a regular basis by the majority of nurses in any setting where nursing care is provided.[16] Using standardized elements is helpful for computerized multicenter studies. NMDS is also useful for management information, quality assurance/quality improvement, and research.

Based on a collaborative approach and driven by standardized treatment protocols, computerized critical paths and algorithms for the emergency department are now being used in the emergency department based on standards of care.[17] These paths are invaluable in achieving clinical resource management within the department, as well as quality patient care.

Policies and Procedures

Policies and procedures need to be written by the project coordinator or system administrator before going live. The policies must be part of the staff's education and computer training. Policies and procedures include (1) general information, (2) password usage, (3) system security, (4) troubleshooting the system, (5) charting, (6) printed reports, (7) systems maintenance, and (8) the process for making configuration changes to the system. Boxes 29-6 and 29-7 illustrate a sample policy on Accountability/Passwords/Security and the Access Code Agreement Form. Before approving policies and procedures, the forms should be reviewed in relation to

BOX 29-7

COMPUTER ACCESS CODE AGREEMENT TEMP# ____________

(Please Print)
EMPLOYEE NAME ____________ **DATE** ____________
(Last) (First) (MI)

SIGNATURE ____________ **TITLE** ____________
(RN/RT/Unit Sec/Tech)

SOCIAL SECURITY # ____________ **DEPT or AGENCY** ____________

PASSWORD ____________ (8 character limit)

I have received my **personal** sign on/password, which gives me access to the computer system. I understand that this password is linked to my legal signature and, therefore, that there is no differentiation between my written signature and my electronic signature for charting of patient data.

I recognize that this system contains confidential clinical and financial patient information. I also recognize and **accept the responsibility** that comes with having access to the system and agree to:

1. Protect **all** patients' right to privacy by ensuring that information that appears on the screen or in printed form as a result of my using the system is seen or accessed by only those people in the hospital's employ who have a "need to know."
2. Maintain my personal signon/password access code in **the strictest confidence; not sharing it with *anyone* at *any* time.** This is done to:
   a. prevent others from charting patient data in my name.
   b. prevent untrained/unauthorized persons from harming the system through inappropriate use.
   IF FOR **ANY** REASON I FEEL THE SECRECY HAS BEEN BREACHED I WILL REQUEST A NEW PASSWORD FROM THE SYSTEM ADMINISTRATOR (or designee) IMMEDIATELY.
3. I **understand and agree** to the following procedures:
   a. I will sign all data I have entered in the system with the signon/password access code I have been assigned.
   b. I will notify the System Administrator (or designee) of changes required of my legal signature necessitated by changes in job class, assignment, and/or termination from the hospital.
4. I will be subject to **disciplinary action, including termination,** if I give out my signon/password access code to anyone *or* if I use another person's code to sign clinical data.
5. I will adhere to the **specific policies** set forth relating to the use of the system and all its related equipment.
6. I will adhere to the **hospital-wide data processing password policy.**

JCAHO requirements and by the medical records and information systems departments.

Project Team Training

One of the most important aspects in the implementation phase of a clinical information system is adequate hands-on training time. Some vendors allow end users to practice with the system after their training but before the day of system activation. It also gives the vendor an opportunity to see whether the system has been properly tested to avoid "crashes" on the day of activation.

Another important aspect of training is the development of super users. These are staff members who are chosen, on the basis of interest and background with computers, to act as resources to other staff nurses in real-time on the unit.[18] These individuals are invaluable when it comes to day-to-day troubleshooting. They may be given greater levels of security access and the responsibility of entering passwords. Additionally, super users are an asset when it comes to training new employees. This train-the-trainer concept is especially helpful after system installation because these individuals act as "champions" of the system. One super user should be chosen to represent staff on the computer committee. They also become configuration specialists with the ability to configure screens and flowsheets over time.

Use of the change process for system implementation is necessary to gain system acceptance and long-term buy-in. Change theory states that individuals will maintain the status quo and that creating a controlled disequilibrium is a necessary element of the change process. The role of the change agent, usually the advanced practice nurse or system administrator, cannot be underestimated for making and keeping the change. The change agent also may be an emergency physician or nurse manager.

Going Live

The term *going live* is used for the actual day that a system is brought forth to the end user. *Show stoppers* (Box 29-8) is the term used for any events that may prevent the system from going up. Box 29-9 provides tips for the day of going live.

Date/time	Problem identified	Background information	Intervention performed	Reported by	Logged in by	Was customer service called?

FIGURE 29-1 System problem log.
(Courtesy EMTEK System 2000, Tempe, Ariz.)

BOX 29-8

SHOW STOPPERS BEFORE GOING LIVE

1. Are there any hardware, software, or connectivity issues that have not been resolved?
2. Has there been adequate training time for all system users?
3. Is there adequate vendor support on the day of going live?
4. Is there adequate information systems support within the hospital?
5. Is there adequate staffing for this day (around the clock)?
6. Have all policies and procedures been approved and are staff knowledgeable?

BOX 29-9

TIPS FOR THE DAY OF GOING LIVE

1. Pick a time of day that is least disruptive (e.g., low census, nights) for go live.
2. Have problem log/enhancement available for staff to write in, and have a forum for staff to vent (computer committee).
3. Prepare staff at training/staff meetings for system downtime. Overestimate the time.
4. Provide adequate staffing. Staff up! Use super users to circulate throughout the unit to assist with documentation needs the first few days.
5. Plan troubleshooting coverage throughout the night by the vendor and the system administrator.
6. Notify key personnel and departments that will be affected by this implementation.
7. Provide refreshments on the day of going live.

FROM SELECTION TO DIRECTION: POSTIMPLEMENTATION

Configuration Changes

After going live there are usually screen configuration changes. Plan for these changes. A request process can be used through a problem log for system failures (Figure 29-1) or through the use of an enhancement log for configuration requests (Figure 29-2). The approval process should create a multidisciplinary subcommittee, which includes end users.

Ongoing System Maintenance

System maintenance is important for long-term system viability and acceptance. On-call support with a knowledgeable

Date	Enhancement suggestion	On which screen (?) (if applicable)	Your name and title (RN, MD, etc.)

FIGURE 29-2 System enhancements log.
(Courtesy EMTEK System 2000, Tempe, Ariz.)

system administrator is a key component to the success or failure of a clinical information system.

System Acceptance

System success depends on choosing a reliable information system and on the participation of staff during the process. Adequate training and an understanding of all the policies and procedures, especially the troubleshooting policy, are crucial before implementation occurs. Empowering staff to troubleshoot the system after going live gives them a sense of control and autonomy.

Continuous dialogue through a computer committee and ongoing support by both the department and the vendor are other key success factors. System failure occurs when either the system architecture lacks performance or the staff perceive there is no forum for problem solving. Inadequate training leads to frustration and is perceived as lack of ongoing support. The role of the change agent cannot be underestimated at this time. The change agent can mean the difference, at times, between system acceptance or system failure.

SUMMARY

No hospital department will be affected more by shifts in U.S. demographics than the emergency department. The American Hospital Association predicts that the emergency department will generate more than 50% of all hospital admissions by the mid 1990s.[19] Whether emergency departments continue tobe the primary care provider or the observation/holding unit for the hospital, they will need to manage clinical, financial, and management information for the 90 million patients seen in emergency departments across the country each year.[14]

Hospitals must develop or reinforce a corporate culture that rewards long-term efforts in technology. Emergency departments must look toward the future with creative vision. As hospitals change the way they do business, the use of patient information systems in the emergency department will be an important part of that future.

REFERENCES

1. American Hospital Association—Society for Ambulatory Care Professionals (SACP): Emergency services, *Trendlines* p. 6-7, 1996.
2. American Health Information Management Association (AHIMA): *In confidence,* 1:1-3, 1993.
3. Gagnon L: Automating emergency department aftercare instructions. In Hoyt K, Bradley V, Taylor T editors: *Topics in Emergency Medicine* 18(1):74, 1996.
4. Gardner E: Get the computers right, and physicians will get with the program, *Mod Healthc* 23:35,38,40,44,46,50, 1993.
5. American College of Emergency Physicians: Clinical pediatric fever policy, *Ann Emerg Med* 1993.
6. Lumsdon K: The clinical connection, *Hospitals* 16, 1993.
7. Joint Commission on Accreditation of Healthcare Organizations: *1996 accreditation manual for hospitals,* Oak Ridge Terrace, Ill, 1996, Joint Commission.
8. CPRI Demonstration Projects Work Group: *CPRI survey,* Chicago, 1993, Computer-Based Patient Record Institute.

9. Paul R: Voice-controlled computer software in emergency medicine. In Taylor T, Bradley V, Hoyt K editors: *Topics in Emergency Medicine,* Frederick, Md, 1995, Aspen.
10. American College of Emergency Physicians: *A view of the emergency department of the future: computers in emergency medicine,* 1993, ACEP.
11. American College of Emergency Physicians: *Emergency medicine practice committee. Emergency department medical record elements,* 1993, ACEP.
12. Simpson RL: Technology: nursing the system—how to survive the next decade, *Nurs Manage* 21:24-25, 1990.
13. Rantz MJ, Miller TV: Change theory, *Nurs Clin North Am* 22:887-897, 1987.
14. Meyer C: Bedside computer charting: inching toward tomorrow, *Am J Nurs* 38-44, 1992.
15. Hoyt K: Clinical information systems: writing the winning proposal, *ENA Etcetera* 1(1)3-4, 1993.
16. Leske JS, Werley HH: Use of the nursing minimum data set, *Comput Nurs* 10:259-263, 1992.
17. Nelson MS: Critical pathways in the emergency department, *J Emerg Nurs* 19:110-114, 1993.
18. Burkes M: Identifying and relating nurses' attitudes toward computer use, *Comput Nurs* 9:190-201, 1991.
19. Matson T: Ambulatory care to drive hospital services in 1990's, *Health Care Strateg Manage* 1991.

30 Observation Units in the Emergency Department

Louis G. Graff

OUTLINE

Traditional emergency department patient evaluation and management has certain shortcomings. Emergency physicians in their initial evaluation may miss 4% to 13% of acute myocardial infarctions,[1,2] 10% to 40% of acute appendicitis,[3,4] and 40% of ectopic pregnancies.[5] Improvement in emergency physician performance is needed. In former times emergency physicians admitted most of the patients they could not successfully diagnose or manage in the initial several hours of care. Patients and third-party payors now expect as many patients as possible to be managed on an outpatient basis with hospitalization the recourse of last resort. Given these expectations patients with acute asthma, congestive heart failure (CHF), and other conditions often fail outpatient therapy and return to the emergency department for admission.[6,7] In many of these situations a longer observation and treatment period during the initial visit might have prevented the subsequent patient admission.

REASONS FOR OBSERVATION UNITS

Observation medicine has developed over the past two decades to address many of these problems. With emergency department (ED) observation units, emergency physicians have improved their diagnostic accuracy.[3,8] Patients with a difficult diagnostic syndrome (e.g., abdominal pain, chest pain, or grand mal seizure) are not discharged home until the physician has a high degree of certainty that they do not have a serious disease. With ED observation units, emergency physicians have also improved their therapeutic success rate. Most patients who fail an acute trial of clinical therapy (such as those with asthma or acute congestive heart failure) can be successfully managed with the use of ED observation beds. With the evolution of these units, emergency physicians have assumed a greater role in providing acute care to the patient. Given the relatively short time available to make a definitive disposition in traditional emergency practice, many patients have to be admitted for further evaluation because they have the potential for serious disease or have not been adequately stabilized. If these patients can be evaluated over 24 hours in ED observation beds, diagnostic and therapeutic yield increases and many such patients can be discharged home. Savings to the health care payers can be substantial, ranging from $1000 to $3000 per patient.[9] Through the use of observation units, not only can the emergency physicians provide high-quality, cost-effective patient care, but also patient satisfaction is often enhanced by the avoidance of a hospital admission.

IMPLEMENTATION STRATEGY

An emergency department needs to substantially change its infrastructure to successfully introduce an ED observation program (Box 30-1). In the first place, the mission of this unit needs to be clearly defined after collaboration with various hospital departments, the medical staff, and emergency department personnel. Observation is a service provided in addition to traditional emergency department evaluation and treatment. The patients are in the department for a mean 12 hours rather than 1 to 2 hours. The emergency department needs to develop additional space and staff to provide the services for these prolonged stays. Because the complexity of patient care is increased by the prolonged patient stay, patient care policies and procedures need to be developed and implemented specifically for observation patients. For instance, mechanisms to provide food, medications, and physician oversight must be defined. The quality management program needs to be expanded to evaluate and continuously improve the processes of patient care for these patients. Responsibility for the various management entities needs to be clearly delineated. In addition, the department should have a utilization review program to prevent inappropriate admissions to the unit.

DESIGN OF FACILITY

The design of the ED observation area should be consistent with the function of the ED observation area (Box 30-2). Patients are in the observation area for 12 to 24 hours and need appropriate amenities such as a sink, table, cabinet, and bathroom. Suggested national architectural guidelines for such a unit include a centralized nursing station, 100 square feet of clear floor space per treatment area, a nurse call bell, oxygen, vacuum, and air.[10] Most emergency departments with observation units have one or two beds per 10,000 patient

BOX 30-1

IMPLEMENTATION STRATEGY

Design of facility
Staffing
Policies and procedures
Management of observation unit
Funding and reimbursement

BOX 30-2

FACILITY DESIGN

One to two observation beds per 10,000 ED visits
100 square feet of clear floor space per observation room
Centralized nursing station
Monitored beds for patients with selected conditions
  Diagnostic evaluation—chest pain, syncope, palpitation, chest trauma, overdose, dizziness
  Treatment—CHF, allergic reaction, hypertensive urgency
Nonmonitored beds for patients with other conditions
  Diagnostic evaluation—abdominal pain, flank pain, confusion, weakness, fever, gastrointestinal/genitourinary bleed, abdominal trauma
  Treatment—pneumonia, asthma, dehydration, hyperglycemia, hypoglycemia, pyelonephritis
Oxygen outlet
Vacuum outlet
Air outlet
Nurse call button
Electrical outlets
Phone outlet
Sink
Table
Bathroom availability

BOX 30-3

STAFFING

Physician
  One FTE for 1500 to 3000 patients per year
Nursing
  One nurse for four monitored observation beds (4.2 FTE per year)
  One nurse for eight nonmonitored observation beds (4.2 FTE per year)
Aides/Techs
Secretary

visits.[11] This number may vary based on local medical staff practice, hospital resources, and institutional case mix.

The need for monitoring capabilities in the observation unit depends on the types of patients treated in the unit.[12] Monitoring is not needed for patients free of cardiovascular risk or hemodynamic instability. Examples of such patients are those being evaluated for abdominal pain or treated for asthma. In such cases, the observation unit bed functions similar to a hospital ward bed. Monitoring is needed for patients at risk of sudden cardiovascular events or hemodynamic instability. Examples of such patients are those being evaluated for chest pain, syncope, or new atrial fibrillation. The observation unit bed then functions similar to a step-down unit. Monitoring capabilities for such patients may include arrhythmia alarms, oximetry, blood pressure, pulse, respiratory rate, and advanced monitoring techniques such as ST-segment analysis.

The use of observation units may allow the emergency department physician to significantly increase his or her ability to diagnose acute myocardial infarction in patients with chest pain. Only 50% to 60% of patients with acute myocardial infarction have a positive creatinine phosphatase isoenzyme (CK-MB) or positive electrocardiogram (ECG) on presentation. On the other hand, given 12 hours of observation, 95% of patients with acute myocardial infarction will have a positive CK-MB or positive ECG.[8,13] These monitored ED observation units have been called chest pain EDs, short-stay coronary units, and heart EDs, and there has been a rapid growth of them nationally.

STAFFING

Additional nursing staff are needed to staff an ED observation unit (Box 30-3) because services are provided in addition to those normally provided in traditional emergency department evaluation and management. In general, one nurse is needed for every eight nonmonitored beds. This equates to 4.2 nursing full-time equivalent (FTE) to provide service 24 hours per day for 7 days per week. Minimum nurse staffing for monitored beds is one nurse for every four beds.

Additional physician staff are needed as well for an observation program. Observation patients require on average 58 minutes of physician service per patient.[13] This is considerably more than the average for patients requiring nonselected ED services (22 minutes per patient).[14] Approximately one additional FTE of physician staffing will be required for every 1500 to 3000 patients observed.

Additional ancillary staff are needed for an observation program. Need for additional aides, secretaries, and physician assistants depends on the type of staffing desired for the department, the apportionment of patient care tasks, and the number of emergency physicians.

POLICY AND PROCEDURES

Policies and procedures are needed for the observation unit beyond those required for usual emergency department patient services. They should be consistent with the goals of the observation unit in providing continuing care in contrast with the episodic care provided in the traditional emergency department. Documentation and orders should be written so that the multiple personnel providing services to the patient over a prolonged time are clearly directed in what should be done for the patient and what is expected in the patient's ultimate disposition.[15]

BOX 30-4

EMERGENCY DEPARTMENT OBSERVATION UNITS STANDARDS SET BY THE JOINT COMMISSION ON ACCREDITATION OF HEALTHCARE ORGANIZATIONS

Written policies and procedures addressing type of patient use
Maximum time for care
Mechanism for providing appropriate surveillance
Type of nurse/patient system

BOX 30-5

QUALITY ASSURANCE/UTILIZATION REVIEW

Services provided
- Number of observation patients
- Number (%) of observation patients admitted

Delays in providing services
- Time to see physician
- Number of patients leaving against medical advice

Complications/problems
- Death
- Codes
- Complaints

Staff to provide services
- Physicians—FTE
- Nurses—FTE
- Aides—FTE
- Secretary—FTE

The Joint Commission on Accreditation of Healthcare Organizations (JCAHO) has set four standards for ED observation programs (Box 30-4).[16] The American College of Emergency Physicians has published guidelines for managing ED observation services since 1988.[17] A textbook has been published as a reference source on most of the conditions managed in an ED observation unit.[18] Policies in the emergency department should address the issues discussed in these authoritative publications.

UNIT MANAGEMENT

An active continuous quality improvement (CQI) and utilization review (UR) program needs to be developed to ensure high quality of patient care (Box 30-5).[19-21] When emergency physicians provide observation services, they assume additional responsibilities. The processes of patient care need to be carefully evaluated and constantly improved. Useful quality indicators include physician and nursing documentation, timeliness of care, and patient satisfaction. In addition, a utilization review program examining the appropriateness of observation unit admissions is critical to the success of the unit and good patient care.

In general, the admission of patients with high service intensity or high severity of illness may result in unnecessary risk to patients during the period of ED observation. These patients should be admitted to the acute care hospital. It is also inappropriate to admit patients to the ED observation unit who have minor complaints or simply for the convenience of the private physician. The CQI/UR program should examine on a monthly basis the appropriateness of all admissions in relation to the admitting guidelines.

Table 30-1 Reimbursement

Charge	Codes	Relative Value Unit
Facility	99281	0.29
	99282	0.51
	99283	1.67
	99284	2.53
	99285	3.96
Physician	99218	1.86
	99219	2.99
	99220	3.73

FUNDING AND REIMBURSEMENT

Additional services are provided to emergency department patients who are observed, and consequently additional funding must be found to allay the cost of these services (Table 30-1). Observation patients receive frequent nursing services and more than double the amount of physician services than the average patient.[14] Charges for the services depend on whether monitored or nonmonitored care is provided. Nonmonitored service charges are similar to those of hospital ward beds with a similar intensity of service. Monitored bed services are charged similar to those of step-down units because care is most similar to that offered in these units.

Physician charges for observation services are now nationally standardized. Current procedural terminology (CPT) 4 codes specific for observation services have been developed (99218, 99219, 99220) and are used instead of evaluation and management (E&M) codes for emergency department visits (99281, 99282, 99283, 99284, 99285).[22] The charges for these observation codes are similar to the top three E&M codes for emergency department visits.

The economic impact of the observation unit must be viewed from a hospital and physician perspective in terms of the overall cost of both services in a competitive healthcare market.

IMPACT ON EMERGENCY MEDICINE PRACTICE

The development of emergency department observation services is another step in the maturation and development of emergency medicine. Through the 1950s there were no physicians in the emergency department. The private physician would be on call and contacted by the nurse in the department when patients arrived. The on-call physician would decide over the phone whether he or she had to come to the emergency department, call a specialty physician, or triage the patient to a physician's office. The surgeon would be called for lacerations, the obstetric/gynecologic physician for the female with abdominal pain, or the internist for the patient with chest pain. Patients who were seriously ill were admitted directly to the hospital.

Beginning in the 1960s many physicians began to work full-time in emergency departments. They would manage patients who had minor illnesses. They would decide which specialist to call in to the emergency department for certain patients, and they would also contact the on-call physician for patients who required admission. Patients were expected to have a disposition within an hour or two, and extended therapy or evaluation was not commonly performed in the emergency department.

In the 1970s the presence of physicians in the emergency department 24 hours per day, 7 days per week, created the opportunity for the development of observation services.

Prospective payment and hospital admission criteria were implemented in 1983. This created powerful incentives for ED observation services. Patients were not to be admitted to the acute care hospital without clear documentation of the presence of serious disease. Extended emergency department evaluation and therapy were often needed to determine which patients really needed such care. With a 10- to 12-hour period of ED observation, many studies have shown that as many as 80% of potential short-term hospital admission patients can be safely discharged home.

SUMMARY

Emergency department observation services are rapidly becoming a crucial element of the modern healthcare system. The creation of observation units may represent the final stage in the evolution of the emergency department from a nursing triage station to a definitive patient care unit. The creation of observation units may also enhance the image of emergency department physicians as primary caregivers and "gate keepers," which will underscore their importance in the managed care systems of the future.

REFERENCES

1. Tierney WM, Fitzgerald J, McDenny RM et al: Physician's estimates of the probability of myocardial infarction in emergency room patients with chest pain, *Med Decis Making* 6:15-17, 1986.
2. Goldman L, Cook EF, Brand D et al: Computer protocol to predict myocardial infarction in emergency department patients with chest pain, *N Engl J Med* 318:797-803, 1988.
3. Graff LG, Radford MJ, Werne C: Probability of appendicitis before and after observation, *Ann Emerg Med* 18:439, 1989.
4. Cacioppo JC, Dietrich NA, Kogh G et al: The consequences of current constraints on surgical treatment of appendicitis, *Am J Surg* 157:276-280, 1989.
5. Stovall TG, Kellerman AL, Lling FW et al: Emergency department diagnosis of ectopic pregnancy, *Ann Emerg Med* 19:1098-1103, 1990.
6. Murphy DG, Zalenski RJ, Raucci JC et al: The utility of extended emergency department treatment of asthma: an analysis of improvement in peak expiratory flow as a function of time, *Ann Emerg Med* 18:467, 1989 (abstract).
7. Dunbar LM, Dyer TW, Grender J: Congestive heart failure patients: admit or discharge? A prospective study of observation unit care for 101 patients, *Clin Res* 39(4):828A, 1991.
8. Gibler WB, Young GP, Hedges JR et al: Acute myocardial infarction in chest pain patients with nondiagnostic ECGs: serial CK-MB sampling in the emergency department, *Ann Emerg Med* 21:504-512, 1992.
9. Graff LG: Economical service. In Graff LG, editor: *Observation medicine,* Stoneham, Mass, 1993, Butterworth-Heinemann.
10. American Institute of Architects Committee on Architecture for Health with assistance from the US Department of Health and Human Services: *Guidelines for construction and equipment of hospitals and medical facilities 1992-1993,* Washington, DC, 1993, American Institute of Architects Press.
11. Graff LG: Principles of observation medicine. In Graff LG, editor: *Observation medicine,* Stoneham, Mass, 1993, Butterworth-Heinemann.
12. Graff LG, Joseph T: Hospital site of service. In Graff LG, editor: *Observation medicine,* Stoneham, Mass, 1993, Butterworth-Heinemann.
13. Gaspoz JM, Lee TH, Cook EF et al: Outcome of patients who were admitted to a new short-stay unit to "rule out" myocardial infarction, *Am J Cardiol* 68:145-149, 1991.
14. Graff LG, Wolf S, Dinwoodie R et al: Emergency physician workload: a time study, *Ann Emerg Med* 22:1156-1163, 1993.
15. Severance HW: Continuity of care for the emergency department observation unit. In Graff LG, editor: *Observation medicine,* Stoneham, Mass, 1993, Butterworth-Heinemann.
16. *Accreditation manual for hospitals 1991,* vol 1, *Standards,* Chicago, 1990, Joint Commission on Accreditation of Healthcare Organizations.
17. American College of Emergency Physicians: American College of Emergency Physicians Practice Management Committee. Emergency department observation units, *Ann Emerg Med* 17:1348-1352, 1988.
18. Graff LG, editor: *Observation medicine,* Stoneham, Mass, 1993, Butterworth-Heinemann.
19. Brillman J: Intensive managerial review. In Graff LG, editor: *Observation medicine,* Stoneham, Mass, 1993, Butterworth-Heinemann.
20. Kritchevsky SB, Simmons BP: Continuous quality improvement: concepts and applications for physician care, *JAMA* 266:1817-1823, 1991.
21. Graff LG: Utilization review: emergency medicine implications, *Emerg Med Clin North Am* 10(3):583-596, 1992.
22. American Medical Association: Hospital observation services, *CPT Assistant* 3(1):1-4, 1993.

31 The Emergency Department Fast Track

George M. Innes, Jr. and Peter L. Sosnow

OUTLINE

In the last 30 years, emergency departments throughout the United States have seen unprecedented increases in patient volume and utilization. A broad spectrum of patients challenges us to provide appropriate and timely emergency care while maintaining cost effectiveness and patient satisfaction. Emergency department fast tracks have evolved to help meet this challenge and have achieved significant success.

Emergency departments see patients with a wide range of acuity and severity levels. Studies have shown that between 20% and 60% of all patients presenting to emergency departments have urgent yet simple and uncomplicated problems that can be cared for quickly and efficiently in lower intensity settings.[1,2]

Fast track programs allow these patients to be seen in a separately defined "track." This approach avoids the inherent conflict, delay, and gridlock that often occur in the delivery of care in the full-service emergency department. Fast track patients are seen separately in an efficient and continuously flowing area set aside in or adjacent to the emergency department. Patient satisfaction is greatly enhanced by appropriately shortening the turnaround time in the delivery of simple, uncomplicated medical care.[3] In addition, the efficiency and effectiveness of acute emergency care delivery are enhanced by relieving congestion in the "main" department. Staff are free to focus and concentrate their efforts on the more complex diagnostic workups, treatments, and dispositions required by more serious, acute patients in the main department.

IMPLEMENTATION

Fast track programs may operate in any size emergency department. The belief that fast track programs are only for large emergency departments with some specific threshold census number may be shortsighted. A fast track program can be created even in small departments by rededicating existing staff and space to the fast track concept. The designation of even one or two beds in a small department may be enough to create a fast track with all its advantages. Larger emergency departments can accommodate a separate but integrated fast track treatment area. The fundamental requirement for a fast track program is a dedicated treatment area for use by the appropriately selected fast track patient. This area must be continuously staffed despite other demands of the main department. Patient flow and staff stress levels will both be manageable as long as this principle is followed.

The fast track area ideally should be located adjacent to the main emergency department. This geographic configuration allows for shared triage. In addition, enhanced supervision of physician extenders (physician's assistants or nurse practitioners) who may staff the fast track can occur. Sharing of supplies and equipment is also possible. The greatest advantage is the ability to better control patient flow. Physicians or physician's extenders may float between the main department or fast track, depending on specific patient requirements and department census. Many departments have found that when the fast track is removed from direct access of the main department, delays may occur when the fast track is busy and the main department is slow.

The fast track's space requirements can be estimated from the department's overall census. Approximately one third to one half of the total emergency department volume will meet the triage criteria for the fast track (Box 31-1). These patients may be seen in an 8- to 16-hour period as appropriate to accomodate the timing of patient presentation to the emergency department. On average, three to four patients may be easily seen every hour by one practitioner in the fast track.

The ordering of radiographs and laboratory studies by triage will speed assessment and shorten turnaround time. Movement of patients from triage to outpatient laboratory facility, radiography, and then to fast track will give patients a sense of forward momentum, which will lead to increased patient satisfaction. Patients may be brought back to the waiting room if waiting for their laboratory or radiographic studies delays their disposition. This option will free up treatment areas for other fast track patients waiting to be seen. Any patient who requires a more involved workup than originally identified in triage should be transferred to the main department for care.

The need for good primary care should be emphasized to all fast track patients, and appropriate follow-up referrals should be given. The hospital medical staff should be fully informed about these policies to address potential fears of competition with their practices and to ensure their support and cooperation.

Staffing

One of the most important ingredients of a successful fast track program is nursing staff committed to the area. It is the responsibility of that staff to ensure that the fast track flow remains optimal. Continuous nurse staffing should not be in-

BOX 31-1

TRIAGE DIAGNOSES FOR FAST TRACK

1. Minor contusions, sprains, or possible fractures of a stable nature (triage should order radiograph)
2. Musculoskeletal complaints without neurodeficits
3. Minor lacerations or abrasions
4. Insect bites without systemic involvement
5. Sore throats, earaches, URIs without dyspnea or airway compromise
6. Dental problems
7. UTIs, uncomplicated vaginitis, STDs (Triage to send off UA, urine pregnancy, dip stick urine, hold urine C&S)
8. Rash without fever
9. Medication refills
10. Emergency department rechecks and suture removal

URI, Upper respiratory infection; *UTI,* urinary tract infection; *STD,* sexually transmitted disease; *UA,* urinalysis; *C&S,* culture and sensitivity.

BOX 31-2

COMPLAINTS OF PATIENTS WHO SHOULD NOT BE SEEN BY PHYSICIAN EXTENDER WITHOUT PHYSICIAN CONSULTATION

1. Head trauma with loss of consciousness
2. Allergic reactions with systemic symptoms
3. Chest pain
4. Abdominal pain
5. Shock or hemodynamic instability
6. Third- and second-degree burns involving palms or large area of distribution
7. Altered mental status
8. Neurologic deficits
9. Drug overdose
10. Headache with neurovascular signs/symptoms and/or fever
11. Sexual assault

terrupted by "breaks" or by pulling staff back to the main department. A common critical staffing mistake is to place the least experienced or least productive member of the nursing staff in the fast track because it has a lower acuity. By doing nursing staffing this way the effectiveness of the area may be decreased, leading to longer patient waits and decreased patient satisfaction.

Physician extenders are a cost-effective method of staffing the fast track. The lower acuity of the fast track correlates well with the scope of practice of physician extenders.[4] If multiple physicians are on duty, a specific physician should be assigned to supervise and act as backup to the physician extender. This strategy will ensure clarity as to which physician is responsible for the physician extender. A delineation of the physician extender's role and responsibilities must be formally documented. Specific conditions and procedures that may be handled by a physician extender, as well as conditions and procedures that should not be seen, must be defined in department policy and procedure and implemented at triage[4] (Box 31-2). On-site availability of an emergency department physician for appropriate concurrent consultation is essential.[5,6]

In general, the fast track functions best when dedicated staff provide coverage. Rotating staff between the main emergency department and the fast track may not result in optimal staff efficiency or motivation. The fast track should not be an area that staff retire to when they can no longer manage the main department. The high turnaround of these patients requires a well-trained and productive staff if patient flow is to proceed at greatest efficiency.

Triage

A fast track program allows a great opportunity to improve any department's triage capability. The triage nurse is the quarterback of emergency department flow. Accurate and complete triage of patients is vital in selecting the correct patients for the fast track. A nurse should complete a full program of directed readings, in-servicing, and orientation before being allowed to staff triage alone. Box 31-1 lists examples of patients who can be triaged to the fast track.

The triage nurse must have a constant awareness of the delays facing all areas of the department. This information can be shared with the charge nurse and physicians on duty to redirect resources in the best way to maintain flow and level of care.

Finances

The fast track allows more patients to be seen quickly and with greater cost effectiveness. These goals are important if an emergency department is to compete for patients who may be redirected by managed care programs or lost to free-standing urgent care centers. The charge for a service, whether made in the main department or fast track, should be based on the actual level of service for the procedure. The charges for fast track care, therefore, should be lower because of the decreased acuity and lower level of service required.

Fast track programs increase patient satisfaction and decrease patient walkouts substantially, thereby recouping revenue that otherwise would have been lost. The decreased waiting time in a properly run program also can lead to an increase in market share from competing emergency departments that are unable to control their turnaround times.

Healthcare reform may bring many changes to emergency departments. A fast track program will allow these departments to get costs under control, properly positioning them for future changes.

OUTCOME MONITORING

Fast track must be monitored and evaluated on an ongoing basis to improve. Patient turnaround time should be routinely screened and should fall in the 30- to 90-minute range from registration to discharge.

All hospital admissions from fast track should be evaluated for appropriateness of the original triage. Care must be taken to prevent staff from overlooking more serious conditions as a result of an initial fast track triage. These cases should be regularly discussed at staff meetings to maintain a high degree of alertness. All return visits also should be reviewed carefully. Patient satisfaction surveys are invaluable to gauge the success or failure of the program.

SUMMARY

The appropriately managed fast track can be a major boost to the efficiency and cost effectiveness of any size emergency department. It can lead to increased satisfaction of patients and staff, decreased gridlock, decreased walkouts, and improved department competitiveness. With good planning and appropriate implementation, any department can meet this challenge and succeed.

REFERENCES

1. Padgett DK, Brodsky B: Psychosocial factors influencing non-urgent use of the emergency room: a review of the literature and recommendations for research and improved service delivery, *Social Sci Med* 35:1189-1197, 1992.
2. Purnell LDT: A survey of emergency department triage in 185 hospitals: physical facilities, fast-track systems, patient-classification systems, waiting times, and qualification, training, and skills of triage personnel, *J Emerg Nurs* 17:402-407, 1991.
3. Clark RB: Fast track (editorial), *Ann Emerg Med* 17:543-544, 1988.
4. Sturmann KM, Ehrenberg K, Salzberg MR: Physician assistants in emergency medicine, *Ann Emerg Med* 19:304-308, 1990.
5. American College of Emergency Physicians: *Guidelines on the role of physician assistants in emergency departments, Ann Emerg Med* 26:773, 1995.
6. American College of Emergency Physicians: Guidelines on the role of nurse practitioners in emergency departments, *Ann Emerg Med,* 26:772, 1995

ADDITIONAL READINGS

Cardello DM: Implementation of a one-hour fast-track service: one hospital's experience, *J Emerg Nurs* 18:239-243, 1992.

Covington C, Erwin T, Sellers F: Implementation of a nurse practitioner-staffed fast track, *J Emerg Nurs* 18:124-131, 1992.

Henne SJ, Warner NE, Frank KJ: Ambulatory care centers: a unique opportunity for nurse practitioners, *Nurse Practitioner* 13:43-55, 1988.

Koska MT: Urgent care/primary care concept proves profitable, *Hospitals* 63:74-77, 1989.

Meislin HW, Coates SA, Cyr J, Valenzuela T: Fast track: urgent care within a teaching hospital emergency department: can it work? *Ann Emerg Med* 17:453-456, 1988.

Romanelli N: Taking charge: we put ED patients on the fast track, *RN* 55:17-19, 1992.

Snell FI, Jones SL, Yoder L: Factors in choosing an urgent care center versus an emergency department, *J Emerg Nurs* 13:355-358, 1987.

Wright SW, Erwin TL, Blanton DM, Covington CM: Fast track in the emergency department: a one-year experience with nurse practitioners, *J Emerg Med* 10:367-373, 1992.

32 Death in the Emergency Department

Dan Mayer

The situation of an older family member who has multiple medical problems and suddenly arrests at home is often handled well by the family. However, the totally unexpected death of a previously healthy person, sudden infant death, the young victim of accidental death, or the middle-aged or older person who was in excellent health and had unexpected sudden death is always devastating for the family, and sometimes also for the emergency care providers. This chapter discusses the mechanics of telling the living, the process of death notification, and the principles of critical incident stress reduction in crisis situations.

Emergency department staff members are primarily concerned with saving lives. This primacy of the resuscitation effort often reduces the amount of time staff members are willing to spend with family members explaining the death of their loved one and helping them to understand and accept the death. Surveys of survivors of victims of sudden death show that a significant number felt that the emergency department staff lacked warmth, lacked sympathy, and was not reassuring.[1]

UNEXPECTED DEATH—THE MECHANICS OF TELLING THE LIVING

When a patient dies in the prehospital area or in the emergency department, it becomes the responsibility of the emergency department staff to notify the family. Traditionally done by the physician on duty with the assistance of a senior nurse, the most senior person available (an attending or senior resident) should tell the family. Programs for teaching residents the skills of informing the family have been proposed.[2] The process of notifying family and friends is stressful to the physician, and most emergency physicians do not feel well trained for this task.[3] There is a great temptation to delegate this duty to other staff, especially nursing. Nursing staff should be involved in the process as part of a team with the physicians.[4] Notification should not be delegated because it gives the family the mistaken impression that the physician does not feel that the death of their loved one is important. With a proper mind-set, physicians can minimize the stress to themselves, give the family vital information about the patient and the patient's death, and allow the family to get on with the grieving process.

The setting in which this discussion occurs is important. Avoid telling the family over the phone, in the hall, or in another public setting. A quiet room with a phone, some comfortable chairs, and access to coffee and other refreshments should be available in the department. Set aside time to talk with the family. Give the impression that you really care; do not give the impression that the interaction is interrupting your busy day.

The process of notification of family begins during the resuscitation itself. The physician should enter the room, take a brief look around to see who is present, and set the stage for a quiet discussion of the patient's condition with the family. Sit down if possible, and unless you perceive hostile circumstances, move away from the door. It is best not to respond immediately to quick questioning by the family. If asked "Is he dead?" the best initial response is not to answer directly, but to explain your presence in the room and proceed with the interview. If the family knows that the patient is dead (told by care providers or knowledgeable about signs of death) and state "He's dead isn't he?" it is appropriate to tell them directly, "I'm sorry but there was nothing we could do."

Introduce yourself and determine which family members are present. It is usually best to address the closest relative or the one who appears to have the most control over his or her emotions at that moment. However, your conversation should not be limited to the most stable person, and you must deliver the bad news and attempt to make eye contact with all present.

The initial discussion should include a review of the patient's past history and an account of the events leading to and following the sudden collapse. This gives an inventory of the state of the family's knowledge about the patient's condition at the time he or she was taken to the hospital, gives the provider background information about the patient, and helps reduce anxiety and guilt in family members. After reviewing the history from the family, briefly relate the circumstances of the sudden death as you know it, and give the status of the patient in the emergency department up until that time, including the present status of the resuscitation.

If the patient has already been pronounced, tell them he is dead using words that are unmistakable in describing the situation. Words such as "he is dead" or "he has passed away" are much clearer than "he's gone." The use of other terminology may lead to confusion, and you may need to repeat your information to clarify the situation for the family. If the resuscitation is still in progress, tell the family that the outlook is not good. This gives them some time to digest what is happening and prepare for the inevitable bad news.

Once the patient has been pronounced, use words to the effect that "everything possible was done" or that the patient's heart "wouldn't respond to measures to stimulate it, including using adrenaline." Tell the family how much was done during the resuscitation. Allow 30 to 60 seconds for the grief reaction and give physical comfort (if you are comfortable with it), but do not move away. After a brief delay ask the more stable or closest person to the deceased about his or her perception of the event. This reduces abnormal grief response. Reassure the family that no pain was involved, unless of course it is obvious that there was (as in a major trauma).

Showing emotion when telling a family of the death of their relative is a normal reaction to the situation. There is no shame or weakness in the physician crying with the family, and if appropriate, touching to comfort them. A simple touch on the arm is usually appropriate.

Some families will request you to allow them to view the resuscitation in progress. Family requests and reactions to this have been studied and, where implemented, found to be an important part of the grief process for most families.[4,5] This is appropriate in many situations and allows the family to see firsthand that things are going as well as can be expected and that everything appropriate has been done. A plan for accommodating families who wish to be present in the resuscitation room should be included in the emergency department policies and procedures manual. When such a program is in place, the family may be asked early during the resuscitation if they wish to be present in the resuscitation room. All staff should be aware of this possibility at the time the request is made. There must be a staff member who can explain what is occurring with the family member at all times.

Support emergency medical services (EMS) and other physicians involved in the patient's care by letting the family know that everything that needed to be done was done in an appropriate manner. The resuscitation period is not the time to make snap judgments about someone else's care of the patient. If major problems did occur, do not address them with the family. If asked about them and you are aware of potential problems, it is best to explain to the family that you do not have all the information. Offer to evaluate the situation through the emergency department's quality improvement program.

Tell the family and friends that they did everything they could in the situation. This is an important part of notification any time a patient dies with family members present. It is especially important in sudden infant death syndrome (SIDS) cases, where the family is searching for an answer to the unanswerable question of why this seemingly healthy child suddenly died. This helps the family accept the death and reduces later guilt among family members.

Find out who the family's supports are and help them contact other family members and friends. Offer to enlist the aid of clergy if the family desires. Before concluding the conversation, always ask if there are any questions. The family may be in a state of shock over the death and not able to ask appropriate questions at the moment. If there is a hospital bereavement team, notify them to assist the family. Some emergency departments have established their own bereavement teams.

Tell the family that you will contact the patient's family physician, and ask if they want to see their relative. Make sure that this is arranged before viewing by notifying the nursing staff, who can assist the family in visiting the deceased.

Explain the process of notifying the coroner and if a medicolegal investigation is required by law. It is important to be familiar with the laws in your state for which deaths are reportable to the coroner at the time of death. The coroner will make the determination of need for a mandatory autopsy.

Inquire as to potential for autopsy or organ donation, especially bone, cornea, or skin. Do not press the issue, but in the case of an otherwise healthy young person, let the family know that their loss can assist other patients. Reviews of emergency department charts have demonstrated a lack of documentation of requests for organ donation.[6] Know what organs are transplanted at your institution or at nearby institutions and have preexisting arrangements for obtaining consent for donation and for obtaining the organs themselves.

Express your sorrow for loss, and scan the group for anyone who might need assistance with immediate crisis intervention. Let the family know that you have other work and that you must leave. Give them your name, and offer to be available for answering their questions in the future. As you are getting ready to leave, offer to assist the family if they have any other needs.

If other staff members are left with the family, make sure that all healthcare personnel give the same information. It is essential that the grieving family is not further burdened by poor communication among healthcare providers. If you do not personally know relevant information concerning burial arrangements, refer the family to nursing, clergy, or social services. Let the family know that you will be back to answer questions if needed (particularly on autopsy or organ donation), after discussion with the coroner and the family's primary care physician.

Allow the family to grieve. What looks abnormal (tearfulness, sobbing, and even hysterical crying) is probably healthy. Any family members who are having trouble with immediate grief reactions should be left with a staff member in attendance. In general, it is unwise to prescribe medications to "help a person get over the shock." Sedative-hypnotics are not indicated in this situation; they can delay the resolution of grief and convert a normal grieving process into a pathologic one.[7]

Finally, the emergency department staff should assist the family in leaving. Finding hospital exits and getting someone to drive them home become major obstacles that can be facilitated by the staff. Offer to call friends, neighbors, or other family members or call a cab to take the family home.

Some families feel let down by the emergency department experience of the death of their loved one. The most common problems are associated with a feeling of depersonalization caused by lack of adequate and timely information about the resuscitation. Families want explicit details about the hospital and prehospital attempts at resuscitation. This situation requires the emergency physician to spend adequate time with the grieving family.[8]

SUDDEN DEATH IN A YOUNG PERSON

Young people who die suddenly fall into three categories: the infant with SIDS, the teenager or young adult with sudden unexpected cardiac (presumed) death, and the victim of accidental death. Resuscitation of these patients should always be aggressive, until obviously futile. An extended resuscitation indicates to the family that everything was done that could be done. Some families know that their child is dead, feel that the resuscitation should be stopped as soon as it is clear that resuscitation is hopeless, and want to be with their child at the moment of declared death.

The initial reaction of families of victims of sudden death is shock and a feeling of numbness. This begins immediately after death and is the phase usually seen by hospital staff. The intense numbness is emotional protection but may result in impaired decision-making ability and bursts of anger. The family should be cautioned not to drive during this phase.

In the case of infant death, explain what is physically going to happen to the baby's body in the morgue, at autopsy, and at the funeral home. All SIDS babies have autopsies. This is necessary to understand the nature of the disease and to help the family know that it was SIDS and that nothing could have been done to prevent the death. An autopsy release form must be signed in order for the private pediatric physician to get the autopsy results. The autopsy results are discussed with the family during the postautopsy conference. This increases their understanding of the death and assists in the processing of the grief.

Avoid clichés such as "It's for the best," "It's God's will," "You can have another child," and "Be thankful for others." These paternalistic statements cut off grief and do not help the family accept their loss. Referral to one of the many SIDS support groups throughout the country should be made for all SIDS deaths.

Ask if the parents want to see and hold the baby, which is an important part of the grieving process because it helps begin closure, and should be encouraged. Before viewing, all tubes and lines should be removed if possible. Be sure to tell the family what to expect when they see the child. Provide a comfortable and quiet place for the family to sit (e.g., rocking chair), give them as much time as needed, and let them know you will be back to answer questions. The death of a child is also a stressful event for providers. Training and the development of a team approach to the family are needed.[9]

CRITICAL INCIDENT STRESS DEBRIEFING: IMPLICATIONS FOR THE HEALTH CARE PROVIDER

Another victim of death in the emergency department is the staff itself. A high rate of dysfunction among emergency personnel occurs after unexpected sudden death situations. For example, studies of the rescuers at the Hyatt Regency skywalk disaster in Kansas City, Mo, found that the majority had repeated recollections of the disaster, recurrent sadness, fatigue, recurrent nightmares, and guilt.[10]

The immediate goal of critical incident stress debriefing (CISD) is to assist the emergency department staff in accepting the loss of the patient. Critical incident stress debriefing also assists nurses and other staff, EMS, fire, and police personnel in coping with their reactions to stress. Staff should be taught to recognize the symptoms of abnormal adaptation to stress among peers. There is also a need for special groups to teach how to minimize stress and recognize symptoms of impairment in other healthcare workers.

The stress may be a reaction to loss or fear of loss and may range from "normal" grief response to panic (staff member feel they are going to lose control). Stress is characterized by potential for harmful behavior (can lead to homicide or suicide) and opportunity (impels person to seek help and results in personal growth). The crisis is the result of a perception of an event or situation as so intolerable that it exceeds the resources and coping mechanisms of the person. This leads to disorganized thinking, anxiety, and a variety of responses, including solutions, immobilization, and loss of conscious control.

A crisis may resolve on its own accompanied by growth or change in a positive manner (develop strength), resolve on its own without change in the person (crisis will "haunt" the person throughout the person's life), or result in a breakdown without self-resolution. This is an emergency and requires immediate and intensive intervention. Acute stressful crises are usually time limited to 6 to 8 weeks before some sort of conclusion or outcome occurs, but they may become chronic, lasting months to years. Problems may surface during other crises and lead to psychiatric distress or substance abuse.

Stages of crises can be defined using the Kubler-Ross stages of death and dying or those modified by Schneider, which examine the process of grieving. A full discussion of these is beyond the scope of this text.

Treatment and prevention require the recognition of "burnout" in emergency department and EMS workers and use of CISD to help them get early intervention. Most often these crises serve as a painful reminder of the realistic limits of the science of medicine and the skills of physicians. Keller and Koenig[11] studied stress in practicing emergency physicians and found that a majority reported moderate to high emotional exhaustion and depersonalization, but also moderate to high levels of personal achievement. Positive coping mechanisms included drawing on past experience, seeing humor in the situation, taking definite action, and involvement in outside activities. Negative coping mechanisms included cursing, daydreams, use of alcohol, food, and drugs.

Critical incident stress debriefing is crisis intervention for emergency services workers. There are multiple settings for intervention, including sudden death, domestic violence, multiple traumas, and child abuse. Emergency departments should develop teams to conduct stress debriefing sessions to prevent burnout and abnormal stress reactions.[12,13]

An emergency department CISD team should be developed from within the department. Staff members who express an interest in participating in debriefings after "routine" critical incidents should be recruited. Staff members who volunteer for the team require some formal intervention training. This may be provided by local mental health workers trained in crisis intervention. Records of interventions should be kept and reviewed by a mental health professional, the "mental health advisor" for the team. This allows for ongoing assessment and continuous quality improvement of team activities.

Some severely traumatic situations (e.g., multiple deaths) may require more formal CISD intervention. In these cases, an outside CISD team headed by a mental health professional should be called in to assist the counseling resources of the ED.[14] This service may be provided by the mental health staff of the hospital.

Critical incident stress debriefing should occur as soon after the traumatic situation as possible. The emergency staff should be fully aware of the existence of the CISD team and the role of the team in intervening after traumatic situations. These "crisis" situations may be identified by any staff member. The charge nurses and attending physicians should be given additional training to recognize situations that may require stress debriefing. Critical incident stress debriefing should (where possible) occur at a neutral site away from the emergency department, preferably a location away from the hospital and at a generally convenient time.

The goal is to help people vent their feelings. It must be performed by persons knowledgeable in the process and should include a critique of the scene by all persons involved. Group sessions are suitable for most situations, although intense individual therapy may be needed for those emergency department staff who are having severe emotional problems as a result of a death.

Critical incident stress debriefing is a brief process of reviewing the events involved in the patient's death and allowing each staff member to ventilate his or her feelings about the situation. It should be nonjudgmental about the process of the resuscitation and should allow everyone involved to speak.

A well-trained crisis worker is needed to facilitate CISD groups. This person should be attentive, reassuring, and able to analyze, synthesize, diagnose, assess, and refer with the facilitator's help. Each person must gain his or her own perspective of loss, not merely reflect the values of the CISD facilitator.

Discussion usually centers on each person's appreciation of the event and a discussion of the normal response to acute loss. Consultation with a psychiatrist is required to assist staff members who show extreme or bizarre response, who have a history of psychiatric problems, and who show no improvement despite the debriefing efforts.

The message to all emergency department workers is "Take care of yourself by accepting your feelings, asking for help and support, and supporting each other." The emergency department administration must remind each worker, "You did the best you could with the information you had at the time."

SUMMARY

Death in the emergency department is a common experience for the staff. There must be a heightened awareness of the need for sensitivity to the survivors. This includes providing more information, presence of family in the resuscitation room, and provision of postdeath information and instructions. The sudden death of a young person increases the stress involved. There must be an organized emergency department response to "helping the helpers" using techniques of critical incident stress debriefing.

REFERENCES

1. Parrish GA, Holden KS, Skiendzielewski JJ et al: Emergency department experience with sudden death: a survey of survivors, *Ann Emerg Med* 16:792, 1987.
2. Schmidt TA, Norton RL, Tolle SW: Sudden death in the ED: educating residents to compassionately inform families, *J Emerg Med* 10:643, 1992.
3. Schmidt TA, Tolle SW: Emergency physicians' response to families following patient death, *Ann Emerg Med* 18:42, 1989.
4. Mian P: Sudden bereavement: nursing interventions in the ED, *Crit Care Nurse* 10:30, 1990.
5. Doyle CJ, Post H, Burney RE et al: Family participation during resuscitation: an option, *Ann Emerg Med* 16:673, 1987.
6. Riker RR, White BW: Organ and tissue donation from the emergency department, *J Emerg Med* 9:405, 1991.
7. Dubin WR, Sarnoff JR: Sudden unexpected death: intervention with survivors, *Ann Emerg Med* 15:54, 1986.
8. Walters DT, Tupin JP: Family grief in the emergency department, *Emerg Med Clin North Am* 9:189, 1991.
9. Greenberg LW, Ochsenschlager D, Cohen GJ et al: Counseling parents of a child dead on arrival: a survey of emergency departments, *Am J Emerg Med* 11:225, 1993.
10. Wilkinson CB: Aftermath of a disaster: the collapse of the Hyatt Regency hotel skywalks, *Am J Psychiatry* 140:1134, 1983.
11. Keller KL, Koenig WJ: Management of stress and prevention of burnout in emergency physicians, *Ann Emerg Med* 18:42, 1989.
12. Mitchell JT, Resnik HLP: *Emergency response to crisis,* Ellicott City, Md, 1986, Jeffrey T. Mitchell, Ph.D.
13. Swanson RW: Psychological issues in CPR, *Ann Emerg Med* 22(part 2):350, 1993.
14. Mitchell JT: Teaming up against critical incident stress, *Chief Fire Executive* 1:24, 1986.

33 Violence and Security in the Emergency Department

Stephen Colucciello

OUTLINE

SCOPE OF THE PROBLEM

"The growing ranks of aggressive, addictive and deranged people for whom the Emergency Department is the last resort."[1] Not a classified ad for emergency physicians, but a headline from *The LA Times* reflecting the escalating violence in emergency departments. As many as 43% of large teaching hospitals experience at least one assault a month, 80% experienced serious staff injury in the past 5 years, and 7% had a staff member killed in the emergency department.[2] An American College of Emergency Physicians (ACEP) survey noted that 86% of all reporting hospitals suffered a violent event in the previous 2 years.[3] Another study demonstrated that 36% of emergency departments have at least one violent incident a month, and 37% of respondents state that emergency department violence had increased in the last 2 years (results of the ACEP leaders survey, Feb. 1993 "Violence in the E.D.").

Nearly 70% of all emergency nurses are assaulted while on duty at some point during their career.[4] As alarming as these statistics are, up to 80% of all emergency department assaults are not reported.[5,6]

Isolated violent events in the emergency department affect the entire institution.[7] Those dramatic enough to be reported in the lay press devastate a hospital's public image and pose major liability risks. In addition, workplace violence fosters an "us versus them" mentality between healthcare providers and the people they serve.

In response to this growing problem, the American Medical Association encouraged hospitals to "institute and/or maintain appropriate and adequate security measures, such as general identification, patrols, visual monitoring systems, and metal detectors."[8] ACEP mandates a safe environment for patients in its Emergency Care Guidelines, and the Emergency Nurses Association voted unanimously to support legislation to protect the healthcare worker.[9]

Who, What, When, and Where

The greatest risk of assault is from patients with psychiatric illness, drug or alcohol intoxication, and altered mental status, as well as from those in police custody.[5,10]

"Spillover" violence occurs when gang warfare or domestic disputes lead to further confrontations in the emergency department. Both time of day and location in the emergency department influence the risk of assaults. About 60% to 70% of all emergency department violence takes place during the evening and night shifts, usually between 7 PM and 3:30 AM. The locations with greatest risk are triage/waiting room, trauma, and psychiatric areas.[5]

Weapons

Although the incidence of weapon use varies according to the community, between 3% and 30% of all emergency department patients carry concealed weapons. An additional number of patients or visitors have weapons readily available in their cars.[11] Many paranoid schizophrenics carry weapons and are willing to use them. Up to 25% of hospital-related assaults involve weapons.[12] In a single urban hospital, more than 16,000 hazardous objects were confiscated through the use of a metal detector over a 2-year period, with knives being the most common.[13] In some areas, as many as 25% of gunshot victims transported by medic from the scene of a shooting are likely to be armed.[14]

INSTITUTION AND PROVISION OF EMERGENCY DEPARTMENT SECURITY

The degree and nature of hospital security are extremely institution dependent and must reflect individual needs. The risks posed at a small suburban hospital obviously differ from those of an inner city training center. Risk assessment should include the incidence of crime in the community, local drug use and murder rate, and previous incidents in the hospital. All dangerous or potentially dangerous incidents occurring in the emergency department should be documented with a copy to hospital security. The emergency department staff should be obsessive in maintaining an accurate log of all threats, thefts, violent episodes, and detection of weapons. This incident log reflects the nature of the event, any injuries sustained, and hospital security response. The emergency department director, hospital administrator, and security director should review this log on a regular basis and assess the need for increased security. Written requests for increased emergency department security, accompanied by copies of this log, are difficult for administrators to ignore.[15]

Security and Design

The design of the emergency department and its environs plays a major role in security. Parking lots must be well lit and, in high crime areas, encircled by a fence, with a guard posted at the entrance. The hospital security office is ideally located in the most dangerous part of the hospital (i.e., the emergency department). This provides high visibility for officers and the capacity for immediate overwhelming response. Some hospitals either rent or offer free space to the police department for use as a substation, ensuring immediate police back-up. Receptionists and cashiers must have a wide desk to separate them from patients and, in violent communities, partitions with bullet resistant glass serve to protect them. All departments regardless of size must have a well-designed, secure room for the violent or agitated patient. This room, with heavily padded walls, should have a solid ceiling to prevent patients escaping by that route or hanging themselves from beams. A large, shatterproof window mounted in an unbreakable door permits monitoring, while a closed circuit television camera mounted in the ceiling allows remote viewing. The door should be hung to open outward so that staff members trapped in the room may escape. If the door opens inward, the patient may be able to push the door shut. Any furniture in the room, such as a chair, may be used as a weapon unless bolted to the floor.

Access Control

Reducing crime and violence in the emergency department requires tightly controlled access. A security guard should be posted at the entrance between the waiting room and the treatment area and should allow only patients or authorized visitors to pass. A security officer may operate an electronically controlled gate for additional security. All hospital personnel should wear photo identification badges, and security must challenge those not wearing badges, even if they are wearing a white coat and concerned expression. A magnetic stripe encoded on the identification number will activate a magnetic "card key" lock at employee entrances, forcing staff to carry their badges. Security personnel should issue color-coded passes to visitors to ensure that visitors to the emergency department do not wander into the rest of the hospital without being challenged. If the main entrance to the emergency department is well guarded, but other entrances to the hospital are not, emergency department security is easily breached.

TECHNOLOGY AND SECURITY

Metal Detectors

Metal detectors are well integrated in daily life and are common in airports, courtrooms, schools, and hospitals. Walk-through detectors rapidly screen large volumes of patients and visitors, and are generally well accepted.[16,17]

Hand-held detectors are useful for selective screening of high-risk patients such as those who are restrained, victims of penetrating trauma, and patients presenting for psychiatric clearance.

If a hospital is equipped with a walk-through metal detector, a prominent sign should be posted outside the department entrance to warn patients and visitors that weapons are prohibited and that they may be electronically screened. A typical sign would read: "This hospital reserves the right to inspect all visitors and patients for dangerous objects or drugs." In areas of high firearm prevalence, weapon lock boxes should be provided for people who wish to disarm before passing through the magnetometer. In these urban combat zones, armed security should be provided for the detector. Policies should be established to dispose of confiscated weapons or drugs and to manage the rare patient who refuses electronic screening.

Monitoring Devices

Monitoring devices, such as closed circuit cameras and motion detectors, extend security resources for a relatively low cost. Monitored areas should include parking lots, entryways, treatment areas, waiting rooms, and all access doors to the emergency departments. Fixed cameras cost less than panning devices. All cameras must be monitored 24 hours a day, and the monitoring officer must have radio contact with other security personnel. "Dummy" cameras, which are merely external shells with no working parts, have been used as deterrents. They are not recommended, however, because hospitals are liable for events that take place in view of these nonfunctioning devices. Motion detectors should be used in conjunction with cameras to alert security personnel to a particular view screen.

Alert and Alarm Systems

Alarm systems should be convenient, redundant, and unobtrusive. Alarm buttons should be placed in triage, trauma, and psychiatric areas. Pull-type buttons are less likely to be misused than push-type alarms, as the curious or intoxicated patients are more likely to push a button than pull it out. Foot-activated buttons should be located beneath the desk at triage and registration. Small alert devices worn around the neck or arm may be issued to staff who move around frequently, such as the triage nurse. Most emergency department alarm systems are silent and ring only in the security office. Because electronic alarms cannot communicate details of evolving situations, their usefulness is limited. Because electronic alarms ring just as loudly for a belligerent drunk as for a schizophrenic with an Uzi, back-up verbal systems are helpful. Such systems include direct dial telephones that connect to the security office when the receiver is lifted, as well as push button intercoms at strategic locations. A code system allows staff to communicate with each other and security without alerting a violent perpetrator. One common code that enumerates relative stages of urgency is Dr. Armstrong levels 1, 2, and 3.[18] Level 1 alerts security to potential danger, such as a hostile but not overtly violent patient, and a level 2 refers to an uncooperative dangerous patient in need of restraint. Dr. Armstrong level 3 notifies security of a situation in which a weapon is involved, requiring a police response.

SECURITY PERSONNEL

Personnel may consist of hospital-based security or local police officers. Highly visible uniforms may deter violent confrontation. Authorities debate the relative merits of police versus security guards. On one hand police training tends to be more comprehensive, officers have clear arrest powers, and potential liability rests more with the police department than with the hospital. Police officers represent a greater deterrent because of their official status and the fact that they are armed. On the other hand, some administrators fear that a law officer's arrest-oriented mentality may escalate certain situations rather than deescalate them. Other issues involve divided loyalties, crossed chains of command, and firearms. A police officer may be most valuable in a highly visible area, such as a fixed security post near triage, whereas hospital security provides roving patrols. Canine patrols monitor hospital perimeters in some large urban hospitals and have proved valuable in gang confrontations.[19] Each state has different laws with regard to arrest powers and possession of firearms by hospital security. In some locales, they are routinely armed. Great emphasis should be placed on training security forces for the unique environment of the emergency department. Officers must predict and prevent violence, rather than merely react to it. Emergency physicians should help train these personnel to deal with the psychiatric patient, recognize previolent behavior, and deescalate crises.

Armed Security Officers

The issue of armed security officers/police officers in the emergency department is controversial. Although weapons represent an effective deterrent to an armed urban warrior, they pose safety concerns for bystanders caught in the crossfire. Mace contaminates the ventilation system, affecting staff and patients in other areas of the emergency department and hospital.[20] Other irritant sprays, such as pepper gas, have the potential for fatal bronchospasm and upper airway obstruction. The electronic dart gun, the Taser, effectively neutralizes dangerous, uncontrollable patients, but occasional deaths occur in conjunction with PCP intoxication.[21,22] Stun guns are a safe alternative and are gaining acceptance for hospital use.[23] If security officers or police carry firearms, a strict weapons policy must be followed when restraining patients. When an officer restrains a patient, he or she must first remove the firearm and place it in a lock box located in the emergency department. If this policy is not followed, a weapon wrested from the officer during a struggle puts the entire department at risk. To be effective, the commanding officer must instruct the police officer to comply with the written policy.

Restraint Issues

The restraint team plays a central role in emergency department security. The courts mandate that hospitals must provide sufficient personnel to safely restrain patients.[24] Aggressive, combative patients, whether psychotic, intoxicated, or head injured, pose significant risks to themselves, other patients, and staff. The emergency physician must intervene with restraints before the situation becomes dangerous. Restraints should never be used as a threat or punishment, and once the decision has been made there should be no "bargaining" with the patient. The restraint team should be assembled out of view, the restraints made available, and with a show of overwhelming force the patient informed that he or she will be restrained and should cooperate. In an agitated patient, restraining one arm over the head and the other at the side prohibits wild flailing. Patients who are at risk for aspiration may be placed in the left lateral decubitus Trendelenburg position. In this case, both arms are restrained to the same side of the stretcher. Restraints must be soft, unbreakable, and nonconstricting; most physicians prefer to use leather restraints. Specially designed wide plastic restraints are an acceptable substitute, but Kling or Kerlex should never be used to restrain patients, as their tourniquet effect can cause ischemic damage. Patients who violently struggle against restraints are candidates for chemical sedation with neuroleptics or benzodiazepines, as straining may produce significant rhabdomyolysis.[25]

Every patient who is restrained should be searched carefully. A hand-held metal detector may reveal concealed or disguised weapons. A foolproof alternative to a professional search is to strip restrained patients completely, place them in a hospital gown, and lock up their possessions. The reason for restraint should be documented in all patients, the most common indication being that the patient is a danger to self or others. The careless physician who neglects to document indications for restraint may be sued for assault, battery, and false imprisonment.[26] The Joint Commission on Accreditation of Healthcare Organizations requires that all restrained patients have a restraint flow sheet attached to their chart.[27] A sample flow sheet is shown in Figure 33-1.

TRAINING OF EMERGENCY DEPARTMENT PERSONNEL

Poorly trained personnel trigger assaults. Perhaps half of all assaults on staff are unintentionally provoked by the healthcare provider. A healthcare worker who sternly dictates to a paranoid schizophrenic or biker drug lord will be assaulted. Many workshops and videos are available to assist in this training.

Prisoner Protocol

Although any patient in police custody may be dangerous, prisoners who have just been arrested represent a greater risk than the chronically incarcerated. These patients are often intoxicated with cocaine or alcohol and in a high state of arousal. When prisoners are sutured, the suture tray should never be left unattended, as patients may surreptitiously take scissors or scalpel. After suturing, all instruments should be removed immediately from the room.[28,29]

Police guards must constantly remain in sight of their ward. Hospital and police policy must forbid officers from relinquishing custody to hospital security or emergency department staff. Emergency department personnel should not accept responsibility for police duties. If a handcuffed patient requires cuff removal for examination, the alternate limb must be secured to the stretcher. Prisoners should never be restrained in wheelchairs, which may be picked up and used as weapons.

Information given to prisoners should be limited with regard to repeat visits; rather, the information should be written on the jail instruction sheet given to the guard. Advance knowledge of a recheck date allows the prisoner to arrange an escape.

Emergency Department
Restraint Flow Sheet (sample)

Date ____________

RESTRAINT ORDERS:

_____ 1. Patient and possessions searched by security _____ 2. Patient placed in hospital gown _____ 3. Possessions out of recch of patient _____ 4. Physician Restraint Order on chart

_____ 5. Flow sheet imprinted with patient's name _____ 6. Key in designated place if leather restraint

Reason for restraint: ____________

Initial application of restraints ________ (Time) Physician ____________ RN (sig) ____________

Date	Time	Vital Signs q 30 mn x2 then q h	Distal Neurovasc check, q 30 mn	Rotate restraints q 2 hrs	Restraints RA RL C/W LA LL	Bathroom/ Food/ Fluids	Medications	Observations:	Initials

Additional notes: ____________

____

Patient disposition: Restraint removal (time) ________

Time ________ ________ Mental health ________ Discharge home

________ Admit to hospital ________ Other ____________

FIGURE 33-1 Restraint Flow Sheet.

Hostage Situations

Hostage crises are a growing problem for emergency departments. More than 150 hostage incidents have occurred in hospitals since the mid 1980s. Hostage takers are usually disturbed young men with real or imagined griefs against physicians. The hostage should remain quiet, make no sudden moves, and should not cower, plead, or whine, but instead act with quiet dignity. Medical help should be offered either to other hostages or to the hostage taker.[18] When a hostage situation occurs, a level 3 alert should be called for police response. The administrator or emergency physician in charge should make no bargains or promises, but instead tell the hostage taker that someone will come to negotiate soon. Hospital security must clear the area, establish perimeters, and set up a command and negotiation post. Media and family liaisons should be designated. The police will require a floor plan of the emergency department and hospital. Incoming ambulances should be diverted.

Gangs

Gang violence is growing throughout the United States,[30] and up to 30% of all penetrating trauma in some areas may be gang related.[31] Members of gangs can be recognized by insignias or "colors" on jackets or hats. Visitors should be screened with metal detectors in areas of gang activity.

Gang victims should be registered as John or Jane Does to prevent rival gangs from tracking down and killing them in the hospital.[32] Emergency department security should call for additional armed security when gang-related shooting victims arrive. Occasionally, a hospital lock down may be necessary during gang warfare to avoid the emergency department's becoming a battleground.

AFTER THE EVENT

After a violent event, when the perpetrator has been restrained, the victim should be treated, and the entire affair recorded in the incident log. The emergency department should note whether a weapon was involved, the extent of injuries, and the adequacy of security response. A critical incidence stress debriefing (CISD) is useful in cases of traumatic and emotionally disturbing events. This debriefing allows the involved staff to talk about their reactions and "unload." The Department of Psychiatry can assist in setting up the CISD team and provide counseling for the victim. The security director must investigate violent incidents immediately and determine how to prevent future situations.

LEGAL ISSUES

Security-related lawsuits are rapidly increasing, including restraint-related litigation. Up to 16% of emergency departments report a restraint-related lawsuit over the last 5 years; some of these involve injury or death during a restraining process.[26] Additional liability involves patients who are assaulted on hospital property.[33] Such suits have increased 30% over the last several years.

Courts recognized the validity of emergency department restraints in *Youngberg vs Romeo,* 1981, but require the physician to exercise "professional judgment."[34] Only careful documentation demonstrates professional judgment. Uncontrollable, wild behavior should be charted and the way in which patients placed themselves or others at risk described.[35] An important issue in security-related lawsuits concerns foreseeable events (i.e., events that have a reasonable potential for occurring). Historically, the first time a violent incident took place in a hospital, the event was not considered foreseeable because it had no precedent. This was known as the "every dog gets one bite" rule. This rule has been invalidated by the courts.[36] If crime exists in the community surrounding the hospital, it is foreseeable that such crime or violence may overflow into the emergency department.[37]

STRATEGIES TO INCREASE SECURITY

There are several impediments to improved emergency department security, including deliberate ignorance, lack of expertise, financial costs, and image concerns. The "head-in-the-sand" mindset is a dangerous and uninformed response that overlooks the fact that assaults are ubiquitous in emergency departments throughout the country, even in "nice" hospitals.[38] The attitude that it "can't happen here" must be adjusted in light of these statistics. Many hospitals lack the knowledge necessary to improve security, but outside specialists, local police, and publications provide needed direction. Increased security requires financial commitment. However, the cost of merely defending a single lawsuit (apart from any settlement costs) is often far higher than the cost of needed security.[24] Some administrators worry that highly visible security may give the impression that the emergency department is somehow a dangerous place. They do not wish to be the first hospital in a community to have a visible police presence. Yet the paying public expects and deserves a safe environment and is likely to be comforted by a police officer. A dramatic example of bad image occurred after a hostage was killed in an emergency department. The hospital subsequently changed its name because of financially crippling publicity.

SUMMARY

The emergency department is the most dangerous place to work in any hospital and poses significant risk for physicians, nurses, and staff.[12,32] The emergency physician must help train personnel to recognize the dangerous, previolent patient and instruct staff members in deescalation and restraint techniques. Metal detectors are useful in communities in which weapons are prevalent. An incident log should be kept and reasons for restraint documented for every patient. A highly visible officer located at the entrance to the treatment area will go a long way in preventing violent events. Alarm systems and electronic monitoring improve security response. Protocols should be developed to ensure proper handling of prisoners, restraint-related issues, and hostage situations. The emergency physician must insist on adequate security for the department.

REFERENCES

1. Katz J, Spiegel C: Hospitals caught in crossfire, *LA Times,* November 4, 1991.
2. Lavoie FW, Carter GL, Berg RL: Emergency department violence in the United States teaching hospitals, *Ann Emerg Med* 17:182, 1988.

3. American College of Emergency Physicians comment sheet on Violence in the Emergency Facility, *ACEP Leader,* Nov. 20, 1986, pp 11-13.
4. Mahoney BS: The extent, nature and response to victimization of emergency nurses in Pennsylvania, *J Emerg Nurs* 17:282-291, 1991.
5. Pane GA: Preventing and controlling violence in emergency departments, *West J Med* 155:285-286, 1991.
6. Lion JR, Snyder W, Merrill G: Under-reporting of assaults on staff in a state hospital, *Hosp Comm Psychiatry* 32:497-498, 1981.
7. Brantley A: Rising violence in ER's cause hospitals to redesign security, *Mod Healthc* 22(40):44-46, 1992.
8. AMA House of Delegates, Resolution 187, Hospital Security, Chicago, 1987, American Medical Association.
9. Stonis NL: ENA works to prevent violence in emergency departments, Emergency Nurses Association (ENA). *Am Nurse* 26:6, 8, 1994.
10. Lavoie FW, Pane GA, Winiarski AM et al: Aggression directed towards emergency department staff at a university teaching hospital, *Ann Emerg Med* 20:283-286, 1991.
11. Nelson DJ: ED's must address security issues as violent behavior increases: crack use exacerbates long standing problem, *Emerg Med News* 9:11, 1989.
12. Crime in Hospitals 1988, 1989, the latest IAHS surveys, *J Healthcare Protection Mgmt* 7:1-29, 1991.
13. Thompson BM, Nunn JC, Kramer TL et al: Incidents and types of hazardous objects found among patients and visitors screened by magnetometer in an urban emergency center, *SAEM Abstract,* May 1992.
14. Wasserberger J, Ordog GJ, Dolodny M et al: Violence in the community emergency room, *Arch Emerg Med* 6:266-269, 1989.
15. Turner JT, editor: *Violence in the medical care setting: a survival guide,* Rockville, MD, 1984, Aspen Publishers.
16. McCulloch LE, McNeil DE, Binder RL et al: Effects of weapons screening procedure in a psychiatric emergency room, *Hosp Community Psychiatry* 37:837-838, 1986.
17. Thompson BM, Nunn JC, Kramer TL et al: Disarming, department weapon screening, and improved security, to create a safer emergency department environment. U/AEMS, Abstract 92, *Ann Emerg Med* 17:419, 1988.
18. Emergency department violence: prevention and management, *ACEP* Dallas, 1988.
19. Eddinger C: K-9 teams in a California hospital, *J Healthcare Protection Mgmt* 7:1-29, 1991.
20. Lenehan GP: Notes on the "violence in the emergency department" theme issue, *J Emerg Nurs* 17:263-264, 1991.
21. Ordog GJ, Wasserberger J: Electronic gun (Taser) injuries, *Ann Emerg Med* 16:72-78, 1987.
22. Koscove EM: The Taser weapon, a new emergency medicine problem, *Ann Emerg Med* 14:1205-1208, 1985.
23. Waller FS Sr: The hospital emergency room security—the next decade, *J Healthcare Protection Mgmt* 7:1-29, 1991.
24. Rusting RR: Emergency room violence: dealing with the frightening and still growing problem, *Hosp Secur Saf Manage* 10(4):5-12, 1989.
25. Dubin WR: Evaluating and managing the violent patient, *Ann Emerg Med* 10:481-484, 1981.
26. Lavoie FW: Consent, involuntary treatment and the use of force in an urban emergency department, *Ann Emerg Med* 21:25-31, 1992.
27. Joint Commission on Accreditation of Healthcare Organizations: *Accreditation manual for hospitals,* Chicago, 1988, JCAHO.
28. *Clinton vs City of New York.* New York Supreme Court Appellate Division. 528 NYS2D108 AD2 Department 1988.
29. Hayden JW, Laney C, Kellerman AL: Medical devices made into weapons by prisoners: an unrecognized risk, *Ann Emerg Med* 26:739-742, 1995.
30. Hutson HR, Anglin D, Mallon W: Minimizing gang violence in the emergency department, *Ann Emerg Med* 21:1291-1292, 1992.
31. Written testimony of the Emergency Nurses Association, Chicago, IL, by the House Select Committee in Narcotics Abuse and Control. Hearing on the crisis in emergency rooms due to the drug epidemic. Sept. 28, 1990.
32. Hutson HR, Anglin D, Mallon W: Injuries and deaths from gang violence: they are preventable, *Ann Emerg Med* 21:1234-1236, 1992.
33. Colling RL: Hospital security: is the patient at risk? *J Healthcare Protection Mgmt* 7:1-29, 1991.
34. American Psychiatric Association: Seclusion and restraint. Task force report #22, Washington, DC, 1984, APA.
35. Wexler DB: Seclusion and restraint: lessons from law, psychiatry and psychology, *Int J Law Psychiatry* 5:285-294, 1982.
36. *Isaacs vs Huntington Memorial Hospital.* Supreme Court of California, 695P.2d653 (California 1985).
37. Morgan RB: Health facility crime to worsen during 1990's, *Health Facil Manage* 26-29, 1989.
38. Cullen EJ: Violence to staff in the health services, *Br Health Safety Comm* 1-12, 1987.

PART THREE
Contract Management

34 Negotiating

Robert W. Strauss and John G. Keene

I worked for a menial's hire
Only to learned dismayed
That any wage I had asked of life
Life would have paid

Jessie B. Rittenhouse

OUTLINE

Why negotiate? Why can't we just take or leave what is being offered? Few people enjoy the conflict created by trying to get something beyond what is offered. The result is avoidance. The problem is, negotiations cannot be avoided. We all deal with negotiations and negotiators every day. Like it or not, we are regular participants. Every time one interacts with another person to obtain any outcome that does not already exist, a negotiation is occurring.

Negotiation is simply a form of conflict resolution. The conflict is you want something you do not have.

"Everything that we want or would like to own is currently owned by or under the control of someone else."

Roger Dawson

PRECONCEPTIONS

Most people think of one of two scenarios when they visualize a negotiation:

- The Aggressive Salesman—A used car salesman or a merchant in a foreign city haggling over the price of some desired object. After some struggle, the negotiators settle on a price and the deal is made. In fact, once the negotiation begins, if the agreement comes too easily, one party will be dissatisfied, thinking he or she might have gotten a better deal.
- The Monumental Treaty—Representatives from labor, management, or two warring factions in a dispute of national or international importance. Negotiations in this area require remarkable discipline and years of training.

As a result of these preconceived notions, many people perceive negotiating as distasteful, whether it is haggling over price or the perception that years of training are required. In reality, we learn negotiating at an early age at home. Children are master negotiators. They know that success in negotiating is achieved by knowing and caring about what you want.

PHILOSOPHY

Most people want to negotiate a deal that is beneficial for them. If you approach every negotiation with the idea that "I'm going to win and I really don't care what happens to the other side," you will develop a "win-lose" style of negotiation. While this philosophy may be successful in the short term, it runs counter to the development of positive long-term relationships. Insisting on agreements that are beneficial for both parties ensures that everyone will leave the negotiation satisfied. Adopting this "everybody must win" standard will ensure long-term success as a negotiator.

By understanding the process of negotiation and learning some of the techniques and pitfalls, we can become substantially more effective. This chapter (1) defines the five components of negotiating, (2) explains the process of negotiating, (3) introduces the concept of principled negotiations, (4) discusses how to overcome obstacles, and (5) describes techniques used in negotiations.

Study these ideas, learn them, practice them daily, and apply them in ways that communicate your desire to meet the other person's needs, and you will dramatically improve your ability to negotiate.

FIVE COMPONENTS OF SUCCESSFUL NEGOTIATING

Attitude

Mental and Physical Preparation. People who exercise regularly recognize that being in good physical and emotional condition makes them more capable of dealing with day to day stresses (Box 34-1). This is particularly true in negotiating. Negotiating sessions can be intense and occasionally prolonged. Participants who are physically and mentally prepared have a distinct advantage.

Expectation and emotional attitude can play a significant role in the success of a negotiation. If your expectation is favorable, you will project confidence and influence those around you. If you are depressed and anticipate a negative outcome, you will communicate this expectation nonverbally.

Trust and Respect. Management principles provide important lessons about negotiating. When trying to influence people or resolve conflict you must develop an attitude of trust and respect.

A key method of developing trust and respect in a long-term relationship is to create understanding by identification. Management should not distinguish itself as different. Successful management teams do not "send down directives" or concentrate personal amenities about themselves. Rather, they get close to those who deliver the service and inspire commitment to it. Management should be perceived as being like everyone else. A person who identifies with another believes the other person understands his or her issues and is more willing to listen.

The same principle applies during a negotiation. The first step is to be perceived as a peer of the person with whom you are negotiating. Setting yourself apart by declaring that you are "a doctor" or "a nurse" creates a barrier to understanding. Find areas of mutual interest to establish a bond of commonality. When both sides of a negotiation identify with each other, a foundation for understanding exists.

Listening. Another key principle of successful negotiation is to be a good listener. For most people to be mentally receptive to someone else's message, they must feel they have been heard. An axiom for successful negotiating is to remember that the person who does the most talking thinks the most was accomplished. Allowing the other side to have a say lets them establish their point of view, relax, and prepares them to listen to you. By listening actively you let the other parties know that you understand their point of view.

Active listening involves body language and eye contact that communicate your concern and interest in what the other person is saying. Neurolinguistics expert, Suzette Hayden Elgin points out that someone who is actively listening begins to move and breathe in sync with the speaker. In small groups, when we are interested, we tend to mirror the body positions of the speaker. This occurs naturally when we listen intently. Taking notes may help you keep focused. It is important to avoid thinking about your side of the discussion and to stop planning your rebuttle. When you are thinking about your issues, you cannot possibly be listening.

BOX 34-1

THE FIVE COMPONENTS OF SUCCESSFUL NEGOTIATING

1. Attitude
2. Information
3. Aspirations/Goals
4. Time
5. Power

Information

The Value of Information. The more information you accumulate, the better prepared you will be for a negotiation. Understanding what they need allows you to meet their needs while simultaneously meeting your own. Like a game of poker, the side with the most information usually wins in a negotiation. You are more likely to be successful when you know some of the other side's cards. For example, if you are negotiating for a director's position, the following are examples of information that might be advantageous:

- What are the expectations of the position?
- What were the responsibilities and salary of the last director?
- Why did the previous director leave?
- What are other directors being paid for similar positions?
- How quickly must the position be filled?
- Who else is competing for the position?

Information is key in a negotiation. Large corporations spend millions in research before entering major negotiations. Countries may spend tens of millions of dollars before entering international negotiations. By taking the time to gather information, you are doing the "homework" that will lead to success.

Obtaining Information. One of the best ways to obtain information is to ask open-ended questions. By patiently waiting for a response, you allow the person to say what is on his or her mind, which is frequently revealing. You can then probe deeper and gain greater insights.

Another particularly good method of uncovering important information is to take someone with you who will engage the counterpart at the other institution. Nurses relate to other nurses, administrators are comfortable with administrators, and physicians have a natural affinity for other physicians. A physician, nurse, or administrator may be quite willing to share information with another person with whom he or she shares a common professional involvement.

Aspirations and Goals

> "The significance of a man is not in what he attains, but in what he longs to attain."
>
> Kahil Gibran

Aspiration Levels. Negotiating goals are defined by two aspiration levels, your bottom line and your optimum realistic goal. Your bottom line is the set of minimum criteria that you must have to negotiate a deal. Your optimum realistic goal is the set of parameters that would maximize the deal for you and which you believe the other side could still accommodate. These two aspiration levels may be the same depending on the market. Never assume that your optimum realistic goal is unattainable. Once you have established a positive relationship, it does not hurt to ask for something reasonable that is more than they are offering. The worst outcome is that they will say no; however, they may offer you substantially more than your bottom line.

Fouraker's Experiment. Dean Fouraker of Harvard performed one of the classic negotiating experiments. To study the relationship of expectation to outcome in a negotiation, he placed pairs of negotiators at a table with a wall between them. They could neither see nor speak with each other. Their only means of communication was to pass paper beneath the table. There was $10 at stake. The person on the left was told that typically the person on that side got $2.50 and the person on the right was told that typically the person on that side got $7.50.

Although it would have been reasonable to assume that the actual split would be $5.00 and $5.00, the actual split was $2.50 and $7.50. He demonstrated that the negotiators who expected more achieved more.

Karass's Experiment. In 1968, Chester Karass published results of a study in which he paired 120 skilled professional negotiators against each other to negotiate a settlement.[1,2] This was a mock case of a man who was suing a pharmaceutical company because a drug he had taken caused hair loss and blindness. The study compared initial demands (aspirations) with final outcomes. It also contrasted the negotiators' expectations of their opponent's demands with their actual demands. He concluded the following:

1. Higher aspiration levels lead to higher awards.
2. People with high aspiration levels did particularly well against those with low aspirations.
3. Unreasonably high initial demands in this experiment led to the greatest success.
4. Skilled negotiators cannot accurately estimate the aspirations of their opponents.
5. Participants tend to project their own aspirations on the opposition.

"Our level of aspiration is a yardstick by which we measure ourselves."[1] In other words, your level of aspiration represents your intended success. Most people would like to earn a little more money than they presently do. Setting goals just above your present status allows you to achieve success with minimal risk of disappointment. The higher you set your goals, the greater the success that can be achieved and the more difficulty and risk of failure there will be. Karass' experiment demonstrated that expectation has a direct bearing on outcome. Those negotiators willing to strive for higher goals attained more.

Assumptions. This experiment also demonstrated that it is difficult to estimate what the other side will demand. In other words, do not assume you know what they want. Test any assumptions you have to determine the other side's aspirations. Assuming that others want the same things that you want is a projection and is often inaccurate. Your needs and expectations are as unique as theirs. Rather than assuming you know what the other side wants, develop hypotheses and test them as the negotiation progresses. Be prepared to modify your assumptions about their goals and motives as you gather more data.

Feedback and Aspiration Levels. In a negotiation, assumptions about the outcome will go up or down depending on the feedback and data you obtain. Feedback such as yes, that's fine, and a smile are encouraging. Reactions such as stern silence, scowling, laughter, NO! "Are you kidding!" are discouraging. Discouraging feedback tends to lower aspiration levels. Be aware, however, that such feedback may be a ploy designed to lower your expectations.

Time

Time is a powerful tool in a negotiation. It can be used effectively to modify outcomes. The impact of time can be broken down into three primary areas:

1. Planning and preparation time
2. Time during the negotiation
3. Deadlines

Planning and Preparation. A key concept of successful negotiating is to prepare thoroughly for a negotiation. Advanced preparation is both the most important part of the process and the most neglected. Inexperienced negotiators most frequently fail here. Gather as much data as possible to formulate goals and positions. The more clearly you understand and care about what you want, the more effective you will be.

Advance research allows you to establish meaningful goals. For example, if you are negotiating a contract to staff an emergency department, an enormous amount of homework must be done. A few of the details you will need to know are listed in Box 34-2.

Without this information and many more details, you will be unable to make a realistic proposal. You would also be severely limited in your ability to participate in the give and take, trade-offs, and sharing that must occur in such a negotiation.

On the other hand, if you have done your homework, you will be able to create a meaningful, flexible, and collaborative approach that will meet your needs and the needs of the other side. This is critical to success, particularly in a highly competitive market.

When developing your position and strategy, it is equally important to understand the other side's position and strategy. Returning to the previous example, take the time to research the hospital's reasons for negotiating, political pressures, financial position, and likely strategy. The more you know about their position, the easier it will be to formulate a solution that meets both your needs and theirs.

Careful, thorough preparation is also the best way to prepare yourself emotionally for a negotiation. It allows you to adopt a calmly assertive attitude that will help you communicate a sense of confidence and collaboration.

Time During the Negotiation. Understanding the interplay of time during a negotiation is a crucial element for success. Time has tremendous strategic importance. Time can be used to build momentum, facilitate decision making, and increase commitment.

Difficult negotiations requiring concessions by the other side are most often successful when both sides are committed. One effective way to increase the other side's investment in making the deal is to work on all of the easy issues first.

BOX 34-2

DATA RECOMMENDED FOR AN EMERGENCY DEPARTMENT CONTRACT

Volume in the department	Physician availability
Payor mix	Fee schedule
Nonbillable patient details	Pay rates
Registration/data collection	Third-party details
Case mix/acuity	HMO penetration
Charting/documentation levels	HMO contract details
Physician qualifications	

This creates an atmosphere of success and collaboration before tackling the really tough issues. The more time the other side invests in you, the more likely they will feel compelled to complete the process.

Outside time pressures that create quasideadlines can be useful. For instance, if the chief negotiator for the other side is going on vacation in a week, you can use this fact to accelerate the negotiation, even when the real deadline for completing the negotiation may be months away.

The tempo of the negotiation can enhance or limit success. Momentum may be facilitated by properly arranging the agenda and conducting the negotiation. Conversely, if a negotiation starts to drag, momentum is lost and the deal may die. It is critical to avoid long periods of inactivity between sessions. Depending on the needs of the parties, a delay of even a day or two can have a chilling effect.

Time can also be used to defuse an explosive situation. Given a little time, people can calm down and let anger dissipate.

Deadlines. Difficult negotiations usually last to the deadline. Congress makes most decisions just before recess. Labor-management negotiations almost always get resolved just before the strike. This occurs for two reasons. First, the greatest concessions are often made at the last minute. Second, under the theory that easy settlements do not achieve all possible concessions, the rank and file would be both distrustful and disappointed with their leadership if the settlement were made without the appearance of an arduous and vexing process.

Deadlines are powerful tools. They create the incentive to settle because of the possibility of losing the opportunity or "deal" if the deadline is not met. Generally, we set our own deadlines. Be sure you understand the reasons for your deadlines and the cost of going beyond them. Flexibility may be useful. In a difficult and adversarial negotiation, it may be wise to state you have less time than you actually do, allowing yourself a margin of safety and a way to "give the other side more time."

Carefully determine the other side's time limit. Be skeptical about stated deadlines. Some are real but others are not. Because of the fear that a deadline may be used against them, some negotiators do not reveal their true deadlines. It is important to understand the consequences of going beyond a deadline. However, be cautious when considering the use of a deadline or any ploy to "force a deal." Most negotiations are part of a longer term relationship. If you use a ploy to force someone into a one-sided deal, you may create the foundation for a poor relationship.

Power

In many negotiations, both sides feel that the other side has more power. Common worries include not being as tough or as smart as the other side or not having the same leverage. Some negotiators believe the other side can walk all over them because every negotiator is acutely aware of the pressures on themselves but not necessarily those on the other side.

Everyone entering a negotiation has a variety of strengths and weaknesses. There are six power sets in any negotiation (Box 34-3).

Much of the power we wield in a negotiation is "perceived power." How each side perceives their and the other side's power will influence their actions. The degree to which we can alter those perceptions may determine the success or failure of the negotiation.

If you enter a negotiation believing you are in a less powerful position, you will do less to convince the other side of the merits of your case. The converse is equally true. If you think you have a powerful position, you will pursue your goals with more confidence and determination.

Using Power. If you approach the use of power and the developments of power as skills that can be learned and refined, negotiating becomes much less foreboding. Every encounter becomes an opportunity to practice and play with these skills.

The best use of power is to create solutions that will be good for both sides. If we use our power to win at the expense of the other side, we may have the victory today, but we have lost an opportunity to gain an ally and may have an enemy tomorrow. On the other hand, if we seek solutions in which both sides win and we use our power to move toward that goal, then we establish its foundation for a lasting relationship. Using power in subtle, nonconfrontational ways can influence behavior in positive ways.

The Power of Weakness. Sometimes it is better to appear weak. It may be smart to act dumb and dumb to act smart. "The dumber one appears to be, the more relaxed and vulnerable the other side will be."[3]

A phrase such as "could you please go over that again?" will usually slow the other side down and reduce their momentum. It gives you more time to consider your response and may reveal helpful details. Not quite getting it is powerful. In some instances it can even stimulate a concession.

Similar to the power of weakness, the "I need help" approach is valuable. Asking the other side for help compliments them and gives them an opportunity to demonstrate their expertise. This helps develop the lasting relationship most successful negotiators seek. As the other side reviews their position and tries to "help you understand," they may gain new insights that will enhance their understanding of your side. They actually may become your advocate.

The Power of Competition. Creating competition for you or your services enhances your value. A real estate broker uses the power of competition by suggesting there are other serious buyers looking at the house you are considering. Interviewers do this when they tell interviewees how many candidates they have. Conversely, candidates may reveal the names of other prestigious programs that are wooing them.

If you are interested in an opportunity, as one of several options, you can compel the other side to compete for you and hold you in higher esteem by using the power of com-

BOX 34-3

NEGOTIATION POWER SETS

The Power I Have
The Power I Think I Have
The Power They Think I Have

The Power They Have
The Power They Think They Have
The Power I Think They Have

petition. Alternatively, if you are or appear desperate, the value of your position will be diminished, and you will lose bargaining power. For example, how are you affected by the following answers to the question, "are you looking at other positions?"

Response A "Not really, nothing seems very interesting."
Response B "Yes, I'm very excited about my opportunities."

The first response creates the impression that the job seeker has few opportunities and could be hired easily. One might further infer that this candidate is unexcited and disinterested. The second response creates the impression that this candidate has several good offers and is in high demand. It is not clear whether the position being offered is one of those options. You may have to compete and "sweeten" the offer.

Another facet of the power of competition is that people generally are more satisfied with prizes that are earned and victories that are hard fought. A fish caught will seem to taste better than a fish bought. A mountain climbed will seem to have a better view than the same mountain driven.

CONTRACT EXAMPLE. A physician director becomes furious and somewhat threatening when a physician with whom he contracts for emergency department services looks at other opportunities. The director confronts the physician and speaks about allegiance, commitment, loyalty, and disappointment. Nonetheless, the physician goes ahead and contracts with another hospital for part-time work because it decreases the physician's dependence on this institution and is a good business decision.

Future negotiations with the director may actually become easier and more successful because the physician will be less dependent. The physician gains respect and will be pursued by the director rather than at his mercy.

USED AGAINST YOU. The power of competition may be used against you when seeking an opportunity. For example, "There are several others that we are considering." There are several steps or solutions you can use.

SOLUTIONS

1. Gain Information: Find out how much competition really exists. You will then be able to deal more effectively with the situation. If your position, offer, or proposal is substantially stronger and you believe you are the first choice, you will be able to effectively negotiate. On the other hand, if your position is one of many similar options, then you must create new advantages and redefine your position.
2. Describe Your Uniqueness—Let the other side know what makes you different and how you will meet their needs.
3. Develop Your Options—A candidate who has many opportunities will be respected more than one who has few.

The Power of Legitimacy. In every circumstance, outward manifestations of success can lend credibility and legitimacy. In certain business settings, the people with whom you associate, the type of car you drive, and the clothes you wear convey a message. Clients are more likely to hire a lawyer who drives a Mercedes than a beat up jalopy.

Certifications by specialty boards, advanced training, publications, previous recognition, and a well-written resume all authenticate and validate an individual. Using a document to present information confers legitimacy. There are many examples where the written word is meant to convince us of the validity of a claim. Examples include testimonials, a "we will not negotiate price" sign in a store, the price on a side window of a car and "infomercials." A sloppy document, on the other hand, creates a negative impression and undermines the data. An example is the impression created by a photocopied curriculum vitae that has strike-outs and misspelled words.

USED AGAINST YOU. You are negotiating an expansion of your emergency department. You are handed a study of local emergency departments that indicates the current space is more than adequate. It is concluded therefore that the board will not approve funding for additional space. Although most people would assume the data are correct, there may be bias in the sample. Do not accept such a document at face value.

SOLUTION. The solution is to add legitimacy to your side. Create your own documents to demonstrate the legitimacy of your position. Develop a wealth of material that matches or exceeds the other side's in both form and substance.

The Power of Expertise. A corollary to the power of legitimacy is the power of expertise. The appearance of knowledge, experience, and expertise is very influential. It is a powerful tool that we use in our daily practices. We can walk into a room wearing a white coat and a stethoscope, and those present will assume that we know exactly what we are doing. They will allow us to perform invasive and painful procedures on them without question. Then, they will thank us. All this occurs because we have the appearance of expertise. The same phenomenon occurs in business.

USED AGAINST YOU. You develop a proposal to renovate the emergency department. The hospital calls in a "consultant." This firm of architects has substantial credentials and a record of having conducted multiple consultations in hospitals in the past. The consultant draws up plans and makes recommendations that result in a much less costly approach; however, the plan creates an impractical practice environment. Pleased with the new plan, the committee prepares to move ahead.

Further exploration of the consultant's background would have revealed broad experience in developing outpatient clinics and minimal experience in developing emergency departments.

SOLUTIONS

1. Do not be overimpressed by an expert: Have a healthy skepticism for proclaimed expertise. Most experts rely on previous work experience to guide future recommendations. If this approach is taken without thoroughly considering the particular characteristics and nuances of the case, the result will be, at best, ineffective. The solution is to ask experts to show you and the other side exactly how their ideas work.
2. Understand their expertise and use it to your advantage: Determine the experts' relevant experience. Find out from them and others if their past experience has led to the types of results you believe are warranted. The solution is to participate actively and guide the expert. Use their expertise to help meet your needs and the other side's needs.
3. Establish your own expertise early: For example, when negotiating a contract, establish your background and credentials early during the introduction, not during the debate phase so that they are more likely to be accepted. Bring in your own experts as needed.

The Power of Previous Investment. The more time and effort you put into a task, the harder it is to walk away. If you have been working on a project or negotiation and it is not going well, your willingness to continue will, in large part, depend on the previous efforts expended.

Examples of this phenomenon abound. In poker, it is called "chasing." It occurs when you have put a lot of money into the pot and, even though your hand now appears to be a loser, the decision of whether to continue to invest in this hand is based on previous bets, not future potential to win. As the United States lost more lives in Viet Nam, it became harder to pull out. The government became more committed to achieving a victory because of their investment in lives rather than making a rational assessment based on contrasting the benefits of victory with the cost of future investment in lives and resources. Surrogate mothers want to keep the baby they carried for 9 months. These are all examples of the power of previous investment.

CONTRACT EXAMPLE. The more time and effort spent agreeing on contractual issues, the more likely you are to attain compromise on the final issues. If early in a negotiation, a difficult issue, such as money, seems to be heading toward an impasse, it may be wise to postpone discussion of that issue. You can defer it by saying "this is obviously a difficult point for both of us. Let's work on some other issues and come back to it a little later." Then agree on as many issues as you can. Do everything to enhance the relationship and the desire to work together. Replace the frustration of an impending impasse with the elation of accomplishing agreement. When you return to the issue of money you can say, "we have made so much progress, we are virtually done with this contract. Why don't we find a compromise with which we can both live?" At this point, both sides will be more willing to make the extra commitment to complete the deal. This phenomenon explains why incumbency in a contractual relationship is so powerful. A hospital becomes so invested in a group or individual that it is difficult to change.

USED AGAINST YOU. The same approach can be used by either side. Once you have developed a long-term relationship, it may be difficult to walk away from a "bad deal." The other side may string you along so that your commitment of time and resources grows to such an extent that you will make critical compromises.

SOLUTIONS

1. Put off difficult issues: Deal with simpler issues first and develop a relationship built on successes. Delay or postpone issues that create consternation until you and the other side have a fuller understanding of each other.
2. Use incumbency to your advantage: Be prepared to demonstrate the advantages of your continuing presence. Market your successes, on-going projects, and future potential.

The Power of Persistence. Persistence is one of the hallmarks of a good negotiator. This is the quality of sticking to the job until you are successful. It requires mental toughness and discipline. You may need to present a proposal over and over again before it is accepted. The fact that you repeatedly stick to your goal sends the powerful and positive message of commitment.

It is important to be physically and emotionally fit to endure the rigors of persistence. A long and complex negotiating session can be physically exhausting. As the hours stretch on, there is a tendency to give in and say, "okay, enough . . ."

CONTRACT EXAMPLE. You are the director of a busy emergency department. The physical plant is poorly laid out, and the facility is substantially understaffed. To renovate and hire additional staff would be expensive. Your plan meets stiff resistance. You work long and hard and demonstrate the long-term benefit to the hospital and its patients. Eventually the necessary changes are approved. Persistence wins the day.

USED AGAINST YOU. Some negotiators continually reintroduce the same issue even though you have described your inability to meet that need. If they persist, there may be a tendency to concede a little each time or even capitulate completely.

SOLUTION

1. Be well rested and in good physical shape: It is necessary to be physically and emotionally sharp during a negotiation. If you get tired or preoccupied, you will lose concentration and put yourself at a disadvantage. Do not hesitate to take a break to refresh yourself.
2. Take good notes: If you have resolved an issue and it is brought up again in an attempt to wear you down, refer to your notes to remind everyone of this agreement. Publishing notes and having the other side sign off on them is even better.
3. Creatively restate your objectives: Because it may be necessary to persevere on an important issue, learn to restate the issue using different examples and perspectives. This approach demonstrates that the issue is multifaceted and well thought out.
4. Hold your ground: Be willing to persevere in the face of persistent attack.

The Power of Silence. It is tempting to respond emotionally to an obnoxious person and to overpower them by getting angry. The tendency is to fight fire with fire, to snarl back at a snarler. Responding emotionally to an emotional situation is loss of control. Difficult and fiery negotiations often can be successfully handled with complete silence.

Silence has great power; the more tension in a situation, the greater the desire for action. People will invariably become increasingly uncomfortable with silence in a tense situation. Most people have a strong urge to fill the void. Resist the desire to speak and the other side will become uncomfortable and start to move in your direction.

In other words, doing the opposite of our initial impulse may be the better response. Sometimes, when we have the greatest urge to speak, silence is the best action we can take. You may be better off not discussing your limits, your motives, and your time pressures unless they are specifically used to make a point. The less you speak, the more you will hear. The one who talks the most thinks the most was accomplished. The one who talks the most gives away the most information.

CONTRACT EXAMPLE. You are negotiating an emergency department director's stipend. You have been wined and dined. This is your fourth visit, and they have made it clear that you are the candidate they want. You are heavily invested in getting this job. This is a great opportunity for your family and they are excited. In short, you are ready to make the deal. The other side has just made an insultingly low offer. You are livid and disappointed. You are thinking about either yelling at him or walking out. Rather than reacting in angry or negative fashion, remember that the amount offered was *only the first offer.* An alternative response would be to use the power of silence. Simply look at the person and say nothing. The longer you remain silent, the more uncomfortable the representative will become. In all likelihood, the representative will eventually break the silence with another slightly higher offer. You can then show some disappointment on your face and continue to remain silent, which will either result in a further increase or an inquiry such as, "aren't you going to say anything?" If such a question is raised, respond calmly and evenly with "most directors are paid substantially more" or "you'll have to do better than that."

USED AGAINST YOU. Imagine you are negotiating a managed care contract. You have presented all the ways in which your emergency department group can facilitate cost-effective care for the health maintenance organization (HMO). The HMO representative has agreed and has said there would be a natural synergism. You then move on to financial issues and propose that your group is prepared to accept a certain low rate, with an incentive for decreasing the use of ancillary testing. You believe this is a reasonable offer that would meet everyone's needs.

You are greeted with silence and facial expression showing disappointment. As you wait for the HMO representative to say something, you become more anxious. You are concerned about negotiating this deal because you have seen that the HMO is eroding the volume in your emergency department. You are fearful that your group will suffer significantly as the HMO becomes more powerful. You are having the power of silence used against you. What can you do?

SOLUTION

1. Wait comfortably: Take a couple of slow deep breaths and relax the muscles in your shoulders and neck. Focus on a positive outcome and be ready to listen when the other side speaks.
2. Distract with humor: If the other side is intent on winning the battle of silence, allow the victory by speaking first in a way that will not have a negative impact on your position. You can tell a story about a humorous event in the emergency department or something that your child did. The key is to make it light and engaging so that the other person will feel good about reentering the discussion.
3. Give them some time to think: If the other negotiator is unwilling to make a counterproposal or comment on your proposal, simply offer to give the person time to think about it and discuss it with others. Set a time for the next meeting with the express goal of coming to closure on this item.

The Power of Limited Authority. In many situations you may have the desire to display your power and authority. While you deal with the other side's decision maker, it may be advantageous to refer your decision to a "higher authority." There is power in limiting your own authority in the eyes of the other side. The key is not what authority do I have, but rather what authority do I want to avoid.

This technique is commonly used by automobile sales people. After haggling with a sales person, you finally reach a deal. The sales person shakes your hand. You are relieved and psychologically committed to the deal. Then he or she says "everything seems in order, I just have to get the final approval from my manager." You, being the final decision maker for your side, have made a commitment. The sales person has just taken the position of having limited authority and has thereby gained substantial power. After a few moments the salesperson returns saying "well, gee, I'm really sorry, I felt sure my boss would approve the deal. Unfortunately, he said that with the recent increases in overhead, we will lose money at that price. We could, however, do the deal for $300 more." Once you have mentally purchased the car, it is hard to walk away for just $300.

Although it is ideal to deal with the other side's decision maker, it is not always possible. Therefore it may be necessary for you to establish that you have a higher authority to whom you must take the final deal.

This type of power should not be used in a deceitful way or to force the other side into a deal that is not fair. To do so would ultimately erode your long-term relationship. The real purpose is to establish a legitimate power that will protect you from being swept into a deal without time to think about all the ramifications and to make sure it is an agreement with which you can live. In addition, the power of limited authority can be used to move the parties toward a conclusion that is mutually beneficial.

USED AGAINST YOU. After negotiating an HMO deal, the other side could say, "I have to take this back to my Board. I am confident that it will be approved. I will get back to you." After a few days she returns and sadly announces that the Board has been troubled by overutilization and can only approve 75% of the agreed rate. Alternatively, she may phrase it positively, "what a surprise, the Board was really tough but I have good news, they agree to everything except the price. I think if you would just give a little on this issue, we could close the deal now." The other side has effectively brought you to agree on a price and then used the power of limited authority to put pressure on you to accept a lower rate.

SOLUTIONS

1. Establish Authority Early: Determine at the beginning of the negotiation who has final authority to make decisions. If the negotiator indicates he must obtain final approval from someone else, ask to deal with the decision maker.
2. Determine limits of negotiator: If negotiators from the other side are not empowered to make a final decision, determine how much authority they do have and in what areas. Ask them to tell you each time you are discussing something for which they do not have authority. This will prevent you from making a one-sided commitment.
3. The last minute surprise: If representatives from the other side catches you off-guard by their limited authority, it may be helpful to play on pride and gain their commitment by saying, "well, I'm sure they will agree to whatever you suggest, won't they? And you will recommend our agreement, won't you?" It will be embarrassing for the representatives to answer, "no" to either of these questions. If, however, they answer "yes" to both questions, it is more likely that the deal will go through as agreed.[3]
4. Invent your own higher authority: This is the most powerful counter to limited authority. Common higher authorities include your spouse, lawyer, partners, accountant, and family advisor. If the representatives return with a different deal, you can respond by saying, "I am really embarrassed but my accountant said we would have significant financial problems at that rate." If you are negotiating for a job, to refer to your spouse as an objecting higher authority is unassailable. For the other side to attack your

husband or wife puts them in an untenable position. For example, "my wife is unhappy with the deal. She isn't sure she wants to move the family here. She's so happy where we are; it just doesn't seem worth it to her, even though I explained your limitations."

CRITICAL ASPECTS OF THE NEGOTIATION

Several critical aspects of the negotiation clearly influence success (Box 34-4).

The Starting Point

The "starting point" is your initial position in a negotiation. There is a relationship between your starting point and the final outcome. Hovland from Yale[4] demonstrated that when you want to influence people to move from A to X, by starting at Z (unless Z is ridiculous) you get the most movement (Figure 34-1).

Starting High. In the Karass negotiating experiment (pharmaceutical company versus plaintiff who had partial loss of the eyesight and loss of hair), the highest initial demands led to the highest settlements (Box 34-5).[1]

1. Enhances other's perceptions of you. Starting high communicates to others that you place value on yourself and your services. High, not excessive self-esteem enhances other's perceptions of you. Starting high suggests confidence and self-assurance.
2. Allows room for negotiation. Typically, in negotiations each side believes the other side is "starting high" and will work toward a compromise. In this setting you are at a disadvantage when you begin at your desired end point. The other side will assume that your proposal is "padded" and interpret your resistance to concessions as unyielding rigidity. Look for ways to give the other side something.
3. Gets you more. Karass,[1,2] Hovland,[4] and practical experience have shown that starting high gets you more. As long as you are not excessive, you will create an expectation that leads to an improved outcome.

BOX 34-4

ASPECTS OF SUCCESSFUL NEGOTIATIONS

Starting point	Dealing with difficulties
Concession behavior	Breaking deadlocks
Principled negotiations	

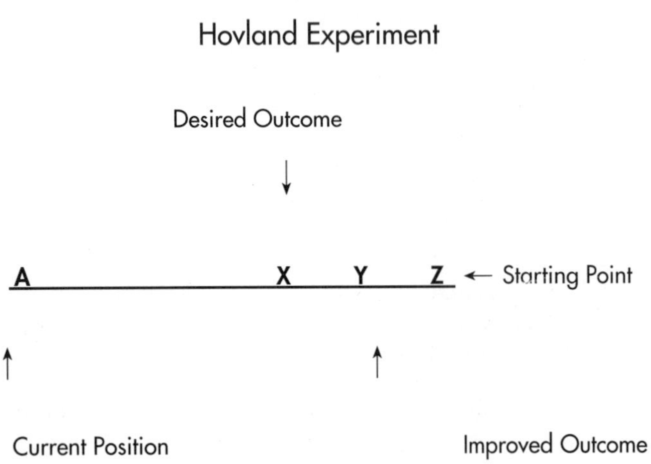

FIGURE 34-1 Hovland experiment.

Starting Low But Implying Flexibility. Starting low is the same concept from the buyer's perspective.[3] In this situation, you are the purchaser rather than the seller of a product or service. Beginning at a low point demonstrates that you do not place great value in the seller's offering. Starting low carries some risk and should be done with sensitivity to avoid the insult inherent in asserting low value to their offer. A low initial offer should convey flexibility.

Perhaps you are in the market for a particular item such as a piece of art or a used car that you believe is worth $7500. You offer a particularly low amount with implied flexibility: "*I'm not exactly sure* what it is worth but given what I see, *I think* that $4200 would be a fair price." This implies flexibility so as not to alienate the seller. Future concessions on your part will allow them to "get something" more than your initial offer and allows you to purchase it for less than their starting point.

Concession Behavior

All negotiations involve compromise. Without compromise, there is no negotiation. Without flexibility you may become trapped in an all-or-none position. Alternatively if you approach all negotiations by simply "giving in" you may close a lot of deals, but they will be very costly. To compromise or adjust your goals in negotiation is referred to as *concession behavior.* How you concede dramatically influences your success as a negotiator.

Two Views of Concession Behavior

1. Give to get: When dealing with conflict or negotiating, the approach of "you have to give something to get something" engenders the belief that both sides should succeed. If they help you attain your goals, it is appropriate to look for ways to meet their needs. This approach builds strong relationships.
2. My way or no way: This strategy is based on the belief that concessions are a sign of weakness and that long-term relationships have no importance at the negotiating table. The ancient Romans maintained peace by demonstrating a readiness to use overwhelming force *(Pax Romana).* They demanded complete concessions and gave none. They were willing to win at any cost.[5] The view of the former Soviet Union was a variation on this theme. The classic Soviet style of negotiation was never to concede. Concessions were not to be responded to with a concession. By this theory, a concession is proof that the other side's position is weak, and more concessions are likely to follow.

BOX 34-5

ADVANTAGES OF STARTING HIGH

1. Enhances other's perceptions of you
2. Allows room for negotiation
3. Gets you more

The Incremental Nature of Concessions. Negotiators communicate their end point by the manner in which they make concessions. Those who concede easily and in large amounts are sending the message that they have great flexibility and little commitment to their initial position. Some people erroneously believe that a large concession will favorably impress the other side and lead them to a deal. Ironically, a large concession usually raises the aspirations of the other side. They will interpret easy, large concessions as a sign that more is available and instead of coming to closure, they may ask for more concessions. Those who concede slowly and in a "stingy" manner reveal strong attachment to their position. This behavior sends the message that there is little room for movement and will lower the aspirations of the other side. Typically, negotiations are a back-and-forth process, with each side making concessions as they draw closer to a deal. The size and relationship of successive concessions influence the endpoint (Figure 34-2).

Karass on Concession Behavior. In the Karass experiment, early large concessions by the plaintiff's side led to the lowest settlements.[1] Early large concessions by the pharmaceutical company (the defendant) led to the highest settlements. Karass found that:

1. Losers tended to make the first concessions and the largest concessions.
2. Winners tended to make the smallest concessions. Those obstinately making small concessions occasionally deadlocked, but if they didn't deadlock, they won. Winners also made smaller concessions as the deadline approached. Deadlines create increasing pressure for both sides. Most deals are made as the deadline nears, not before. The winners made smaller concessions at this point than the losers and, therefore, made better deals.

The Diminishing Value of Concessions. The value of services always decreases rapidly after those services have been performed. Once a concession or favor has been given, its future value decreases. The concept "they will really owe me a lot for this concession" has no place in negotiation. This concept is also referred to as the *Hungry Man Principle*. The wealthy man dying of hunger and thirst in the desert may say he'll give everything he has for water, food, and safety. Once these are provided and he is in the safety of his mansion on his estate, what is the likelihood that he will turn everything over to his rescuer? Because the value of the ser-

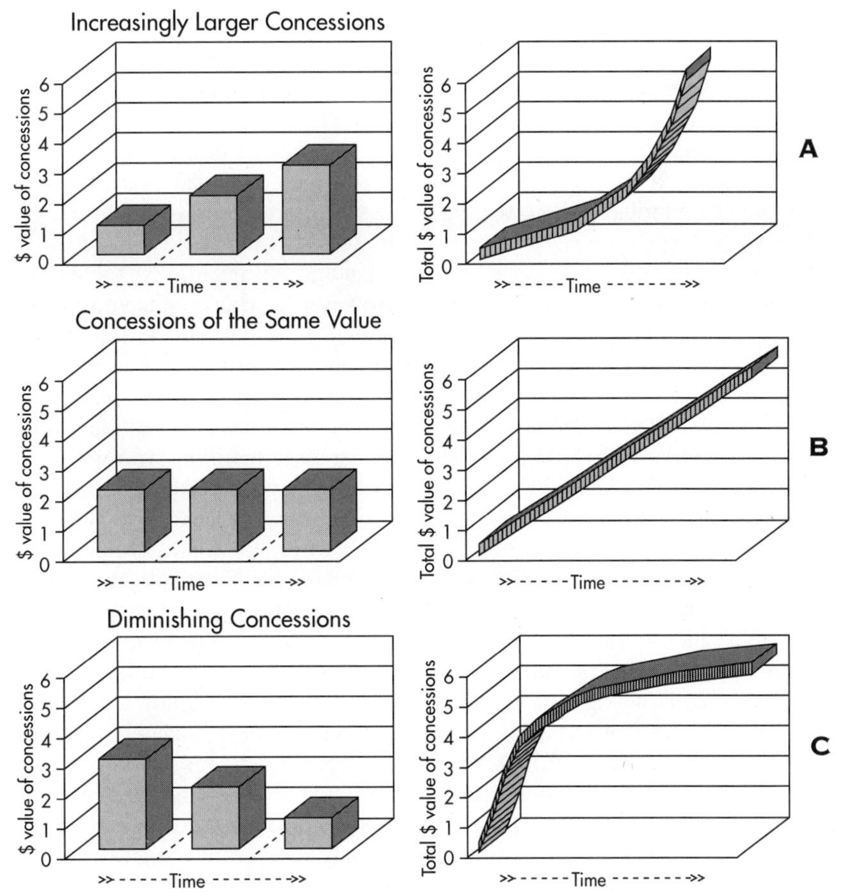

FIGURE 34-2 Concession patterns. **A,** The negotiator gives increasingly larger concessions, perhaps to convince the other side to close the deal. However, this pattern of concessions may have the opposite effect. The unspoken message is that by holding out, the other side can get increasingly larger concessions. **B,** Each of the concessions is similar in size. There is no message to suggest a limit to these concessions. The total value of the concessions is continuing to increase. **C,** This pattern sends a different message. Each successive increment is smaller, suggesting to the other side that you are getting closer to your end point. The total value of your consession is approaching a limit. Your concession behavior demonstrates that you have limits and moves the negotiation toward closure.

vices (concessions) diminishes rapidly after they are provided, when asked for a concession, always get something in return immediately. The following scenario illustrates this point:

> "Well quite frankly I'm not sure that we can concede on this point. I have to ask the group (higher authority). But if we can do this for you, what can I tell them you will do for us?"

In this way, you have elevated the value of the concession. If you continue to give things away for nothing, even unimportant things, you may be setting up a grinding away process. Some negotiators will keep asking for more until you say: "ENOUGH!" Alternatively, if they know that every time they ask for something additional, they have to give up something in return, they will be less likely to continue to ask. By insisting on reciprocal concession, you increase the value of your concessions. The following examples illustrate this approach.

1. The hospital agrees to provide the emergency physicians transcription services if they will forego support for recruiting.
2. The physicians agree to lower the guarantee if the hospital will provide an incentive plan.
3. The group accepts a restrictive covenant prohibiting them from approaching area hospitals if the hospital will accept a long-term contract.

The "Too Easy" Win. It is possible to be unsatisfied with a good deal and more satisfied with a bad deal. This is often the result of a settlement that is reached too easily. People often think, "I could have done better. If they gave me what I wanted without hesitation, then they probably were willing to give a lot more. I really blew it!"

For example, you put your house on the market for $175,000. The first person who looks on the first day says "I'll take it for the full asking price." What happens? You got what you wanted and yet you feel like you made a big mistake. Alternatively, if many offers have been made around the $150,000 to $155,000 range and then someone offers $170,000, you may feel satisfied with an offer less than the original asking price.

When a negotiated purchase is made too easily, the purchaser may think "I could have done better" and "I wonder if there's something wrong." For example, you go to buy a used car that is advertised for $10,000. After inspection, you believe it is worth $8,000. You decide to offer the low price of $4,000, and it is accepted without hesitation. What happens? You immediately wonder what is wrong with the car. Alternatively, if the seller haggles for an hour and eventually you get the car for $5250, you may feel very satisfied. The "too easy" win occurs when commodities and services that are typically negotiated are purchased without any struggle.

Principled Negotiations

Fisher and Ury[6] describe one of the most important concepts of negotiation, principled negotiating, the philosophy of focusing on issues not positions. This philosophy avoids positional bargaining and focuses on meeting the interests of both parties by collaboration.

Positional Bargaining. Unwise agreements often result from positional bargaining. There are two types of positional bargaining: hard and soft.

In hard positional bargaining, the more you try to defend the position, the more strongly committed you become to it. As you continue down this path, relationships deteriorate and inefficient solutions result. Hard positional bargainers typically see the other side as adversaries that must be overcome. The goal is winning; the cost is unimportant. The hard bargainer's demeanor is distrustful, threatening, and insistent.

One response is to acquiesce, to say okay to avoid conflict. This gentle and placating approach avoids confrontation and maintains the relationship. The nice bargainer only gets one need met, an agreement, often at great cost. Soft bargainers see the other side as friends whose relationship must be maintained. The goal is agreement; the cost is unimportant. The soft bargainer's demeanor is trusting, yielding, and solicitous.

Principled Bargaining. Negotiations that are based on merits rather than positions produce wise outcomes. This type of bargaining limits the discussion to problem solving based on objective standards. It avoids getting bogged down in personalities, positions, and narrowly defined solutions. Principled bargainers typically see both sides as problem solvers. The goal is a wise outcome achieved in a cordial environment. The principled bargainer's open-minded approach tries to develop options to meet the needs of both sides. The following example shows the advantages of principled bargaining.

An admitting resident has been quite busy all night with multiple admissions and sick patients. You call and inform him there is another patient in the emergency department ready for admission. The angry response is, "No! I cannot accept another patient. I am overwhelmed with sick patients." If you react to the position and insist that the resident live up to his responsibility immediately and threaten to call the attending physician, you solve the problem in the short run. However, if you ever have to deal with that resident again, he will look for ways to retaliate.

The resident's underlying issue (not the position) is: "I'm exhausted, overwhelmed, and drowning in work." Avoid reacting to the position and search for the underlying issue. By focusing on the issue, you will find many solutions that will meet both your needs and the needs of the resident: "It has been a rough night for you. I'll tell you what. I can hold the patient here for about 45 minutes while you catch up." This response was directed at the issue and away from the position. You met the resident's poorly expressed need without compromising your own.

An example of contract negotiations that involves principled bargaining follows. A group and a physician are negotiating. The physician, eager to join the group, expresses determination to get a certain amount of money and has demonstrated inflexibility. The group, in the present reimbursement environment, cannot afford the requested amount, but the physician would be an extremely desirable addition to the group.

Positional bargaining will lead to frustrating concessions by one or both sides or to deadlock. Alternatively, the group and the physician can work to uncover and address each other's underlying issues. This process may lead to a successful conclusion for both sides. Perhaps offering partnership, helping to secure a loan, finding additional sources of income such as an administrative stipend for helping the hospital in other ways, or enhancing the benefits package will meet the physician's needs.

Conversely, the physician should seek to understand the contract and limitations of the group and be willing to look for creative solutions.

Issues Before Positions. At times there is only one solution to a problems. When a position is essential, describe the issues before stating the position. Tell why you need it before you tell what you need. By putting issues before positions, the other side has an opportunity to listen and understand your reasoning.

For example, the statement "We're going to have to find a way to pay our physicians more because we are unable to recruit doctors for our current needs" thrusts the position, paying more, on the other party. They may focus on this position and overlook the issue, which is recruiting physicians in a competitive market.

Consider this example. "Alice just turned in her resignation. Her husband has a great job opportunity and she will be leaving in 2 months. It is unfortunate because she is an excellent physician who is respected by the medical staff. Some of the attending and prehospital care personnel specifically send their patients here because of her abilities. I am sure you remember that the cost effectiveness program she developed has been the critical factor in our success with the managed care contracts. We have tried to recruit a replacement for Alice, but it is difficult to attract quality physicians like her. In fact other members of the group are considering leaving. To keep the doctors we have and be able to attract a replacement for Alice, we are going to have to find a way to pay our physicians more." By identifying the issue first and providing the other side an opportunity to understand it, you are laying a foundation for collaborative problem solving. When the other side finally hears the position, "paying more," they are more likely to work with you.

Dealing with Difficulties—Overcoming Obstacles

Negotiating does not come easily to many and, at times, is difficult for everyone. Difficulties can come in many forms. Some negotiators adopt an "all or none" attitude. Some become emotional and blaming. Still others resort to ploys to accomplish their end. To effectively negotiate, one must recognize when the negotiations are going off track and initiate methods to realign the discussion. The following techniques may be used to move the discussion forward in a productive manner.

The Set Aside. The set aside is the postponement of difficult issues until later when mutual trust has developed and early successes have been achieved. Deal with easy issues first. If a difficult issue arises, one that is likely to become an impasse, set it aside: "I understand how you feel about that aspect of the deal. I would like to think about it. Let's set it aside and talk about some of the other issues first." Later, when both sides have invested more time and consideration, there will likely be more willingness to compromise to achieve agreement.

The Theory of YES. Acknowledge the other's point of view. Say *yes* and say it frequently. When people respond to a proposal by shaking their head and saying "no" or worse "no-no-no-no-no" (the quintuple no), they are disagreeing and making the value judgment that your idea has no merit. This further suggests a lack of concern or understanding. Saying yes and incorporating the other side's idea into your response validates the other side and demonstrates appreciation of their concern. This approach moves the discussion forward. By repeating their point of view, you recognize their goals and aspirations.

> "So you would like to have triple coverage 24 hours a day for our 12,000 visit emergency department. Yes, I can understand your desire. This would decrease the waiting time and provide excellent customer service for the patients. Let's consider some of the other ramifications."

You do not have to accept their proposal, but you should accept their perspective. By acknowledging their point of view, you put them in a frame of mind to hear your concerns.

Feel, Felt, Found. A variation on the Theory of Yes is the "feel, felt, found" technique.[3] It is another way to avoid arguing. Arguing causes defensiveness and a feeling that you are not listening. Recognizing the other's point of view, even when you believe the other is wrong diffuses the competitive spirit that sometimes enters a discussion. The feel, felt, found technique effectively moves the discussion forward by incorporating the other's concerns as if they are your own.

For example, you say, "I think fee-for-service would create a stir in this community, because the patients would think we're too expensive." The other side responds "I understand how you *feel* because patients would receive two bills. When we started billing at another hospital, they *felt* the same way. We send the bills to the third parties whenever possible and the quality of service has improved so dramatically that we have *found* that this concern has not been a problem.

Breaking Deadlocks

Deadlocks occur. They create great stress, test resolve, and reduce aspirations while jeopardizing a successful outcome. Sometimes during a negotiation there seems no way back to meaningful dialogue. The key is to learn how to walk back in the door without losing face and to let the other side do the same thing.

Deadlock breakers work because they refocus the parties on meaningful discussion. The following methods of breaking deadlocks are often successful.

- **Change the Team:** Bringing in new participants often gives greater objectivity to the negotiations. Different people will be less encumbered by preconceptions and emotional attachment to the previous positions.
- **Reorder the Agenda:** Similar to the set aside, changing the agenda and dealing with different issues often regain forward momentum.
- **Caucus:** Caucus is an accepted part of negotiating. It allows you to review the negotiation in private where you are free to reexamine your position. It is an excellent way to decompress a situation.
- **Take a Break:** Taking a break is different from caucusing because its intent is to allow both sides to stop thinking about the negotiation, cool down, and relax.
- **Ask for Help:** Simply state the problem and recognize the impasse. Then ask for help to get beyond it. Ask the other side, "what would you do in my position?" For example, "To get the type of coverage that you are asking for will require paying more money than is available. What would you do in my position?" By asking for advice, you flatter the other side while helping them to see the situation through your eyes. Further they may help you figure out

how to solve the problem. Third parties are also valuable sources of help.

Deadlock breakers are effective because they allow both parties to begin to move forward together. Once both parties begin to negotiate after a significant deadlock, there is great relief and significant potential for bilateral concessions.

NEGOTIATING PLOYS

There are many negotiating ploys (Box 34-6). These techniques or tricks are used in negotiations. We learn many of them playing in the sandbox as children. Although the term *ploy* has negative connotations, ploys can be used in positive ways to move a negotiation forward. However, they can also be used to gain advantage or "win" at the expense of the other party, resulting in short-term gains, but undermining the long-term relationship.

In most instances, it is best to avoid using negotiating ploys and techniques. Unless you are very adept, most people will recognize them, and be put off by their use. Experienced negotiators may turn your ploy against you. It is necessary to be aware of the techniques so that you can recognize them when they are being used without falling prey to them.

Bait and Switch

The bait and switch technique is common in everyday life. The underlying concept is to lure the potential buyer (prey) with the bait (an attractive offer or a deal that is too good to be true). Once the prey has been enticed to buy or is psychologically committed to the offer, the switch is made. A less attractive or somehow diminished model is substituted, and the buyer makes a less advantageous deal.

For example, a deluxe video camcorder is advertised for a very low price. You have been looking for a camcorder and this is the best deal you have seen. You get excited and arrive eager to buy only to find that they have "run out of the sale model." But for a few dollars more you can get a deluxe store brand. The technique is often successful. You are there, committed to a product, and ready to buy.

Contract Example. You reach oral agreement and commit to joining a group with the understanding that you will achieve partnership within 2 years. The conditions of partnership are never explicitly discussed. You give notice to your old job and move to your new location. The written contract arrives and does not mention partnership.

Solutions

- Take notes assiduously: Take notes when discussing the various points of the deal. Sending a copy of your notes to the other side may be helpful. Having both sides sign off on the notes will demonstrate your understanding and clarify theirs. It is possible that your notes may be the only record of the discussion.
- Get it in writing: The best method of preventing a bait and switch is to document the agreement in writing with explicit details covering all aspects of the understanding.
- Penalties and termination clauses: If you build in penalties or are able to invoke termination based on noncompliance or nondelivery, you can often prevent a bait and switch.

BOX 34-6

COMMON NEGOTIATING PLOYS

1. Bait and switch	5. Nibble
2. Good guy-bad guy	6. Flinch
3. End run/splitting	7. Puppy dog technique
4. Threats/brinkmanship	8. Funny money

Good Guy-Bad Guy

The tough and irate bad guy is aggressive and demanding, perhaps even threatening. The pleasant, soft-spoken good guy intervenes and offers to protect you from the bad guy or to salvage the deal if only you can do something to appease the bad guy. Even if the good guy is not making a great offer, it is much easier to deal with the nice guy rather than have to deal with the jerk again. This is a classic setup to gain key concessions.

For example, the surly cop begins to rough up the suspect. The gentle, brotherly good guy rescues the suspect, temporarily stopping the bad guy. The good guy does not know how long he can hold off the bad guy. He suggests that the suspect cooperate before the other guy loses control completely.

In the family setting, a homemaker mother will say, "if you continue to behave like that I'm going to have to tell your father". The mother is playing the good guy implying "do it my way and it will be easy for you." She casts the father as the bad guy to modify the child's behavior.

Contract Example. Two physicians representing a group are negotiating a contract with a hospital administrator who is desperate to get emergency department coverage. One member of the physician team gets angry over the compensation package and storms out of the room. As the other physician picks up his papers to leave he says "gee, I am really sorry this happened. We were so close to a deal. This is a sensitive issue for him. If there was something you could give, maybe I could get him back.

Solutions

- Recognize it: The good guy and bad guy are on the same team. They are partners with the same goal—to get the best deal from you. Do not be drawn in by it.
- Never respond to anger or threats by trying to appease: If you try to placate them, they have won and will continue to use this technique until it does not work anymore.
- Refer to the issue, not the position: If the bad guy tries to maneuver the negotiation into positional bargaining, remember to refocus the discussion on the underlying issue that is being discussed.
- Identify the ploy and create embarrassment: "Hey, you guys aren't going to use the old good guy-bad guy technique on me are you?" You might also say, "you guys are really good; that is the best good guy-bad guy routine I have seen." Once caught, they will probably smile, deny it, and get back to the discussion in a more fruitful manner.

Splitting Behavior—The End Run

The underlying principle of splitting behavior is to play team members against each other and reduce their aspirations. This technique can create conflict within a group and lead to concessions by individual members of the group. The end run is similar in that it attempts to split the other side by going around the negotiators and appeal to the real decision maker. There are legitimate reasons for the end run, including trying to break a deadlock, bringing a more collaborative person into the discussion and involving the decision maker. There are also deceptive and improper reasons for using the end run and splitting behavior. They may be used as strategies to create conflict to gain an advantage. To successfully counter this technique, it is necessary to recognize it.

Examples. A couple is purchasing a car. The salesman identifies areas of disagreement and weakness. He plays one against the other to enhance his profits. Another common example is a child asking the second parent's permission to do something to which the first parent has said no.

Contract Example. You have been empowered by your group to negotiate for them. The other side goes directly to the group and states it is impossible to deal with you, and the group is at risk of losing the opportunity. If the ploy is unrecognized, you and your group are put at a disadvantage.

Solutions

- Don't get sucked in: Make no decisions apart from the selected negotiator and reaffirm the group's decision-making process.
- Expand the group: Agree to send an additional person, not a replacement. By offering to expand the group, you address their alleged concern without undercutting your side.

The Ultimatum/Threat

The threat of nonagreement is present in every negotiation. The threat becomes a reality if the sides cannot find a mutually acceptable solution. Some negotiators will threaten nonagreement as a ploy to accomplish their objectives.

The key to effective threats is believability. They are meant to lower aspirations and soften the opposition for the kill. The normal response is to get defensive. This ploy should be avoided because it always builds resentment. Threats are the classic game of chicken—seeing who will blink first. If you ever use this technique, make it clear that you mean what you say and preferably make it possible for the other side to give you what you want.

For instance, one side may threaten to walk away unless certain demands are met. This is also called brinkmanship. The threats can be in the form of verbal attacks or veiled in the righteous air of trying to save the deal.

For example, Khrushchev was speaking at the United Nations. In a moment of spontaneous fury, he took off a shoe and said, "We will bury you!" As he pounded the table, people observing this behavior became fearful of this barbarian. When they considered that "he had his finger on the (nuclear war) button," his threat created an intolerable risk. This led many to a policy of appeasement. Interestingly, a picture of the event subsequently revealed that Khrushchev was wearing two shoes while he was pounding the podium with a third. This was a very effective planned event.

Solutions

- *Maintain control:* The normal response is to get upset and feel the need to either acquiesce or get up and walk out. Instead of being thrown off balance, relax and take a deep breath. Ask them to repeat what they said to give you some time to settle down and think.
- *React the opposite way:* If you react in the expected manner, you will become defensive and perhaps angry. Put them off balance by reacting in the opposite way. Respond with a smile and recognize their point of view. "Yes, I understand you feel strongly about this issue." You could even ask them to explain it in more detail or really catch them off guard by agreeing with them (the "theory of yes").
- *Use the power of silence:* Let the room fill with silence. They will become increasingly uncomfortable. They may recognize how obnoxious they have sounded and begin to retreat.
- *Focus on the issue, not the position:* Their threat is a position. Identify the issue and seek to solve it.

The Nibble

The definition of the nibble is to chew off a little more after the deal is completed.[3] This technique is successful because once agreement is achieved, both sides become psychologically committed to the deal; you've lost your walk-away power and let your guard down. We do things to reinforce our decisions. (Therefore if someone asks for a little more after a deal has been struck, he or she usually gets it. Recognizing this phenomenon, the other side can add more and more, slowly changing the deal.)

The nibble will generally be preceded by: "of course you are including . . ." or "and by the way . . ." or "just one more minor detail. . . ."

For example, you have been negotiating with a couple to sell your house. They have just agreed on the price and have shaken hands. They say, "Of course, you are leaving the refrigerator." You agree and they add, "Just one more minor detail, we assumed you will fix the fence." This nibbling process could continue until you stop it. Each time you acquiesce to an additional request, you reinforce the behavior.

Contract Examples. You have recruited a person to work in your group. The deal is completed and you shake hands, at which point, the recruitee says: "Oh, by the way, to whom should I give the bill for my moving expenses?" "Of course you will be paying for my license and dues, won't you?" This ploy works because you have achieved psychologic commitment. To say no might undo the deal you have struggled to close.

Solutions

- *Recognize the ploy:* The most important step in protecting yourself against the nibble is to recognize it. You can congratulate them on the deal they have already negotiated and point out the nibble. "You negotiated a fantastic deal. You're not going to nickel and dime me now, are you?"
- *Just say no:* Some people will continue to nibble until you say enough. "We've made a deal. If you would like to discuss additional items, I would be happy to reopen the negotiations."

The Flinch

The flinch is a physical reaction demonstrating strong rejection of a proposal. It is designed to create embarrassment and concession. This is an extraordinarily powerful ploy. The more dramatic the flinch, the more effective it becomes. On hearing the offer, the flincher responds immediately with a look of astonishment and disbelief while simultaneously uttering, "You want what?!"

Some would never flinch, believing it to be beneath their dignity or improper. This attitude may make one side particularly susceptible to a flinch. Further, appropriately used, the flinch may provide an excellent opportunity to bring a ridiculous first offer closer to an acceptable level.

For example, you are in an antique shop looking at an early American desk. You ask the price, When the dealer tells you, you flinch. Your jaw drops, you throw your arms up in the air and you angrily claim, "That's ridiculous!"

Contract Example. Your group is presenting a proposal to staff the emergency department. Upon stating the financial requirements, the other party suddenly stands up, throws her arms in the air and with a stunned expression yells, "You've got to be kidding! There is no way we can do this deal." There is a sinking feeling in your stomach and your expectations begin to drop. Your immediate reaction is to try to figure out how you can change the deal to make it more appealing.

Solutions

- *Recognize the ploy:* Avoid responding defensively or in a way that tries to appease this apparently upset person.
- *Calmly reassert value:* Be prepared to restate calmly and clearly the value of the product or service.
- *Ask for a reciprocal concession:* If you feel obliged to respond to the person flinching, couch your response in terms of your willingness to change if he or she will reciprocate with something of equal value.

Puppy Dog Technique

The puppy dog technique or trial offer is a classic sales technique. It is a successful way to close a deal. "Why don't you take the puppy home over the weekend and show it to the kids. If you don't like it you can bring it back next week." Once the puppy dog is home, the kids will naturally fall in love with it and the deal is closed. This ploy is the same as the 30-day trial period. It is rare for the purchaser to return something within the trial period.

The trial offer is frequently used in television commercials. A good example is the company that promises a complete refund of your money if you are not completely satisfied. Once purchased, the equipment may be used a great deal initially. Even if you are not using it at the end of the 30-day trial period, you may rationalize that you will start using it soon.

Solutions

- *Know what you want in advance:* The less advanced planning you do, the more likely you are to fall prey to this technique.
- *Predetermine your return criteria:* Before the trial period begins, determine exactly how you will evaluate and base your decision to keep or return the product or service.

Funny Money

Funny money is a term used to describe reducing the cost down to unreal or small increments. By not recognizing the true value, we are encouraged to spend more. We are confronted every day with examples of funny money.

For example:

- Mortgage interest is spoken of in percentages rather than actual dollars. The 8½% in interest seems a lot smaller than $24,000 per year.
- Payments for subscriptions or products may convert this cost to a daily amount. For only 23 cents a day you can enjoy our product. The funny money ploy tries to create this perception that something is inexpensive, when it is not.
- For example, you are looking for a house and the realtor has shown you a place that is out of your price range. He may say, "it only costs a dollar more a day. Are you really going to let a dollar keep you from your dream house." It is considerably more than one dollar that stands between you and this house. It is $10,950 in increased principal plus approximately $23,800 in interest (at 10%) or $34,750 in additional cost to you.

Contract Example. The hospital foundation comes to your group and says. "You have been very successful here. The hospital campaign is asking your group to donate only $1 an hour for each year of the contract. It does not seem like a lot at $1. However, $1 per hour × 8760 hours per year × 5 years equals $43,800.

Solution

- *Determine the true cost:* Before making the deal, determine the true total cost by translating it into real money—not pennies per hour, but dollars per year.
- *Correct the time frame:* In considering the cost, use the time frame for which you will have to write a check.

SUMMARY

This chapter has provided basic negotiation theory and a few practical applications. The skill to negotiate results from practicing and studying the process. To prepare effectively for negotiation, one must recognize his or her own needs while gathering extensive information about the other party's history, strengths, weaknesses, and goals.

The success of negotiation should not be measured by short-term gain at the expense of the other side. Rather it should be measured by the development of a long-term and mutually beneficial relationship that is built on trust and the desire to achieve common goals. In a successful negotiation, both parties feel they have achieved their goals and want to do business with each other in the future.

REFERENCES

1. Karass C: *The negotiating game,* New York, 1992, Harper Collins.
2. Karass C: *Give and take: the complete guide to negotiating strategies and tactics,* New York, 1993, Harper Collins.
3. Dawson R: *Secrets of power negotiating,* Hawthorn, NJ, 1995, Career Press.
4. Hovland CI et al: Order of presentation in persuasion, New Haven, Conn, 1957, Yale University Press.
5. Cohen H: *You can negotiate anything,* New York, 1982, Bantam Books.
6. Fisher R, Ury W: *Getting to yes,* Boston, 1981, Houghton Mifflin.

ADDITIONAL READINGS

Levin E: *Negotiating tactics: bargain your way to winning,* New York, 1980, Fawcett Columbine Books.

Nierenberg GI: *Negotiating the big sale: super strategies for smart dealmakers,* New York, 1993, Berkley Books.

35 General Contract Principles

David Kalifon

OUTLINE

Emergency physicians are confronted with diverse incomprehensible contracts that may profoundly affect their finances and practice. These diverse contracts may involve employment or independent contractor relationships with practice groups, arrangements with hospitals to provide administrative or clinical services in an emergency department or urgent care center, relationships with billing and collection companies, or arrangements with managed care plans or independent practice associations (IPAs). Physicians should negotiate or sign a contract only after consulting knowledgeable legal, accounting, and other advisers. Physicians, nonetheless, should be familiar with certain contracting fundamentals. This chapter describes some of those fundamentals:

- The formation and purpose of contracts
- The organization of the written document
- Provisions important to emergency physicians
- Who should draft the written document
- The role of an attorney in the contracting process
- Common errors in drafting

CONTRACTS AND HOW THEY ARE FORMED

I promise to do something for you and, in return, you promise to do something for me. The mutual exchange of promises creates a contract. Contracts may be oral, in fact, or written.

Oral Contracts

Many physicians believe that enforceable contracts must be in writing; this is not true. Oral contracts generally are enforceable, although their terms can be difficult to prove, and disagreement about such terms often is central to a dispute. Certain types of oral contracts are not enforceable in some states, such as those involving personal services contracts extending beyond 1 year.

In Fact Contracts

An enforceable contract (or contract provision) may even be established by actions. For example, if a group paid the continuing medical education (CME) tuition and expenses for all of its physicians over the last 5 years even though the group never promised to do so, a physician could credibly claim that the group breached its contract by suddenly refusing to pay the physician's CME costs.

Written Contracts

When discussing contracts, physicians generally envision a written agreement. Most of this chapter discusses this common form of a contract.

PURPOSE OF A CONTRACT

People make contracts to get things done: buy property, sell services, and so forth. Legally, contracts are meant to define the expectations of the parties and to allocate the risks.

As a result, a contract helps focus the parties' attention on the terms of a relationship. Writing a clear statement of what each party expects to give and to get is the best way to ensure there has been a meeting of the minds. Preparing a contract encourages the parties to resolve foreseeable potential disputes in advance, while their relationship is good. Hopefully the contract will be stored in a drawer and never have to be referred to again. However, if a dispute arises later, a contract can help refresh the parties' memories; often that will be enough to resolve the problem. If not, the contract should show what the parties agreed to do in the face of an unresolvable dispute.

The clearer, more detailed and more comprehensive the contract, the more protection the parties are likely to have. However, the negotiation or drafting of such a contract should not unnecessarily undermine the parties' relationship. An unreasonable negotiating stance, including inappropriately pushing for an ever more protective document, may sour the relationship. The most finely crafted contract is no substitute for an excellent relationship with the other side, especially if the contract calls for the parties to work together. Any business deal requires each side to intelligently balance its risks and benefits. Neither side should expect a contract to make a deal risk free.

ELEMENTS OF A CONTRACT

All that is required to create a written contract is a promise to do something, "consideration" (payment or its equivalent—the promise by the other party), and a signed document. Most written contracts go further, sharing certain common elements. Although these elements may not always appear in the same order, being able to recognize them reduces the mystique of a contract and allows the physician to use it more easily. The overview that follows should allow you to find your way around the written document. The subsequent conceptual discussions explain the importance of including selected provisions in the written agreement; specific language for these provisions is presented in other chapters. The selection reflects the provisions about which emergency physicians most often inquire.

Although every part of a contract is potentially important, in most cases, the term/termination, exclusivity (where applicable) and compensation provisions are typically the most important parts of emergency physician contracts. If these provisions are acceptable, the parties usually find ways to come to terms on other differences.

An Overview

Usually, an introduction and recitals identify the parties and the reasons for entering into the contract. Then the rights and obligations of the parties are delineated, typically including the duties of each party and the compensation to be paid. The contract usually contains a set of business provisions applicable to both sides. These include general issues, such as the creation, storage, and ownership of records; matters of confidentiality and proprietary information; insurance and indemnity; and dispute resolution (such as court versus arbitration). The term of the agreement and the grounds and means for termination are stated. Toward the end of the document is the classic "boilerplate," which deals with general legal provisions, such as how notice is given, whether the contract can be assigned, how it can be amended, and similar formal but important concerns. The contract should end with signature blocks providing for the proper parties to sign in the correct capacities. Finally, many contracts refer to exhibits and schedules, all of which should be attached before the agreement is executed. Blank spaces also should be filled in before the agreement is signed.

Obligations

A contracting party should ensure that it can reasonably perform its obligations, that its needs are satisfied by the other's obligations, and that the costs of performance are properly apportioned. Consider the following examples.

A contract between a hospital and emergency group obligated the group "to comply with all the hospital's administrative regulations, policies, and procedures." Unfortunately, the group forgot that the hospital unilaterally controls revisions and therefore could unilaterally amend some of the group's obligations. Six months into the contract, the hospital revised its policy for emergency department screening and triage. The group disliked but was contractually obligated to accept the revision, which the group believed might violate federal patient transfer law and increase its malpractice risks.

In a second example, a draft contract between a hospital and an emergency group stated that "At its sole cost, the hospital shall provide all usual, ordinary and customary personnel, supplies, equipment and services reasonably required for the *proper operation* of the emergency department." Does this general statement satisfy the emergency physicians' need for timely transcription of medical records? Transcription substantially reduces the physicians' paper work; fewer physicians are needed to staff the department. Transcription also results in more comprehensive medical records, reducing malpractice risks and improving reimbursement.

After difficult negotiations, the hospital added a new, separate contract provision that stated, "Hospital shall arrange for timely transcription of the emergency department physicians' medical records." Unfortunately, this new provision did not state who would pay for the transcription and, in these times of skyrocketing costs, the hospital felt pressured to pass the cost through to the group. The hospital stated it was only obligated to pay for "usual, ordinary, and customary" services. The hospital also stated that "timely" transcription for the emergency department required a more rapid turnaround than its existing transcriptionists and equipment could provide and thus entailed "extraordinary, new" costs for which the group must pay.

Term and Termination

The term and termination provisions of an agreement should always be considered together. The term is the duration of the contract; the termination provisions provide grounds for ending the contract before its term expires. As an example, consider that the following appears in a group's agreement with a billing and collection company: "This Agreement is for two years and automatically renews for successive two year periods, unless either party gives advance notice of termination." "Either party may terminate this Agreement, with or without cause, upon 90 days' written notice." Together, these provisions effectively turn an ostensible 2-year contract into a rolling 90-day agreement. Sometimes this arrangement is desirable. In our example, if the group discovers within 1 month that its billing and collection company is performing inadequately the group need not fear being locked into a 2-year agreement. On the other hand, the billing company might find the "90 day notice" contract provision desirable if the billing company wishes to terminate the agreement because it made a bad deal and is undercharging for its services.

Always review a contract carefully and determine whether it allows termination under circumstances that might be significant and adverse. Consider the following scenario: The wing of the hospital building in which the emergency department is located is severely damaged by fire or other catastrophe, and the hospital will not be able to repair and reopen it in less than 120 days. The emergency physicians might well decide to relocate permanently rather than just for the duration of the repairs. If so, would the physicians be in breach of their contract(s) if they decided not to return to the damaged department once it were restored?

Exclusivity

The right to be the exclusive provider of emergency services in the emergency department is an essential provision of an agreement between an emergency group and a hospital. (Such exclusivity generally should not preclude private attendings from caring for their own patients in the emergency department.) The exclusivity preferably should extend to any services or facilities in which the hospital has an ownership interest or managerial control and which might compete for the emergency department's patients.

Without such a grant, an emergency group might find its patient load carved away, as the following story illustrates: One group saw 32,000 visits in its department during the previous year. As is typical of many departments, about half these visits involved patients with nonemergent problems that could have been treated elsewhere. The hospital opened an urgent care center on its campus, about 150 feet from the entrance to the emergency department, and for political reasons arranged for a family practice/internal medicine group to provide the center's physician coverage. The hospital also stationed a triage nurse at the entrance to the emergency department to redirect many of the nonemergent patients to the urgent care center. Within 1 month, the emergency group lost 15% of its volume and had to terminate one of its full-time physicians.

Compensation

Because the methods of compensation are myriad, this chapter can do no more than urge that a party to a contract thoroughly understand its compensation provisions. The following anecdote illustrates the harm that can befall the unwary. A single hospital emergency group signed a capitation contract with a managed care plan. For a certain fee (a fixed dollar amount per month for each enrolled member residing in the hospital's cachement area), the group would provide all the physician care for plan patients seeking medical care in the hospital's emergency department. Unfortunately, the overworked, office-based primary care physicians started referring to the emergency department patients they previously would have seen on short notice in their offices. The emergency group soon was seeing 60% more plan patients than it anticipated and found its capitation fee woefully inadequate. Additionally, in accordance with the capitation agreement, the plan deducted from the group's fees any amounts it paid to non-plan on-call specialists the group called in to treat the patients. Unfortunately the group did not understand its compensation arrangement and the extent of its risk. At the least, the group should have had a "stop loss" provision.

Records

Contracts often state that the medical records of emergency department patients belong to the hospital and that groups and physicians must maintain, for a minimum of 4 years, certain records to support claims for reimbursement by the Medicare and Medicaid programs. The 4-year retention is required by federal law.

Contracts also can ensure groups and physicians that they have access to records (medical, billing, or other) after their contract terminates. These records might be important in peer review proceedings, licensing actions, demands by third-party payors for return of alleged overpayments, medical research, and other actions. Without a specific contract provision, access might be denied. (In malpractice cases, records generally are available by subpoena or a demand for production.)

Confidentiality

Whether or not restated in the contract, an emergency group and physician must comply with existing state and federal laws protecting the confidentiality of certain medical records and patient information and prohibiting their improper disclosure or redisclosure. The contract also might prohibit disclosure of the terms of the contract (unless required by law) to maintain one party's bargaining position. For example, consider a hospital that is renegotiating all its hospital-based physician group contracts and is willing to pay the emergency group, but not the radiologists or pathologists, an administrative fee. Assume that the hospital could not politically resist paying the radiologists an administrative fee if it were generally known that the emergency physicians received one. The hospital might agree to pay the emergency group only if the terms of their contract remained confidential.

Insurance

In addition to malpractice insurance, emergency physicians and groups should seek protection and coverage for work premises, nonphysician personnel, and administrative services, including quality assurance (QA) or continuous quality improvement (CQI), utilization review (UR), and an emergency department physician director's sundry duties. See Common Drafting Errors for comments on malpractice insurance.

To protect from unknowingly practicing "bare," insist that the contract obligate the purchaser of insurance to provide certificate(s) of coverage and statements from carriers that the insureds will be notified at least thirty (30) days before any cancellation, nonrenewal, or change in the specified coverage.

Dispute Resolution

Always consider including in the contract a method for resolving disputes short of resorting to the courts. For example, a dispute might be submitted to arbitration by a professional society, the American Arbitration Association, or some other group organized for the purpose. (In California, one commercial group specializes in providing retired judges to settle disputes.) Arbitration is less expensive and quicker than litigation, but does not have all the protections of a court proceeding. Most physicians elect to include an arbitration provision in their contracts. The advantages and disadvantages of arbitration should be discussed with a knowledgeable attorney.

Consider a bifurcated mechanism for resolving disputes. All disputes about patient care issues might be settled through the medical staff process or by a medical society. All other disputes might be submitted to third-party arbitration by laypersons. Generally, the medical staff is not an appropriate forum for resolving political or business disputes; the staff is not expert in these areas, and some staff members may be competitors of the emergency physicians. Avoid allowing a hospital's board of trustees or directors to make the final decision about a dispute between administration and an emergency group; the board generally will be biased in favor of the hospital's administration.

Breach and Remedy

A party breaches a contract when it fails to carry out an obligation or condition of the agreement. If the breach is material—a legal term that roughly means substantial and important—the injured party might use the breach as grounds for terminating the contract and seeking monetary damages or an injunction. The injured party wants to avoid additional harm and to be compensated for the injury it suffered.

Many emergency groups, physicians, and hospitals include in their contracts a provision that may preserve a relationship: The breaching party is allowed a limited time in which to "cure" or correct a breach brought to its attention. Consider the following example: A contract between a group and a physician states, "Either party may terminate this agreement on 90 (ninety) days notice with or without cause." It also states, "Group may terminate this agreement immediately, or at any time thereafter, if physician breaches this agreement, which breach continues uncured for a period of seven (7) days after written notice of such breach is provided by group to physician." After night shifts, the physician goes home to sleep and returns 8 to 16 hours later to finish the charts. On several occasions, no medical information was available when patients returned for unscheduled revisits. The group sends the physician a letter stating that (1) the contract requires him or her to complete patient records before leaving the hospital and (2) the group will terminate the contract at the end of 1 week unless he or she reforms. The physician reviews the contract, reassesses his or her behavior, and reforms. The formality of the serious letter, the attention it drew to the issue, the threat of dismissal on short notice, and the opportunity to cure allows the group and physician to preserve their relationship.

Other Provisions

Other chapters in this book discuss many of the other provisions commonly appearing in emergency physician contracts.

WHO SHOULD DRAFT THE WRITTEN DOCUMENT?

There are advantages and disadvantages to being the party responsible for drafting a written agreement. A disadvantage is the cost. Precise legal writing is difficult and time consuming. It can even be expensive to prepare documents that appear simple or to make straightforward revisions of preexisting documents. Also, a court is likely to construe any ambiguities (inadvertent or otherwise) against the drafter.

On the other hand, the drafter of a written agreement has control. To use a military analogy, the drafter has the high ground and the other party must fight uphill. Although the parties always negotiate the few more important provisions, they often tire and execute an agreement before the less important and finer points are negotiated. Consequently, these points tend to favor the drafter. A party should analyze whether the advantages outweighs the disadvantages of drafting. The result should guide the party's negotiations about which side will draft.

THE ROLE OF THE ATTORNEY

An experienced, quality attorney can do more than review and analyze a written contract. An attorney might participate in direct negotiations with the other side or only provide behind the scenes advice on strategy, tactics, and options for resolving problems. An attorney with extensive experience with emergency practitioners should be familiar with the usual and customary business practices of the specialty and might provide invaluable background information for structuring a deal. When negotiating particularly contentious issues, a party can blame the conflict and the outcome on an attorney; the parties may thereby preserve their relationship.

Remember that the attorney's role generally is (and properly should be) limited to that of advisor. As stated previously, any business deal requires an intelligent balancing of risks and benefits, the legal risks and benefits being only a part of the equation. Even when kept well informed, the attorney rarely can evaluate the nonlegal aspects of a deal as well as the client can. If business benefit substantially outweighs legal risk, a client might reasonably choose to override an attorney's advice.

COMMON DRAFTING ERRORS

The text of a contract always should be drafted as clearly as possible. Where necessary, the contract should be revised to eliminate redundancies, inconsistencies, and ambiguities and to define words and phrases having special meaning for the contract. In case of a dispute between the parties, such clarity may help an arbitrator or judge interpret the agreement as the parties intended.

For example, consider the following provision in an agreement between a physician and an emergency group:

> Group shall provide Physician with malpractice insurance covering Physician's practice at Hospital during the term of this Agreement. Such insurance shall have limits no less than one million dollars for any one incident and three million dollars in the aggregate for any one calendar year.

Malpractice insurance, in this example, is "claims-made" and covers only those lawsuits filed during the policy year. If the physician leaves the group, who is responsible for paying the considerable cost of "tail" coverage for any lawsuits filed after departure but based on malpractice occurring before departure? Generally, courts construe ambiguities against the party who drafted the document. (Although a tail may be superfluous if the group remains intact and continually renews its claims-made policy, such stability cannot be assumed.)

Be sensitive to language that is broadly and vaguely drafted and expansively defines obligations. Try to clarify and limit such phrasing by expressly limiting obligations or stating that only what is "reasonably" required must be performed. For example, consider the obligations if the following appeared in a contract between a physician and a practice group: "Physician shall provide such back-up or on-call coverage as Group assigns." If more senior group physicians decide they want easier schedules, might the physician be assigned a disproportionate amount of night and weekend on-call coverage?

Also watch for and eliminate unachievable guarantees. Although a physician or group may intend to provide exemplary service at all times, should a contract ride on such aspirations? Consider the following provision in a contract to manage a hospital's emergency department: "Group shall at all times assure the highest quality of care in its services at the Hospital." Might this create a laudable goal that the group may not be able to achieve at all times? If the group is understaffed and hires a competent but not outstanding physician, does it risk breach and possible loss of the contract? Finally, consider whether a malpractice plaintiff could argue that the group should be held to a higher standard in a malpractice case brought by a patient.

Be attentive to who has the authority to make a decision and what standard applies to the decision making. If sole authority cannot be retained, perhaps decisions can require "mutual agreement." As a practical matter, mutual agreement allows either party to veto any change from the status quo. If the other side has the right to make a decision, it should have to be "reasonable." In some cases, the parties can create a short list of predetermined options. For example, if an emergency group and a managed care plan's utilization review committee disagree about the necessity of evaluating and managing a plan patient in the emergency department, how will the matter be resolved? Will the group not be paid? Will repeated refusals to pay effectively pressure the group to transfer plan patients to the plan's after hours clinic? Would such transfers be against the group's better judgment, possibly violate Consolidated Omnibus Budget Reconciliation Act (COBRA) and state antidumping laws, and perhaps risk a malpractice suit?

SUMMARY

Physicians are confronted with diverse contracts that may profoundly affect their practices, both economically and professionally. Because of the importance of these contracts, they should be reviewed by knowledgeable attorneys and, perhaps, other advisors such as accountants and business managers. Nonetheless, physicians should be familiar with the fundamentals of contracts, including their formation, purpose, organization, most important provisions, and drafting.

ACKNOWLEDGMENT

The author wishes to thank Hilary Huebsch Cohen, Esq. for her assistance in coauthoring an earlier version of a portion of this material.

36 Contracting with Hospitals: MONETARY AND LEGAL ISSUES

John G. Keene and Stephen J. Dresnick

OUTLINE

A contract defines the essential elements of a business relationship, establishes the relationship between the parties, and provides them an opportunity to grapple with difficult issues before there are problems. It is important to define the business relationship as clearly and thoroughly as possible to facilitate a smoothly running operation. This process also establishes appropriate expectations, which helps to avoid a conflict. This chapter is divided into two sections: financial issues and key contract clauses.

PHILOSOPHIC APPROACH

Establishing a Relationship

Negotiating a contract can be the first major test of a relationship or a major challenge in an established relationship. How the parties approach the task and resolve the areas of conflict leaves an indelible stamp on the relationship. In many ways it sets the tone for almost all future interactions.

If resolving areas of conflict is difficult and stormy, the parties will fear this type of interaction for all future conflict resolution. On the other hand, if the parties are able to engage each other in collaborative problem solving, everyone will expect that type of interaction when future issues arise.

Because contract negotiation is such an important part of developing a successful long-term relationship, it is worth taking the time to establish a collaborative interaction. This does not mean that one constantly has to concede points to the other side. It does mean that the other side should be given plenty of time and opportunity to communicate their issues and identify their needs.

Once the other side is certain their issues will be understood, they will be much more receptive to hearing yours. This process of careful listening and seeking a full understanding develops trust and rapport, which will allow for dissecting each side's true needs from their positions. Only then can energies be devoted to finding creative, synergistic solutions where both parties' needs are met.

Seek Win-Win Solutions

Because a contract negotiation is only part of establishing a successful long-term relationship, it is important to approach the process with the attitude that both sides' needs must be met. With this approach there is no longer the attitude of "winning a negotiation." To successfully operate an emergency department requires a team effort. In contracting with a hospital, you are joining forces to deliver a product to the public. The product is emergency medical services. The goals of the hospital and the physician group are the same.

Even when you find yourself embroiled in a difficult dialogue with regard to the amount of the subsidy or the need for a revenue guarantee, there are areas of mutual interest that can lead to a successful solution. On the surface it might appear that one side was arguing for a higher subsidy to afford higher quality physicians whereas the other side was trying to save a significant amount of money. If each side's goals are distilled down to providing that product, you have laid a foundation on which a solution can be reached. On one hand, if a hospital insists that it is only interested in saving a lot of money (this is their position). If the hospital must give up its reason for existing, which is to provide quality medical care, to achieve this goal, it may be time for serious reevaluation. To insist that only money matters is incongruent with the mission of a healthcare institution. On the other hand if one accepts the tenet that it is important to provide the services in the most cost-effective manner, with a caveat that a certain baseline quality is essential, then it is simply a matter of going to the marketplace and defining the costs of providing those services. Going through this analysis reframes the situation and allows both sides to work together to find the best solutions. This win-win approach is critical for long-term success.

Defining the Details

The last philosophic concept essential for writing a contract is defining the details. That is, what each side is expected to do must be defined with sufficient clarity and detail so that there is little if any chance for misunderstanding or unmet expectations. It is always easier to sort through issues and define terms beforehand than to put the pieces back together after a major conflict develops. Not every contingency can be defined, but the major aspects of running a department, such as the medical credentials for the physicians, the hours of coverage, required leadership activities, and equipment and space to be provided can be specified.

FINANCIAL CONSIDERATIONS

Cost of Doing Business

It is important for both parties to have a clear understanding of the costs incurred in providing emergency care. Armed with a clear understanding of all the costs involved in providing emergency care and a reliable feasibility study to define the revenue available, one can then make a reasonable assessment of the financial parameters necessary to make the emergency department successful. To understate the costs, to expect providers to work for below-market rates, or to fail to build in some profit with the contract are all formulas for failure. The oldest saw, "you get what you pay for," is equally true in this circumstance. If people feel they are being inadequately compensated then it is likely that they will provide services that you perceive are inadequate.

It is always better to overestimate expenses and underestimate revenue. If a contract is workable under those circumstances, if either more revenue is generated or less expense is incurred, everyone will be pleasantly surprised. Emergency services costs can easily be broken down into four main categories (Box 36-1):

Provider Costs. Provider costs, whether for physicians, physician assistants, or nurse practitioners, can be broken down to salaries and benefits. If one develops an independent contractor relationship with the providers, then compensation should be equal to the sum of the salaries and benefits in an employee-employer relationship if the opportunities are equivalent. The salaries are straightforward. The only hidden costs that may be considered are the cost of producing the payroll.

On the other hand, benefits can be complex and entail many hidden expenses. Box 36-2 lists the typical items that can be part of a benefits package.

The decisions of whether to have independent contractors or employees and what to include in a benefits package for employees are largely determined by the market for emergency providers. To remain competitive, the offer must compare favorably with that of competitors. In some settings it may be necessary to have an on-call system. This system may add additional expenses in the form of pagers and payments for being on call.

Leadership Costs. Modern emergency departments require significant administrative input. It is important to create leadership positions commensurate with those responsibilities. An important part of defining these positions is creating the compensation packages. The director should not be expected to carry out administrative tasks during clinical shifts. The amount of time required to accomplish the administrative tasks should be estimated and the time compensated separate from clinical responsibilities. This approach allows for a direct relationship between the administrative expectations of the director and compensation for those responsibilities. To weave the director's administrative compensation into increased remuneration for clinical hours or increased vacation time creates incentive for doing additional clinical time or taking vacation rather than carrying out administrative duties.

Depending on the size of the emergency department, additional leadership and administrative positions may be required. As a rule of thumb, emergency departments with a volume greater than 30,000 visits a year should have an associate director. It is not unreasonable, however, to have an associate director at an emergency department with a smaller patient volume.

Emergency departments with major teaching involvement may require an educational director or a residency liaison. Depending on the department's mission and goals a quality assurance director, an emergency medical services (EMS) director, a marketing specialist, or community outreach director and/or risk manager may be recruited. In creating each of these positions, the needs of the department should be balanced against the time and compensation they will require.

It is important to build compensation for the contract

BOX 36-1

FOUR CATEGORIES OF EMERGENCY DEPARTMENT CONTRACT COSTS

Provider Costs
Leadership Costs
Malpractice Insurance Costs
Business/Administrative Costs

BOX 36-2

TYPICAL BENEFITS PACKAGE

Statutory benefits (varies slightly state to state)	Optional benefits
Employer contribution to FICA	Pension plan
Employer contribution to medicare	Life insurance
Workers compensation	Health insurance
State unemployment insurance	Dental insurance
Federal unemployment insurance	Disability insurance
Short-term disability	Paid time off
	Vacation
	Holidays
	Sick days
	Personal days
	CME time
	CME stipend
	Books/dues and licence fees

FICA, Federal insurance contributions act; CME, continuing medical education.

holder into the budget. That individual is responsible to ensure that all of the requirements of the contract are met. To hold that person responsible, in a legal sense, he or she must receive something of "good and valuable consideration." When attempting to hold someone responsible for something, it is always helpful to create a written document detailing the agreement; however, an even stronger argument is made when the person is paid to carry out certain responsibilities.

Malpractice Insurance Costs. All hospital contracts should include a clause that requires all providers to carry malpractice insurance. The coverage limits of the malpractice insurance policy should be specified in the contract. The minimum amounts are usually specified in the medical staff bylaws, the hospital's policies, or state statute.

The contract holder should have the freedom to choose the malpractice insurance carrier provided the carrier is duly licensed and in good standing with the appropriate state regulatory agency. If the contract holder is using independent contractors rather than employees, the contract should specify that the contract holder will require the independent contractors to have the appropriate malpractice insurance rather than purchase it for them. A provider must be completely responsible for his or her own benefits to be considered a truly independent contractor.

In some settings it may be reasonable to factor the cost of an umbrella policy to extend the coverage limits beyond the basic amounts. Just as with a basic malpractice insurance policy, it is important that independent contractors pay for their own umbrella coverage.

In the past, plaintiff lawyers have focused primarily on the physician of record; however, is seeking to cast their net as widely as possible they are now sueing contract holders and groups. Under the doctrine of *respondeat superiore,* the contract holder or agency is ultimately responsible for the acts of its employees and therefore bears some liability in malpractice cases. The contract language can materially affect the strengths of that contention. The bottom line is that the contract holder should build the cost of corporate coverage into his or her budget.

Business Costs/Administrative Costs. An emergency department contract is in essence a document governing the provision of services by a small business. There are numerous business overhead expenses. They vary in amount from place to place and generally represent a sizable amount of money. Box 36-3 lists some of the business expenses that someone is likely to encounter.

BOX 36-3

TYPICAL BUSINESS EXPENSES

Legal counsel
Bookkeeping
Accounting
Recruiting agency fees
Recruiting-travel and lodging
Billing costs
Collection agency fees
Office rent
Secretarial/staff salaries
Secretarial/staff benefits
Equipment costs
- Office furniture
- Computers
- Copier
- Fax

Computer software
Books and tapes
Office supplies
Telephone
Postage
Beepers
Payroll expenses
Bank charges
Electricity/water/janitorial service
Debt service
Contributions
Educational program costs
Marketing costs

Every practice should have legal counsel in developing a contract. The day-to-day needs for legal counsel vary from place to place. The type of advice that may be needed falls into three main areas: (1) contract law, (2) healthcare law, and (3) labor law.

Tax law and pension law also come into play. In every case, it is critical to have an attorney or firm that you trust and who will be available whenever you need them.

Sound bookkeeping and accounting are essential in running a small business. The cost of these services is money well spent. An accountant can actually be helpful with initial budget expectations.

Recruiting expenses should not be underestimated. The success of an individual advertising effort is highly variable. At the same time, the fees charged by the recruiting agencies are high. The attrition in emergency medicine has been estimated at 10% to 12% a year compared with all other specialties, where the attrition rate is less than 2½% a year. A given contract may produce a stable physician force for several years; however, one could easily see periods of significant turnover or a continuous low level of turnover. Because recruiting costs can be substantial, they must be considered in the budget.

Billing for emergency providers' services is expensive, ranging between 8% and 16% of gross revenue. In some settings with particularly poor payor mixes, the cost may be even higher. To maximize revenue, a collection agency should be engaged to pursue those bills not collected in the first 6 months. Most feasibility studies include a small portion of the revenue stream as being generated by a collection agency. Therefore the cost of that service must be included in the budget. Box 36-4 details some of the expenses encountered in the billing process.

A frequently overlooked cost is debt service. When a group starts a fee-for-service contract, the group will need to borrow money, unless the hospital is providing the start-up funds or there is a guarantee. With proper planning, there are ways to reduce that amount to a minimum. If a loan is taken out, however, the interest on that loan will need to be included in the cost of running the contract. Paying down the principal also must be calculated.

Many other items are likely to be part of running a con-

BOX 36-4

BILLING EXPENSES

- Billing company fees
- Legal fees for contract development
- Post office box
- Lock box
- Bank lock box
- Secretarial time
  - Chart processing
  - Data entry
  - Patient inquiries
  - Insurance forms
  - Physician enrollments
- Telephone service
- Courier service
- Forms
- Photo copying
- Physician time
  - Problem solving
  - Quality assurance
  - Interdepartmental issues
  - Educational programs

BOX 36-5

KEY SERVICE ELEMENTS

1. Definition of triage
2. Triage ordering
3. Standard for triage time
4. System for back up triage
5. Maximum Time before initiation of physician evaluation (except in extraordinary circumstances)
6. Maximum "through-put" time
   a. For 90% of discharged patients
   b. For 90% of admitted patients
7. Maximum turnaround time for laboratory
8. Maximum turnaround time for radiographs
9. Maximum time from decision to admit to patient being moved to the floor
10. Chart documentation
11. Chart flow

tract. Most of these items are self-evident. Some facilities may have needs that are particular to their environment.

Elements of a Business Plan

A business plan is a document that defines business goals, nature of the product/service, competitors, marketing/sales plans, expense/revenue projections (for 3 years), and educational needs. Going through the process of preparing a business plan enables one to approach the process of developing the contract with the hospital in a much more pragmatic way. The business plan is also the road map for moving the business to success. Because everything has been defined in advance, measurable parameters are available by which to judge success.

As the business plan is developed, extra time should be devoted to incorporating the hospital in defining services. This process can help set appropriate expectations with regard to the way in which the department will operate. For instance, the elements of the quality improvement program could be defined to get the hospital's commitment to involve the nurses and administration in this program. It is useful to spell out all the elements of this program including the standards used in assessing the various monitors.

By taking time to define with the hospital all the elements of patient flow, appropriate standards for turnaround time of the patients in the emergency department can be established. Box 36-5 lists some of the key elements of the service, which can be defined in advance and will require commitment of both the physician group and the hospital.

In attempting to address elements such as those listed in Box 36-5 two goals are sought (1) to gain the commitment of both the hospital and the physician group to provide services in a high-quality, customer-friendly manner and (2) to develop a series of mutually acceptable and measurable parameters by which both parties can determine whether the provision of services is meeting expectations. Some items on the list will be controlled by the physician group and others will be controlled by the hospital. The two parties would essentially be trading commitments to provide high quality service to customers and to cooperate in that process. It is important to be thorough and detailed. The process of setting up the budget and business plan can be time consuming, particularly when mutually acceptable performance parameters are considered. The result of being thorough, however, is better understanding about the business and realistic expectations of what can be accomplished.

Costs always turn out to be higher than expected. By assuming the worst and planning for "unexpected expenses," cost overruns and disappointments can be avoided. At the same time, it is important to avoid rosy revenue projections. It is best to base projections on solid data. Whenever an estimate is involved, project on the low side.

In building the budget, a cushion or buffer should be established in case the malpractice rate increases, unanticipated salary demands are made, or revenue is reduced. Most businesses add a 5% to 15% buffer.

Finally it is important to plan ahead. It is always wise to project expenses and revenues for at least 3 years to anticipate factors such as inflation, changing payor mix, employment patterns, and the influence of managed care.

Reimbursement Formulas

Fee-For-Service

CONCEPT. A fee-for-service contract is one in which the revenue to support the contract is generated, for the most part, by the physician group billing for services of the physicians and allied health professionals. If the revenues from the fee-for-service billing are inadequate to cover the budgetary expenses, a subsidy from the hospital is required. When a subsidy is necessary, the hospital can recoup at least part of this through Part A reimbursement for administrative services. Generally by switching to fee-for-service billing, a hospital can save money or afford higher quality service, or both, even when a subsidy is required.

As the healthcare industry has sought to control costs, hospitals have seen shrinking revenues. One way of reducing costs is to move the emergency physicians out of the hospital. By taking them off the payroll and developing either a new group or contracting with an existing group, the hospital will incur little or no cost from running those services.

The emergency physicians now assume the risk that revenues will not meet expenses, but at the same time gain the potential for profit if revenues exceed expenses (Table 36-1).

START-UP COSTS. The lag time from issuing a bill to receiving payment in the healthcare industry is generally 60 to 90 days. In some practices it is even longer, but this usually results from poor billing practices. Because of this delay in payment, there will be substantial cash shortfalls when starting a new fee-for-service contract. There will be almost no cash in the first 2 months; thereafter it will gradually increase to reach a steady state somewhere at between 6 and 9 months. This cash shortfall is roughly equivalent to the budget for 4 to 4.5 months. In entering into a fee-for-service contract this cash flow issue must be considered and arrangements made to subsidize this period. Box 36-6 lists some of the options for subsidizing the start-up.

All of the loan options involve paying off the principal and interest and must be added to the budget. This becomes somewhat problematic if the fee-for-service revenues are insufficient to meet the budgetary needs. In these situations a subsidy is required. The subsidy would have to be large enough to include payments against that start-up loan. Depending on the makeup of the group and their financial conditions, some of the other options may be more appealing. It may be difficult to forego income for 4 to 6 months, and variations could include paying as much as possible based on the revenue that is generated or paying at some modest base rate so that the budget during the start-up phase is substantially less than the budget during steady state. If the fee-for-service revenues are large enough so that there will be profit beyond the budgeted amounts, any shortfalls in payments during the start-up phase could be made up from later profits.

Table 36-1 Fee-For-Service Model

Advantages	Disadvantages
1. Hospital usually saves money	1. Creates potential for overzealous charging
2. Creates incentive for better documentation	2. May place excessive emphasis on procedures
3. Creates incentive for improved customer service	3. No incentive for cost effectiveness, unless capitated
4. Places emphasis on high quality services	
5. Involves physicians in the business of running the department	

BOX 36-6

START-UP OPTIONS

1. Bank loan
2. Providers (partners) work without pay
3. Partners contribute to start-up fund
4. Hospital subsidy
5. Hospital loan
6. Trade start-up subsidy for ownership of accounts receivable
7. Private loan

ACCOUNTS RECEIVABLE. If the contract stops, money will still come in against outstanding balances. The sum of this money is referred to as the accounts receivable. The value of the accounts receivable is roughly equivalent to the shortfall in the start-up phase.

The accounts receivable may have substantial worth and should not be given up unless something of equivalent value is provided. For example, if the group's gross revenue at steady state are expected to be $100,000 a month, the value of the accounts receivable will be between $400,000 and $450,000. If the cost of billing is subtracted from this gross amount, the result is the amount of cash the group would receive in the 12 months after the termination of the contract. Because of the value of the accounts receivable, they can be used as collateral for a start-up loan or as collateral on other business ventures.

In general the accounts receivable are slightly larger than the start-up costs because of inflation, fee increases, volume increases, and improved collections. Therefore if the accounts receivable is traded for start-up monies, the pay back should be limited to the actual dollar amount of the start-up monies. It would also be prudent to include a stop loss statement so that if the accounts receivable are less than the start-up costs, in no event will the group owe the hospital money beyond the value of the accounts receivable. It is also important to note that in determining such a pay back, the value of the accounts receivable would be net of the cost of billing.

FEE SCHEDULE. In a fee-for-service contract, the physician group must maintain control of the fee schedule. The group will be relying on the revenue from their billing to pay the physicians and other costs. It is appropriate therefore for the group to determine those fees.

Not infrequently hospital administrators may fear that the physicians will be overzealous in charging the patients, and the net result will be a drop in the emergency department census. If the physicians are relying on that patient base for their revenue, however, then they have exactly the same concern and it would be an unwise business decision to overcharge and drive away business.

The hospital should insist that the physicians control the fee schedule for another practical reason. Most hospitals seek to have the physicians characterized as independent contractors when they employ a fee-for-service contract. If the hospital insists on controlling the fee schedule, they risk having the Internal Revenue Service challenge that independent contractor status. The hospital owns the facility, provides the equipment supplies, and hires all of the other personnel. The more tightly the hospital retains control over the physicians, the more likely they will be determined to be employees in the case of an audit.

It is important to remember that the hospital and physician group are partners in running the emergency department. They have exactly the same goal of providing high-quality service. Part of providing high-quality service is charging an appropriate amount. Prudent business sense therefore would dictate that the hospital and the physicians work together to ensure appropriate hospital and physician fees, as well as the best possible service.

COST OF LIVING ADJUSTMENTS (COLA). All businesses are faced with keeping pace with inflation. At the very least, an employer or contractor needs to give his or her employees or independent contractors compensation increases that will keep pace with inflation. Beyond that, market pressures will generally determine what other increases will be necessary. To accommodate such increases, a physician group must increase its fees. Unfortunately with a third-party payor system there, is a variable response to fee increases. In some cases where the fee schedule is established by the government or other entity, fee schedule increases will make no difference in the revenue stream. It is important therefore to carefully analyze the impact of the increase based on the payor mix.

In a contract with a hospital, if there is any subsidy or stipend, a COLA mechanism should be included so that all subsidy, stipends, and party mony are increased appropriately. At least, the COLA mechanism should mirror the increase in the consumer price index (CPI).

REGISTRATION DATA. Collecting good insurance and other demographic data is essential for a fee-for-service contract. and for the hospital to send out its bills. Unfortunately, many times, insufficient attention is paid to the registration efforts. It is important both for the emergency physician group and for the hospital to commit to optimizing the data collection at registration in the emergency department. The specific requirements should be detailed in the contract. This will clarify expectations and allow the hospital to measure for itself whether it is gaining adequate information for billing. Box 36-7 lists some of these registration specifics. It would be appropriate to spell out in the contract a specific quality assurance mechanism whereby the physician group and the hospital could measure the effectiveness of the registration efforts.

It is important to establish in the contract that the acceptable standard for compliance on obtaining this data is 100%. The only exception would be when the patient is unable to provide the information, and there is no one with the patient from whom the data may be obtained. It also important to establish a mutually acceptable policy for dealing with patients who do not have their insurance card. If they are registered as *self-pay patient,* it is possible that the data will never be collected and that the bills will be sent to the patients rather than to third-party payors. In general, this is not good for public relations and usually results in lower reimbursement. It is essential to establish a follow-up system to contact these patients and obtain the appropriate insurance information. Unless both parties commit to complete and accurate billing data collection, it is likely that both the physician group and the hospital will be incompletely compensated for their services.

NONBILLABLE VISITS. It is important in assessing the feasibility of fee-for-service contracting to identify how many and what kind of nonbillable visits occur in the emergency department. This may substantially reduce the revenue-generating population in the emergency department. Box 36-8 lists the major classes of nonbillable visits.

Patients leaving before examination (LBE) result in lost revenue. It behooves both the physician group and the hospital to make substantial efforts to remedy the problems that cause this phenomenon. Fortunately, this is an area over which some control can be exerted, thereby improving the bottom line. It would be reasonable for both parties to be contractually obligated to reducing the number of patients leaving before examination. This is particularly true if the physician group will be relying on the revenue of those patients to make ends meet.

Patients being seen in the emergency department by their private medical doctors (PMD) is potentially a politically charged issue. If a large number of visits are generated by private medical doctors, it may be the result of inadequate care that has led to a contract change. If this is the case, then it may be possible to convert a substantial number of these patients to billable patients as the medical staff becomes acquainted with the new physician group and develops a level of trust.

BOX 36-7

REGISTRATION DETAILS TO BE INCLUDED IN THE CONTRACT

1. Patient demographics
   Name, address, telephone number, Social Security number, date of birth
2. Guarantor's demographics
   Name, address, telephone number, Social Security number, date of birth
3. Patient's employer
   Name, address, telephone number
4. Guarantor's employer
   Name, address, telephone number
5. Primary insurance data
   Company name, group number, policy number, individual identification number.
6. Secondary Insurance Data
   Company name, group number, policy number, individual identification number.
7. Tertiary Insurance Data
   Company name, group number, policy number, individual identification number.
8. Photocopy of both sides of insurance card.
9. Photocopy of drivers license and/or employee identification card.
10. Signature authorizing release of information to insurance companies (original for both hospital and group)
11. Signature authorizing payment directly to the physician and hospital (original for both hospital and group)
12. Authorization of services by HMOs

HMO, Health maintenance organization.

BOX 36-8

MAJOR CLASSES OF NONBILLABLE EMERGENCY DEPARTMENT VISITS

1. Left Before Examination (LBE)
2. Private Medical Doctor Visits (PMD)
3. Nonbillable Services

It also may be the result of financial pressures, particularly from health maintenance organizations (HMOs) pressing primary care physicians to reduce the cost of emergency care and avoid admissions. It is important that the hospital and physician group work together to limit or eliminate the visits generated by private medical doctors. One way is to develop a collaborative relationship with the members of the medical staff so that he or she will be perceived as a partner in dealing with patients. Specific contracts for medical screening examinations or capitation may need to be negotiated for HMO patients.

Significant numbers of physician-referred visits also can expose the hospital and physician group to a significant malpractice risk. Critically ill patients waiting to see their private medical doctor are at great risk for untoward events that may be preventable. Specific criteria for immediate evaluation of these patients by the emergency physician must be developed. Depending on the political climate, those criteria may or may not need to be included in the emergency services contract.

Some services, particularly follow-up services, may be included in the fee for the initial service. This is generally true with surgical procedures such as a wound repair. A subsequent visit for suture removal is not a separately reimbursable service. This is important only to the extent that significant follow-up care is being provided in the emergency department and that follow-up care inflates the volume in the emergency department.

When negotiating the financial provisions of an emergency services contract with the hospital, it is critically important to identify these nonbillable services, as they may substantially affect the financial viability of the contract. The contract negotiation is an ideal time to have both parties commit to making the necessary changes relative to nonbillable services, such as taking steps to reduce patients leaving before being examined and developing a collaborative environment with the medical staff.

COURTESIES. It is customary for hospitals and physician groups to write off the charges for emergency care for certain groups of patients. This may come in the form of a professional courtesy to members of the medical staff, board of trustees members, or hospital employees. A number of different special groups that may be considered for courtesies are listed in Box 36-9.

It is important to delineate in the contract the groups to whom a courtesy will be extended. In addition the parameters and limitations on such courtesies should be detailed. Spelling out these details will define everyone's expectations and eliminate future problems.

It is important that the decisions on courtesies be made mutually and that the financial impact be defined in advance. When the financial impact on the physician group is large and potentially too great of a burden, the hospital may choose to underwrite all or part of that cost. For example some hospitals use the emergency department as an extension of their employee health program. Because the hospital believes that this is an important benefit for their employees, it actually encourages use of the department. Because the volume of visits may be very large, it may be unfair for the hospital to insist that this be provided gratis. A fair and reasonable formula for compensation should be sought in such cases.

HEALTH MAINTENANCE ORGANIZATION (HMO) CONTRACTS/GLOBAL RATES. Frequently hospitals negotiate global fees or capitation for emergency services either alone or as part of a larger package with a managed care organization. It is critical in a fee-for-service contract that all such agreements be shared with the physician group. A fair and reasonable formula for compensating the physician group should be created.

When dealing with global rates, it is important to remember that multiple factors may go into establishing an emergency department rate. For instance a hospital may give an HMO a "below cost" emergency rate to secure additional admissions. Because the hospital gains significantly from such an arrangement, it is important to find a reasonable formula for the physicians' services.

The key in dealing with these issues is working together. The hospital and emergency physicians are clearly on the same team and should seek to develop a synergistic relationship for working out these arrangements.

SPECIAL SERVICES AGREEMENTS. To solve problems, meet special interest needs, or increase business hospitals will sometimes negotiate special services agreements with either physicians or businesses. Such agreements can affect the emergency departments in several ways. For example, a hospital might have an agreement with the orthopedic surgeons that would allow them to essentially have "cast clinic" in a portion of the emergency department. Depending on how those cases are registered, it may influence the volume in the emergency department. In addition, such an agreement will use emergency department resources such as personnel and supplies.

Another example would be the provision of physical examinations for groups such as volunteer firefighters or camp physicals for the Boy Scouts and Girl Scouts. Some of these contracts are aimed at getting additional business such as an agreement for services with a local college or university.

It is important to understand the nature and impact of such special services agreements. Sometimes it is necessary to address these agreements in the contracts between the hospital and the emergency physicians to delineate things such as responsibilities and payment. The keys to success in dealing with such issues are openness and a proactive approach.

DOCUMENTATION/TRANSCRIPTION. This element is not essential in a contract for emergency services; however, it is such an important aspect of the provision of modern emer-

BOX 36-9

SPECIAL GROUPS

- Members of the medical staff
- Hospital staff
- Hospital employees
- Board of trustees members
- Members of the clergy
- Emergency medical services providers
- Firefighters
- Police
- Graduates of nursing
- In house nursing/residency program

gency medicine that it is worth exploring. It is reasonable to expect the emergency physicians to provide appropriate documentation on the care of emergency department patients. At times, however, it is difficult to specify standards in a contract because of the variability of patient presentations.

On the other hand, it is easy to specify that the hospital will provide and the physician will use a transcription system. Such a system could be real time transcription or voice activated computer transcription. Carefully documented and legible charts are important to the quality of patient care, limiting malpractice risk, and marketing the sophistication of the emergency department to the medical staff. It is also highly likely that reimbursement for physician services in the emergency department will be improved because transcription tends to reflect more accurately the level of services provided.

MARKETING. If you are improving services or offering new services, it is reasonable to communicate this fact to customers. It is reasonable to commit to a marketing program in a contract. It would be ideal to specify the types of marketing activities and the budget. At the very least, the physician group should be free to market if it exists under a fee-for-service contract.

CONTROL OF BILLING AND COLLECTIONS. In a fee-for-service environment, the physician group must be free to choose its own billing company and collection agency. If the physician group is relying on the revenue from fee-for-service billing to pay for services, it must be free to select the billing company that will provide them the best service.

Guarantees

CONCEPT. Under this arrangement, the hospital provides a revenue guarantee so that if the income from fee-for-service billing is inadequate to meet the budget, the hospital will make up the difference. This is a particularly useful concept when dealing with a particularly poor payor mix and in situations where there is significant question about the payor mix. Using a guarantee, the hospital can provide security for the emergency physicians. Assuming that the hospital is contracting with a quality group, this helps to ensure delivery of quality emergency care.

PARAMETERS. The guarantee should be for net revenues. To do business, the emergency physicians will need spendable cash. Therefore a guarantee must address that need.

A guarantee of gross charges is a meaningless construct in this context. To achieve a desired charge level, one can simply manipulate the fee schedule. Because many of the third parties work off their own payment schedules, fee increases may only marginally increase revenue. For example, some HMOs will only reimburse physician services based on their predetermined payment schedule. A physician could double his or her charges without affecting the payment from the HMO.

Setting the level of the guarantee is a matter of establishing a mutually acceptable budget. In doing this, it is important to include the cost of billing, if it is not covered by a "net revenue" guarantee, as this is usually the second largest expenditure for the physician group after the physicians' salaries. As with any business, it is appropriate to build in some cushion to cover expenses that exceed projections. An alternative would be to include a mechanism by which the guarantee could be increased if there is a significant and precipitous increase in the cost of doing business. This puts the physician group somewhat at a risk. Depending on the nature of the mechanism put in place, the hospital could be in a position to block all such increases. Fairness and good business sense must drive such decisions.

PAYMENT CAPS. To generate some risk sharing and limit their downside risk, some hospitals may seek a cap on the total amount they would pay out under a guarantee in any given year. This is a reasonable concept as long as the payment cap is large enough to cover the projected shortfall. It is a prudent business practice to include a cushion when determining the size of the cap.

CASH VERSUS ACCRUAL ACCOUNTING. To pay its physicians and other overhead, the physician group needs to operate on a cash basis. Therefore month to month guarantee payments and annual reconciliations also must be on a cash basis. Most hospitals use accrual accounting, but that only comes into play if the hospital owns the accounts receivable. In that case the hospital must use a method acceptable to its auditors to establish a value for those accounts receivables.

OWNERSHIP OF THE ACCOUNTS RECEIVABLE (A/R). Under a guarantee whereby the hospital payments to the physician group cover the start up costs, it is not unreasonable for the hospital to demand ownership of the A/R. On the other hand, the value of the services, particularly over a long time, might make it worth allowing the physician group to retain ownership of the A/R.

Certainly under a guarantee construct that includes a payment cap, such that the physician group must underwrite the start up costs, the physician group should own the A/R. If the physician group must take out a loan to obtain the start up monies, the financing charges may be a substantial cost, which must be added to the budget.

RECONCILIATION. When a hospital provides a guarantee for the physician group, there is usually a reconciliation at the end of the year to make sure the hospital is neither underpaid nor overpaid. The details included in the contract are listed Box 36-10.

FEE SPLITTING. In some instances, particularly when the volume increases in the emergency department, the revenue from the fee-for-service billing may exceed the guarantee amount. The hospital may insist on being paid all or part of the excess. This could be construed as a kickback or fee splitting. Guarantee payments can be repaid only up to the amount that was paid by the hospital. Beyond that amount, payments by the physician group back to the hospital would be considered kickbacks or fee splitting. Some hospitals have sought to characterize these as facility fees (rent) or payment for

BOX 36-10

GUARANTEE RECONCILIATION DETAILS

1. Clear definition of guarantee amount.
2. Clear definition of what makes up net revenue.
3. Time frame for delivery of reconciliation statement.
4. Details to be included in reconciliation statement.
5. Time frame after submission of reconciliation statement within which any payments due must be made.
6. Consider interest on late payments.

goods or services. Such transactions are legal only to the extent that they are consistent with local pricing and are documentable.

RELATIONSHIP TO VOLUME. To establish a guarantee level, a mutually acceptable budget must be created. Staffing will be related to the projected volume. Ideally, the contract would contain language allowing for additional income to offset increased staffing requirements. This arrangement could be as simple as an hourly rate for overtime or increased staffing or as complicated as a volume-driven formula that increases the guarantee. To be completely fair, such a formula should deal with both increases and decreases in volume.

COST OF LIVING ADJUSTMENT/INCREASES. At the very minimum, a guarantee should be increased to adjust for inflation. If such a factor is not incorporated into the contract the group would end up working for less each year.

To maximize the effectiveness of the emergency department team, it is appropriate to develop a system of incentives. These incentives must comply with federal and state laws. For example, incentives for increasing admissions would be a violation of federal regulations. Federal law specifically prohibits hospitals from paying individuals to admit patients. Incentives could be created for reducing throughput time and other customer services issues.

Flat Rate Contracts

CONCEPT. Flat rate contracts compensate the emergency physician group at a fixed rate, usually at a specified number of dollars per hour. Under this construct, the hospital is purchasing emergency physician services for a defined amount of money. The hospital is then responsible for billing the third parties for those services. This type of contract works particularly well for hospitals that either want to clearly define their emergency physician costs or believe it would be a significant advantage for them to bill for the emergency physician services themselves. Hospitals with emergency departments with low volume often find this approach advantageous.

PAYMENT TIMING. Because the payment from the hospital is the sole source of revenue in these contracts, it is critical that the contract spells out exactly when a payment will be due. This schedule should coordinate with the physicians' payroll. Because a late payment can create significant difficulties for the physician group, it is appropriate and probably essential to create a penalty for a late payment. Interest with some form of minimum penalty payment is appropriate.

COST OF LIVING ADJUSTMENTS. In a multiyear, flat rate contract, it is appropriate to include a COLA so that at the very least, the rate keeps pace with inflation. To build in some form of incentive may be productive in meeting the goals of the emergency department.

OVERTIME AND ADDITIONAL COVERAGE. There should be a provision in the contract for payment for hours worked beyond the scheduled coverage. In many smaller emergency departments, this is not an issue. In some cases, however, having the ability to pay the emergency physicians for staying late or coming in early may be the most cost effective way to deal with bottlenecks resulting from volume surges.

Percentage of Gross Charges Contracts

CONCEPT. In a percentage of gross charges contract, the hospital pays the physician group a fixed percentage of the charges generated each month. This approach generally works in situations in which the payor mix allows the hospital to generate at least enough revenue to defray the payments to the physician group. It can also be an effective tool for obtaining outstanding physician staffing for the emergency department.

CODING. Coding for the services under a percentage of gross charges contract, as in a fee-for-service contract, is critically important. The physician group should be in charge of the coding to ensure that all of the services it renders are being billed. Because there is a substantial incentive to overcode, it would not be unreasonable for the hospital to insist on some form of oversight or quality assurance on the coding. The hospital should have the right to audit that coding. The coding, may be done by the physician group or someone it hires as long as it is accurate and fair.

FEE SCHEDULE. Control of the fee schedule can also be a break point in negotiating a percentage of gross charges contract. The pitfalls include the possibility that the hospital could defer reasonable fee increases if it is seeking to reduce payments to the emergency physicians. Alternatively, the physicians could unfairly increase fees to increase their income. Mechanisms that can be used to control such potential abuses include the following:

1. Place the physician group in charge of the fee schedule, but require a review by the hospital at least 1 month before implementation.
2. Contractually oblige the physician group to have its fees consistent with usual and customary charges in the area.
3. Hire an unbiased consultant to set fees.
4. Place a cap on the amount of an increase with the caveat that increases above that level require hospital approval.

In the end, the fee schedule must be fair to the physicians and a reasonable charge for the services being rendered.

Fee schedule should be reviewed and updated at least once a year. Most businesses are conscientious about optimizing their pricing structure. They take into account their cost of doing business, changes in the economy, and competitors' fees.

COST OF LIVING ADJUSTMENTS. Because revenue is predictable and tied to charges, a COLA will be achieved through the annual fee schedule increases. COLAs are critical to stay competitive in recruiting for emergency physicians.

ACCOUNTS RECEIVABLE. Because the physician group is essentially being paid immediately after rendering the services, there is no build up of accounts receivable for them. On the other hand, the hospital will be sending out bills for the physician services to offset the payment made to the physician group. In this case, the accounts receivable would belong to the hospital.

TIMING OF PAYMENTS. Just as in flat rate contracts, it is critical that the payment by the hospital be timely so that the physician group can meet its payroll. The majority of all businesses define a late payment penalty. Providing emergency physician services is a business; therefore it is reasonable for a contract between an emergency physician group and a hospital to contain such a provision.

Subsidies

CONCEPT. Subsidies are payments by a hospital to a physician group for specific services outside the provision of physician coverage for the emergency department, or they may be provided to make up a shortfall in a fee-for-service arrangement. Subsidies can cover a wide variety of services and activities ranging from management of the department to provisions of special services such as occupational medicine.

Subsidies are ideal for smaller emergency departments that would like to take advantage of fee-for-service billing and would like to control their costs. A thorough feasibility study to estimate the revenue that fee-for-service billing would generate and a detailed look at the cost the emergency physicians will incur allows the physician group and the hospital to work together to determine an appropriate subsidy. The key advantages are that the hospital defines and limits its cost for their provision of emergency physician services and the emergency physician group has a reliable source of funds, which should make up any shortfall. An incentive is created such that if the volume in the department increases, the emergency physicians will generate additional revenue.

TIMING OF PAYMENTS. Just as with other payments by the hospital to the physician group, subsidies must be paid on a timely basis. The exact time frame should mirror the timing of the payroll or other costs to the physician group.

COST OF LIVING ADJUSTMENT (COLA). This subsidy is no different than any other payment made by the hospital to the physician group. The value of that subsidy should at least keep up with inflation.

KEY CONTRACT CLAUSES

Definitions

The contract should contain certain definitions to make the contract language as clear as possible. Frequently a variety of somewhat interchangeable terms are used in a contract negotiation. Box 36-11 lists examples of terms that are frequently defined in an emergency department contract.

Relationships of the Parties

It is important to define the nature of the relationship of the parties for Internal Revenue Service and malpractice issues. Historically, emergency physicians were employees of the hospital. When a hospital contracts with a group, it is important to define that relationship so that the hospital will not be held liable for income taxes and benefits for the physicians. As a corollary, the other provisions of the contract must be worded to support the independence of the physician group. The more tightly the hospital controls the physician group through measures such as controlling the manner in which the physicians practice, their fee schedule, and their work schedule, the better the possibility that the Internal Revenue Service will disqualify the physicians' pension plan and hold the hospital liable for their income taxes.

Most hospitals would like to separate themselves from the emergency physicians and from the medical malpractice liability of the physicians. In an employer-employee relationship, the legal concept of *respondeat superiore* holds that the employer is responsible for the actions of its employees and agents. Because of the historical precedent that emergency physicians were hospital employees, it is difficult to eliminate the public's perception that emergency physicians are still agents of the hospital. Carefully crafted contract language can be helpful in this area. The emergency physician group must be truly independent.

Responsibilities of the Group

This section of the contract specifies the duties and responsibilities of the emergency physicians. It is typically related to the provision of a director, the provision of medical care, the maintenance of medical records, and other critical functions of the emergency physicians. Box 36-12 lists some of the typical items found in a duties and responsibilities section.

Writing admitting orders, responding to cardiac and respiratory arrests, evaluating patients on the floors, and pronouncing patients are some of the controversial items that may appear in this section.

Responsibilities of the Hospital

This section defines the duties and responsibilities of the hospital. The duties and responsibilities sections can be helpful in setting the stage for collaboration. By indicating that the group and the hospital will share some of the duties and responsibilities important expectations are created. Box 36-13 lists some of the duties and responsibilities that may appear in this section of the contract.

To promote team work and collaboration, many of the items such as quality improvement, risk management, and utilization review should be mirrored in the hospital responsibility section. At the very least, the hospital should be held responsible for those activities as they relate to their employees; however, the collaborative approach is preferable.

The duties and responsibilities sections can also be the ideal format for setting standards of performance in areas such as laboratory turn-around time, radiograph turn-around time, speed of moving admitted patients to the floor, and time for triage and overall through-put time. By discussing and

BOX 36-11

FREQUENTLY DEFINED TERMS

Emergency department
Emergency physicians
Medical director
Hospital policies
Emergency room
Hospital

BOX 36-12

EMERGENCY PHYSICIAN DUTIES AND RESPONSIBILITIES

1. Provision of a director
2. Quality improvement program
3. Complaint management
4. Customer services
5. Utilization review
6. EMS participation
7. Evaluating and treating patients

BOX 36-13

DUTIES AND RESPONSIBILITIES OF THE HOSPITAL

1. Provide adequate space for the evaluation and treatment of patients
2. Provide adequate space for the administrative function of the department
3. Provide appropriate nursing and other staff
4. Pay the salaries and benefits of the nurses and staff
5. Provide adequate equipment and supplies
6. Provide electrical service, water, and telephone
7. Provide janitorial and maintenance services
8. Provide registration services

BOX 36-14

FOR CAUSE TERMINATION PROVISIONS

1. Bankruptcy, insolvency, or receivership
2. Breech
3. Adverse reimbursement changes

agreeing on such standards and responsibilities, the hospital and physician group take the first important steps toward dramatically improving services in the department. It is relatively easy to espouse the ideals of customer services and efficient care; it is a substantially more significant step to commit to those ideals contractually.

Term

The start date and time of day as well as the ending date and time of day should be specified in the contract. To deal with issues such as reconciliations, it may be necessary to specify the "contract year."

Termination

Both parties must be able to terminate a contract under certain significantly adverse conditions. Termination provisions fall under two broad headings: For cause terminations and Not for cause terminations. Box 36-14 lists some of the common for cause termination provisions.

Bankruptcy, Insolvency, or Receivership. Each of these terms refers a situation in which one of the parties to the contract is financially distressed. Bankruptcy refers to the legal definition of insolvency. Insolvency is the state of being unable to pay one's obligations. Receivership is being placed in the hands of a court appointed financial manager because of bankruptcy. It is only reasonable that a contract can be terminated in such situations.

Breech. A for cause termination for breech of a contract gives the nonbreeching party the ability to terminate the contract because the other parties did not keep their end of the bargain. Typically, termination for breech clauses include a "cure." This cure period is a specified amount of time, usually 30 days, in which the breeching party will have an opportunity to correct the deficiency. The clock usually starts running on the cure period once the breeching party has been notified of the breech in writing.

The length of the cure period is negotiable and may vary based on the severity of the breech. For example, in an emergency department contract, if the physician group staffing the emergency department leaves the emergency department without a physician for even a short time, the hospital should have the right to terminate the contract immediately.

Not for Cause Clauses. A not for cause termination clause provides that either party can terminate the contract with a specified amount of advanced written notice without specifying the reason. Typically in emergency services contracts, not for cause clauses require 90 to 180 days advanced notice.

There are two schools of thought with regard to no cause terminations. One suggests that it is better not to have such provisions as a means of providing some sense of security for the physicians over the life of the contract. The other believes that it is a prudent business step to have this type of clause as a safety valve. It is easy to imagine situations in which even though no one has breeched the contract, significant problems may still exist that erode the relationship and quality of care. A no cause termination may be the only way out of such an awkward situation. Alternatively, a situation may not be profitable for one or the other partner, and if there is no financial provision for termination, a not for cause termination is essential.

Indemnification and Hold Harmless Clauses

To indemnify is to secure or protect against hurt, loss, or damages. As indemnification applies to emergency services contracts, if one of the parties indemnifies the other, that party is protecting the other or holding the party harmless from financial damages that may arise out of the events or issues for which the indemnification is being provided. For example, an emergency services contract may have a hold harmless clause in which the physician group and a hospital indemnify each other from loss related to their own malpractices cases. On the surface, this arrangement may make sense. If an emergency physician made a mistake, why should the hospital suffer financially? Therefore it would seem fair for the physician group to protect the hospital by giving it an indemnification holding it harmless in such instances.

In practice, however, malpractice cases are rarely that simple. When a malpractice problem occurs in the emergency department, there are frequently multiple contributing factors. As a malpractice case proceeds, the involved parties often deny responsibility and blame each other. Such arguments form the basis for invoking a hold harmless clause and having the emergency physician group or hospital ask the other party to reimburse any payment they may have to make, including legal fees.

To make things even more complicated, if there is a settlement, the insurance company for the party receiving the indemnification may argue that it is a de facto beneficiary of that indemnification and ask for reimbursement. Some malpractice insurance companies indicate in their policies that the provision of an indemnification will result in loss of coverage. Alternatively, for an additional premium, some companies will extend their insurance to cover that indemnification.

In general, where there is a significant discrepancy in the size of the parties, such as the difference between a small physician group and a hospital, the larger entity gains a greater advantage, and the smaller entity is less capable of dealing with the financial repercussions of such a clause. For this reason, hold harmless clauses should be avoided in emergency services contracts. In some instances, a potential liability may be foisted on one of the parties by the other, and the party at risk has little ability to influence that risk. In that situation, it may be reasonable for the at-risk party to be protected by a hold harmless clause. An example of this situation is a private medical doctor who sees patients in the emergency department without the involvement of the emergency physician. Malpractice case law has found the emergency physician responsible for all of the patients in the emergency department, including those waiting to see their private medical doctor. A hold harmless clause may be appropriate in such instances, particularly if the hospital encourages this type of practice.

Restrictive Covenants

Definition. There are three forms of restrictive covenants: noncompete, nonsolicit, and nondisclosure. A noncompete restrictive covenant prohibits parties doing business together from establishing a separate business that would be competitive with that business. A nonsolicitation restrictive covenant prohibits the parties from soliciting each other's employees or clients. A nondisclosure restrictive covenant prohibits the parties from releasing or transferring proprietary information. Depending on the setting, all three of these covenants may be applicable in an emergency services contract.

Noncompete Restrictive Covenant. Noncompete clauses are important in emergency services contracts. During the course of the contract and perhaps for some limited time thereafter, a noncompete clause would protect against the possibility of one party opening an urgent care center across the street from the emergency department. Noncompete clauses make a great deal of sense from a business standpoint. If two parties are going into business together it is reasonable to have contractual protection against one of those parties using the information and expertise gained in that relationship to set up a separate business. These covenants are generally much more enforceable when they apply to businesses rather than individuals.

There are usually time and geographic components to a noncompete restrictive covenant. A well-drafted noncompete clause would prohibit the parties from competing during the course of the contract and for sometime thereafter. It would also be necessary for that clause to define the geographic boundaries for the restriction. This would generally be related to the catchment area for an emergency department. It also depends a great deal on the marketplace. The criteria used in judging whether a restrictive covenant will hold up in court includes the following: (1) Is it reasonable? (2) Is it fair? (3) Is it consistent with the good of the community?

The longer a restrictive covenant extends beyond the termination of a contact, the less reasonable it appears. The parameters for such an evaluation vary among businesses; however, for emergency services, contracts that prohibit competition for 5 years after their termination would probably be difficult to enforce. A noncompete clause that covers the duration of the contract and for 1 or 2 years thereafter is common in emergency department contracting.

The geographic component of a noncompete clause can be highly variable. The restriction that prohibits either party from practicing emergency medicine or opening a walk-in center within 10 miles of an emergency department in upstate New York may be a reasonable geographic boundary. For an emergency department located in New York City, however, that restriction would be completely unreasonable.

Controversy continues about noncompete clauses as they relate to individuals. In many states, the courts will not enforce these clauses based on the concept that to restrict an individual would take away his or her ability to earn a living. This is most common in contracts between individual physicians and a physician group. The physician group would seek to restrict the individual from working for the hospital to prevent a mutiny. Enforceability also may be an issue in a contract between a physician group and a hospital if that physician group has only one hospital contract and is owned by a single physician rather than a small group of physicians. It could be construed that the physician group or a small group of physicians will be deprived of their livelihood through such a restriction. In addition, what is best for the communities' interest must be considered. If enforcement of a restrictive covenant would deprive a community of much needed medical services, it is doubtful that such a covenant would be upheld.

Nonsolicitation Restrictive Covenants. A hospital may want protection from the physician group hiring away its best employees. Conversely, the physician group may want to be protected from the hospital employing its physicians, which could lead to staffing problems and substantial recruiting expenditures. Similar to a noncompete restrictive covenant, a nonsolicit restrictive covenant should protect during the term of the contract and for a reasonable period of time after its termination.

Nondisclosure Restrictive Covenants. Nondisclosure restrictive covenants are most applicable in industry where product specifications, chemical formulas, or other manufacturing secrets may have cost the company a great deal of money to develop and are the key to that company's success. Emergency services have few trade secrets that need to be protected. It might be reasonable, however, to protect knowledge of financial terms, quality assurance materials, and other custom designed materials.

Liquidated Damages Clauses

A liquidated damages clause imposes a self-executing monetary penalty when a party to a contract violates a restrictive covenant. For example, a physician group and a hospital may form a contract, which is later terminated. The physician group may decide to open a walk-in center in the area. If there were a restrictive covenant in the contract prohibiting this move by the physician group, a liquidated damages clause would make enforcement much easier. The liquidated damages clause for violating the restrictive covenant could specify that the physician group would have to pay the hospital $250,000. This type of contract clause will give teeth to a restrictive covenant in a form that is easily adjudicated. The monetary penalty must not be too severe, or a court may rescind it as unconscionable.

Specific Performance Clauses

When monetary damages cannot compensate for a particular situation, a specific performance clause is created to indicate that both parties agree that this is true and that the damaged party should be granted "equitable remedies or injunctive relief" by the courts. For example, if a hospital was planning to open a walk-in center across the street from its own emergency department and this would result in several physicians in the physician group losing their jobs, simple monetary damages might not adequately compensate for that restrictive covenant violation. A specific performance clause would allow the physician group to seek a court injunction to prohibit the hospital from opening the walk-in center. These types of clauses may be helpful in resolving issues about the violation of a restrictive covenant; however, they are not indisputable and are subject to interpretation by a judge.

SUMMARY

In contracting with hospitals to provide emergency physician services, it is important to have a thorough, well-thought-out, detailed contract. In this way, appropriate expectations are created for the delivery of those services and the working relationship with the hospital.

The process of negotiating a contract begins the building of a working relationship embodied in that contract. It is important to strive to find solutions with which both parties are comfortable. Look for ways to use the contract development process to enhance collaboration and team work. Before signing a contract, have it reviewed by competent legal council familiar with healthcare and contract law. A good contract is the first step in building a strong positive professional relationship.

ADDITIONAL READINGS

American College of Emergency Physicians: *Contracts: a practical guide for the emergency physician,* Dallas, 1990, ACEP

McAdams RW: *Hospital contracts manual,* Frederick, Md, 1996, Aspen Publishers.

37 Contracts with Physicians

Leslie S. Zun, Robert W. Strauss, and David Kalifon

OUTLINE

Hospitals and emergency physician groups generally enter into a contractual relationship with physicians to provide emergency services. The success of the contractual process is contingent on consideration of critical issues and steps found in the process. This chapter addresses the pertinent contractual issues between physician and hospital or groups. These include the following:

- Necessity of a contract
- The negotiation process
- Role of legal counsel
- Letter of intent
- Key contract clauses
- Pearls and pitfalls

CONTRACT NECESSITY

There are several important reasons to develop a contract between physicians and physician groups or hospitals. Some physicians provide emergency services without a contract. One arguable advantage of a relationship without a contract is that it may allow a party to sever the relationship with no more than a few days notice.

In most other circumstances, a contract between the physician and hospital or group is recommended. The contract protects interests, clarifies discussions, and provides details for services and compensation. The contract generally contains a number of provisions to protect the physicians and groups or hospital in case of disputes relating to promised services, compensation, responsibility, and other covered provisions. The written contract supersedes and replaces all discussions that precede signing of the agreement.

Another reason to clarify the intent of the parties with a written contract is to satisfy inquiries by the regulatory authorities. They may request a copy of the contract in order to verify the relationship between the parties.

Although the contract addresses the expectations of the parties, it will not cover all of the eventualities that may arise during the life of the contract. Successful contracts are based on mutual respect, understanding, and trust. This will provide a foundation of understanding when an issue arises that is not contained in the contract.

CONTRACT NEGOTIATION PROCESS

The negotiating process is a critical aspect of contracts. The approach that each party takes in the negotiation will influence the success of the process. This section briefly outlines several practical issues of the negotiation process.

The negotiations should be performed by the decision makers. This may be the medical director/president of the group, hospital president/management, or legal counsel. It is problematic to negotiate with a person who may defer decision making to a higher authority.

The negotiation process should use productive strategies and avoid adversarial approaches. Use techniques that deal with issues, not personalities or power positions. Both parties should search for mutually beneficial solutions or options and agree on objective criteria and predetermined time frames. Avoid tactics such as take it or leave it, get the best deal at their expense, bidding process, and secret deals.

The negotiation process may take weeks to months to complete (Table 37-1). Realistically, 2 weeks to 30 days is a short time frame, whereas greater than 3 to 4 months is long. It is likely that if the parties do not agree to terms after this time, they will not agree at all.

It is important in contract negotiations to clarify the important issues early in the process (Box 37-1). These may include salary and benefits, clinical versus nonclinical time, start dates, and time off.

Editor's note: Example language is used several times in this chapter. Its only intent is to familiarize the reader with types of language that may be used to convey contractual intent. The example language is not meant to be definitive or used in a contract by the reader. Before accepting any contract language, consult advisers with expertise in contract law in the state in which the contract is to be executed.

BOX 37-1

PHYSICIAN AND HOSPITAL/GROUP EXPECTATIONS

- Physician expectations
  - Clinical
  - Nonclinical
  - Nursing/ancillary personnel
  - Compensation/benefits
  - Professional/personal growth
- Hospital/group expectations
  - Clinical
  - Nonclinical
  - Quality improvement
  - Education/research

Table 37-1 Contract Relations—Time Frame

Activity	Time	Weeks
Initial interview	0	0
Second meeting	4 wk	4
Letter of intent	1 wk	5
Review issues	2 wk	7
Legal counsel drafts document	2 wk	9
Review document	2 wk	11
Revise document	2 wk	13
Sign document	1 wk	14

Courtesy Emergency Resources Group, Chicago, Ill.

The best way to begin a negotiation is to be thoroughly prepared. This entails substantial planning. Proceed in a systematic manner by determining goals in advance. (This information is covered in detail in Chapter 34, on negotiating skills.)

LEGAL COUNSEL

Legal counsel generally performs the essential legal functions of contract review and modification. Legal counsel also can provide the gamut of services for physician contracts. It can assist in contract negotiations, contract composition, and even establishment of the practice. This expanded role for legal counsel can be costly.

Consider whose counsel should prepare the contract. Generally, the hospital or group may have a "boilerplate" contract that is used for most physicians. However, either party may elect to prepare the contract. Contract preparation usually involves substantial legal cost and time, but it provides the advantage of first presentation of terms and conditions.

Use legal counsel experienced in the issues of emergency medicine contracts. As in medicine, the legal profession has many areas of specialty (healthcare law) and subspecialty (emergency medicine contract) expertise. The search for legal counsel can be performed by word of mouth and personal references. The American College of Emergency Physicians or state chapter may be a referral source for legal services. Obtain the legal counsels' references, and determine their level of expertise in emergency medicine contracts.

BOX 37-2

KEY CONTRACT CLAUSES

- Requirements
- Status/relationship of the parties
- Compensation and benefits
- Payment clause
- Physician duties and responsibilities
- Hospital duties and responsibilities
- Group duties and responsibilities
- Restrictive covenants
- Bylaw, policy, and procedures
- Indemnification
- Hold harmless
- Breach
- Dispute resolution
- Term
- Termination
- Miscellaneous issues

Legal counsel costs can vary depending on geographic location, size of the firm, and hours of work. Small firms or solo practitioners may charge between $75 and $150 per hour for their time. Hourly charges by large and national firms may be in the $200 to $300 per hour range. The preparation and review process can take from a few hours to hundreds of hours. Do not choose the firm by its hourly rate alone. It is more important to find an efficient attorney who understands the issues and deals effectively with your concerns. Money well spent early in the process may prevent contractual and monetary losses later.

LETTERS OF INTENT

Many times during the contract process, a letter of intent is drawn up by the involved parties. A letter of intent is an agreement by the parties laying the groundwork for the negotiations by describing the general terms. It suggests that both parties are sincere about moving the process forward and signing a formal contract.

Letters of intent are usually short, briefly delineating the basic issues of the relationship. Letters of intent usually reference issues such as compensation, benefits, start dates, duties, and responsibilities. It may give an approximate time frame for contract completion.

If a formal contract is not forthcoming, the letter of intent may serve as an enforceable document. Most often, the formal contract will contain language that supersedes prior discussions and documents, including letters of intent.

KEY CONTRACT CLAUSES

Box 37-2 contains many of the key provisions that may be found in a contract between a physician and hospital or group. The list in Box 37-2 is meant to be representative of the contractual relationship. It is critical to understand these elements and how they pertain to the responsibilities of the parties.

Requirements

Requirements stipulate what a physician must possess to work for the group or hospital. They may include medical license, Drug Enforcement Administration membership, board certification, special training, academic appointment, medical staff membership, and privileges.

Some groups or hospitals may require a physician to have board certification or acquire it by a certain date. To be eligible for a position, the physician may need special training, such as fellowship in research, emergency medical services, or administration. The physician generally must obtain and maintain medical staff membership and perhaps an academic appointment for the contract to remain in force.

EXAMPLE LANGUAGE

The physician represents and warrants that to carry out duties and responsibilities hereunder, he/she shall:

A. Hold a currently valid and unlimited license to practice medicine in the State of ______________.

B. Apply for, be awarded and maintain in good standing, membership on the Staff with clinical privileges in emergency medicine, or have received and maintain temporary privileges, all in accordance with Hospital Policies.

C. Be board certified or board prepared in emergency medicine or have completed ______________, ______________, ______________.

Table 37-2 Compensation and Benefits: Employee versus Independent Contractor

	Employee	Independent contractor
Paid hours worked	1,840	1,840
Paid hours not worked		
Vacation	160	0
Continuing medical education	40	0
Holidays	40	0
Hourly rate	$68.50	$89.00/hr
Benefits		
Insurance		
Malpractice	15,000	0
Health	3,500	0
Disability	1,000	0
Life	400	0
Dues	1,000	0
Subscriptions	250	0
Continuing medical education	850	0
Pension (3% salary)	4,280	0
Total value (approximate)	163,760	163,760

Status/Relationship of the Parties

The relationship of the parties may be that of independent contractor or employer/employee. Each arrangement has significant ramifications for both sides regarding compensation, benefits, responsibilities, Internal Revenue Service (IRS) rules, and so forth. These differences must be clearly understood when entering a contractual relationship.

EXAMPLE LANGUAGE

Independent Contractor. The independent contractor and its provided physician(s) shall perform all obligations imposed by this agreement as an independent contractor. Nothing in this agreement shall be construed to create the relationship of employer and employee between Hospital/Group and the independent contractor. The independent contractor shall not be entitled to receive employee benefits. The Hospital/Group shall not have or exercise any control or direction over the manner, means and methods by which Independent Contractor shall perform work pursuant to this Agreement. Independent Contractor shall have the exclusive right and obligation to direct the manner, means and methods used to provide service pursuant to this Agreement. Independent Contractors, at all times:

A. shall not have authority to bind the Hospital/Group in any manner;

B. shall not hold themselves out as officers, agents or employees of Hospital/Group.

There may be an additional relationship or status beyond that of employee or independent contractor, such as partner, stock owner, or profit sharer. If any additional relationship exists, it is imperative that the terms and conditions are unambiguous at the outset. This may take the form of an optional buy-in period and amount after meeting distinct criteria. Some partnership agreements are expressed in vague terms, such as "After satisfactorily completing two years of employment, the physician may be offered shares in the partnership." The terms are so ambiguous that both sides may in good faith have separate interpretations of "satisfactory," "may," and "shares," creating eventual disappointment, dissatisfaction, and hostility.

Compensation and Benefits

Compensation and benefits depend on the relationship of the parties, that is, employee versus independent contractor. Employees receive a salary and benefit package; an independent contractor receives an hourly compensation inclusive of the cost of benefits. Theoretically, the independent contractor receives a higher hourly rate to compensate for the cost of benefits.

When considering an employee or independent contractor relationship, it is important to calculate the value of the benefits. The cash value of the total packages can then be compared.

Both employee and independent contractor relationships may be structured to incorporate bonuses, incentives, and profit sharing. Profit sharing and incentives can be a powerful motivating tool. The amount and timing of the disbursement of the bonus, incentive, or profit sharing should be defined in the contract. The determination should be based on objective and measurable criteria such as productivity, quality, and contributions to the emergency department. These incentives should be tied to an annual or biannual evaluation.

Benefits specific to employee relationships may include insurance (liability, life, health, dental, unemployment, and disability), paid time off (vacation and continuing medical education [CME]), license, dues and fees (professional membership, journals, hospital dues), and vestment in a pension plan.

Vacation and time off may include personal time, sick time, paternity/maternity leave, professional development time, and military leave. Some parties contractually define required minimum hours of work.

The contract usually specifies compensation increases and timing. The compensation increase may take the form of salary raise, bonus/incentive, or hourly rate increase. These increases may be based on performance evaluations, which include personal characteristics, duties and responsibilities, clinical abilities, and disciplinary action. The increase may also be tied to the financial performance of the group or department (Table 37-2).

Payment Clause

The payment clause describes the timing and method by which the physician will be paid. It should be clear and without ambiguity.

EXAMPLE LANGUAGE

Compensation shall be payable to the physician monthly, in arrears, on or before the fourteenth (14th) day of the month following the month in which service is rendered by the physician.

Physician Duties and Responsibilities

The duties and responsibilities of the physician may vary according to the job description. These may include clinical duties (on-call, in-house coverage/in-house emergencies), administrative duties (scheduling, quality assurance, budgeting, reports, and records), education (students, residents, attending staff, nurses), research/grants, and publications.

It is preferable that each of these duties and responsibilities be clearly delineated in a contract. These may include such issues as how many hours of research are required or how many manuscripts must be published each year. These duties may be tied to a bonus and incentive system or may stand alone as a requirement for employment.

In today's changing healthcare environment, the duties and responsibilities should be reviewed annually and updated or modified as necessary.

EXAMPLE LANGUAGE

When scheduled for service, the physician will provide emergency medical treatment to patients in the department, such service to include:

A. The evaluation of the medical needs of all patients presenting themselves to the Department for medical care;

B. The generation and maintenance of medical records in form and content consistent with policies and procedures of the Hospital, established from time to time, for all patients treated in the Department.

Hospital Duties and Responsibilities

The hospital has responsibilities to the physicians for personnel, equipment, and services. The contract may specifically describe the type and number of personnel, including clerical, nursing staff, and administrative staff. Equipment, maintenance, supplies, fixtures, and utilities are generally the responsibility of the hospital. The contract may designate meeting and office space. The hospital also has the responsibility for insurance of the premises.

EXAMPLE LANGUAGE

The Hospital shall provide and maintain for the physician suitable office space, equipment, supplies, and utilities as shall be necessary for the proper functioning of the Emergency Department.

The Hospital shall, at its own expense, furnish usual and customary mail service, laundry service, gas, water and electricity for light and power and telephone, as may be required for the proper operation and conduct of the Emergency Department.

The Hospital shall provide, at its own expense, staff including technicians, clerks, registrars, nursing personnel and other employees, as are required for the efficient and proper operation of the department. All salaries, benefits and other obligations attributable to such employees shall be paid by the Hospital in accordance with its usual personnel policies.

Group Duties and Responsibilities

The group has certain responsibilities when contracting with individual physicians. These responsibilities include the operations of the group scheduling, quality improvement, hospital contract fulfillment, and financial management of the group (payroll, taxes, bonus/incentive dividend disbursement).

Restrictive Covenants

Restrictive covenants are common in emergency physician contracts. The enforceability of these covenants varies greatly from state to state and even within states. Certain states allow only limited restrictive covenants. There are three basic types of restrictive covenants: noncompete, outside practice, and hiring restrictions.

Noncompete. Many contracts restrict physicians from working within a set distance from the hospital for a set time period in the event the physician leaves the group or hospital if the present contract is terminated. The language in the contract may state that the physician agrees not to provide services to other hospitals within a specific radius for a specific time period. A group or hospital that spends significant sums of money to recruit and relocate the physician to its locale may be particularly supportive of this type of restrictive covenant.

EXAMPLE LANGUAGE

The physician covenants and agrees that he/she will not, for a period of one year after termination of this Agreement, whether by expiration of the Term or by earlier termination in accordance with the Termination Section of this Agreement, directly or indirectly engage in, solicit or perform any work for the Hospital or any affiliate thereof, or engage in the practice of medicine within 7.5 miles of Hospital. This restrictive covenant survives the termination of this Agreement.

Outside Practice. Many contracts restrict a physician from working in an outside practice or hospital. This clause may be intended to prevent physicians from building a competing practice. In university teaching hospitals, this clause prevents physicians from moonlighting in other settings. It may include other sources of outside income, such as consulting or expert testimony. The clause commonly is worded as follows: "The physician may not engage in teaching, consulting or practice of his or her specialty outside the Hospital."

Hiring Restriction. Hiring restrictions prevent the hospital from hiring physicians working with the current group after termination of the contract. From the point of view of the group, this may prevent a hospital from terminating the contract and keeping the physicians.

In particular circumstances, this clause may seem overly restrictive to the physician. The following example will demonstrate a particularly restrictive situation. The hospital, which has the only emergency department within a radius of 50 miles, is unhappy with the contract. The hospital exercises its right to terminate the contract. Several of the emergency physicians and their families who are committed to the area may now have to move to seek employment.

Tortuous Interference. Tortuous interference is a legal concept describing a process in which a person obtains a contract by interfering with the present contractual relationship. For example, a physician under contract with a group may not interfere with the group's contract with the hospital to obtain the contract for himself or herself. This covenant can have the effect of reducing the competition in the marketplace on one hand and stabilizing a work situation on the other.

Policies and Procedures

The contracting physician should be provided with all pertinent bylaws and policies and procedures before the contract is signed. There may be hospital, group, medical staff, and department policies and procedures. An example of this clause is worded as follows: "Physicians hereby agree to follow established procedures to assure the consistency, quality and appropriateness of all Emergency Services." The physician will be held to these standards and should review and understand them.

Dispute Resolution

A mechanism for dispute resolution should be established in the contract. Without a specific dispute resolution process, unresolved issues may involve the court system with its attendant consumption of time and psychologic and monetary resources. Options include arbitration, grievance procedures, and specific dispute resolution policies. The mechanism should specify the process, cost, timing, and method of resolution.

Term

Contracts may be for 1 year or several years. Some contracts contain an "evergreen clause," which allows continual renewal unless one party gives notice or requests renegotiation within a predetermined time frame. Typically this occurs 60 to 120 days before the end of the current contract. An evergreen clause may be advantageous for any party that may not want to go through a contract renegotiation. If terms need to be altered, they are for practical purposes limited to this window.

EXAMPLE LANGUAGE

Hospital/Group hereby contracts with physician. Unless terminated in accordance with Section (Termination Section), this Agreement shall remain in full force and effect for a term of three years commencing on (date). Unless either party shall give notice of intent not to renew this Agreement to the other party ninety (90) days prior to the termination date of this Agreement, this Agreement shall automatically be renewed for (number) year(s) on the terms and conditions set forth herein.

Termination

Many contracts contain a "no cause" termination clause. This clause entitles the hospital or group to terminate the physician without cause within a certain time frame, usually 90 days. One problem with this provision is that the hospital or group can terminate a physician arbitrarily—without due process. However, this clause is commonly reciprocal, so the physician also may terminate the relationship with 90 days' notice.

All contracts should contain language whereby the contract can be terminated "for (reasonable) cause." For the hospital or group, the cause may be impairment, loss of license, professional misconduct, disability, and so on. For the physician, the cause may be breach of contract, nonpayment of monies, or change in the working conditions.

EXAMPLE LANGUAGE

Either party may terminate this Agreement, for any reason or for no reason whatsoever, upon ninety (90) days written notice. Notwithstanding the foregoing, this Agreement shall terminate as follows:

A. If physician becomes disqualified to practice the specialty of emergency medicine in (state), Hospital/Group may terminate this Agreement immediately upon notice to physician;

B. If physician loses staff/clinical privileges at the Hospital, Hospital/Group may terminate this Agreement immediately upon notice to physician;

C. If physician fails to comply in any material respect with the terms of this Agreement and such failure continues for thirty (30) days after written notice thereof to physician, Hospital/Group may terminate this Agreement immediately upon notice to physician;

D. If Hospital/Group fails to comply in any material respect with the terms of this Agreement and such failure continues for thirty (30) days after written notice thereof to Hospital/Group, physician may terminate this Agreement immediately upon notice to Hospital/Group.

Failure of Performance—Breach

In the termination example language (C and D) there is reference to both failure of performance (breach) and cure. Breach in this example is material, or serious and significant. If departmental policy required physicians to dress neatly and conservatively with a white coat and a tie and a physician wore a "loud" tie, this would not be a material breach. On the other hand, a physician who refused to complete medical records may be materially breaching the contract.

Note in the example language that a 30-day cure period, or opportunity to resolve the material breach without immediate termination, is available. With change in behavior, this clause allows a continuation of what may be an otherwise mutually beneficial contractual relationship.

Miscellaneous Issues

Many other boilerplate clauses may be seen in contractual relationships between physicians and hospitals or groups. The following definitions include typical examples of some of these other clauses.

Definitions. Defines the terms that will be used subsequently in a contract.

EXAMPLE LANGUAGE

Agreement. The term "Agreement" shall mean this Emergency Service Agreement and any amendment(s) hereto as may be from time to time adopted as hereinafter provided.

Department. The term "Department" shall mean the emergency department of the Hospital, including, without limitation, the Emergency Treatment Area and the administrative offices for the Department.

Insurance. Defines the types and limits of insurance that must be kept in force by the parties to enter into and continue the relationship.

EXAMPLE LANGUAGE

Physician shall maintain and keep in full force and effect throughout the term of this Agreement professional liability insurance coverage in the minimum amounts of (One Million/Three Million Dollars ($1,000,000.00/$3,000,000.00) or such other amount as may be specified by Staff regulations. Physician shall provide a documentation of such insurance to the Hospital/Group.

Effect of termination: A "clean-sweep" clause commonly exists in the contract between the physician and the hospital or group that defines the relationship once termination has occurred. It is common for physicians to be required to immediately resign their staff membership and clinical privileges. Such resignation is without regard to provisions in the bylaws alluding to due process.

Modification: Describes the method by which the agreement may be modified or amended and generally requires the mutual written agreement of both parties.

Maintenance of records: By federal mandate, certain books, documents, and records must be maintained and accessible for review for a minimum period of time, often 4 years. This type of clause in a contract stipulates each party's responsibility to comply with these mandates.

Obligations to comply with laws: This "catch-all" clause obligates the parties to comply with "all" applicable federal, state, and local statutes.

Notice: Designates to whom and the method by which formal notices and demands permitted in the contract may be delivered.

Assignment: Defines the degree to which the parties may transfer the responsibilities described in the contract to another nondesignated party.

Entire agreement: Defines the agreement to be the understanding of the parties and usually includes a statement that the present agreement supersedes previous representations and agreements.

Severability: A legal concept used in a contract to allow the remainder of the agreement to remain enforceable if any provision within it is declared invalid, illegal, or unenforceable.

Addenda: Any and all additions, appendices, or addenda should be referenced in the body of the contract, understood, and present at the time of signature.

PEARLS AND PITFALLS

The following are a few key concerns that should be considered.

Fraud Alert of May 1992

The May 1992 Fraud Alert of the Healthcare Financing Authority attempts to restrict hospitals from directly or indirectly paying physicians for hospital admissions.

The application of the fraud alert to emergency medicine regards the issue of payment. Any relationship between the hospital or group and the physician that can be interpreted as an incentive to admit patients is subject to this Medicare fraud and abuse statute. Alternatively, a hospital that performs billing and collecting services in the name of the physician caregiver and keeps a portion of that money greatly in excess of the normal reasonable cost of billing may also be subject to scrutiny under the fraud and abuse statute.

BOX 37-3

RIGHT QUESTIONS

License—suspended, revoked, or limited
Medical privileges—suspended, denied, revoked, or reduced
Specific clinical privileges—granted with limitations or denied
Medical liability—claims or cases pending

References

Before the agreements are signed, both sides should obtain references. It is advisable and important to both request a letter in writing and personally phone the references. The personal phone call permits commentary that a person may not be willing to put in a letter of reference. The physician should provide professional and residency recommendations. The hospital or group should provide a list of physicians who currently work or have previously worked at the institution for the interested parties. The National Practitioner Data Bank and state medical society should be queried.

Right Questions

It is appropriate to ask some difficult questions about a physician's or hospital's background early in the negotiation process. Physicians should be asked about their malpractice history and "skeletons in their closets" (Box 37-3). Physicians should ask hospitals and groups about unhappy physicians or clients, pending or settled lawsuits, and reasons that physicians have left.

SUMMARY

Many emergency physicians are intimidated by contracts and do not take the time to understand them. The contract process should be positive and collaborative. Physicians need to establish their goals, understand contract terms and conditions, review the contract, and work closely with legal counsel. This process can ensure a satisfactory contract that remains in force for many years.

BIBLIOGRAPHY

American Academy of Medical Directors: *Physician managers and the law, Tampa, FL,* 1987, American College of Physicians.

American Hospital Association: *Management advisory: contractual relationships with physicians,* Chicago, 1991, AHA.

Freeman CK: *Physician employment contracts,* Denver, 1989, Medical Group Management Association.

Strauss RW: *Contracts: a practical guide for the emergency physician,* Dallas, 1990, American College of Emergency Physicians.

Zismer DK: Hospital-physician negotiations: a focus in productive success, *Minn Physician* 2(9):11-12, 1989.

38 Employee versus Independent Contractor

Stephen J. Dresnick

OUTLINE

Internal Revenue Service
Common-law tests
- Instructions
- Training
- Integration
- Personal services
- Hiring and paying assistants
- Set hours of work
- Full time
- Order or sequence set
- Oral or written reports
- Employer's premises
- Payment by the hour
- Payment of business or travel expenses
- Furnishing of tools and materials
- Significant investment
- Profit/loss potential
- Working for more than one group
- Available to work other places
- Right to discharge
- Right to terminate without liability

Section 530 relief
Contractual issues

Before the development of a contract between a physician and a contract group or hospital, it must first be determined whether the physician will be treated as an employee or as an independent contractor. It is important to realize that this distinction is critical to establish the tax status of the physician. The major difference between the two classifications lies in how taxes are paid, who pays them, and what the benefits are. Regardless of the physician's classification, the amount of money available for compensation and benefits combined is usually the same after deduction for professional liability insurance and group overhead. Additionally, emergency physician responsibilities are often the same regardless of the classification.[1]

Emergency physician compensation is commonly based on an hourly rate. Over the years this has been found to be an easy method of calculating payment because of the disparity of hours that various physicians have worked. In the traditional employee setting, working 40 hours a week, 52 weeks a year, the typical employee would work 2080 hours. Many physicians work either more or less than this amount, and thus traditional calculations become more complex. Additionally, calculating the value of business expenses, such as those for continuing medical education, travel, and automobile expenses, becomes more difficult.

There are major differences between employees and independent contractors as to who is responsible for various items (Table 38-1). Business expense deductions are handled differently between the two designations. Independent contractors are permitted greater individual flexibility with business deductions than are employees. Independent contractors may develop individualized benefit plans that include pension and various types of insurance. An employee may take advantage of the premium reductions offered with group benefit plans, but he or she will be confined to the precise benefit plan to which other members of the group are entitled. The restrictions of a group plan may or may not be advantageous to an individual. On the other hand, the discounted group rates available to an employee may not be available to an independent contractor.

Choosing the most appropriate designation is not simple because various physicians within a group will have different financial needs. For example, an unmarried physician with few expenses may prefer to maximize contributions to a pension plan, whereas a physician who is married with a large mortgage and a large family may need his or her entire paycheck to make ends meet. Such a physician may be unable to put money into a pension plan at the current time.

It is precisely because of the issues of disparity of hours and diverse financial needs that many emergency physicians have elected treatment as independent contractors over the years. Surveys performed indicate that over 60% of emergency physicians are currently classified as independent contractors.[2] The switch from employee to independent contractor may present some problems if physicians have been treated as employees in the past. Any group of physicians is recommended to seek tax planning before making any decisions regarding this complex issue.

INTERNAL REVENUE SERVICE

In recent years, the Internal Revenue Service (IRS) has turned attention to the issue of employee versus independent contractor, particularly within the medical field. It has placed greater scrutiny on independent contractor designation and has even challenged the use of this designation by various contract management groups. The IRS is interested in this issue because its goal is to maximize revenue for the federal government. The IRS believes that treatment as an employee generates more tax revenue. This is generally true because tax is paid on all of an employee's income, whereas tax is paid only on an independent contractor's income after several large deductions are taken. Such deductions include car lease payments, continuing medical education, and health benefits.

Table 38-1 Differences Between Employee and Independent Contractor Status

	Responsibility of employer/employee	Responsibility of independent contractor
Withholding for income tax	Each payroll period	Quarterly
Employment tax	Employer contribution	Self-employment tax
Employer benefit plan	Yes	No
Employer pension plan	Yes	No
Business deductions	In excess of 2% of gross revenue	All
Reporting	W-2 940 (quarterly)	1099 annually

Employees have taxes paid on their behalf throughout the year based on actual income generated, whereas independent contractors make quarterly payments based on reasonable estimates of income; therefore independent contractors retain greater use of their money throughout the year and leave the government with less revenue and less interest. A 1977 IRS report indicated that reclassification of all independent contractors to employees would result in a federal revenue increase of $100 million.[3] Although physicians make up only a small portion of this group, they have higher visibility and therefore have been targeted by the IRS for greater scrutiny.

COMMON-LAW TESTS

Emergency physicians must understand the criteria used by the IRS to determine whether a physician should be treated as an employee or an independent contractor. Although the election of independent contractor status will not present any initial problems, it is only on an IRS audit that the designation could be challenged. An IRS audit with an adverse outcome could result in payment of significant penalties and interest by both the group and the physician. To determine the appropriate designation, the IRS has developed a number of common-law tests that it uses to evaluate individual cases (Box 38-1). The physician, the emergency management group, and their legal advisors should address these issues when developing contract language. One common mistake, for example, is to claim independent contractor status even though the contract is titled "Employment Agreement."

A casual review of the common-law tests would suggest that emergency physicians rarely comply with all of them. Fortunately, the IRS does not expect 100% compliance; rather, it looks for what it deems "substantial" compliance. There is no formula that is used when applying these common-law tests to arrive at a final decision. Only an IRS audit, which considers all of these factors, will determine the outcome.

The 20 common-law tests used by the IRS cover a broad spectrum of working relationships, and obviously some are not applicable to the practice of emergency medicine. Criteria carry different weights; however, the weighing of each one is somewhat arbitrary from case to case. Although there are numerous IRS rulings regarding designation, the courts have determined that IRS rulings do not set precedence, as do legal cases; therefore an IRS investigator is in no way obligated to rely on determinations made in other cases. Following are the common-law tests and the explanations as to how they might apply to emergency medicine in several contract language is included.

Instructions

Does the party receiving the benefit of the service, that is, the hospital or group, have the right to control the details, manner, and method of the work? The contract should state: "The physician will be responsible for the method and manner in which care is rendered."

Training

If training—rather than orientation—is provided, it generally indicates that the physician is an employee. An independent contractor should already possess the skills necessary to render appropriate care. The contract should state: "The physician possesses the skills and training necessary to perform the services described herein."

Integration

Integration of a particular worker's services into a business operation suggests that the worker is an integral part of the business and is therefore an employee. When drafting the contract, avoid stating that the group provides "physician staffing" of the emergency department. Instead, state that the group provides "physician recruiting and scheduling services."

Personal Services

A contract requiring the contracted individual to provide the work himself or herself suggests that the worker is an employee. The contract should avoid the use of the phrase "personal services agreement." However, this section usually is not given significant weight because many independent contractors provide services on an individual basis.

Hiring and Paying Assistants

A worker's practice of hiring assistants and paying them out of personal funds usually is interpreted to indicate that the worker is an independent contractor. Although it is not common practice for emergency physicians to hire and pay their own assistants, the contract should state: "The physician shall have the right to hire any assistants necessary to carry out the duties of this contract as long as the cost is borne by the physician and as long as the presence of such an assistant is in compliance with the rules and regulations of the hospital." This prevents the use of unauthorized assistants.

Set Hours of Work

Set hours of work usually indicate an employer-employee relationship. The contract should contain language stipulating that there are no set hours of work. The contract may specify

BOX 38-1

INTERNAL REVENUE SERVICE COMMON-LAW TESTS

- Instructions
- Integration
- Hiring, paying assistants
- Set hours of work
- Order or sequence set
- Employer's premises
- Business/travel expenses
- Significant investment
- Other work
- Right to discharge
- Training
- Personal services
- Continuing relationship
- Full-time
- Oral or written reports
- Payment by hour
- Tools furnished
- Profit or loss potential
- Available to work other places
- Right to terminate without liability

that, for the convenience of scheduling, the physician will submit, in advance, a list of unavailable work days.

Full-Time

A full-time worker generally is considered to be an employee rather than an independent contractor. Avoid the use of this term anywhere in the contract. However, the contract may state the minimum or maximum number of hours that the physician will work.

Order or Sequence Set

A worker usually is considered to be an employee when the group is allowed to determine the order or sequence in which the work is performed. This does not apply to emergency physicians because the individual physician determines the order in which patients are seen. The same contract language suggested in the instructions section is applicable here: "The physician will be responsible for the method and manner in which care is rendered."

Oral or Written Reports

If the group requires the worker to provide reports, the worker may be considered an employee. Many groups do, in fact, require reports from their medical directors. These responsibilities should be delineated in a separate document and not listed in the contract. Medical director stipends should be made separately from clinical stipends and should be clearly designated on payment vouchers.

Employer's Premises

Performing work at the employer's premises usually indicates employee status. Emergency physicians contracting directly with a hospital—the owner of the premises—are more likely to be considered employees. The contract, then, should state that the group has contracted to "recruit and schedule" physicians at the hospital and that the physician is "desirous to provide services" at that hospital.

Payment by the Hour

Workers paid by the hour usually are employees. Workers paid a percentage of collections, with potential for both profit and loss, usually are independent contractors. Most physicians are compensated on an hourly rate; this should be noted in the contract as a "minimum guarantee." Then, if the physician receives compensation higher than the guaranteed amount, this would suggest independent contractor status.

Payment of Business or Travel Expenses

The IRS has, in the past, paid particular attention to this common-law test. Payment of travel and continuing medical education expenses and malpractice premiums by the worker suggests that the worker is an independent contractor. The contract should state that "the physician is responsible for any business and travel expenses he or she incurs." Ideally, the physician should pay the group monthly or quarterly for the cost of malpractice insurance. An intermediate alternative is possible: the group makes a deduction of a certain amount per hour for malpractice insurance. Many groups pay the expenses for their medical directors, but this should not be referenced in the physician-group contract.

Furnishing of Tools and Materials

The provision of one's own tools and equipment usually is an indication of independent contractor status. The contract should clearly state that "other than the equipment that will be provided by the hospital, the physician will be responsible for providing personal equipment."

Significant Investment

A significant investment in the business or facility suggests independent contractor status. Emergency physicians usually do not invest in the particular facility in which they practice; however, the contract may reference the "significant investment" the physician has made in securing training and equipment. If an office is to be provided to the physician, this should not be mentioned in the contract because the physician is not "investing" in the acquisition of the office or the ongoing maintenance of such an office.

Profit/Loss Potential

This is an important factor in distinguishing between an employee and an independent contractor. The IRS tends to agree with the physician's designation as an independent contractor if the physician has the potential to realize a profit or a loss from the work performed. When possible, the physician's contract should state that the compensation will be based on a percentage of the receipts rather than strictly on an hourly rate.

Working for More Than One Group

Physicians who work for more than one group usually are independent contractors. Those who work for a single group run the risk of being classified as employees. This is a difficult test to satisfy. Most groups prefer that physicians work only for them. Depending on the group's philosophy, compliance with this criterion may require the contract to state that the physician is free to perform services at other places when not scheduled to work at the designated hospital. A group with multiple practice sites may establish each as a separate legal entity and sign separate contracts and paychecks with the physician for each.

Available to Work Other Places

This common-law test is similar to the preceding one. Again, the contract may contain specific wording that allows the physician to make independent decisions regarding places of work.

Right to Discharge

The group's right to fire a physician implies an employer-employee relationship. Avoid contractual language stating that the group or hospital can terminate the physician. Instead, the contract may include a provision that gives the hospital or the group the right to request that the physician not be scheduled.

Right to Terminate without Liability

A worker who can terminate a contract without liability is, in some circumstances, considered an employee. This is not a major criterion as it pertains to emergency physicians.

SECTION 530 RELIEF

In the event that an IRS audit determines that a physician is an employee rather than independent contractor, the decision can be appealed by seeking "relief" under Section 530 of the Internal Revenue Code. Section 530 relief, if granted, permits independent contractor designation to stand even though there may not be substantial compliance with the common-law tests. To gain relief under Section 530, the taxpayer must have had a reasonable basis for not treating individuals as employees. A reasonable basis is said to exist if either a letter ruling or previous audit defines the workers as independent contractors or a long-standing practice within a particular industry recognizes workers as independent contractors.

To obtain Section 530 relief, the taxpayer must also have treated all individuals in similar positions in the same manner and must have treated them since 1978 or since inception. Additionally, all tax returns since that time must have been filed as if the individual workers were, in fact, independent contractors (Box 38-2). There have been several emergency physician–related cases in which Section 530 relief has been granted. Assuming that the other conditions to obtain Section 530 relief are met, the major argument has been that a significant segment of the industry treats emergency physicians as independent contractors. Although this has been upheld in numerous cases, there have also been cases in which Section 530 relief has been denied. It is critically important that all of the issues discussed in this chapter be considered when drafting a contract.

BOX 38-2

CONDITIONS OF OBTAINING SECTION 530 RELIEF

Taxpayer must have had "reasonable basis" for not treating individuals as employees.

- Judicial precedent, published ruling, or letter
- Past audit
- Other individuals in similar positions also not employees
- Long-standing, recognized practice of a significant segment of the particular industry
- Treatment the same since 1978
- All tax returns filed as if individual not an employee

CONTRACTUAL ISSUES

When the IRS challenges an emergency physician's independent contractor designation, it will closely examine the physician's contract, that is, the physician's written agreement to provide services to a group, hospital, or other entity. To this end physicians who claim independent contractor status should address these major issues of concern within their contracts. Of particular importance is a delineation of the nature of the relationship, as well as addressing the issue of payment of taxes. The contract should clearly state that the physician is an independent contractor and will be treated as such under the Internal Revenue Code. Any reference to or use of the word "employee" should be avoided. The contract should additionally state that the physician is personally responsible for any and all payroll taxes, including state and federal unemployment tax. The IRS's major concerns are that all applicable taxes are paid and that someone is responsible for paying unpaid taxes.

The decision to designate an emergency physician as an independent contractor rather than an employee is frequently a complex one, and any group that chooses the independent contractor status must be aware of the potential for an adverse ruling by the IRS.[4] Internal Revenue Service audits are more likely to be favorable if the common-law tests are substantially addressed within the physician-group/hospital contract. Although the IRS will, if requested, issue a ruling on the request of the group before an audit, this is not a recommended way to proceed.

Emergency physicians should realize that the goal of the IRS is to increase tax revenue and that, as well-paid professionals, emergency physicians and physicians in general will continue to be targeted for close scrutiny. Such decisions require both a thorough working knowledge of the issues and advice from the appropriate legal, financial, and tax advisors.

REFERENCES

1. Dresnick SJ, Crook PL: Employee versus independent contractor status. In Strauss RW Jr, editor: *Contracts: a practical guide for the emergency physician,* Dallas, 1990, American College of Emergency Physicians.
2. Henry GL: *Emergency medicine risk management: a comprehensive review,* Dallas, 1991, American College of Emergency Physicians.
3. Clousson JP: Key contract clauses. In Strauss RW Jr, editor: *Contracts: a practical guide for the emergency physician,* Dallas, 1990, American College of Emergency Physicians.
4. Rothenberg MA: *Emergency medicine malpractice,* New York, 1994, Wiley & Sons.

39 Equity, Parity, and Group Structure

Thom A. Mayer, Joel A. Stettner, Charles L. Zeller, Jr., and Samuel J. Kiehl

OUTLINE

Emergency medicine is by nature a group practice of affiliated physicians, because staffing the department on a 24 hour per day, 365 day per year basis requires multiple physicians, even in a single-coverage environment. For patient management reasons alone, this requires a minimum of three to four full-time emergency physicians, plus those needed for part-time or double coverage. The evolution of emergency medicine into a mature specialty has created numerous models of the group practice of emergency medicine, including individual physicians employed by the hospital, small single-hospital democratic physician groups, sole proprietorships, regional or local groups, and large, multihospital national groups. By nature a group practice environment exists in emergency medicine, and there are protean models of group structure; nonetheless there has been little analysis of the specific types and more important the factors underlying the choice of a specific structure. The type of emergency department group at an individual hospital varies widely, often because of factors such as the history of the emergency department at that institution, geographic factors, preferences of the chief executive officer, board, or medical staff, and availability of emergency physician resources within a given geographic area. Although it is clear that emergency medicine requires some sort of group structure (even if the specific type is not a consciously chosen one), the taxonomy of emergency medicine groups have been poorly defined and inadequately articulated.[1]

Woven into this group structure concept is the notion of emergency medicine as not only an art and a science, but also as a business (Figure 39-1).[2] Without question, the primary goal of emergency medicine and the physicians who practice it should always be quality patient care. Nonetheless the definition of quality patient care itself has become a moving target. In the past, it was presumed that making the right diagnosis and providing the right treatment constituted "quality," at least in the minds of the providers of emergency department care. However, emerging concepts in the healthcare environment[3,4] have made it clear that the definition of quality involves a careful understanding of the diverse customers involved in the delivery of healthcare. These customers include the family, payers, emergency medical services (EMS) providers, medical staff members, administration, and the hospital board, as well as the internal customers of the process—the emergency physicians, emergency nurses, technicians, and other ancillary staff. As the definition of quality patient care continues to undergo revision, it becomes clear that factors such as interaction with the family, communication with the private physician or managed care plan, turnaround times, and cost efficiency are all elements of the sometimes frustrating nature of defining quality patient care in the 1990s and beyond. When the factors of maximizing potential revenues and providing care on a cost-efficient basis are added, "quality patient care" begins to look like a confusing, confounding witches' brew rather than a clearly defined entity.

As emergency medicine has continued to develop both as a clinical specialty and as an important aspect of the overall healthcare environment, it has become increasingly clear that the application of sound business principles to clinical practice in emergency medicine is a *requirement* for the successful practice of emergency medicine, not an attractive option provided by some providers but not others. In the best tradition of the old adage, "Be careful what you wish for—you might get it," emergency medicine has effectively educated the healthcare community, and to a large extent the public, that the emergency department is the front door, not the back door of the hospital. As understanding of the importance of emergency medicine has grown, so too have the demands on emergency physician groups, seemingly at an exponential rate.

In addition to realizing that emergency medicine is by nature a group practice to which sound business principles must be applied, it is also critical to recognize existing marketplace issues affecting healthcare. The landscape of healthcare is changing at an extraordinary rate, independent of legislative reforms intended to restructure the marketplace (Figure 39-2). Even basic definitions of the building blocks of healthcare provision are undergoing rapid change. For example, in the recent past, the hospital was the primary unit of measure in healthcare. The institution was governed by a board, administration, and medical staff structure that focused its time, effort, and energy almost exclusively on "inpatient days" as the primary product produced. It operated on a simple, economically attractive "cost plus" basis with well-defined payers, including indemnity insurance and government payors, and provided a certain percentage of indigent care. Cataclysmic changes in the healthcare environment have resulted in fundamental structure alterations in the way healthcare is

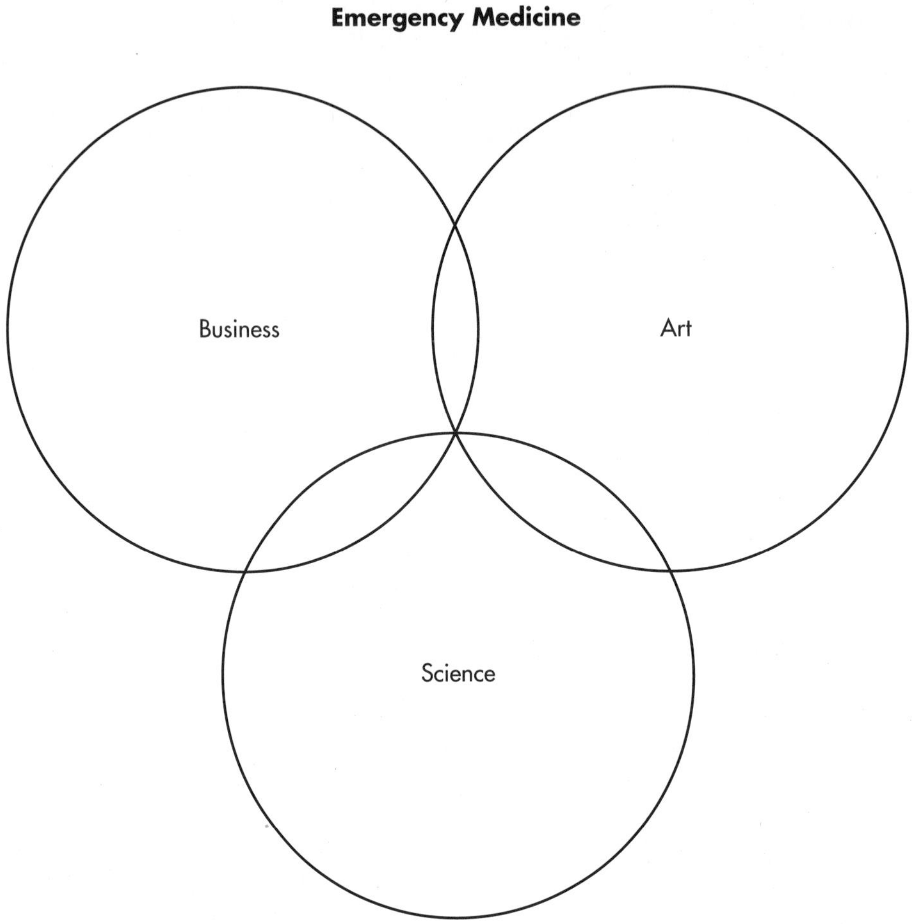

FIGURE 39-1 The evolving notion of emergency medicine involves the intersection of the practice as an art, a science, and a business. Elements of all three aspects must be addressed for a practice to be successful.

planned, organized, financed, and delivered in the United States. This was only partially driven by potential legislative changes, with the major drive coming from the marketplace and the participants themselves.

As Figure 39-2 illustrates, the taxonomy, units of measure, and driving forces in healthcare are substantially different than they were several years ago. The key issues for the next 10 to 20 years will include consolidation, affiliation agreements, buying power and leverage, and aggressive (sometimes desperate) growth in numbers of covered lives and services that were not traditionally under the purview of hospitals. Those services include providing comprehensive, efficient, and coordinated healthcare services, documentably superior outcomes, customer-driven and customer-defined quality, superior cost efficiency, and a "single-signature" marketplace interface, all within a defined geographic area of adequate size to help support the infrastructure for such services. Management or acquisition of physician office practices, contract negotiations, integrated billing services, employee and benefit management, and other physician support services are but a few of the new product lines that hospitals and other healthcare service providers find themselves offering at a frightening pace. Concepts of risk sharing and capitation have also radically changed the mental models that have been traditional in planning and implementing healthcare services.

For the emergency department, the change in healthcare structure has created an even more important need for a sound understanding of business principles, as well as for a new set of expectations. These expectations include an expanded definition of quality, the need for physician stability in a changing market, cost-effectiveness, managed care experience, responsiveness in changing emergency department group operations to meet required changes in the healthcare structure, and the ability to function effectively in a team model, as opposed to an independent environment.

These three bedrock issues—the essential nature of emergency medicine as a group practice, the necessity of recognizing the business aspects of emergency medicine, and the rapid changes in the healthcare marketplace's structure and function—all speak to the need for a clearer understanding of how emergency department practices are structured and how these structures can best be positioned to adapt to a changing environment. Because of this, the goals of this chapter are as follows:

- Define the terms group structure, equity, vesting, parity, and stock.
- Describe group structure alternatives.

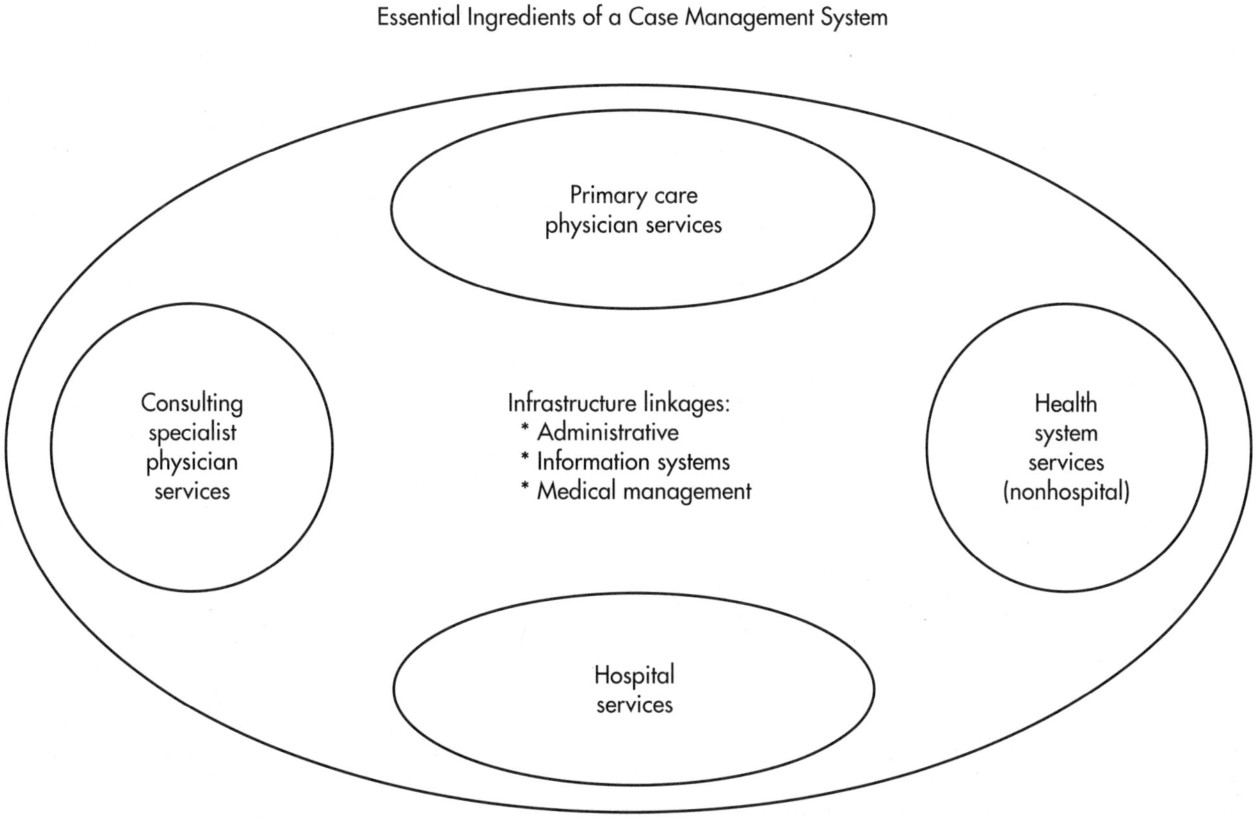

FIGURE 39-2 Independent of legislative healthcare reform, the landscape of physician services is changing to the development of care management systems, designed to provide comprehensive coverage to large groups of "covered lives." As this landscape changes, emergency medicine must adapt and anticipate future models of care delivery.
(Adapted from William Carter, M.D.)

- Address factors to be assessed in determining appropriate group structures.
- Define advantages and disadvantages of each alternative.

DEFINITIONS

Group structure refers to the functional and structural elements of emergency medicine at a given institution, including diverse professional, personal, financial, and fiduciary elements. It concerns the organization and interrelationship among the emergency physicians themselves, as well as their contractual relationship with the institution that they serve. Specific definitions for types of group structure are included in the following section, including hospital employees or individual independent contractors, "pure" democratic groups, democratic groups with defined equity structures, sole proprietorships, partnerships, and multihospital groups.

The word *equity* is derived from the Middle English term meaning fair or reasonable. The current definition is a fascinating one: "1. The quality, state, or ideal of being just. 2. The money value of a property beyond any liability associated with it."[5] The etymology of words is instructive in that the term *equity* is often associated simply with "ownership" in the current context of emergency medicine practice. To say that one wants "equity" usually means that one wants ownership or a "piece of the action." Too often, it is assumed that this simply means a share of the profits, whereas the definition clarifies that any money value associated with ownership can only be taken into consideration with the *liability* contingent on it. More important, the derivation of the term *equity* with regard to fairness, justness, and equality raises important issues with regard to emergency medicine group structure. Emergency physicians by nature want to be in an environment that is considered to be fair, reasonable, and just. In clinical practice this is manifested by decisions being made based on consideration of what is best for the patient in the individual circumstance as the patient is treated clinically in the emergency department, not on seniority, training, or committee chairmanship. A classic example of this is the "debate" early on in the evolution of thrombolytic therapy as to whether the decision to use lytic drugs should be in the hands of the emergency physician or the cardiologist. In a short period of time it became clear from a quality of care and fairness standpoint that the decision to institute therapy should be made at the earliest possible time, and therefore resided with the emergency physician, not the cardiologist. This was not a turf, training, or ego issue; rather, it was an issue of being just and fair to the patient from a clinical standpoint.

In applying this doctrine of fairness to the concept of equity in emergency medicine group structure, it is important to recognize that emergency physicians desire a situation in which their voice can be heard in a fair and reasonable fashion, particularly in the midst of the massive changes in healthcare described earlier in this chapter. Thus as emergency physician groups begin to address the issue of equity, as it pertains to "the money value of a property beyond any liability associated with it," it is also important to ensure that consideration is given to the issues of fairness and justice as well. For example, it is important to weigh the time, energy, effort, and dollars that were initially spent in building the emergency medicine practice at the institution. For physicians who have spent many years in helping develop the practice, the concept of providing equity for junior partners requires careful thought with regard to how best account for the "sweat equity" expended in developing the contract. Conversely, completely closing the equity pathway for junior physicians simply because they were not present at the initiation of the contract also appears unjust.

Vesting is Latin in origin, from the word meaning "to clothe or place in vestments." In current use, vesting usually refers to a time, performance, commitment, or financial schedule by which new members are assimilated into the equity structure of an existing group. Such vesting schedules not only apply to emergency physicians, but also to other physicians, accountants, lawyers, architects, and other professionals. However, the origin of the term is again instructive and fascinating in that the inclusion of new members into a group certainly does involve clothing them or placing them in vestments with regard to their assuming a higher position in the group, as well as the substantial responsibilities that pertain thereto. *Parity* is also Latin in origin and has a simple meaning—"equality." Although the terms *equity* and *parity* are often used in conjunction, in fact the very nature of the concept of a vesting schedule or growth to senior physician status speaks against the concept of true parity, at least at the outset of the relationship. In essence, the term *parity* simply refers to a situation in which individuals at certain levels of a group are treated in an equal fashion. However, application and interpretation of the term is certainly subject to substantial variation. For example, the concept of parity may be applied to senior partners to say that each of them should be paid in exactly the same fashion and at exactly the same level, because of the driving force of equality. However, many groups have used either direct fee-for-service or fee-for-service bonus arrangements to recognize variable productivity among different physicians at the same level of the group structure. Although this is a concept that cuts across the principle of strict equality, some may well interpret that it addresses the issue of fairness, justness, or parity in a more reasonable fashion.

The roots of the term *stock* are Middle English, the origin of which refers to a tree trunk. The more commonly accepted definition of this term relates to the actual shares of a given corporation that are offered according to specified purchase or transfer plans in attaining equity status with the group. Yet the unavoidable analogy of the tree trunk as the foundation on which the tree exists has important connotations as it relates to our current understanding of stock in emergency department groups.

Goals

The goals of emergency physician groups vary somewhat and are as difficult to classify in a generic fashion as it is to create the ideal emergency physician group structure. Nonetheless the following points would generally be considered as appropriate goals for an emergency physician group, regardless of the specific structure:

- Provide quality patient care.
- Provide quality service to diverse groups, including the patient's family, medical staff, administration, and emergency medical services.
- Provide personal and professional growth opportunities for individuals in the group.
- Provide a practice opportunity that is intellectually stimulating.
- Provide the ability for the group to be responsive to rapid changes in the healthcare environment.
- Provide a practice that is economically viable and fiscally sustainable.
- Provide a fair and equitable practice opportunity.
- Provide an environment in which the opinion of the emergency physician can be voiced in a meaningful fashion.

The importance of each of these goals will vary among individual emergency physicians and across different emergency department groups, regardless of their structure. However, *quality patient care* is an absolute, bright-line distinction that should form an essential benchmark for any emergency department group. For example, does the group hire only board-certified emergency physicians, or is it more interested in simply "filling shifts" or "warm bodies"? How does the group determine its patient care objectives, and how are protocols for such care developed and disseminated? Whether in a single- or double-coverage environment, it is important to emergency physicians to ensure that the care that they are providing can be handed off during shift changes to colleagues of similar background, training, and experience. The *concept of quality of service* also extends to other internal and external customers of the emergency department environment. Does the group and its structure address the needs of these diverse interests? Does the definition of quality for the group include a high degree of professionalism with family members, nurses, medical staff, and EMS?

Providing *personal and professional growth opportunities* for the emergency physicians in the group is an area of increasing importance to emergency physicians. Does the group have a recognized structure for ensuring that the individual can develop his or her personal and professional career goals and objectives? Or is the physician going to be considered a full-time equivalent (FTE), whose very function is to accede to the dictates of the senior management of the group? Are there defined administrative paths that the physician can pursue as his or her knowledge and experience expand? Does the group have a philosophy of growth into other contracts, which might allow the individual an opportunity as a medical director or chair? Is the personal growth of the individuals comprising the group and issue of central importance to the group's leadership?

An *intellectually stimulating practice environment* is important to most emergency physicians. Particularly for those just out of residency, practicing in an environment where multiple ill or injured patients are seen can be helpful in preparing for and passing the board examination in emergency medicine. To what extent does the group and the structure help provide the emergency physician the opportunity to update the skills, abilities, and expertise in recent developments in emergency medicine? It is also important for the group to have the ability to be *responsive to the rapid changes* occurring in the healthcare environment. For example, the group's structure must be such that it is able to rapidly and efficiently adapt to changes in the managed care environment, including negotiating favorable contracts that allow the hospital to participate in obtaining its objectives of managing specified levels of covered lives in a certain geographic area. Similarly, as the ebb and flow of practice diversification carry ideas such as fast track services and chest pain emergency departments through this specialty, the group must have the ability to determine which, if any, of these practice diversification opportunities to pursue.

One of the most often ignored aspects of emergency department group structure is the necessity of *providing a practice that is economically viable and fiscally sustainable*. For example, an emergency physician may be drawn to a purely democratic group; however, if it turns out that that group does not have the knowledge, expertise, or inclination to apply sound business principles to its practice, it may be doomed to failure. Regardless of the specific structure, each emergency physician group must ensure that the business knowledge and expertise required for successful practice are attained and maintained throughout the life of the group. In many cases this expertise will reside with individual group members, but in others it must be sought either through consultants, advisors, or affiliation agreements.

The last two goals for an emergency physician group—*fairness* and *ensuring that the voice of each group member is heard*—have become the source of substantial controversy in emergency medicine. One of the most important questions that an emergency physician asks is, "Does my opinion matter?" Will the emergency physician's voice be listened to with regard to departmental operational decisions, group structure changes, long-term development, and financial issues? And yet even this seemingly straightforward issue of fairness can be a difficult and confusing one. What constitutes fairness for one person may seem grossly unfair to another. For example, a recent graduate from an emergency medicine training program may feel that he or she should have the same voice in departmental structure and financial disbursements as the senior partners in the group. Conversely, those senior partners may feel that the 10 years that they have spent building the practice and strengthening its integration into the hospital and the community speak toward a more long-term vesting schedule, at least with regard to financial disbursements. Those same partners may feel comfortable ensuring that the "new" group member should have an equal voice with regard to departmental operations, and yet insist on a more graded integration of that new member into the business and financial structure of the group.

Each of these issues must be looked at carefully as one accesses the various group structure alternatives. For ease of consideration, the following areas help encompass the aforementioned goals: ownership, control, responsibility, profits, and liability/investment.

As emergency physicians approach practice opportunities, it is incumbent on them to determine which structure best meets the professional, personal, philosophical, and financial needs of the individual. In many cases, groups may have certain features of more than one of the following structures.

GROUP STRUCTURE ALTERNATIVES

In the past there have been no clear-cut classifications of emergency department groups. By nature, any such classification is of necessity somewhat arbitrary. The intention of the following classification is to list not only structural categories, but *functional* categories that allow the creation of a taxonomy of emergency physician groups. What we call such groups is far less important than how they *operate*. Although we will attempt to classify such groups, framing the advantages and disadvantages of each, it is far more important to determine how the organization works and operates on a daily basis because that determines its success.

Ideally, this taxonomy should allow emergency physicians to classify existing groups, as well as look creatively at the formation of new emergency department groups when those opportunities present themselves. In many cases, elements to be shared between structures and precise classification of either existing or newly created groups may be difficult. The primary goal in such a classification is simply to help clarify alternative structures and the way these structures function on a day-to-day basis. Again, how the organization works for the emergency physicians and for those the emergency physician group serves is far more important than the precise form or structure of the group. Without exception, functionality, not strict taxonomy, determines the success or failure of the emergency physician group.

Hospital Employees or Independent Contractors

Emergency physicians may be contracted directly with the hospital in either employment relationships or as independent contractors. In employee relationships, the hospital has a detailed employment contract, usually with terms and benefits clearly defined. The hospital withholds taxes, specifies hours of service, and is responsible for establishing the parameters of practice for the physician. This differs from an independent contractor relationship, in which benefits are not provided to the physician, there is less control over the hours of work and precise parameters of practice, and yet the physician is still contracted directly to the hospital.[6] In such relationships, the multiple emergency physicians required to staff the department are directly contracted by the hospital, which handles recruitment and recontracting with the individual physicians. In most cases, one of the individual emergency physicians is also contracted, either as an employee or independent contractor, to perform certain duties and tasks as medical director or chair. In some cases, the hospital may have some emergency physicians under employment contracts and others as independent contractors (usually for reasons relating to the physician's preexisting benefit package before affiliation with the hospital). However, these "mixed" employee–independent contractor relationships are becoming far less common, at least partially because of recent Internal Revenue Service (IRS) directives on employee and independent contractor issues.

In some respects such a structure is simple in that each of the physicians is contracted directly with the hospital and the terms of employment or independent contractor agreement are clearly spelled out. However, it also represents an extremely complex relationship in other respects, particularly because the individual emergency physicians have no clearly specified relationship to each other and the terms of the contracts with the hospital can vary widely from physician to physician.

Advantages. Nonetheless there are some advantages to such relationships. First, such a relationship results in less competition between emergency physicians, with each of them presumably having the same basic relationship with the hospital as the others, except perhaps the medical director or chair. Second, it creates a single taxable entity per physician, which can be of theoretic and practical significance to the hospital, the physician, and the IRS. Third, there is no "middleman" involved in the transaction or relationship, so that there is a more or less direct passage of revenue to the physician. (However, as will be detailed under the section on disadvantages, this does not necessarily mean that revenue for the emergency physician is maximized, because revenues depend solely on the hospital's ability to bill and collect for emergency physician services.)

For many emergency physicians, such direct employee or independent contractor relationships offer the advantage of "independence," in that the emergency physician does not "work for" another physician or contract entity, but directly for the hospital itself. For many emergency physicians, this offers an aspect of power and control because they are responsible only for their day-to-day practice of emergency medicine. Further, while the physician may feel independent from other physicians, such direct relationships with the hospital place the physician at the mercy of whoever the contracting officer or administrator is for emergency services. In this sense, it is difficult to construe such a relationship as a truly independent one. An additional potential advantage is that the physician is able to make rapid decisions with regard to contracting with the hospital. For example, if the hospital offers a change in the compensation rate, required hours of work, or benefit package, physicians need only consult themselves, their business advisors, and their family to determine whether to continue in that relationship.

Disadvantages. The disadvantage of direct employee or independent contractor relationships are many and seem to be increasing in number. First, hospitals have increasingly found these relationships to be labor intensive, involving multiple and frequent negotiations with individual physicians. Second, in attempting to meet the needs of a diverse group of physicians, the hospital often finds itself with multiple employee or independent contractor relationships, which are difficult to justify from the standpoint of the corporate structure of the institution and its IRS responsibilities. Indeed, the trend in recent surveys conducted by hospital administration publications indicates a strong trend toward outsourcing, contracting with specific defined entities to provide hospital-based physician services.

Third, there is usually little group cohesiveness among the emergency physicians under such a structure. Instead, the emergency physicians are perceived to operate in an independent fashion, with their primary reporting relationship being an individual one to the hospital and its administration. This can result in a less collegial interaction among the emergency physicians, due in part to this lack of group cohesiveness.

Fourth, a substantial disadvantage to direct contracts with the hospital is that the emergency physician "group" is by nature without substantial leverage and power in contract negotiations with the hospital when it comes to adding additional resources, increasing hours of physician coverage, responding to market pressures, and so on. Whether intentionally or not, it puts the hospital administration in a strong position with regard to a "divide and conquer" strategy with its hospital-based physicians. Under such circumstances, it is extraordinarily easy for the hospital administration to replace emergency physicians, particularly on very short notice. This is true both of the individual physicians and of the overall "group" itself.

In looking at issues of practice diversification or additional contracts, a structure as employees or independent contractors puts the emergency physicians at a position of having limited capital and access to resources to diversify their practice. Thus, if the emergency physician group wishes to diversify its practice, either internally (fast track services, chest pain emergency departments, trauma center verification, etc.) or externally (off-site freestanding clinics, additional emergency department contracts, etc.), it is strictly limited by the hospital's dictates and its lack of access to capital and resources.

One of the most important potential disadvantages to such a relationship is that hospitals are notoriously untrained and unskilled at billing and collecting for emergency physician professional services. In this sense, as hospitals find themselves under increasing financial pressure, it is likely that the emergency department physician group will be seen as a "loss leader" instead of a revenue center for the hospital. Even in circumstances under which the emergency physicians assign and code for charges, the collection procedure from the hospital is often inadequate to build a substantial revenue base for the emergency physician group practice.

Variations of the emergency physician as employee or independent contractor with the hospital are often seen in academic medical centers. In most centers, emergency medicine faculty are employed by the institution and have a reporting relationship through a designated chair of the department. Many such departments have a combined structure that involves aspects of being hospital employees, as well as indirect relationships as are represented in faculty practice plans. (The academic emergency department structure is addressed in Chapter 3.)

Assessment. In assessing the hospital employer independent contractor group structure as an alternative, there is no *ownership* per se in that the structure does not have a discrete contract or accounts receivable that are owned by a specific individual or group of individuals. Instead, ownership, to the extent that it exists, resides with the hospital itself. The issue of *control* is an interesting one, because majority of the control in such a relationship actually resides with the hospital or the administrator. There is usually a director or chair identified as having responsibility for overall operations, but in reality the contractual structures vary so widely that it is often difficult to tell where control lies in such a situation. On the one extreme are academic medical centers, where the chair of the department has a discrete aspect of control, even though the physicians are contracted more or less directly with the institution itself. At the other extreme are medical directors or chairs whose contracts do not give them substantial control over the individuals for whom they are responsible. There may or may not be a team or democratic approach in employee and independent contractor structures because this depends much more on the personalities involved than on the actual structure itself. Similarly, the *responsibility* for the provision of services varies widely under such circumstances. On the one hand physicians may have a responsibility solely to themselves and their patients, and on the other the contractual structure may be such that there are much broader responsibilities implied in the relationship.

Profits are a far less distinct issue in most such circumstances, particularly because the very nature of the contractual structure often results in a cash shortfall for the hospital. In those circumstances in which there are faculty practice plans or percentage of gross arrangements, profits may be distributed based solely on the numbers of patients seen and the revenue generated. However, percentage of gross arrangements is becoming far less common as hospitals increasingly realize that such contracts almost inevitably force them to operate at a loss with respect to emergency physician billings and collections.

With regard to *liability and investment,* such issues are usually addressed in the contractual relationships themselves. Because there is a single taxable entity in most cases, liability is usually limited to the individual physician's professional liability, which is often covered under the hospital's master malpractice insurance policy. However, in circumstances under which physicians operate as independent contractors, there is at least the theoretic business liability for the individual physician or the corporation that contracts as an independent contractor with the hospital. This business liability can also be addressed by insurance policies but is less commonly covered under the hospital's master policy. The issue of investment of time, energy, and effort into the development of the practice is rarely addressed under such relationships. Instead, as physicians come and go during the course of their careers, another physician simply replaces them as an employee or independent contractor with the hospital.

In summary, although there are advantages to physicians working as employees or independent contractors with the hospital, particularly in academic medicine, and there are institutions in which this model has operated successfully, the future for such contractual relationships appears limited. As reimbursement becomes an increasing issue, it is likely that it will be difficult if not impossible for individual hospitals to have the expertise that is necessary to bill and collect for the emergency department physician component in a fashion that maximizes revenue for the services provided.

Democratic Emergency Physician Groups

The essential feature of democratic physician groups ("pure" democratic groups and groups with defined equity) is that all members (after a certain trial or probation period) share in the decision-making efforts of the group. This usually applies not only to decisions on the type, number, and specific emergency physicians to be hired, but also extends to financial decisions, group expansion, contractual relationships with the hospital, and policies and procedures. Many of such groups rotate or elect the chair or medical director of the department on an ongoing basis. However, this feature is not essential to be considered a democratic group. The most common description of such democratic groups is summarized by the concept of "equal voice, equal pay, and equal responsibility." Most democratic groups contract as a discrete contractual entity with the hospital to provide emergency physician staffing and management services, rather than acting as hospital employees or independent contractors. However, there may be substantial similarities between this practice model and the one listed previously, at least in certain circumstances.

Advantages. The advantages of small democratic groups certainly begin with the capacity for shared decision making and investment and with motivation on the part of the emergency physicians to make the practice successful. Because each individual within the group has the capacity to guide its direction (within the group's overall structure), there is strong reason to believe that there is incentive for the individual to perform at the highest possible level to ensure the success of all. Similarly, in most circumstances ownership of the group is also shared in a democratic or quasi-democratic fashion.

A theoretic advantage of the democratic group is that there should be higher compensation for the individual physicians because of the elimination to the "middleman" concept. However, as indicated in the previous section, this presupposes that there is the business and financial expertise available within the group to maximize potential revenues. In circumstances in which such expertise is available (either internally or externally), elimination of middlemen or corporate entities can result in higher compensation. However, such expertise is often not available, and this may actually result in lower revenues for the group members, even if revenues are equally distributed. Another advantage of such a democratic structure is that it is usually easier to ensure that there is a defined team approach to decision making and to adapting to the environment because each group member is heavily invested in the need for overall success of the group. Recruitment may be easier for such groups because at least some data suggest that board-certified or residency-trained emergency physicians may prefer such a practice option when it is available within the geographic area that they desire. In addition, it is also possible that there is better retention of emergency physicians with such a group structure, which may be of advantage to the group, the medical staff, and hospital administration.

Disadvantages. The disadvantages of democratic groups begin with the labor intensity of such a group structure. Rather than having a single person or entity who is responsible for making "bottom-line" decisions, the hospital administration must rely on what can be a long and difficult process of debate and decision making among group members. In some cases, when consensus cannot be reached, this can create substantial conflict among the emergency physicians. The group must also decide how administrative responsibilities will be handled. Will there be a single medical director or chair, or will the duties be split up among the members? Does the office of the chair or medical director rotate, or does it reside with a single individual over a prolonged period of time? Decision making can result in so-called analysis paralysis. For example, if a hospital administrator believes that additional physician coverage is necessary to reduce waiting times and that the physicians should fund such coverage, can the data be analyzed quickly or will the group be paralyzed by dissension among members about the need for additional coverage?

One of the potential disadvantages of a democratic group may also be construed as an advantage—a long-term commitment is needed to ensure the continuity and consistency required for such a group to function effectively. The disadvantage is that the physicians may have limited ability to leave the group and move to other practice opportunities. The advantage is the assurance that there is substantial incentive for group members to remain at the facility on a long-term basis. Structuring the group in such a way that physicians have long-term commitment is an important part not only of democratic groups but also of all emergency department practice opportunities.

In some small democratic groups, there is limited capital and access to resources for practice diversification, as was discussed with hospital employee and independent contractors. In other democratic groups, a physician with substantial business expertise may be available, which can offer the availability to capital and revenues that might otherwise be impossible. Further, many small democratic groups have formed alliances or affiliations, which allow them far broader exposure to business expertise, access to capital, and sharing of resources such as recruiting, quality improvement, and physician billing services.

As hospitals move rapidly to managed care contracting models, some democratic groups do not have the ability to develop so-called single signature capability with regard to rapidly contracting with such entities. In other words, if the emergency physician group has to debate every managed care contract, including the specific language contained therein, this may paralyze the group and the hospital with regard to its ability to move quickly into managed care relationships. Some hospital administrators do not react well to dealing with a group decision-making process, whether in the managed care or some other environment. Another potential disadvantage to democratic groups is the limited amount of personal and financial reserves available to them. Is the group able to provide physician coverage in the event of illness, injury, or death to an emergency physician in the group? Is the group able to recruit new physicians when necessary? Can the group enter into new business ventures when the opportunity presents itself?

Assessment. With regard to *ownership,* democratic groups by their very nature usually ensure a true sense of parity in ownership. Thus partners with the group usually have an equal share and an equal voice in department operations. In most cases such groups have defined structures for junior physicians to progress to senior physician status, including various types of cash buy-ins, "sweat equity," deferral of bonus payments, and increased hours of clinical coverage.

Similarly, the concepts of *control* and *responsibility* are also equally distributed within a democratic partnership. Shared decision making, with its concomitant strengths and weaknesses, is an essential part of a democratic group. In most cases, responsibility for ensuring that the group's contractual and philosophic obligations are met is also shared among group members. For most emergency physicians seeking a democratic group, a central issue is equal distribution of *profits.* Although the distribution of profits may not be precisely the same for each member of the group (as in a strict fee for service relationship), a clear understanding that profits will be openly discussed and debated is an important feature of such groups. Similarly, the *liability/investment* is usually also equally shared among members of democratic groups.

Partnerships

A partnership is an association of two or more persons as co-owners of a business for profit. This bedrock definition is the simplest and most practical one for a partnership and applies whether it is a single hospital or a multihospital group. Partners share in the profits and losses of their business and participate in management according to a predetermined agreement or formula. That agreement simply reflects what the partners have agreed to, establishes the culture of the organization, sets a tone of collegiality and respect, sets forth guidelines for running the business, and, in the best of circumstances, delineates ways in which the partnership can be dissolved or modified to meet the needs of the partners. Partnerships pay no income tax directly, and profits and losses are passed on to the individual partners. Partners are generally liable for the acts of their partners, although individual partners can also incorporate for business purposes to limit liability. In some states only licensed professionals can participate as partners in a professional practice, but in others both professionals and nonprofessionals can legitimately act as partners in the provision of professional services.

A partnership agreement delineates the purpose, definitions, and terms of the organization and lays out specific capital contributions and accounts. Partnership documents should also address the governance of the organization, including reporting lines of authority and limitations, compensation, distributions, and liabilities. Noncompetition clauses and terms for dissolution of a partner's participation should also be part of a complete partnership agreement. The agreement itself does not make the day-to-day management decisions of the group, and its existence does not obviate the need to have ongoing, hands-on work by partners to make the organization succeed. Compensation can vary according to the dictates of the partnership agreement and often requires changes over time, particularly when additional hospitals are added.

Advantages. The advantages of a partnership as an emergency department group structure include a lack of legal encumbrances of more formal corporate structures, the lack of a separate tax structure, and the avoidance of double taxation on profits generated by the business. In addition, when properly conceived and implemented, the partnership can establish a firm culture of the organization based on collegiality, respect, and adaptation, formalized through written guidelines for resolving differences among physicians. A partnership offers both an important long-term perspective on emergency medicine and an opportunity for growth for individuals within the partnership as it expands. When a partnership reaches a certain size (the precise level of which is open to debate) it may also offer advantages through financial leverage, including substantial benefits, contracting flexibility, development of related business entities for professional liability insurance, billing, and the ability to absorb partners elsewhere in the group should an individual hospital contract be lost.

Disadvantages. The disadvantages of the partnership agreement primarily reside with the need to have a clearly defined decision-making structure and partnership agreement in place before signing the initial hospital contract. Too often, emergency physicians have a verbal partnership but have not done the difficult negotiations among themselves that are necessary to have a legal entity delineating the precise aspects of the partnership in some detail. Ideally, the partnership agreement should also delineate carefully how new partners will be advanced into the group, perhaps based on longevity, hours worked, financial contribution, attainment of board certification, and so on. Appendix A lists details of a sample partnership model developed by California Emergency Physicians Medical Group, one of the nation's oldest and most recognized partnerships in emergency medicine.

Assessment. With regard to *ownership,* the partnership is clearly owned by the partners as defined in the agreement itself. Similarly, *control* resides with the management structure as defined by partners in their preexisting agreement. In most circumstances, the partnership has a specific structure delineated both at the individual hospital level and, in cases of partnerships covering multiple hospitals, with a central governing board of directors or management team. This entity usually has the *responsibility* for ensuring that the obligations of the partnership are met in a timely and appropriate fashion. *Profits* may be disbursed in a number of different ways, but, again, always according to the relationship delineated in the partnership structure.

Corporate Models

A corporation is a legal entity that is separate and independent from its stockholders. Emergency medicine corporations are usually structured as professional or personal services corporations similar to those in law, engineering, architecture, accounting, actuarial sciences, and consulting. Corporations are usually characterized by the principle of limited liability, meaning that individual shareholders are not liable for the acts of other shareholders or for the debts or liabilities of the corporation, although of course individual shareholders are liable for their own negligence or wrongdoing. Corporations are generally subject to the laws of the state in which they legally reside and are subject to stipulated accounting requirements. If corporate profits are not "zeroed out" at the end of the year they are subject to appropriate taxation before distribution to the shareholders. However, in most cases corporations bonus out profit before the end of the year to avoid this double taxation issue.

The majority of corporations providing emergency physician services do not specifically limit the number of shareholders, but most require a specific stock repurchase agreement to allow for buyback of stock in the event that a shareholder leaves the group. The precise language regarding these stock repurchase agreements should be determined in advance to ensure that there is a legitimate stock valuation procedure to be followed in the event that the corporation is liquidated or that shareholders leave the corporation to pursue other career opportunities or retire. Corporate models with specified buy-in arrangements offer a number of advantages, which are similar to those of a partnership arrangement. Physicians usually have strong incentive to pursue stock purchase agreements and ensure that the corporation is successful. Profits are usually distributed according to a predetermined formula, presumably a reasonable one. Liability is limited for stockholders, and the corporate structure avoids risks of double taxation. Disadvantages include the need for certain legal and accounting fees to meet state and local regulations, the possibility of the need for corporate licensing fees in certain states and jurisdictions, and the need for the shareholders to abide by corporate bylaws (or revise them to meet their needs). In general, corporations are often structured similar to partnerships in many fashions, with the choice of one structure versus another usually residing with the individual physicians who form the original partnership or corporation. Appendix B describes the corporate model developed for Southwest Emergency Physicians.

Sole Proprietorship

A sole proprietorship in emergency medicine usually consists of an individual physician who holds a personal services contract (whether as the individual directly or a corporation operated as a sole proprietorship) with the hospital or healthcare system. The sole proprietorship simply means that 100% of the ownership of the corporation resides with a single individual who is responsible for staffing and managing the emergency department with qualified emergency physicians. The contract may also involve varying degrees of specificity regarding additional services provided to the hospital, including quality assurance, risk management, nursing inservices, occupational health, and direction of air medical services. In some circumstances limited proprietorships may closely approximate sole proprietorship by having two or three physicians responsible for the ownership and management of the contract, with multiple other physicians contracted to the corporation. However, for the purposes of this discussion we will focus on true sole proprietorship. Under this model, the individual assumes the risk and the management responsibility for ensuring that the contractual obligations are met. There may be substantial financial risk at the outset of the contract, particularly if the terms are fee-for-service, where start-up costs can be considerable, depending on the size of the contract.

Although sole proprietorships share at their essence a single individual who is responsible for the overall staffing and management of the emergency department, the structure that is used by this sole proprietor can vary extremely widely. Some sole proprietors hire emergency physicians as employees and others as independent contractors. In some cases sole proprietorships operate as either benevolent or nonbenevolent dictatorships, in which all ownership, control, responsibility, profit disbursement, and liability resides with a single individual. In other cases, sole proprietors have structured their practice so that, while ownership resides with a single individual (as does liability), control, responsibility, and profit disbursement are structured in such a way that the employees of the corporation are treated not only with parity, but also as "near-equity" players in the contract. Thus sole proprietorships encompass a wide range of structures, from dictatorships to benevolent dictatorships to groups that operate with principles of a democratic group structure but in which ownership and liability are held by a single individual.

Advantages. The primary advantage of the sole proprietorship is that the hospital administration has a single, clearly identified individual with whom to work to reach decisions. Similarly, in managed care contracting, this single signature approach can be helpful in ensuring that the physician group will participate in prescribed agreements. Similarly, sole proprietorships have clear lines of authority and, presumably, structure of the emergency department group. At least at the management level, there is a long-term commitment on the part of the sole proprietor to continue to provide service at the institution, provided that the contract is a well-structured and successful one. In the best of circumstances, sole proprietorships have the capacity to adapt and change their structure to meet the needs of the individuals within the group, provided that the sole proprietor recognizes the need and has the capacity to do so. Finally, sole proprietorships can be operated in such a way that they incorporate the best features of democratic groups.

Disadvantages. The disadvantages of a sole proprietorship are that both the hospital administration and the physicians "have all their eggs in one basket." If the sole proprietor should become disabled, die, or become incapacitated or incapable of providing service in any way, the structure of the contract falls under serious question. Under certain circumstances, sole proprietorships can be abused or abusive in a number of different ways, not the least of which are financial, fairness, and undue exercise of power by the individual holding the contract. In this regard, the structure of the sole proprietorship is in many ways the most critical aspect of the relationship. That structure should be clear, fair, equitably applied, and able to be changed according to the consensus of the emergency physicians in the group. To the extent that the sole proprietorship is unable to react to these changes, these may be disadvantages.

Assessment. In a sole proprietorship, both the *ownership* and *liability* clearly reside with the sole proprietor. However, *control* may vary widely, from a situation in which the sole proprietor exercises complete dictatorial control to one in which he or she has developed a structure and mechanism to ensure that individual physicians have a voice in management decisions, application of business principles, recruiting, and so forth. Similarly, the *responsibility* for meeting contractual obligations could also either be handled by a single individual or be shared among many of the physicians within the group. Finally, *profit* disbursement can be highly variable, from "none" to formulas tying compensation to a fee-for-service or modified fee-for-service approach, based on billing and collection information. Appendix C lists the sole proprietorship structure used at Fairfax Hospital's Department of Emergency Medicine.

Multihospital Groups

Although partnerships and corporations may each operate at multiple sites, the term *multihospital groups* is restricted here to large corporations in which emergency physicians have little or token ability to obtain either partnership or meaningful shareholder status. Although this is an arbitrary distinction, it has extremely practical significance when compared with the other emergency physician group structure alternatives listed previously. In essence, a physician working for a multihospital group is an employee or independent contractor but is rarely able to participate at the most senior levels of management. Multihospital groups vary widely in their size, sophistication, and commitment to the emergency physicians who staff them.

In the best of circumstances, such multihospital groups of emergency physicians can truly help offer "economies of scale" in that they are able to offer substantial programs involving risk management, quality improvement, benefit packages, continuing medical education opportunities, and practice diversification that might not ordinarily be available with a smaller group. When the resources of the group are truly brought to bear to help strengthen the practice of emergency medicine, substantial benefit may result for both the patient and the emergency physician. However, in the past both reality and perception have been that some multihospital groups have in fact not delivered on their promises to bring substantial services to the individual hospital or the physicians in the emergency department group. High profit margins, inability to deliver promised services, poor recruitment, and inadequate scheduling have at times been the norm for certain hospitals and physicians contracting with multihospital groups.

Advantages. The advantages of the multihospital group are that the hospital has a single contractual entity to deal with that is capable of replacing emergency physicians, including the director, usually on relatively short notice. Single signature contracting is easily obtainable and is usually a part of the standard contractual relationship with a multihospital group. The advantages for the physician include relatively short contract lengths in case the physician chooses to change practice, as well as the potential ability to relocate to other locations with the same multihospital group, depending on recruitment opportunities. In addition, most large multihospital groups do offer some form of career advancement for physicians as quality assurance coordinators, regional medical directors, continuing medical education coordinators, and so on. For some physicians, multihospital groups offer the opportunity to relocate to a geographic location of interest to them without substantial investment of capital.

Disadvantages. Some would say that the disadvantages of multihospital groups are legion. In fact, each of the groups operate off of a recognized profit margin, the fairness of which is up to the individual emergency physician to decide. For a physician who desires a strong sense of equity or ownership in his or her practice, multihospital groups are, in general, limited with regard to such options. There are rare exceptions when senior physicians or long-term physicians with the group are offered equity positions, but in general these are not the norm for multihospital group structures. However, as many multihospital groups have undergone public stock offerings (thereby raising capital), acquisition of smaller emergency physician groups has presented the principles thereof with cash or stock buyouts. Some maintain that multihospital groups encourage turnover, exploitation of the emergency physician, and the use of physicians who are not either residency trained or board certified in emergency medicine. However, there are also emergency physicians who are well qualified in emergency medicine who have had long and distinguished careers with multihospital groups.

Several multihospital emergency department groups have lately diversified substantially into managed care and primary care practice product lines. Such a philosophy recognizes that control of "covered lives" may help guide the future of United States medicine in general and emergency medicine in particular. In this regard, publicly traded companies have substantial access to capital and therefore diversification opportunities that are not available to their smaller, undercapitalized counterparts. Whether such a development is positive or negative is the subject of intense debate but must be decided by each individual seeking a practice opportunity within a specific location.

Assessment. The issues of ownership, control, responsibility, profits, and liability with multihospital groups are clearly with the group itself, not the emergency physicians providing the service. However, some groups have developed attractive career advancement positions such as emergency department chair in large hospitals or regional medical directors to whom substantial management duties are assigned.

SUMMARY

The elements of group structure and function are essential to an understanding of practice opportunities in emergency medicine. Although no specific taxonomy has previously existed regarding emergency medicine group structure, there have been attempts to help identify ways in which emergency medicine practices respond to the needs of their constituents. This chapter has attempted to offer a classification based on structure and functionality, which broadly represents the ways in which emergency medicine may be practiced. Understandably, some groups will not easily fit within one category and may span several.

In choosing a setting in which to practice emergency medicine, analyzing the group structure according to the precepts entailed here may be of some assistance. However, it is important to recognize that the most important factor regarding the choice of a practice opportunity is, has been, and most likely will be *location*. In this regard, if physicians have a specific location in which they choose to practice, their choices will be understandably limited to types of practice available within that setting.

Over 10 years ago Mayer and Cohen[7] offered four essential questions to help address whether an emergency physician should affiliate with a group:

1. Is the group's primary commitment to quality medical care?
2. Are the principals of the group practicing emergency physicians?
3. Does the group foster growth and development for individual emergency physicians, as well as the practice of emergency medicine as a whole?
4. Is the distribution of resources and compensation fair?

These questions are as pertinent today as they were 10 years ago, and they constitute a reasonable checklist by which an emergency physician can begin to assess practice opportunities. The taxonomy offered here is intended to be functional in nature, and it is always the responsibility of the individual emergency physician to determine how best to choose between practice opportunities to meet his or her own needs, those of the profession, and those of his or her family.

REFERENCES

1. Larsen LC, Allegra JR, Franaszek J: Equity buy-in structures of emergency medical group practice, *Am J Emerg Med* 11:28-32, 1993.
2. Mayer TA: Emergency department staffing. In Schwartz GR, Cayten CG, Mayer TA et al, editors: *Principles and practice of emergency medicine,* ed 3, Philadelphia, 1992, Lea & Febiger.
3. Berwick D: Managing quality: the next five years, *Qual Lett Healthcare Leaders* 6:1-7, 1994.
4. Camp RC, Tweet AG: Benchmarking applied to healthcare, *Jt Comm J Qual Improve* 20:229-238, 1994.
5. *Webster's II New Riverside University Dictionary,* Boston, 1984, Riverside Publishing.
6. Dresnick SJ: Contracts in emergency medicine. In Schwartz GR, Cayten CG, Mayer TA et al, editors: *Principles and practice of emergency medicine,* ed 3, Philadelphia, 1992, Lea & Febiger.
7. Mayer TA, Cohen RL: Entrepreneurism and benchmarks of emergency medical practice, *Ann Emerg Med* 13:1161-1163, 1984.

APPENDIX

A Partnership Model

Emergency Medicine and Ambulatory Care Group Practice Structure and Organization*

CLINICAL PRACTICE

California Emergency Physicians Medical Group (CEP) is a partnership of emergency medicine and ambulatory care specialists. Since 1973, the Group has provided quality medical care and comprehensive management services to emergency departments and ambulatory care centers throughout California.

California Emergency Physicians offers a wide variety of practice opportunities, from trauma centers to teaching institutions and community hospitals. We have an excellent reputation with our clients in over 40 communities. Many of CEP's client hospitals have been contracting with the Group for as long as 16 to 20 years, with the average being 15 years.

CEP has achieved broad recognition in California for its leadership role in emergency medicine, its commitment to quality medical practices, and its high percentage of Board Certified physicians. The more than 300 physicians now associated with the Group see approximately one million patients annually. CEP is uniquely positioned to use its size to advantage in the increasingly complex emergency medicine market, while offering its Partners control through its democratic structure and culture.

ORGANIZATIONAL STRUCTURE

As a democratic organization, CEP is structured to provide leadership and support at the local level, as well as participatory opportunities at the group management level.

Group Management

The CEP Board of Directors is responsible for establishing overall operating policy for the Partnership. There are nine physician Board members who meet on a semi-monthly basis. Three members are annually elected by the voting Partnership to three-year terms.

The Executive Committee is comprised of the Chairman of the Board, the Managing Partner, and two other members elected from the Board. Committee members serve one-year terms. The Committee meets monthly to resolve issues delegated to it by the Board and make recommendations to the Board regarding policies and procedures.

The Managing Partner, appointed by the Board, is responsible for implementation of Board policy and overall management of operations, including interactions with contracting hospitals, potential business associates, and physicians within CEP.

Standing committees have been established by the Board to identify and implement projects and programs that will benefit the Partnership. Interested physicians may seek to participate in the committees' work. Current committees include Credentials and Partnership Affairs, Quality Improvement, Retirement and Benefits, Practice Management and the Managed Care Task Force.

Local Support

The Regional Directors are responsible for 1) implementing CEP policies and procedures in their regions; 2) assuring the clinical quality and continuity of their facilities; 3) maintaining the excellence and effectiveness of services throughout their regions; and 4) directing regional marketing and public relations functions, all with the assistance and support of the CEP administrative staff. At the present time, CEP clusters its practice sites into eight geographic regions. The regional concept promotes local identity for the physicians and hospitals.

Regional Directors are also available to provide back-up to emergency department and amulatory care center medical directors in areas such as marketing, contract maintenance, billing and reimbursement, development of new services, staffing, and educational programs. They are appointed by the Managing Partner, subject to Board approval.

Medical Directors have on-line responsibility for the operation of their facilities and management of their contracts. At many of our sites, the duties are shared among physicians, with the medical director maintaining overall responsibility for the quality and effectiveness of services, medical administration, supervision of the physician staff, in-service education for nursing personnel, community involvement and education, quality improvement and risk management.

Staff physicians are first and foremost responsible for providing quality medical care. They are expected to become involved members of the local medical community, with the extent of their activities depending on the individual situation.

BENEFITS

Employees

- Group-supported malpractice insurance.
- Health Plan (optional).

Partners

- Group-supported malpractice insurance.
- Group health plan with "state of the art" coverage; choice of deductibles, dependents and PPO option, dental and vision plans.
- Disability Insurance.
- Retirement plans, including both 401(k) and defined benefit elements.
- Dependent Care assistance program.

*Appendix A courtesy of California Emergency Physicians® Medical Group.

Table A-1 Partnership Categories

To attain this level of partnership you must:	To maintain this level of partnership you must:	To advance to the next level of partnership you must:	Benefits at this level of partnership are:
Level 1			
• Complete 500 hours of service • Have current credentials on file • Have positive evaluations and recommendations from medical and regional directors	• Continue to work on a full or part-time basis • Maintain current credentials • Partners not working any hours for 6 months will be considered voluntary terminations	• Work full-time a minimum of 1,728 hrs/yr (or 1,440 and treat 4,000 pts.) Year is counted from *first month* in which you worked full-time. Up to 18 months to complete • Maintain current credentials • Have positive evaluations from medical and regional directors • Attend a New Partner Orientation meeting—mandatory • Complete one year as a partner	• 5% share of profit distribution • 1 vote in Partnership matters excluding Board elections, Amendments to the Partnership Agreement, and Recall & Referendum measures • No taxes withheld • Health insurance benefits —mandatory participation • May attend Partnership Meetings
Level 2			
• Complete 1,728 hrs of service in preceding year (or 1,440 + 4,000 pts.) • Have current credentials on file • Have positive evaluations, recommendations from medical/regional directors • Complete 1 year as a partner	• Continue to work 1,728 hrs/yr (or 1,440 + 4,000 pts.) • Maintain current credentials	• Continue to work full-time a minimum of 1,728 hrs/yr (or 1,440 + 4,000 pts.) Up to 18 months to complete • Maintain current credentials • Have positive evaluations from medical and regional directors • Complete 2 years as a partner	• 17% share of profit distribution • 1 vote in all Partnership matters
Level 3			
• Complete 1,728 hrs of service in preceding year (or 1,440 + 4,000 pts.) • Have current credentials on file • Have positive evaluations, recommendations from medical/regional directors • Submit $3,000 Capital Contribution • Complete 2 years as a Partner	• Continue to work 1,440 hrs/yr • Maintain current credentials	• Continue to work full-time a minimum of 1,440 hrs/yr. Up to 18 months to complete • Maintain current credentials • *For ED:* Demonstrate ABEM or AOA ED certification or a primary care specialty. *For ACC:* Board certification in EM, FP, IM, Peds, Occupational Medicine or Osteopathy GP boarded. • Obtain outstanding evaluations and recommendations from medical/regional directors • Complete 3 years as a Partner	• 33% share of profit distribution • 1 vote in all Partnership matters
Level 4			
• Complete 1440 hr of service in the preceding year • Have current credentials on file • Have outstanding evaluations and recommendations • Maintain Board Certification • Complete 3 years as a partner	• Continue to work 1440 hr/yr • Maintain current credentials	• Continue to work full-time a minimum of 1440 hr/yr. Up to 18 months to complete • Maintain current credentials • Maintain Board Certification. *For EDs:* attain Emergency Boards if not ABEM or AOA ED certified • Obtain outstanding evaluations and recommendations • Complete 4 years as a Partner	• 50% share of profit distribution • 1 vote in all Partnership matters

Continued.

Table A-1 Partership Categories—cont'd

To attain this level of partnership you must:	To maintain this level of partnership you must:	To advance to the next level of partnership you must:	Benefits at this level of partnership are:
Full partner			
• Complete 1440 hr of service in the preceding year • Have current credentials on file • Have outstanding evaluations and recommendations • Maintain Board Certification • Submit proportionate Med-America stock share buy-in • Complete 4 years as a partner	• Continue to work 960 hr/yr • Maintain current credentials • Maintain Board Certification	• Continue to work full-time a minimum of 960 hr/yr • Maintain current credentials • Maintain Board Certification • Complete 10 years as a partner	• 100% share of profit distribution • 3 votes in all Partnership matters • Eligible to run for Board seat
Senior partner			
• Complete 10 years as a partner, working the required number of hours in each of these years • Have current credentials on file • Maintain Board Certification	• Continue to work 750 hr/yr • Maintain current credentials • Maintain Board Certification	• N/A	• 100% share of profit distribution • 3 votes in all Partnership matters • Eligible to run for Board seat • Receive a total of $12,000 once every 5 years for a 60 to 180 day sabbatical • Employment guarantee after a sabbatical at same facility if CEP retains contract and you return full-time

- Profit-sharing, etc. (see Table A-1).
- An equity position in the Group.
- Senior Partners may receive a total of $12,000 once every 5 years for a 60- to 180-day sabbatical.

GENERAL INFORMATION

- CEP maintains physician credentials; a complete physician record contains the following:
  —A completed application
  —Copies of current California license, DEA registration, ACLS certification and Board certification
  —ACEP membership verification and documentation of other appropriate professional affiliations
  —Three letters of reference
  —Verification of medical training
- Work schedules are prepared monthly by the medical director of each facility in concert with staff physicians.
- Staff physicians assist in maintaining practice statistics, which are compiled monthly by the medical director for submission to the CEP office.
- Physicians use fee schedules that have been approved by CEP. Each physician is instructed in the most appropriate use of the fee schedule.

APPENDIX

B Corporate Model

Southwestern Michigan Emergency Services, P.C.*

Mission Statement

- Promote and provide quality physician services to the patients and the institution it serves.
- Develop and maintain optimal working and growth environments for physicians and staff.
- Establish policies, procedures, and circumstances to enhance the working longevity of SWMES, P.C. physicians.

Southwestern Michigan Emergency Services, P.C.

Advancement Tree

I. Base Salary
II. Health Insurance
III. Medical Liability Insurance
IV. Additional Reimbursement Distribution and Benefits

1st Year	10%	Regional Hospital Dues & Application Fees AMA & ACEP Dues
2nd Year	25%	Educational Stipend Regional Hospital Dues & Application Fees AMA and ACEP Dues
3rd Year	50%	Educational Stipend Term Life Insurance Regional Hospital Dues & Application Fees AMA and ACEP Dues

BENEFITS

	Independent contractor	Employee	Stockholder
Medical Liability	✓	✓	✓
Health Insurance	✓	✓	✓
Dues/Membership	✓	✓	✓
Educational Stipend	✓	✓	✓
Medical Reimbursement		✓	✓
FICA		✓	✓
Taxes—Fed/State		✓	✓
Auto Allowance		✓	✓
Merit System	✓	✓	✓
Profit Sharing Program		✓	✓
Additional Reimbursement	✓	✓	✓
"Corporate Profit"			✓
Accounting Fee Allowance		✓	✓

*Appendix B courtesy Southwestern Michigan Emergency Services, P.C.

STOCK BUY-IN VALUATION METHOD

I. The subsequent formula was designed to determine a dollar amount per share for purposes of a new doctor to buy into the corporation.
   The philosophy of the formula is meant to reflect the benefits inured to the new stockholder. Otherwise, a new owner pays a price to obtain future earnings and benefits.

II. Formula
   A. Obtain the past year-end financial statement.
   B. Schedule the following:
      1. Gross revenue for the year.
      2. Less all expenses and deductions except federal income tax and Michigan income tax.
      3. Add back salary amounts of the owners in excess of $100/hr worked the year.
      4. Add back for the stockholder doctors the auto allowances, life and disability insurance, medical reimbursement, business promotions and accounting allowances.
      5. Recompute and deduct the applicable Michigan single business tax.
      6. Recompute and deduct the applicable federal income tax.
      7. Add to this new income number (#1-#6) the beginning of year stockholders equity.

The result obtained in step seven above gives a market value of the stock for computation purposes.

This number is then divided not by the current number of outstanding shares, but by the number of shares to be issued and outstanding immediately after the buy-in.

This number is averaged with similar computations of the past three years to obtain an average per share. The per share average is used for the buy-in at that time and until next year end.

STOCK VALUATION

The purchase value of the stock is set by a formula. The cost gives the stockholder the following benefits and responsibilities:

A. Prorate share of hard assets—cash receivables, furniture, etc.
B. A formal voice in the direction of the corporation.
C. Vote by share for Board of Directors.
D. Right to other corporate earnings.
E. Right to be elected to the Board of Directors.
F. Share of fiduciary responsibilities of corporation.
G. Share of all corporation liabilities (medical malpractice, trustee, employer/employee Internal Revenue Service).
H. Right to attend the annual shareholders meeting.
I. Enhanced commitment to corporation.

Stock Valuation
Southwestern Michigan Emergency Services
December 31, 1991

	Nine months 1991	1990	1989	1988
INCOME	3,246,492	3,620,087	3,435,963	2,886,934
EXPENSES (less SBT & FIT)	3,318,125	3,624,819	3,417,286	2,840,190
	(71,633)	(4,732)	18,677	46,744
ADD BACK				
Salaries in excess of base amounts paid to Stockholders	371,590	530,581	456,559	286,184
Auto allowance	24,197	28,387	26,999	17,990
Life & disability insurance	9,376	7,835	9,990	11,974
Medical reimbursement	9,771	16,005	19,039	7,340
Business Promotion	22,290	24,868	21,849	18,156
Accounting allowance	0	900	0	
TOTAL	365,591	603,844	553,113	388,388
12 MO TOTAL	487,455			
LESS				
Recomputed SBT	38,146	42,536	40,373	33,921
Recomputed FIT	152,765	192,454	178,280	120,519
ADD				
Beginning equity	82,253	84,361	120,482	117,494
TOTAL	378,797	453,215	454,942	351,442
TOTAL AVERAGE	409,599			
OUTSTANDING SHARES	120	160	200	240
VALUATION PER SHARE	3,413	2,560	2,048	1,707
TOTAL COST	136,520	102,400	81,920	68,280
STOCKHOLDERS	3	4	5	6

SWMES, PC Facts

- The bylaws do not limit the # of SWMES, PC stockholders.
- The stock valuation procedure effectively decreases the cost of stock as the # of existing and incoming members increases.
- As the profitability of the corporation increases the cost increases.
- An executed stock/repurchase agreement calls for a buy back system and must be signed upon receipt of first shares.

SWMES, PC
ORGANIZATIONAL CHART

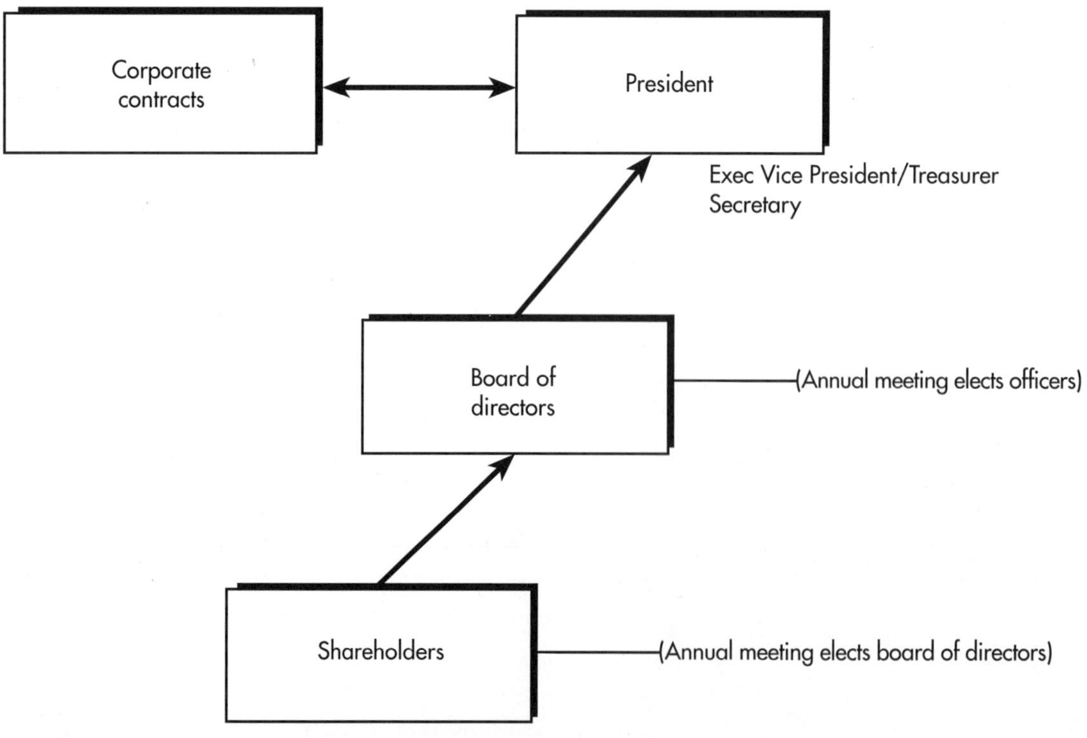

SWNES, PC
FUNCTIONAL ORGANIZATIONAL CHART

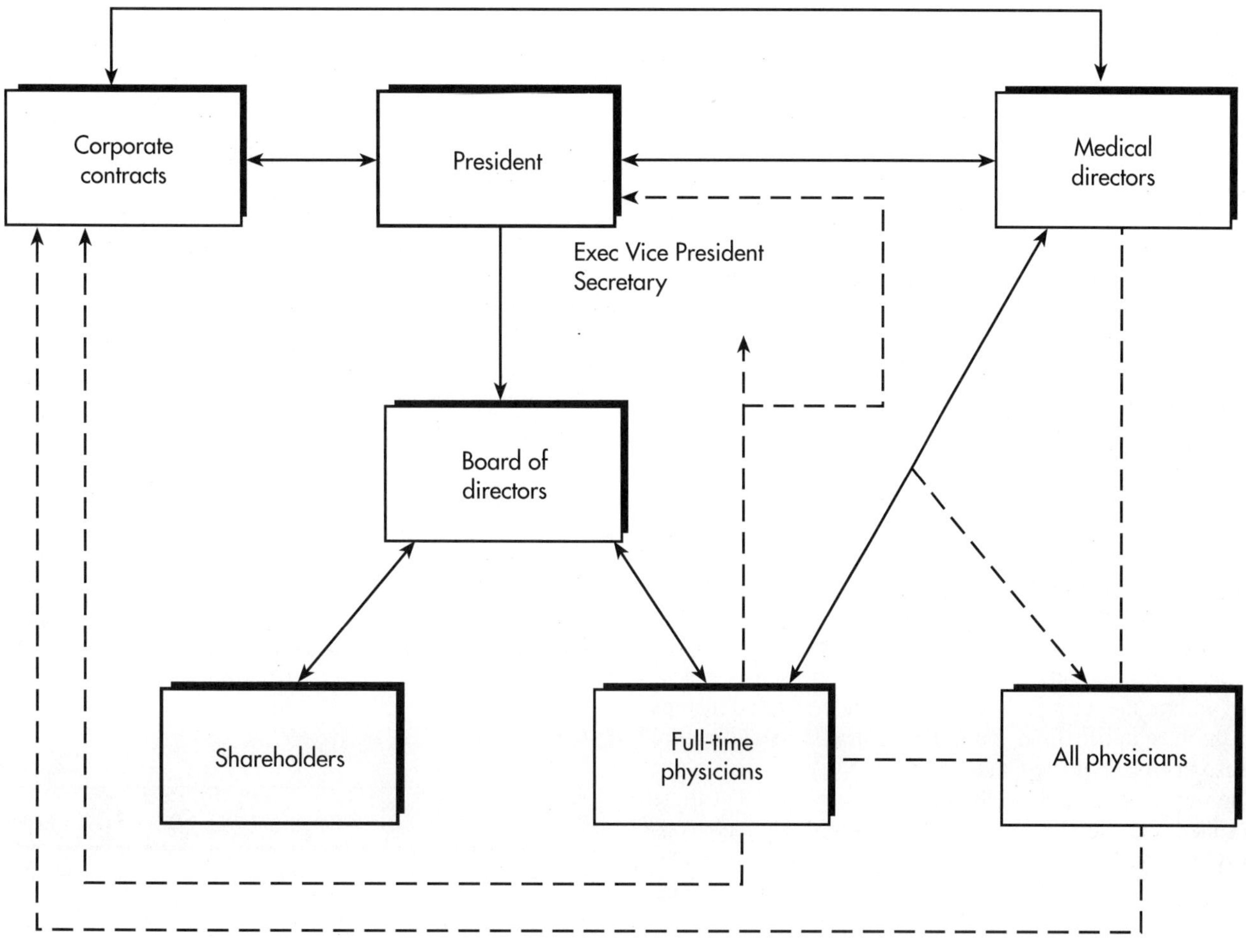

ACKNOWLEDGEMENT REGARDING
SOUTHWESTERN MICHIGAN EMERGENCY SERVICE, P.C.
STOCK PURCHASE AGREEMENT

I acknowledge that I am acquiring shares in Southwestern Michigan Emergency Services, P.C., a Michigan professional corporation, that I have received a copy of the Southwestern Michigan Emergency Services, P.C. Stock Purchase Agreement dated _______________, 1991, that the Agreement binds me, as well as existing and future shareholders, in the P.C.

I commit to observe and be bound by all terms and conditions of the Agreement as a condition of the additional consideration for the sale of shares in the P.C. to me.

Dated: __________________, 1992 ______________________

APPENDIX

C Sole Proprietorship Structure

The Department of Emergency Medicine at Fairfax Hospital is structured as the sole proprietorship, but with a structure that enables each emergency physician to have a clearly specified progression to senior emergency physician status, as well as an equal voice in departmental affairs. Emergency physicians work with the group with a clear understanding that there is a progression based on time and experience with the group, which progresses from an initial entry level of 40 hours per week of service to an eventual 32 hours per week of service, with a commensurate raise in compensation during that time frame. Physicians are hired with a 6-month probationary period, after which they receive an assessment from the senior physicians in the group.

In addition to compensation increasing over a specified period of time, participation in the fee-for-service bonus plan also progresses over a specified period of time to allow for an equity buy-in process for the group.

With regard to the business of the emergency department, the physicians in the group have an equal voice and equal vote in all departmental affairs, including policies and procedures, adding additional physician coverage, and nursing staff interrelations.

Administrative positions within the group are chosen by the Chair, with the advice and consent of the senior physicians within the group. Separate contractual relationships with the hospital to fund these administrative positions are the responsibility of the Chair.

The overall objective of the group is to ensure that there is a stated and clearly defined progression to senior physician status, with incentives built in for the emergency physicians to improve services, reduce turnaround times, and increase patient satisfaction.

EPNV BONUS PLAN

- 1/4 Participation after 1 year
- 1/2 Participation after 2 years
- Full Participation after 3 years
- Each Physician's Share is met by working equivalent hours for his/her level of participation

Example

Level	# Hours
Full	1472
3	1656

- Additional hours would be paid and credited on a proportional basis

EXAMPLE

A full partner working 1600 hours would have 1.09 shares (1600/1472)

- Extra nights and weekends would be weighted 30% (1.3) in the calculation of total shares
- Physicians with decreased contracted administrative hours would be calculated versus full partner hours.

EXAMPLE

900 hours/1472 = .61 share

- Total bonus paid is equal to the total pool/number of shares
- Minimum Bonus amount set prior to Bonus year; additional monies as profits allow

EPNV LEVELS OF PARTICIPATION*

	Hours	
	Per week	Per year
Full	32	1472
Level 3	36	1656
Level 2	40	1840
Level 1	40	1840
Interval	**Compensation**	**Bonus**
1 year	100%	Full Share
1 year	100%	Full Share
1 year	85%	Full Share
	75%	No shares

Bonus Calculation*

Amount	Criteria
45%	Number of clinical hours
45%	Volume patients/revenue generated
10%	Discretionary Bonus

40 Joint Venture Contracts

Kelvin P. Quan and James B. Wieland

OUTLINE

The joint venture has become a popular vehicle in healthcare delivery to allow two or more parties or legal entities (participants) to come together for a single business purpose without necessarily having to completely merge their legal identities. The joint venture draws on selected assets and activities from its participants to offer to the market a product or service that its participants might not otherwise offer individually. As a general public policy, this strategy is socially desirable because the market, defined as the community and patients, benefits from a greater selection of services. Demands for alternative healthcare delivery services, systems, and cost efficiencies have led to new joint ventures among physicians, hospitals, and other healthcare providers. Many collaborations are beneficial because they provide financial and operational economies of scale. Others are attractive because they engender an atmosphere of cooperation and dialogue. The goals of joint ventures are furthered when the hospital seeks to avoid competing with its own medical staff physicians for outpatient services.

Since the 1980s, free-standing emergency clinics have grown in number and popularity. These facilities are sometimes known as *urgent care centers,* or *ambulatory care centers* to avoid some state regulations that apply when the term *emergency* is part of the facility's name. Free-standing emergency clinics are generally open longer hours than physicians' private offices, do not require appointments, usually have short waits for service, and charge less than hospital emergency rooms.

Four general organizational models of free-standing emergency clinics exist. In the first model, a single physician, a physician partnership, or a physician group may form a private practice model in which the physician is in complete control of all aspects of the operation. This model is little more than that of an expanded traditional office practice. In the second model, physicians may contract with a management services company for specific administrative services such as site and equipment selection, building design, operating policies and procedures, staff training, accounting, billing, and advertising. Although the physician-owners in this model purchase certain services, they retain ultimate control over all aspects of the practice. In the third model, the facility may be owned by an investor-owned corporation or hospital that contracts with independent physicians or professional corporations to provide medical services. Here, the physicians have control only over medical issues, and the corporation retains control over all other matters. The final model is the joint venture model, in which the participants are of equal standing. This chapter discusses a contract model joint venture in which a hospital and a group of emergency physicians jointly operate a simple free-standing emergency clinic.

Today's healthcare delivery system is evolving rapidly in an era of discounted reimbursement, risk sharing, capitation, and withholds. Physicians are being asked to provide coverage and professional services for less than their usual, customary fees or based on entirely new forms of reimbursement. In the entrepreneurial marketplace, these alternative payment methodologies represent an increasing portion of the relevant payment sources. Therefore physicians must carefully evaluate the joint venture in which they will provide professional services and subject their income to the risk of the overall profitability of the venture.

JOINT VENTURES MODELS

Joint venture is an imprecise term, and definitions vary depending on the context. State laws differ with regard to the definitions and legal consequences of a joint venture, and legal counsel familiar with the laws of each individual jurisdiction should be consulted on any joint venture enterprise. Notwithstanding the differences in state statutes and the literature, the following elements are shared by all joint ventures.

The interests of the participants of the joint venture are merged through a sharing of economic rewards and risks, the profits and losses. The management rights, including the right to direct and control each participant's activities with regard to the venture, are allocated among the participants. The participants are governed by a duty of "good faith" and "fair dealing" with each other, which are legal obligations given serious consideration by the courts. Other common, although not singularly determinative, characteristics include the development of a new product or entry into a new market, the establishment and marketing of an entity separate from the participants, a common location of operation, and the performance of administrative functions such as billing, collections, credentialing, and utilization review.

A joint venture can be structured as a partnership, a corporation, or a contractual relationship between multiple parties. Whereas the first two organizational models create new formal legal entities, the last creates a comparatively more flexible, legal relationship between the parties.

Partnership Model

A partnership is an unincorporated association of two or more parties doing business as co-owners. The partners may be individuals, corporations, or other partnerships. Unless stated otherwise in the partnership agreement, each general partner is entitled to reimbursement of his or her initial investment, and each general partner shares in the profits and losses equally, regardless of the time and money contributed by each.

Joint venture partnerships also may be limited (or silent) partnerships, rather than general partnerships. Although specific aspects of limited partnerships vary from one jurisdiction to another, all limited partnership have at least one general and one limited partner. The general partners conduct the everyday business affairs and are ultimately responsible for all debts and liabilities arising from the partnership activity. Unless a written agreement states otherwise, disputes over ordinary business matters are decided by a majority vote among all partners. The limited partners typically contribute cash toward the capital of the partnership, and their liability for the debts of the partnership is limited to the amount contributed. Limited partners cannot have management responsibilities or authority over operations.

A contract model joint venture and a partnership are treated similarly under the laws of most jurisdictions, particularly as they relate to the rights and liabilities of the participants between themselves and third parties. A partnership, however, usually relates to general business activities of a particular type and is frequently not limited in its duration and scope. Partnerships are often formed by physicians as their medical practice entity to provide emergency medicine on an ongoing basis at various hospitals. In contrast, a joint venture is limited in its scope and duration by contract. Physicians and a hospital might form a joint venture to establish an outreach urgent care clinic. The more limited scope and duration are preferable for those who want to avoid a deeper commitment of their future and fortunes given the newness of the venture and the vicissitudes of the healthcare industry.

Corporate Model

In the corporate model of the joint venture, a new and distinct legal corporate entity is formed and owned by the participants. Participants typically become shareholders and receive shares of stock to represent their ownership interest in a general business corporation. Corporations may issue different classes of stock, allowing the parties to tailor control and financial expectations. The advantage of this model is that it provides limited liability to participants with respect to the corporation's debts and obligations. The primary disadvantage is that income is taxed twice, once at the higher corporate level and again at the personal level after dividends have been distributed to the shareholders. Besides the additional tax liability, there is the added expense of preparing and filing two sets of income tax returns. Management in the corporate model through a board of directors is more formal and, as a result, may be more cumbersome, more expensive, and less flexible.

Contract Model

The contract model should be considered when four factors are present (Figure 40-1). First, the contemplated activity is *simple and limited in scope*. Second, *no significant capital expenditure* is required. Third, the business environment allows for some form of *profit and risk sharing* between the participants; and finally, the nature of the enterprise permits payment on some basis *other than fee-for-service*. An example of these factors can be found when the operation of the joint venture requires staffing by only one physician group, and the facility is a former clinic or other form of outreach site of the hospital. Further, the joint venture provides services to beneficiaries of a managed care program to which both the physicians and hospital belong and share in a capitated risk pool. This chapter focuses on this contract model.

The written contract defines the joint venture and commits each participant to contributing certain resources to the operation of a joint enterprise of a limited duration. The contract model joint venture must be distinguished from an independent contractor arrangement to provide professional services. In the independent contractor arrangement, the physician group provides staffing and professional services, and the hospital provides facilities and equipment. Each party bears the comparatively limited rewards and risks of its own individual commitments. In a joint venture model, those risks and rewards are pooled, and the emergency physicians share in the overall profits or losses of the joint venture. The financial results of the joint venture are allocated according to the terms of the contract.

The main advantage of the contract model is simplicity. No new legal entity is created. The enterprise can be established with a single document, similar to a professional services contract between a hospital and a hospital-based physician. Federal and state securities laws, which regulate the offer and sale of interests in most limited partnerships and corporate entities, are not likely to apply. As a result, the participants are free from potentially cumbersome and expensive compliance procedures, and the relationships are more straightforward than those in a limited partnership.

The federal and state income tax consequences also are straightforward. The participants are liable for income tax attributable to their own entities. Contributions of property to

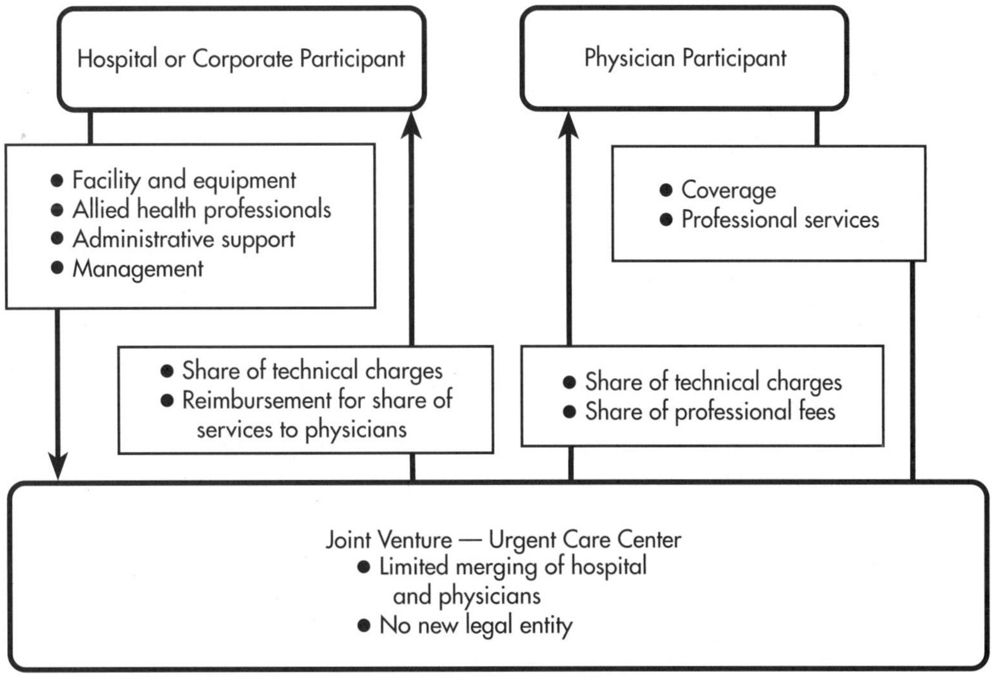

FIGURE 40-1 Contract model joint venture for emergency physician service.

the venture do not ordinarily generate a gain or loss recognizable for tax purposes. However, when the contribution is credited to another venture participant or when it is made in payment for services of another participant, there may be reportable tax.

A disadvantage of the contract model is that significant tax benefits, such as deductions for depreciation, cannot be shifted among participants. Facilities and equipment used in the venture must remain the property of the contributing participant because no new partnership or corporate entity is created through which the tangible assets of the joint venture can be owned.

In most states, each participant in a joint venture is fully and personally liable, as a general partner would be, for any debts or liabilities that arise within the scope of the joint venture. Specific legal and regulatory restrictions are discussed later in the chapter.

JOINT VENTURE CONTRACT

Although there is no single type of joint venture contract, it is strongly recommended that it be written even though an unwritten agreement is legally sufficient. An activity as complex as the provision of medical care in a joint venture contract should be memorialized in a single, integrated, written document. Creating this document will minimize the possibility of misunderstanding and furnish a reference point for the participants by which any disagreement will be resolved. It will also document the parties' relationship for regulatory, tax, and liability purposes. Properly drafted, a written contract will control the participants' individual responsibility for liabilities of the venture by carefully defining the scope of the venture. Equally important, a written contract compels the participants to focus on the important principles underlying the venture and enables them to come to a clearer and more complete agreement.

Especially if it is presented by the hospital, the proposed draft of the contract should be considered completely negotiable. Strategically, however, it is probably best for the physicians to take the initiative and submit the first proposal. Throughout the negotiations and in the spirit of fair dealing, the physicians must consider the needs and resources of the hospital, as well as their own requirements.

Recitals

Although they begin most contractual arrangements, the recitals are often not given enough attention by the contracting parties. The "whereas" clauses articulate the intent and reasons for the respective parties entering into the contract. These opening clauses provide background information that will help interpret the component parts of the contract itself. In a joint venture contract, this background may be important in distinguishing the joint venture relationship from a general partnership and in helping to describe the scope and limits of the joint venture activity. Still, the parties' own characterization of their relationship is not binding on courts or third parties if it is challenged. Substance will prevail over form. However, the contents of the written joint venture contract furnish important evidence of the parties' intent.

Identification of the Participants

The legal name of each participant must be stated in full to adequately affix responsibility for compliance with the contract. This can be particularly important when a participant such as a healthcare delivery system functions through a complex structure with discrete corporate entities for its hospitals, clinics, ancillary services, and for-profit ventures. Generally, persons and entities that are not a party or a signatory to the contract cannot be bound by the terms of the contract. Consequently, physicians negotiating with entities composed of multiple components should make sure that the entity with authority and financial assets is legally bound to the contract.

Name of Joint Venture

The same regulatory and licensure requirements that affect hospitals, physicians, and urgent care facilities usually govern the determination of the joint venture's name. Some states require physicians practicing through a joint venture to include the name of one or more of the physicians in the legal name of the enterprise. Generally, names other than the physicians' themselves must be filed with the state as a fictitious name. Some states require accreditation, minimum staffing levels, and minimum hours of availability when an enterprise uses words such as *emergency* or *urgent care* in its name.

Description of the Joint Venture Activity

This description defines the scope of the venture activity in sufficient detail to permit clear understanding by a third party or a court. Each participant is fully liable for legal obligations or liabilities arising from the venture, even when those liabilities arise solely through the conduct of another participant. Therefore the contract must clearly establish the limits of the joint venture, including the nature of the venture, its location, and its precise services.

The qualifications of allied health personnel should be specified. Even if the hospital participant actually employs the support staff, the physician should have the opportunity of comment on the staff's selection, retention, termination, and compensation. This approach will reduce the possibility of problem personnel being transferred into the venture or of poorly qualified support staff hampering the venture's performance. Although the hospital will likely seek these controls, at a minimum, the physician should retain appropriate independence to designate qualified physician personnel.

Physician coverage issues such as the hours of coverage, the number of physicians present during specified hours, on-call or backup coverage and the overall commitment of full-time equivalent coverage should be carefully defined. The contract should describe the hospital's obligations to provide and maintain a facility, equipment, supplies, and support staff. Budgetary constraints must not be allowed to excuse the proper acquisition or maintenance of necessary equipment and supplies. The contract also should define the hospital's obligation to market the joint venture to potential patients, physicians, and other referral sources.

Contributions to the Joint Venture Activity

The financial, property, and service obligations provided by each participant should be carefully described along with a mechanism to resolve any failure to provide a required contributions. One possibility is that the failure by one party to make a required contribution would permit the other participant to obtain substitute performance at the expense of the venture. This provision, however, should not unduly restrict the physician's ability to declare a contract breach and seek appropriate remedies.

Management Responsibilities

The management responsibilities of each participant should be specified. Typically, responsibilities in a joint venture contract for an urgent care center are allocated according to the expertise of the parties. The physician should participate actively in management decisions. The reverse, however, is not necessarily true; the joint venture contract should specifically recognize the right and obligation of the physician participant to make independent professional judgments in matters relating to patient care (see Corporate Practice of Medicine and Fee-Splitting).

Marketing materials should be approved in advance by the physician participant, especially if it includes his or her name. Particular care must be taken to comply with medical ethics and licensure requirements. Marketing zeal must be tempered to avoid expectations of a higher standard of care than the law would otherwise require. For example, advertising "state-of-the-art facilities and care" may attract patients, but it may also obligate the venture to provide standards of medical practice that may not be available.

Liability and Insurance

Under the theory of cross liability, one individual is liable for the acts of another based on some special relationship between the two individuals. Generally, all parties to a joint venture are individually and jointly liable for all debts or obligations arising within the scope and operation of the joint venture activity, regardless of the absence of any active participation in the event giving rise to the liability. By creating a joint venture through a contract, partnership, or corporation, however, the participants are demonstrating that they contemplate an exchange of duties and obligations greater than a reasonable duty of care between unrelated parties.

The physician must recognize the potential liability and then determine the appropriate level of malpractice, premises, and other types of liability insurance coverage. In many states, the courts and insurance carriers may find that by entering into a joint venture contract, the emergency physician assumed liability for an act or omission by the nonphysician participant if it arises within the scope of operations of the joint venture. Professional liability and other forms of insurance specifically exclude coverage for risks of such loss deemed to be "liability assumed by contract." As a result, the physician would not be covered under the primary malpractice policy. A specific addendum or rider may have to be purchased to extend existing coverage to the joint venture activities.

Some jurisdictions and insurance carriers consider the creation of a joint venture by contract as the creation of a new entity. In these cases, it is necessary either to purchase a separate liability insurance policy for the joint venture or to make certain that the joint venture is named as an additional insured on the appropriate policies of all the venture participants. The joint venture contract should be submitted to legal counsel and, perhaps, to the insurance carrier for a written determination.

Emergency physicians typically practice medicine in settings where the safe condition of the physical premises is the legal responsibility of the hospital. As such, the individual physicians may not have premises insurance to cover liability for injuries that occur on the premises. Because each participant in a joint venture may be fully liable to a patient or visitor who is injured on the premises, appropriate insurance coverage must be obtained. Workers' compensation insurance coverage also must be considered where applicable.

Indemnification

Indemnification is reimbursement by one party for a loss, in whole or in part, incurred by another party. The hospital may request that the physicians indemnify the hospital against losses resulting from negligent or intentional acts or omissions by members of the physician group. This kind of indemnification should be avoided because this type of liability would not be covered by professional malpractice policies because it amounts to "liability assumed by contract." Insurance carriers should be consulted with regard to questions of coverage for contractually assumed liabilities by the group for peer review and administrative "malpractice," which are excluded from most liability insurance policies.

Allocation of Profits and Losses

Physician compensation in a joint venture goes beyond reimbursement for professional services. Otherwise, a professional services agreement similar to that between a hospital and a hospital-based physician would be all that would be required. As with the other points of negotiation, the allocation of profit and loss is a balance of considerations. The hospital argues a favorable allocation on the basis that it has invested capital, personnel, goodwill, and management expertise. In turn, the emergency physician promotes the importance of his or her own contribution of goodwill and medical skill. Indeed, it can be argued that the everyday medical decisions made by the physician are more determinative of the quality of care, the presumed correlative of success of a venture, than any other single factor. After the parties have negotiated the allocation of risk and reward and profits and losses, the terms must be clearly defined. All possibilities from the disastrous to the optimistic must be considered. Confronting these issues in advance allows the participants to negotiate them with the greatest degree of objectivity. Advanced planning also may encourage the incorporation of operational safeguards to protect against their undesired occurrence or to promote their desired benefit. Finally, the distribution of profits and losses also may be affected by state laws prohibiting fee splitting.

As managed care becomes increasingly popular, some joint ventures may enter into capitation arrangements whereby the provider of emergency medical services assumes financial risk for inappropriate or overuse of such services. By receiving a prepaid amount per beneficiary a month, an incentive is created to manage efficiently the delivery site and to channel patients to the most appropriate venues for medical care. There should be an advanced agreement for the distribution of the profits and losses of such capitation arrangements. In some states, there may even be prohibitions against providers sharing in the risk of services that they do not themselves provide. In the context of joint ventures, an objection may arise from the emergency physician benefiting from surpluses in a the hospital's risk pool receiving capitation that covers emergency care in toto.

Termination

Termination of the joint venture, either at the end of its planned duration or during its term, may be the most important part of the contract. A balance must be struck between the need to provide an orderly mechanism by which obligations can be ended and the need to secure a commitment for the continuity of the arrangement.

Contract terminations may be *for cause* based on a material breach by one participant, or *without cause,* which may be invoked by one participant for no reason at all. Although definitions of "cause" will vary, they may include anything that is a material failure by one participant to fulfill the contractual obligations. An example of a cause is a clear failure by the hospital participant to provide adequate levels of trained personnel. A process for the review of termination for cause may be developed in the contract, and an arbitration clause may be included to resolve disputes between the participants.

Deciding on whether to accept terminations without cause must be weighed against the risk that the coverage and services commitment of the emergency physician to the joint venture will not generate sufficient financial return. This suggests that terminating the arrangement on short notice without cause may be desirable. On the other hand, many joint ventures take time to become profitable because they involve new, expansion-oriented provisions of services. The emergency physicians may have provided services and made commitments during an unprofitable start-up period. After profitability has been established, the hospital could terminate without cause on short notice and bring in another party to take over. Alternatively, the hospital could renegotiate significant portions of the joint venture contract under a threat of termination without cause.

The hospital and emergency physician group should have the same rights to terminate without cause. This right appears equitable, but on closer examination the emergency physicians are at a marked disadvantage. Generally, termination with short notice without cause for the emergency physicians means an abrupt loss of employment and direct personal income. An abrupt termination of a contract for a hospital requires it to simply call a *locum tenens* while it awaits for bids from a new group. The ease of termination without cause must be balanced against the desire for security. Otherwise, termination should be limited to *for cause* and only then with sufficient due process and notice to provide for an opportunity for correction. A detailed *for cause* termination could relieve some pressure when bargaining for the rejection of a termination *without cause.*

Some new joint ventures are contracted before they acquire the necessary license or certification, and the date of initial operations may be made contingent on regulatory approval. If approval is not obtained by a predetermined date or within a specified reasonable period of time, the participants would then have the right to withdraw from the joint venture. This right would allow the participants to reevaluate their commitments if significant problems or unanticipated developments result.

Term

The term of the contract is closely tied to the termination provisions. One, two, and three year terms are not uncommon. Many contracts provide an automatic renewal clause to automatically extend the contract on expiration of the original term for an additional defined term, subject to the termination provisions of the contract. Without this clause, the contract will expire at the end of the term, leaving it to the parties to affirmatively take steps to renegotiate the contract. As a practical matter, the term will be significant because it creates a time for review and assessment of the contractual arrangement. The term must be read in conjunction with the contract's termination clause. For example, if the term is 3 years, but terminable by either party ". . . without cause at any time upon ninety (90) days' notice. . . ," it is functionally a 90-day contract, not a 3-year contract.

Hospitals with tax exempt bond funding and public hospitals frequently have specific limits on the maximum allowable term of contracts with mandated rights to terminate without cause. Previously, the Internal Revenue Service (IRS) required a 90-day termination *without cause* for all percentage of fees service contracts in order for interest to be tax exempt on a facility's bond. Even contracts in which the hospital did not pay the physician anything and instead allowed the physician to bill the patient directly were consider by the IRS to be percentage of fees contracts in which the percentage was 100%. This requirement was changed in 1993. Currently, physician compensation for professional medical services is based on a percentage of fees charged; the term of the contract, including renewal options, may not exceed 2 years; and the contract must be cancelable by the hospital without cause or penalty on reasonable notice at the end of the first year. This term is also required if the physician bills patients separately for the professional component. If physician compensation is based on a per-unit fee or a combination of per-unit fee and periodic fixed fee, the term may not exceed 3 years, and it must be terminable without cause by the hospital at the end of the second year. Finally, if physician compensation is based on capitation or a combination of capitation and a periodic fixed fee, the term may not exceed 5 years, and it must be terminable without cause by the hospital at the end of the third year.

Covenant Not to Compete

Covenants not to compete are common in partnership agreements and typically prohibit a departing party, whose partnership relationship is terminated, from engaging in any activity that is competitive with or adverse to the interest of the protected activity within a certain geographic area and for a specified period of time. Although these contractual provisions are generally enforced in many states, the laws of 28 states do not *expressly* enforce a noncompetition requirement to professions and instead only prohibit such practice limitations to business, trade, and commerce. The enforceability of noncompetition agreements in these jurisdictions is governed by the "rule of reason."

In the context of a joint venture, the rule of reason first asks whether the joint venture has a legitimate interest that warrants the court's protection. Here, the party seeking enforcement of the noncompetition clause most commonly asserts that the "protectible interest" is the need to prevent patients from following a departing physician. This argument is further strengthened if the departing physician was provided with confidential business information, training, or patient contacts. Most states regard a practice's patient base as a protectible asset and may support the joint venture's right to prevent the departing physician from soliciting its patients. On an individual patient basis, however, this right would not likely be supported because the conflicting right of the patient to select his or her own physician generally has priority over the practice's business rights. The distinction may lie in whether the departing physician actively solicited the patient of the previous practice or whether the patient took the initiative to seek care from the departing physician.

The second query in a rule of reason analysis is whether the limitations of time, geography, and scope of practice are broader than necessary to protect the employer's interest. The time duration of the covenant not to compete should be no longer than is necessary for the joint venture to recruit replacements and for the replacements to have a reasonable opportunity to demonstrate their effectiveness. Durations between 1 and 3 years are generally found acceptable by most courts. The appropriate geographic scope of the limitation is designed to protect the area in which the joint venture markets its medical services to the public. Although specific distances from a site of service are frequently cited, the unique characteristics of each situation require individual consideration. Generally, a departing physician is permitted to practice medicine within the restricted area as long as the departing physician's specialty is not offered by the former employer. For example, an emergency physician would still be able to provide urgent care within the time and geographic limitations as long as urgent care services were not provided by the joint venture.

A final consideration is whether the enforcement of the limitation would harm the public. For example, if a departing emergency physician in an underserved community was barred from practicing for 3 years within many miles of the joint venture, the court could determined that the community's need for an adequate number of emergency physicians outweighed the public interest in upholding a contract freely agreed to by private parties. In balancing the public interest in competition in the healthcare market against the public interest in freedom to contract, the court could hold the limitation unenforceable.

Medical Staff Privileges

Some hospital participants propose that the emergency physicians agree that their medical staff membership and privileges in emergency medicine terminate simultaneously with the contract. This "clean sweep" provision should be rejected. Although this practice may have operational practicality and legal standing in hospital-based exclusive arrangements, it is unlikely to serve any justifiable purpose in the context of the joint venture.

Title to Assets

The contract should state who holds title to any tangible assets used or developed by the venture both during and after its term. The contract also should define rights to intangible assets such as accounts receivable; forms, processes, and procedures developed as a part of the venture; and trade or business names when the venture terminates. As mentioned, deductions for depreciation cannot be shifted from the hospital to the physician participant. The contract must recognize that the facilities and equipment remain the property of the contributing participant because no new entity is created through which the tangible assets of the joint venture can be owned. Subsequent purchases of tangible assets can have shared ownership only to the extent that participants contributed capital for its purchase. If income from the joint venture is used for the acquisition, ownership of the asset is allocated in the same proportion if the income had been distributed to those participants.

Right to Audit

Each participant should have the right to inspect the books and records of the joint venture at his or her own expense. Although authorization of the participant implies that this right extends to the participant's accountant, attorney, or agent, it is recommended that the language clearly refer to the "participant or designated agent."

Other Contractual Issues and Terms

The legal terms of art throughout the contract and the "standard" provisions at the end of most contracts often receive insufficient attention until the participants need to resolve a dispute. The term *representation* refers to a statement of truth as of the date of the contract. A *warranty* is a guarantee that the statement will remain true in the future. An *assignment or transfer* of the rights or duties from one participant to a party not contemplated in the contract is nearly always prohibited without the written consent of the other party. The Social Security Act requires a provision that allows the Department of Health and Human Services, the Comptroller of the United States, or their representative access to any books or records necessary to verify the cost of services rendered to Medicare beneficiaries under the contract.

Joint venture contracts may include provisions such as the state law that will govern the contract, the jurisdiction where any dispute will be litigated, the manner in which the contract may be modified, and language of arbitration and other special dispute resolution. These issues and terms should be understood with the same depth as the other substantive provisions of the contract.

SPECIFIC LEGAL AND REGULATORY PROBLEM AREAS

Antitrust

Antitrust laws are designed to protect free competition in the marketplace. Since their first passage in the 1890, antitrust laws have not historically been applied to healthcare delivery, partly because of a belief that competition did not apply to the medical professions and partly because healthcare has been viewed historically as more akin to a charity or a public utility. This serene backdrop changed in the last few decades with two dramatic developments. In 1982, the Supreme Court ruled that the medical profession is not immune from the enforcement of antitrust laws. Then, increased social demands and technologic advances infused the healthcare industry with tremendous growth and financial opportunities and vaulted it into a rapidly evolving era of competition, commercialization, and regulation. Although much joint venture activity in healthcare delivery is recognized to be efficiency enhancing, special care must be given to those circumstances in joint ventures that may run afoul of antitrust laws.

Violations of the federal antitrust laws embodied in the Sherman Act, the Clayton Act, and the Federal Trade Commission Act may be charged by the Federal Trade Commission, the Department of Justice, or aggrieved private parties. In addition to these federal laws, many states have adopted their own antitrust statutes, which are commonly referred to "Little Sherman" acts. Antitrust issues are complex, and their analysis depends on the particular facts of each situation. The focus is whether a collaborative arrangement qualifies as a bona fide venture and is not a sham designed to accomplish otherwise unlawful cartel behavior. This section introduces the general principles and some potential antitrust violations particularly applicable to joint ventures involving emergency physicians.

The courts will apply one of two standards in judging the wide array of possible anticompetitive behaviors and settings. The *per se* rule applies to antitrust behavior that has no plausible procompetitive justification. These "naked" restraints on trade are considered pernicious and deserving of criminal prosecution. Under the strict *per se* standard, the court will find an antitrust violation if the basic elements of the prohibited violation are present and will give no consideration to extenuating circumstances. If conduct is judged under the *per se* test, even the legitimate intent of the joint venture to promote innovative, lower cost methods of delivering care will not protect the venture. Increasingly, however, conduct alleged to violate the antitrust laws is judged under the "rule of reason." This standard permits the effects of an activity to be balanced against the harm to competition. If the conduct is judged under the rule of reason test, the venture's activities are balanced against its anticompetitive effects and may help bolster a finding that the venture activity is reasonable under antitrust principles.

Section 1 of the Sherman Act prohibits conduct that constitutes a "contract, combination, or conspiracy in restraint of trade." A joint venture is particularly vulnerable to this kind of antitrust scrutiny because it involves a concerted, planned activity by two or more parties who have only joined together to affect the competitive marketplace. A joint venture may involve competing (e.g., multiple emergency physician groups) or noncompeting (e.g., an emergency physician group and a hospital) participants. Generally, antitrust risk is greater when the participants are competitors.

An express or implied agreement among the participants of the joint venture exists to refer patients to the joint venture to the exclusion of its competitors may a violation of Section 1 of the Sherman Act. For example, the primary care physician participants of a free-standing emergency clinic may agree to refer their patients to that facility rather than the hospital emergency room or other emergency facilities. As long as the agreement does not involve price-fixing or market allocation (an agreement among competitors not to compete in certain market sectors), the rule of reason is applied. Assuming that such an agreement existed, a court would weigh the proportion of physicians involved from the community and nature of the restraint—limiting referrals only to the venture—against any possible market efficiencies that could be achieved only by such an agreement.

Joint ventures among actual or potential competitors in which there is a price-fixing agreement to set maximum or minimum prices or to stabilize prices will likely be scrutinized under the stricter *per se* test. Price-fixing conduct distorts the natural market force that sets prices based on the quality of and the demand for the service or product. It controls the market pricing mechanism by exerting pressure on competitors to artificially lower their charges. Illegal price-fixing conduct also may be found in manipulative advertising or the exchange of price information among competitors.

There may be an illegal "nonhorizontal potential competition merger" violative of antitrust laws if the participants are a hospital with an emergency facility and an emergency physician group. Here, the joint venture is organized in a market where one participant already provides the service. A court would consider (1) whether the hospital already had a significant share of the market (generally more than 30%); (2) whether the market for emergency facilities was highly concentrated among few providers; and (3) whether the hospital, the physician group, or another party would have entered the market independently and deconcentrated the market had the joint venture not been formed.

Generally, antitrust concerns raise questions of the market power held by the joint venture during its operation and the market power held by the participants at the time of its formation. Theoretically, when the percentages of market share and concentration are high during the operation of the joint venture, market competition in terms of quality and price would lessen as a result of fewer competitors. When the percentages are high at the formation of the joint venture and the participants become even more entrenched in the market, the fear is that barriers to entry will result for other potential competitors. In response, it is argued that the emergency services would not have been provided at all, if not for the formation of the joint venture because of the large requirement for capital investment or the high degree of risk.

Medicare Reimbursement for Services

Emergency physicians are typically organized in integrated group practices from which they receive salaries and through which they bill for their services. In a joint venture, the fundamental issue is whether legal identity of the billing individual or group is the emergency physician or the joint venture. Ideally, a contract model joint venture bills the patient's insurance carrier and receives payments in its own name. Although this plan simplifies the control and the allocation of payments and may be important for tax purposes, it is not always possible to carry out. State license laws may dictate that only an entity licensed in certain categories (e.g., hospital, clinic, or physician) may bill for services within the scope of licensure. In addition, governmental programs such as Medicare limit the ability of physicians to transfer the right to bill other entities.

The Medicare program is an indemnity insurance, in which the physician bills the patient for services and the patient submits the charge to Medicare for reimbursement. Medicare allows the patient to "assign" payment to the individual physician who provided the treatment. That is, the physician may bill Medicare directly for the service in the patient's name. Attention should be given to the Medicare limitation of the right of the physician who accepts assignment to *reassign* this right to bill and to receive payments to other entities (such as a joint venture). Medicare limits this reassignment to the physician's employer, an inpatient facility in which the services are rendered, an entity referred to as an "organized health care delivery system," or, under certain circumstances, a billing agent. An entity accepting reassignment is required to have a separate Medicare provider number.

Local Medicare representatives (i.e., the Medicare carrier) may have discretion in designating the contract model joint venture as an "organized health care delivery system," issuing a separate Part B Medicare provider number, and permitting reassignment from the individual physician or group to the joint venture. Their determination is based on the joint venture's structure, local laws, and local Medicare policy. The local Medicare carrier and other insurance carriers should be consulted before a joint venture is formed to ensure in advance that third-party benefits are reassigned to the joint venture.

Other issues related to Medicare billing include the requirement that physicians participating in Medicare are obligated to accept Medicare assignment on *all* eligible claims. Medicare participation agreements bind all signatory physicians to accept assignment at all delivery sites at which they practice. Failure to do so may result in serious sanctions. Notwithstanding, possible exceptions may exist if the physician practices through different legal entities at different sites. A physician who intends to decline Medicare assignment for services rendered through the joint venture and accept Medicare assignment through another entity must analyze the Medicare implications carefully. In addition, governmental payer billing rules for the use of the physician extenders as an incidental part of physician services must be considered. Medicare's "incident-to" billing rules, for example, require that the physician employ the physician extender or that they have a common employer.

Prohibitions against Payment for Referrals

In a joint venture, the allocation of the financial proceeds to nonventure participants must be structured carefully to ensure compliance with prohibitions against the payment for patient referrals. Laws prohibiting payment for patient referrals are designed to prevent abuses related to overutilization and unnecessary referrals. Fear of these abuses arises when the referring physician has a financial interest in providing a high volume of referrals to the joint venture. Although this may make business sense in other industries, in medicine there is a conflict of interest between the referring physician and patient, which may lead to unnecessary referrals. Although a joint venture may market to physicians for patient referrals, it cannot pay for those referrals. The distribution of joint venture funds and profits cannot be based on the revenue generated from referrals by any participant. Rather, funds and profits must be distributed by ownership and equity considerations documented in the joint venture contract. Nonparticipants cannot be compensated, directly or indirectly, for referring patients to the venture.

Federal Medicare regulations prohibit the knowing and willful solicitation, receipt, offer, or payment of any remuneration in return for the referral of an individual for a service covered by Medicare. Many states have similar laws. Remuneration is broadly defined to encompass virtually anything of value that may be made directly or indirectly. As of 1993 the federal government published "safe harbors" from the fraud and abuse laws that prohibit, among other things, the payment for patient referrals. Because no safe harbor expressly covers a contract model joint venture, whenever a provider has a financial relationship with another provider involving the referral of patients to one of those providers, there will be a factual question as to whether there is any violation of the fraud and abuse laws. Although individual states may have their own particular requirements, general guidelines for avoiding violations of fraud and abuse laws include the following:

- Payments to venture participants cannot be tied to a requirement to refer patients. Payments cannot be "volume sensitive"—tied directly or indirectly to the number of referrals or to the revenue generated from those referrals. Payments should not be dependent on admissions, referrals, or a percentage of revenues or profits.
- Payments made to any referral source, whether or not a participant, can be made only for valid services actually rendered. Charges for "processing" must be bona fide.
- The services for which a referral source is compensated must have been medically or administratively necessary. The value and the actual performance of the services must be documented accurately.
- Payment should be made only for those services that are commonly performed in the medical community under similar circumstances, absent the joint venture.
- Payment made to a referral source for additional services must be appropriate for the qualification of the referring individual and reasonable in amount when compared with payment for similar services in the locality.

To the extent that a particular joint venture departs from the simple contract model, other more complicated factors must be analyzed to avoid state and federal referral payment sanctions. Violations can result in serious administrative and criminal penalties.

Prohibitions Against Self-Referral

Physicians are often in a unique position to identify an unmet medical need in their community, to participate in some form of a joint venture to serve this need, and to ensure quality by their own participation in the provision of service. Unfortunately, these valid justifications are accompanied by the same risks of abuses described in the prohibitions against payment for referrals. When patient referrals involve an ownership interest in the joint venture, the nexus between the number of referrals and the physician's financial return raises the familiar concerns that the referring physician may be motivated by the financial profit rather than the best interests of the patient. As a result, many states have regulations that prohibit any form of self-referral without notice to the beneficiary of the referring physician's beneficial or ownership interest.

The federal law known as "Stark II," which became effective on January 1, 1995, prohibits referrals of and claims for Medicare and Medicaid covered services for a designated health service by physicians who are involved through ownership interests, compensation arrangements, or both. Although the designated health services do not include emergency departments, urgent care centers, or ambulatory surgical centers, it does include outpatient hospital services. The ownership or investment interest is broadly defined and could be debt, equity, or any compensation arrangement between the entity and the physician. The remuneration can be direct or indirect, overt or covert, cash or in kind. The indirect remuneration specifically refers to an ownership interest in the parent of a designated health entity subject to Stark II. It is arguable whether this includes other situations such as ownership of an entity that invests in a designated health entity.

Generally, the federal self-referral laws prohibiting physicians participation in emergency services joint ventures probably should not apply because of exemptions for emergency departments. (42 U.S.C. § 1395nn) The joint venture also may be exempt if its geographic area is "rural" or if the referring physician personally provides the service. Nonetheless, given the complexity of the exceptions, legal counsel should be sought to ensure compliance with the federal and individual state self-referral prohibitions.

Corporate Practice of Medicine and Fee-Splitting

Many state have laws that prohibit the corporate practice of medicine and bar a physician from rendering professional services as an employee of a nonphysician enterprise on the theory that the nonphysician employer might interfere with the physician-patient relationship. Concerns about potential violations of this doctrine arise most often when the joint venture involves a nonphysician corporate entity such as a hospital. Although the corporate participants of the joint venture argue that they exert no control over the physicians' medical decisions, there is a fear that much lay influence remains. Because emergency services joint ventures are typically operated for profit, physician loyalty is confronted with the occasionally competing interests of the patient's welfare and the venture's commercial motives. Technically, when the corporate participant contracts for physician services, the corporate practice prohibition laws are avoided. Still, the physician must take care not to allow the corporate participant in the joint venture to exert inappropriate control over the physician and thereby practice medicine.

Many state laws prohibit splitting fees for professional services (as distinguished from the technical component) between a physician and a nonphysician. Aside from allocation of the joint venture's proceeds, these laws typically recognize that the emergency physician may pay a fee for actual and necessary administrative services such as billing, personnel, marketing, contracting, and accounting. The amount charged must be within the range of the demonstrable market rate for such services, and the services must be of a type that is customary and usual in the field.

Retirement Plan Issues

Certain joint ventures may have a detrimental effect on the tax-qualified status of retirement plans maintained by emergency physician participants. Joint venture arrangements constituting an "affiliated service group" within the meaning of Section 414(m) of the Internal Revenue Code are at risk. An "affiliated service group" is defined as a group in which all employees of each participant within the affiliation are treated as having one common employer, thereby requiring a single retirement plan. If a joint venture is an affiliated service group and does not meet certain guidelines such as the minimum participation test, the retirement plans of joint venture participants who have only a few employees will likely fail the test and be disqualified.

Disqualification results in immediate taxability of the vested benefits of all participants and loss of tax deductibility for plan contributions. These considerations will be of significant concern for emergency physicians evaluating any proposed joint venture.

SUMMARY

The merits of the joint venture deserve the serious attention of physicians who practice emergency medicine. The unique structure of a contract model joint venture dictates that special care must be given to thorough negotiations and accurate drafting. Even after the joint venture is operational, its ramifications must be carefully scrutinized because the dynamics and economics of healthcare delivery are increasingly complex and rapidly changing.

41 Contracting with Managed Care

Thom A. Mayer and Stephen J. Dresnick

OUTLINE

The emergence of managed care represents a fundamental change in the funding and operational management of healthcare. Like all major changes, this one has been variably greeted by healthcare providers, including physicians and hospitals, with everything from denial and antipathy to enthusiasm. The transition to managed care as a primary funding and operational strategy has been driven by several sources. First are employers, who are painfully aware that the cost of healthcare insurance premiums per employee doubled between 1984 and 1992, from $1800 to nearly $4000.[1] From a macroeconomic standpoint, healthcare costs accounted for 14% of the gross national product in 1994, a percentage that will grow to 17% to 18% by the year 2000 unless such costs are reined in.[2] For many employers, every dollar saved in employee healthcare costs translates to an additional dollar in pretax profits. As American business and industry struggle to remain competitive, such savings in healthcare costs assume increasing importance. The initial experience of employers with managed care organizations (MCOs) and other prepaid healthcare options has resulted in stabilization and, in some cases, actual reductions in employer costs for healthcare benefits. Overall, between 1991 and 1995 annual premium increases for health maintenance organizations (HMOs) have been 35% to 40% less than increases for preferred provider organizations (PPOs) and indemnity insurance plans.[3]

Managed care is not a new concept, dating back nearly 65 years. The earliest efforts at prepaid group practice plans include the rural farmers cooperative in Oklahoma in 1929, Group Health Association in Washington in 1937, Kaiser Permanente's medical care programs in 1942 in California, the Group Health Cooperative of Puget Sound in Seattle in 1947, the Health Insurance Plan of Greater New York in 1947, and the Group Health Plan of Minneapolis in 1957.[4,5] However, despite the fact that HMOs have a long history, their most explosive growth has occurred in the last 10 years. In 1980, less than 10 million people were covered in HMOs, a figure that has grown to over 50 million in 1995[6] (Figure 41-1). The growth of managed care plans has largely come at the expense of commercial or indemnity insurance markets. As the insurers themselves develop strategies that transfer some or all financial risk to the healthcare provider, most have developed prepaid healthcare alternatives to their indemnity insurance products. Most major insurers now offer several different healthcare plans, ranging from straight, fee-for-service indemnity insurance to fully developed HMO products.

An additional source of growth for managed care as a funding strategy has been legislative in nature. Legislative initiatives that presaged the managed care movement include the 1995 Congressional enactment of title XVIII and XIX Medicare and Medicaid legislation, the 1982 Health Care Financing Administration (HCFA) implementation of diagnosis-related groups (DRGs), and the 1992 HCFA use of the Resource-Based Relative Value Scale (RBRVS). Despite the cataclysmic change that each of these pieces of legislation represents, however, none in and of themselves constituted eroded essential fee-for-service structure under which American Medicine has operated for decades. In 1973, Congress enacted the HMO Act, which ostensibly did little more than allow HMOs to enter the Medicare and Medicaid markets. States such as Minnesota and California, however, quickly followed this legislation with similar state statutes that at least allowed (and most would agree encouraged) enrollment of patients into prepaid healthcare options. Finally, the raging healthcare debate in 1992 and 1993 focused even more attention on HMOs, PPOs, and other forms of prepaid healthcare options. In particular, the concept of managed competition, as espoused by the Jackson Hole Group, received par-

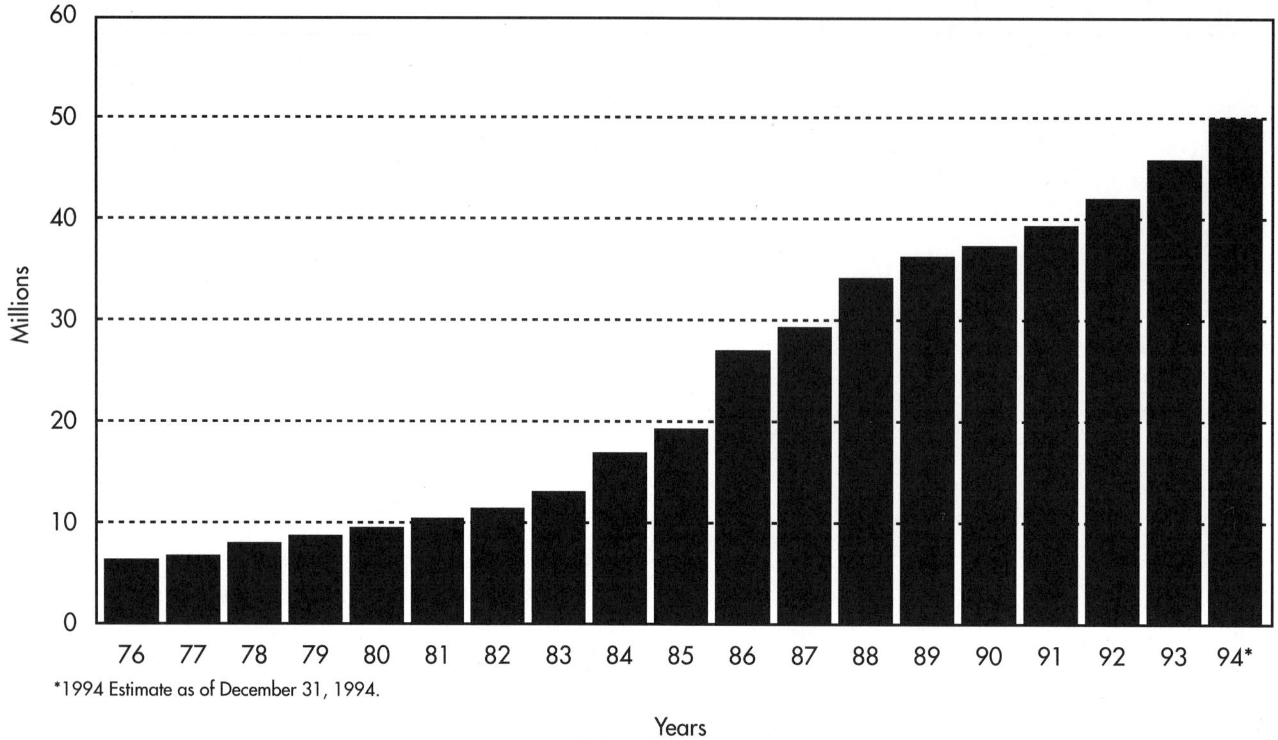

FIGURE 41-1 Number of people receiving their care in an HMO (1976-1994).* *1994 estimate as of December 31, 1994.

(From: Health Affairs (Summer 1988) (1976-1987), CHAA's National Directory of HMO's database (1988-1993), CHAA's 1994 Market Position Report (1994).)

ticular attention and discussion.[7] Although legislation at the federal and state levels have not mandated a move towards managed care, they have caused employers and others to consider managed care as an option to lower overall healthcare costs. Whatever form healthcare reform takes, the primary healthcare progress (government and employees) will continue to shift responsibility for managing healthcare costs onto private healthcare plans, just as the plans will shift costs and expenditures onto the providers through capitation or fixed price contracts and onto the subscriber through cost-sharing, co-payments, and other strategies.

Perhaps the strongest force in the growth of managed care has been the effect of managed care providers capturing large market segments and its subsequent effect on hospitals, physicians, and other healthcare providers. As employers have discovered that there are potential cost savings in employee health benefits with MCOs, hospitals and physicians have recognized that MCO payors wield substantial clout in most healthcare markets. The economic impact of MCOs are particularly important at a time when the hospital industry has felt additional pressure with regard to lowering costs. Hospitals are attempting to increase market share and keep available beds occupied. Hospitals will then increase their participation in managed care plans to capture a larger market share.

DEFINITION OF MANAGED CARE

Although *managed care* is a widely used term, it encompasses an extraordinarily wide range of healthcare funding alternatives. These alternatives are defined later, but there are certain common features to each that cause them to fall under the managed care rubric. Managed care contracting is a healthcare funding mechanism that transfers healthcare risk by contracting selectively with healthcare providers to whom patients will be preferentially referred, in return for which the provider agrees to participate in less costly, more efficient patterns of care. Thus, the essential features of a managed care organization are the following:

1. Transfers risk to the provider
2. Contracts selectively
3. Preferentially refers patients to less costly providers

Each of these elements deserves some discussion.

The transfer of risk from the plan to the provider is in many respects the most important aspect of managed care organizations. The precise form of this transfer of risk varies widely according to the type of MCO, maturity of the plan in the specific market, and other factors. Regardless of structure, however, MCOs need to transfer risk to the provider through disincentives to overuse. Under indemnity insurance plans, the insurer assumed virtually all risk and providers were paid on a fee-for-service basis. In managed care plans, this risk is shared and/or transferred from the plan to the providers, including hospitals and physicians.

MCOs contract selectively both with their patients and with providers who will deliver or manage the care of such patients. With certain exceptions, MCOs, like most insurance companies, prefer to contract with populations that have a specified (low) risk for the development of disease and consumption of healthcare resources.[8] However, as MCOs have matured, establishment of risk pools and acceptance of risk for elderly and low income patients have become more widely accepted. MCOs contract selectively with providers as well and in all cases attempt to establish a group of hospitals, physicians, and other healthcare providers who agree contractually to accept patients who are preferentially referred, and to do so in exchange for acceptance of certain risks on the part of the provider. Precisely how selective the managed care organization is in its contracting depends on both the MCO itself and on local factors. For example, a given MCO may contract with all emergency department providers within a given area, or it may choose to affiliate with either a smaller number, or in some cases, a single emergency department. The ability of the MCO to direct patients to a specific emergency department is questionable, but is an important factor in understanding the essential relationship between the MCO and the emergency department group.

The third aspect of the relationship, the ability to preferentially refer patients to the provider, is much different for an emergency department than it is for either primary care physicians or specialists. Although there are often similar relationships with regard to co-payments or deductibles for patients who seek services (emergency or otherwise) outside of the plan, the ability of an MCO to specifically direct its patients to an emergency department is difficult except in mature managed care markets in which highly controlled preauthorization procedures have been put into place between the MCO and the patient.

TYPES OF MANAGED CARE ORGANIZATIONS

MCOs vary widely in their essential structure, mode of operation, and mechanisms for transfer of risks, incentives, and funding. The taxonomy of such organizations is necessarily somewhat arbitrary, but the following definitions provide a general framework through which plans can be characterized.

Indemnity Insurance

Traditional indemnity insurance is practiced under a fee-for-service model, in which providers (both physicians and hospitals) bill the insurance company for the specific services provided to the patient. Patients often have deductibles or co-payments associated with indemnity insurance, but the essential feature is that providers are paid on a fee-for-service basis according to the volume of patients seen. Indemnity insurance plans therefore take into account the risk profile of the patients insured and pay to the providers those fees agreed to for services deemed as covered under the contractual relationship between the insurance carrier and the patient and the insurance carrier and the provider. Indemnity insurance is subject to utilization review and quality assurance, but these have traditionally had little impact on either the total cash outlay from the plan to the providers or in altering practice patterns of physicians. For understandable reasons, insurance companies have moved away from offering indemnity insurance as their sole product because it is extremely difficult to control costs, referral patterns, or physician practice patterns in such a plan.

Managed Indemnity

As healthcare funding mechanisms have evolved, some indemnity plans have changed their operational details, while retaining the essential structure of a fee-for-service relationship. Managed indemnity plans usually involve some discounts by the provider, as well as more stringent utilization review and quality assurance. In some cases, managed indemnity has begun to develop clinical pathways, but these are rarely contractually agreed to. The managed indemnity option is a relatively small, first step toward risk sharing and control of the healthcare dollar.

Preferred Provider Organization

PPOs are managed care entities that contract with providers for discounted services, in return for which the PPO preferentially directs enrollees to those providers. In most cases, the discount is from the fee-for-service schedule (whether the PPO's schedule or the provider's schedule), as opposed to a strict capitation agreement. In most PPOs, the providers have agreed to a negotiated charge level and are prevented from balance billing patients at a higher rate. Patients are encouraged to select providers from within the plan by disincentives such as co-payments, deductibles, or balance billing directly to the patient by physicians who are "out of plan."

Patients typically have a wider selection of physicians in PPO arrangements as opposed to HMO arrangements. In the past, the majority of PPO contractors were not technically insurance companies, but rather entities that contracted with insurers or self-insured employers and with providers in an effort to help negotiate reduced costs for services. The distinction between PPOs and HMOs, however, is decreasing in many markets as PPOs have required enrollees to use specified primary care physicians (PCP) as gatekeepers to specialty referral and utilization.

Point of Service Plans

Point of service plans encompass features from both PPOs and HMOs. In most cases, these plans attempt to blend the strengths and weaknesses of PPOs and HMOs. Point of service plans use financial incentives to encourage enrollees to remain in network for care through the use of gatekeeper PCPs. For those patients who stay within the network, the PCP manages all care, controls subspecialty referral, and thereby reduces cost. The majority of point of service plans continue to allow patients to self-refer outside of the network, but with higher deductibles, co-payments, lower benefit schedules, and/or the ability of the out-of-network physician to balance bill. Many point of service plans thus represent one further step in the evolution toward increasing control and transfer of risk than PPOs or managed indemnity options. Although utilization management, quality assurance, and quality improvement are used in point of service plans, the very nature of the contractual relationship does not allow for total control of healthcare costs.

Independent Practice Association

The independent practice association (IPA) concept allows individual physicians or physician groups to participate in managed care, while retaining their practice in their own office. An IPA is typically an entity collectively contracting with employers or insurers and with physicians who provide both primary and specialty care services. Early on, IPAs were similar in many respects to managed indemnity plans in that they rely on discounted fee-for-service systems, but most have moved aggressively toward risk-sharing contracts, including fully capitated contracts. Currently, most PCPs in IPAs are paid a capitation payment for primary care case management. Specialists are paid in variable ways, from capitation arrangements to discounted fee-for-service contracts. Because of the wide variation in utilization rates, it has been more difficult to establish capitation rates for specialists, as opposed to primary care physicians, in which the average number of office visits and inpatient hospital days can be calculated more easily.[9] In some cases, IPAs have further developed into so-called "clinics without walls," in which the contracting entity allows physicians to practice independently, but in which it assumes variable control over the assets of the physicians' practices. In some cases, the clinic without walls owns the physicians assets, including buildings, equipment, and accounts receivable, while providing all necessary administrative support to the practice. In other cases, physicians have retained control of their assets while relinquishing contractual negotiating authority to the entity itself.

Health Maintenance Organizations

HMOs represent a more fully integrated financial, administrative, and medical delivery system, including aligned incentives for the providers, increased risk transfer as the primary reimbursement strategy, and establishment of more fully developed healthcare networks to deliver care while minimizing risk. There are four main types of HMOs:

- *IPA Model HMO:* These entities contract with individual physicians to deliver services to specified enrollees, but physicians continue to practice in their own office settings and can also contract with other providers, including, fee-for-service plans and other HMOs. IPA model HMOs typically contract with several health plans and providers. In most cases, IPAs are not strictly considered HMOs in the sense that there is less control, less aligned incentives, and less acceptance of the full risk transfer concept. However, some plans still refer to themselves as IPA model HMOs, so this classification is included here. Over time, it is likely that such plans will evolve into more fully controlled, risk transfer payment mechanisms.
- *Network Model HMO:* The network model HMO is similar to the IPA model, but differs in that the HMO usually contracts with several multispecialty medical groups in an effort to help establish a specified "network" through which patients can be selectively referred in a more predictable fashion. In general, network model HMOs are further along in the risk transfer concept, including capitation for primary care physicians and/or specialists.
- *Group Model HMO:* A group model HMO involves a single, multispecialty physician group contracting with the insurer to provide more comprehensive services. The group typically agrees to establish case management and patient care protocols, quality assurance and peer review, utilization management standards, and, in most cases, at least limited clinical guidelines and practice standards. Many group model HMOs contract with multiple insurers.
- *Staff Model HMOs:* The staff model HMO is in many respects the most developed of HMO models, including salaried physicians who agree to deliver services exclusively to the patients of the staff model, usually in hospitals and/or clinics owned by the HMO. Staff model HMOs have strong incentives for physicians to decrease the cost of utilization and therefore are among the most cost-effective HMO models. In many cases, there may be specified "carve-outs" for highly specialized services such as cardiac surgery, transplants, mental health, pediatric intensive care, etc.

Integrated Delivery Systems

The development of integrated delivery systems (IDS) in some respects arose as a result of the development of HMOs. Simply stated, HMOs have as their core business managing and contracting for the delivery of comprehensive healthcare services in a given healthcare market. IDS were developed in response to the success of many HMOs in capturing substantial market share.[10] The IDS is a group of affiliated organizations that attempts to provide a full continuum of care, including hospital, physician, home health, long-term care, and related ancillary services through specified contract providers. The most sophisticated of such systems include substantial aspects of preventive medicine, home healthcare, hospice care, skilled nursing, rehabilitation, and long-term care, as well as the more traditional provision of office-based hospital services for patients. In many cases, the IDS does not own all of the assets or resources within its system, but instead relies on affiliation and/or contractual relationships to ensure that the continuum of healthcare can be provided cost efficiently. At its essence, the development of an IDS requires strong cooperation among primary care physicians, hospitals in healthcare organizations, and subspecialty physicians and strong administrative systems that allow for contractual, administrative, and operational networks to deliver care. Integrated delivery systems involve both horizontal (among physician providers) and vertical integration, including inpatient, outpatient, long-term care, and home health systems. Figure 41-2 illustrates one structure of an IDS. The evolution of integrated delivery systems represents several opportunities for emergency medicine (Box 41-1).

First and most important, it is important for emergency physician groups to assess the value of participating in an ownership role in the IDS, because this is the level at which control, decision making, and financial arbitrage occur. In such arrangements, the level of reward is usually strictly commensurate with the level of risk. Second, participation in an IDS facilitates emergency department group practice diversification (see Part 8) in areas such as observation services, ICU coverage, pediatric emergency medicine, telephone triage, and transport medicine. Third, emergency physicians will find themselves participating in the critical role of gatekeeper for many elements of the IDS, including after-hours and weekend services. For all of these reasons, emergency physician groups need to begin to put programs and systems in place today to be prepared for the evolution of integrated delivery systems of tomorrow. This includes assumption of risk sharing contracting, developing financial and information services, and structuring payments to realign incentives.

THE CONTINUUM OF RISK AND CONTROL

From a practical standpoint, healthcare funding mechanisms have evolved from systems with low control, unaligned incentives, and little in the way of transfer of risk from the

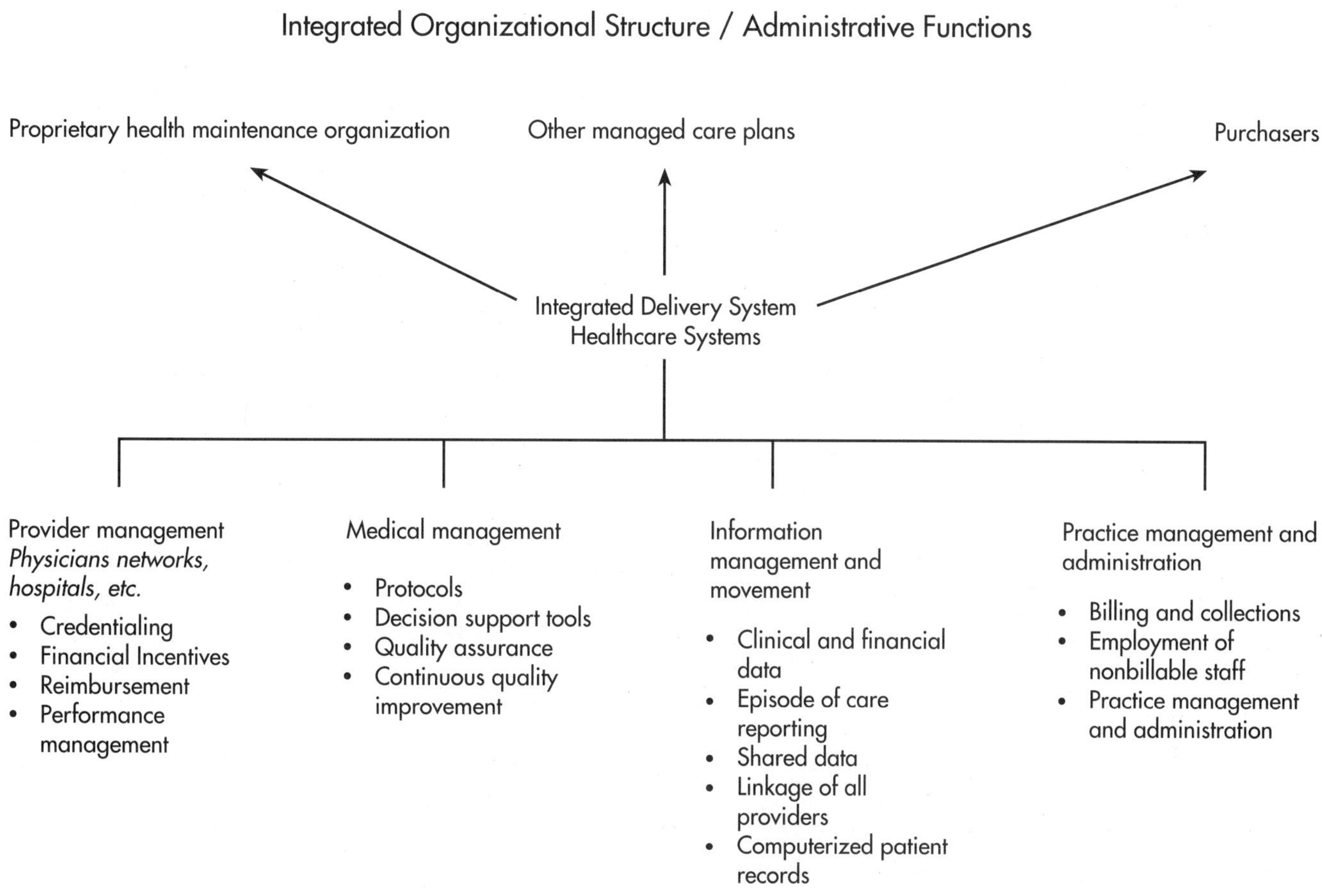

FIGURE 41-2 Integrated delivery system (IDS) involves horizontal integration (among physicians) and vertical integration with other areas of the healthcare system.

BOX 41-1

OPPORTUNITIES FOR EMERGENCY MEDICINE AND INTEGRATED DELIVERY SYSTEMS

1. The future is having an ownership stake in integrated delivery systems to participate in savings arbitrage.
2. The level of reward will be commensurate with the level of risk.
3. The control of additional services will translate to additional income (e.g., observation units, inpatient services, ICU coverage, telephone triage, transport medicine, pediatric emergency medicine).
4. Emergency medicine will participate as gatekeepers, responsible for significant savings to the integrated delivery system.
5. Emergency medicine must develop programs and systems today and be prepared for the integrated delivery systems of tomorrow.
6. Information systems must be put in place to measure savings and/or differences in outcome.
7. Payments should be structured to realign incentives.
8. Start small to minimize failure and build on success.

insurer/payor to the provider. Similarly, there has traditionally been little in the way of quality improvement, clinical pathways, preventive services, use of data acquisition to augment risk transfer, and coordination of networks of healthcare into integrated systems. As healthcare markets have progressed, MCOs have horizontally and vertically developed healthcare funding and operational patient care systems that have fully aligned incentives, full risk transfer, and substantial control over healthcare expenditures. Figure 41-3 illustrates continuum of risk and control among the types of MCOs listed previously.

CONTRACTING WITH MANAGED CARE: THE HOSPITAL ADMINISTRATION VIEW

For most hospitals, contracting with MCOs forms an essential part of their strategic plan. The growth and leverage that MCOs have undergone wield a substantial financial power in most healthcare marketplaces. As hospital-based physicians, emergency physicians should be well aware of the views of the hospital administration and hospital governance with regard to contracting with MCOs. In all cases, emergency physician groups should prospectively meet with members of administration to discuss the overall strategy for managed care, including a clear understanding of which plans are viewed as key strategic partners for the hospital. Emergency physicians should be aware of the number of covered lives

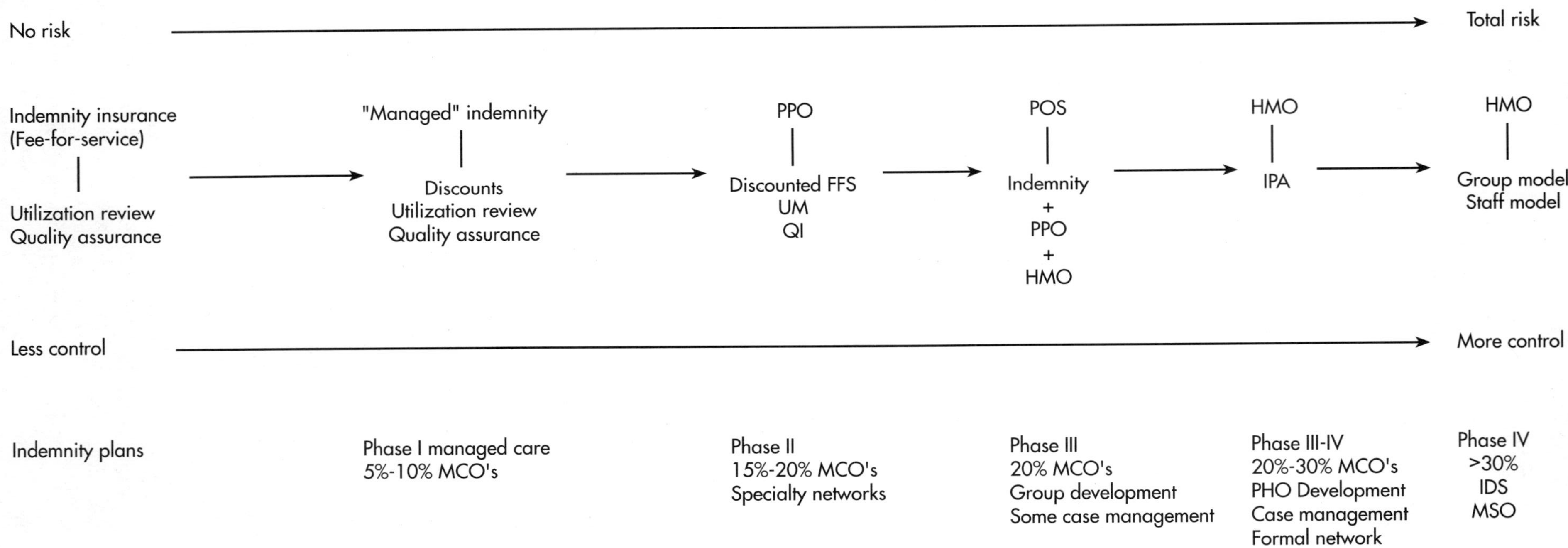

FIGURE 41-3 A continuum of risk and control in managed care organizations. Managed care organizations represent a continuum of control and risk, ranging from indemnity insurance plans to fully capitated HMO models. Each MCO should be assessed independently to determine its place on this continuum. Managed care markets are graded in phases I to IV depending on percentage of market share, transfer of risk, and increase in control through development of PHOs, MSOs and IDS.

(PPO, Preferred provider organization; POS, point of service; IPA, independent practice association; HMO, health maintenance organization; PHO, physician hospital organization; MSO, medical/management services organization; IDS, integrated delivery system.)

held by each specific plan and any additional details regarding their contractual relationships with the hospital that would be of importance in negotiating a managed care plan. Many healthcare organizations now have specific divisions of managed care, with administrative personnel who focus their efforts nearly exclusively on managed care issues. The emergency physician group should become familiar with these individuals and meet with them regularly to help understand their perspective on the growing managed care market.

Whenever possible, discussions with administration should help establish a relationship in which the emergency department group is given the opportunity to negotiate in good faith directly with the MCO, as opposed to having the hospital complete all such negotiations. By stressing common ground, the emergency physician group can usually negotiate a fair and equitable relationship with managed care, but which also helps protect the interest of the hospital in contracting with specific MCOs. For example, emergency physicians need to stress several important points in the course of such discussion.

First, the emergency department is the "front door" to the healthcare system for many patients and therefore represents an excellent opportunity for the emergency physicians to act as representatives of both the hospital and the MCO in dealing with patients. For that reason, it is to the advantage of the emergency physician group, the MCO, and the hospital to ensure that negotiations are handled in a mutually beneficial fashion.

Second, it is often useful to point out to hospital administrators and representatives of MCOs that the total cash outlay for emergency department professional fees is actually quite small compared to fees for anesthesia, radiology, and pathology, much less those of subspecialty groups that may be consulted. This is an important aspect because the emergency physician is in a position to control and/or substantially affect use of other resources, including ancillary services, referral to subspecialists, and fee-for-hospital admissions.

By stressing that emergency physicians have strong principles of group management, application of sound business principles, cost-containment measures, and a history of cooperation with managed care, emergency department groups can gain substantial leverage in the course of contract negotiations. For example, if the emergency department group has developed asthma treatment protocols that allow for aggressive outpatient treatment of patients with reactive airway disease, this can be an important bargaining point in assuring managed care that the emergency physician group will have incentives that help avoid admission to the hospital, unless patients fail the existing protocols. By taking these approaches, it can usually be demonstrated that the emergency physician group, the MCO, and the hospital can develop reasonable contractual alternatives that can be of mutual benefit.

MANAGED CARE'S VIEW OF EMERGENCY MEDICINE

Although most emergency physicians and the American College of Emergency Physicians have traditionally taken the position that the patient defines the emergency and the need for emergency care,[11] managed care fundamentally disagrees with this view. One of the primary goals of managed care plans is to ensure that patients are referred only for those illnesses or injuries that require the evaluation and expertise of specialists, including emergency physicians. Managed care programs tend to view the emergency department as an extraordinarily expensive place to provide care that, in their view, should be handled in alternate settings in 40% to 50% of cases.[12] Although examination fees for emergency physicians and primary care physicians may be similar, the emergency department typically has a facility and ancillary services component, which can result in an overall fee two to three times that of a physician's office. Similarly, MCOs often believe that emergency physicians order too many tests, which is largely driven by the lack of history and previously established healthcare relationship with the patient, as well as real or imagined risk management concerns.

Further, in addition to viewing the emergency department as the locus of high cost care for many low acuity patients who have sought the emergency department largely for convenience, MCOs tend to view the emergency department as uncontrolled in their overall operations. Most managed care organizations have the perception that emergency departments lack understanding about the use of PCPs as gatekeepers, the importance of limiting referrals, the necessity of keeping referrals within the network, and general concepts of risk transfer that form the bedrock of the MCOs structure.[13] For that reason, many managed care organizations have tried to implement effective disincentives for what they consider to be the "inappropriate" use of emergency departments. These include co-payments, preauthorization, and transfer of patients from nonparticipating hospitals to those that participate in the plan.[14]

Co-Payments

For more than 30 years it has been well accepted that patients who are responsible for a percentage of their bill (co-payment) are more aware of the cost of their services than patients who have total coverage for their illnesses or injuries. MCOs have generally had a significantly larger co-payment for emergency department visits than have more traditional indemnity markets. For example, if the co-payment for an office visit in a MCO is $5, it is not unusual to see copayments of $25 to $50 for emergency department visits, even when such visits are deemed to be a covered service. Indemnity plans have also relied on the concept of co-payments as a disincentive for emergency department care.

Preauthorization

Most MCOs recognized that co-payments have limited success in reducing emergency department visits and therefore implemented preauthorization for payment of services as an essential strategy of disincentive for patients to come to the emergency department. Patients are given a telephone number to call if they believe that they may have a condition warranting emergency department evaluation. Typically, these telephone numbers are staffed by nurses or other healthcare providers who question the patient about the nature of their illness or injury to determine whether they can be referred to alternate levels of healthcare. These alternatives include seeing the managed care physician the next day or using urgent medical care centers. In many cases, patients do not bother to call the number and simply come to the emergency department seeking care, only to be told that they must have preauthorization approval to ensure coverage for their care. The requirements of the COBRA/EMTALA act require hospitals to provide a medical screening examination to any patient presenting to the emergency department. HCFA has specified that the hospital must define who the "qualified medical person" is who is responsible for providing this screening examination (although HCFA does not have to accept this determination as meeting the requirements of the statute).[15] Preauthorization is a related but separate issue to the medical screening examination. Many hospitals have interpreted it to be met by the functions of the triage nurse. The issue of preauthorization is addressed in some detail later (see Preauthorization).

Transfers to Nonparticipating Hospitals

The cornerstone of cost savings for managed care programs is negotiated discount of fees, whether with specified physicians and hospitals, or through staff model HMO arrangements. Hospital admissions account for nearly 50% of an MCO's total cost; therefore it is important to ensure that patients are admitted only to participating hospitals. In addition to the preauthorization requirement for treatment in the emergency department, most plans also require additional authorization if the patient needs admission, including transferring stable patients to participating hospitals.

In summary, managed care organizations tend to view emergency departments as costly alternatives to physicians' offices or urgent care centers for the care of a large number of low acuity patients seeking convenient medical care. Further, managed care tends to view emergency medicine as lacking a full understanding of the need for use of the PCP as gatekeeper, referring patients sparingly and selectively to specialists, keeping patients referred within the MCO's network, as well as lacking an understanding of the concepts of risk transfer essential to the structure of the MCO itself. Nonetheless, to the extent that emergency physician groups can prospectively address these concerns, there is a substantial opportunity to create successful relationships with MCOs.

Many managed care plans, particularly those in mature environments in which the plan has been successful, also tend to appreciate the level of expertise provided by well-trained emergency physicians in the evaluation, stabilization, and treatment of acutely ill and injured patients. Many such plans have recognized the significant risk management effect that participating with a qualified group of emergency physicians can provide to them and to their patients. Although many wags refer to MCOs as organizations that manage money, not healthcare, many emergency physician groups have cooperated successfully in negotiating mutually beneficial arrangements with MCOs.[16]

GOALS OF MANAGED CARE FOR EMERGENCY MEDICINE

The first goal of managed care for emergency medicine is to ensure that the emergency care providers with which they contract are available and accessible and have sufficient expertise to care for the acutely ill and injured patients that the MCO believes "truly need" emergency department evaluation and treatment. The credentials and experience of emergency physicians are important to ensure managed care plans, as they evaluate emergency departments with whom they will affiliate. Second, plans clearly intend to reduce access to and the cost of emergency services for the plan and its enrollees. As indicated previously, traditional wisdom has held that emergency services are costly compared to other alternatives and that emergency departments have a large percentage of patients who could be cared for in other settings. Although the validity of this assumption has been substantially challenged in the literature and the concept of the marginal costs of covering emergency care has been developed,[17] the emergency physician group will have to recognize the existence of this assumption when negotiating with managed care plans. Third, managed care plans want the emergency department to recognize the need to use the primary care physician as the gatekeeper, or essential contact for guiding the care of the patient through the healthcare system. The gatekeeper role includes, in many cases, the initial evaluation in the emergency department, the decision for admission or discharge, and the referral of patients to subspecialists on an outpatient basis. Fourth, in addition to wanting to use the primary care physician as the gatekeeper, MCOs are also sensitive to the use of "in network" physicians to provide both inpatient and outpatient care. Simply using the "on-call" physician for the emergency department often results in denial of payment, increased cost to the patient, and ill feeling among physicians who have been called to care for patients who have an insurance plan in which they do not participate. Fifth, many plans prefer to negotiate an arrangement that allows the emergency physician to perform a primary screening examination of the patient for a specified (reduced) fee, but either refer them for more definitive care to the MCO's physicians or obtain approval for further diagnostic and therapeutic interventions. Finally, managed care plans strongly believe that emergency physicians and other hospital-based physicians should cooperate carefully in negotiating ongoing relationships with the MCO. As funding mechanisms for healthcare change, MCOs insist on a high level of cooperation from hospital-based physicians in this regard. This insistence on cooperation varies from stringent demands to more cooperative, collegial relationships in which the MCO and the emergency physicians can mutually negotiate in good faith.

ESSENTIALS OF MANAGED CARE CONTRACTS

A contract is a written document that outlines the duties and responsibilities of the parties involved. Most contracts with managed care organizations are two-way in nature, naming the MCO and the emergency physician group as principals of the contract. The document must be *written;* verbal commitments hold virtually no weight when a written contractual document exists. In the event that a written document is in place, all verbal subsequent conversations should be committed to writing, preferably by specific contractual amendment. The assistance of qualified contract attorneys is essential in negotiating effective contractual relationships with managed care organizations. In many cases this assistance is needed not so much for the attorney's negotiation skills but to ensure that qualified legal advice is obtained with regard to the validity of specific contractual clauses. When seeking legal advice, one should access the expertise of a firm with documented experience in dealing with contract law, healthcare issues, and specifically managed care experience. It is usually not advisable to use the hospital's attorney because of potential conflict of interest issues. However, qualified contractual legal advice can usually be obtained from local firms.

Although the emergency physician group should always insist on a written contract with the MCO, it is also important to recognize that the contract itself is only as good as the integrity of the parties involved. *All managed care contracts should be viewed as negotiable.* In many cases, managed care plans will arrive with preprinted contracts, creating the image that they cannot be changed and that it is "our policy" not to change our contract. Nothing could be further from the truth. All contractual relationships should be viewed as open to negotiation at the outset. If in the course of negotiating the agreement, the inflexibility or integrity of the opposite party comes into question, details of a written contractual agreement will be of scant recompense if there is no trust in the organization. Similarly, it is important to ensure that the negotiations are taking place with someone who has the authority to effect needed changes in the contract. This authority should preferably be established before any meetings are held to discuss the contract. If changes need to be made in the contractual relationship, the emergency physician representative should be speaking directly with the person who will make the decision about the change. Contracts should be as specific as possible with regard to the issues delineated below. Ambiguities, lack of definition, and lack of clarity can all result in extreme difficulty and contentiousness unless these issues are resolved during the course of contract negotiations.

Contract Term

All contracts with MCOs should have a specified term, including a beginning and ending date. Failure to ensure the contract has a beginning date can result in disputes about fees and obligations under the contract. In most cases, a 1-year contract term is preferred if any form of fee schedule, negotiated rate, discounted fee-for-service system, or capitation rate is to be utilized. The essentials of the MCO involves transfer of risk. In contracting with the MCO, the emergency physician group should be aware that it is entering into a relationship of risk, which may involve financial risk, risk of increased patient flow without increased compensation, and others. For that reason, in most cases the term of the contract should be restricted to 1 year, unless the emergency physician group has substantial experience either with the specific MCO or with MCOs in general that allow it to predict the risk of entering into the relationship.

Similarly, in many cases it is wise to insist on automatic termination of the contract, subject to timely negotiations to update and/or renew the relationship. In most cases, this is a better strategy than automatic renewal because substantial risk may be involved for the emergency physician group in entering into the relationship. For example, if the emergency physician group has incurred more financial risk than was anticipated under the agreement, it is far easier to have the contract terminate automatically than to have to issue a letter of termination. In many cases, canceling an existing contract with a MCO can cause dismay and consternation among hospital administrators, who feel it may reflect on their overall relationship with an MCO. In these circumstances, the negotiating leverage is substantially more with the emergency physician group if the MCO is under a position of automatic termination of the contract at the end of the contract term because the fee schedule reverts in most cases to the original fee-for-service mode. If possible, in addressing the contract term, it should be clearly specified that the fees to be used on termination are the usual and customary fee schedule, as opposed to continuing the schedule listed in the contract.

"Evergreen" or "forever green" contracts have a clause that continually perpetuates the contract, so that there is, in essence, no term of the contract, and in many cases no termination clause. It is essentially a contract that automatically renews forever, unless specifically terminated. In many cases, evergreen contracts allow termination only for material breach of the contract. Although managed care organizations and hospitals often prefer evergreen contracts, it is essential to understand the risk transfer concept in the MCO's strategy before agreeing to any such relationship. The more the emergency physician group is put at risk in the contractual relationship, and the less experience the emergency physician group has in negotiating managed care contracts, the less likely it is to be beneficial for the physician to agree to an evergreen contract. Potential exceptions include contracts that involve favorable discounted fee-for-service relationships without clauses for downcoding denials. Thus in certain, clearly specified circumstances, it may be beneficial to have an evergreen contract. However, to the degree that the emergency physician group is put at risk, financially or otherwise, by the details of the contract, an evergreen contract should be scrutinized carefully, and in most cases, avoided.

Facility-Specific Contracts

Contracts with MCOs should specify the specific facility or facilities in which the contract will be effective. In most cases, facilities should be limited to the single emergency department that the group covers. With some local, regional, and multihospital groups, however, the MCO may be contracting for additional service sites as well. Extreme caution should be taken in agreeing to a contract that covers other facilities because the financial aspects of the negotiations are almost always facility specific. Payor mix and average patient charge differences alone can account for huge differences in reimbursement between hospitals, even within a specific geographic area. Listed below are specific areas that need to be addressed from a financial standpoint when entering into any such contract, but this financial analysis must be performed on a facility-specific basis to allow for a clear understanding of the financial impact on the physician group.

Further, contracts should clearly specify that the plan cannot transfer, broker, or extend the terms of the contract to other managed care plans without the express written approval of both parties. At a time when there is a great deal of consolidation of MCOs, it is entirely possible that they could acquire other prepaid healthcare options and insist that the details of contract be extended to other patient groups included in the acquisition. This should be addressed as specifically as possible in the contract. In some cases, MCOs have actually attempted to broker their fees to other MCOs for financial reasons, which should be precluded in the contract.

Covered Benefits

Contracts should clearly specify the benefits covered by the MCO. In addition, this section of the contract should specify that benefits cannot be changed without prior consideration and consent of the emergency physician group. As more and more plans use capitation and other strategies to transfer risk to the emergency department, specification of covered benefits and its extension to other areas needs to be addressed.

Equally important, the contract must specify that the emergency physician group should be able to bill the patient directly for any noncovered or denied charges. This issue is completely separate from balance billing patients for charges over and above those allowed by the managed care plan. However, in cases in which the MCO denies payment because it is not a covered benefit (usually because it is not deemed to be an emergency), there must be clearly specified permission for the emergency physician group to bill the patient directly for such charges, preferably at full as opposed to discounted charges.

Preauthorization

Preauthorization constitutes the single area of most concern and confusion between MCOs and emergency physician groups. The contract should have a defined mechanism for preauthorization, so that all parties involved understand it. MCOs prefer to ensure that some mechanism of preauthorization is required for emergency care. Although this option is theoretically attractive for the MCO, in many cases the MCO has little effective mechanism for ensuring that patients comply with this requirement, except to deny payment, which results in the enrollee being billed directly by the emergency physician group and/or hospital. In Virginia and Maryland, state statutes have defined emergencies by a prudent layperson definition and have precluded MCOs from denying payment and/or services in such circumstances.

The need for authorization, however, has clearly led to inappropriate delays in the treatment of many patients presenting with urgent complaints that are not necessarily true emergency medical conditions.[18,19] Virtually all emergency departments have put policies into effect that exclude the need for preauthorization in patients who present *in extremis*. Ideally, MCO contracts should include a preapproved list of authorized presenting complaints, for which preauthorization is not necessary. Box 41-2 lists common symptoms and/or presentations that may be included as an appendix to the contractual language. These include not only patients *in extremis,* but those who are likely to need immediate evaluation and/or intervention within a specified time frame (e.g., 30 minutes).

In addition, the contract should specify that if the plan does not respond to the request for preauthorization within a reasonable time period (usually 30 minutes) an authorization should be deemed to have occurred. Many plans object to such authorization clauses, primarily because of the difficulty in providing accurate documentation that the plan did not respond within that time period. The issue of preauthorization is sensitive for MCOs because they believe so strongly that patients are seeking convenience care in the emergency department. However, this issue often can be balanced in the negotiation process by ensuring the MCO that the emergency department group is sensitive to this issue, wishes to ensure that the plan is well represented to its patients, and is willing to help cooperate to the best extent possible. One alternative is to agree to a specified charge for medical screening examinations on patients presenting to the emergency department. For example, some physician groups have negotiated substantially discounted rates to MCOs for a medical screening examination on patients who present with minor upper respiratory illnesses, abrasions, and other minor problems.

Specific contractual language should be included to indicate that, once authorization has been granted, it cannot be retrospectively denied. To the best extent possible, the contract should differentiate medical screening examinations from evaluation and treatment with regard to this preauthorization issue.

BOX 41-2

POTENTIAL PROSPECTIVE AUTOMATIC AUTHORIZATIONS BY MCOS

1. All patients presenting by ambulance
2. All patients with unstable vital signs
3. All patients with shortness of breath
4. All patients with chest pain
5. All patients with active hemorrhaging
6. All patients with altered mental status or obvious neurologic deficits
7. All patients with cardiac dysrhythmias or palpitations
8. All patients with obvious fractures or dislocation
9. All patients with severe pain
10. All pregnant patients with contractions
11. All patients with systemic allergic reactions
12. All patients with drug overdose
13. All patients with lacerations requiring sutures
14. All patients under 3 years with fever $\geq 38.3°$ C
15. All patients with acute eye injuries

Billing Issues

The section Financial Analysis addresses billing issues in some detail. The contract should clarify in what specified period of time submission of claims must occur. Many MCOs prefer to have claims submitted within 30 to 60 days, after which the plan can reject the claims. To begin with, the term *submission* needs to be clearly defined, preferably by ensuring weekly and/or monthly reports with regard to specific claims that have been submitted. In the past, many physician groups have had difficulty with documentation of specific submission times on claims. In general, it is to the physician group's advantage to submit the claims as early as possible, although in some cases submission of those claims within a 30-day period can be difficult, particularly if there are multiple contractual and operational requirements with regard to submission of the claim. Chief among these requirements is that it be submitted on a plan-specific form. In most cases, emergency physician groups should request that they be able to submit claims on the HCFA 1500 form rather than on plan-specific forms. Further, contractual language should detail the MCO's responsibility for documenting receipt of submitted claims in a timely fashion. In general, physician groups should attempt to have 120 days for submission of claims from the emergency department.

Two of the most common ways for MCOs to reduce their cost in emergency department claims are downcoding and retrospective denials. MCOs frequently downcode emergency physicians charges under the pretense that adequate documentation to substantiate the original level of service has not been provided. Adherence to the Resource-based Relative Value Scale (RBRVS) guidelines has assisted somewhat in this regard, but downcoding continues to be an issue for some providers. In general, downcoding issues should be specified in the contract, and it should be clearly stated that service codes cannot be downcoded further than one Evaluation/Management code level. Providing the managed care plan and its review agents with a dictated copy of the medical record can help simplify review of such claims. It is helpful to ensure that the hospital cooperate in providing a dictated medical record, particularly given the importance of documentation in the RBRVS system.

The other area of concern under the contractual billing language is retrospective denials. To the best extent possible, language should be included that ensures that any preauthorized patient cannot have a retrospective denial. In the event that denials do occur, it is important to ensure that the hospital and the emergency physician group retain the option of billing the patient directly for denials or "uncovered services."

The emergency physician group must have any managed care contracts reviewed carefully by their billing agency before the contract is implemented. The billing agents should be of benefit in analyzing the financial impact of the contract (see Financial Analysis). The physician group should request the billing agency to develop the capability of aging accounts receivable by individual managed care plans, rather than by simply classifying them under the single financial class *HMO*. This information is essential to ensuring that the collections can be monitored and that appropriate contractual clauses are developed to protect the physician group from delays in payment. Systematic collection procedures should be in place for any balances of more than 60 to 90 days, including a mechanism for ensuring that follow-up calls are placed to the MCO's billing office.

In some cases in which medical screening examinations have been agreed to for a specified fee, it may be cost effective to simply submit a list of such patients directly to the managed care plan, as opposed to incurring the costs of billing through the billing agency itself. However, if such a tactic is undertaken, the data must still be collected with regard to utilization by the managed care plan. In some cases, billing difficulties with MCOs have required the development of weekly, biweekly, or monthly batch billing procedures, with documented delivery of the claims, including backup documentation to the MCO billing office. The physician group should review managed care payment trends at least quarterly to monitor compliance with the contractual obligations.

When disagreement arises with regard to the use of service codes, the contract should clearly specify the mechanism for changing such codes. The American Medical Association's Common Procedural Terminology-4 (CPT)[20] should be the standard definitions. Discrepancies on physician group coding policies should be based on specified audit criteria, including methods for settling differences. If possible, an attempt should be made in serious disputes to get independent reviewers to assist in reviewing the codes and settling disputes.

The issue of medical necessity review documentation also needs to be addressed within the contract. The emergency physician group should attempt to insert a clause indicating that the managed care plan will obtain, at its own expense, all documentation needed for prepayment and postpayment on medical necessity reviews. It is important to place the financial and operational onus for such reviews with the managed care plan, as otherwise it would be easy for the plan to "tie up" the physician group and its billing agency with requests for medical necessity review documentation. If possible, contractual language should indicate that the managed care plan will pay reasonable copying and handling charges ($.50 to $1.00 a page) to supply copies of medical record documentation to the plan for review.

Prompt Payment

The contract should specify clearly the time of payment on covered benefits in the claims process. In general, this time of payment should be no more than 30 to 60 days, but in no case should it be longer than the time allowed for submission of claims. For example, if claims need to be submitted within 30 days, they should be paid within 30 days. In some cases, managed care plans will indicate that this is sometimes not possible, in which case the physician group should request a monthly penalty of interest of 1% to 1.5% on claims that are not paid promptly. In some cases, it may be beneficial to have an outside limit for claim payment, beyond which the claim will be paid at 100% of charges, as opposed to the previously negotiated discounted rate.

Plan Insolvency

The rapid proliferation of managed care plans has resulted in several plans with limited financial capacity. Truly the growth of this industry has in some cases vastly outstripped certain managed care plans' ability to deliver on their contractual obligations. On the other hand, there are numerous managed care providers with extremely strong financial statements, in which insolvency is unlikely. Regardless of the financial stability of the plan or its reputation, however, the managed care plan should have reinsurance to cover the contingency of insolvency. In the event reinsurance is not provided, the plan should have adequate cash reserves set aside pursuant to state insurance regulations to meet the obligations of the contract with the emergency physician group. In cases in which the physician group is unfamiliar with the plan and has concerns that they may be undercapitalized, it is not unreasonable to request proof of reinsurance or audited financial statements to determine the financial stability of the organization. In all cases, it is essential to avoid contractual language that requires the continuation of treatment to plan enrollees in the event the plan becomes insolvent.

Most-Favored Nation Clause

Favored nation or most-favored nation clauses allow for a managed care plan to ensure that it is given the best possible discount that is being offered to any other plan with which the provider contracts. Such clauses typically ensure not only that the existing rate is adhered to, but that if any deeper discount or more favorable terms are negotiated with *any* other managed care provider, then the same terms will apply in this contract. These clauses should be avoided whenever possible when dealing with managed care plans. The most common problem is that many hospitals agree to such clauses within their contracts with the managed care provider, thereby creating strong leverage for the managed care plan to insert a most favored nation clause into the physician agreement. In coordinating carefully with the administration (see below), it is imperative to attempt to avoid such language whenever possible. If such clauses are included, it again needs to be made clear that the discount is for plan enrollees only because some MCOs are now selling their favored nation status to other plans. Such brokerage of discounts is highly questionable from a legal standpoint, but should still be specifically precluded in the contractual language.

Dispute Resolution

With any contract, sometimes parties cannot resolve their differences through negotiation. The contract should specify a mechanism for dispute resolution, preferably impartial arbitration. Arbitration should apply to medical necessity issues, utilization review, and fee adjustments, preferably according to the rules of the American Arbitration Association. An odd number of arbitrators should be selected, usually three, one selected by each party and a third agreed to by both parties. In many cases the inclusion of an arbitration clause in the contract can be an incentive for the parties to resolve their differences through negotiation. Finally, decisions of the arbitration panel should be subject to judicial review, although such language is not essential.

Contract Amendments

All contracts with managed care providers should include specific language indicating that amendments to the contract shall be allowed only with the mutual consent of *both* parties. This provision precludes either party from unilaterally changing the terms of the agreement and encourages negotiations in a setting of mutual benefit. Similarly, language should specify that the contract cannot be assigned or delegated without the prior written consent of the other party. This helps ensure that the terms of the contract cannot be extended to other managed care plans. In some cases, specific language can be included with regard to acquisitions and/or transfer of stock.

FINANCIAL ANALYSIS

The most important factor to keep in mind in undertaking contracts with managed care plans is that the essential nature of their contractual relationship is intended to transfer risk to the provider, whether in the form of discounts for fees, incentives for seeing additional patients, or fully capitating the provider. For that reason, the physician must have a clear understanding of both the types of reimbursement methods available and the methods for analyzing each contractual arrangement in a detailed fashion. For that reason, this section details both specific reimbursement models, as well as giving a framework through which financial analysis can occur.

Reimbursement Methods

While the basic premise of managed care contracting is to transfer risk, the specific methods under which this is accomplished vary widely, including fee-for-service, discounted fee-for-service, fee schedules, risk pools, withholds, and full capitation. Definitions of each of these options are offered below.

Fee-for-Service. Direct fee-for-service relationships are largely the province of indemnity plans or "managed" indemnity plans at the current time. In some cases managed care organizations agree to a fee-for-service relationship utilizing the Current Procedural Terminology (CPT) codes and Evaluation and Management (E/M) codes, but stabilizing rates at a preset value according to the *plan's* as opposed to the *physician group's* fee schedule. However, fee-for-service emergency medicine as a primary contractual relationship with managed care providers is increasingly a thing of the past.

Discounted Fee-for-Service. Discounted fee-for-service (DFFS) plans are an entry level relationship with managed care organizations, in which the physician group agrees to a discount (ranging from 20% up to 50%) from the fee schedule. That fee schedule might be provided by the managed care plan or by the emergency physician group, depending on the negotiation strategy of the MCO. In most cases, the emergency physician should carefully compare the fee schedules provided from the MCO with their own, but in most cases the emergency physician fees will be higher. For that reason, it is usually preferable to discount from the emergency physician group fee schedule as opposed to the managed care plan. The degree of discount varies widely, from requests for discounts across the board to specifically negotiated discounts by the level of care or even by CPT codes. In the section Financial Analysis it is important to pay close attention to sources of revenue for the group, including the distribution of E/M codes and the generation of revenue from specific service codes themselves. In analyzing whether a proposed relationship is profitable, this approach is essential.

The reason that DFFS arrangements are less attractive to managed care is that discounts alone cannot effectively control either utilization or physician practice patterns. Traditionally, such contractual relationships also do not effectively control increases in costs from year-to-year, because they do not affect utilization significantly. The primary advantage of a DFFS contract for an emergency care provider is that the negotiated discount does provide specified compensation for volume increases, even though it may be at a reduced rate. Such contracts are certainly easy to implement and to understand.

The disadvantages of DFFS contracts include the usual requirement that the MCO will require the physician group to submit their fee schedules for approval of any future increases. (However, *increases* in fee schedules are highly unlikely in negotiating with managed care at any time in the near future). Perhaps the major disadvantage of DFFS is that they fail to control utilization and costs in the manner in which the MCO desires. As costs rise, the MCO typically focuses on uncovered services, denials, and other mechanisms to decrease their costs. Over time, discounted fee-for-service relationships will also begin to give way to reimbursement methods that allow for more effective transfer of risk to the provider. However, at the present time DFFS relationships can be profitable to the emergency physician group and acceptable to many managed care providers during this transition phase in the healthcare market.

Fee Schedules. Physician fee schedules have been used for many, many years in the generation of physician charges. The specification of specific fee schedules in the emergency medicine environment, however, is undergoing transition as risk is transferred to the provider. The most commonly recognized physician fee schedule has been the concept of "usual, customary, and reasonable" (UCR) fees, which basically reimburse in full for many services, depending on the comparison between UCR and the physician group's fee schedule. These systems have essentially been set up to pay the lower of either the billed charge or the fee schedule for a specific procedure. As managed care contractors have become more aggressive in their transfer of risk, fee schedules have been used to lower reimbursement to the provider. For example, whereas a UCR fee schedule in the past may have paid 85% to 90% of physician charges, current fee schedules typically pay in the 50% to 80% range, depending on the competitiveness of the market, availability of alternate providers, and aggressiveness of the MCO. The fee schedules themselves are either fixed fee schedules that assign a specific dollar amount to each procedure, or some variant of a relative value scale (RVS) concept. Using an RVS system involves assigning each procedure a unit value, which is then multiplied by a fixed dollar amount. In negotiating such arrangements, agreement must be made on both the fee schedule and the conversion factor that will be used.

Three specific fee schedules are commonly in use by MCOs:

- *Harvard Resource-Based Relative Value Scale (RBRVS):* This fee schedule was developed by Harvard University at the request of the Medicare Program and has been used by many managed care payors. This scale can be fairly complicated to use because it has relative values, geographic adjustment factors, malpractice adjustments, as well as both surgical and medical conversion factors. The figures are adjusted annually by HCFA in February or March.
- *California Relative Value Study (CRVS):* This scale was originally used for California Workers' Compensation reimbursement, but is still used by many West Coast MCOs. It is not a preferred mechanism of use, particularly because it does not have unit values assigned for emergency department level IV and V codes, which is a serious drawback.
- *McGraw-Hill Relative Values for Physicians:* This fee schedule was developed in 1984 and has been updated annually, but has been used less frequently since the RBRVS system was developed.

When using the RBRVS scale as a basis for managed care contracting, it is important to specify the conversion factors in some detail. For example, in 1995, a 99283 emergency department visit code had a Medicare RBRVS fee schedule unit value of 1.6. If the managed care organization offers a dollar conversion base rate of $15 (for a unit value of 1.0), the approved fee would therefore be $24. In addition, the contract should specify that in using the Medicare Economic Indicator update whether the surgical or medical factors will be utilized. If possible, it is preferable to negotiate an arrangement that uses the surgical factor for surgical codes and medical factors for all other codes. The contract should also specify the time at which the conversion factors will go into effect. The Medicare updates usually come out in February or March, so it is usually a good idea to ensure that updates go into effect no later than April or May.

In some managed care environments, the payor prefers to negotiate either a global professional fee or case rates for emergency physicians. Such fees do not compensate separately for both visits and procedures, but rather bundle the payment into an entire physician professional fee component. The first type of global fee is a simple flat professional fee regardless of patient acuity. Most emergency physician groups avoid such a payment because there is a substantial degree of acuity-related risk to such a plan. It is particularly risky when the emergency physician professional fee component and hospital facility component are bundled together because physicians are often penalized for such an acuity-related risk under such a program. Further, under such an arrangement, the managed care plan could divert its lower acuity patients to a different provider, such as an urgent care center, leaving the emergency department with a fixed flat fee arrangement for selective higher acuity patients.

A second type of global fee arrangement includes a specified reimbursement for the five E/M service codes (99281-99285), with a separately negotiated fee for each of the levels. However, no additional charges can then be billed to the plan or to the patient, regardless of the additional procedures provided. Although such a fee can be administered easily, there is still potential for lost revenue in this environment. For example, the five E/M service codes usually account for 75% to 80% of all charges generated out of an emergency department. Depending on the level of fee negotiated, 20% to 25% of the available revenue is at risk to the provider.

The third type of global fee involves the hybrid where there is a set reimbursement for specific categories of care, usually set by the E/M code levels or by the categories of emergent, urgent, or nonurgent. However, this third type also allows for billing for procedures performed in the emergency department at a rate to be agreed to by the managed care plan and the physician group. This third type then represents a hybrid between the global fee and unbundled, procedure-related coding system.

Capitation. Capitation agreements constitute a major step in transferring risk to the provider, most noticeably for primary care physicians, but also for emergency physicians. Capitation agreements constitute a major change in reimbursement strategy by MCOs. Capitation systems contract prospectively to pay providers a fixed amount based on numbers of plan enrollees, regardless of utilization. Most plans pay a specific amount per member per month (PMPM). Many managed care plans prefer such an agreement because they are able to transfer risk effectively to the emergency department provider under such a system. In a capitated contract, the physician exchanges utilization risk for collection and cash flow guarantees. Thus the advantage to the emergency physician is a dependable cash flow from the managed care plan, as well as the opportunity to decrease billing costs for plan enrollees. However, the risk that they take is one of utilization, in which the managed care plan preferentially can direct patients to the emergency department because they are already "paid for." In a discounted fee-for-service environment, managed care plans implement disincentives to emergency department use because utilization equals increased cost. In a capitation environment, however, the managed care plan has already reimbursed the provider for care, in which case utilization risk is transferred to the emergency department physician. For example, some managed care plans have closed their after-hours clinics or extended hours at facilities after the implementation of a capitation agreement, with the patients preferentially sent to the contracted emergency department. This results in decreased cost for the managed care provider (e.g., in the form of overhead, physician salaries) and can result in substantial flow-related problems for the emergency department. Most managed care organizations negotiate rates separately for Medicare and commercial populations because the Medicare population base is older, has more acute illnesses, and requires increased resources. In general, the PMPM for Medicare tends to be two and a half to three times the commercial rate for emergency services, whereas Medicaid rates tend to be 65% to 75% of the commercial rate.

When entering into a capitated contract, the emergency physician should ensure that there is some protection in the form of volume stop-loss arrangements. In such an arrangement, the emergency physician group would agree to receive a specified capitation agreement based on a PMPM basis, but with a specified volume level, above which visits would be reimbursed on a discounted fee-for-service or fee-for-service basis. Such a stop-loss clause prevents primary care physicians and the plan from flooding the emergency department with excessive patients to decrease their cost and/or utilization.

Clearly, the major advantages of a capitated contract for an emergency physician group are financial in nature. As indicated previously, the first advantage is a guaranteed cash flow within a specified period of time. This advantage can have an important impact on protection of cash flow for the emergency physician group and, in some cases, can alleviate a lag in accounts receivable days, particularly if the payment times are negotiated so that they are paid on a routine, upfront basis. In addition, the second advantage is decreased billing costs. Emergency physicians have typically had extremely high bad debt rates, which are often reflected in an increased per patient billing costs. By eliminating the need to submit individual bills for capitated patients, these costs can be decreased. It is essential, however, to analyze each and every financial situation to determine whether a capitated agreement is beneficial. This process is presented in detail in the section Financial Analysis. It is essential in calculating capitation rates to look not only at the utilization per thousand members, but also at the acuity of services within that patient group.

When capitation arrangements are in place, it is still important to continue to monitor and code charts with regard to acuity of care and level of service codes to assist the group in negotiating with the managed care plan in the future. In some cases, utilization review committees, including members of the emergency physician group and managed care plan, can be instituted to help monitor trends in the changing healthcare environment. If possible, it is preferable to arrange for a direct billing relationship to the managed care plan for any stop-loss billings because this approach can further reduce billing costs.

In some highly advanced managed care markets (Minnesota and California), the concept of true global capitation for emergency services has developed. Under these systems, the emergency physician group accepts a true global capitation for all risk of emergency services that the plan enrollees may encounter. For example, if a patient under the plan were to seek emergency medical care at a facility not covered by the emergency physician group, the group would be at risk for paying that healthcare provider for the emergency services delivered. In such settings, some emergency physician groups have actually developed their own preauthorization procedures, including telephone numbers staffed by nurses, to ensure that patients are triaged to emergency departments that are "within the plan." However, such true global capitation arrangements are at the present time uncommon in emergency medicine, outside of certain geographic areas.

Similarly, concepts such as percentage of premium reimbursement, risk pools, risk sharing, and risk corridors and withhold amounts are aspects of emergency medicine-MCO contracting that have not yet been used widely.[21] Percentage of premium reimbursement has been used for primary care physicians and relies on a strategy wherein the physician receives a percentage of premium dollar and vests him or her in the interest of ensuring that the marketing and underwriting skills and strategy of the organization are successful. Typically such arrangements do not extend to specialists who are hospital-based specialists such as emergency physicians. Risk pools, risk sharing, and risk corridors are devices to help ensure that utilization is controlled to the best extent possible, usually by the PCP and the MCO. In some cases, risk pools and risk sharing have extended to specialists and the hospital, although it is uncommon for emergency physicians to participate in such pools. As the emergency physician community increasingly identifies itself as "after-hours gatekeeper," however, this concept of risk pools and risk sharing may extend, at least partially, to such emergency physicians. Most emergency physician groups avoid the concept of withholds within their contracts, primarily because they can easily persuade the managed care provider that they cannot control the volume of services to which they are exposed.

To summarize, capitation involves a major step in the risk transfer spectrum. Before entering into such a contract, the emergency physician group and hospital should assess several factors, including the following:

- What is the existing culture of the physician group or emergency department? How major a cultural change will capitation represent? Are the physician and nonphysician leaders of the department prepared to undertake this major change?
- What are the mutual responsibilities of the contracting partners and what is the degree of risk associated with the contract? Are these risks either predictable or avoidable?
- Are sufficient information systems in place to allow for adequate prediction of resource utilization, financial reimbursement, and operational impacts?
- What is the reputation and history of the payor? Does the

BOX 41-3

FINANCIAL ANALYSIS OF MANAGED CARE CONTRACTUAL OFFERS

Step One: Calculate Payor-Specific Average Charge.
a) Run Procedure Code use report for Payor-Specific Patients

E/M code	Charges	# Pts	E/M code continuation
99281	a	v	(a × v)
99282	b	w	(b × w)
99283	c	x	(c × x)
99284	d	y	(d × y)
99285	e	z	(e × z)

Total Payor Specific Patients—n

b) Calculate Payor-specific average patient charge

$$\frac{(a \times v) + (b \times w) + (c \times x) + (d \times y) + (e \times z)}{n} = \text{Average Patient Charge}$$

Step Two: Calculate Payor-Specific Average Collection.
a) Determine Payor-Specific collection per procedure code

E/M code	Charges	Allowable/collection	# Pts
99281		A	a
99282		B	b
99283		C	c
99284		D	d
99285		E	e

Total Payor-Specific points n

b) Calculate Average Payor-Specific Collection

$$\frac{Aa + Bb + Cd + Dd + Ee}{n} = \text{Average Payor-Specific Collection}$$

Step 3: Compare Current Payor-Specific collections to Proposed Contractual Offer.

Current collections		*Proposed Contract*
Average Payor-Specific Collection	versus	Proposed Contractual Allowance
less—Billing Costs		less—Billing Costs (if applicable)
Average Net Collection		Average Net Collection

payor have a track record of meeting contractual obligations, reviewing and paying claims in a timely fashion, diverting urgent care patients to contracted emergency departments?

- What are the incentive and penalty methodologies of the contract?
- Does the hospital assign strategic importance to contracting with the specific plan? What is the political downside of failing to negotiate an acceptable agreement with the MCO?

Financial Analysis

To assess the financial impact and relative risk of entering into a managed care contract, the emergency physician group must understand several key factors. First, the five E/M codes typically account for 75% to 80% of all revenues generated by the emergency physician group. Further, the top 20 E/M codes account for 90% to 92% of all revenue generated by emergency physicians. The emergency physician group should carefully monitor these trends, analyzing trend data so that it is clear that the group understands how the revenue of the practice is generated. Trends should be analyzed both for overall payor mix changes and for changes in reimbursement within specific payor mix and MCO payor categories. As indicated previously, the billing agent should be able to break out managed care plans by specific contractual entity, rather than simply lumping all HMOs together. Each specific managed care plan should be analyzed carefully, and according to its own terms, to determine whether it is beneficial to the group to enter into the contractual relationship.

Box 41-3 lists the specific steps that should be taken in the financial analysis of each of these plans. First, the specific facts of the financial arrangement should be specified. What payor mix and type of service are under discussion? Is the relationship proposed a discount off of usual fees, a fee schedule, a case rate, or a capitation agreement? How will billing be handled; will the billing agent be required to submit usual charges to the managed care plan? How many patients will this arrangement affect, and what has been the historical experience with payment?

Detailed financial analysis should be provided on each of the plans. The first step in this process should be to calculate the average patient charge *for that specific payor category.* In calculating this charge, it is necessary to run the procedure code use report for all patients within that payor category, after which a calculation should be made to determine the average charge overall, based on the numbers of patients within each specific E/M code category. This calculation will result in an accurate representation of the overall average patient charge for that specific payor category.

The second step in that process is to calculate the average collection for the specific payor mix. The collection per procedure code should be calculated for the payor mix category, after which the average collection can be calculated, similar to step one.

The third step is to carefully compare the average collection rate under the current system of the collection rate offered by the managed care plan. Only when these steps are followed in a careful fashion with each managed care offer can specific information be determined with regard to the advisability of entering into the plan.

Case study 1—discounted fee-for-service

A Medicaid HMO offers a 50% discount from the normal physician fee schedule. Is this a good deal or a bad deal? Facts:

- Medicaid HMO
- Discount Off Physician Fee Schedule
- Billings with one statement listing charges, date of service for all patients during the month.
- Currently Seeing 500 Medicaid Patients Per Month

Step 1 Calculate *Medicaid* Average Charge

a. Run procedure code use report for all Medicaid patients

	Charges	#pt	% of pts Seen
99281	$38	25	5%
99282	$50	125	25%
99283	$75	200	40%
99284	$100	75	15%
99285	$150	75	15%

b. Calculate average Medicaid charge

$$\frac{(\$38 \times 25) + (\$50 \times 125) + (\$75 \times 200) + (\$100 \times 75) + (\$150 \times 75)}{500} = \$81.90$$

Step 2 Calculate Average *Medicaid* Collections

a. Determine Medicaid collection per procedure code.

	Charge	Medicaid allowable
99281	$38	20
99282	$50	30
99283	$75	40
99284	$100	50
99285	$150	70

b. Calculate average Medicaid collection

$$\frac{(\$20 \times 25) + (\$30 \times 125) + (\$40 \times 200) + (\$50 \times 75) + (\$70 \times 75)}{500} = \$42.50$$

Step 3 Compare Average Medicaid Collection to MCO Offer Applied to Medicaid Patient Charges

Medicaid		MCO	
Average Collection	$42.50	Average Collection (.50 × 81.90) =	$40.95
Billing Costs	(7.00)	Billing Costs	0
Average Net Collection/pt.	$35.50	Average Net Collection/pt.	$40.95

Conclusion: MCO offer of 50% discount is really a good deal.

At the outset, the concept of taking a 50% discount from the normal fee schedule on Medicaid patients would seem to be unattractive. However, when the detailed financial analysis is performed, it is apparent that there will actually be some increase in reimbursement under this system, assuming that the billing cost for the patients is actually zero. In fact, some billing costs are always associated, but in fact individual bills and/or codes are not specifically generated in this scenario.

Case study 2—discounted fee-for-service

Facts:

Commercial MCO
Discount is off usual fees
Regular billing
Currently seeing 1000 patients/month

Step #1 Calculate *Commercial* Average Charge

a. Run procedure code use report for all commercial patients

	Charges	#pts	% of Pts seen
99281	38	25	5%
99282	50	125	15%
99283	75	400	40%
99284	100	250	25%
99285	150	150	15%

b. Calculate average Commercial charge

$$\frac{(\$38 \times 25) + (\$50 \times 125) + (\$75 \times 400) + (\$100 \times 250) + (\$150 \times 150)}{1000} = \$84.70$$

Step #2 Calculate Average *Commercial* Collections

a. Determine commercial collection

	Charge	Commercial allowable	#pts
99281	38	38	50
99282	50	45	150
99283	75	75	400
99284	100	90	250
99285	150	140	150

b. Calculate average commercial collection

$$\frac{(\$38 \times 50) + (\$45 \times 150) + (\$75 \times 400) + (\$90 \times 250) + (\$140 \times 150)}{1000} = \$80.15$$

BOX 41-4

CASE STUDY 1—DISCOUNTED FEE-FOR-SERVICE

MCO would like 50% discount from normal fees

Average Charge	$95/pt.
Collection Percent	61%
Average Collection	$58
(billing cost)	(7)
Average Collection	$51

MCO offering (.50 × avg. charge) = $47.50/pt.

Good Deal or Bad Deal?

BOX 41-5

CASE STUDY 2—DISCOUNTED FEE-FOR-SERVICE

MCO would like 30% Discount from Usual Fees

Average Charge	$95/pt.
Collection Percent	61%
Average Collection	$58
(billing cost)	(7)
Average Collection	$51

MCO offering (.70 × avg. charge) = $66.50/pt.

Good Deal or Bad Deal?

Step #3 Compare Average Commercial Collection to MCO Offer Applied to Commercial Patient Charges

Commercial Collection		MCO	
Average collection	$80.15	Average Collection (.70 × 84.70) =	$67.00
Billing Costs	(7.00)	Billing Costs	(7.00)
Average Net Collection/pt.	$73.15	Average Net Collection/pt.	$59.29

Conclusion: MCO offer of 30% discount is really a bad deal.

In this scenario, because of the specifics of the commercial patients involved and their acuity, accepting a 30% discount would not be a financially attractive deal for the emergency physician group.

Case study 3—fee schedule (see Box 41-6)

Step #1 Calculate Effect of Fee Schedule on Commercial Patients

a. Determine current collection per procedure code

	Charges	Commercial allowable	100% of RBRVS	# pts
99281	38	38	35	50
99282	50	45	40	150
99283	75	75	70	400
99284	100	90	80	250
99285	150	140	135	150

b. Calculate average collection

$$\frac{(\$35 \times 50) + (\$40 \times 150) + (\$70 \times 400) + (\$80 \times 250) + (\$135 \times 150)}{1000} = \$76$$

Step #2 Compare with Commercial Collections

Commercial collection		Fee schedule collection	
Avg. Collection	$87	Avg. Collection	$76
Billing Costs	(7)	Billing Costs	(7)
Avg. Net Collection/pt.	$80	Average Net Collection/pt.	$69

Conclusion: Fee Schedule using 100% of RBRVS represents 15% discount off usual fees.

In this example, using a fee schedule approach with 100% of RBRVS reimbursement actually represents a 15% discount off of the usual fees. Unless this percentage were offset by increased emergency department volume, the emergency physician group would receive less reimbursement.

Case study number 5—capitation model

Conversion to capitation models from traditional commercial or Medicare professional billing arrangements requires careful consideration. The first step in such a process is to differentiate the numbers and percentage of members who fall into the traditional "commercial" model from senior citizens who would fall under the Medicare population base. To begin to evaluate such relationships, it is important to consider the number of members in each category and the percentage that they represent.

Thus the historical review with this plan under a capitation model indicates that the group has actually been paid a total of $1.23 PMPM in reimbursement. If the capitation model presented is for a lower reimbursement, the group will probably lose money on this contractual arrangement. It should be kept in mind that the emergency physician group should know both the commercial and senior reimbursement because the risk for utilization is much higher in the senior

BOX 41-6

CASE STUDY 3—FEE SCHEDULE

MCO is offering to contract using RBRVS as basis of fee schedule
100% RBRVS for Commercial patients
80% RBRVS for Medicare patients
Good Deal or Bad Deal?

BOX 41-7

CASE RATES

- As managed care markets mature, MCOs may negotiate case rates.
- Case rates may be for all patients or may be split between outpatients and those requiring admission.
- Case rates are also popular when employers direct contract.

BOX 41-8

CASE STUDY 4—CASE RATES

MCO would like to contract for $80/patient for all patients

Average Charge	$95/pt
Collection Percent	61%
Average Collection	$58
(billing cost)	(7)
Average Collection	$51

Good Deal or Bad Deal?
Facts: Commercial MCO
Billing: One bill at end of each month
Step #1 See Case Study #2—Step #1
Step #2 See Case Study #2—Step #2
Step #3 Compare average commercial collection with case rate

Commercial collections		Case rate	
Average Collection	$87	Case Rate	$80
Billing Costs	(7)	Billing Costs	0
Average Net Collection/pt.	$80	Average Net Collection/pt.	$80

Conclusion: Case rate collections are the same as commercial collections.

BOX 41-9

CASE RATES

- Determine whether case rates apply to all patients or just a segment.
- If MCO has Medicaid, commercial, and Medicare products, negotiate rate for each.
- Monitor periodically to determine effects of volume and acuity.

BOX 41-10

CASE STUDY 5—CAPITATION MODEL

Membership	#	%
"Commercial" Members	42,000	76.36
Senior Members (≥65 years)	13,000	23.64
Total	55,000	100%

Next, the billing company should generate a report that reviews the *actual* visits per month by plan members in the commercial and senior categories.

Historical review of billing experience

Visits Per Month	#	%
"Commercial"	504	51.85
Senior	468	48.15
Total	972	100%

After calculating the number of visits per month on historical experience, the *actual historical reimbursement* should be calculated based on historical review from the billing company.

Billing history of covered lives: ED professional fees

Total Reimbursement		
Commercial	$30,240	45.27%
Senior	$37.440	46.63$
Total	$67,680	100%

This total reimbursement then needs to be divided by the numbers of covered lives proposed under the contract. These again need to be broken out by commercial and senior levels.

Historical payments converted to PMPM rates

Commercial Reimbursement/Commercial Lives = Per Member Per Month Reimbursement
$30,240/42,000 members = $.72 PMPM
Senior Reimbursement/Senior Lives = PMPM Reimbursement
$37,440/13,000 lives = $2.88 PMPM
Total Reimbursement/Total Lives
$67,680/55,000 = $1.23 PMPM Reimbursement

age group. In some cases, managed care organizations actually prefer to negotiate specific rates for senior- and nonsenior-age group patients.

SUMMARY

Managed care represents the largest single area of growth among healthcare payors.[4-6,22] This growth arises because of cost imperatives placed by employers, as well as the impact of MCOs on hospital utilization. Emergency department physician groups must cooperate carefully with representatives of hospital administration to identify key strategic partners in the managed care market with whom they will affiliate. Prospective discussion about these partners, the need for contracting with MCOs, and the parameters of such relationships should be a firm foundation of the relationship between the emergency physician group and the hospital. The structure of MCOs and the payment mechanisms they use are under constant evolution, but all of them share the common denominator of transferring risk to the provider. Emergency department physician groups should carefully assess those risks to each contractual relationship. The change to contracting with managed care and providing emergency department operations is a major challenge to the specialty of emergency medicine. In most cases, emergency departments are well advised to begin to educate themselves aggressively with regard to the information systems that will be necessary to provide data to support both contracting and operations with MCOs.

REFERENCES

1. Foster Higgins survey, *The Wall Street Journal,* March 2, 1993.
2. Waldo D: Health spending through 2030: three scenarios, *Medical Benefits* 10:23-31, 1992.
3. Shaw E et al: *Capitation strategy,* Washington, 1994, The Advisory Board, 1994.
4. Luft HS: *Health Maintenance Organizations: dimensions of performance,* New York: 1981, John Wiley and Sons,
5. Nelson A: The History and spirit of the HMO movement: the early years, *HMO Pract* 1:75-85, 1987.
6. Goldsmith JC, Goran MJ, Nackel JG: Managed care comes of age, *Healthc Forum J* 38:14-24, 1995.
7. Eiglehart JK: Physicians in the growth of managed care, *N Engl J Med* 331:1167-1171, 1994.
8. Manning W et al: A controlled trial of a prepaid group practice on the use of services, *N Engl J Med* 310:1505-1510, 1984.
9. Iglehart JK: The American health system: managed care, *N Engl J Med* 327:742-747, 1992.
10. Rodwin M: Conflicts in managed care, *N Engl J Med* 332:604-607, 1995.

11. American College of Emergency Physicians Board of Directors: Managed healthcare plans in emergency care, *Ann Emerg Med* 17:97-98, 1988.
12. United States General Accounting Office: *Emergency departments: unevenly affected by growth and change in patient use,* Gaithersburg, Md, 1993, US General Accounting Office.
13. Karpiel M: Managed care in emergency medicine: understanding the new economics and opportunities, Dallas, 1995, American College of Emergency Physicians.
14. Dresnick S: Managed care systems in the emergency department. In Schwartz GR et al, editors: *Principles and practice of emergency medicine,* ed 3, Philadelphia, 1992, Lea and Febiger.
15. Schulman RD: ACEP comments on interim final regulations, *Patient Transfer News,* 2:1-4 1994.
16. Dresnick S: Emergency departments in the integrated healthcare system. Presented at the ACEP Management Academy, May 18, 1995, Boston, Massachusetts.
17. Williams RW: The image of emergency medicine: overcoming the myths by emphasizing the realities. Presented at the American College of Emergency Physicians Scientific Assembly, September 12, 1995, Washington, DC.
18. Shaw KN, Selbst SM: Indigent children who are denied care in the emergency department, *Ann Emerg Med* 19:59-62, 1990.
19. Baker DW, Stevens CD, Brooks RH: Patients who leave a public hospital emergency department without being seen by a physician, *JAMA* 266:1085-1090, 1991.
20. American Medical Association CPT Editorial Panel: *American Medical Association current procedural terminology*—95, Chicago, 1994, American Medical Association.
21. Krohn RW: Achieving the best—and avoiding the worst—of capitation contracting, *Group Pract J* 44:18-24, 1995.
22. Young GP, Sklar D: Healthcare reform in emergency medicine, *Ann Emerg Med* 25:666-674, 1995.

42 Professional Liability Insurance

John D. Dunn

OUTLINE

Professional liability insurance is the highest single professional expense for emergency physicians. Because the hospital component of liability coverage is usually obtained through the hospital's insurer, this chapter focuses on professional liability insurance for physicians. General principles are applicable to all insurance arrangements for hospitals, as well as for other professional liability coverage.

PRIMER ON INSURANCE LAW

Generally insurance coverage is obtained and maintained through insurance contracts. Although insurance law is a modification of contract law, some esoteric concepts of insurance are peculiar to the nature of arrangements to indemnify.

The basic concept of a contract is an exchange of promises of performance for consideration. Consideration is a legal term that means *something of value*. The terms of the contract contain the specifics of the performance and the consideration.

In the case of an insurance contract, the insurer, usually an insurance company, agrees to protect the insured in exchange for money. The terms of that protection are laid out in the insurance contract or policy.

Contract law specifies that the written words will control the agreement. If the agreement is silent or ambiguous, courts commonly will rely on the most reasonable interpretation of the words of the contract. The insurance company usually controls the language of the insurance policy and the terms of coverage. Therefore the courts place a greater burden on the insurance company than on the insured and will interpret any ambiguity in the policy in favor of the insured and coverage. This basic rule of insurance law is critical to the discussions hereafter.

REGULATION OF THE INSURANCE INDUSTRY

When selecting an insurance provider, the physician/group must understand the regulations that govern the insurer's activities. These regulations may have important implications in the areas of solvency and accountability. One important law is the Federal Risk Retention Act (RRA).[1] The RRA preempts state law and provides an alternative to state insurance regulations for specialty insurance programs.

Generally insurance companies are allowed to sell insurance to the residents of a state if they are an admitted or a nonadmitted carrier. Admitted carriers are required to contribute to state insurance insolvency funds and submit to regular financial reviews by the insurance commissioner's office. Investigation of any complaints about an admitted carrier's denial of coverage or business practices are referred to the state's insurance commission. Violations of civil or criminal law are referred to the attorney general of the state, and prosecutions are pursued by a cooperative effort between the insurance commission and the attorney general. The admitted carriers contribute to an insolvency fund, which is provided for the victims of a loss of coverage as a result of an insolvency of the insurance company. The insurance commission is required to try to prevent insolvencies by investigation and audit activities.

Nonadmitted carriers are exempt from these contributions and financial reviews unless an investigation by the state insurance commissioner is undertaken because of specific problems. Most states allow only admitted carriers to sell insurance in their state. Nonadmitted carriers are subject to varying amounts of regulation or tolerance.

The RRA allows another exception. Nonadmitted carriers may come into a state to insure professional groups with a common interest in a certain type of insurance coverage. The insured professionals are then called risk retention act groups and may insure as a nonadmitted insurance carrier as long as that program is admitted in at least one state.

A significant percentage of emergency physicians across the country are insured through Risk Retention Act insurance entities, and many of the insurance programs, particularly those developed by large contract groups, have at least at one time insured themselves with risk retention groups or captive insurance companies or other combinations of arrangements. Emergency physicians/groups should be aware of these various kinds of insurance companies and insurance entities because nonadmitted insurers may not be participants in insolvency funds and therefore not provide liability protection in the case of insurance company insolvency.

THE INSURANCE POLICY

The insurance policy is simply a contract that sets out the terms of an exchange of promises for consideration. An insurance policy contract includes the following basic elements.

The Parties

The parties include the insurance company and the insured physician. The parties may also include those who are employed or supervised by the practitioner. It may also include other physicians or a hospital with which the physician is associated.

Additional Insured. Frequently entities such as groups, partnerships, and corporations are named as an additional insured. This is intended to clarify any potential ambiguity of the relationship. Named additional insureds should be considered any time a professional with quasi-independent authority is involved, for example a physician assistant or a nurse practitioner.

In an independent contractor's agreement with a group that includes provisions for malpractice insurance, the independent contractor and the group should be certain that their names are added to the list of additional insureds. Usually the parties are specified on the face sheet. In addition to the principal insured, additional insured such as groups, corporations, and individuals also should be specified. An exception to this practice occurs if other insureds are designated in the policy in generic terms, such as allied professional personnel supervised by the physician, or employees of the physician.

Channeling. This insurance concept involves adding physicians to an institutional malpractice insurance policy as additionally insured. The programs may vary in size and strength from the Harvard Risk Management Foundation to one hospital programs. Some hospitals offer low cost channeled programs to attract additional staff and to encourage loyalty.

The advantages of channeling are financial security and or availability of coverage in a bad market. There are also disadvantages to channeling. A *unified defense* may not be advantageous. The obligation to report settlements or judgments to the National Practitioner Data Bank or the State Licensing Board may create a conflict of interest.

The best national example of a cooperative channeled program is the Harvard Risk Management Foundation, which insures several hospitals and all the physicians of the staffs of these hospitals in the Boston area affiliated with Harvard. The benefit is a cooperative program that encourages risk management, reduces overhead costs, provides easy access to malpractice coverage for physicians who are credentialed to practice at those hospitals, and encourages a cooperative venture in risk management and quality assurance. The Harvard Risk Management Foundation, in addition to providing basic insurance coverage for a very large group of physicians and hospitals, does research and educational programs designed to reduce professional liability problems.

Insurance Types

Occurrence Policies. Occurrence policies provide coverage indefinitely for anything that happens during the policy coverage period, that is for the time during which premiums are paid. These policies apply for a claim made after the term of the policy for an incident that occurred during the term the policy is covered.

Claims-Made Policies. A *claims-made* policy is more complex. This type of policy provides for coverage during the term of the insurance policy only for those claims brought during that term. If an incident occurs during the policy term and the claim is brought after the term of the policy, coverage is not provided unless the coverage is continued or a "tail" or "nose" is purchased.

Tail Coverage. *Tail Coverage* must be purchased to get coverage for claims that are brought after the end of the claims-made policy term. This effectively converts the claims-made policy to occurrence (see Cost of Insurance below).

Most emergency physicians are covered by a claims-made policy, the most prevalent form of insurance available for physicians today. When a contract terminates or a physician leaves the group, tail coverage must be purchased to protect the rest of the group and the emergency department for claims arising from incidents that occur during the covered term. The prudent emergency physician/group should make arrangements for tail purchase if an individual leaves the group.

In a contract between a hospital and a group, the hospital may require the group to provide a tail if the contract is terminated. Without this contractual guarantee, the hospital may have the only insurance coverage for a claim filed after the group has left, creating greater liability for the hospital.

Avoidance of Tail Coverage. Under certain circumstances some insurance companies and policies provide automatic tail insurance for the insured. These exceptional circumstances may include retirement or disability. Some policies provide tail coverage in the event of a group's no cause (no fault) loss of the contract. These cases are rare exceptions and are applied only in special circumstances where the insured is blameless and the purchase of a tail would create significant burdens. Whenever liability for buying a tail can be avoided, the insured should look for these rare but valuable escape hatches.

Nose Coverage. When terminating an insurance agreement on a claims made policy, future claims arising from prior incidents can be covered either by purchasing a tail from the original insurance company or buying nose coverage from a subsequent insurer.

Nose policies are similar in coverage to tail policies. Both involve purchasing coverage for past incidents that may be claims in the future. A tail policy purchases insurance from the old insurance company for the period after coverage has ceased. A nose policy purchases insurance from the new insurance company for previously unreported incidents that occured before the new policy is in place.

Coverage Disputes. Coverage disputes may arise in a claims-made policy. Language in some insurance policies defines a claim as a formal demand or a filed lawsuit. These policies specifically exclude incidents that might result in a malpractice claim or lawsuit until legal action is initiated by the patient or patient's family. This distinction is particularly important for those insured by a claims-made policy who are changing insurance coverage.

For example, suppose you have a claims-made policy with insurance company A in 1992 and a patient has a bad outcome. In 1993 you change to insurance company B and buy nose coverage from company B, which may specify coverage except for incidents already known. You reported the incident to company A, which did not accept it as a claim because its definition requires filing of a lawsuit or receipt of a demand letter or complaint letter. The incident is not covered by company A even though the incident was known and reported because company's definition of a reported claim was not met. Company B also refuses to cover the incident because according to company B's definition of a claim, it was known and reported as an incident to company A. Although this situation may seem unfair and confusing, the courts probably would rule in favor of coverage one way or the other because the courts, when possible, rule in favor of coverage for the insured. However, be wary of the problem and potential for no coverage based on conflicting language in policies.

Coverage Issues

The usual and customary activities of the identified insured are covered activities under the insurance policy. The courts will interpret an emergency physician's professional liability insurance policy to include the reasonable expectations of an emergency physician unless specific exceptions are carved out by the insurance company.

Because the usual practice of an emergency physician includes radio control of prehospital care personnel, it would be unreasonable for an insurance company to deny coverage for this activity, particularly if the patient is coming to that emergency department. On the other hand, the insurance company reasonably might not expect that an emergency physician would be responsible for medical control of a 10 county area. However, rural emergency physicians might be expected to provide supervision for prehospital care services in a wide service area.

Although the court will generally interpret insurance policies in favor of coverage, it is important not to stretch the limits too far. In questionable situations, it is necessary to specify coverage of exceptional activities with a rider to the policy. Nonetheless, it is unlikely that an emergency physician will be able to get a rider covering procedures far outside the general practice of emergency medicine such as performing epidural anesthetic procedures in the emergency department for patients with chronic pain.

The rule of thumb is that the reasonably anticipated practice of the specialist is insured. The specialty and the area of practice are also used to determine what is expected of a practitioner. In equivocal situations, the courts generally find in favor of coverage. The insurance policy will be controlling on specific exclusions in the coverage sections.

Compensatory Damages. Compensatory damages are a legal means to return a person to the state or condition that he or she existed before the injury caused by the negligent or intentional act. Returning a person to the previous state could include compensation for lost wages, medical expenses, and measured pecuniary losses of all kinds, which are called special damages. General damages may be difficult to measure, but they are recognized by the courts to include pain and suffering, loss of companionship, loss of marital consortium, and other intangible compensable damages. Insurance policies always cover or indemnify for compensatory damages.

Punitive Damages. Insurance in most states is restricted to coverage for negligence. Most insurance policies as a matter of law cannot provide coverage for intentional acts, violations of criminal or regulatory law, or other compensable acts or omissions that fall outside the umbrella of negligence law. Therefore punitive awards may not be covered. In a medical malpractice case, the condition on which punitive damages are usually awarded is gross and flagrant disregard for patient safety.

Although a few states do not recognize punitive damages, the majority of states do allow punitive damages in many circumstances, including professional liability negligence actions. If a jury awards damages above and beyond those legally considered compensatory, insurance coverage is doubtful.

Although much is made of the problem of punitive damages, they are rarely awarded in a professional liability case. Frequently they are pleaded by the plaintiff's attorney who may want to scare the insurance company and especially the defendant. It is easy to imagine that a plaintiff's attorney will include many forms and amounts designed to psychologically affect the defendant. In addition, the insurance company is obligated to advise a defendant that the insurance policy does not cover punitive damages. The defendant physician not only is initially frightened by the plaintiff attorney's pleading, amounts of damage alleged, and the punitive damages included, but also is then further unnerved by a letter from the insurance company saying that the punitive damages are not covered under the policy.

It is important to understand that the insurance company is obligated to defend on these cases even though state policy prohibits insurance companies from indemnifying the losses that result from punitive damages. A personal attorney should be consulted on these problem coverage situations.

Examples of acts or omissions clearly not covered by professional liability insurance coverage or professional liability policies would usually be listed in the exclusions of the policy. Exclusions include violations of the medical practice act. Examples are unethical, immoral, or unprofessional behavior; misuse of the patient-physician relationship; misuse or abuse of chemical substances; prescribing or therapeutic practices that fall outside the accepted standards of care as outlined in the medical practice act; and other violations of regulatory law.

Types of uncovered activities for which professional liability insurance would be unavailable include the following examples: (1) a physician inappropriately employs a nurse to practice medicine without supervision, (2) a physician takes sexual advantage of a patient, or (3) a physician abuses chemical substances, impairing his or her ability to provide proper medical care.

Contract Indemnification Clauses. Many contractual relationships include indemnification of the hospital for the negligence of the emergency physician. In other words, the emergency physician's/group's liability insurance will provide coverage to the hospital for liability arising from the physician's/group's negligence. Often these indemnification agreements are bilateral so that the emergency physician/group is covered for any negligence on the part of the hospital staff.

Insurance companies consistently will not indemnify an organization that is not party to the policy. If an emergency physician group has agreed to indemnify the hospital and the group's insurer does not agree, the group/physician could have a problem obtaining irreconcilable contract/coverage conflicts.

In the real world, however, the legal process will assess liability according to accepted legal principles. Neither an insurance policy nor an emergency department contract will modify the actual legal liabilities arising from a negligent action. Moreover, an indemnification contract between a hospital and an emergency physician group does not create an insurance obligation. State law and court decisions disallow any illegal effect of indemnification agreements. Therefore indemnification clauses are not as important as they might seem and do not nullify the law of liability. They involve clauses written by overzealous lawyers trying to prove their worth to their clients. In a lawsuit, the courts impose liability and indemnity analysis that ignores any contract impositions.

Violations of Regulations. Although professional liability insurance generally does not cover intentional violations of criminal law, there are a few gray areas where coverage may be provided. An example is violation of Section 1867 of the Social Security Act referred to as COBRA or Emergency Medical Treatment and Active Labor Act (EMTALA).[2] There are negligence provisions in regulatory law, and legal action can be taken against a physician for negligent violation of the law. As a result, in some circumstances the damages covered by a malpractice insurance policy may include fines and assessments, as well as awards and judgments based on a negligent violation of the regulations. There is no easy answer on this complex coverage problem.

Section 1867 provides for action by a patient who alleges damages as a result of failure to comply with Section 1867. State law provides remedies under professional liability actions. In addition, the Office of the Inspector General of the Department of Health and Human Services also has the authority to pursue physicians for violations. Specifically Section 1867 allows for fines of up to $50,000 and/or termination from the Medicare program. Most insurance companies would assert that they are not obligated to pay these fines and would exclude the fines and civil penalties from coverage. If specific inclusion language is not written in the policy, however, it is advisable for the defendant threatened by such potential losses to obtain personal legal counsel and explore the obligations of the insurance company.

Amounts of Coverage

Amounts of coverage are stated on the face sheet of an insurance policy. Usually there are two amounts of coverage. The first amount is the per incident total available and the second amount is the aggregate total available for the period of coverage, usually 1 year. For example, a policy that has coverage limits of $1/$3 million has coverage of $1 million for each incident and a total of $3 million for the period of coverage.

The declaration of coverage on the face sheet may be modified by other contract provisions in the insurance policy. For example, the cost and expense of investigation and defense may be subtracted from the total amounts available for indemnity coverage, the money available for compensating a patient.

Awards and Judgments in Excess of Insurance Coverage. One of the great psychologic games of professional liability litigation occurs when the plaintiff's attorney initially asks for a huge award and then offers settlement within the coverage limits. The defendant may be quite distraught when he or she realizes that the policy falls short of the potential award and his or her personal assets may be at risk. The defendant then may be both relieved and eager to settle within the limits of coverage when this offer is subsequently made.

Plaintiff's attorneys are reluctant to try to collect by execution on the property of the defendant physician if the award, judgment, or settlement exceeds the insurance coverage. It is much easier for plaintiff's attorneys to deal directly with the insurance company, collect the cash, and walk away rather than attempt to acquire a defendant's personal assets and possibly instigate a bankruptcy action. As a result, plaintiff's attorneys are inclined to settle cases within the policy coverage limits with few exceptions. In addition they create a psychologic and legal advantage with the insurance company and the defendant physician on offers of settlements within the coverage limits.

For example, a defendant agrees to a settlement within the coverage limits. The insurance company refuses the settlement and the case goes to a jury. If the jury then awards the plaintiff an amount in excess of the policy limits, the insurance company may be liable for the entire amount. This outcome could be considered failure to properly defend and indemnify the insured physician. This principle of law requires that insurance companies settle cases within the policy limits for the benefits of their insured or take the risk that they will be, as a company, separately and independently liable for the award in excess of the insurance policy limits. This concept of "good faith" provides that the insurance company defend and indemnify the insured. It creates pressures to settle and offers real advantages for the plaintiff in a case that has some merit.

OBLIGATIONS OF THE INSURANCE COMPANY

Obligations of the insured and the insurer are outlined in insurance policies and should be reviewed.

Defend and Indemnify

The requirements to defend and indemnify create significant legal obligations for the insurance company. First, the insurance company is required to provide adequate defense and investigation of a claim. It must provide an unfettered defense with a competent attorney. The defendant has the right to demand another attorney and a better defense if he or she finds that an attorney is incompetent, unwilling, or restricted in investigating and defending the professional liability action. If the insurance company refuses, it may be liable for damages. These damages are usually awarded in multiples. For example if the insured shows that the insurance company's bad faith resulted in a loss of a certain amount of money, many states allow for the insured to recover three to four times that amount.

Obligations of the Lawyer

Common law and tradition require that the attorney, even though hired by the insurance company, is obligated to provide uncompromised representation of the insured policy holder.[3] This stipulation prohibits insurance companies from interfering with defense of a case, and it obligates attorneys to be clearly responsible to the insured and not to the insurance company. In the real world of insurance, the insurance company pays the bills and has substantial influence over the defense attorney's actions. However, when that influence compromises the interest of the defendant, insurance law clearly states that the attorney has as his or her primary obligation the interests of the insured.

OBLIGATIONS OF THE INSURED

The insured physician has three basic responsibilities. The first is to maintain licensure and comply with the laws of the state. Any voluntary or negligent violation of the law potentially can invalidate coverage.

The second responsibility is to immediately notify the insurance company on receipt of a notice that a lawsuit is being filed. On receipt of a complaint or any significant threat of a lawsuit, the defendant is obligated to consider whether the insurance company should be notified. It is always better to notify the insurance company, even when uncertain, particularly if there are significant potential damages involved. This notification allows the insurance company to develop a timely defense. If an insured physician fails to properly and immediately report receipt of the lawsuit notice, several things can happen—all of them negative. The defense can be compromised by a finding of default judgment. This finding may occur because one must respond to a lawsuit within 20 to 30 days or, in most jurisdictions, a default judgment is entered. In the case of default judgment, the insurance company could refuse to pay on the default. Late hiring of an attorney may occasionally reverse a default judgment if the court is convinced that it would serve the interest of justice. If the default judgment is not reversed, however, the amount of damage is all that can be litigated because liability is already decided. If a jury is instructed that the question of liability is already settled, it can then focus only on the amount of money to be awarded, creating the potential for a generous verdict. The insurer will refuse payments.

The third obligation of the insured is to cooperate with the defense of any malpractice case from beginning to end.

After notification or filing of a suit, the insured physician or group must cooperate with the investigation and defense of the case. The defendant should be available for deposition, for discovery response to interrogatories and questions, to help the lawyer research the records and the medical issues of the case, and for the trial. The defendant must not act in a way that would compromise the defense of the case. For example, communication about the case should be restricted to confidential and privileged inquiries such as by an investigator or the lawyer assigned to the case. Talking with individuals in a way that might compromise the defense of the case could result in the insurance company issuing a notice of possible noncoverage based on failure to cooperate.

Just as the insured physician has the right to object to the insurance company's failing to provide an adequate attorney and an adequate defense, the insurance company has the right to object to the defendant's unwillingness to cooperate and provide assistance in the defense of the case. This two-way street of cooperation is essential. It obligates the defendant physician to be informed about the case, to protect the files and the records of the case, to restrict conversations and communications about the case to the insurance company and its representatives, and to cooperate with the discovery and trial process.

Although insurance companies may tolerate some lack of cooperation from a busy physician, it is the physician who as a result of a loss is injured the most and whose name goes into the National Practitioner Data Bank. These are serious matters and require substantial and continuing attention. The defendant physician/group and their partners in the defense of the case, the lawyer, and the insurance company, must cooperate and demand a comprehensive and thorough effort.

PRACTICE PARAMETERS AND RISK MANAGEMENT PROGRAMS

Most emergency physicians are aware that the American College of Emergency Physicians (ACEP) and others have published practice parameters and guidelines on the management of high risk medical problems. These problems include febrile infants, chest pain, blunt trauma, and seizures. Others will be developed by ACEP, the Agency for Health Care Policy and Research of the Department of Health and Human Services, and other medical specialty societies.

Some insurance programs have incorporated those practice parameters into their guidelines for healthcare practitioners. In Maine, a special program has been developed that provides for the defense of emergency physicians if they follow a practice parameter approved by the participating specialties of emergency medicine, radiology, and obstetrics and gynecology.[4] Practice parameters may become more important if current healthcare reform efforts succeed in their attempt to outline efficient and scientifically accepted methods of management of various conditions.

Specialty insurance and professional liability companies in emergency medicine are increasing their level of preventive and educational activities to reduce repetition of previously recognized problems. They encourage physicians to participate in risk management programs with discounts and favorable premium structures. It is likely that many insurance companies with active risk management programs will require that their insured participate in risk management education and audit programs.

As a corollary to risk management education and preventive practices, many insurance companies are now surcharging physicians with bad experience. Further, insurance companies that promote practice parameters may penalize physicians on any claims paid where the physician failed to comply with the practice parameter. Watch for the appearance of these clauses in malpractice policy language.

The risk management program of ACEP is based on an actuarial analysis of risk and the dollars and frequency of malpractice losses by emergency physicians. After many years of analysis, it is now well recognized that the vast majority of risk management problems involve patients who are discharged from the emergency department.

Several areas of diagnosis account for more than 50% of malpractice dollar losses for emergency physicians. These categories are nontraumatic chest pain in the adult, febrile infants, abdominal pain, and trauma. Specific missed diagnoses include acute myocardial infarction or unstable angina, ectopic pregnancy, appendicitis, fractures of the cervical spine or pelvis associated with major trauma, and wound management with foreign bodies and infections. Because the list for emergency physicians is so short, risk management programs have been designed specifically to improve the management and documentation of these cases.

A special program initiated by the Massachusetts College of Emergency Physicians and in cooperation with the Massachusetts Joint Underwriting Authority provides discounts and special treatment for physicians who participate in a comprehensive risk management program. This is one of many developing programs that encourage increased attention to managing malpractice risks. Insurance companies involved in these programs deserve consideration by the potential purchaser. These companies demonstrate a higher level interest and professionalism and take a proactive role in reducing malpractice risks and controlling costs.

EVALUATING THE INSURANCE COMPANY

Stability

It is difficult in the professional liability market to be certain about the financial stability of the insurance company providing coverage. It is particularly difficult to assess when layered coverage is involved (see the following discussion). Further, the risk retention act groups (see earlier discussion) admitted under special law are so new that many do not have a track record that allows a financial rating.

The general rule on financial stability is to look for the "Best" rating,[5] which is an industry report describing the financial strengths of the insurance company. A "Best" rating of at least "A" is usually recognized as the cutoff for financial security. Many companies have higher than an "A" rating. Companies that have a rating below an "A" are considered to be on shaky financial ground.

Longevity of the company or the entity in the malpractice area is certainly important. Many commercial insurance companies have jumped in and out of professional liability markets, which creates inconsistent and potentially troubling coverage problems.

Ultimately it is difficult to take the time and muster the resources to evaluate an insurance company. Therefore some basic strategies are advisable for managers of groups or individuals trying to decide on the purchase of professional liability insurance. Check with your professional association. ACEP may have information about the insurance entity you are considering. The state medical association or society may have similar information and also access to the insurance commissioner's information about an insurance company. In addition, a professional broker may have contacts and resources that will help to reduce the chance of a mistake. If insurance is purchased through a broker, the broker's errors and omissions policy of insurance may provide extra protection if the primary insurance program chosen is compromised.

Claims Management and Other Services

The company's claims management and litigation resources should also be evaluated through a review of company brochures or pamphlets or other company information. Reputation of the company, particularly in a relatively close business such as emergency medicine, is usually available from other professionals in emergency medicine.

The quality of an insurance company's defense is directly related to the quality of the attorneys engaged for that defense. Therefore the quality of the law firms and attorneys that an insurance company uses in your area is another excellent measure of the competence of the insurance company and its willingness to provide good faith defense.

Other insurance company benefits such as consulting on risk management and educational programs should be used as resources for improving risk and decreasing loss experience for the emergency medicine group. These are measures of expertise and company commitment.

Layered Insurance

Within the insurance policy coverage, there may be many layers. The insurance coverage may involve not only the insurance company mentioned on the policy, but also other insurance entities participating at one or more levels.

For example, in a $1 million policy for a physician, the policy may appear to be with the Summa Company of the United States of America. However, a close look at the insurance treaties and arrangements reveals that for a $1 million award, Summa may pay only the first $100,000. The second $200,000 might be paid by an on-shore excess insurance carrier. In this example, the umbrella coverage above $300,000 may be put together in US domestic and in foreign excess insurance markets such as Germany, England, and France.

Captive and special interest excess insurance companies may participate at various levels for various amounts. The policy written on the paper of an admitted carrier may represent the financial security of multiple companies. This fact may seem unimportant, but the insolvency of excess insurers off shore in particular may leave the insured physician or group without part of its coverage. In circumstances where excess insurance layers are lost because of insolvencies, the state insolvency funds may not guarantee backup. For example, a state insolvency fund may guarantee a maximum payout of $300,000 for anyone insured by an insolvent company. Major disputes may arise, particularly if one of the excess insurers is off shore and not admitted. In that case, the only access to the insolvency fund may be through the "fronting" or stated company.

When purchasing malpractice insurance, the wise buyer seeks reputable companies that can be readily and adequately evaluated. Major contract group insurance policy purchases are complex and usually involve piecing together insurance packages that take advantage of market opportunities and the resources of the insured group. The face sheet of a large group's policy may not reveal the complexity of the insurance structure. If the fiscal integrity of the group and the insurer are marginal, the group itself may not be able to guarantee malpractice insurance, potentially leaving the contracted physician uncovered.

Some bankruptcies of professional liability companies have had impact on groups and individuals. Several years ago a syndicate from the Lloyd's of London insurance programs suffered bankruptcy because of extraordinary international losses. This syndicate participated in a number of medical professional liability programs, leading to some compromises to coverage for physician groups in the United States. These purchasing decisions are more than routine and have long-range implications.

COST OF INSURANCE

Price

Shopping for malpractice insurance requires an evaluation of price. Although price is important, it should not be the controlling factor. Choose a company with the intent of maintaining a long-term relationship, particularly when purchasing a claims-made policy, since switching claims-made policies carry with them substantial "tail" costs.

There are two mechanisms for pricing emergency department coverage. The first is a single policy held by a named physician; the second is per visit coverage for a location. Single policy cost varies from state to state and regions of various states because of malpractice experience. Also, the nature of the emergency department and its type of practice will affect price. More sophisticated approaches to underwriting are usually available within the specialty companies that focus on emergency medicine coverage.

ACEP Endorsed Professional Liability Insurance Program. The best analysis is the experience of the ACEP-endorsed emergency physician professional liability program from 1976 to 1984. This closed program and actuarial analysis has resulted in many of ACEP's risk management programs including the risk management publication *Foresight*.

The ACEP-endorsed program had total indemnity losses of about $.50 per visit on a 55 million visit insurance exposure. Adding in defense costs, which in most insurance companies is 20% to 30%, and administrative costs of 5% to 10%, the basic cost of this program endorsed by ACEP was $1 to $2/visit of exposure. In the early 1980s emergency department coverage was being sold by various insurers for about $2 to $6/visit.

Per Visit Policies. Per visit coverage is more flexible than malpractice policies purchased for the individual physician. Per visit arrangements cover the emergency department and the group irrespective of its composition. Members of the group may change and include part-time practitioners without changing the premium. The part-timers are named as additional insureds.

Contemporary prices for per visit policies cost from $4 to $8 or more/visit, depending on group size and location, coverage, amount of self-insurance, and the attractiveness of the business to the insurance companies. Because typical full-time physicians work about 2000 hours/year, and an average physician sees 2.5 patients/hour, a $15,000 premium would be the equivalent of about $3/visit. The cost is based on the number of visits and adjusted as census changes.

The price is affected by the insured groups' previous malpractice loss experience. If the malpractice claims and loss experience exceeds 1 claim/10,000 to 20,000 visits, the insurance company may add a surcharge to the emergency group for bad experience. It is appropriate to compare costs of insurance obtainable in the independent market.

Tail Costs. Specialty insurance companies offering per visit coverage generally offer claims made policies only. Typically the claims made policy starts at a low premium and matures over 5 years to a higher level premium. The low initial cost of premiums is offset by the "maturation" of the policy. The cost of the tail necessary to terminate the coverage with the insurance company by converting it to an occurrence policy can be expensive, usually one and one-half to two times the last annual premium. Further, tail coverage may provide variable tail coverage, sometimes as short as 3 years.

Remember that even though claims made insurance looks attractive during the first year, after the third or fourth year it matures to be equivalent to the cost of occurrence policy, and the tail still has to be paid on termination of the policy. Whenever considering entering into an insurance arrangement, the cost of nose or tail must be included as part of the total calculation.

In a group per visit policy, coverage is provided for the whole group, which requires a single aggregate tail to be purchased when the coverage is terminated. This is an advantage for an individual physician and a stable group, as it is unnecessary to purchase individual tails whenever a physician leaves the group. For hospitals employing physicians, this plan also creates a stable insurance arrangement.

Self-Insured Groups

Some emergency medicine groups have become large enough to self-insure a significant portion of their business. They then find excess insurance to prevent catastrophic losses. There is no method to clearly determine the per visit costs for self-insurance programs. To maintain independent contractor status, most major groups make a book entry for malpractice coverage. The contractor physician is well advised to check the amount deducted per visit for malpractice to make sure that book entry reflects a realistic cost.

SUMMARY

The basic rule in insurance, as well as other purchases is, "If it sounds too good to be true, it probably is." Even though the basic rules of insurance law are designed to provide protection, there are times when insurance coverage will be disputed, leaving the insured frustrated, upset, and worried.

Professional liability coverage for the emergency department is an important and costly expense for hospitals and emergency physicians. A competent manager should consider professional liability insurance coverage carefully, review insurance policies for the details mentioned in this chapter, and evaluate the insurance program for fiscal soundness, adequate coverage arrangements, and value. Competent legal advice is well worth the cost.

REFERENCES

1. Risk Retention Act: 15 U.S.C.A. Sec. 3901-3906, West Supp, 1993.
2. 42 U.S.C. 1395 (dd).
3. *Employers Casualty Co. v Tiley,* 496 S.W. 2d 552, 558, Texas, 1973.
4. Maine Medical Liability Demonstration Project, Maine Laws, Ch 24, Sec 2971-2978, 1989.
5. *Annual Report Rating Insurance Companies,* Oldwick, NJ, A.M. Best Co.

43 Common Contract Problems

Jay W. Edelberg

OUTLINE

During the life of a contract between an emergency physician group and a hospital, problems arise that may affect the security of the contract or, at least, the relationships among the various people. It is necessary to build these relationships to ensure smooth operation and effective management of the emergency department. This chapter discusses a variety of common problems that arise in the evolving relationships among key people and various approaches to resolve them. Techniques are presented to prevent issues from becoming crises.

ISSUE IDENTIFICATION

Many problems can be identified before initiation of the contract. During the exploration and negotiation phases, emergency physician managers should ask probing questions. They should get clear direction from the administration about existing and potential problems and the short- and long-term goals of the administration. This precontract time provides a golden opportunity for the physician group to begin to develop a plan to resolve many of the identified problems.

These early problem identification discussions should include dialogue with the emergency department nurse manager, staff nurses, attending physicians, and, in certain circumstances, the emergency physicians currently working in the emergency department. Input from these key people is invaluable and provides direction to the incoming group about its mission and management responsibilities.

Once the contract is initiated, the emergency physicians have an opportunity to directly experience problems in the working environment. Even if many of the issues previously identified were addressed and resolved, some problems will inevitably emerge that were not adequately identified or resolved. New problems will continue to arise, and old problems previously thought to be resolved will reappear in the same or an altered form. Managing an area as complex as an emergency department is a dynamic process.

Typical Problems

Many of the issues facing the emergency physician group are generic and often predictable. Long waits for laboratory tests, difficulty getting patients admitted to the intensive care unit, and prolonged delays caused by attending physicians are some examples of problems that plague most emergency departments.

A good example of a recurring problem is patients leaving before examination. Typically this problem is resolved by adding staff or streamlining patient flow in some manner. When the problem recurs months later, it must be reexamined to see whether the causes are the same or if new causes require new solutions.

Prevention

The best way to deal with problems is to prevent them from happening. Good physician managers can use several effective techniques to prevent potential problems.

Emergency Services Committee. Regular meetings with administration, medical staff members, and nursing should be a routine part of the physician manager's monthly regimen. An Emergency Services Committee should be established as a standing committee of the medical staff and chaired by the chief of the emergency department. The membership may include staff emergency physicians, the emergency department nurse manager, and key members of the medical staff from other disciplines such as pediatrics, medicine, surgery, orthopedics, psychiatry, and obstetrics/gynecology. The agenda of this monthly meeting should include both quality and operational issues and also should allow opportunity for open discussion during which medical staff members can bring issues directly to the committee.

Medical Staff Meetings. Another effective method of problem prevention with the medical staff is to have the chief of emergency medicine or one of his or her designees attend medical staff departmental meetings. Because medical staff meetings are always open, it is reasonable for an emergency physician to sit ex-officio at the regularly scheduled meetings of the departments of medicine, surgery, pediatrics, etc.

Issues related to the emergency department arise spontaneously at these meetings, and emergency department representation prevents these issues from growing out of proportion. The emergency physician can address the issues either immediately at the meeting, or as follow-up to the meeting. Concerns can be voiced by both parties and emotions kept in check. Working relationships will be strengthened, and friendships and respect can evolve.

Emergency Department Operations Meeting. The emergency department requires a monthly operations meeting. The physician group, nurse management, and a representative from administration should meet regularly to review issues raised internally, or by members of the medical staff, nursing staff, administration, or patients. Quality improvement programs should be instituted and come under the purview of this committee.

Feedback/Surveys

It is critical for the physicians to receive feedback on a routine basis. Surveys may be developed and specifically designed for administration, nursing, attending physicians, and patients. These surveys may be sent out on a regular, perhaps quarterly, basis so that the physicians and other members of the department can receive written feedback from these essential audiences. The emergency department management then can keep a finger on the pulse of the department's performance and develop solutions such as policy modification to problems identified through these surveys.

Expectation Management

A common failing of physicians, administrators, and nurses is inadequate determination of reasonable end points and outcomes. For example, an administrator who assumes that the new physician group will reduce patient complaints to zero has unrealistic expectations. If three or four patient complaints have been received weekly, it might be reasonable to try to reduce that number by 50% or 75%, but it is unreasonable to expect that complaints can be permanently eliminated.

Another problem involves patients leaving before physician examination. A reasonable number of patients in this category may be less than 10 or 20 patients a month, or a percentage of total visits, for example 1% of monthly volume. Once there is agreement that a problem exists, information must be gathered and data analyzed. In this example the number of these patients should be tracked by month, day of the week, and hour of the day. The charts of these patients should be analyzed for trends, including types of presenting complaints, payor mix, and risk management issues. Improvement may be based on consideration of historical statistics and realistic operational changes.

Once data have been gathered and analyzed, an action plan must be developed. All stakeholders should be involved in the process including representatives from registration, triage nurses, the nurse manager, administration, and emergency physicians. In the example of unacceptable waiting times for laboratory tests, the laboratory director, nurse manager, emergency physician director, and a representative from management information services (MIS) might be the key individuals to assess the data and develop the plan to resolve problems.

After an action plan has been prepared and implemented, the problem-solving team should agree to reevaluate the data at appropriate time intervals to ensure that the intended results are achieved.

CONTRACT ISSUES—FINANCIAL ARRANGEMENTS

A common source of contract problems between a hospital and a group are the issues related to financial arrangements. The broad variety of arrangements including guarantees, subsidies, and billing services can become a source of irritation or even distrust. Once a contract has been initiated, monetary issues may surface by either the administration or the physician group.

Guarantee Arrangements

Monetary issues commonly arise in arrangements in which the hospital pays the emergency physician group a set sum of money. The root of this problem is that the hospital is taking all the financial risk while the emergency physician group may have none. As hospital finances are being squeezed by the shrinking healthcare dollar, the administrator may see the cost of emergency physicians as a large expense item. As such, he or she may attempt to renegotiate the contract with the existing group, with the intention of having the group work for less money, or at least share some of the financial risk.

A typical reaction from an emergency physician group to this type of renegotiation is to react with anger and cries of "foul play." In today's healthcare economic environment, however, it may be reasonable for emergency physicians to assume financial risk, which can result in either more or less money, depending on the final negotiation.

Billing Arrangements

Some hospitals may advocate the elimination of the guarantee arrangement and insist that the group be responsible for their own billing. Groups that bill and collect for the first time may realize greater revenues and discover opportunities to further enhance their reimbursement. Alternatively, the group may not recover the amount necessary to adequately compensate the physicians. A compromise is to develop contract options that enable physicians to achieve their financial goals while markedly reducing the capital outlay by the hospital. One option would be a combination of independent billing by the group and a limited guarantee by the hospital. The proposal could include a cap on the monthly amount that the hospital would have to provide the group (a floor/cap contract). Another option is to provide a flat rate subsidy every month to supplement the group's collections. This amount can be fixed each month, or it can vary according to a sliding scale based on monthly or quarterly volumes.

Additional Programs/Service

The administration may desire more service for the money. In such situations, the group may be able to provide added value to the contract. The emergency physicians may hire transcription services at their own expense, may add additional coverage during peak volume hours to improve service, or may opt to work additional shifts to improve coverage and add value to the contract without increasing cost.

The emergency physicians and administration may want to start a new service, such as a fast track or a pediatric emergency area. Both hope to attract new customers to enhance revenue and eventually offset the cost of this new service. In such an instance, it is reasonable for the hospital to provide temporary monetary support to the physicians for additional staffing. This negotiation may be accomplished by limiting the money by time and volume. In other words, the group and the hospital might enter into a financial arrangement for 1 year during which if a certain volume of new patients is achieved, the financial support will be discontinued.

CONTRACT ISSUES—PHYSICIANS

Problems related to physicians and physician performance are a frequent cause of conflict between the hospital and the emergency physician group. These problems can be related to lack of leadership, ineffective screening of physicians, mediocre clinical performance, poor attitude, and complaint management.

Physician Leadership

An emergency department is a difficult and complex environment for a physician leader to test out his or her skills. Working with other emergency physicians, nurses, administration, and the attending medical staff requires special skills in collaboration. The root of this potential problem is often related to the physician medical director's lack of leadership skills. In fact, many physicians are poor leaders, despite their years of hard work and success in life. Some physicians do not understand why others around them do not live up to their expectations. A good leader understands the strengths and limitations of those around him or her and works within these confines to get the most out of everyone involved.

Leadership does not require knowing all the answers. Instead leaders must make sure that the right things get done. They should be able to motivate people, not through arrogance and intimidation, but through understanding and empowerment. The interaction between leaders and followers is critical for the ultimate success of any project or process.

When administration is unhappy with leadership in the emergency department, the group is faced with a serious challenge. The leader may be the owner of the contract or the most senior ranking member of the group. In many instances, that physician is well integrated into the power structure of the medical staff.

When administration or staff express frustration that is due to lack of leadership exhibited by the director, the best solution may be to expand the leadership within the group. By sharing and collaborating on some of the essential operational tasks, the group can help solve departmental problems, improve relationships, and support the leadership role of the physician director.

For example, one physician may assume the continuous quality improvement functions for the department; another might work with the nursing leadership of the department to help resolve physician-nurse issues; still another might work to improve communications between the emergency department and the ICU and the management of in-house codes. Ideally, the director and/or administrator will reward these motivated physicians for their time and effort. In any case, collaborative leadership will motivate others to recognize and implement the goals of improving the day-to-day operations of the department and enhancing relationships with others.

Physician Credentials

Emergency physician credentialing issues can arise during the initial contract negotiation or during the contract term. In an ideal world, all emergency physicians would be residency trained and board certified in emergency medicine. However, there is an insufficient number of physicians with these credentials, so many hospitals allow physicians who are residency trained in other primary care specialties to be credentialed to practice emergency medicine. Some hospitals require physicians to have only "some experience" in emergency medicine to be credentialed to work in the emergency department.

Problems may arise from overly strict or permissive credentialing criteria. If the contract demands all residency trained board-certified emergency physicians and the group is unable to meet this requirement, a renegotiation is necessary. The emergency physicians will advocate staffing flexibility, such as incorporating other primary care physicians, residency trained and board certified in their specialty. An agreement to keep the number of these physicians to no more than a certain percentage of the coverage may be a reasonable compromise. Alternatively, the physicians may have to negotiate additional money from the hospital enabling them to pay top dollar and attract board-certified emergency physicians.

From another perspective, attending physicians on the medical staff may want to take shifts in the emergency department. This puts the emergency physicians on the other side of the issue. In this case, the emergency physicians may argue that only board-certified emergency physicians be credentialed to work in the emergency department.

Physician Competence

It is uncomfortable to deal with questions of clinical competence. First, the problem must be recognized. Second, there should be due process and a process by which the physician demonstrates improvement. Third, there must be a reevaluation in a given time frame to reassess clinical competence.

When faced with the perception that a physician's clinical competence does not meet expectations, the emergency physician manager is faced with the difficult task of assessing the level of clinical deficiency and determining the remedy. Assuming that the problem is not impairment or attitude, but rather true clinical deficiencies, the emergency medicine director must evaluate the deficiencies. Discourse with those who hold these negative perceptions, including nursing staff, other emergency physicians, and attending medical staff, is mandatory. The CQI evaluation process should include the review of charts, patient complaints, and any serious incidents.

Isolated Deficiencies. If the physician has isolated areas of clinical deficiency, such as heart disease, multiple trauma, or eye injuries, there is a greater chance in improving the physician's skills and successfully resolving the problem. For example, if the deficiency is determined to be the assessment of patients with potential myocardial infarctions, then perhaps the physician can participate in a review course in this clinical area. Further, the physician could spend time with the cardiologists reading electrocardiograms. Review literature can be provided. The physician can even participate in some type of preceptorship to help improve knowledge and assessment skills in the area of deficiency.

Poor Judgment. If the deficiencies are broad based, the problem may not be a deficiency in knowledge, but rather a deficiency in judgment. Because judgment cannot be taught easily, there is a much greater likelihood that the physician will not be successfully rehabilitated. Judgment comes from being a good listener, recognizing the implications beyond the words, and having a high degree of suspicion on all patients, regardless of appearance or presenting complaint.

If the problem with the physician's clinical competence ultimately is rooted in poor judgment, it may be in everyone's best interest to terminate that physician quickly. Groups make the self-destructive error of desperately defending physicians to bide time when termination of a physician creates emergency department coverage problems. When the group acts in this arbitrary manner, the physician, group, and hospital are more susceptible to medicolegal problems. Further, the nursing staff loses confidence in the physician group and its leadership for making the wrong decision and exposing them and the patients to risk. Even when the group subsequently terminates the physician, the lengthy delay may create the distrust and disrespect of administration because of the lack of appropriate action.

Physician Attitudes

The medical director of the emergency department is again faced with a difficult task when he or she receives several complaints from patients, nurses, administration and/or attending staff about an emergency physician's attitude. An investigation may reveal that the physician has a problem with drugs or alcohol and is in fact impaired. In such cases, immediate action must be taken to remove the physician from the emergency department and report him or her to the appropriate impaired physician program.

However, when the attitude problem is not impairment, the solution may be even more difficult. Some physicians are arrogant and condescending. Others are hostile. Many do not like to "take orders" from nurses or have things suggested to them by patients or their family members. Other physicians appear disheveled and unkempt. In such cases, the physician's behavior may not be in question, but his or her appearance can create a poor image to the patients and staff. This poor image can create a lack of confidence in the physician's ability and lead to complaints.

A consistent pattern of these types of complaints will create a serious problem for the emergency physician group. Peer group counseling sessions may be helpful. In these sessions, the emergency physician meets with the other emergency physicians and the nurse manager to discuss observations and suggestions. These interventions may lead to temporary improvement; unfortunately, it is common for the original attitude to resurface. Some physician groups cling to the fact that the physician practices competent medicine and advocate continuation of the physician's privileges in the emergency department. This problem becomes serious when others demand the physician's removal from the schedule.

At some point, depending on the strength of the feelings of administration and the commitment of the group to the individual physician, a decision will be reached. In general, physicians with inappropriate attitudes tend to move from group to group and do not stay in any one place for a long time. If a physician has good clinical skills and is worth keeping, however, the emergency physician group should work hard not only to provide peer counseling but also arrange for professional counseling to improve the physician's attitude as much as possible. This support and commitment may help the physician function appropriately in the emergency department on a long-term basis.

Patient Complaints

Every emergency department experiences patient complaints from time to time. These complaints can be raised by the patient, a family member, or the patient's attending physician. The complaints can come through administration, the nursing staff, the patient's private physician, or directly to the emergency physician.

Regardless of the source and routing of the complaint, physician leadership in the emergency department must have an effective program in place to deal with complaints (see Chapter 66). A follow-up form should be developed on which to document discussions with the complaining party. A copy of the patient record should be included with this follow-up form. The physician and nursing directors should determine whether the complaint is related to nursing and/or physician personnel.

If the complaint is related to the physician or the physician's care, the medical director of the department must take charge of the investigation and the resolution. The treating physician should be contacted and questioned about the patient interaction and care. It may be necessary to interview nursing staff involved in the care. Once the data are gathered, the medical director should contact the patient and listen carefully to the complaint. If there is some fault with the care rendered by the treating physician, the medical director should seek an opportunity to meet the patient's need, which may include permitting the patient to speak directly with the treating physician. If the patient's complaint seems to have no clinical merit, the problem probably lies with the interpersonal relationship between the physician and the patient. The medical director should then apologize for any miscommunications or attitude problems.

The physician medical director should not attempt to dismiss the physician's comments or actions, or make the patient feel that there is nothing wrong. Rather, the director should accept the perception of fault or error and promise to address the problem with the treating physician. Even if no fault or error is found by the physician director on review of the complaint, the patient should still be advised that the complaint will be discussed with the treating physician. Sometimes patients just want to know that they have been heard and that someone has responded to them.

CONTRACT PROBLEMS—ATTENDING MEDICAL STAFF

Although emergency physicians are granted privileges at a hospital like other physicians and undergo specialty training like other physicians, there is often remarkable disparity between the treatment afforded emergency physicians and other physicians on the medical staff. This disparity is particularly evident when the emergency physicians are expected to cater to the demands of the medical staff. The administration may encourage the emergency physicians to please the admitting physicians because the hospital is competing with other facilities for patients. As a result, emergency physicians sometimes are asked to do things that are not in the patient's or the department's best interest.

Emergency physicians may be asked to write admitting orders. They may be asked to allow telephone orders for narcotic injections for patients who are not seen by a physician in the emergency department. In many hospitals emergency staff must provide prolonged care to patients while waiting hours for the arrival of the admitting or consulting physician. Some attending physicians, despite COBRA law, insist that the emergency physician arrange transfer for patients because they are unwilling to come in and provide care to patients. These actions result in poor patient care and create risk for the patient, hospital, and physicians.

Admitting orders are the responsibility of the admitting physician. Although emergency physicians can agree to help with temporary orders, the American College of Emergency Physicians (ACEP) has made it clear in its position statement that the responsibility falls on the shoulders of the admitting physician.

Giving narcotic orders by telephone is inappropriate. Patients should not be allowed to come to the hospital and receive narcotic injections without being examined by a physician. A condition that sounds benign to the private physician over the phone may, in fact, be much more serious on examination in the emergency department. Stories abound about patients with an intracranial bleed, dissecting aneurysm, rupturing appendix, and ectopic pregnancy who have come to the emergency department for narcotic injections per phone orders from the attending physician. ACEP has developed a position paper on the issue of telephone orders. It suggests all patients should be seen before receiving treatment in the emergency department.

Some medical staff members keep patients waiting in the emergency department for hours. The emergency physicians should work with the medical staff leadership to develop policies and procedures that enable patients to get timely care. The policies should describe the timely management of patients needing consultation, admission, or evaluation by private physicians in the emergency department. If policies are unclear, inconsistent, or nonexistent, departmental operations and the emergency physicians themselves will be seen as arbitrary. The loss of respect engendered by this perception may put the contract at risk. Conversely, if emergency physicians work with the medical staff to establish clear and consistent policies, the patients, staff, physicians, and administration will benefit from better service and gain a deep respect for the emergency physicians.

CONTRACT CLAUSES

Restrictive Covenants

No other clause in emergency medicine contracts stirs as much emotion and controversy as the restrictive covenant. Debate rages as to whether these clauses are fair and enforceable. Logic prevails on both sides of the issue. Because these clauses commonly appear in contracts, emergency physicians should understand their use and abuse.

Hospital-Group Restrictive Covenant. This clause often appears in the contract between the hospital and the emergency physician group. It restricts the group and its physicians from competing with the hospital. The hospital may be particularly concerned that a group or one of its physicians might set up competing free-standing clinics or work in a competing emergency department in the community.

It may be reasonable for the hospital to restrict the group or its physicians from directly competing with the hospital for its emergency patients. It may also be reasonable for the hospital to restrict the group from taking over other emergency contracts in the community, thereby sharing what may be a competitive advantage in the marketplace. However, it maybe unreasonable to restrict individual physicians from doing occasional shifts in other local emergency departments. The physicians may avoid absolute restriction by including language that allows individual emergency physicians to perform limited part-time work in other emergency departments as long as the physician has prior written consent from the hospital.

Group-Physician Restrictive Covenant. A more limiting restrictive covenant clause is often found in contracts between groups and individual emergency physicians. Some jurisdictions do not uphold restrictive covenants while others accept them broadly. To be upheld, a restrictive covenant must have reasonable limitations of time and place. For example, it might be unreasonable to restrict a physician from working in another local hospital once that physician leaves the group. A court might not uphold a restrictive covenant that forces a physician to move out of the community, particularly when it would be difficult to prove the physician's presence at another hospital would adversely affect the business of the group.

It is unreasonable for a group to restrict a physician from working at a hospital for a prolonged period of time (e.g., 5 years). Various jurisdictions have upheld 6 months to 2 years as reasonable. A time limited restrictive covenant gives the group reasonable protection from a physician who might otherwise attempt to obtain the contract while still employed by or contracted to the group. In other words, courts are likely to uphold a restrictive covenant that prevents a physician from using insider status to steal the contract from the group.

On the other hand, what happens if the group loses the contract with the hospital and the hospital wants to keep certain physicians? It can be argued that the restrictive covenant is unfair to physicians who have been working at the hospital when they had nothing to do with the contract termination and were not involved in any way with competing for the contract. For instance, the cause for termination may have been related to financial issues, poor leadership, or inadequate staffing. In these circumstances, it probably is not reasonable to restrict those physicians who want to stay on at the hospital and are desired by the medical staff and administration. One way to deal with such a problem would be to have language in the contract stating that the restrictive covenant will not be enforced if there is no evidence that the individual physician competed for the contract.

Another approach to managing restrictive covenant clauses

is to consider the four reasons that a contract between an emergency physician group and a hospital would be terminated: the hospital terminates for cause, the hospital terminates without cause, the group terminates for cause, and the group terminates without cause. In these scenarios, it is reasonable to put language in the contract stating that if the group terminates without cause or the hospital terminates with cause, the individual emergency physicians would be released from their restrictive covenants. In other words, if the group decides to leave without cause, whether for personal, financial, or political reasons, the physicians should have the option to stay, if they so choose. Alternatively the hospital may terminate "for cause," because the group has breached the contract. In this situation the hospital may want the right to retain some or all of the existing emergency physicians. Terminations for cause are usually rapid and may not allow enough time to find another group.

The other two instances for which a restrictive covenant would apply occur when the group terminates the contract for cause, or the hospital terminates the contract without cause. In both cases the physician group will argue for enforcement of the restrictive covenant in its negotiations with the hospital. Enforcement would prevent the hospital from reaping the benefit (physicians) of acting capriciously or in bad faith. However, it may still be appropriate to develop language that voids the restriction when there is no evidence that the physicians played a role in the termination of the contract or in any way competed with the group.

Some maintain that restrictive covenant clauses are not appropriate in contracts between emergency physician groups and its individual physicians. They contend that this is unfair restraint on the physician's ability to practice in the community and therefore should not be enforceable. They believe that the burden of maintaining the contract and satisfying the physicians lies with the contract group, not with the contract. This issue is quite controversial. Certain restrictive covenants are enforceable if they are reasonable. Restrictive covenants protect legitimate business interests of a group and may protect the physician members of a group from a ruthless administrator. Conversely, they may be unreasonable and used inappropriately to control physicians. Each case is different. The individual physician, the group, the circumstances of the contract between the hospital and the group, and the particular community all must be considered when evaluating whether restrictive covenant clauses are reasonable, enforceable, or desirable.

Hold Harmless

Many hospitals encourage the inclusion of "hold harmless" language in the contract. This language states that the group will hold the hospital harmless and indemnify it for any actions taken by physician members of the group that result in financial loss for the hospital. This situation arises if the emergency physician is found negligent and the hospital is not. A hold harmless and indemnification clause would obligate the group to pay the hospital for any expenses incurred in defending itself.

Even if such terminology is stated to be mutual, so that the hospital also holds the group harmless, these clauses should be eliminated from contracts between emergency physician groups and hospitals. Mutual hold harmless clauses are biased toward hospitals. In addition many professional liability (insurance) companies will not honor a hold harmless clause, leaving the physician personally responsible for all costs attributable to this clause. The best solution is to avoid inclusion of a hold harmless clause in the hospital/group contract. Legal advice should be sought when any such clause appears in a contract.

Concurrent Termination

Many contracts between emergency physician groups and hospitals contain concurrent termination or co-terminus clauses. These clauses state that if the group contract with the hospital is terminated, whether with or without cause, all emergency physicians working as part of the group must automatically resign their medical staff privileges, without due process. Although this type of contract language may be distasteful, it is fairly standard. The hospital reasons that at the time of contract termination, it must be able to retain new physicians so that it can maintain continuous emergency department coverage.

These clauses are thought to be reasonable and have been upheld by the courts. However, when the emergency physician's group is terminated, the physician may request reinstatement of privileges at the time of termination so that he or she can continue to practice emergency medicine at the hospital. Reinstatement may be accomplished easily when there is no restrictive covenant to prevent the physician from staying at the hospital. Even when a restrictive covenant clause exists, it would be reasonable for the group to release the physician from the restriction if the physician had nothing to do with the termination.

SUMMARY

A myriad of contract issues can arise during the life of a contract between a group and a hospital, as well as between individual physicians and a group. Proactive techniques for issue identification and preventive strategies are recommended. These techniques and strategies, along with a commitment to problem solving and consensus building, are the key elements to a successful contractual relationship. If the management of a contract is always viewed as a dynamic process that requires constant attention and fine tuning, and the parties are committed to resolving the contract problems as they arise, the longevity of the contract and the stability of the relationships will be maintained.

BIBLIOGRAPHY

Allison EJ et al: *Managing the emergency department: a team approach,* Dallas, 1992, American College of Emergency Physicians.

American College of Emergency Physicians, Policy statement on medical staff responsibility for emergency department patients, Dallas, 1993, American College of Emergency Physicians.

American College of Emergency Physicians: Policy statement on telephone orders in the emergency department, Dallas, 1992, American College of Emergency Physicians.

American College of Emergency Physicians, Policy statement on writing admission orders, Dallas, 1993, American College of Emergency Physicians.

Kotter JP: What leaders really do, *Harvard Business Review* 68(3):103-111, 1990.

Strauss RW: *Contracts: a practical guide for the emergency physician,* Dallas, 1990, American College of Emergency Physicians.

PART FOUR
Financial Management and Reimbursement Issues

44 Developing a Business Plan

Marc V. Weiner

OUTLINE

In today's healthcare environment being a visionary alone is simply not enough. To meet the multitude of challenges facing the industry, the successful emergency department team must be able to implement well-thought-out solutions. Such solutions must identify and address the various components that, when well planned, will use available resources in an effective and efficient manner.

The frustrations and negative outcomes resulting from a lack of planning can be found in all industries, not just health care. Most top managers and CEOs of health care and non-health care companies alike would attest to the need to plan and the importance of planning. In many organizations, however, the actual steps to develop a plan and the requisite corporate culture integral to planning may not be fully realized, followed, implemented, or have management's commitment. For some, skepticism has replaced enthusiasm as planning processes have dragged on for months or years without results, and voluminous "Business Plans" lie on corporate shelves gathering dust while operations continue as usual. For others, unrealistic expectations of what a Business Plan can do have left planners and implementors taking the heat for unsuccessful plans doomed for failure.

If planning has so many potential vulnerable points, then why plan? Because when understood and done properly, it works. And without planning, only bona fide miracles or consistent good luck can maintain, let alone improve, health care institutions' market and financial position in today's health care environment.[1]

The development and implementation of a business plan are valuable processes that can successfully change vision into reality. A complete business plan addresses a variety of important issues and functions. The business plan:

- Details the scope of a proposed project.
- Identifies all required resources.
- Determines key time frames to be met.
- Identifies specific priorities.
- Defines organizational goals and objectives.
- Improves collaboration and team involvement.
- Analyzes and proactively manages risk.
- Acts as a catalyst for improved communication.
- Provides a means for ongoing feedback.

When complete, a business plan should serve a variety of needs. The written document can ensure that all members of the team completely understand the various activities involved in implementation of an idea. It can be used as a presentation tool to a wide variety of audiences including, but not limited to, boards of trustees, other physicians, financial institutions, regulatory and licensing authorities, and investors. When used for these purposes, a well-written plan can be used in its entirety or abbreviated by presenting appropriate components taken from the entire document.

Remember, the actual document is not what makes the strategic plan work. A plan that sits on the shelf, lacks flexibility, and places unrealistic demands on employees is sure to fail. The planning process is practical not theoretical. The document is a flexible working reference that provides direction, realistic goals, and a workable implementation schedule.[1]

COMPONENTS OF A BUSINESS PLAN

A complete business plan consists of sections, each fully addressing a specific major component of the plan. These sections are consolidated and organized to achieve a thorough analysis and plan of action for the proposed project.

Box 44-1 presents a recommended order for the presentation of components of business plans relevant to emergency department projects.

Each of these components is discussed in detail to coordinate the efforts of team members in the development of a comprehensive business plan for any proposed major project.

EXECUTIVE SUMMARY

An executive summary is the first component of the plan. It is used to summarize and emphasize the major aspects of the proposed project. Its primary purpose is to provide anyone reading the plan the ability to gain an overview and understanding of the project.

The summary statement should be concise and should precisely convey the nature of the proposed project. It is an es-

BOX 44-1

BUSINESS PLAN COMPONENTS RELEVANT TO THE EMERGENCY DEPARTMENT

Section	Purpose
Executive summary	Fundamental overview of the project
Mission statement	Philosophies and values of the organization
Vision statement	Organization's vision of itself in the future
Strategy statement	Overall methods of achieving the plan
Goal statement	Benefits of a successful business plan
Organizational background	Description of organization's history
Service area description	Overall and target market
Program description	Detailed project description, including: Provided services Hours of service Scope of service Site selection Site description Site access Parking Descriptive capacity analysis Capital equipment Organization and management Information management Professional and consulting support Legal structure Insurance requirements Training and education
Risk analysis	Strategies to assess and minimize risk
Marketing strategy	Inform and create desire with target audience
Financial analysis	Financial translation of assumptions/plans
Implementation plan	Action items organized to effect plan
Appendices	Supporting documents referred to in main text

sential method for developing a vital first impression. One of the major reasons for preparing a business plan is to cultivate support. The executive summary is the primary means of building a foundation toward the achievement of this objective.

Whenever possible, this summary should be limited to a single page, and it should never be longer than two pages. When preparing the executive summary, it is helpful to think of this section as the descriptive advertisement for the entire business plan. The trick is to inform readers while piquing their curiosity to delve into the entire document.

It is often best to write this portion of the plan after all other components are complete. As each section is being prepared, keep track of significant items that should be included in the executive summary. Then review the list of significant items and further narrow the choices until only the key elements remain. This list will be the outline for the preparation of the executive summary. By following this procedure, the executive summary provides meaningful information and conveys to the reader a sense of well-organized thought.

MISSION STATEMENT

The mission statement outlines the particular philosophies and values of the organization. A clearly stated mission enables the reader of the business plan to specifically and/or intuitively understand why the particular project supports the overall objectives of the sponsoring group.

Properly written, this section permits the reader to better understand the "Why?" questions pertaining to the proposed project. Without establishing a clear foundation demonstrating how this project fits within the mission of the sponsoring organization, the entire proposal may be suspected of being unnecessary or inappropriate to the organization's key strategies.

The mission statement should be brief and to the point. The language and phrases should be clear, concise, and convey specific meaning. The reader should understand the purpose and values of the sponsoring organization.

VISION STATEMENT

This brief statement describes what the sponsoring organization wants to be at some stated time in the future. By identifying this vision, it should be obvious and/or implied how and why the proposed project contributes to the realization of this vision.

A well-written vision statement should be no longer than two or three sentences. The reader should be able to understand where the organization sees itself going and what it plans to be when it gets there. A specific time frame for accomplishment of this vision, if known, should be included.

It is not necessary or appropriate to specifically state why this specific project supports the vision. If the vision statement is written properly, it will be implicitly understood.

STRATEGY STATEMENT

The strategy statement details the methods by which the overall objectives of the business plan are to be accomplished. It is important to tie the objectives and goals of the sponsoring organization's existing operations into the objectives of the proposed project. The fundamental question of this section is: "Why is this initiative vital to the sponsoring organization?"

It is not necessary to know the final strategy at the time the business plan is being written. If different strategies are being considered, but a final choice has not yet been made, the pros and cons of each strategy and the conditions necessary for a final strategy to be selected should be identified.

This section should be less than two pages long, and if a final strategic approach has been selected, one page. A concise outline form can be used. It is not necessary to identify every component that will be involved in implementing the strategy. This will be addressed later in the implementation section of the business plan.

GOAL STATEMENT

The goal statement describes the benefits that will be achieved when the proposed project's business plan is successful. It is desirable to include a time frame. The goals (benefits) should be meaningful, clear, and measurable.

The variety of audiences that may review the business plan should be kept in mind when preparing the goal statement. The statement must be comprehensive enough to be meaningful to every reader. It is important to remember that goals, particularly appealing to a staff member, may be unattractive to a potential equity provider or loan officer.

The entire goal statement should be no more than three to four paragraphs. A lengthy statement can begin to lose impact, as the reader may question whether the goals are too broad and, therefore, unachievable.

The key to the goal statement is that it must be based on attainable realistic achievement founded on visionary concepts.

ORGANIZATIONAL BACKGROUND

A written description of the background of the sponsoring organization is necessary only if the business plan is going to be read by individuals and/or groups unfamiliar with the organization. It should include at least the following descriptive information:

- A brief history of the sponsoring organization.
- A description of the purpose of the sponsoring organization, both when it was formed and at the current time.
- A description of the current organizational structure with identification of key personnel and their relevant credentials.
- An operational description of the organization providing measurable information regarding how the organization has changed over time.
- A financial history of the organization providing measurable information pertaining to the financial performance of the organization over time.

All text pertaining to these items should be concise and directly intended to leave the reader with a solid understanding of the organization. In one sense, it is a narrative advertisement.

Information provided in this section can often be presented effectively by incorporating charts and graphs. However, the charts and graphs should not be included in the text of this section. Instead a brief explanation of the information portrayed by them should be included, and the actual chart or graph is displayed and referenced in an appendix.

Following the logic that this section is a descriptive advertisement, it is important that the reader not be distracted from the main focus of the business plan itself. Each reader will relate to this section differently. Some will read the text without referring to the appendix. Others may scan both sections. A third group may spend quite a bit of time with the appendix looking for specific areas of interest. The goal is to present the information in a way that accommodates a variety of audiences and their particular approaches toward reviewing the information.

SERVICE AREA

The service area is the first section of the business plan that focuses on the proposed project. It provides an important foundation for the volume projections that will be presented in a later section. It also sets the stage for the reader's determination of credibility of the plan. If the service area is poorly defined, too limited, or grandiose and unrealistic, the reader will discount the validity of the entire plan. A well-conceived and written description of the service area builds trust in the reader and can stimulate curiosity and further interest in the plan. Areas to be addressed include the following:

- A description of the market size. The methods for identifying the market size should be stated clearly and should be statistically based whenever possible. They must be based on generally accepted statistic data. Without readily accepted data, the reliability of the plan can be undermined.
- A description of the target market. The description must make clear why the proposed target market is correct. It is often helpful to specify if and how the target market may increase over time based on staged successes of the business plan. A staged approach demonstrates realistic and well-rounded thinking.
- A description of the current state of technology in the proposed target market. This description is necessary because the proper use of technology plays a major role in the success of any venture. The goal is to identify how the proposed project is new and innovative and/or builds on successful and proven approaches.

This critical section of the business plan must convince the reader beyond a reasonable doubt that the market to be served is the right one. It is often valuable and appropriate to include detailed information to support the conclusions presented in this section. This supportive information should be summarized briefly in the text and detailed in a supporting appendix. It is vitally important that the information included in the appendix be derived from standard published data such as that made available by federal, state, and local governments; local and regional health planning agencies, or comparative data prepared by recognizable and respected consulting firms.

PROGRAM DESCRIPTION

The program description describes the proposed project in detail. In addition to the traditional description of a project, it is necessary to include information about requirements for the proposed use of clinical staff, buildings, and equipment.

This section should flow easily and not get bogged down in detail. Appendices should be used liberally to delineate information summarized here. Minutia should not be included, as it may distract the reader from the overview of the program.

These areas should be addressed:

- *Service description.* Include timing and phasing of the implementation of these services. Also include an explanation how these services will differ from those offered by other providers.
- *Hours of service.*
- *The scope of service.* Will this be a free-standing operation? Will it be provided using service contracts with other providers? Will this service be offered to other providers under contract? (If the scope will change over time, this should be acknowledged.)
- *Site selection.* Identify proposed location(s) and include information about the advantages or disadvantages of the site. (If the final site[s] has not been determined, the advantages and disadvantages of the potential site[s] should be described.) In addition, identify the specific conditions and timing that will lead to site selection.
- *Site description.* A schematic diagram showing offices, square footage, diagnostic and treatment areas, etc. should be included as an exhibit in the appendix and described briefly here.
- *Capacity analysis.* A selected site may need conversion and/or renovation for use in the healthcare environment. If this is the case, describe the "preferred capacity", as well as the "rated" capacity. A good method of portraying a capacity analysis is to include a graph comparing preferred and rated capacity in the appendix.
- *Capital equipment.* Include a detailed listing of the major equipment needed for this project. The listing should include vehicles, office machinery, medical equipment, furniture, furnishings, and fixtures. Identify whether new or existing items will be used. Estimate the purchase price of new items. Detail the age and condition of existing items. Finally, indicate the expected useful life of the equipment and specify those items that will require upgrading and/or replacement during the first 3 years of the project. This detailed exhibit should be placed in the appendix and referred to in the body of the text.
- *Site access and modes of transportation.* Describe both private and public means of transportation. It is particularly important to demonstrate that the transportation plan ensures full access to the proposed project by the target population. If this section is brief, it can be included in the text; if it is lengthy, summarize it in the text and include a detailed description in the appendix.
- *Parking at the proposed site.* A site diagram should be included as an appendix and referred to in the text. Identify any special parking arrangements such as an outside contract with a commercial parking service.
- *Organization and management.* Include a descriptive summary in the text. The appendix should include:
  - An organizational chart showing lines of authority.
  - Position descriptions that include a detailed listing of the number and type of staff required and delineation of duties and responsibilities.
  - Staff compensation program including benefits and incentives.
- *Information management.* Describe the type and extent of computerization, identifying both software and hardware requirements. Describe how existing systems, can be extended, modified, or expanded to meet the needs of this project. Identify any special contracts that will be required.
- *Professional and consulting support.* Describe the type and form of consulting support that will be needed, as well as the timing of the support.
- *Legal structure.* Identify the legal relationship of the project to its participants.
- *Insurance.* Describe the directors and officers liability, professional liability, and general liability insurance needs of the participants.
- *Training and education plan.*

RISK ANALYSIS

Assessment of risk is critical. In the broadest sense, risk takes two forms, financial and business. Financial risk is the variability of net revenue induced by leverage. Business or economic risk is the variability of net revenue induced by the general economic conditions of the industry. Assessment of business risk requires answering questions such as: Are we going into the right business? Is the market ready for us? What do we do if we do not succeed with this effort? How do we get out if necessary? Assessment of financial risk requires answering questions such as: How will we meet our loan payments if interest rates change? In general, assessing business risk means asking where we might be wrong, and assessing financial risk means asking how much it will cost us to be wrong.[2]

Many significant factors must be addressed when assessing risk in the business plan. An important place to begin is an evaluation of the competition. The factors used in the analysis of the competition are not standard and should be developed to fit the particular project. If several individuals are participating in the preparation of the business plan, a team approach should be used to prepare this analysis.

An effective means of presenting this evaluation is to include a table describing the organization's competitive position. This table identifies the competitor, the bases of competition, the critical success factors, and critical failure factors. Consider using an easily understandable system such as +1 for strong competitor, 0 for no impact, and −1 for weak competitor. Rank each competitor for each factor using the proposed project as the benchmark. Table 44-1 shows an example of this type of chart.

Table 44-1 shows that Competitor A is the stronger of the two. However, as a result of compiling this information in this form, it is clear that neither competitor has effective pricing or convenience. Thus paying particular attention to these two factors could be of strategic advantage to the proposed

Table 44-1 The Organization's Competitive Position

Factors	Competitor A	Competitor B
Image	+1	−1
Historic growth rate	+1	0
Range of services offered	+1	−1
Price of services offered	−1	−1
Convenience	0	−1

project. The new project should also establish a positive image and fill perceived voids in the target market.

Other areas that must be addressed in the risk analysis section include the following:

- A review of the political climate that may have an impact on the proposed project.
- Planning and regulatory requirements, processes, and impediments, if any.
- Reimbursement ceilings and/or limitations.
- Anticipated changes in payment practices and/or arrangements.
- Public perception of the sponsoring organization and of the leadership of that organization.
- Competitive or collaborative position relative to other providers.
- Impact of ongoing changes in the healthcare industry.
- Availability of appropriately skilled staff.
- Impact of seasonality.

After the various risk factors have been identified and analyzed, it is critical to outline plans and strategies to minimize risk. An excellent method for minimizing risk is to identify and address both the critical success factors and the critical failure factors. The critical success factors describe what must be accomplished for the project to succeed. Conversely, the critical failure factors identify what must not occur. Failure to identify and address the critical success factors will lead to less than full success and possible failure of the project. Not knowing and planning for the critical failure factors generally will result in a failed project.

This section should emphasize minimizing, but not eliminating, risk. Because risk is inherent to any project, it would be unrealistic to detail a plan that eliminates it completely. However, communicating a strategy to address the various components of risk can itself become a critical success factor.

MARKETING STRATEGY

When contemplating a new product or line of business, it is vital to ascertain what the consumer wants, how to package it, and how to competitively price it. It is important to outline clearly the approaches that will be used to inform the target group of the availability of the proposed project. When preparing this strategy, consider the following issues:

- The geography of the target group including the size and density of population.
- The demographics of the area including age, sex, family size, income, range of occupations, education, and religious, cultural, and social class issues.
- The psychographics of the area including lifestyle characteristics, personality types, preferred reasons for selection of products and services, benefits sought, satisfiers, expectations, and activities that result in customer loyalty.
- Verification that the provided services will be in demand. This can be accomplished by surveys, focus groups, and targeted meetings with community leaders, representatives, and members. In some cases it may be necessary to retain the services of a professional consulting service to complete this analysis.
- Pricing decisions. Consumers generally prefer quality services for the lowest possible cost. In the healthcare field, some pricing decisions are complex. A multitude of regulations may complicate and/or prohibit discount pricing strategies. It may be necessary to consult financial advisors who have knowledge of healthcare pricing and reimbursement issues to determine the latitude available when pricing decisions are made.
- Determination of the sales tactics. There are many different sales approaches, and it is important to select the correct approach. It may be necessary to consult with a professional marketing service.
- Assessment of the need for sales and marketing personnel. What style, background, and experience are best suited for the project? It is necessary to determine the best method of compensation, perhaps incorporating some form of incentive.

After addressing these issues, the marketing strategy must focus on advertising and public relations. The resources available for advertising must be determined. The goal is to reach the target audience while staying within the constraints of available financial resources. Once the strategy of reaching the target audience is determined, a method of evaluating whether the target group was reached and which form of advertising was most effective must be developed. The purpose of this strategy is to ensure that future advertising dollars will be spent in those areas that achieve results.

FINANCIAL ANALYSIS

The financial analysis of the plan should be prepared and presented *only after* the vast majority of conceptual and operational concepts have been determined and fully explored. In essence, the financial plan is a financial translation of all the statistic and operational assumptions that have been made relative to the proposed project.

The overall goal in this section is to determine the financial requirements to break even and the time frame for reaching this point. The secondary goal is to make sure that the project has sufficient working capital and cash flow. New initiatives often fail because they are undercapitalized, capitalized at the wrong time, or inappropriately overcapitalized using debt financing. In these situations, volume does not grow quickly enough to outpace the fixed expenses of the project. Therefore it is essential to prepare a careful and comprehensive financial plan.

The financial analysis should project for 3 years. A shorter period does not demonstrate effective planning. A longer period is not necessary because the financial plan will be updated and adjusted on a regular basis. The analysis should include a profit and loss statement and a statement of cash flow.

Although not every profit and loss statement incorporates the same components, the following is a list of common

Table 44-2 Break-Even Analysis

Cases/year:		200		Charge:	$5,000.00
Revenue:					
	Payer	%	Cases	Net revenue per case	Total revenue
	Medicare	25%	50	$3,500.00	$175,000.00
	Medicaid	10%	20	$3,625.00	$ 72,500.00
	Commercial	15%	30	$5,000.00	$150,000.00
	Managed care	35%	70	$3,250.00	$227,500.00
	Self pay	5%	10	$1,250.00	$ 12,500.00
	Charity	10%	20	$ –	$ –
	Total revenue:	100%	200		$637,500.00
Expense:					
	Salaries				$382,000.00
	Benefits				$ 95,500.00
	Medical supplies				$ 35,000.00
	Office supplies				$ 10,000.00
	Utilities				$ 22,000.00
	Insurance				$ 16,000.00
	Fees				$ 10,000.00
	Interest				$ 12,000.00
	Contracts				$ 35,000.00
	Depreciation				$ 10,000.00
	Contingency				$ 10,000.00
	Total expense:				$637,500.00

areas that should be considered when preparing this statement:

Revenues:

- Number of admissions
- Number of discharges
- Patient days
- Length of stay
- Payor mix
- Charges for services
- Discounts, uncollectibles, charity care, and bad debt
- Impact of regulation on reimbursement levels

Expenses:

- Salaries
- Full-time equivalents (FTEs)
- Employee benefits
- Professional fees
- Office supplies
- Medical supplies
- Food
- Utilities
- Contracted services
- Interest
- Insurance
- Operating fees
- Depreciation
- Allowance for contingencies

It is also necessary to include a detailed list of the major assumptions that have been used in preparing this statement.

The profit and loss statement should be prepared in two ways: break-even and probable. The break-even analysis portrays the exact volume required to match revenue expense. This information is critical because it identifies the type and level of volume necessary to prevent financial losses. The probable analysis portrays the expected profitability of the project if all assumptions hold true. When compared with the break-even analysis, it also identifies the incremental differences in volume, revenue, and expense that are required to achieve a profit.

Table 44-2 shows an example of the type of information that should be included in the break-even analysis (in an inpatient hospital setting). In this case it takes a volume of 200 cases based on the stated payor mix and schedule of expenses to break even.

With this baseline knowledge, financial modeling can be accomplished and the impact of changes in pricing, payor mix, volume, and items of expense estimated. For example, assume that everything was to stay the same except that the payor mix was to change slightly. Table 44-3 shows the possible result. The result is improved profitability and a lower number of cases to break even.

This modeling is important. It can help determine marketing strategy and gives the project managers the ability to monitor financial results on an ongoing basis.

The financial reports are simply a financial translation of operational activities. Whatever happens operationally will ultimately be translated to the balance sheet, the profit and loss statement, and the cash flow statement.

A cash flow statement also should be included in the business plan. For any proposed project, it is vital to understand the sources for working capital and when capital will be needed.

In the healthcare field, cash for services rendered is almost always received after the actual delivery of services. However, a substantial portion of the cash outlay to meet ongoing expenses of operation must be paid on a regular basis

Table 44-3 Break-Even Analysis

Cases/year:		200		Charge:	$5,000.00
Revenue:	Payer	%	Cases	Net revenue per case	Total revenue
	Medicare	20%	40	$3,500.00	$140,000.00
	Medicaid	20%	40	$3,625.00	$145,000.00
	Commercial	15%	30	$5,000.00	$150,000.00
	Managed care	30%	60	$3,250.00	$195,000.00
	Self pay	10%	20	$1,250.00	$ 25,000.00
	Charity	5%	10	$ –	$ –
	Total revenue:	100%	200		$655,000.00
Expense:					
	Salaries				$382,000.00
	Benefits				$ 95,500.00
	Medical supplies				$ 35,000.00
	Office supplies				$ 10,000.00
	Utilities				$ 22,000.00
	Insurance				$ 16,000.00
	Fees				$ 10,000.00
	Interest				$ 12,000.00
	Contracts				$ 35,000.00
	Depreciation				$ 10,000.00
	Contingency				$ 10,000.00
	Total expense:				$637,500.00

and during start-up expenses will outstrip revenues. This gap must be anticipated and provided for, or the new venture will fail. Even sound projects, efficiently operated, may fail without adequate consideration of working capital. This usually occurs when the venture is undercapitalized and insufficient working capital is available for the period of time it takes for cash receipts to exceed cash expenditures. The cash flow statement then is used to verify that adequate resources will be available to meet ongoing cash requirements.

A 3-year projection of the financial statements will help minimize unexpected financial surprises. If some expectations are unmet, the project managers can use the plan's financial statements to make informed course corrections.

These statements and the associated financial projections should be updated on a monthly basis for at least the first year of the proposed project. This approach avoids the unexpected financial jolts that can occur at the end of the first year if only annual reviews are performed.

IMPLEMENTATION PLAN

This section of the business plan describes the various action items required to gain approval for implementation of the proposed project. The implementation plan delineates the tasks to be performed, the sequence in which the tasks are to occur, the expected time frame required to complete the tasks, the assignment of responsibility for achievement of the tasks, and identification of budgeted financial resources.

In essence, the implementation plan takes all the previous areas of the business plan and converts them from philosophy to action. It serves as a map to take the proposed project from design to full implementation.

In the healthcare environment it is particularly important to be cognizant of the review and approval process necessary to achieve success. Specifically, approval from administration, individual physicians and physician committees, the governing board, and external regulatory agencies may be required. The approval process should be included in the implementation plan.

A tracking diagram called a Gantt chart is an excellent method for outlining the specific steps required during the implementation phase and for keeping track of progress. Figure 44-1 presents an example of a Gantt chart for the implementation of a proposed project.

The actual chart is more detailed and includes a greater number of steps and related actions. It should be comprehensive, but not so detailed that it becomes impractical.

It may be appropriate to use a series of charts with individual Gantt charts for each major phase of the overall project. A detailed subchart for the implementation phase is usually necessary and quite helpful.

Another advantage of this management tool may be seen when actions occur ahead of or behind schedule. A project manager can quickly ascertain the effect of an implementation delay on any other area of the plan and institute immediate corrective action. The converse is also true: if an action occurs sooner than expected, the entire plan can be viewed easily and adjustments made.

This section should include a brief description of the major activities of the implementation plan. However, the actual charts should be placed in the appendix to the plan.

Task Name	Duration	Start	End	Responsible	Cost
BUDGET CYCLE:	20.0 d	02/Jan/96	30/Jan/96		$0.00
Complete assumptions	5.0 d	02/Jan/96	08/Jan/96		$0.00
Prepare statistics	5.0 d	09/Jan/96	16/Jan/96		$0.00
Revenue forecasts	5.0 d	17/Jan/96	23/Jan/96		$0.00
Expense forecasts	5.0 d	17/Jan/96	23/Jan/96		$0.00
Final budget reviewed	5.0 d	24/Jan/96	30/Jan/96		$0.00
Budget approved	0.0 d	30/Jan/96	30/Jan/96		$0.00
SECURE FINANCING:	22.0 d	26/Feb/96	26/Mar/96		$0.00
Prepare presentation	7.0 d	26/Feb/96	05/Mar/96		$0.00
Present to equity partners	5.0 d	06/Mar/96	12/Mar/96		$0.00
Present to financing group	10.0 d	13/Mar/96	26/Mar/96		$0.00
Financing secured	0.0 d	26/Mar/96	26/Mar/96		$0.00
IMPLEMENTATION:	53.0 d	26/Mar/96	07/Jun/96		$0.00
Program A	30.0 d	26/Mar/96	06/May/96		$0.00
See GANTT - Program	30.0 d	26/Mar/96	06/May/96		$0.00
Program B	40.0 d	12/Apr/96	07/Jun/96		$0.00
See GANTT - Program	40.0 d	12/Apr/96	07/Jun/96		$0.00

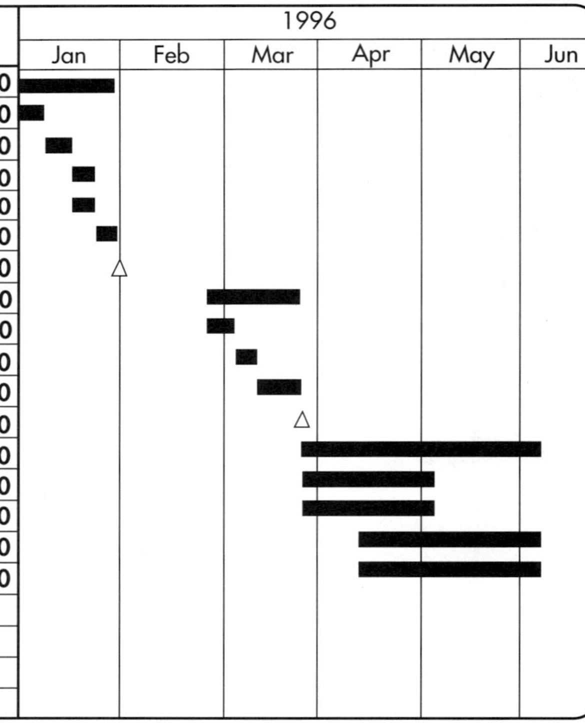

FIGURE 44-1 Gantt chart example.

APPENDICES

The appendix section of the business plan contains all of the supporting schedules, exhibits, graphs, and other documents. It also should include resumes of key individuals, product information, market research, technical information, etc.

Each item in the appendix must be mentioned in the text of the plan document, with a reference to the appropriate section of the appendix. Any items not mentioned in the main text should not be included in the appendix. Extra presentation material creates confusion.

Items included in the appendix should be able to stand on their own and, in a sense, convey a story. For example, if a survey is used to determine consumer need, a copy of the survey instrument and a summary of the findings should be included. Unanalyzed or raw data such as completed surveys and/or tally sheets should not be included.

Charts and graphs should be used in lieu of text wherever possible. When these formats are well designed, information is easily and quickly understood.

SUGGESTIONS FOR A SUCCESSFUL BUSINESS PLAN

Although different business plans will have some components that are the same, each individual plan will develop a personality all its own that distinguishes it as a customized model intended to address and deliver the unique activities of the proposed project. However, several suggestions can be used with virtually any plan during its development, which will make the document a useful tool:

Commitment

- Obtain management commitment to the plan at all stages of development.
- Seek and obtain consensus from all interested parties. The key here is to make sure that all participants are working on and implementing the same project.
- Identify and foster advocates for the proposed project. Seek out opportunities to turn adversaries into advocates.

Team Participants

- Use the right talent at the right time.
- Overcome participants' natural resistance to change.
- Ensure that action-oriented members of the implementation team try to focus their activities on confronting real problems.
- Include representation from all interested parties. Pay particular attention to ensuring that each specific representative carries the correct weight in the organization.
- Consider linking bonus compensation to the plan's success.

Preparation Process

- Conduct major planning sessions in a "retreat" format at an offsite location without the disturbances of daily routine.
- Consider visits to other programs that may be similar to the project being proposed. Benefit from their successes and learn from their mistakes.
- Focus on specific operational details and activities; generalities without explicit steps for implementation often result in a weak plan.
- Remember the purposes of the plan: to establish direction, define the business, improve communication, heighten teamwork, develop staff, help measure performance, improve profitability, and serve as a process to manage change.
- Stress implementation. Include specific objectives and describe how each will be accomplished. Include realistic and achievable time frames with each objective. Assign a specific individual specific responsibility for the completion of tasks.
- Use the plan primarily as a guide to implementation. Although it can also serve as the first operating and capital budget, it must be more than just a document to arrange financing or prove that the financial aspects of the plan will work over time.
- Recognize that the plan is an evolving process. Do not attempt to obtain "perfect" information. The use of appropriate sensitivity analysis techniques eliminates the need for perfect information and allows the planning process to move forward.
- Concentrate 90% of the implementation section on year 1. Later revisions will be based on actual experience.
- Plan for the unexpected and provide for both positive and negative contingencies. A business plan must be much more sensitive to variation than a normal budgetary process. Ask lots of "what-ifs" and make sure to provide for them in the plan.
- Measure progress of the plan effectively. Select objective, measurable milestones.
- Develop the plan concepts fully before developing the financial aspects of the plan. Outside investors will be more interested in substance than the financial components. They are more likely to contribute equity to a substantive venture.

Presentation

- Produce a refined document. Remember a good plan can be used in multiple settings for a variety of audiences.
- Distill major goals to 1-page understandable summaries.
- Display performance information in graphics that are easy to understand.
- Allow all participants in the plan a chance to discuss and understand these graphics before presenting them to any audience.

Plan Revision and Feedback

- Schedule regular meetings to discuss the plan and nothing else. This approach will make follow-up planning easier.
- Update the plan as implementation takes place. Consider a major update of the plan at least 6 months into implementation. Let it become an ongoing tool with a continued useful life.

VISION INTO REALITY

Business planning in the healthcare industry is complex, difficult, and necessary. It can be a cumbersome, disappointing exercise or a productive, enjoyable, and ultimately profitable undertaking. When accomplished properly and with realistic expectations, the business plan becomes the framework for all of the operations of the organization, and the ongoing process becomes the test of the framework that ensures that it remains sound.[1]

Successful business plans anticipate roadblocks to success and identify key strategies to implement real solutions. Merely coping with complexity and change will not bring about favorable outcomes. Today's emergency department leaders must communicate a vision and have the means of translating this vision into reality.

Managing the multitude of activities necessary to achieve these goals requires the use of a reliable methodology. This chapter has identified the business plan process as a tried and proven tool to accomplish this objective. The discipline involved in following this process ensures that all areas of a proposed project are reviewed in a thoughtful and orderly manner. The ability for a number of individuals to work collaboratively better ensures that the project will enjoy a successful outcome. For the emergency department leader, this process ensures that he or she will be viewed and known as a positive thinker who can identify needs, coordinate resources, solve important problems, and turn strategic thinking into realistic outcomes.

REFERENCES

1. Worthem JC: Business planning: who, what, when, where, why and how, *Top Healthc Financ* 1992.
2. Pink GH, Deber RB, Lavoie JN, Aserlind E: Innovative revenue generation, *Healthcare Management Forum (Wash)* (4):38, 1991.

ADDITIONAL READINGS

Abrams, RM: *The successful business plan: secrets & strategies,* Grants Pass, Ore, 1993, The Oasis Press.

Arkebauer JB: *The McGraw-Hill guide to writing a high-impact business plan,* New York, 1995, McGraw-Hill.

Bangs DH: *The business planning guide,* Dover, NH, 1992, Upstart Publishing.

Burton JE, McBride WB: *Total business planning,* New York, 1991, John Wiley & Son.

Covello JA, Hazelgren BJ: *The complete book of business plans,* Naperville, Ill, 1994, Sourcebooks.

Edmonstone J, Havergal M: Business planning: new wine in old bottles?, *Health Serv Manage* 87(1):33-35, 1991.

Hyypia E: *Crafting the successful business plan,* Englewood Cliffs, NJ, 1992, Prentice Hall.

Kohn D: The role of business process reengineering in health care, *Top Health Info Manage* 14: 1994.

Kravitt GI: *Creating a winning business plan,* Chicago, 1992, Probus Publishing.

Langland-Orban B, Krasik ER: Successful business planning for new programs in health care organizations, *Eval Health Prof* 18(1):61-78, 1991.

Lasher W: *The perfect business plan,* New York, 1994, Doubleday.

Malburg CR: *All-in-one business planning guide,* Holbrook, Mass, 1994, Bob Adams.

Mancuso JR: *How to write a winning business plan,* New York, 1985, Simon & Schuster.

Mancuso JR: *How to prepare and present a business plan,* New York, 1983, Simon & Schuster.

McKeenen M: *How to write a business plan,* Berkeley, 1992, Molo Press.

Pinson L, Jinnett J: *Anatomy of a business plan,* Dearborn, Mich, 1989, Dearborn Publishing Group.

45 Financial Statements

Don B. Cohen

OUTLINE

Whether we like it or not, the practice of medicine is also the business of medicine. Because of events from the changing of standards that allow advertising by professionals to the efforts at all levels of government to control the costs of medical care, we are becoming more and more reliant on the use of sound business practices to make a success of our medical practice. To that end, we need to understand the financial data on which we make decisions.

THE BALANCE SHEET

Most physicians when asked to review a set of financial statements will jump to the income statement and look to the bottom line—how much income was made. Not a bad idea, but most will not go any further because of lack of interest or lack of understanding of the statements.

Theoretically, there is only one financial statement, the balance sheet (Figure 45-1). Unfortunately, the title, balance sheet, adds nothing to a reader's knowledge except to know that the two sides are equal or in balance. A better name would be a statement of assets, liabilities, and owner's equity: admittedly, a longer title, but a real description of what it represents.

Assets are things of value that your practice owns. They include many different types of things with monetary value. When we list assets in a balance sheet, we like to know how "liquid" they are or how easy they may be converted into cash to pay our bills. The most liquid is cash itself, either in the form of a checking or savings account. Probably the next most liquid category includes government bonds or stocks in companies listed on a stock exchange; these have a ready market.

The most important asset is accounts receivable (A/R). This is the money that insurance companies, Medicare, patients, and the other third parties owe to the practice.

The A/R are not all equally collectible in full or in part. Various government insurers, such as Medicare and Medicaid, do not fully reimburse medical services. In addition, discounted care is given to many large purchasers of care and HMOs. Many people are uninsured and some patients have no domicile even to send a bill for services rendered. Although these amounts due from various sources are not equally collectible, they rank high on the list of assets and are almost always listed under the subheading of current assets.

Current assets are assets that are cash, cash equivalent (e.g., stocks, bonds), or can be readily converted into cash. There are people who will buy accounts receivable from businesses at a discount. They pay a percentage of the value of A/R and keep the balance as their fee for going through the problems of collecting the money. This would not be a good business move for a medical practice, as it could create havoc with your professional relationship with your patients.

The next major division of the asset side of the balance sheet is fixed assets. This section includes assets whose value is relatively fixed, such as land or buildings. The price of land can fluctuate over time as the economy changes. By convention, however, the value used for land is the cost of purchase.

Other items that could appear in the fixed assets section are any buildings or equipment owned. Unlike land, these items tend to lose value over time because of wear and tear or changing technology. The old business machines have been replaced by the spectacular memories and utilities of computers. The old machine may still work but it will not be used and cannot be sold. This is recognized in the balance sheet. A building with a 30-year useful life will lose 1/30th of its original value every year. At the end of 30 years, the balance sheet will list its value as zero.

The last section in the asset side of the balance sheet is called other assets. It can be a mixture of many things. For example, security deposits and prepaid expenses could be listed here. When a professional corporation is formed, all the expenses of the organization are not deductible for federal income tax purposes in the first year of business. The part the Internal Revenue Service allows to be expenses over a fixed period of time could be carried in this section. The total of current assets, fixed assets, and other assets is the total assets owned by the practice.

The amount owed to others is listed in the section called liabilities. In a manner similar to assets, they are also divided according to when they are due and are therefore called current liabilities and long-term or fixed liabilities. Current liabilities could include what is owed to the billing service, wages, Social Security, and income taxes owed to different governments. It could also include amounts owed to utilities, stationery stores, or anyone else from whom a purchase was made. If money was borrowed to start the practice, the amount owed due in less than 1 year to the bank or other lenders is also a current liability. The long-term liability section usually includes only those portions of the loans to be repaid in over 1 year.

The last section of the balance sheet is the owner's equity.

Emergency Medicine Corporation
Balance Sheet
December 31, 199X

ASSETS		LIABILITIES & OWNERSHIP	
Cash	10,000.00	Accounts payable	15,000.00
Accounts receivable	150,000.00	Taxes payable	30,000.00
Current assets	160,000.00	Current liability	45,000.00
Land	50,000.00		
Building	100,000.00	Common stock	100,000.00
Fixed assets	150,000.00	Retained earnings	170,000.00
Other assets	5,000.00	Total ownership	270,000.00
Total assets	315,000.00	Total liability & ownership	315,000.00

FIGURE 45-1 Balance sheet.

The title of this section depends on the legal type of organization. A partnership will list partnership accounts; a corporation will list stock and accumulated retained earnings.

This statement is a balance sheet because the liability section plus the owners section equals the sum of the asset sections. The two sides are in balance. Balance sheets are always dated. The heading reads "As of Month 31, 199x." It represents the status of the business as of a moment in time, usually the end of a month or year.

Preparation of the balance sheet at the end of the year can be time-consuming. It will take time for a billing service to put dollar values on the services delivered the last week of the year. If employees are paid every 2 weeks and the next pay period is in January, there is a legal liability to compensate them for work done in December. This along with the taxes owed is shown as part of current liabilities. The bill from the billing service will not come until mid-January and so forth.

At the end of the next year, another listing of the assets, liabilities, and owners' equity sections can be made. This is the basis of the other financial statements in common use. For example, if we wanted to know what happened to the cash account during the year, we would start with the cash on January 1, add all the deposits, and deduct all the checks written. The resulting figure would be the cash on the December 31 balance sheet. The title for this statement could be: Statement of Cash Receipts and Disbursements for the year ended December 31, 199x.

Most of us like to know what happened to the owner's part of the balance sheet. In a similar fashion, if we add all the additions to it (fees generated) and subtract all the expenses, the portion as of January 31 will equal the owner's portion on December 31st.

Balance sheets are as of a specific date. The other statements are reconciliations of amounts in cash or owner's equity over a period of time, with balance sheets made at the beginning and end of that period.

ACCRUAL AND CASH BASIS

To most nonaccountants accrual and cash basis are the hardest concepts to grasp. Simply stated, accrual basis recognizes income when earned and expense when it is incurred. Cash basis recognizes income only when it is received and expense only when it is paid. Income can be earned only once and expense can be incurred only once. It sounds quite logical but is the cause of almost all the confusion. A few examples will help illustrate the difference. A patient is seen on December 31. On a cash basis we have income not in the year ending but in the next March when the account is paid, but only to the extent paid. If $80 of a $100 fee is paid in March, no income is recorded in the year ending and only $80 is recorded in the following March. On an accrual basis, income is $100 in the year ended. If we collect $80 the next year, no income is recorded but a $20 bad debt is recorded. The cash basis practice has no accounts receivable on its balance sheet, so it is unable to write off a bad debt. The accrual basis practice had $100 on the December 31 balance sheet and can write off $20 when only $80 dollars is collected. The net result is exactly the same, $80 of income, regardless of the methodology. Using the accrual basis, the effect is to overlap two accounting periods.

Expenses can be evaluated in the same way. The billing service sends us a bill in January for December's work. On a cash basis, this has no effect on our December statement because we did not pay it until late in January. The accrual basis lists it as an account payable or "liability" as of December 31 and reduces income by the same amount. Here is

Accounts	Total	Current	30-60 days	60-90 days	90-120 days	>120 days
Insurance company	100,000	60,000	30,000	10,000		
HMOs	50,000	9,000	8,000	7,000	9,000	17,000
US government	75,000	10,000	10,000	15,000	15,000	25,000
No insurance	25,000	10,000	7,000	4,000		4,000
Total	250,000	89,000	55,000	36,000	24,000	46,000

FIGURE 45-2 Aged trial balance report.

where the confusion enters. When it is paid in January, it is not considered an expense, because we reduce income in December. When we pay the bill in January instead of "paying an expense" we are reducing our liability.

The accrual method of accounting may seem confusing, but is does have practical value. Assume we go into practice in November and bill $100,000 each month. On the cash basis, because the third parties will not pay us for 60 to 120 days, we have no income and therefore no income taxes. Using the accrual basis, we have $200,000 of accounts receivable and $200,000 of income. We also have no cash, but have a liability for federal and state income taxes. This is not a desirable position to be in. On the positive side, however, the accrual basis allows for the recognition of the value of the accounts receivable, which can be useful in establishing lines of credit.

Both of the accounting methods described previously have a basic similarity; all entries or transactions have two parts. Every entry must affect two accounts equally, which results in the two sides (assets and liabilities) of the balance sheet always adding up to equal numbers.

The following examples involve the accrual basis of accounting:

1. Services of $100,000 are delivered. Accounts receivable on the left side of the balance sheet increases by $100,000 and owner's equity on the right side also increases by $100,000. Because the entries are equal, the balance between the assets and liabilities remains zero.
2. Insurance payments of $75,000 are received. Cash on the left (asset) side is increased. Because the cash was received, the value of the accounts receivable, also on the left side, decreases by $75,000.
3. A payment of $25,000 is made to the bank that lent money to start the practice. Cash on the left (asset) side of the balance sheet is decreased by $25,000, and notes payable on the right (liability) side of the balance sheet are also decreased by $25,000.

In all three illustrations, the totals of the balance sheet on the left and right sides remained equal. This is true for absolutely every transaction that can occur in business. The balance between the assets and liabilities forms the basis for keeping track of the thousands of transactions that occur for a business such as managing an emergency department.

AGED TRIAL BALANCE

Usually, the largest dollar value asset owned by a practice is the amounts owed to it by its patients and third parties, the accounts receivable. Earlier in this chapter, we assigned this account to current assets, assuming that they would be collectible in full in a reasonably short time. Practically, we know this is not true. Some will never be paid, some will be paid late or in installments, and some will only be partially paid. The orderly collection of these accounts is the lifeblood of a practice.

Billing and collection work may be performed by a commercial billing service or in-house. Part of the monthly billing report should be an aged trial balance or accounts receivable. This listing shows who owes money on the vertical axis and when it was billed on the horizontal axis (Figure 45-2).

An aged trial balance can include a great deal of detail. It could include data such as the number of patients in each payor group, a listing of each individual insurance company or HMO, and even a listing of individual patients names. Reviewing this report supplied by the billing service teaches the basics of cash management. This review and analysis must be accomplished by the physician, not the billing service.

The insurance companies appear to be paying on time and all is well. The HMOs, however, show a problem. Most bills are paid on time, but a significant number seem to stretch out, and 34% of the dollar value is more than 4 months old. This problem requires a call to the HMO to determine how it can be solved. The problem may be that this HMO needs a code that is not being captured. Simply having registration clerks record another insurance code when the patient registers could be all that is needed. The problem could be more complex and involve negotiations about billing codes, authorizations, or elements of their retrospective chart review.

John Q. Doctor, MD	June 30	Year to Date
Salary		
Overtime		
Bonus		
Miscellaneous income		
Total earnings		
FICA withheld		
Federal withholding		
State withholding		
Medicare tax		
Salary advance		
Miscellaneous deductions		
Total deductions		
Net pay		

FIGURE 45-3 Typical pay stub.

Medicare appears to have a similar problem that requires investigation. Most states are in financial crunches, but these bills eventually get paid. Our "No Insurance" patients appear to pay on time except for a few stragglers. Perhaps a phone call program should be used to see whether payment is forthcoming.

Obviously, many other problems and solutions can occur. The totals and percentages need to be watched carefully each month to detect trends. Data that do not appear on an aged trial balance of accounts receivable pertain to the number of days between a patient appointment and the billing for that appointment. The faster the bill is rendered, the more likely it will be paid when dealing with private pay or noninsured patients.

Another important concept relative to the aging of the accounts receivable is the "average days in receivables." This variable is a measure of how long, on average, it takes for an individual or third party to pay the bill. Most businesses insist on payment within 30 days before interest starts to accrue. In medicine, however, because of involvement by government and insurance companies, payment time frames are lengthened.

The length of time that accounts remain in receivables is a measure of the effectiveness of the billing service. Generally speaking, the average days in receivable should be less than 90 days and closer to 60 days. This time will vary by payor type (e.g., commercial insurance, Medicare). If the average days in receivables is higher, the billing service needs to be more aggressive in collecting A/R. For example, if the average days in A/R is 120 d, by reducing this time to 90 days cash flow will improve dramatically. More money will be available to run the business.

PAYROLL SYSTEMS

Many banks and payroll services will do all the work of paying employees each pay period, including making deposits to the bank for federal taxes and to the state if there is state income tax. For reasons of security or convenience, many groups opt to do payroll accounting themselves. Effective payroll software programs such as Intuit Quickpay or DacEasy Payroll cost less than $100. Another alternative is to use a spread sheet program such as Lotus 1-2-3 or Microsoft Excell and design a personalized payroll program. Whatever system is chosen, certain data must be supplied to each employee every payroll period. The categories of income and expense for the current pay period and year-to-date totals are necessary. Figure 45-3 illustrates a typical pay stub with this data.

This payroll stub is a sample and can be edited to fit any circumstance that is unique to a practice.

SUMMARY

Understanding financial statements is critical to managing the business aspects of an emergency medicine practice. Reviewing them and the reports generated by a billing service should provide an understanding of the financial position of the practice. Physicians must be involved in the analysis every month to ensure that decisions are made that directly influence the financial success of the practice.

46 The Budget Process

Linda Greenberg

OUTLINE

The management of an emergency department has become increasingly complex, paralleling changes in the healthcare industry over the last 5 to 10 years. Before then, managers concentrated on clinical issues and rarely paid attention to fiscal matters. Hospitals did not have to worry about reimbursement issues because they were always reimbursed at the rate they charged. In this climate of decreasing reimbursement and cost containment, attention to fiscal matters is important to the viability of an emergency department.

The budget process sets goals for expenses and revenue and then measures how well those goals were met. Goal evaluation is the on-going piece of the budget cycle. If the goals are not met, operational adjustments are made to meet the goals that were identified. If the budget targets are not met, the department will lose money and may experience cutbacks in staffing or services to meet fiscal constraints.

The actual process to set budget targets starts long before the end of the fiscal year. The fiscal year may or may not parallel the calendar year. The first step in this planning process is to do volume forecasts for the next year. These volume forecasts are used to set salary, operating expense, and productivity targets. Projections for changes in service delivery, such as funding for new programs, are considered at this time. At the same time, requests for capital and minor equipment are placed. All of these factors are built into a budget for the department for the next year. This chapter provides an overview of basic budgeting concepts and their application to the emergency department setting.

ELEMENTS OF A BUDGET

A budget has three main components: the personnel budget, the operating budget, and the capital and minor equipment budget. Each of these distinct budgets are based on the strategic plan for the department, including projected growth and projected revenue.

Personnel or Salary Budget

The personnel, or salary budget as it is sometimes called, consists of the expenses related to department personnel. The nursing and ancillary staff are usually budgeted for in a separate line item from the physician staff. Both productive and nonproductive time are calculated to derive an overall salary expense for the department. Definitions and sample calculations for productive/nonproductive time are discussed later in this chapter.

Operating Budget

The operating budget details all of the expenses related to the general operations of the department, excluding salary and capital/minor equipment expenses. Costs are grouped in a variety of line items that summarize all of the projected and actual expenses for a group of items. A sample of line items that may be found in an operating budget is presented in Box 46-1.

An operating statement is sent to the department manager once a month. Under each line item the statement compares the budgeted amount with the actual expenses. Both the month and a year-to-date summary are compared. In some facilities, the salary expense may be displayed on the operating statement as a separate line item; however, the budget planning process to derive the salary and operating budgets is completed in two separate phases.

Capital and Minor Equipment

The budget for capital and minor equipment is completed separately from the operating budget. Capital equipment is usually considered to be items that cost more than $500; minor equipment is considered to be any items less than $500. Minor equipment includes items that are not routine patient care supplies (e.g., pacemaker pads, disposable pulse oximeter sensors). The other difference between minor and capital equipment is the depreciation of the cost of the equipment. Capital equipment is depreciated over a longer time than minor equipment. The concepts of amortization and depreciation are discussed later in this chapter.

Box 46-1

OPERATING BUDGET
Emergency Department IMSick Hospital

Cost center/line item	Description of line item
7230-8320	Supplies nonbillable
7230-8360	Drugs
7230-8390	Supplies billable
7230-8420	Food—direct costs
7230-8452	Computer supplies
7230-8461	Incident reports
7230-8450	Office supplies
7230-8495	Repair parts—materials
7230-8570	Telephone
7230-8620	Repairs and maintenance
7230-8780	Rental equipment
7230-8830	Dues
7230-8840	Travel expenses and meetings
7230-8872	Patient education, printing
7230-8891	Transportation expense

Requests for equipment fall into the categories of new, replacement, and remodel. The purchase of new pieces of equipment should be justified by volume increases, new technology, the opportunity to increase staff productivity, or to generate additional revenue. If a piece of equipment is being replaced, administration will want to know the fate of the old equipment (e.g., trade-in, use on another unit with less intense needs, the garbage). Justifications based on increases in productivity or billed revenue should be accompanied by a summary of the amount of projected increase in billed revenue or time saved.

FIXED VERSUS VARIABLE AND SEMIVARIABLE COSTS

In determining the department budget, the various costs must be defined as either fixed or variable. Fixed costs remain constant over time. Variable costs change over time, largely in relation to the activity level of the department.

Fixed Costs

Fixed costs are incurred regardless of the activity level of the department. The expense is not related to the volume of patients treated in the emergency department, nor the acuity of those patients. An example is the salary of the nurse manager. Other examples of fixed costs are listed Box 46-2.

Variable Costs

Variable costs fluctuate with the changes in volume and acuity of patients. An example would be the number of intravenous (IV) catheters needed; as volume of patients needing an IV increases, the number of catheters used will increase. Likewise, if the volume is below budget, these expenses should be below budget at a comparable percentage. If the volume is over budget, then the expenses in these areas should be over budget but in line with the volume increases. Other examples are listed in Box 46-3.

Box 46-2

FIXED COSTS

Nurse manager salary
Clinical nurse specialist/educator salary
Furniture at nurses station and in examination rooms
Cost of telephones and base monthly line charges
Medical director salary/stipend
Rental equipment
Uniforms
Office supplies
Routine fees for equipment maintenance
Marketing

Box 46-3

VARIABLE COSTS

Number of chart forms needed
Patient care supplies (i.e., IVs, splints, crutches)
Telephone charges (i.e., volume of calls beyond monthly fee; long distance service)
Patient food
Patient medications
Equipment repair secondary to equipment failure

Semivariable Costs

Semivariable costs are partially fixed and partially variable. They tend to be fixed over a certain range of volume and variable up to the next range of volume. An example of this type of cost would be staff salaries. If the patient/nurse ratio is 7:1, the eighth patient triggers a change in staffing. That additional registered nurse (RN) will cover the eighth patient, as well as up to the sixteenth patient. The seventeenth patient will require the addition of one more staff. If only one additional patient is included, revenue does not increase in proportion to the staff costs. However, if seven additional patients come in, the increase in revenue compensates for the increase in costs.

Certain pieces of equipment are a semivariable cost. The number of cardiac monitors is volume dependent. If the department has eight monitors and once a month needs a ninth monitor, it is not cost effective to add another monitor and central station. A portable monitor may be used to provide safe care in those few instances. If routinely more patients require monitors than there are monitors in the department, it is not only cost effective but a quality of care issue to purchase additional monitors. The number of computers needed for patient registration is another example of a semivariable equipment cost.

This information is important in projecting costs and productivity in an emergency department. When assessing semivariable costs, the benefit versus the disadvantage of adding additional staff or other semivariable units must be weighed carefully to ensure that the outcome is cost effective and productive.

Box 46-4

FACTORS TO DETERMINE FEASIBILITY OF A NEW SERVICE OR PURCHASE

Personnel costs to implement the program or run the equipment
Cost to train personnel on new program/equipment
Annual routine maintenance costs
Projected downtime and cost of alternative processes
Installation costs
Projected repair costs
Effect on staff productivity
Life span of equipment
Projected volume increase/decrease
Other equipment/supplies needed to operate the program/equipment

Amortization

The concept of amortization is to spread out a cost over time. The term *depreciation* is a special type of amortization and refers to the wearing out of equipment or physical plant. Finkler[1] describes the depreciation process:

> The cost of an asset, less its salvage value, is depreciated over the asset's useful life. The cost is the fair market value at the time of an acquisition, plus cost to put the asset into service, plus the costs of improvements made to the asset. . . The asset may be depreciated on a straight-line basis, taking equal amounts in each year, or by an accelerated basis, which results in greater depreciation in the earlier years of an asset's life.

This process may be accomplished by the department manager or through the purchasing department.

Cost/Benefit Analysis

Whether considering a new program or service, purchasing new equipment, or implementing new levels of staffing in the department, a cost/benefit analysis should be performed. This type of analysis can help quantify the results that a new purchase or program will have on the department. The department must calculate the expected volumes, implementation costs, annual costs, and projected revenues to determine whether the idea/purchase is feasible.

When making the calculations, the factors in Box 46-4 should be considered. Ideally, these factors should be balanced to ensure that the program will increase volume, revenue, and/or productivity before implementation. At the least, these factors should be identified so that the benefits of the new program can be weighed against the disadvantages. Statistic equations can be used to calculate cost/benefit ratios.

PERSONNEL COSTS

Personnel costs are based on productive and nonproductive time worked. These costs are then summarized as the number of full-time equivalents (FTEs) needed to staff a unit. Salary dollars are calculated based on FTEs.

Box 46-5

EMPLOYEE BENEFITS/NONPRODUCTIVE TIME EARNED

Vacation	Average 15 days/year	= 120 hours
Sick time	Average 4 hours/pay period	= 104 hours
Holiday time	Average 6 days/year	= 48 hours
Educational days	Average 3 days/year	= 24 hours
Mandatory education	Average 3 days/year	= 24 hours
		320 hours

Productive Time

Productive time is time actually worked by the staff performing direct patient care.

Nonproductive Time

Nonproductive time is time the staff is paid for, but not actually involved in, direct patient care. Vacation and sick time, out of house educational time, bereavement leave, and inservice training are considered nonproductive time.

Calculating Hours Worked/Paid

The actual hours that an employee works vary based on the personnel policies of the facility, union contracts, and the educational policies of the department. A full-time equivalent is the time equivalent of 40 hours a week times 52 weeks a year. This amounts to 2080 hours, the amount a full-time person is paid for over the course of 1 year. However, this person is not on the unit for all those hours so consideration must be given for the hours worked versus the hours paid. For example:

> A typical full-time employee at the IMSick Hospital is paid 2080 hours a year. The employee accrues the benefits/nonproductive time as shown in Box 46-5.
>
> If the nonproductive time is subtracted from the total paid hours, the balance is the actual hours worked:
>
> 2080 total paid hours − 320 nonproductive hours = 1760 actual hours worked

If nonproductive time is not subtracted, the department will not have enough hours/people to meet its staffing requirements. The following example illustrates how to make the transition of FTEs to the required staffing hours so that the proper number of staff are hired to staff the department.

The emergency department at the IMSick Hospital has the following staffing standard, and all shifts are 8 hours long:

944 hours for one week × 52 weeks = 49088 RN hours

Thus 49088 hours are needed to staff the department for 1 year at the staffing level denoted in Box 46-6.

Once the required staffing hours are calculated, the number of FTEs needed to fill those hours should be calculated. The total number of required hours should be divided by the number of hours a full-time equivalent actually works to arrive at the number of FTEs needed by the department:

49088 required hours ÷ 1760 hours actually worked = 27.89 or 28 FTEs

Box 46-6

SAMPLE STAFFING STANDARD

Days	= 5 RNs	Monday-Friday	(5 RN × 8 hour × 5 days)
	6 RNs	Saturday-Sunday	(6 RN × 8 hour × 2 days)
Evenings	= 7 RNs	Monday-Friday	(7 RN × 8 hour × 5 days)
	8 RNs	Saturday-Sunday	(8 RN × 8 hour × 2 days)
Nights	= 4 RNs	Sunday-Thursday	(4 RN × 8 hour × 5 days)
	5 RNs	Friday-Saturday	(5 RN × 8 hour × 2 days)

TOTAL of the above multiplication = 944 RN hours required for staffing one week

Table 46-1 Sample Position Control: Department Summary

Position	Full-time equivalents: Approved	Filled	Vacant
Director	1.0	1.0	0.0
Nurse manager	1.0	1.0	0.0
Educator	1.0	1.0	0.0
Registered nurse	28.0	27.0	1.0
Secretary	7.0	6.5	0.5
Total positions:	38.0	36.5	1.5

Table 46-2 Sample Position Control: Subgroups

Position numbers	FTEs	Shift	Name
RN Positions			
001	1.00	Day	Joann Jones
002	0.75	Evening	Mary Smith
003	0.50	Evening	Lynn Hasbeen
004	1.00	Night	Peter Deer
Secretary positions			
101	1.00	Day	John Kiley
102	1.00	Evening	Chris Beck
103	0.50	Night	Sue Reese

Each department should have a position control form that details all approved FTEs, the number of filled FTEs, and the number of vacant FTEs. Some facilities keep more detailed reports by job category (e.g., RN, technician) with a list of all of the employees filling those positions (see samples in Tables 46-1 and 46-2).

BUDGET VARIANCE

Budgets represent a projection of the expected expenses over a period of time. During that time the manager must compare the actual expenses with the budgeted ones. This comparison is known as the budget variance. Both expenses and revenue should be evaluated against the projected figures. The variance can be favorable (under budget) or it can be negative (over budget). When calculating the variance, the manager should explain the reason for the variance.

Table 46-3 Monthly Budget Statement for IMSick Hospital Emergency Department

Line item	Budget	Actual	Variance
Salaries	$12,000	$13,200	<$1200>
Supplies	$ 1200	$ 1272	<$ 72>
Drugs	$ 750	$ 825	<$ 75>
Education	$ 895	$ 949	<$ 54>
Volume	12,000	12720	720

Volume changes can cause fluctuations in expenses and revenue; however, the manager cannot assume that the variance is always related to volume. The monthly budget statement for the IMSick Hospital emergency department showed the variance depicted in Table 46-3.

The volume for that time period was 6% over budget. Those items that are volume related (i.e., salaries, supplies, drugs) should be *no more* than 6% over budget. In this case, salaries were actually 10% over budget, so the manager must explore why there was an increase in salary expense that month. On investigation, the manager found that there were three concurrent maternity leaves. Overtime was needed to cover those staff on leave, since the emergency department only has two supplemental RNs. The supply line item was exactly 6% over budget. Drugs were 10% over budget, which was related to an increase in the acuity of the patients during that month, as well as the increase in overall volume. The education line variance should not be volume related. This line item should be within the budgeted amount. The hospital had started a new timekeeping system whereby staff had to attend mandatory inservices. This class time was not anticipated when the budget was prepared.

If the volume was under budget, then the variance seen in expenses should also be under budget. Let's assume the same operating expenses as above were noted for the next month but the volume was only up 4% over the previous year. The projected volume increase was 6%, so the department was actually under the projected volume by 2%. Expenses should then also be 2% under budget. The salaries were 10% over budget when they should have been 2% under budget because there were fewer patients. Maternity leave would account for some overage but would not justify the entire difference. On inspection of the staffing patterns, an on-call schedule was implemented whereby staff were sent home on-call. They were paid a flat on-call fee and then only paid their regular wages if called in to work. This saved the department $5000 a month.

Volume projections should be based on historical data from the emergency department. Patient census for prior years, calculated per shift, per day of week, week of month, and per month, provides valuable information in making future year volume projections. Acuity also should be factored into staffing needs. Initial budget calculations should be based on those volume and acuity projections.

CASE MIX AND ACUITY IN RELATION TO BUDGETING

As mentioned earlier, patient acuity can affect the budget in terms of resource consumption. Sicker patients require more staff time and more supplies than less acute patients. All of these factors must be considered in the budget process.

Patient census and acuity data should be trended to allow the manager to match staffing patterns to patient activity. An on-going monitoring system can allow for adjustments in staffing on an as-needed basis rather than on a reactive basis. Analysis of visit types can then be matched with overall volume patterns to help the manager determine the mix of licensed to nonlicensed care providers.

The acuity level of patients is the other aspect that needs to be factored into staffing patterns. Numerous software programs, books, and consultants are available resources for selecting and developing a patient acuity or classification system (PCS) (e.g., Emergency Nurses Association [ENA] PCS manual). All of the systems have the common element of performing time-flow/motion studies or work sampling to assess the time required to deliver care. These time studies are then compiled by patient types to classify patients according to nursing and supply resource consumption. This information is then used to further define resource and staffing needs in a prospective and retrospective process. See Chapter 24 for more information on this topic.

CRITERIA FOR STAFFING LEVELS

A national standard for nursing and physician staffing does not exist. The future may yield a computer simulation model that will enable managers to simulate the patient and systems flow in their emergency department and to assess the impact on staffing patterns (see Chapter 23).

The Emergency Nurses Association revised its staffing position paper to address this issue. The revised paper, *Staffing and Productivity in the Emergency Care Setting,* advocates the use of key criteria that should be addressed when determining staffing requirements (Box 46-7). These key criteria address the unique but essential features of each emergency department that can affect the acuity of patients and the resources available to care for those patients. Staff issues, patient issues, and departmental issues are discussed.

Numerous staffing and acuity factors can have an impact on the budget. The turnover rate at the IMSick emergency department is very high. Each year for the last 5 years, 12 of 35 RNs have left the department. This turnover is costly in terms of training and orienting new staff, as well as in the overtime required to cover the vacant positions until replacement staff have completed orientation.

Physician staffing is also very complex. The number of physicians needed to staff is also based on patient volumes and acuity. Nurse practitioners or physician assistants may be used to assist the physician. Resident physicians staff many emergency departments but should be supervised by the attending emergency physician on duty. Residents can increase the average length of stay for emergency department patients because they may not be as efficient as the attending physicians. These factors can have a negative impact on the nursing staffing by increasing patient length of stay and the number of diagnostic tests/interventions performed on patients. Residents are also required to have the signature of the attending physician on the chart, further increasing the workload of the attending physician.

Departmental factors relate to specialty programs in place (e.g., minor care treatment area, trauma center, rape crisis center), the physical plant, technology available, and the work flow processes used by both the emergency department and the hospital. Specialty programs may require extra staffing. A minor care treatment area can enhance patient flow by separating nonurgent patients into a different treatment area. If that area is physically located in another part of the hospital, however, additional staffing may be needed. If the minor care area were in the same location as the main emergency department, staff can be more flexible in covering the minor area. Only one nurse may be needed with a technician if the area is within the main emergency department. During sudden increases in census, additional staff may float from the main emergency department to assist in the minor care area. If the minor care area is located across the street, the staffing requirement of the minor care area must meet the majority of the patient volume fluctuations without relying on assistance from the main emergency department.

COMMON EMERGENCY DEPARTMENT BUDGET CONTINGENCIES

Just as the clinical nature of an emergency department is complex, so are the factors that affect the department budget. Many of these factors interact to produce distinct effects. This section describes several of the more common factors affecting budgets and contingency plans for dealing with their impact.

Volume and Acuity Fluctuations

These fluctuations were addressed in earlier sections of this chapter, but are mentioned here to highlight their significance. The manager must track volume and acuity to plan for resource consumption. Numerous commercial products are available to track patient flow. Once patterns and trends are noted, adjustments in staffing and budgets should be made.

Regulatory Agencies

State, federal, and other regulatory agencies can have a negative impact on the budget. These agencies mandate that certain requirements must be met, requirements that often cost money to comply with. The COBRA legislation requires that all patients have a medical screening examination regardless of their ability to pay for care. Emergency departments that did not have triage nurses were forced to add triage nurses

BOX 46-7

EMERGENCY NURSES ASSOCIATION POSITION STATEMENT STAFFING AND PRODUCTIVITY IN THE EMERGENCY CARE SETTING

Staffing model determination factors

The following elements should be considered when addressing staffing and productivity issues.

Staff
Skill mix (i.e., RN, LPN, technician, clerical)
RN staff (i.e., relief, per diem, agency, float, on call, cross trained)
Scheduling patterns (i.e., flexible shifts and schedules)
Physician staffing (i.e., number, type and response time)
Mandatory educational requirements
Turnover/vacancy rate
Management structure
Nursing intensity time (i.e., sick time use, longevity, paid time off)
Indirect productive time (meetings, inservice education)
Specialty programs (i.e., shared governance, TQM/CQI, QA/QI)
Use of advanced practitioners (i.e., CNS, Nurse Practitioners)

Patient
Volume (i.e., total, trends, census fluctuation)
Patient flow
Length of stay
Patient mix (i.e., pediatric, geriatric, OB, psychiatric, cultural diversity)
Patient acuity (i.e., nursing/medical diagnosis, percentage of admissions)
Payor mix
Patient satisfaction survey results

Emergency Department
Type of care delivery system
Physical plant
Number of beds
Type of Triage System
Specialty programs (i.e., toxicology, trauma, observation centers, chest pain center, fast track, sexual assault, flight programs, burn centers, base station, psychiatry)
Technology
Computerization
Systems (i.e., work flow analysis, admissions process, inpatient bed availability, access to and availability of ancillary services)
Managed Care/Contractural Issues

Organizational Structure
Size of operation
Union/non-union
Academic affiliation
Mission statement
Expectations of emergency care setting (i.e., direct admission, employee health, in-house code response, drug screening)
Regional referral capability
Interfacility transport

Regulatory Agencies
JCAHO
HCFA
OSHA
State or local regulatory boards
State Board of Nursing

From Emergency Nurses Association: *Staffing and productivity in the emergency care setting: position statement,* Chicago, 1995, ENA.

to "examine" patients before registration and collection of financial information. The Joint Commission on Accreditation of Healthcare Organizations (JCAHO) is another example of a regulatory agency that can cause budgetary impacts through policy development. JCAHO requires that each level of emergency department have certain pieces of equipment. If the emergency department and the hospital are not in compliance, they can lose accreditation, perhaps causing lost revenue from patients who will no longer use that facility.

Changes in Reimbursement

Reimbursement has changed dramatically in the last 5 years. Managed care is becoming commonplace. There are stricter rules for reimbursement from the majority of third party payors. Preauthorization for admission is required by most insurance companies. Many managed care plans also require authorization to treat in an emergency setting. This requirement to get reimbursed for care provided increases the workload of the emergency department and the billing staff. Often, additional triage nurses or secretaries are needed to place the preauthorization phone calls.

The payors are also stricter in terms of what charges they will reimburse. In the future, ambulatory patient groupings will be used for emergency departments, similar to the diagnostic-related groups for inpatients settings. These groupings will reimburse based on set fees schedules for certain types of procedures.

Physician Staffing

As mentioned earlier, the type of physician staffing used in an emergency department can have a negative impact on the nursing staffing and patient flow. The use of board certified emergency physicians is the optimal physician coverage. In departments where residents provide the staffing, the length of stay for patients will usually increase. This effect can be minimized through the use of close supervision by attending emergency physicians, who can screen cases and prevent the ordering of unnecessary tests and interventions. When private physicians see their patients in the emergency department, length of stay can increase. These physicians may come to see their nonemergent patients after they finish office hours. The longer the length of stay for patients, the more nursing time required. Beds/examination space is also tied up, causing delays for other patients waiting to be seen.

SUMMARY

The budget process for an emergency care setting is complex and challenging. Proper use of volume statistics, along with operating and salary budget projections, can set useful budget parameters. Variances should be calculated, with corresponding adjustments made as needed. Careful attention should be paid to changes in healthcare reimbursement and regulations that affect emergency care.

REFERENCES

1. Finkler SA: *The complete guide to finance and accounting for nonfinancial managers,* New York, 1983, Prentice Hall.

47 Cost Containment

Linda Greenberg

OUTLINE

Problem areas of cost control in an emergency department
- Standard operating procedures
- Salary costs and staffing patterns
- Type of care delivery system
- Use of diagnostic testing
- Use of supplies and equipment
- Assessing the problem

Practice methods to contain costs

Long-term benefits of cost containment

Cost containment affects both the clinical and the business side of managing an emergency department. To implement an effective cost containment program, all levels of personnel in the department must be actively involved in assessing problem areas, as well as proposing and implementing solutions.

The nature of an emergency department lends itself to disorganization. Many different and often opposing activities occur at any one point in time. Sudden volume fluctuations, varying levels of patient acuity, and the wide number of care providers (e.g., attending physicians, residents, ancillary personnel) require constant coordination. The department manager and the medical director collaborate to develop operating systems that will lend organization and consistency to the department operations. The standardization of basic operating procedures will allow the staff to focus on the unique needs of their patients with the flexibility to distribute resources based on the needs at that time.

Variable operating costs, as the name implies, reflect the level of activity in the department for the period of time being measured. Having established systems in place to ensure that the right people and the right supplies are available at the right time can decrease costs in an emergency department and enhance the quality of care.

PROBLEM AREAS OF COST CONTROL IN AN EMERGENCY DEPARTMENT

Many interactive processes in an emergency department can have a negative impact on cost containment measures. These factors include lack of standard operating procedures, staffing patterns and salary costs, type of care delivery system, use of diagnostic testing, and supplies and equipment. Each of these factors is discussed in relation to costs in an emergency department setting.

Standard Operating Procedures

Standard operating procedures affect the budget in a variety of ways. Industry has embraced quality improvement concepts for many years. Hospitals are just now moving into the quality improvement arena. One of the basic tenets of most quality improvement theories is that people come to work to do a good job. Frequently, the operating systems they work with do not support them in doing a good job. Therefore the use of standard operating procedures can enhance staff productivity and decrease costs.[1] An example of these procedures is the process for ordering stat laboratory and radiology tests for trauma patients. A standardized trauma battery of tests that can be ordered using one test number will minimize errors and ensure that all major trauma patients at that emergency department undergo the same evaluation.

Quality improvement concepts can actually save money, not increase costs.[2] The underlying theory is that it is less expensive to perform a task or make a widget correctly the first time than to go back to correct deficiencies later. An environment that has an organized system of standardized procedures to guide workers and that teaches all staff problem-solving skills will promote zero defect production.

There are numerous examples of work in an emergency department that would benefit from standard operating procedures. The handling of abuse and rape cases are good examples. A comprehensive sexual assault examination can take up to several hours to complete and encompasses obtaining numerous specimens of evidence. Without a detailed and well-organized procedure to follow, staff may not gather critical pieces of evidence that may be needed for both legal and medical reasons. Staff may also complete the examination in a random fashion, increasing the amount of time that the staff and physician spend with one patient. The remaining patient assignments must be covered by other staff in the interim. Clinical practice guidelines to ensure adequate evaluation and diagnosis are another example. The process for handling authorization for managed care also lends itself to standardization. One aspect of that process is assigning responsibility to contact the private physician or health maintenance organization (HMO) for authorization to treat. Ensuring that no acutely ill patients leave the department without proper evaluation minimizes risk and liability for the department. A malpractice lawsuit or COBRA violation can be costly to the department.

Salary Costs and Staffing Patterns

Salary costs are the largest expense item for an emergency department after capital equipment expenditures. Both nursing and physician costs should be examined closely and monitored for efficiency, productivity, and cost-effectiveness.

Patient volume and acuity should be trended to identify patterns as a basis for staffing the department. The staffing patterns and patient activity should be aligned wherever possible. This alignment will minimize the need for overtime, calling in extra staff, or holding over staff from a previous shift. The use of per diem or on-call staff can also help to fill in for unplanned illness and unexpected sudden influxes of patients. The base number of full-time equivalents should be adequate to meet the base staffing requirements and to cover the majority of vacation and illnesses.

Having an adequate number of staff with the right qualifications and on duty at the right time applies to nursing and medical personnel. A shortage of either group can cause delays in patient flow. These delays can range from delays in being triaged by a registered nurse, being evaluated by a physician, and administration of medications. Both disciplines should use the volume and acuity patterns discussed previously to plan their staffing schedules.

Emergency physician staffing can be a major cost item for an emergency department. Several factors should be weighed when evaluating this cost. Emergency physicians are better trained to diagnose and treat emergency cases than a family practitioner or specialist who may treat and evaluate based on either too many or too few tests. Resident physicians can increase the cost of patient care if they order excessive amounts of tests. They can also increase the length of stay for patients if they do not have the experience to perform a focused evaluation. The use of board certified emergency physicians and certified emergency nurses may decrease liability risks, as these providers have demonstrated competency in emergency care and therefore are more likely to have correct focus for the emergency care setting.

Type of Care Delivery System

The type of care delivery system can affect the budget significantly, both for medical and nursing personnel. Medical coverage should be dependent on the volume and acuity of the patient population served. The use of supplemental caregivers can also decrease costs. One example is the use of nurse practitioners or physician assistants to help evaluate patients. Residents can also decrease the physician/patient ratio but may increase patient care costs through previously addressed issues. Guidelines for the recommended physician/patient ratio have been explored by the American College of Emergency Physicians but are not included here.

Nursing care delivery systems vary greatly. All RN staffing will increase costs but can also increase patient satisfaction and provide continuity of care. The use of nursing assistants and technicians to help stock items, transport patients, and perform certain procedures can enhance the efficiency of the department.

Use of Diagnostic Testing

Physicians can control the costs of patient care through the appropriate use of diagnostic testing. Ideally, a quality improvement study should be performed to trend the types and quantity of tests for each major patient type (e.g., clinical diagnosis). This information can be used to develop case management or practice guidelines for care of those patient types. Historical data from the emergency department are needed to determine adequately the present practice patterns and serve as a baseline for future planning. This method reduces the use of tests in cases where the index of suspicion for an illness is relatively low, but the tests are ordered to reduce malpractice liability.

Tracking the ordering patterns of individual physicians, nurse practitioners, and physician assistants reveals whether some practitioners order more or fewer tests than the rest of the practitioners in that group. A wide disparity in ordering practices should be examined in light of clinical concerns, as well as fiscal issues. Residents should be supervised by the emergency department attending physician on duty to ensure that excessive tests are not ordered. Using an organized systems approach to the monitoring of ordering practices can decrease both the number of tests ordered and costs.

The use of standardized practice guidelines, clinical pathways, or case management strategies will help decrease costs and ensure that a certain standard of care is met. These guidelines are developed collaboratively with nursing and medical staff. Each patient within a diagnostic patient type is evaluated similarly based on historical data from that facility.

Use of Supplies and Equipment

Supplies and equipment affect the budget of an emergency department. Lack of proper equipment and supplies causes waste and inefficiency. Staff may substitute with more costly items in the interest of providing care in a timely fashion. Many products are available that can increase the efficiency of staff and enhance patient flow. Emergency department tracking (constant monitoring of patient flow and progress through the department) and productivity systems are one example. Clinically focused products, such as the use of special wound irrigation systems, can decrease the amount of time needed to irrigate major wounds such as extensive dirty abrasions. The machine also makes the process less painful than the old method of scrubbing the wound. These new technologies can enhance staff productivity, decrease patient costs, and increase patient and staff satisfaction.

New and improved products are available every day. The medical and nursing staff should collaborate to evaluate new products for their proposed cost savings and increased efficacy. Some of the new products are fancy versions of older models and products that still perform adequately and cost significantly less to operate.

The cost of inservice for staff to teach new technologies and pharmacologic agents should also be explored. Deciding which staff should receive the inservice training (i.e., all staff or only full-time employees) depends on the frequency of use anticipated and the complexity required to operate the equipment. Alternative methods of instruction can enhance employee learning skills, and make the learning experience pleasurable. Videotaped lectures, articles, books, bulletin board displays, and self-guided learning modules are readily adapted to an emergency department setting.

Assessing the Problem

The warm body theory is not found in formal research anecdotes but is a phenomenon that most managers are familiar with. It states that by throwing more bodies at a problem, the problem will disappear. In reality, this theory does not work. Often a systems issue, not a personnel issue, causes a problem. The use of quality management principles and tools to assess problems is critical to avoiding sticking Band-aids on a major wound that requires surgery.

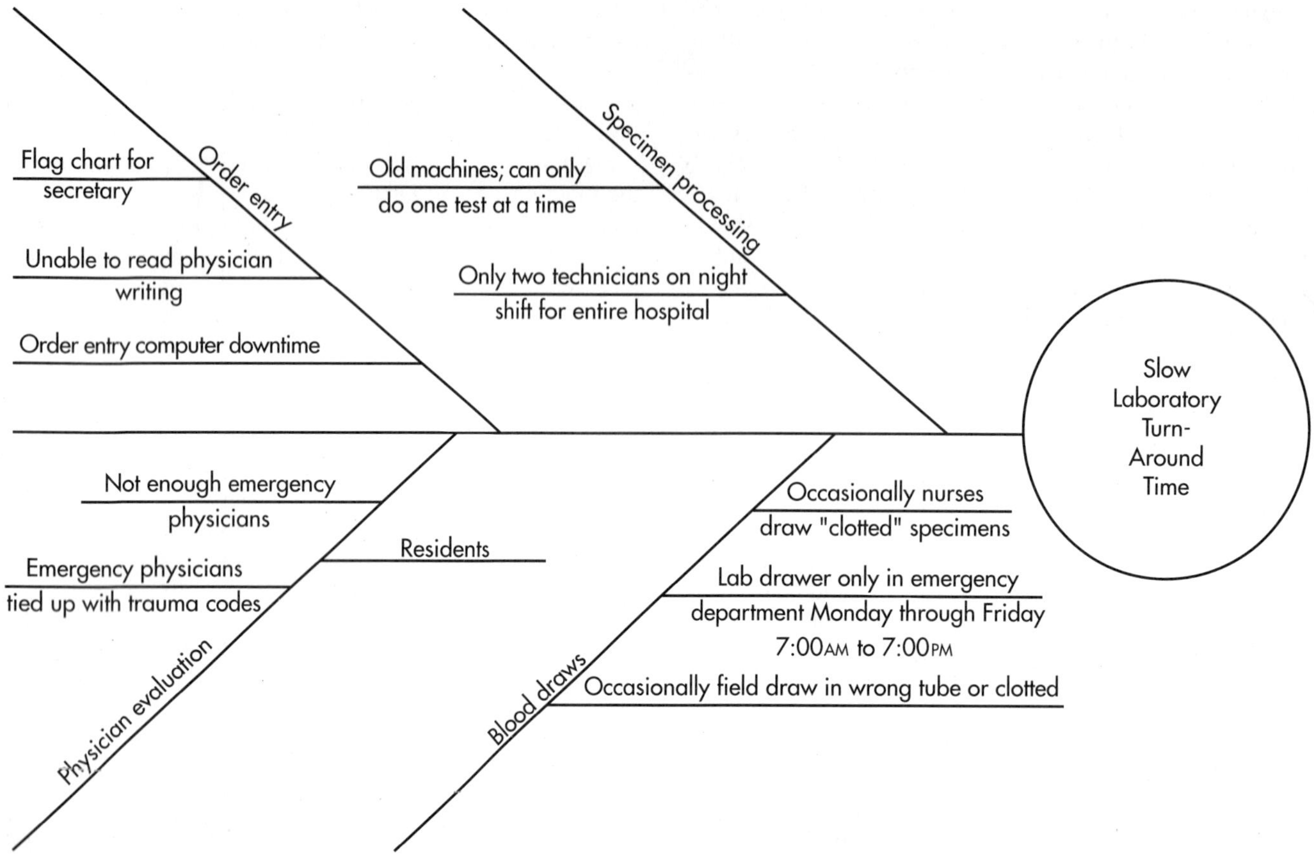

FIGURE 47-1 A fishbone (cause and effect) diagram identifying causes of slow laboratoty turn-around times.

Problems that appear to be simple on the surface may have deeper roots that are unrelated to the surface manifestation of the problem. Flow charting the problem can help uncover hidden causes. If a lack of appropriate or volume of personnel resources is the underlying issue, adding additional staff is appropriate.

The turnaround time in an emergency department is an example of an issue for which people often apply the warm body theory in an attempt to resolve problems. Additional physician staffing will not alleviate delay in radiology or laboratory turnaround time (Figure 47-1). The extra physician would only see more patients, who would wait for diagnostic test results anyway. The problem must be evaluated carefully for any system deficiencies that could be corrected before more staff are added.

PRACTICE METHODS TO CONTAIN COSTS

Physicians can use several additional methods to decrease healthcare costs. This section explores practice options that can be implemented.

Emergency physicians are trained to expect the worst. This training is intentional to minimize the misdiagnosis of life- or limb-threatening conditions. To ensure that the worst case scenario is not occurring, numerous tests are ordered that may not be necessary. Constant diligence is needed to remember that some common symptoms are really just common problems and not all cases are potentially life- or limb-threatening.

Another area of practice relates to patient follow-up referral patterns. Patients should be referred to lower cost, alternative care settings for follow-up unless other alternatives are not available. It is more cost effective to remove stitches in a clinic setting than in an emergency department. Primary care is also difficult to practice in an emergency department, so referral to a primary care provider is crucial.

Defensive medicine is costly. Careful attention to risk management issues is important and should be balanced with the clinical requirements of the patient population. Clinical pathways, practice guidelines, and case management can be based on clinical and risk management data by the emergency department. These tools allow physicians and nurses to use their skill, training, and experience to diagnose and treat patients as a common collective voice unless deviations occur in the patient's progress that suggest another possibility.[3] This approach reduces the ordering of tests to look for a condition that only occurs 0.5% of the time.

The use of medications, both within the emergency department and after discharge, can have budgetary implications. The costs of medications should be shared with physicians, so that suitable alternatives can be compared in terms of cost and efficacy. Generic medications also help minimize costs. Filling discharge medications may or may not increase costs. In some areas, this service is important if commercial pharmacies are not open after hours. Other areas may use this service to cater to customer needs so that patients do not have to go to the pharmacy after they leave the emergency department. In instances where patients repeatedly use the emergency department for primary care, filling only the minimum amount of medication necessary to help the patient until a primary care provider can be seen encourages the patient not to use the emergency department in this way.

Care planning is not traditionally performed in an emergency department setting; however, collaboration among medical, nursing, social service, and private attending staff can be helpful in providing appropriate, cost-effective care to persons who regularly use the emergency department. By working together to find alternative sources for care and working together to consistently encourage and refer patients to those sources, clinical care is improved and cost savings can be realized.

Urgent care centers within the emergency department setting can be promoted as revenue-generating programs. These programs are not a substitute for a primary care physician; rather the program is designed to provide emergent care when the primary physician is unavailable. Once treated in the urgent care center, the patient is usually referred back to the primary care physician for ongoing follow-up. Occupational medicine programs are another area in which the urgent care center can collaborate with community businesses to provide urgent care and work physicals in a cost-effective manner. The emergency department already pays the overhead operating costs and can frequently accommodate more patients without having to provide additional space beyond that of the original urgent care center. The business may have to provide space, staff, and equipment to provide the same services for their employees. Referrals can often be made to the hospital's physical and occupational therapy departments, generating additional revenue for the facility.

LONG-TERM BENEFITS OF COST CONTAINMENT

There are numerous benefits to building cost containment practices into everyday practice. Appropriate use of resources conserves the resources for areas where they are truly needed. As reimbursement decreases, operating budgets will become leaner, requiring resource utilization to be as efficient and cost effective as possible. If the healthcare industry is able to follow the examples of the manufacturing industry, performing the service or making the product right in the first place will decrease costs and increase provider satisfaction. The key to success is collaboration between nursing and medical staff to enhance efficiency and decrease costs.

REFERENCES

1. Frank IC: *Managing emergency services,* Rockville, Md, 1989, Aspen Publications.
2. Juran JM: *Juran on quality by design,* New York, 1992, The Free Press.
3. Etheredge ML: *Managed care: controlling costs, guaranteeing outcomes, New England Medical Center, Boston,* 1988, The Center for Nursing Case Management.

ADDITIONAL READINGS

Klein AR, editor: *Emergency nursing core curriculum,* Philadelphia, 1994, Saunders.

Matson TA, editor: *The hospital emergency department: a guide to operational excellence,* Chicago, 1992, American Hospital Publishing.

Matson TA, editor: *The hospital emergency department: returning to financial viability,* Chicago, 1986, American Hospital Publishing.

Strasen L: *Key business skills for nurse managers,* Philadelphia, 1987, JB Lippincott.

Walton M: *Deming management at work,* New York, 1990, GP Putnam's Sons.

48 Reimbursement and Legislative Issues in Emergency Medicine

Dieter Lehnortt

OUTLINE

Restructuring the financing and delivery of medical care in the United States has been the major focus of the public policy agenda for the last several years. The primary goals guiding policy makers' efforts in health system reform have been to constrain rising costs, increase access, and ensure the quality of care. Ultimately, the success or failure of health system reform will be judged by its success in achieving each of these goals.

According to the United States House of Representatives' Committee on Ways and Means, growth in national spending for healthcare has exceeded spending in the overall economy in 29 of the last 32 years. In 1992 national health expenditures grew to more than $800 billion and accounted for 14% of the gross domestic product (GDP).* Compared with other developed nations, the United States devotes a much larger portion of its national resources to healthcare. Without any significant efforts to curtail healthcare expenditure growth, the Congressional Budget Office (CBO) projects that healthcare spending will reach almost $1.7 trillion by the year 2000.

*Gross domestic product (GDP) is defined as the gross national product (GNP) less net property income from abroad.

Approximately 90% of national health expenditures fall into the category of personal health spending, which includes all spending directly related to patient care. According to the CBO, the portion of personal health expenditures devoted to physicians' services rose from 19.4% in 1983 to 21.5% in 1992. During these 10 years, spending on physicians' services increased 11% a year, from $61 billion to $153 billion. Increases in expenditures for physicians' services have consistently outpaced the growth in both GDP and personal health expenditures.

Paying for approximately 25% of all hospital and physician services, the Medicare program is the fourth largest category of federal expenditures after defense, social security, and interest payments on the national debt. As the nation's largest single payor for healthcare services, the Medicare program has borne much of the responsibility of being a leader in healthcare reform.

To a large extent, Medicare has met its leadership responsibility. In fact, the U.S. Department of Health and Human Services (DHHS) predicts that the Medicare and Medicaid programs will grow more slowly and cost less than previously expected, primarily because of decreased medical prices brought about by system reform. DHHS predicts that Medicare's rate of growth will continue to rise, peaking at 13% in 1995 but then slowing to about 7% in 1998. Medicaid spending will slow more dramatically and is expected to be 11% higher in 1994 than in 1993, slowing to 9% in 1995 and 5% in 1996.

Many other third-party payors will continue to follow the federal government's and Medicare's lead in healthcare reform. The benefits from containing costs and increasing efficiency in the healthcare marketplace are considerable for individuals and the nation. Judging from recent trends in healthcare spending, attaining health system reform that achieves these worthwhile goals will be extremely formidable. However, federal policies aimed at restructuring financial incentives to promote the cost effective use of medical services, restrain the growth in system capacity, and encourage more rational decision making about the focus and use of technology are now being debated.

With respect to the emergency department and emergency physicians, it is likely that major reimbursement changes still lie ahead. Providers should expect increased scrutiny of utilization from payors jolted by skyrocketing outpatient bills. The incentives, created by the current reimbursement climate, for medical care being delivered on an outpatient basis will change dramatically as the federal government continues development of an outpatient prospective payment system. In addition, ongoing review of the emergency department's role in providing nonurgent, primary care services will continue to result in the federal government seeking ways to move patients into less costly sites of service.

Hospitals and other providers of healthcare services will have to become much more aware of the range and scope of costs involved in providing services to patients in outpatient settings to survive. Hospitals and physicians will be forced to work much more closely to ensure that the most appropriate, cost effective care is rendered to patients in the emergency department setting. In the future, it is likely that emergency physician groups will be awarded hospital contracts based on the group's ability to provide cost effective care to emergency department patients, as well as the group's ability to provide high quality care to these patients.

This chapter describes recent initiatives in national healthcare reform. The information is intended to help hospital administrators, emergency physicians, emergency nurses, and other individuals involved in the delivery of emergency care better prepare for the myriad reforms that are likely to evolve during the next decade. Armed with this information, perhaps these individuals can also work together more closely to ensure that emergency departments, emergency physicians, and other providers of emergency care continue to be the healthcare safety net for the nation's citizens.

THE FEDERAL ROLE IN HEALTHCARE POLICY

Before the end of World War II, healthcare was little more than a cottage industry. The delivery of healthcare and efforts to coordinate and plan health services were primarily initiated by private, voluntary, nongovernmental agencies at the state and local levels. Voluntary health agencies, such as the American Cancer Society, were frequently the only entities initiating healthcare delivery or planning services. Studies or planning efforts were generally disease oriented and fragmented in their approach. Personal healthcare was provided by the private sector, predominantly in a one patient-one physician relationship.

From the 1920s to the mid-1940s, domestic unemployment, economic instability, and World War II dominated federal concerns. However, after the conclusion of the war, the federal government had more time and more money with which to examine those healthcare issues raised by the private sector. At this point in our nation's history, the face of healthcare changed forever.

Hospital Survey and Construction Act of 1946

The first sustained governmental infusion of cash and involvement in national healthcare coordination and planning was the Hospital Survey and Construction Act of 1946, known as the Hill-Burton Act (PL 79-725). To receive funds, states had to establish Health Planning Councils responsible for assessing the need for new hospital construction. For the next 30 years, the Hill-Burton Act supplied partial funding for hospital construction projects, providing \$4 billion in grants to approximately 4000 hospitals and \$1.9 billion in loans to 300 facilities.

In 1954 the Hill-Harris amendments to the Hill-Burton Act revised and expanded the program to include funding for modernization and replacement of public and nonprofit hospitals. Emphasis shifted from providing hospital care in rural areas to improving urban hospitals. More significantly, however, the amended Hill-Burton Act now served as a model for federal grants-in-aid and began the government's involvement in ensuring healthcare for its citizens. Because state Health Planning Councils now had to impose a new formula for assessing hospital bed need (incorporating utilization data, projected population, and occupancy factors), these amendments also shifted the federal government's emphasis from construction to health service planning. The federal government had become a firm and irreversible part of the American healthcare system.

Hospitals began to ride a wave of growth that was bolstered by federal dollars from Hill-Burton and other programs. Health insurance money, increasingly secured as job benefits by unions and then offered by most companies in the 1950s and 1960s, also supplied inducements for further healthcare expansion.

Medicare and Medicaid

At this point, the federal government took an idealistic turn, seeking to provide health insurance for the nation's elderly and poor. The passage of the Social Security Act in 1935 had earlier marked the federal government's acceptance of public responsibility for designated categories of the needy, deprived, and handicapped. By the end of World War II, the nation had become somewhat conditioned to disbursements of tax dollars by the federal government for social purposes. Social Security provided the philosophic rationale for protecting the elderly and the medically indigent in a federally administered program. These efforts culminated in the enactment of Titles XVIII (Medicare) and XIX (Medicaid) of the Social Security Act in 1965.

The early versions of Medicare and Medicaid provided for payment of "reasonable" and "allowable" costs. This system, which maintained the highly esteemed fee-for-service system and the private practice of medicine, was a concession to the strong lobbying efforts of the American Medical Association. As a result, however, healthcare expenditures skyrocketed because the system provided no incentives for either provider efficiency or cost containment. Although efforts to curb the inflationary cycle of healthcare spending were initiated almost immediately after the passage of Medicare and Medicaid, most had little impact. For instance, in the early 1970s, the federal government attempted to constrain healthcare spending through a series of price freezes. However, this effort conflicted with providers' rising costs for labor and medical equipment.

National Health Planning and Resources Development Act of 1974

On January 4, 1975, the National Health Planning and Resources Development Act of 1974 (PL 93-641) was created. This Act established health systems agencies in an effort to improve the delivery of healthcare services while cutting costs, primarily through oversight of construction and service expansion. The Act also placed an emphasis on consumer-provider partnership, comprehensive planning, and regulation and evaluation, and it encouraged a closer relationship among regional, state, and federal governments. For the first time, national health priorities were established, requiring area-wide and state health plans.

Unfortunately, healthcare providers quickly became adept

at challenging or circumventing the Act's intended results. Increased legal and planning costs associated with obtaining Certificates of Need (CON) contributed to rising healthcare costs. Conversely, many projects were not approved and many more were never attempted, thus reducing some of the potential increase in healthcare costs. Overall, the National Health Planning and Resources Development Act of 1974 did little to stem the tide of explosive healthcare expenditure growth of the 1970s and early 1980s.

Prospective Payment for Medicare Inpatient Hospital Services

Healthcare costs during the 1970s and 1980s grew at almost twice the rate of the GNP, consuming an increasingly larger share of domestic resources. During this time, pressure intensified to control surging healthcare costs, rising at their own dizzying speed and further propelled by double-digit inflation rates. By 1982, the Reagan administration realized that existing policies were not effectively controlling costs. Along with deregulation and competition, the Administration persuaded Congress to implement massive reforms in America's healthcare policy. On October 1, 1983, Title VI of the Social Security Amendments of 1983, Prospective Payment for Medicare Inpatient Hospital Services, became effective. Patterned after a system developed by researchers at Yale University, this system set hospital prices prospectively on 470 diagnosis-related groups of illnesses.

Physicians' Medicare Fee Schedule

As America moved into the late 1980s and early 1990s, medical price inflation had abated only slightly. Turning its attentions to physicians, the federal government enacted a massive reform in the way in which Medicare reimburses physician services. The Omnibus Budget Reconciliation Act (OBRA) of 1989 (PL 101-239) amended Title XVIII of the Social Security Act by adding a new section 1848, "Payment for Physician Services." This new section contained three major elements:

- Establishment of volume performance standard rates of increase for Medicare physician services expenditures
- Replacement of the reasonable charge payment mechanism used by Medicare to reimburse physicians with a fee schedule for physicians' services
- Replacement of the maximum allowable actual charge (MAAC) mechanism, which constrains the total amounts that nonparticipating physicians can charge Medicare patients for covered services, with a new limiting charge mechanism.

On January 1, 1992, the Physicians' Medicare Fee Schedule, based on the Harvard Resource-Based Relative Value Scale (RBRVS), was implemented.

In 1994 the focus on cost containment shifted slightly to ensuring universal access to needed healthcare services. However, the federal government's focus on healthcare expenditures continues to play an important role in the current health system reform debate. After being linked with the nation's flagging economy in the early 1990s, healthcare reform became a key plank in the election of President Clinton in 1992.

As Congress' review of healthcare reform proposals slowly marches on, however, other important federal initiatives continue at the Prospective Payment Assessment Commission (ProPAC), the Physician Payment Review Commission (PPRC), the Health Care Financing Administration (HCFA), and the Graduate Medical Education National Advisory Committee (GMENAC) levels. Although overall health system reform remains the primary focus today for much of society, one cannot adequately review the federal government's role in healthcare policy without addressing the incremental reforms and initiatives currently being debated by these administrative agencies and commissions. This chapter is dedicated to bringing several of these important initiatives to light.

OUTPATIENT PAYMENT POLICY REFORM

Since 1980 the number and type of services that can be provided in the outpatient setting have increased dramatically. Between 1980 and 1990, the proportion of personal health expenditures attributable to outpatient hospital care almost doubled, increasing from 4.8% to 8.7%. During this same period, growth in Medicare payments for outpatient services averaged about 15% annually, compared with 12% and 8% for physician and inpatient services, respectively (Table 48-1).

Four basic factors contributed to the growth in expenditures for outpatient services. Between 1985 and 1990, inflation and population growth accounted for approximately 27% of the increase in hospital outpatient spending. Intensity (the frequency and complexity of services provided) and increased utilization each accounted for approximately 31% of the growth in outpatient spending. In this respect, the expanding use of new technologies and changing medical practice are major factors that helped fuel this growth.

Numerous policy changes during the last 10 years have also encouraged more outpatient spending. Expanded coverage for many outpatient services, additional incentives to curtail inpatient services, and more aggressive inpatient utilization review mechanisms all contributed to the explosive growth in outpatient service spending. These policies not only resulted in increased utilization of outpatient services, but also created a complex and fragmented payment environment for these ambulatory services.

The Need for Reform

Currently, outpatient payment policies vary by site and type of service. This fragmentation often results in conflicting in-

Table 48-1 Percent Distribution of Personal Healthcare Expenditures, by Type of Service (1980-1990)

Type of service	1980	1985	1990
Hospital care	46.9%	45.7%	43.7%
Inpatient revenue	31.7%	30.8%	28.1%
Outpatient revenue	4.8%	6.3%	8.7%
Other revenue	10.5%	8.7%	7.0%
Physician services	19.2%	20.1%	22.5%
Other professional services	10.6%	10.8%	10.9%
Drugs	9.2%	8.8%	8.2%
Nursing home services	9.2%	9.3%	9.1%
Other personal services	5.0%	5.2%	5.5%
Total	100%	100%	100%

Data from: Health Care Financing Administration, Office of the Actuary.

centives that undermine efforts to control costs and increase provider efficiency. For instance, Ambulatory Surgery Centers (ASCs) are paid prospectively set rates and therefore are rewarded for efficiently provided services. Conversely, hospital outpatient payments are based on the lesser of the hospital's reasonable costs or charges, or a blended rate composed of 42% of the hospital's reasonable costs or charges and 58% of the ASC prospective payment rate for the service rendered. Under this method, payments to hospitals are reduced when the facility's costs are lowered, eliminating much of the incentive for hospitals to improve their efficiency.

During this same period, the growth in hospital outpatient service expenditures far exceeded expenditures for hospital inpatient services. Medicare payments between 1980 and 1990 for hospital outpatient services increased annually by about 15%, compared to an 8.3% annual growth in inpatient hospital service expenditures. Even after adjusting for inflation and growth in the number of program beneficiaries, the annual change in Medicare outpatient expenditures has surpassed the annual change in Medicare inpatient expenditures.

This rapid growth in the outpatient sector has been the primary motivation behind the federal government's interest in reforming the payment methodology for outpatient services. OBRA of 1986 included a legislative mandate for the HCFA to investigate the feasibility of developing and implementing a prospective payment approach for the facility component of outpatient care. OBRA 1986 also called for the design and modeling of a prospective payment system for all outpatient services, including emergency departments, same-day surgery units, outpatient clinics, and physicians' offices.

Ambulatory Patient Groups

In 1988 HCFA granted a contract to the 3M Health Information Systems Group in Connecticut for the development of an outpatient prospective payment system (PPS). The major objectives of the 3M project were:

- To apply and test the basic concepts of the inpatient PPS in the outpatient setting
- To develop an outpatient payment system methodology that could provide the basic structure for an outpatient PPS while also accommodating a wide range of policy options
- To evaluate the effectiveness of an outpatient PPS by using historical Medicare payment data

Although various systems for classifying ambulatory patients already existed in 1988, each system had proved ineffective in dealing with the complexities of outpatient service payment. In response to the needs dictated by an effective outpatient PPS, 3M developed a patient classification scheme that became known as Ambulatory Patient Groups (APGs).

Under the APG classification system, a patient is described from a list of 297 APGs that correspond to each service provided. Patients in each APG have similar clinical characteristics and involve similar resource use and costs. Unlike Medicare's inpatient PPS, the APG system can involve the assignment of multiple APGs to a single patient. This difference in inpatient and outpatient methodologies is intended to reflect the diversity of services that can be rendered to patients in the outpatient setting.

APGs were initially developed to encompass the full range of ambulatory settings in which services could be provided to Medicare beneficiaries, including emergency departments, outpatient clinics, and same-day surgery units. However, APGs do not address phone contacts between and among providers and patients, home visits, nursing home, or inpatient services. Although the initial application of APGs focused on Medicare patients, they were ultimately developed to represent patients across the entire spectrum of third-party payors.

The data elements used to define APGs were limited to the information routinely collected on Medicare claim forms. They consisted of the patient diagnosis (coded in ICD-9-CM format), physician procedures (coded in Physicians' Current Procedural Terminology, or CPT, format), and patient age and sex. The patient characteristics used to define APGs were restricted to those elements that were readily available in these formats to ensure the quick implementation of the APG system once a final decision had been made to convert to this new outpatient payment methodology.

To better comprehend the payment approach of the APG model, one must understand that four basic characteristics are inherent in any PPS:

- Payment rates are established in advance and are fixed for the fiscal period to which they apply.
- Payment rates are not determined by providers' past or current actual costs involved in rendering the services.
- Prospective payment rates serve as payment in full for the services rendered by the provider.
- The provider retains the "profit" or suffers the "loss" resulting from the difference between the actual payment rate and the cost of providing the service.

In an outpatient PPS model, each APG is assigned a standard payment rate. The payment for services rendered by a provider to a Medicare beneficiary is computed by adding the payment rates for all APGs assigned to a particular patient. However, to create incentives for cost control and to minimize opportunities for APG upcoding or code "creep," not all services provided to a patient under the APG model are assigned an APG. The APG system uses several methods for grouping or packaging similar services provided during the same patient encounter into a single payment unit or APG. These methods include the use of a significant procedure consolidation, an ancillary service packaging process, and a multiple significant procedure and ancillary service package discounting process. The combination of the APGs and the individual rules for procedure consolidation, ancillary packaging, and discounting are collectively referred to as the APG payment model.

Significant procedure consolidation refers to the collapsing of multiple related significant procedure APGs into a single APG to determine the appropriate payment. When a patient has multiple significant procedures, some of the significant procedures may require minimal additional time or resources from the provider. For example, if both a simple laceration repair and a complex laceration repair are performed on the same patient, only the complex laceration repair would be used in the APG payment computation.

Ancillary packaging refers to the inclusion of certain ancillary services into the APG payment rate for a significant procedure or medical visit. For example, a chest radiograph would be packaged into the APG payment for a service provided to a patient with pneumonia.

Discounting refers to a reduction in the standard payment rate for an APG. When multiple unrelated significant procedures are performed or when the same ancillary service is performed multiple times, a discounting of the APG payment rate is applied. Discounting recognizes that the marginal cost of providing a second procedure to a patient during a single visit is less than the cost of providing the procedure by itself.

According to the 3M researchers, a visit-based APG PPS with significant procedure consolidation, uniform ancillary packaging, and multiple APG discounting would have many advantages over the current outpatient payment methodology:

- Many similar units of service are aggregated together (by significant procedure consolidation).
- The need to establish separate payment rates for minor differences in the unit of service is eliminated.
- The number of units of service is greatly reduced.
- The opportunity for unbundling the units of service is greatly reduced.
- There is a financial incentive to providers to use ancillary services effectively.
- There is a financial incentive to providers to not repeat tests.
- Multiple procedures performed during a single visit are reasonably compensated, but not excessively rewarded.
- The costs of atypical visits are recognized in the APG system.

An additional advantage of the APG payment model is its considerable flexibility. This flexibility means that the incentives in the system could be altered to achieve specific policy objectives. The APG patient classification scheme also appears to provide the basic building blocks that can accommodate a wide range of payment system designs.

Because of its ability to adhere to the essential objectives identified by Congress and by HCFA in implementing an outpatient PPS, the APG model has become the favorite approach of many health policy makers intent on revising outpatient payment policy.

Prospective Payment Assessment Commission's Role in Outpatient Payment Policy Reform

OBRA 1990 required the Prospective Payment Assessment Commission (ProPAC) to analyze and comment by March 1, 1992 on HCFA's recommendations for outpatient payment policy reform. The HCFA recommendations were to be submitted to Congress by September 1, 1991. Although the 3M Ambulatory Patient Group system design and evaluation was completed in 1990, HCFA has not, yet, provided its recommendations to Congress. ProPAC, absent the HCFA report, prepared its own interim report and recommendations for Congress in March 1992 *(Outpatient Payment Policy Reform)*.

Because most ambulatory services are furnished in settings outside the hospital, ProPAC recommended that outpatient payment reform must extend to all providers of outpatient services, such as hospitals, physicians' offices, and free-standing ambulatory surgery centers. In ProPAC's view, prospective payment methods should be used for all ambulatory services, regardless of provider or setting. This approach would allow the payment system to control cost increases more effectively and establish a consistent system of behavioral rewards or penalties for all providers.

ProPAC also recommended that, to the extent possible, all outpatient services should eventually be packaged or bundled together for payment purposes. ProPAC believed that bundling would help control the volume and therefore the costs of outpatient services. However, because of data and other constraints, the Commission also realized that an incremental approach to reforming outpatient payment would be necessary. Therefore, it adopted a short-term strategy for outpatient payment policy reform until these limitations could be overcome.

As required by Congress, ProPAC initially focused exclusively on outpatient hospital-based service payment reform. In this vein, the Commission recommended that payment reform begin with and concentrate on ambulatory surgery and radiology services. It recommended that ambulatory surgery and radiology services be paid based on national, fully prospective rates adjusted for variations in area wages and other justifiable cost differences. The Commission also recommended that the level of payments should be based on a blend of average hospital costs and free-standing payment rates.

With respect to physician services, ProPAC recommended that outpatient payment reform should provide neutral incentives for physicians and beneficiaries in choosing the site of care. The Commission also recommended that outpatient payment reform should be consistent with the incentives and disincentives created by the Medicare Physicians' Fee Schedule. Although the Commission was unwilling, at least at the time of its March 1992 report, to expand the outpatient PPS methodology to include outpatient physicians' services, it did choose to continue investigating the feasibility of packaging all outpatient services into this type of system.

In its March 1994 report and recommendations to Congress, the Commission continued to push for a prospective payment system for hospital outpatient services. It has subsequently developed and performed a demonstration project. HCFA's proposal to bring all outpatient radiology, diagnostic, and surgical procedures under a single blended PPS is currently in final clearance within the agency, but would still require Congressional approval before being implemented. Although it is expected that outpatient prospective payment would see quick action by Congress, HCFA would still require 12 to 18 months to develop the needed rates and regulations.

The implications for emergency medicine of Medicare implementing an outpatient PPS are unclear. Although it appears that early efforts to incorporate the emergency department into an APG or some other type of outpatient PPS met with mixed results, one cannot assume that emergency medicine will be left out of the fray after HCFA's recommendation is presented to Congress. Emergency departments have presented some unwieldy problems to PPS researchers with respect to the complexities of effectively categorizing the broad range of services provided in this setting into neat, clearly distinguishable groupings for payment purposes. However, as was the case in the passage of the hospital inpatient PPS, Congress is not always swayed by the argument that additional research and data are necessary before a payment system is put into place. Based on the continuing upward spiral of outpatient costs being experienced by the Medicare program, Congress may likely implement a PPS for all outpatient hospital services, including emergency department services, leaving the HCFA, hospitals, and providers to figure out the details of surviving under such a system.

HEALTH SYSTEM REFORM

Refining Medicare Physician Payment Policy

With the advent of the Physicians' Medicare Fee Schedule (MFS) in January 1992, the federal government embarked on an aggressive journey to change the structure of physician payment in this country. From the federal government's perspective, overall the implementation of the fee schedule has gone quite well. The major fears raised during the implementation of the fee schedule—on the one hand that many physicians would no longer treat Medicare beneficiaries and on the other hand, that program costs would increase sharply because of physicians' increasing volume of services—have been unfounded. In addition, Medicare's resource-based relative value scale has also been well accepted by many private third-party payors and state Medicaid programs.

The Congress, HCFA, and the Physician Payment Review Commission (PPRC) continue to look at ways of further refining the fee schedule. Although several important refinements in the MFS have already been implemented (e.g., elimination of the "new physician/practitioner" adjustment, creation of a primary care service category for the volume performance standards process, and elimination of the prohibition against payment for electrocardiogram interpretations performed in conjunction with a visit service or consultation), further refinement in the MFS is likely. Thus far, plans for these additional refinements are being focused in three primary areas:

- Refinement of the methodology for establishing practice expense and professional liability expense relative value units (RVUs)
- Continued refinement of relative work values for physicians' services
- Enhancing Medicare's Volume Performance Standards (MVPS).

The MFS consists of three components that correspond to the principal types of resources used to provide physicians' services. The physician work component was developed by Harvard University researchers through a study designed to measure the relative time and effort required to furnish different physician services. The other two components, practice expense and professional liability expense, were calculated from historical charge data through formulas that were specified by Congress in OBRA 1989.

The PPRC and HCFA have begun to question the appropriateness of these charge-based practice expense and professional liability expense relative values as part of the MFS. In fact, the PPRC has been working since 1989 to develop alternative methods for calculating practice expense and professional liability expense relative values that are more consistent with the reform goals of resource-based payments.

In its 1993 annual report to Congress, the PPRC recommended that Congress and HCFA revise the practice expense and professional liability expense components of the MFS so that they are resource-based. The PPRC also recommended that, beginning in 1997, practice expense relative values should be based on data about the direct costs (e.g., medical staff time, equipment, and supplies) incurred in delivering each service, with an incentive-neutral formula for allocating indirect (e.g., rents and utilities) costs. The PPRC also recommended that, beginning in 1997, professional liability expense relative values should be based on data about the relative malpractice risk incurred in delivering each service.

It is difficult, at this time, to predict what effect these changes in the relative value units for practice expense and professional liability expense would have on physicians providing emergency department services. Clearly, under the original MFS calculations, emergency physicians fared relatively well in terms of HCFA's assignment of practice expense and professional liability expense factors for emergency department evaluation and management (E/M) services. Because it was unable to segregate emergency department visits provided by emergency physicians from emergency department visits provided by other types of physicians, HCFA set the practice expense and professional liability expense "factors" for the emergency department E/M services at 41% and 4.8%, respectively. It is likely that at least one result of the MFS moving to a resource-based methodology for establishing relative values for these two components would be a decrease in the relative values assigned to emergency department evaluation and management services. The fact that few emergency physicians have any concept of the magnitude of the expenses or costs involved in providing emergency department services does not bode well for the specialty.

The second area in which additional MFS refinements are being focused is the continued updating of physician work RVUs. Two recurring activities currently require establishing new or refined relative work values or reviewing existing ones in the future. One is the yearly publication of new and revised codes in the American Medical Association's *Physicians' Current Procedural Terminology* (CPT). Relative work values must be assigned to each of these new or revised services for Medicare payment purposes. Second, relative work values for existing codes must be reviewed periodically to ensure that they accurately reflect physicians' efforts. For instance, the relative work value for a particular service may need to be refined because its physical or decision-making components may change over time. OBRA 1989 requires HCFA to recalibrate the entire relative value scale at least once every 5 years.

Two processes have been used thus far to accomplish the yearly refinement of relative work values included in the MFS. First, HCFA has used the public comment process (resulting from the publication of the MFS notice in the *Federal Register* each year) in combination with a small-group process (multispecialty panels consisting of Medicare carrier medical directors and physicians nominated by specialty societies) to identify the need for adjustments in the relative work values of specific services. Second, the American Medical Association has implemented a refinement process through the creation of an Relative Value Update Committee (RUC). The RUC was formed in November 1991 and grew out of a series of discussions between the American Medical Association and the major national medical specialty societies. The RUC comprises 26 members, with 22 members representing major specialty societies. This process uses a small group survey method to produce work RVUs that are voted on by the RUC. Approved relative work values are then submitted to HCFA for review.

One of the unintended results of the MFS review and recalibration process, which is perhaps of the most significance for emergency physicians, is devaluation of E/M services as the result of HCFA's "budget neutrality" adjustments in relative work values. OBRA 1989 required that adjustments in RVUs may not cause total fee schedule payments to differ by more than $20 million from what they would have been had the adjustments not been made. The biases towards upward valuation of services that characterizes the current HCFA and American Medical Association refinement processes has caused physicians' evaluation and management services to be inappropriately devalued in the last 2 years. The 1992 relative work value refinement process demonstrated that, if substantial numbers of codes are reviewed and upward bias exists in the review process, the effects on E/M services can be significant.

Over the next several years, each process will continue to evolve as the MFS is reviewed and updated. Continued pressure will be applied by Congress and by the PPRC to ensure that these processes include:

- Mechanisms to promote consistent decision making from year to year
- Fair methods and representation of involved parties
- Means to identify overvalued and undervalued services
- Mechanisms to ensure public accountability
- Feedback to the CPT Editorial Panel when codes need revision to achieve accurate resource-based payment.

The third area in which MFS refinements are being focused is the enhancement of MVPS process. Constraining growth in the volume of services is one of the most important goals of Medicare cost-containment policy. The MVPS system has been the Medicare program's principal tool for moderating the growth in service volume. The MVPS sets annual expenditure targets through Congressional action or, if Congress does not act, through a default formula. The differences between these expenditure targets and actual Medicare physician service expenditures is used to determine future MFS conversion factor updates.

The Administration has proposed three significant modifications to the MVPS default formula: modifying the default volume and intensity allowance, cumulating the MVPS over several years, and eliminating the limit on the size of fee reductions in any year. On one hand, each of these proposals would strengthen the MVPS process by improving the linkage between volume/expenditure growth and fee updates; on the other hand, these changes would likely further reduce Medicare payment rate updates relative to current law, thereby reducing physicians' willingness to treat Medicare patients. Medicare actuaries have estimated that these modifications in the MVPS default formula would reduce Medicare expenditures by approximately $8.9 billion between 1996 and 2000.

Again, although it is difficult to predict the exact effect these proposed modifications would have, it is likely that they would reduce the yearly updates applicable to emergency physician services. Unless additional allowances were to be continued for primary care services, including emergency department evaluation and management services, emergency physicians would likely experience decreases in their payments for services provided to Medicare beneficiaries.

Curtailing Inappropriate Emergency Department Use by Medicaid Recipients

During the last decade, Congress has continued to mandate expansions of Medicaid's covered population and services. From 1988 to 1992, federal Medicaid costs rose from $30 billion to an estimated $65 billion. State Medicaid agencies, feeling the financial pinch of the mandated program expansions, have sought to control program costs through various approaches while attempting to maintain quality care. One method that has become extremely popular among state Medicaid agencies is placing tighter controls on the use of Medicaid services, including emergency department services.

The use of emergency departments by Medicaid recipients for nonurgent problems has long been seen as a problem for the program. In September 1983, the DHHS Office of Inspector General (OIG) released a report (OAI—Non-Urgent Use of Hospital Emergency Departments by Medicaid and Medicare Beneficiaries), which estimated that at least 50% of Medicaid emergency department visits were nonemergency and could have been adequately treated in other, less expensive settings. However, the OIG's report also found that factors such as inadequate access to other outpatient settings and the refusal by many nonemergency physician providers to accept Medicaid recipients were significant contributors to this problem.

In March 1992, the OIG released another report on the use of emergency departments by Medicaid recipients (Report No. OEI 06-90-00180, March 1992, Use of Emergency Rooms by Medicaid Recipients.). In its report, the OIG found that Medicaid recipients often lack access to primary care during or after office hours and thus surpass the general population in hospital emergency department misuse. The OIG estimated that nearly one half to two thirds of visits made by Medicaid recipients to hospital emergency departments were for nonemergency treatment. To combat this problem, the OIG recommended that the following steps be taken:

- Each state should develop a comprehensive initiative to reduce costly nonemergency use of hospital emergency departments. These initiatives could address:
  - Increased use of managed care/prepaid options to improve overall care access and quality
  - Community based access to after hours care
  - Increased reimbursements to physicians and clinics who see Medicaid recipients after hours
  - Defining different levels of emergency department care and providing corresponding tiered pricing and reimbursement levels
  - Triage payments to providers for screening patients not treated in the emergency department.
- The HCFA should encourage states to develop initiatives to review and reduce nonemergency use of emergency departments by Medicaid recipients and should assist states by:
  - Providing instructions on access and use of emergency department data in conducting annual reviews of emergency department utilization.

- Encouraging development of managed care/prepaid programs and expediting the review of state applications for waivers to implement their managed care efforts and emergency department controls.
- Disseminating annual reports on effective practices for reducing nonemergency use of emergency departments by Medicaid recipients.

States attempting to control nonemergency use of hospital emergency departments must consider several federal requirements before proceeding. Medicaid recipients must have the right to freedom of choice of a healthcare provider as stated in Section 1902(a)(23) of the Social Security Act. However, the Social Security Act has provided for exceptions to this ruling if access to care of adequate quality is not denied. When recipients are restricted in their choice of provider by state action, a waiver must be obtained. Several states have used waivers to implement programs to reduce nonemergency use of the emergency department.

Additional concerns with regard to patient access to care are expressed in antidumping legislation adopted by Congress. OBRA 1989 (P. L. 101-239) restricts hospital emergency departments from refusing treatment to patients who lack the ability to pay for services. It also requires hospitals to provide medical screening examinations to patients presenting for care in the emergency department. The antidumping legislation has caused many state Medicaid agencies to proceed carefully when developing programs to limit nonemergency use of the emergency department.

Over the next several years, state Medicaid programs will continue to focus many of their cost-cutting efforts on emergency department services. It is likely that most states will adopt some type of managed/prepaid care arrangement to reduce program costs and to further restrict Medicaid recipient access to hospital emergency departments for nonemergency care. In the face of these challenges, it will become crucial for emergency physicians and hospitals to work together to provide states with additional options for ensuring appropriate access to needed healthcare services, including emergency department services, for Medicaid recipients. Unless state Medicaid programs work to add additional providers to the healthcare system who are willing to treat Medicaid recipients at all hours of the day, these patients will continue to use the emergency department as their sole source of primary care.

Cost Containment and Expenditure Limits

Many policy makers believe that, as Congress considers the various options for health system reform, the opportunity to expand access and maintain an affordable, high-quality health system depends on developing policies that will result in effective cost containment. The high cost of healthcare threatens the ability of both individuals and society to pay for needed health services. Escalating costs also place additional pressures on federal and state budgets. Therefore the critical issue on which the success of any long-term cost-containment measures will eventually be judged is the growth rate of healthcare spending relative to the growth of the GDP.

Two broad approaches to achieving healthcare cost containment have emerged during the last several years. One approach depends on the ability of market pressures to encourage cost containment by organized health plans and providers. The other approach emphasizes government-set limits on provider payments or health plan premiums. To review the healthcare reform proposals currently being debated, the Administration's plan starts from the first approach (by structuring markets to achieve savings) while also incorporating a system of premium limits and fee schedules (to guarantee that savings are achieved). Other plans, such as the Stark Medicare-for-all bill and the McDermott-Wellstone single-payor bill, depend primarily on rate setting to control healthcare costs. Finally, several other plans, such as the Chafee-Thomas, Cooper-Breaux, and Gramm-Santorum bills, rely totally on market mechanisms to control healthcare costs.

Markets can control costs primarily by encouraging providers and consumers (patients) to join health plans that are structured as organized systems of care and by having these plans compete. Individuals in the managed care industry, for instance, point to an improving record of cost containment in recent years as a result of aggressive management. Unfortunately, limited scientific evidence of these successes exist. Recent reviews by the CBO, the GAO, and the PPRC found only limited evidence in the research literature that staff-model and group-model managed care organizations can reduce costs somewhat and that costs were lower in markets with high managed care organization penetration. However, advocates and detractors of the market forces approach could probably agree that today's markets are not structured to maximize their effectiveness and that a restructured market might lead to better results.

Expenditure limits, on the other hand, can be used to address both the price of services and the volume of services that patients receive. Proponents of this approach point to successes of cost-containment initiatives in state all-payor systems, in Medicare, and in various national systems in other countries. For example, implementation of Medicare's prospective payment system led to a reduction in the annual growth rate for hospital inpatient expenditures from 9.1% before reform to 2.5% in the first 6 years after reform. In addition, Medicare payments to physicians have recently slowed because of price constraints (the physicians' MFS).

The real issue for the federal government is how to strike a balance between the two approaches to enforcing expenditure limits and between fee-for-service and managed care delivery systems. Expenditure limits could play a critical role in controlling the price and the volume of services, especially in a fee-for-service market. Stronger market mechanisms might also be helpful in achieving national cost containment goals. Large businesses, for example, point to their success in bringing cost "discipline" to the market by moving more employees into managed care plans. However, structural reforms such as community rating, risk adjustment, open enrollment seasons, and the creation of mandatory purchasing entities for certain market segments would also need to be implemented to allow markets to operate more effectively by removing the major impediments to stronger competition.

It is still unclear which approach the federal government will take in controlling healthcare costs. It is likely that national healthcare policy makers will attempt to take advantage of both market mechanisms and expenditure limits to achieve cost containment. It is also likely that complementary initiatives such as constraining physician supply, reforming the medical malpractice system, supporting outcomes research and practice guidelines, and pursuing a national data strategy will be implemented.

Professional Liability Reform

The importance of professional liability reform is underscored by its inclusion in nearly all of the major health system reform proposals being considered by Congress. The most important goal of today's professional liability system is to reduce the rate of medical injury. A second goal of today's system is to compensate fairly those patients who experience a medical injury. Most healthcare policy makers believe that the current professional liability system fails to meet either of these goals. In addition, the current system likely promotes the practice of defensive medicine and impedes efforts to improve the cost effectiveness of medical care. Further, inefficiencies inherent in the system result in high administrative costs and long delays in claims resolution.

Indicative of Congress' interest in making improvements in the current system, OBRA 1990 directed the PPRC to make recommendations about professional liability system reform. The federal government's interest in this area is derived from the overall aims of healthcare system reform: ensuring that healthcare systems deliver high-quality care, constraining the costs of healthcare, and ensuring access to needed healthcare services. Unfortunately, the PPRC viewed the problems plaguing the existing professional liability system as being so complex and intractable that piecemeal or limited reforms were unlikely to have any major effect. The Commission, therefore, formulated recommendations for a profoundly different system that would require a completely new approach to preventing injury and compensating patients.

In making its recommendations, the PPRC realized that reforming the current professional liability system would entail considerable developmental work. The components of the reformed system would be developed in an evolutionary manner and implemented one at a time. The focus of the Commission's recommendations was on:

- Improving the functioning of the current system.
- Developing and using efficient alternative dispute resolution mechanisms for compensating injured patients.
- Formulating and testing more reliable standards for compensation decisions.
- Collecting better data on medical injuries and improving systems to prevent injuries and improve quality of care.

With respect to improving the functioning of the current professional liability system, the Commission analyzed various proposals, including tort reforms, according special legal status to practice guidelines and enterprise liability. Tort reforms are changes in the legal rules governing malpractice lawsuits and comprise the bulk of the reforms commonly proposed. The tort reforms analyzed by the PPRC included:

- Schedules for noneconomic damages (to reduce the unpredictability and inconsistency of unreasonably high awards).
- Schedules for attorneys' contingency fees (to discourage those claims that have little chance of success and to ensure that more of a large award goes to the patient).
- Modification of the collateral source rule (to be consistent with the compensation function of the current professional liability system and to ensure the affordability of the internal costs of a future, more inclusive administrative system for compensating medical injuries.
- Restrictions on joint and several liability (to ensure that a defendant pays for only his or her share of the fault without coming at the expense of adequately compensating injured patients).
- Periodic payments of large awards (to meet continuing needs resulting from permanent injuries).
- Reductions in statutes of limitation (to eliminate the uncertainty, delay, and expense in insuring against professional liability claims).
- Reductions in or diversion of punitive damages (to use the money from these awards directly for injury prevention or quality improvement activities).
- Requirements for certificates of merit (to screen out frivolous claims before a formal lawsuit can be filed).

More attention is being focused on the relationship between practice guidelines and the existing professional liability system. The treatment of practice guidelines in the professional liability system has important implications for their success in promoting the delivery of appropriate, cost-effective care. However, revisions in the practice guidelines by the judicial system (by explicitly rejecting the content of the guideline or by carving out exceptions to the guideline) could render these guidelines ineffective in helping to reduce costs and improve quality. In response to this concern, numerous states are providing or planning to provide special legal status to practice guidelines to facilitate their use by defense attorneys and physicians.

Empiric research conducted on the use of practice guidelines in malpractice litigation has enabled the federal government to draw several conclusions. First, practice guidelines are playing a modest but increasing role in malpractice litigation. Obstetric guidelines are most frequently being used, probably because they are among the oldest and best known to physicians and attorneys. Guidelines are being introduced more frequently by plaintiff rather than by defense attorneys, and the use of guidelines by either side is usually, but not always, successful in malpractice litigation. Therefore, although the effects of guidelines on the litigation process are varied, overall they appear to be positive.

The final area in which the PPRC recommended reforms in the current professional liability system was enterprise liability. Enterprise liability refers to the situation in which a healthcare organization, rather than an individual practitioner, assumes financial responsibility for all negligent injuries to patients under its care. This approach relieves individual practitioners of all personal tort liability for such injuries. Enterprise liability is thought to offer two benefits over the existing system of professional liability coverage. First, it results in clear savings in administrative costs because the enterprise serves as the single defendant in malpractice cases (thereby eliminating the need for separate lawyers, investigations, and malpractice insurance policies). Second, enterprise liability is believed to result in fewer medical injuries because the burden of injury detection and prevention is placed on the entire entity or system that delivers care.

Enterprise liability may be an inevitable result of legal trends and the inherent incentives induced by increased competition in the medical marketplace. The formation of accountable health plans under proposed system reform would also likely accelerate the trend toward integrated delivery systems and other entities that increasingly look like unified enterprises. In many respects, enterprise liability already exists for hospitals owned and staffed by one organization (such as health maintenance organizations) or a typical university or county hospital. As vertical integration spreads through the healthcare delivery system, enterprise liability is likely to follow for reasons of efficiency.

The components of a future professional liability system (alternative dispute resolution systems, alternative standards for patient compensation, and better prevention of medical injuries) envisioned by the PPRC would utilize an efficient administrative system to resolve claims on the basis of a standard for compensation that is more reliable than the current negligence standard. Such a system would also be helpful in monitoring quality of care and implementing programs to prevent medical injuries.

In the future, it is likely that the federal government will take steps to ensure that practitioners, hospitals, and healthcare organizations engage in effective efforts to reduce injuries resulting from inpatient and outpatient care. It is also likely that these efforts will be a required part of quality assurance and improvement programs of practitioners and healthcare organizations and will focus on both inpatient and outpatient care. The federal government will also likely continue its support of research on the etiology, classification, and prevention of medical injury, as well as the development of the necessary databases to reduce the incidence of medical injury.

Emphasis on Managed Care

Whether one is discussing health policy makers, group purchasers, healthcare providers, or the insurance industry, managed care has been proposed regularly in recent years as a key part of healthcare reform. Numerous proposals before Congress would create special incentives or preferences for managed care arrangements. The result is that managed care has become one of the standard "buzzwords" in healthpolicy circles.

Despite all the rhetoric to the contrary, managed care remains an elusive concept. It is a term used to describe many different approaches or arrangements that seek to improve quality and efficiency or to control costs. Much of what currently falls under the heading of managed care is better described as the private regulation of healthcare focused on the limited goal of containing costs. For this reason, a number of health policy makers have begun to ask how to push managed care toward a more extensive management role. These policy makers tend to envision scenarios in which physicians, patients, insurers, and managed care organizations share accountability for improving patient care outcomes and for meeting cost-containment objectives.

According to the Group Health Association of America (GHAA), the trade association that represents health maintenance organizations (HMOs), the number of individuals receiving healthcare from managed care plans increased 9.2% in 1993, reaching 45.2 million by the end of the year. This compares to 41.4 million managed care plan subscribers from year-end 1992. By year-end 1995, 59 million individuals were being treated under some form of managed care.

As the numbers grow, however, uncertainty continues to reign in the managed care marketplace. Critics of managed care arrangements argue that these organizations offer no more than "managed costs" or price discounting. Any costs savings these plans are able to achieve, according to these critics, are nothing more than lower prices. Little, if anything, is done to reduce service utilization or to manage the delivery of healthcare. To the insurance industry and policy makers, both in Congress and the Administration, however, managed care remains the "magic bullet" that will contain costs and improve quality of care.

The Health Insurance Association of America (HIAA), which represents traditional insurers, identifies four common elements in managed care plans:

- Arrangements with selected providers to furnish a comprehensive set of services
- Explicit standards for selecting providers
- Formal programs for ongoing quality assurance and utilization review, including case management and the use of primary care "gatekeepers"
- Significant financial incentives for members to use the plan's providers

In addition, whether the term is *managed care, coordinated care,* or *managed competition,* three approaches to managing care exist:

- Selecting providers
- Restricting clinical choices
- Inducing changes on the part of providers

Totally unrestricted freedom of choice in selecting providers in today's insurance market is quickly becoming a thing of the past. More commonly, today's consumer is offered some form of panel or network of providers from which to choose, and is required to seek care from only those providers. Strong financial incentives to stay within the network are frequently part of today's managed care plan. Because consumers are required to choose from the managed care organization's panel or network of providers, many policy makers believe that it is now time to move toward more rigorous grounds for selecting the best providers. Tools such as profiling provider practice patterns and researching patient outcomes appear to offer the best potential for managed care plans implementing rigorous, data-based criteria for selecting and retaining physicians.

The use of rigorous profiling and credentialing standards is somewhat more common on the hospital side. Criteria such as mortality, morbidity and infection rates, rates of accidents and iatrogenic diseases, employee attitudes about and utilization of different hospitals, and opinions of local medical societies on hospital quality are being used more frequently by today's managed care organizations to select hospitals for their networks.

Once the group, staff, or panel/network is in place, the next issue addressed by managed care organizations is how to influence the practice patterns of providers included in the network. The most common approach for accomplishing this strategy is review before or after the course of treatment or an admission to determine whether the procedure or course of care is appropriate. Procedures or courses of care deemed inappropriate are denied payment. These prospective or retrospective utilization management approaches primarily focus on specific clinical decisions.

Other methods for restricting clinical choices focus on limiting the use of specialists or specialist services. Unfortunately, this method all too frequently places emergency physicians or emergency departments at odds with managed care organizations. The principal mechanism for limiting the use of specialists or specialist services is the use of primary care physicians as gatekeepers. For this method of restricting clinical choice to work optimally, gatekeepers must be able to deliver a broad range of primary care services and to know when and where to refer patients for more specialized care, when appropriate.

The final issue addressed by managed care organizations is inducing changes in practice patterns on the part of providers. Traditionally, this was accomplished by appealing to professional standards while preserving the individual practitioner's clinical autonomy. More recently, however, practice guidelines have moved to the forefront as the prescribed method of influencing physician behavior in a managed care environment.

The federal government first became involved in managed care with the creation of the Federal Employees Health Benefits Program (FEHBP) in 1959. This program permitted participation by comprehensive medical plans, the predecessors of modern-day managed care plans. The growth of managed care plans was further encouraged in 1973 with the passage of the Health Maintenance Organization Act. This law included federal funds for the development and operation of new HMOs, as well as standards for HMOs that wished to be federally "qualified" or approved. Although most experts would agree that neither of these two laws ever stimulated the enormous growth envisioned by some, it did contribute to significant growth and development of the industry.

The Carter and the Reagan Administrations viewed managed care (or, at least HMOs) as providing a potential means for injecting competition into the Medicare program and reducing program expenditures. A series of demonstration projects (The Medicare Capitation Demonstrations from 1980 to 1981 and the Medicare Competition Demonstrations from 1982 to 1984) ensued. Evaluation of these demonstration projects found that, generally speaking, the HMOs were successful in enrolling Medicare beneficiaries, that the overall satisfaction level of enrollees was high, that the quality of care provided was at least satisfactory, and that HMOs had only a small effect on hospital use.

During the last several years, a new Medicare managed care program has been undertaken. The HCFA, concerned that many beneficiaries are simply unwilling to enroll in HMOs and give up their existing physician relationship, has established several Medicare Preferred Provider Organization (PPO) demonstration projects. In 1990, Congress authorized the establishment of Medicare Select Plans in 15 states. Under these plans, beneficiaries buy a traditional fee-for-service Medigap policy in which coverage is limited to the designated preferred providers. Beneficiaries who obtain in-network services receive Medicare benefits plus full payment of deductibles and coinsurance.

During this same period, the federal government also encouraged state Medicaid programs to experiment with the development of managed care initiatives. According to 1991 data, approximately 2.6 million Medicaid recipients were enrolled in managed care plans. Some states (under their Medicaid waivers) can mandate participation in managed care, which has helped to push the market share for Medicaid managed care higher than that for Medicare. Within the last several years, several states have enacted legislation to expand enrollment in Medicaid managed care dramatically.

Although the philosophic commitment to managed care by the federal government has persisted, the rhetoric has shifted from managed care to coordinated care to managed competition. New initiatives being developed by HCFA include a point-of-service option. Under these initiatives, Medicare would contract with new contracting entities that would develop a network of preferred providers in an area. Selected on the basis of quality assurance systems, outcomes measures, and negotiated prices, these providers would be expected to manage the care they provide to patients. Beneficiaries would have the option of choosing between these providers or out-of-network providers, with financial incentives offered for choosing in-network providers. A special feature of these initiatives would be the bundling of Part A (hospital) and Part B (physician) payments for the specific services offered by the point-of-service contractor.

It is likely that the growth of managed care will continue in the years ahead, regardless of the outcome of national healthcare reform. Because managed care emerged as a tool to combat rising healthcare costs, and not as a result of healthcare reform, the healthcare market will continue its trend toward managed care through the end of the decade. The further development of point-of-service plans, increased self-funding and direct contracting of employers, continued development of managed care workers' compensation programs, the formation of new purchasing arrangements, and the expansion of electronic claims administration will continue to push managed care into the twenty-first century.

GRADUATE MEDICAL EDUCATION PAYMENT REFORM

During the 1950s and 1960s, several major reports expressed concern that a shortage of physicians existed in the United States. The Surgeon General's Consultant Group on Medical Education (1959), the Association of American Medical Colleges (1965), and the National Advisory Commission on Health Manpower (1967) all noted that physician supply was not keeping pace with population growth and increased demand for physician services. These reports called for direct federal assistance to medical schools as a means to increase regional physician/population ratios.

In 1963 the Health Professions Educational Assistance Act provided the first substantial direct federal assistance to medical education by offering construction grants to medical schools that agreed to increase enrollment. Subsequent amendments to this legislation, including the Health Manpower Act of 1968, further increased grants and expanded loan and scholarship programs.

In the 1970s the policy focus of graduate medical education shifted, fueled in part by a 1970 Carnegie Commission

Report on Higher Education. This report called for a more equitable geographic and specialty distribution of physicians. To respond to these shifts in policy focus, the federal government began encouraging primary care and rural health and improving minority representation in medicine. Many policy makers believe, however, that despite some small successes, the larger goals of slowing growth in aggregate physician supply and shifting specialty distribution toward primary care have not been achieved. In addition, although the need for more ambulatory training has been discussed at great length, residents continue to spend most of their time in inpatient settings.

Today, graduate medical education is largely financed through patient care revenues generated by hospitals. The federal government is the largest single explicit financing source for graduate medical education through the Medicare program. According to the GAO, the Medicare program pays for approximately 29% of the total direct costs of graduate medical education. In 1992 Medicare paid $1.46 billion to compensate hospitals for the program's share of costs associated with training physicians. Another $180 million went toward nursing and allied health training programs, and approximately $3.56 billion in Medicare payments were made for indirect costs associated with graduate medical education activities.

According to the GAO, approximately 60% of interns and residents were training in nonprimary care specialties and approximately 40% were training in primary care specialties (family medicine, general internal medicine, and general pediatrics). However, some interns and residents in primary care training will ultimately complete their residency training in nonprimary care and enter practice as nonprimary care physicians (often referred to as "branching"). When branching is considered, the GAO reported that the proportion of interns and residents categorized as primary care was reduced from 40% to approximately 25%. Without considering the effects of branching, approximately 55% of Medicare direct graduate medical education payments were associated with the training of nonprimary care interns and residents. Considering the effects of branching increased this percentage to approximately 72%.

Since the 1980s, Congress has enacted three changes to the payment method used for calculating direct graduate medical education costs. Among the reasons cited for these changes in payment methodology is the desire to enhance the incentives for training in primary care. Congress perceived that Medicare payments were being used to provide greater support to nonprimary care training. Despite these legislative changes, however, barriers to primary care training persist in Medicare's payment methodology for the direct costs of graduate medical education.

The specter of broader system reform brings the potential of developing more effective solutions to the graduate medical education funding dilemma by including all payors in new financing strategies and by developing new systems of service delivery for uninsured patients who historically have relied on teaching institutions as their usual source of care. The health system reform debate also provides an important opportunity that was missing in the past to coordinate supply and training policies with those affecting payment for physicians' services, access to care, and cost containment. Many national policy makers believe that the success of reform to rationalize the delivery of medical care and slow the growth in national health expenditures may actually be undermined unless accompanied by limits on system capacity. These policy makers, as well as numerous interest groups, have issued policy statements that support the creation of a national commission to develop and implement physician work force policy changes and the creation of a national graduate medical education financing pool to which all payers would contribute.

Virtually all of the major health system reform proposals introduced in Congress include provisions that would affect the financing of graduate medical education. For example, the Administration's healthcare reform proposal would establish a new system for managing the supply of specialty training for physicians. Over a 5-year phase-in period, at least 50% of new physicians would be trained in primary care, defined as family medicine, general internal medicine, and general pediatrics. This goal would be accomplished by increasing the number of filled primary care residency slots by 7% each year, while decreasing the number of filled specialty training slots by 10% annually. The Secretary of the Department of Health and Human Services would determine the number of residency slots in each specialty based on recommendations from the National Council on Graduate Medical Education. The Council would also be responsible for apportioning residency positions to regions. Funds to support graduate medical education would be pooled from Medicare's direct graduate medical education fund and from a surcharge on health plan premiums from other insurers. These funds would be allocated directly to approved training programs, including non-hospital-based training programs. Additional measures to support primary care would include a loan forgiveness program and a program to retrain physicians for primary care specialties.

Because the federal government's current definition of primary care physicians does not include emergency medicine, graduate medical education payment policy reform will likely shift funds away from emergency medicine residencies. From a political perspective, the 50-50 policy goal (in which 50% of physicians will enter practice as primary care physicians) espoused by the government, coupled with anticipated cuts in residency positions, has touched off efforts by a number of physician specialty societies (including the American College of Emergency Physicians) to protect their programs by being designated as primary care. This scramble for federal designation appears to have become even more intense because the Administration included obstetrics-gynecology in its definition of primary care specialities. Thus far, however, these efforts have been unsuccessful.

To better comprehend why emergency physicians are not considered primary care physicians by the federal government, but emergency department services *are* considered primary care services by Medicare, one can examine the rationale used by the PPRC in defining primary care specialties. The PPRC bases its definition of primary care specialties on the idea that providing primary care services or being an entry point into the healthcare system is not the defining characteristic of the primary care physician. Instead, the Commission has argued that primary care physicians are distinguished by their training as generalists who do not limit their practice by type of condition or organ system, *and* who provide both continuous and comprehensive services. Although emergency physicians meet most of the characteristics included in this definition, the issue of providing continuous services (as in continuity of care) is the most likely suspect precluding the federal government from accepting emergency physicians' desire to be considered primary care for graduate medical education funding purposes.

This important debate will continue over the next several years as healthcare reform moves forward. The federal government will continue to believe that there is a need for national policies that lead directly to reductions in resident supply and changes in specialty mix. A process that restricts the total number of residency positions and links the clout of public financing with informed decision makers within the medical profession will ultimately be used to achieve these goals.

HEALTH DATA INITIATIVES

A key element in healthcare system reform is the development of a national data strategy. Much of this strategy is currently focused on standardizing data elements, forms, unique identifiers for providers and for patients, and confidentiality and privacy. Some recent progress toward standardization has been made, including reports in the last year by the Workgroup for Electronic Data Interchange (WEDI), the Institute of Medicine (IOM), and the National Committee for Quality Assurance (NCQA).

Perhaps the most important work being undertaken in this area has been by the WEDI, which was created in 1991 in response to a forum convened by the Secretary of Health and Human Services. It is a voluntary, public-private task force that is attempting to standardize health data, particularly the electronic communication of these data across the industry. By using existing technologies, the WEDI has moved forward to bring a host of vital health administration functions (e.g., claims processing, outcomes data collection and reporting, and physician practice profiling) under a common set of guidelines. Through the use of common data formats and standards, the WEDI believes that insurers, hospitals, and physicians and other healthcare providers can achieve significant reductions in administrative costs while greatly enhancing the quality of services that are provided.

In July 1992, the WEDI issued a report to the Secretary of Health and Human Services that laid out aggressive but achievable goals to propel the healthcare industry toward the use of electronic data interchange more quickly. The report made several recommendations to promote full implementation of electronic data interchange within the next 5 years. These recommendations included the following:

- *Adopt standards:* The insurance industry should define and publish standard formats through the American National Standards Institute ASC × 12 Insurance Subcommittee. Standard formats for enrollment, eligibility, claims submission, and payment/remittance advice should be developed first. Formats for other major business transactions, such as claims inquiry and referrals, should also be developed.
- *Provide incentives:* Public and private third-party payors should create incentives for increased use of electronic data interchange. Among the incentives that should be considered are low- or no-cost software and maintenance support, quick payment incentives for electronic claims, and technical assistance. Furthermore, providers and other participants should be urged to explore opportunities for partnerships to reduce development and implementation costs. For instance, hospitals could provide electronic links to physicians to facilitate access to automated coding.
- *Unify data content:* All participants should be committed to full use of standardized billing content for claims submission (including data elements and codes), as developed and/or revised by the National Uniform Billing Committee and the Uniform Claim Form Task Force.
- *Create accreditation for data clearinghouses:* Clearinghouses should be required to meet minimum performance standards to protect the business, confidentiality, and security of electronic data interchange customers.
- *Protect consumer confidentiality and privacy rights:* Congress should enact federal preemptive legislation governing confidentiality and should ensure the uniform, confidential treatment of identifiable information in electronic environments.
- *Simplify healthcare for consumers:* A clear process for the application of coordination-of-benefit rules in electronic environments should be developed. In addition, options for using electronic health insurance cards within the healthcare environment and the types of electronic card alternatives (such as magnetic stripe or smart cards) should be investigated.

In the current national healthcare reform debate, several proposals have been introduced that address data strategies. The overall approaches used in several of these proposals include the following:

- The establishment of a national board to develop and implement a health information system. The national board would oversee establishment of a regional network of electronic data centers to collect, compile, and transmit data. Data would be collected on enrollment, clinical encounters, financial transactions, and other aspects of patient-provider encounters.
- The creation of national standards for health plans to report data to a national board. The board would perform and distribute analyses that illustrate levels and trends in expenditures, rates and trends in the provision of individual provider services, and price levels.
- The establishment of a federal administrative panel to create a healthcare data interchange system to make healthcare data electronically available on a uniform basis to all participants in the healthcare system.
- The development, by each state health plan, of a uniform patient record database that uses standard software and ensures patient confidentiality. The database would be used to collect information on patient medical records to allow for quality review and outcomes analysis.

It is clear from these activities and others that the federal government intends any future healthcare system to revolve around some type of electronic data interchange process. In particular, the WEDI and the PPRC continue to develop recommendations aimed at reducing the administrative costs and paperwork burdens associated with healthcare delivery in this country.

Finally, the HCFA has also taken steps to consolidate its current fragmented Medicare claims processing system and make it easier to detect fraud and abuse. HCFA has awarded a 6-year, $19 million contract to GTE Government Systems to design and help implement the agency's Medicare Transaction System (MTS). The contract award marks the first concrete step in HCFA's plan to eventually process all Medicare Part A and Part B claims at a small number of sites instead of through the current system, which involves 14 different computer systems operated by 79 carriers and fiscal intermediaries at 62 sites.

Under the HCFA plan, when a provider electronically transmits a claim to Medicare, the MTS, rather than the local Part B carrier or Part A intermediary, will determine whether the claim should be paid. The MTS system will also automatically bill any Medigap policy. Because all information on a patient will be in one centralized data bank, physicians and other providers will be able to obtain information about patient eligibility, other insurance policies, and pending claim status. At least in the beginning of its development, the MTS system will be designed to accommodate both encounter data transactions now used in certain managed care settings and the traditional fee-for-service transactions that constitute Medicare's current physician reimbursement system.

Although local carriers and intermediaries would no longer be responsible for processing claims and payments, they will monitor the medical necessity of physician services for which claims are submitted, audit hospital cost reports, investigate fraud and abuse situations, and respond to beneficiary concerns.

SUMMARY

The numerous national legislative and regulatory issues facing emergency medicine will present emergency care providers with both pitfalls and opportunities. The need has never been greater for emergency department staff and hospital administrators to understand and practice the principles of effective management within their institution. Only by making the best use of their available resources can hospitals create efficient and productive emergency departments that provide quality patient care and enhance the level of services offered by the entire facility.

In the emergency department, successful delivery of healthcare services depends on the cooperation and coordination of a team of several dozen individuals and key ancillary services. Unfortunately, the emergency department frequently consists of multiple, conflicting chains-of-command rather than a single, structured chain-of-command. In addition, great demands are placed on the emergency department by several different environmental factors. Patient populations served by the emergency department frequently have no regular source of healthcare outside of the department. Lack of needed inpatient beds or other inpatient services often disrupts efficient patient flow through the emergency department. Other healthcare professionals sometimes become disillusioned with the emergency department and its mission. Examining these factors, one becomes painfully aware of the management nightmare that all too often challenges the department's staff and administration.

To be successful, all organizations must define their mission and their vision of themselves. This definition should include accountability, leadership, motivation, the coordination of resources, and an eye toward the future. Nowhere is this more true than in the complex organizational unit known as the emergency department. If the essence of management is the ability to deliver, in an efficient and productive manner, a superior result in the face of scarce or limited resources, emergency medicine may well be the management challenge of the nineties and beyond.

To create an emergency department management system and a patient care environment that will be prepared to meet the challenges posed by anticipated payment and healthcare system reforms, today's emergency care providers must understand the complex issues being addressed at the national level. Only by understanding the directions for the future can these emergency care professionals prepare for the changes that will have to be made in the present.

BIBLIOGRAPHY

1. Ayres W: GHAA reports 9% jump in HMO enrollment, *CCH Monitor, The Newsletter of Managed Care* 2(10):3, 1994.
2. Deleted in proofs.
3. Department of Health and Human Services: *Medicare program: fee schedule for physicians' services,* 42 CFR Parts 405, 413 and 415, Baltimore, Md, November 25, 1991.
4. Department of Health and Human Services: *Medicare program: revisions to payment policies and adjustments to the relative value units under the physician fee schedule for calendar year 1994,* 42 CFR Parts 405 and 414, Baltimore, Md, December 2, 1993.
5. General Accounting Office: *Graduate medical education payment policy needs to be reexamined,* Report No. HEHS-94-33, Washington, DC, May 5, 1994.
6. General Accounting Office: *Medicare: further changes needed to reduce program and beneficiary costs,* Report No. HRD/91/67, Washington, DC, May 1991.
7. Lehnortt D: Outpatient prospective payment, *Medical Management Resources Reimbursement Report,* Fall:1-7, 1992.
8. Lutz S: Ambulatory care keeps patients, hospitals on the move, *Mod Healthc* Dec:20-32, 1989.
9. Office of Inspector General: *Controlling emergency room use: state Medicaid reports,* Report No. OEI 06-90-00181, Washington, DC, March 1992.
10. Office of Inspector General: *Use of emergency rooms by Medicaid recipients,* Report No. OEI 06-90-00180, Washington, DC, March 1992.
11. Physician Payment Review Commission: *Annual report to Congress,* Washington, DC, 1992.
12. Physician Payment Review Commission: *Annual report to Congress,* Washington, DC, 1993.
13. Physician Payment Review Commission: *Annual report to Congress,* Washington, DC, 1994.
14. Prospective Payment Assessment Commission: *Outpatient payment policy reform: interim Congressional report (C-92-02),* Washington, DC, March 1992.
15. Sikora P: *Trends and transitions in health care financing,* Palo Alto, Calif, 1987, Market Intelligence Research Company.
16. Workgroup for Electronic Data Interchange: *Report to the secretary of the U.S. Department of Health and Human Services,* Washington, DC, July 1992.
17. 3M Health Information Systems: *Design and evaluation of a prospective payment system of ambulatory care,* Wallingford, Conn, 1990, U.S. Department of Commerce National Technical Information Service.

SUGGESTED READING LIST

Commerce Clearing House (CCH): Medicare & Medicaid Guide
Commerce Clearing House, Inc.
4205 West Peterson Ave
Chicago, IL 60646

Part B News
United Communications Group
4550 Montgomery Ave, Suite 700N
Bethesda, MD 20814

Health Legislation and Regulation
Faulkner & Gray's Healthcare Information Center
1133 Fifteenth Street, NW, Suite 450
Washington, DC 20005

Medical Economics
Box 55
Oradell, NJ 07649

CCH Pulse: The Health Care Reform Newsletter
Commerce Clearing House, Inc.
4025 W. Peterson Ave
Chicago, IL 60646

Medicine & Health
Faulkner & Gray's Healthcare Information Center
1133 Fifteenth Street, NW, Suite 450
Washington, DC 20005

Physician Payment Review Commission Annual Report
2120 L Street, NW, Suite 200
Washington, DC 20037

Medicare Compliance Alert
United Communications Group
4550 Montgomery Ave, Suite 700N
Bethesda, MD 20814

Physician's Payment Advisory
American Health Consultants, Inc.
60 Peachtree Park Drive, NE
Atlanta, GA 30309

ACEP News
American College of Emergency Physicians
PO Box 619911
Dallas, TX 75261-9911

Modern Healthcare
Crain Communications, Inc.
740 Rush Street
Chicago, IL 60611-2590

American Medical News
American Medical Association
515 North State Street
Chicago, IL 60610

Reimbursement Report
Medical Management Resources, Inc.
9550 Regency Square Blvd, Suite 1200
Jacksonville, FL 32225

CCH Monitor: The Newsletter of Managed Care
CCH Incorporated
4025 W. Peterson Ave
Chicago, IL 60646

Physicians' Medicare Guide Newsletter
CCH Incorporated
4025 W. Peterson Ave
Chicago, IL 60646

49 Preparing for Fee-for-Service: FEASIBILITY STUDIES

Robert Burleigh

Medical practices, like most businesses, are sometimes faced with important, sometimes critical, decisions that affect the way they conduct their business and their future. The same is true for fee-for-service billing; practices that were formerly compensated via salaries, percentage of gross charges, monthly/annual stipends, or hourly rates will eventually be faced with the prospect of independent billing.

The initiative for the change may be proposed by the practice or the hospital. Today the hospital is more often the initiator, although in the past the opposite was true. We believe the change in initiative is attributable to the physician-driven switch to fee-for-service in the mid-to-late 1980s and early 1990s for those practices in which the economic opportunities are self-evident and likely to succeed. Indeed, practices faced with challenging payor/patient mixes often resisted fee-for-service proposals on the basis that they would be economically damaging to the practice without a subsidy that the hospital was unwilling to provide.

As hospitals are repeatedly squeezed by the constantly changing reimbursement and regulatory evolution in the healthcare industry, however, many hospitals that previously resisted or even refused to permit fee-for-service are now proposing, or imposing, this change in financial arrangements. While the prospect of broad, federal level changes has caused a countertrend *back* to compensation (usually salaries) arrangements *from* fee-for-service, hospitals are continuing to propose/impose fee-for-service billing on emergency practices even though they acknowledge that the change may be reversed in the foreseeable future. As hospitals are forced to make tough fiscal decisions such as staff reductions and layoffs, cutbacks in services, salary freezes, and other belt-tightening measures, they have begun to view physician payroll as an expendable item. Often, they are simultaneously insensitive to, or at least resistant to, requests for financial support from practices that are not financially viable under fee-for-service.

To satisfy themselves that fee-for-service billing is or is not potentially successful, hospitals and/or practices should conduct or secure from a reliable and independent source a feasibility study to assess the economic potential of fee-for-service billing. If conducted by hospital staff, this review should be audited by the practice and an outside advisor because the hospital has an unavoidable conflict-of-interest, as well as limited or no expertise in conducting a feasibility analysis for fee-for-service billing.

Implementation of fee-for-service billing will typically take 60 to 90 days from the time a billing arrangement is chosen (i.e., select a billing company, establish a practice billing office). Selection of a billing service bureau will typically take 30 to 60 days and double that if the practice will do its own billing and is setting up its own office. Billing provided by hospitals, practice plans, or Management Service Organizations (MSOs), may lengthen or shorten these estimates. The feasibility study should be completed 60 days before beginning the billing decision process, assuming that billing is feasible. If a stipend, subsidy, or other economic support must be negotiated, however, add at least 30 days (we recommend 90) for negotiation. Preparation of a reliable feasibility study typically takes about 30 to 45 days.

Generally, from the beginning of the feasibility study to implementation of fee-for-service requires a minimum of 5 months and can take up to 1 year. Although all of these processes can be accelerated, most often accuracy and attention to detail, breadth of choices, and care in structuring the financial arrangement with the hospital are sacrificed. Many billing services are capable of a "quick-start" initiation of billing, but prefer to have the opportunity to work at a more deliberate pace.

Feasibility studies are appropriately named. They are studies, or forecasts, rather than absolute calculations. Even if the study is performed by the biller who is chosen to handle billing, their calculations are, at best, estimates of anticipated results. Nevertheless, it is possible to prepare an estimate that is accurate within ±5%, assuming that billing will be performed by a biller who is at least competent, if not expert. Studies performed by independent organizations (not by billing companies with a vested interest in securing a new client) will usually include caveats that the results actually achieved depend on the skill and expertise of the billing provider, as well as the absence of significant change in the practice's environment, patient acuity, payor mix, managed care participation, and superseding federal program changes. These factors are equally, if not more, applicable if you perform your own feasibility study.

KEY FACTORS

Determining the feasibility of fee-for-service billing is a process of identifying and accounting for all of the factors that will inhibit or contribute to the success of independent billing. In this discussion feasibility should be viewed as the ability of the emergency practice to fully support itself from the proceeds of fee-for-service billing, net of the cost of billing, and collection expense. In addition, there are several general rules that usually apply to most practices with respect to the likelihood of successfully supporting a practice through independent billing.

The financially successful emergency department practice depends on a wide variety of favorable factors; the deficiency of any one or more is potentially devastating to the financial health and self-sufficiency of the practice. Many practices, however, are able to tolerate deficiencies in numerous factors, provided the deficiencies are not too severe. Each combination of circumstances tends to be unique, often with compensating benefits to offset the deficiencies.

In practices contemplating a fee-for-service arrangement, many factors must be favorably addressed.

Patient Volume

Gross Volume. The typical, minimum annual patient volume required to permit a financially independent emergency practice is 18,000 visits, although practices with twice (35,000) this volume have been unsuccessful because of a poor payor mix, as well as practices with volumes as low as 15,000 that were self-sustaining because of a very favorable payor mix and an unusually high average charge and collection ratio. In approaching an analysis, annual volumes between 15,000 and 18,000 should be considered marginal, volumes between 18,000 and 22,000 potentially problematic, and volumes greater than 24,000 generally able to support fee-for-service billing.

Billable Volume. Every emergency department has a certain volume of "meet-me" patients who are seen by their private physicians in the department. These cases, if too numerous, can be distracting or disruptive to the smooth operation of the department, as the nurses suddenly have new "bosses" who must be accommodated on a priority basis. In addition, these cases subtract from the equations used to estimate physician staffing levels, practice revenue and cash results, as well as nursing staff levels.

The estimates should be prepared based on billable volume. To the extent that these volumes change in the future, estimates must be adjusted accordingly.

Physician Staffing Levels

The level of current or planned staffing is a critical factor when considering the feasibility of fee-for-service billing, because you will be spending what is collected, and what is collectible/collected affects what you can budget for salaries. Accordingly, determination of the appropriate or necessary minimum level of staffing and the costs of staffing is an integral part of the feasibility process. To the extent that the level of staffing is affected by external obligations (e.g., contractual commitments, academic/teaching duties, dual locations, department management responsibilities), these additional obligations may adversely affect the practice's ability to support itself through independent billing alone. In addition, some financial support is available through the Medicare program for the so-called "A.S. & T."—Administration, Supervision and Teaching—services provided by practices to the hospital. The latter funding is available only through the hospital's Medicare Cost Report.

The following points outline various methods used to determine *typical* staffing levels for emergency departments.

Annual Visits Model. Emergency physician staffing levels are usually based on one full-time physician per 3500 to 5000 annual visits, with the variation based on the level of patient acuity—the higher the acuity (such as a level I Trauma Center), the lower the ratio of visits to physician.

Operation of a fast-track or convenience clinic often adds staffing requirements, independent of volume, merely because of the physical separation of the two functions. Fast-track staffing with physician assistants or certified nurse practitioners may help control cost.

Hours of Coverage Model. Full-time staffing of an emergency department requires 8760 hours of coverage (24 hours × 365 days) a year. Depending on how shifts are allocated and their duration (8, 10, 12, or 24 hours), departments using as many full-time personnel as possible for coverage require 4.3 to 4.5 full-time physicians.

Another "rule of thumb" for estimating *clinical* staffing levels is to assume 1 hour of coverage a day for each thousand annual visits. Note that this level of staffing may not be deployed evenly, because patient traffic is often clustered around certain hours of the day and/or days of the week, sometimes demanding triple coverage at some hours and single coverage at others.

Full-time emergency physicians are typically scheduled for approximately 1800 clinical hours a year, with the remaining time devoted to continuing medical education (CME), administrative time, inservice training, and holidays and vacation. Although this number varies somewhat from region to region, most practices should fit closely into a range of 1640 to 1840 clinical hours a year. To illustrate this fact, full-time physician coverage can be estimated by using the following formula for a hypothetical 34,000 visit/year practice:

1. 34,000 annual visits ÷ 1000 = 34 hours/day
2. 365 days × 34 hours/day = 12,410 hours/year
3. 12,410 hours/year ÷ 1800 hours/M.D. FTE = 6.9 physicians plus a full time Director. (See 3., below)
4. Variable: If a "Fast Track" is operated, it will probably be a part-time service (less than 24 hours/day), but will require a separate physician or P.A./C.N.P., adding additional coverage hours to be accounted and paid for.

Director and Assistant Director. For departments with more than 30,000 visits, a full-time director is usually indicated, with a part-time assistant director for departments with volumes above 40,000, and a full-time assistant when volume exceeds 60,000. These positions are **in addition to** the clinical staff.

Physician Assistants and Certified Nurse Practitioners. As an alternate to physician staffing for all shifts, physician assistants (PAs) or certified nurse practitioners (CNPs) can be used as part of double coverage. Provided they are *employees* of the practice and are supervised according to Medicare and Medicaid requirements, their services can be billed on a fee-for-service basis, even though they require much lower salaries. In other words, a shortage of physician candidates, cash flow, or both can be addressed with PAs or CNPs. These employees are, of course, equally well qualified to perform their duties.

Payor Mix

The mix of insurance coverage sponsoring patient care is also a critical issue for successful fee-for-service billing. This is important for at least two reasons: (1) the actual amounts paid for services and (2) the ease or difficulty of submitting claims to third parties, as this affects promptness of cash flow and the cost of billing. Hospital-supplied data can be helpful, but must be confirmed by an independent study in most cases. Hospitals may not identify their emergency services payor mix separately. Frequently, hospitals lump all departments into "inpatient" and "outpatient" categories. Outpatient statistics may be diluted with elective diagnostic examinations, physical therapy, dialysis, outpatient surgery, and other nonemergency services. Consequently, use of the generic outpatient statistics will portray the payor mix more favorably than is true for emergency patients alone.

Another factor diminishing the accuracy of hospital payor mix data is the common practice of emergency registrars to default patients who do not supply explicit proof of coverage to "self-pay." Generally (exception should be made for high indigent areas), self-pay percentages reported at greater than 13% to 18% are inaccurate.

Each market is different. For example, as of this writing in Minneapolis/St. Paul, managed care accounts for 65% to 75% of cases, whereas in Idaho managed care has taken less than 3% of cases. Typical payor mix ranges are shown in Table 49-1.

As healthcare reform evolves, increases in managed care and other reduced payment programs will further challenge the fee-for-service practice, particularly capitation arrangements applied to emergency services. It will be important, therefore, not only to determine the payor mix at present, but to look forward and estimate the changes that will/may occur in the following 2 years. Groups have already found themselves in the uncomfortable position of accepting a fee-for-service contract based on present data, only to be unpleasantly surprised by radical changes in payor mix that might have been foreseen or predicted with more careful evaluation. At the least, a safety valve should be part of any fee-for-service contract, calling for renegotiation or cancellation by the practice if the payor mix adversely changes by more than 10%.

Table 49-1 Typical Payor Mix Ranges

	Low	Mid	High
Medicare	15	22	28
Medicaid	8	15	21
Managed Care	5	12	20
Commercial	11	17	25
Blue Cross/Shield	9	16	23
Workers Compensation	3	9	16
Auto/Tort Liability	3	8	12
Self Pay*	9	14	19

*Note: These norms are for "true" self pay cases. Hospitals *frequently* default insured patients to self pay when they cannot "prove" coverage upon registration, or if the registrars are poorly trained or supervised. Any self pay mix above twenty percent should be viewed with strong skepticism; a 200-300 case audit may be warranted unless the hospital is in a highly indigent community. Current federal data reports that 16% to 17% of the population are uninsured.

Billing Arrangement

The provider of billing services plays a key role in the success of a fee-for-service emergency practice. Emergency medicine is affected by a greater share of uninsured patients and noncovered services ("nonemergencies" determined after-the-fact by the insurer) than other specialties. Billers must be specially skilled and properly equipped with systems that will optimize their management of the myriad details that divide success from average or mediocre performance. A poor billing performance can undermine or destroy an opportunity that would otherwise be an unqualified success. Important hallmarks of a successful billing arrangement are resident or acquired skill in emergency medicine coding and billing, highly effective and timely performance reporting and results analysis, close coordination and communication with the physician/client, a sense of partnership with and service to the physician/client, and effective problem identification and solving skills of the staff involved at the "hands-on" level.

Start-Up Considerations

Cash Flow "Ramp-Up". A new fee-for-service practice will rarely reach steady state cash flow for at least 4 months, and more often 6 months from the initial service inception. In percentage of gross arrangements, this shortfall is borne by the hospital. In independent arrangements, the new practice must secure interim funding from the hospital, a bank, or other sources, or do without compensation for up to 6 months. Remarkably, the latter option has been chosen by some practices who planned ahead or had members who could arrange to be self-sufficient for an extended period. Most practices, however, will have to secure some sort of interim funding or sponsorship.

A complete feasibility study should include a cash flow "ramp-up" estimate from the organization who will provide billing services. In most cases, the cash flow will increment monthly, up to the level that will become steady-state, along the pattern shown in Box 49-1.

Provider Enrollment. In the event a new practice is created, provider numbers must be secured from Medicare, Medicaid, Blue Cross/Blue Shield, and some managed care organizations. This process typically takes up to 6 weeks after the practice first secures a taxpayer identification (TID, also known as the Federal Employer Identification Number [FEIN]) from the Internal Revenue Service and signs a contract with a participating hospital. Delays in these steps can significantly impair the cash flow ramp-up described previously.

Banking Relationship. The new practice will need to establish a banking relationship so that its funds can be deposited by the billing provider. This is often accomplished with a "lockbox" arrangement, through which all funds are received and deposited by the bank, with only the attachments, enclosures, and check copies forwarded (usually daily) to the biller. Although this practice does not directly affect billing results, failure to establish banking arrangements in a timely manner can delay access to funds. If interim funding is required, a banking relationship will be essential, regardless of who provides the funding, but particularly if the bank is providing some or all of the funds.

Accounting and Payroll Service. The practice will need to arrange for routine bookkeeping and payroll processing (assuming physicians are not independent contractors). This is an operational cost. Most practices use their accountant or a payroll service, which should be accounted for in the fee-for-service budget. Estimates of $.50 to $1.00 per check are reasonable.

Coding

Assignment of appropriate CPT-4 and ICD-9 CM codes, from a full schedule of billable services is necessary to ensure optimal financial success. The appropriateness and accuracy of coding are extremely important. Too low coding forfeits earned income, but too high coding places the practice at risk for federal and state audits and, ultimately fraud and abuse liability. Both professional services and diagnosis coding should be performed by specialists with skill and training in emergency medicine billing. Coding by the physicians should be subjected to intragroup self-assessment and semiannual or annual external audit.

Accounting for the effect of coding is important to estimating feasibility of independent billing. A billing change is often the event that causes coding to change as well. Physicians may begin to code their own services or may hire a coder to work for the practice. It may be handled by (the new) billing company or a coding service may be engaged. Or some other resource may be used. Because estimates are often based on history, adjustments must be made for coding changes, which also may be affected by other operational changes, such as initiating dictated charts, and/or providing charting and coding training for the physicians.

BOX 49-1

INCREMENTAL CASH FLOW

Month 1	0 - 5%
Month 2	10 - 20%
Month 3	40 - 60%
Month 4	60 - 80%
Month 5	80 - 100%
Month 6	100%

Fee Schedule

Professional fees charged by the practice should be sufficient to produce a reasonable and fair charge for the valuable services performed on demand. In 1995 the national and major metropolitan average charge per visit was $150 to $160, with an average charge per CPT-4 code of $125 to $130 (20% to 30% of emergency patients receive more than one billable service, with an average of 1.1 to 1.25 charges per visit). Lower average fees may undermine the practice's ability to pay competitive salaries (unless a subsidy is provided) in a specialty that has experienced atypically high salary inflation over the last 5 years primarily because of the supply shortage.

Issues such as changes in state laws regulating professional fees or fee increases, contractual limitations, or right of review/approval imposed by the hospital on professional fees (these should only be accepted in exchange for a back-up guarantee and/or subsidy) may have a significant effect on the practice's ability to succeed. Control by the hospital over the fee schedule should be accepted only in exchange for a backup guarantee and/or subsidy. Approximately 80% of emergency professional service fees are for Evaluation and Management (E & M) services; professional fees are largely derived from a short list of CPT-4 codes: 99281, 99282, 99283, 99284, 99285, 99291, 99292, 99218, 99219, and 99220. It is extremely important that these fees are high enough to produce an appropriate average charge based on the average acuity and payor mix of the patient population served.

Documentation

CPT-4 code definition changes made as part of Resource Based Relative Value Scale (RBRVS) have placed extraordinary importance on the chart documentation of all physicians, especially emergency physicians. The highest levels of evaluation and management codes—the so-called "E & M" codes, which make up about 80% of all emergency services—cannot be adequately documented by a handwritten chart. Because the highest level of care carries with it the highest charge and payment, dictated charts have a higher potential value than the same chart if handwritten. Handwritten charts not only reduce potential income, they produce a less useful clinical record, increase medicolegal risk, shortchange the attending physicians who take over admitted patients, and generally weaken the treatment process when compared with dictated and transcribed charts.

Data show that a dictated chart contains five times the amount of data as a handwritten one, based on the same amount of time devoted to documentation. To be truly useful to the clinical process, turnaround times for emergency charts should be within 2 hours, and more appropriately 30 minutes or less.

Typical costs for commercial transcription service are currently $5.00 to $8.00 per chart, with the higher costs based on either lengthy dictation styles or additional services, such as coding and/or clinical databases. Although fees are most often quoted on a "per line" basis, each formula is different (e.g., characters per line, definition of a character, lines per page), making cost-per-chart, plus or minus extra services, the most reasonable approach to cost comparisons. Quality, user friendliness, and dependability are the most important factors, followed by cost. In the last year, industry growth and increased competition have begun to lower the average cost per chart.

Data Quality

Some patients seen in emergency departments arrive unprepared for the registration process, some know how to manipulate or navigate the system to avoid financial responsibility, and others have old, out-of-date data perpetuated by a duplication/reregistration process that blindly copies previous (and invalid) addresses, employment, and/or coverage. Fee-for-service emergency practices are particularly vulnerable to this problem, even though it injures the hospital at least as much as the emergency practice. The completeness and accuracy of patient registration data can often control the difference between success and failure, particularly in practices with marginal payor mixes, patient volumes, or atypically high salary costs. Because data collection is rarely under the direct control of the practice, this ingredient can be volatile in a fee-for-service relationship.

Preparation of a feasibility study should frankly assess (ideally by direct audit and data verification) the overall completeness, quality, timeliness, and accuracy of patient biodemographic data. Frequently omitted information includes insurance coverage for physician services (which often differs from the hospital coverage), signatures authorizing information release and assignment of insurance benefits to physicians, and accurate emergency contact telephone numbers (especially useful for clinical follow-up, as well as completing or correcting billing information). Apparently good information can often deteriorate as a result of personnel, supervisory, managerial, and/or computer systems changes.

Poor data quality, with limited or no hope of improvement, should be accounted for in the collection estimates by diminishing the success rates expected from all payors, particularly self-pay, indigent, and poorly covered patients, whose payments are highly dependent on accurate information and who are least likely to provide it.

Time of Service Payment Collection

Completing the financial transaction with emergency patients should involve a check-out process that estimates their financial liability and provides a variety of methods to collect deductibles, co-payments, or uninsured services. Ideally, this should also provide an opportunity to collect, or at least discuss, previous balances from past encounters owed to the practice as well as the hospital. As a by-product of this activity, patients are more likely to cooperate by providing insurance information in lieu of, or in addition to payment.

Not only is this process becoming more common, its success has been well documented, even in challenged circumstances. The existence of, or prospective agreement to implement, such a program by a specific date related to fee-for-service billing will counter the problems discussed in the preceding section or will further enhance the results where registration data collection is currently acceptable. When properly implemented and managed, these programs do not deter patients from selecting an emergency department, since COBRA* compliance causes this to be a check-out, rather than a check-in process.

DATA REQUIREMENTS

To prepare a complete and accurate estimate, a variety of data must be assembled. As much as possible, these data should be actual, rather than estimated. Each item that must be estimated or "guesstimated" further diminishes the overall reliability and certainty of the outcome. Nevertheless, it is possible to develop estimates that are sufficiently reliable to permit rational decision making. Box 49-2 shows all of the ingredients needed to prepare a fee-for-service feasibility study, along with a short discussion of its importance and alternate sources or methods for estimating unavailable data.

Service and Acuity Mix

Service mix refers to the array of CPT-4 utilization (e.g., 99281 is 3% of patient volume, 99282 is 15% of patient volume). This will include the array of billable procedures (per-

*Comprehensive *O*mnibus *B*udget *R*econciliation *A*ct of 1986. Refers to the so-called federal "anti-dumping" regulations, which prohibit transfer of patients based on their ability to pay or determination of a patient's financial resources or ability to pay prior to performing a "qualified" medical screening examination. Experts disagree as to whether a nurse, or only a physician, can perform the requisite exam.

BOX 49-2

DATA REQUIREMENTS FOR A FEASIBILITY STUDY

1. Service and activity mix
2. Fee schedule and average charge
3. Physician documentation quality
4. Demographics data timeliness, quality, and access
5. Patient volume
6. Payor mix
7. Coded chart sample
8. Target budget
9. Hospital payments policies
10. Billing arrangements
11. Billing history
12. Recent payment voucher
13. Managed care contracts
14. Coding (future)

formed and documented by the emergency physician) commonly provided by the practice. This information may be available from the current biller of professional services, often the hospital's business office. They will usually have a "Revenue and Usage Report," "Service Volume Report," or listing of billed services, by CPT-4 code with another name. This may be useful, depending on whether they have been using all of the codes you will use prospectively and on who is presently doing the coding. (Coding by hospital Medical Records, Emergency Department Registrars, or Business Office coders should be considered *highly* suspect.)

Absent reliable historic data, service mix can be estimated in several ways.

Chart Review. The most reliable means of determining service mix is by conducting a review of historic charts using care records documented in previous charts. Many philosophies and approaches are used to develop data considered statistically reliable. Sample reviews are recommended because the review of an entire year's data would be extremely time consuming without increasing the accuracy of the resulting estimates.

In most cases, a review of 5% to 8% of the previous year's activity is sufficient, provided the sample covers at least 100 charts for each full-time physician who will be serving the department when fee-for-service is implemented. The goals of the review are to (1) develop a pattern of services for use in developing gross charge and income estimates, (2) evaluate the treatment patterns and the quality of *billing* documentation (if it was not documented, it cannot be billed), and (3) identify whether there is opportunity for improvement in documentation, coding, or both.

In cases where the physicians who will staff the department are not the same as those who have been staffing the department, such as in a contract turnover, the validity of past charting patterns is not relevant. In this instance, the review of approximately 700 charts will usually provide a sufficiently useful sample. Obviously, the charting habits of the future physicians must be anticipated, because there is no history available. The assumed level of documentation and coding should be stated as a condition of the resulting estimates.

Most emergency departments in the United States experience seasonal variances in the acuity and services provided to their patients. The case mix generally involves more medical cases in the winter and more accident/injury cases in the summer, although the opposite may be true for ski resorts or "snow bird" resorts. The seasonality of the practice should be accounted for in the sample reviewed by selecting charts from each month, or at least every other month to diminish the possibility of skewing the resulting forecast by using an atypical sample. The estimates should be reality tested against the department's intuitive perception of "how many times per month we perform a (certain) service."

Patient acuity can be indexed several ways: by the admission rates, the procedure ratio, the average age of patients, and the hospital's trauma rating, if any. Average admission rates are calculated two ways: percent of hospital admissions admitted via the emergency department [admissions via the ED ÷ total admissions]; and percent of emergency department patients admitted [admissions via the ED ÷ total ED visits]. The former typically ranges between 30% and 50%, with higher or lower percentages indicating higher or lower acuity. The latter typically averages 18%, with higher or lower percentages indicating higher or lower acuity.

Use of admission rates as an index assumes that the emergency physicians are fully managing the patient's care up to the time of admission. Practices that function as a triage service for the Medical Staff cannot be credited with the "value" of the admission rate. This will be evident where the number of patients seen solely by a private physician is greater than 5%. A similar offset must be made in teaching hospitals if patients are seen by residents without *legitimately documented* supervision by an attending physician, as unsupervised and undocumented cases are unbillable.

National Averages. In some cases, it is not possible to conduct a chart review because of lack of time, lack of access (you may be taking over for an incumbent who is unaware of the imminent change), or lack of resources. In these cases, it is possible to use national average data available from the American College of Emergency Physicians (ACEP) (in some states the local ACEP chapter has state data), HCFA (Health Care Financing Administration—a.k.a. Medicare/Medicaid), or private sources.

Use of national averages must be adjusted for your "best guess" or intuitive estimate of how the practice will vary from the national average. Use of admission rates will help, as will acuity indices or abstract statistics that may be provided by the hospital's medical records department.

State, Area, or Regional Averages. Some Medicare, Medicaid, Blue Cross/Blue Shield, or major payor Claims Departments will share their data on charge profile patterns for emergency medicine. Because this specialty uses a relatively exclusive set of CPT-4 codes, useful conclusions can be drawn from their data. If they are reluctant to provide the data, it is usually because they are concerned that the information will be misused to pattern your claims to conform to the expected or typical pattern, even if your patients are less acute.

Fee Schedule and Average Charge

The fees charged by a practice can be pivotal to their financial success because "you are never paid more than you charge.[1]" As payment discounts, managed care, RBRVS* and other market forces diminish the amounts paid for professional services, the practice's fee schedule and average charge remain important for now.

Physician Documentation Quality

The implementation of RBRVS cemented a historically necessary part of the CPT-4 coding into an absolutely relevant, critical variable in estimating and maintaining the value of a fee-for-service practice. Regardless of the level of care provided, only the services *documented* should be coded and billed. There is no harm in providing more care than is documented, provided that billing is limited to what is supported by the chart.

The billable CPT-4 codes that emanate from a patient population are predicated on all of the following: (1) clinical acuity and the care received, (2) care documented in the chart, and (3) evidence that the patient was treated by an emergency

*Resource Based Relative Value Scale. The system used by HCFA and other payers to assess value and determine payment for professional services.

physician, rather than another member of the medical staff. Do not expect to bill more than is supported by documentation. In developing the data to estimate fee-for-service income, existing documentation quality should be assessed unless all or most of the incumbent physicians will be replaced. In that case, a realistic judgment should be made about the initial and eventual quality of documentation.

Because it is rare for more care to be documented than is (or will be) billed, care should be taken to ensure that estimates are based on a realistic assessment of the "codeable" quality of the practice's charts. Generally, dictated charts are 10% to 20% more "valuable," because transcribed charts contain more information, are easier to read, and more easily meet the criteria for supporting a particular level of CPT-4 code.

The importance of documentation is rooted in the *severe* penalties that have been imposed by Medicare, Medicaid, Blue Cross/Blue Shield, and some commercial payors for "upcoding" (billing a higher level CPT-4 code than is supported by the chart documentation), which the federal programs construe as violations of the False Claims Act, various Fraud and Abuse regulations, and as mail fraud. Federal penalties are routinely triple the amount overpaid (the difference between what you were paid and what they determine should have been paid), plus per-claim or per-line-item penalties of between $2000 and $10,000. They may also impose the ultimate penalty of barring individual physicians from participating or treating federally sponsored patients for from 5 years to permanently.

Payment is not validation of correct coding or sufficient documentation because charts are not routinely submitted with claims. Federal payors have a 7-year statute of limitation during which to retrospectively audit paid claims and recover overpayments and/or establish that a violation occurred. Intent need not be proven for penalties to be assessed. It is no longer enough to get paid; it is equally important that "audit-proof" charts allow you to keep the money paid.

Demographic Data Timeliness, Quality, and Access Method

Emergency medicine billing relies entirely on second-hand information—information collected from patients by hospital staff and entered into the hospital's billing system. For a fee-for-service practice to be successful, prompt, cost-efficient access to accurate information is essential. Although it is difficult for patients who are true emergencies to readily and accurately provide all of the required billing information, it is unacceptable to make the common extrapolation that getting accurate information from all emergency patients is not possible. It is critical for the hospital and the emergency physicians to obtain the best possible data.

Evaluating and anticipating a fee-for-service outcome should include a frank assessment of registration data. The data should be available within 24 hours, which is the industry standard. The accuracy of the data should be >80% based on a *verified* sample.* Completeness is crucial. Hospitals frequently fail to collect the insurance coverage information needed to submit a professional fee claim (hospital coverage + physician coverage). The data access method, whether it is piles of paper forms to be *rekeyed* by a billing staff (yours or the billing company's) or computer-to-computer transfers, is important. In the latter case, the keypunch cost of reentry of data will be between $.60 and $1.00 per case, and the cost will be accounted for in the biller's charge or your budget, if you elect to handle your own billing.

*Verification should be based on selection of all inpatient and outpatient charts from two recent dates and direct telephone verification (reregistration) of the data provided.

Patient Volume

Generally, minimum patient volumes can be used to initially benchmark the potential for fee-for-service success. Departments with patient volumes below 18,000 patients are at increasing risk or certainty of financial nonviability. Although there are financially viable practices with volumes as low as 15,000, they are "blessed" with highly favorable payor mixes, above average acuity, or lower than average costs.

Conversely, practices with volumes >30,000 may be nonviable because of extremely high indigence, low acuity, high physician costs, or other combination factors. Opportunities with low volume or high indigence should be approached with caution and require greater care in forecasting the expected outcome.

Payor Mix

Payor mix is a major factor in the success of fee-for-service emergency practice. Be *sure* of the accuracy of the payor mix for the emergency department when making a projection. Many hospitals aggregate all outpatients together; the data accuracy may be suspect because of your registration audit, and this factor is extremely critical to financial success.

Coded Chart Sample

The most precise method of estimating fee-for-service results is to perform a chart review of actual department charts. This process will provide information about charting habits (assuming the same physicians will remain), patient acuity, and actual CPT-4 code level data about the overall service and payor mix. Generally, a chart sample of 4% of annual volume is sufficient, although smaller samples may be adequate in cases where time or resources restrict this effort.

If a chart review is conducted, be sure to select charts that

1. Represent all of the physicians who will remain.
2. Cover all seasons of the year. In practices that are significantly affected by season—resorts, weather extremes, volume changes, etc— a weighted sample is recommended.
3. Represent the charting method(s) that will be in effect when fee-for-service is implemented.

This is not the time to assume that a switch to dictation will immediately improve charting and enhance coding.

Target Budget

As discussed earlier, a carefully developed, realistic projection of staffing costs is essential. Staffing costs are the major component of a budget. Some of the other costs that must be considered are listed in Box 49-3. A feasibility study must be compared with a target budget number.

Hospital Payment Policies

Hospitals are gradually returning to the practice of requesting payment at the time of treatment, although COBRA now

BOX 49-3

PARTIAL LIST OF BUDGET ITEMS

1. Secretarial and other support
2. Billing costs
3. Banking costs
4. Bookkeeping/accounting
5. Legal fees
6. Recruiting costs
7. Office supplies
8. Rent/maintenance costs
9. Furniture/equipment
10. Telephone
11. Training costs
12. Beepers
13. Books and dues
14. Computer and software
15. Postage

forces the request to be made at discharge, rather than in advance. If a time-of-service payment policy is implemented, an additional allowance can be made for self-pay (add 30% to your estimated self-pay results) and deductible/co-payment (add 25% to your estimate for this category) collections, provided physician charges will be represented in the request for payment. An appropriate formula for dividing partial payments will be required.

When this issue is raised during negotiations, hospitals will often accede to the request, then fail to implement the promised program. If it is not already in place, do not account for the additional income, or secure a "replacement guarantee" from the hospital in the event they postpone implementation.

Billing Arrangement

As part of the data collection and decision-making process, it is important to think about what billing arrangement will be implemented because the "biller" will have to deal with the variables identified during your review. In some cases the variables and "unchangeable" factors can significantly affect the decision as to who should and will perform the billing. If the source of billing is predetermined, such as when a hospital announces they will provide the billing, this answer will materially affect how you interpret the findings in the study.

Billing History, If Available

In some cases, staffing contracts turn over; you may be evaluating a department that has been fee-for-service. Although competitive practices will withhold prior performance information, other changes may provide access to past results. Alternatively, if the hospital has been handling the billing, information may be available. Caution should be exercised in applying data from hospital billing because the "actual" results may be estimates or data from assumptions applied to more global statistics for all outpatients. Reporting historical gross charges is relatively easy, but hospital billing software can rarely isolate and report actual payment data because the receivable and payments are all comingled with the hospital's data.

Recent Payment Vouchers, If Available

If any fee-for-service claims are being submitted, the biller/payment recipient will have current payment vouchers, sometimes called EOBs (Explanation of Benefits) that list the amounts paid by various third party payors such as Medicare, Medicaid, Blue Shield, Workers Compensation, etc. This **actual** information can be extremely useful in verifying the amount of payment to expect from each payer for the most common CPT-4 codes.

Managed Care Contracts, If Volume Greater Than 5%

Despite press reports about the managed care "revolution" that is "sweeping the country," managed care (HMO, PPO, IHS, etc.) plans and their impact are still very much a local market factor. In some areas managed care is significant; in others, managed care is not now, and may never be, a major factor. It is critical, however, to determine what is locally true and to try to estimate the amount and rapidity of change toward more managed care.

If the current volume of managed care patients is >5%, copies of all significant contracts should be reviewed to determine the billing requirements and reimbursement rules and amounts for each plan. In researching the future of the arrangement about to begin, you should also determine the local trends in managed care evolution, and how, or if, they will affect your billing implementation. Rapid volume/mix changes are common in the sometimes explosive managed care growth, and attention should be paid to the potential impact on a fee-for-service arrangement.

Coding (Future)

The importance and dynamics of assigning CPT-4 codes often change as part of a transition to fee-for-service billing. In developing the data for a feasibility study, the future approach to coding should be considered as part of the overall forecast and implementation plan. Specifically, the estimation of practice income assumes that a certain pattern of charges will evolve, producing payments of predictable value. Not only must those future charges rely on well-documented charts, they must also be coded appropriately using a competent process. The physicians may code their own cases using a checklist, a practice-employed coder may be used, a coding service may be hired, or the billing office (your own, the hospital's or a commercial billing service) may code. Regardless, the coding should be consistent and correct; accounting for the coding process is an important part of the feasibility process.

METHODS FOR ESTIMATING FINANCIAL RESULTS

Chart Review

The most accurate method of forecasting future financial results is to base the estimates on historical, actual case data. This approach firmly establishes the patient acuity, physician charting habits, payor mix, and data quality of the cases that will be billed in the future. Appropriate adjustments should be made to compensate for environmental changes that you know will occur, such as initiating dictation/transcription of charts.

Several methodologies are used by organizations and practices that regularly perform feasibility studies for themselves or others. The first example is the selection of a chart sample. Below are a few of the more common approaches and a discussion of their strengths and/or weaknesses.

A Week of Recent Charts. This approach is certainly one of the easiest for the reviewer. Providing a recent week's charts is often the easiest to access, particularly if the review is to develop a proposal to replace an incumbent group/contractor/staff. The hospital's medical records staff can often set the charts aside with little extra effort, although inpatients (emergency cases that were admitted) may still be in-house, reducing access to a full array of cases.

This is a relatively small sample (1.9% of 1 year) on which to base a multiyear forecast. In addition, it ignores seasonal variations and absences (the "best" or "worst" physician(s), transcriptionist(s), and/or registrar(s) may be on vacation) and may be vulnerable to aberrations such as flu outbreaks, ICU/CCU overloads, or even emergency vehicle breakdowns.

100 Charts. Regardless of the department's volume, if only 100 charts are used, this method represents an inappropriately small sample on which to base a decision as important as fee-for-service billing, unless a very clear guarantee, subsidy, stipend, or other financial support arrangement is provided by the hospital. One hundred charts is 1.3% of 8000 annual visits, 0.6% of 18,000 visits, 0.4% of 24,000 visits, etc. This method should be considered symbolic, as the estimates of billing outcome will have to be based on a pro forma or rough estimate method.

A variation of this method is a 100 chart sample for *each physician*. Depending on the timing of the selection (the last week, the last month, or the entire year) the department's annual volume, and the number of physicians involved, this approach can produce a sample of sufficient size and accuracy.

Cross-Year Sample. This method selects charts from across the previous year using a variety of techniques: a week or more from each season (however defined), 1 to 3 days from each month for the past 12 consecutive months, a defined number of admitted and discharged patients for each physician over the last year, or other randomized selection methods. In most cases, this method establishes the most accurate and complete illustration of the scope, acuity, and variety of the department's practice. It is also the most labor intensive and expensive for whomever sponsors the review. If data are developed in conjunction with using the review to evaluate risk management factors, charting habits, treatment protocols, or other purposes, the review can serve multiple agendas.

Rough Estimates

The RBRVS-based system for coding the Evaluation and Management (E & M) services (the former "visit" or "encounter" services that make up the majority of emergency services) condenses roughly 80% of all patient charges into only five CPT-4 codes—99281 through 99285. Because there are millions of emergency visits each year, there are now well-established national data on the pattern of code utilization for Medicare cases, as well as others. Admittedly, the data are predicated on the (possibly incorrect) inference that the codes have been used appropriately for all cases. Nevertheless, the pattern of code utilization is well known and is used by Medicare and others to identify practices that may be "overcoding" by auditing providers whose patterns are one or more standard deviations outside the normal distribution. Of course, they only audit or suspect those who are "too high," without discarding data on practice that are one or more standard deviations "too low."

If the practice to be forecast is treating a "normal" mix of patient acuity, the national pattern of code distribution can be used to develop a rough estimate of financial outcome, particularly for practices that are operating in a hospital with sufficient volume (>20,000 visits/year) an average payor mix, and without unusual or abnormally high costs. In using this method, the annual volume is arrayed in a "normal" distribution of E & M codes; procedures such as laceration repairs, lumbar punctures, and intubations may or may not be accounted for separately.

The risks of using this method include (1) creation of a billing expectation that cannot be realized because of poor documentation and/or coding, (2) overestimating the "averageness" of the practice; adoption of a fee schedule that is materially lower than the one used to develop the estimate, (3) assumptions that the practice will remain stable when it does not, and (4) poor execution of billing for a practice that is correctly reflected in the estimates (the latter two are not flaws in the forecast or the method).

Average Charge, Average Payment

The simplest and most straightforward technique is to base estimates on an average charge and an average payment for each visit. Across the United States, most fee-for-service emergency practices in a given geographic area produce an average charge and an average payment that is within a reasonable and predictable range. As a result, an admittedly rough, but often reasonable estimate of results can be produced by multiplying annual patient volume times the area's average charge-per-patient-visit and the area's average payment-per-patient-visit. You will then know what your practice should produce (assuming it is average) in gross charges and net revenue.

This technique ignores all actual data, or must "guesstimate" the impact of both favorable and unfavorable factors such as above average acuity, a poor payor mix, and poorly documented, handwritten charts. Nevertheless, if time constraints, budget, or lack of access to the real data are impediments to developing a more accurate estimate, this method will at least produce an answer that can be compared and contrasted to other estimates and suppositions.

As with rough estimates, the limitations of this technique are least dangerous with a practice that fits a pattern of "normal" characteristics. If volume, payor mix, documentation, data collection, or coding and billing are marginal, use of this method and the rough estimate method can become problematic.

PERFORMING THE CALCULATIONS

Developing the financial estimates for fee-for-service can be performed readily using spreadsheet software or, if necessary, old-fashioned columnar (accounting) ledger sheets (Tables 49-2 and 49-3. Table 49-2 illustrates how an estimate or actual measurement of patient volume is allocated among the five E & M levels. This could be the result of careful chart reviews and coding or from rough estimates and "guesstimates" of presumed arrays of utilization.

Table 49-2 St. Anywhere Hospital Smallville, USA: Estimated Emergency Physician Patient Volume by Payor and Level

Payors/levels	Blue Cross	Commercial	Medicaid	Medicare	Self pay	Workers comp.	Total	%
1	16	280	1236	95	304	50	1981	8.4
2	70	1120	2880	323	900	100	5393	23.0
3	140	2245	3286	589	1496	465	8201	35.0
4	82	1288	496	532	560	255	3213	13.7
5	40	672	328	361	350	150	1901	8.1
Procedures	55	840	826	285	550	205	2761	11.8
Totals	403	6425	9052	2185	4160	1225	23,450	100
%	1.7	27.4	38.6	9.3	17.7	5.2		100

Table 49-3 St. Anywhere Hospital Smallville, USA: Estimated Emergency Physician Professional Fee Income

Level/fee	Blue Cross	Commercial	Medicaid	Medicare	Self pay	Wrk. Cmp.	Total	%
1	# 16	# 280	# 1236	# 95	# 304	# 50	# 1981	8
$38	608	10,640	146,968	3610	11,552	1900	75,278	3
	365	7980	44,090	1877	3466	1235	59,013	5
2	# 70	# 1120	# 2880	# 323	# 900	# 100	# 5393	23
$51	3570	57,120	146,880	16,473	45,900	5100	275,043	11
	2142	42,840	44,064	8566	13,770	3315	114,697	9
3	# 140	# 2245	# 3286	# 589	# 1496	# 465	# 8201	35
$84	11760	188,580	276,024	49,476	125,664	39,060	688,884	27
	7056	141,435	82,807	25,728	37,699	25,389	320,114	25
4	# 82	# 1288	# 496	# 532	# 560	# 255	# 3213	14
$178	14,596	229,264	88,288	94,696	99,680	45,390	571,914	23
	8758	171,948	26,486	49,242	29,904	29,504	315,842	25
5	# 40	# 672	# 328	# 361	# 350	# 150	# 1901	8
$219	8760	147,168	71,832	79,059	76,650	32,850	416,319	17
	5256	110,376	21,550	41,111	22,995	21,352	222,640	18
Procedures	# 55	# 840	# 826	# 285	# 550	# 205	# 2761	12
$175	9625	147,000	144,550	49,875	96,250	35,875	483,175	19
	5775	110,250	43,365	25,935	28,875	23,319	237,519	19
Total # (%)	403 (2)	6425 (27)	# 9052 (39)	# 2185 (9)	# 4160 (18)	# 1225 (5)	# 23,450	100
Gross $	48,919	779,772	774,542	293,189	455,696	160,175	2,510,613	100
Net $	29,351	584,829	232,363	152,458	136,709	104,114	1,239,824	100
Avg. fee	121	121	86	134	110	131	107	
Avg. pmt.	73	91	26	70	33	85	53	
Collection %	60%	75%	30%	52%	30%	65%	49.4%	

NOTE: Line 1 of each block = *Patient Volume*, Line 2 of each block = *Gross Charges*, Line 3 of each block = *Net Collections. Collection %* = Gross Payments ÷ Gross Charges.

Note that the array of code utilization varies by payor, producing a weighted average service mix for this hypothetical practice. This is important because Medicare patients are usually sicker and receive higher levels of treatment, whereas Medicaid patients are usually the least sick and require and receive the lowest average level of care. Although a generic mix can be used for purposes of estimating, it further dilutes the accuracy of the forecast.

Once the patient volume has been arrayed, the next calculations are developed on the basis of a fee schedule for each of the five levels and an estimated average charge for procedures. The estimated volumes are multiplied by the fees for each level to establish the gross charges for each level and payor, as shown in Table 49-3.

Gross charges represent the amount billed for a service, not the amount paid. Fewer and fewer payors pay the actual charge for a service, instead basing their payment on a preestablished payment schedule, as Medicare does; on a percentage of charges, as some commercial payers still do; or on another of many different methodologies. Some payors, such as Blue Shield in many states, follow a "secret" payment schedule, refusing to publish or report on the amounts they pay, although current providers are certainly aware of the amounts. These data can be estimated, sometimes, by indexing Medicare's payment values and adding about 20%, although in some areas Medicare pays more than the premium charging payor.

Determining the amount to expect in payment is a payor-by-payor exercise in research and/or verification. It is possible to accurately forecast the amounts that will be paid by many, if not all of the payors. Absent code-specific data, a percent-of-charge method can be used to approximate the amounts to be paid. This is demonstrated by the last line in the chart and the last note in Table 49-3.

Additional levels of accuracy can be added by accounting separately for collection of deductibles and co-payments from Medicare (the Part B deductible for Medicare is currently $100 per year, with a 20% obligation by the patient), commercial payors, Blue Shield (if applicable), and managed care programs. Some states require a "nuisance co-payment" by Medicaid beneficiaries of $2.00. It should be assumed that the payments are never made because the hospital rarely requests the payment at the time of service, and billing costs make even one request for payment cost prohibitive.

Finally, there are bad debts. Bad debts are amounts owed by patients (*not* contractual discounts given to Medicare, Medicaid, etc.) that are not collected by the initial biller that, for the most part, are subsequently given to a collection agency. In most emergency practices, bad debts range from about 8% to as much as 15% of gross charges. Although lower amounts are sometimes found in affluent and/or well-managed practices, bad debts that exceed 15% of gross charges are more often the result of poor data collection (by the hospital's staff) and/or poor billing by the biller. Either or both of the latter will dismiss higher bad debt results as "going with the territory," but it is seldom true.

When bad debts are managed properly, they are identified and transferred to a collector within 4 months of the initial service date; waiting longer only decreases the collector's chances of success, without increasing the biller's probability of collecting. A collection agency should be expected to recover approximately 15% to 23% of the amounts referred to them for collection. Collection agencies have become much more automated and competitive in the last 5 years, lowering their fee rates to 25% to 35% of collected dollars.

Thus, bad debt recoveries can be accounted for by adding the result of:

Estimated bad debts (8% to 15% of gross charges)
× Estimated bad debt recovery rate (15% to 23% of bad debts)
Bad debt recoveries (Dollars)
− Collection Agency fees (Dollars)
Net Bad Debt Collections

Using the data in Table 49-3, the results might produce the following:

[$ 2,510,613 × 10%] = $ 251,061 bad debt write-offs
× 20% bad debt recovery rate
$ 50,212 bad debt recoveries
[$ 50,212 × 30%] = $ − 15,064 collection agency fees
$ 35,148 net bad debt recoveries

The result is *approximately* 1.5% of gross charges ($ 35,148 ÷ $ 2,510,613 = 1.4%) that can be added to the total estimated cash results from the practice associated with bad debt recoveries. Timing of the estimated recoveries should be delayed to the last quarter of the first 12 months of fee-for-service billing, because bad debts will typically not be recognized until the end of the first 4 months, followed by up to 6 months of efforts by the agency to establish a regular pattern of recoveries. In most cases, the results of bad debt recoveries are significant only as an accounting matter; a practice's financial viability should not rest on the differences in bad debt recoveries and the costs of collection. Although bad debt recoveries should be expected and received, the results will not make an unviable opportunity viable.

Finally, a cash flow estimate should be prepared. Because payments from the first month's charges will not be collected in the first, or even in the second month, a conservative and reliable estimate of the "ramp-up" of cash flow will be another critical step in assessing the financial viability of a practice. In most cases, physicians and other staff members will expect to be paid according to an agreed-upon basis from the start, even though cash flow for the practice will not reach "steady state" for 5 or 6 months.

Covering this interim period requires financial planning. Some practices have prepared themselves by preparing a start-up fund to cover the interim period. In most cases, however, the interim funding is produced by a grant or loan from the hospital (care should be taken to comply with all self-referral and anti-kickback regulations that may apply), or borrowing from a bank or business lender. In the latter case, an officially prepared feasibility study can often be used to demonstrate to a lender that the loaned funds will be secured by accounts receivable and are subject to a predictable cash flow.

The cash flow pattern for every practice will vary as a result of many variables that can accelerate or inhibit practice income. These include whether the practice is incorporated and already has federal and state tax identification numbers, provider numbers for Medicare, Medicaid, Blue Shield, and other payors; a biller capable of starting up "day one"; approval to submit electronic claims to all payors (this can reduce payment turnaround times by *weeks*) capable of receiving them; and the overall quality of patient data, whether payments are collected at the time of a patient visit, and so forth. As in most critical endeavors, it is prudent to be overprepared for the worst outcome, regardless of your confidence or the assurances of a prospective biller.

Generally, the cash flow ramp-up for an emergency practice will follow a pattern that will fall into a range, depending on the number of favorable and/or unfavorable variables that apply to the circumstances (Box 49-4).

Note that the first month of "normal" cash flow is not achieved until the fifth, sixth, or seventh month, although the latter is low performance and should not be considered acceptable. In addition, the recovery of cash flow shortfalls in the earlier months are not demonstrated by large excess cash months later on because of the establishment of an accounts receivable that will exist (hopefully under reasonable control) until the end of the practice. The so-called "bubble" of cash flow is usually experienced in months 6 through 9.

In all practices, cash flow is the result of charges, which are the result of patients seen by emergency physicians.

BOX 49-4

PERCENTAGE OF "NORMAL" MONTH CASH FLOW COLLECTED

Interval	Low	Mid	High
Month 1	2	4	10
Month 2	10	15	30
Month 3	25	40	60
Month 4	40	60	80
Month 5	70	85	100
Month 6	85	100	110
Month 7	100	110	115
Month 8	110	115	100
Month 9	115	100	100
Month 10	100	100	100

Variations in monthly patient volume, acuity, physician coverage, data quality (vacation coverage of registration), and payor mix can cause additional fluctuations in billing and, therefore, cash flow. The expected billing-to-cash-flow lag is 4 to 6 weeks, once "steady state" is achieved.

Month to month, cash flow will continue to vary for many inevitable, as well as preventable reasons. Normal reasons can include the timing of regular weekly payments from contractual payors such as Medicare, who routinely aggregate payments into one weekly "remittance," rather than paying each claim separately; the day of the week on which a month ends may cause a weekly check to fall into the subsequent month. Likewise, seasonal holidays, extreme weather (preventing billing and/or claim processing), payor budget or staffing cutbacks, or software problems may interrupt cash flow that is otherwise predictable.

Preventable reasons include billing and payment posting backlogs (only epidemics and natural disasters are acceptable excuses), software problems in the billing operation, lost charts and/or paperwork, billing staff vacations (planning is expected and assumed), and lack of surveillance. The biller should not discover, for the first time, in the last few days of the month that cash flow is "short."

SUMMARY

After a projected revenue stream is calculated the final step in a feasibility study is to compare the revenue to the projected budget. This step is helpful in determining the need for a subsidy or guarantee. The accuracy of the entire process depends on the reliability of the data used and the depths to which the analysis is taken.

OPERATING BUDGET

Another critical step in the development of a fee-for-service feasibility study is preparation of a practice budget. The estimated billing and collection results may or may not be highly accurate. The operating costs budget must be highly accurate. Developing a practice budget should be based on several different models to ensure that the estimates are correct and realistic.

Physician Staffing Versus Patient Volume

The first calculation to consider is the volume of patients to be covered, which will produce a minimum number of physicians or physician hours. As discussed earlier in this chapter, the full-time coverage of an emergency department requires at least 4.3 to 4.5 full-time physicians regardless of the patient volume. As patient volume passes 16,000 to 18,000, additional staff coverage is often needed, depending on acuity and volume clustering, which is typical of weekends.

The predicted number of physicians needed may change during the year because a volume threshold is crossed, normal seasonal fluctuations, CME and conferences, and vacations, plus an allowance for illnesses, possible staff turnover, and volume spikes. This determination will be more accurate in the second and later years, assuming that there is no reliable history on which to base estimates, a typical scenario for a new practice.

Cost Per Hour of Coverage

After the number of physicians (include PAs and CNPs) is determined, a staffing budget can be prepared. It should be based on the compensation program that is in place when fee-for-service billing begins. Regardless of the accounting methods used to compensate physicians, PAs, and CNPs (employee, independent contractor, Professional Corporation/Association, Locum Tenens, etc.) a total cost for each can be determined. This number should account for *all* costs, including liability insurance, fringe benefits, paid time off, and reimbursed expenses. This total can, in turn, be calculated into a cost per hour of coverage. [Total staffing costs ÷ total hours of coverage] = Cost per staffed hour.

The latter value is sometimes referred to as the *direct cost per hour,* because other indirect costs are associated with operating the practice and staffing an emergency department. If you prepare estimates on a month-by-month basis, you will also be able to compare estimated expenses with anticipated cash flow, thus allowing for a combined cash flow and expense projection.

Charges and Cash Per Hour

By budgeting hours of coverage, you will be able to calculate gross charges and cash flow by hours of scheduled coverage. The latter value is the most important, as cash flow controls the financial viability (or lack of it) of a department's practice. These calculations are very straightforward:

[Gross charges ÷ hours of coverage] = Gross charges per hour.

[Cash ÷ hours of coverage] = Cash per hour of coverage.

Billing Costs

Regardless of who performs the task of billing, a cost is associated with billing. Even when a hospital provides billing services "free of charge" there is often a cost (usually in lost results and/or lack of actual data on which to base comparisons). The typical billing service charges a fee based on a percentage of collections of between 10% and 13%. Practices who perform their own billing typically incur a cost that approximates the same cost as a billing service. Billing costs can also be expressed as $6.50 to $8.50 per case.

In preparing a fee-for-service feasibility study, be sure to account for the cost of billing. It will reduce your monthly cash flow (cash flow net of billing costs) and is usually your second highest cost, after staffing costs. If the hospital provides billing services "free," you can impute a billing cost by assuming that independent billing would produce at least 10% to 12% higher cash flow. If the latter is consistent with your feasibility study estimate, you can assume that the hospital is providing a commercially equivalent service. If the hospital's results are higher or lower, you can assess these results accordingly.

Start-Up Costs and Administrative Expenses

In addition to the routine monthly costs of staffing an emergency department and operating an emergency practice, a number of additional expenses should be accounted for. These include both one-time and recurring expenses associated with the administration of the Department and the practice.

Examples of one time expenses include the following:

- Legal services for incorporating and registering the practice, development, and negotiation of the contract with the hospital; review and negotiation of the billing contract; and individual physician contracts.
- An accountant to establish the tax structure of the practice (may overlap with the attorney) and set up the books. Your accountant can also advise on banking arrangements, cash management, tax planning for the practice and its members, and assist with preparing and presenting an application for interim financing, if funds are to be borrowed from a lender.
- Consulting assistance to perform the feasibility study, if you do not prepare it yourself, or to review yours/theirs if you prepare it yourself or receive free studies from prospective billing companies or the hospital.
- Initial administrative supplies, such as business cards, stationery, computer, furniture for a practice office, and miscellaneous costs.

Examples of recurring practice costs that should be budgeted include the following:

- Support staff costs (most practices should consider a part- or full-time secretary), including payroll and payroll taxes (if applicable), fringe benefits, CME and conference costs, payroll service charges for preparing payroll checks, liability insurance, and reimbursed dues, such as ACEP and AMA memberships and certification/recertification costs.
- Billing costs. The budget should be based on actual proposals from billers you are likely to engage, or a realistic estimate of the cost of your own billing office. For budgeting purposes, an allowance of $7.25 to $8.50 per visit can be used if more accurate estimates are not available. If your annual patient volume will be less than 25,000, costs will be higher if you do your own billing.
- Loan repayments, if interim funding was provided by a commercial loan or a loan from the hospital or members of the practice.
- Bank service fees for the practice's checking account, lockbox charges, etc.
- Monthly or quarterly accounting expenses, including tax return preparation.
- Secretarial support (may be provided by the hospital).
- Reference and textbooks and periodicals purchased by the practice for use by the staff.
- Dues and membership fees for professional organizations joined by the president or elected leader of the practice in his/her official capacity.
- Semiannual or annual legal services to assist with officially required corporate meetings, Board of Directors meetings, maintenance of corporate minutes books, officially required corporate filings, etc.

Examples of variable and as-needed costs include the following:

- Legal assistance to review contracts presented to the practice by managed care programs, review and negotiate modifications to the hospital contract, and assist with the contractual arrival or departure of physicians.
- Consulting assistance to review the billing service's performance, update your fee schedule, and provide general and strategic advice.
- Training programs for the physicians (and coders, if the practice elects to hire a coding staff) in "billing" documentation and CPT-4 coding. In addition, many practices arrange for annual or semiannual coding audits by an outside auditor to ensure that their coding support and coding are reasonable and appropriate.

SUMMARY

A feasibility study is a critical aspect of preparing for fee-for-service reimbursement. A well-designed and meticulously executed study can prevent many of the pitfalls in managing the business aspects of an emergency department. This study must be performed by individuals who are unbiased and possess the expertise to provide data on which you can rely in making your practice management and contractual decisions.

50 Coding for Emergency Services

Caral Lynne Edelberg

OUTLINE

The codes and associated rules contained in the *Physicians' Current Procedural Terminology (CPT)* and the *International Classification of Diseases, 9th Revision, Clinical Modification (ICD-9-CM)* are constantly evolving. Third-party payors such as Medicare, Medicaid, and Blue Shield have individual requirements with regard to reporting procedure and diagnosis codes by emergency medicine specialists. Compounding the problem of different rules being applied to the same codes by different payors is the fact that, within an individual hospital or emergency physician group, no two physicians are likely to interpret coding guidelines in the same way. The result is often a general sense of confusion, a tendency to surrender to the complexities of the system, and a greater potential for third-party payor scrutiny.

Coding for emergency department services, in particular, presents many specialized challenges to coders and to payors, alike. In most cases, the CPT and ICD-9 codes reported by emergency physicians and emergency departments do not readily convey the acute nature of services rendered in this setting. In addition, most payors have limited knowledge of the unique problems associated with coding for emergency physician and emergency department services. As a result, extraordinary pressures are being placed on the coder to follow a coding process that adequately describes the nature of services rendered in the emergency department setting without straying too far from coding policies established by individual payors.

This chapter explains the basic principles involved in the accurate reporting of procedures and diagnoses in the emergency department setting. It also describes the relationship between the CPT and ICD-9 coding systems, and the way in which this relationship translates into appropriate payment for services rendered.

AMERICAN MEDICAL ASSOCIATION PHYSICIANS' CURRENT PROCEDURAL TERMINOLOGY

Physicians' Current Procedural Terminology (CPT) is a standardized numeric and descriptive coding system for physicians' services that the American Medical Association (AMA) has published since 1966. CPT neither endorses any particular therapeutic procedure nor contains suggested values for those procedures. The inclusion of a description and its associated five-digit code number in CPT is generally based on the premise that the service is consistent with contemporary medical practice and is being performed by physicians in clinical practice in many locations.

Before 1966, many third-party payors had developed and were using their own lists of physician services and corresponding codes. These multiple lists of numeric codes and descriptions made it extremely difficult for physicians to effectively describe their services for billing purposes. The CPT was developed as a result of an effort by the AMA to standardize these codes and descriptions.

The first edition of CPT was published in 1966. Three subsequent editions were published in 1970, 1973, and 1977; and in 1983, the fourth edition (CPT-4) was published. This particular edition of CPT has been revised annually ever since. The 1992 and later editions of CPT underwent major revision to improve consistency in assigning the proper code to the service provided. The current CPT manual is organized into the following chapters, appendices, instructions for using the CPT index, and the index itself:

- Introduction (Explanation and Instructions)
- Evaluation and Management (E/M) Services Guidelines
- Evaluation and Management Services
- Anesthesia
- Surgery
- Radiology
- Pathology and Laboratory
- Medicine
- Appendix A—Modifiers
- Appendix B—Summary of Deletions, Additions, and Revisions
- Appendix C—Update to Short Descriptors
- Appendix D—Clinical Examples Supplement
- Index

Each year, members of the AMA's CPT Editorial Panel meet to discuss needed code and/or description changes. The 14-member Editorial Panel, made up of representatives of various medical specialty societies, insurers, and the federal government (Health Care Financing Administration), bears the ultimate responsibility for revising CPT. The AMA's CPT Advisory Committee, along with other organizations such as the Physician Payment Review Commission (PPRC), provides input into the CPT revision process. The American College of Emergency Physicians (ACEP) is currently represented in the CPT revision process through its representative to the AMA's CPT Advisory Committee and its designated member of the CPT Editorial Panel.

With the 1992 adoption of dramatic changes in the way physicians report their evaluation and management (E/M) services, CPT has embarked on an ambitious approach to describe more objectively services provided by physicians. A great deal of work remains, however, as the CPT Editorial Panel continues its efforts to define more adequately many of the terms associated with these revised definitions. In addition, the work of the Editorial Panel is now much more closely linked with the efforts of the AMA's Relative Value Update Committee (RUC), at least with respect to addressing changes in code descriptors resulting from modifications in assigned relative work values. Finally, third-party payors such as Medicare continue to pressure CPT to reduce the number of codes describing physicians' services to patients and to create more objective, standardized descriptions for the remaining codes.

CPT STRUCTURE AND USE

Evaluation and Management (E/M) Services

As indicated in the previous section, CPT is organized into various types of physician services. The evaluation and management (E/M) section of CPT is probably of the greatest importance to emergency physicians.

Emergency department E/M services are defined by the following five levels of service:

- 99281 Problem focused
- 99282 Expanded problem focused, low complexity
- 99283 Expanded problem focused, moderate complexity
- 99284 Detailed
- 99285 Comprehensive

Each E/M service includes the following services:

- Examinations
- Evaluations
- Treatments
- Conferences with or concerning patient
- Preventive health supervision

In 1994 a joint committee of the AMA and the Health Care Financing Administration approved and released formal guidelines for use in establishing requirements for documentation used to support the E/M levels. These guidelines establish a higher level of objective criteria to be used by providers and payors in determining E/M levels. In the 1996 edition of CPT, language was added to the *Evaluation and Management Services Guidelines* section to facilitate recognition of screening services as a potential component of each evaluation and management service. Thus the "levels of E/M services include examinations, evaluations, treatments, conferences with or concerning patients, preventive pediatric and adult health supervision, and similar medical services, such as the determination of the need and/or location for appropriate care. Medical screening includes the history, examination, and medical decision-making required to determine the need and/or location for appropriate care and treatment of the patient (e.g., office and other outpatient setting, emergency department, nursing facility, etc.)

The following components are encompassed in E/M codes as required for prevention or diagnosis, treatment of illness/injury, and promotion of optimal health:

- Skill
- Effort
- Time
- Responsibility
- Medical knowledge

Seven components are listed in the descriptions for all E/M levels:

Key components:

- History
- Examination
- Medical decision making

Contributory components:

- Presenting complaint
- Counseling
- Coordination of care
- Nature of presenting problem

Emergency department evaluation and management codes are the only codes listed in the E/M section of CPT that do not include physician attendance time requirements for each level, because these services are provided on a variable intensity basis.

To select the appropriate emergency department E/M service code, *all* of the key components must be met or exceeded for the particular level of service chosen, which is determined by:

- The extent of patient history
- The extent of physical examination
- The complexity of medical decision making.

History. History is the first of the three key components that determine the level of service provided. Four types of history have been established by CPT:

- Problem focused—chief complaint; brief history of present illness or problem
- Expanded problem focused—chief complaint; brief history of present illness or problem; pertinent system review
- Detailed—chief complaint; extended history of present illness or problem; pertinent system review extended to include a review of a limited number of additional systems; pertinent past, family and/or social history directly related to the patient's problems.
- Comprehensive—chief complaint; extended history of present illness; review of systems, which is directly related to the problem(s) identified in the history of present illness plus a review of all additional body systems; complete past, family, social history.

DOCUMENTING THE ELEMENTS OF HISTORY. History has three components: history of present illness (HPI), review of systems (ROS), and past medical, family and/or social history (PFSH). The level of history selected must meet or exceed each required element unless the documented patient's condition or circumstance prevents obtaining the required information. Boxes 50-1 to 50-3 indicate the level of documentation required for each emergency department E/M code:

REMINDERS. The emergency physician often must request and review records from a previous encounter. When reviewed, relevant information should be entered into the current record and updated by the emergency physician. This information often is obtained by ancillary emergency department staff. In either case, information obtained by these means is used to determine the extent of ROS and/or PFSH.

BOX 50-1

HISTORY OF PRESENT ILLNESS

99281 Problem Focused	99282 and 99283 Expanded Problem Focused	99284 Detailed	99285 Comprehensive
Brief, one to three elements	Brief, one to three elements	Extended, four or more elements	Extended, four or more elements

Elements of history of present illness (HPI)

( ) Location (where, radiation to)

( ) Quality (sharp, burning, dull, radiating, tearing, etc.)

( ) Severity (recognized pain scale of 1-10, severe, mild, worst, progressing, etc.)

( ) Associated signs and symptoms (swelling, nausea, can overlap with system review)

( ) Timing (course of symptoms, start, steady, intermittent, etc.)

( ) Context (activity at onset, causation, etc.)

( ) Duration (length of episode, time of presentation, length of overall problem, etc.)

( ) Modifying factors (what helps, how relieved or worsened, how affected and by what, etc.)

BOX 50-2

REVIEW OF SYSTEMS

99281 Problem Focused	99282 and 99283 Expanded Problem Focused	99284 Detailed	99285 Comprehensive
No review of systems required	Problem Pertinent	Extended (2-9 systems)	Complete (10 + systems)

BODY SYSTEMS RECOGNIZED FOR REVIEW OF SYSTEMS (ROS)

A review of systems (ROS) is an inventory of body systems obtained through a series of questions seeking to identify signs and/or symptoms the patient might be experiencing or has experienced.

Constitutional symptoms (fever, weight loss, etc.)
Eyes
Ears, Nose, Mouth, Throat
Cardiovascular
Respiratory
Gastrointestinal
Genitourinary
Musculoskeletal
Integumentary (skin and/or breast)
Neurologic
Psychiatric
Endocrine
Hematologic/Lymphatic
Allergic/Immunologic

If this information cannot be obtained because of the patient's condition or circumstances, the reason should be indicated in the record. Information from both the ROS and the PFSH may be contained in the HPI but also considered as separate history elements.

Physical Examination. Physical examination is the second of the three key components that determine the level of service provided. Box 50-4 lists the four types of physical examination that have been established by CPT.

DOCUMENTING THE PHYSICAL EXAMINATION. The physical examination is determined by the extent of body area(s) and/or organ(s) reviewed by the physician. Box 50-4 indicates the level of documentation required for each emergency department E/M code.

Medical Decision Making. Medical decision making is the third of the three key components that determine the level of service provided. Medical decision making is the process of combining subjective data obtained through the history with objective data collected during the physical examination and/or testing to formulate a diagnostic and therapeutic plan. The amount of medical decision making (complexity of establishing a diagnosis and/or selecting a management option) is measured by the following:

- Number of possible diagnoses and/or the number of management options that must be considered
- Amount and/or complexity of medical records, diagnostic tests, and/or other information that must be obtained, reviewed, and analyzed
- Risk of significant complications, morbidity, and/or mortality, as well as comorbidities associated with the patient's presenting problem(s), diagnostic procedure(s), and/or possible management options.

Box 50-5 illustrates each component's effect on the level of medical decision making.

NATURE OF PRESENTING PROBLEM. Although only a contributory element, the nature of presenting problem (reason

BOX 50-3

PAST, FAMILY AND/OR SOCIAL HISTORY (PFSH)

99281 Problem Focused	99282 and 99283 Expanded Problem Focused	99284 Detailed	99285 Comprehensive
None	None	Pertinent (one item from any of three hx areas directly related to problem(s) identified in HPI)	Complete (review of one item from two history areas)

Past history includes patient's past experiences with illnesses, operations, hospitalizations, current medications, allergies, age-appropriate immunization status, age-appropriate feeding/dietary status, injuries and treatments.

Family history is a review of medical events in the family including diseases that may be hereditary or place the patient at risk.

Social history is an age-appropriate review of past and current activities including marital status and/or living arrangements; current employment; occupational history; use of drugs, alcohol and tobacco; level of education; sexual history; and other relevant social factors.

BOX 50-4

TYPES OF PHYSICAL EXAMINATION

99281 Problem Focused	99282 and 99283 Expanded Problem Focused	99284 Detailed	99285 Comprehensive
Limited examination, affected body area or organ system	Limited examination, affected body area or organ system, and other symptomatic or related organ system(s)	Extended examination of affected body area(s) and other symptomatic or related organ system(s)	Complete examination of single organ system, or general multi-system examination (8 + organ systems)

Body areas

Head, including face
Neck
Chest, including breasts and axillae
Abdomen
Genitalia, groin, buttocks
Back, including spine
Each extremity

Organ systems

Constitutional (vital signs, general appearance)
Eyes
Ears, nose, mouth
Cardiovascular
Respiratory
Gastrointestinal
Genitourinary
Musculoskeletal
Skin
Neurologic
Psychiatric
Hematologic/lymphatic/immunologic

BOX 50-5

MEDICAL DECISION MAKING

Number of diagnoses and/or management options	Complexity	Complications	Level of medical decision making	Evaluation and management code
Minimal	Minimal or None	Minimal	Straight-forward	99281
Limited	Limited	Low	Low complexity	99282
Multiple	Moderate	Moderate	Moderate complexity	99283 or 99284
Extensive	Extensive	High	High complexity	99285

for encounter) also plays an important role in determining the appropriate emergency medicine E/M service level. Presenting problems may categorized as follows:

- Minimal: may not require presence of physician but with physician supervision
- Self-limited or minor: definite and prescribed course, transient in nature, not likely to permanently alter health status or has good prognosis with management/compliance
- Low severity: risk of morbidity without treatment is low; little to no risk of mortality without treatment; full recovery without functional impairment is expected
- Moderate severity: risk of morbidity without treatment is moderate; moderate risk of mortality without treatment; uncertain prognosis or increased probability of prolonged functional impairment
- High severity: risk of morbidity without treatment is high to extreme; moderate to high risk of mortality without treatment or high probability of severe, prolonged functional impairment

CPT Definition of Emergency Department E/M Codes

Emergency department evaluation and management codes are defined by CPT as follows:

99281

- Problem-focused history
  - chief complaint
  - brief history of present illness or problem
- Problem-focused examination
  - examination limited to affected body area or organ system
- Straightforward medical decision making
  - minimal number of diagnoses or management options that must be considered
  - minimal to no amount and/or complexity of medical records, diagnostic tests and/or other information that must be obtained, reviewed, and analyzed
  - minimal risk of complications and/or morbidity or mortality, as well as comorbidities
- Counseling and/or coordination consistent with nature of problem(s) and patient's and/or family's needs
- Presenting problem(s)
  - self limited or minor: definite course, transient in nature, not likely to permanently alter health status or has good prognosis with management and compliance

Examples of E/M code 99281 include:

- Suture removal (well healed, uncomplicated laceration)
- Several uncomplicated insect bites
- Tetanus toxoid immunization

99282

- Expanded problem-focused history
  - chief complaint
  - brief history of present illness
  - problem pertinent system review
- Expanded problem-focused exam
  - a limited examination of the affected body area or organ system and other symptomatic or related organ system(s)
- Low complexity medical decision making
  - limited number of diagnoses or management options that must be considered
  - limited amount and/or complexity of medical records, diagnostic tests, and/or other information that must be obtained, reviewed, and analyzed
  - low risk of complications and/or morbidity or mortality as well as comorbidities
- Counseling and/or coordination of care with other providers or agencies are provided consistent with the nature of the problem(s) and the patient's and/or family's needs.
- Presenting problem(s)
  - usually are of low to moderate severity: risk of morbidity without treatment is low, little to no risk of mortality without treatment, full recovery without functional impairment is expected.

Examples of E/M code 99282 include:

- Child with localized impetigo on face
- Infected sclera, purulent discharge from both eyes (no pain, visual disturbance or foreign body in eye)
- Rash on both legs from poison ivy
- Painful blistered sunburn
- Red, swollen cystic lesion
- Minor traumatic extremity injury with localized pain, swelling, and bruising

99283

- Expanded problem-focused history
  - chief complaint
  - brief history of present illness
  - problem pertinent system review
- Expanded problem-focused examination
  - a limited examination of the affected body area or organ system and other symptomatic or related organ system(s)
- Medical decision making of moderate complexity
  - multiple number of diagnoses or management options that must be considered
  - moderate amount and/or complexity of medical records, diagnostic tests, and/or other information that must be obtained, reviewed, and analyzed
  - moderate risk of complications and/or morbidity or mortality, as well as comorbidities
- Counseling and/or coordination of care with other providers or agencies are provided consistent with the nature of the problem(s) and the patient's and/or family's needs.
- Presenting problem(s)
  - usually are of moderate severity: risk of morbidity without treatment is moderate, moderate risk of mortality without treatment, uncertain prognosis or increased probability of prolonged functional impairment

Examples of E/M code 99283 include:

- Afebrile female with vaginal discharge, no abdominal or back pain
- Inversion ankle injury, unable to bear weight
- Blunt head injury, local swelling; no confusion, loss of consciousness, or memory deficit
- Well-appearing child with fever, abdominal cramps, no vomiting, tolerating fluids
- Acute pain from suspected foreign body in eye

99284

- Detailed history
  - chief complaint
  - extended system review
  - extended history of present illness
  - pertinent past, family and/or social
- Detailed examination
  - extended examination of affected body area(s) and other symptomatic or related organ system(s)

- Medical decision making of moderate complexity
  - multiple number of diagnoses or number of management options that must be considered
  - moderate amount and/or complexity of medical records, diagnostic tests, and/or other information that must be obtained, reviewed, and analyzed
  - moderate risk of complications and/or morbidity or mortality, as well as comorbidities
- Counseling and/or coordination of care with other providers or agencies are provided consistent with the nature of the problem(s) and the patient's and/or family's needs.
- Presenting Problem(s)
  - usually of high severity: risk of morbidity without treatment is high to extreme, moderate to high risk of mortality without treatment, or high probability of severe, prolonged functional impairment
  - require urgent evaluation by the physician but does not pose an immediate significant threat to life or physiologic function

Examples of E/M code 99284 include:

- Child who fell off bike with head injury and brief loss of consciousness
- Female with lower abdominal pain and vaginal discharge
- Elderly female who has fallen and complains of hip pain and inability to walk
- Patient with flank pain and hematuria

99285

- Comprehensive history
  - chief complaint
  - extended history of present illness
  - complete system review
  - complete past, family, and social history
- Comprehensive examination
  - complete single system specialty examination or general multisystem examination
- Medical decision making of high complexity
  - extensive number of diagnoses or management options that must be considered
  - extensive amount and/or other information that must be obtained, reviewed, and analyzed
  - high risk of complications and/or morbidity and/or mortality, as well as comorbidities
- Counseling and/or coordination of care with other providers or agencies are provided consistent with the nature of the problem(s) and the patient's and/or family's needs.
- Presenting problem(s)
  - usually of high severity: risk of morbidity without treatment is high to extreme, moderate to high risk of mortality without treatment, or high probability of severe, prolonged functional impairment
  - immediate significant threat to life or physiologic function

Examples of E/M code 99285 include:

- Active, upper GI bleed
- Rapid heart rate requiring IV medication
- Victim of automobile accident with intraabdominal injuries or multiple extremity injuries
- Acute onset of cerebral vascular accident
- Aggressive management of complicated overdose
- Patient with "worst headache of her life," complaining of stiff neck, nausea, inability to concentrate
- Adult with acute febrile illness, shortness of breath, altered level of consciousness

Critical Care Services. Critical care services include the following:

99291 Critical Care, evaluation and management of the unstable critically ill or unstable critically injured patient, requiring the *constant attendance* of the physician; first hour

99292 Each additional 30 minutes.

The AMA made significant changes in the critical care descriptors in 1996. The 1996 CPT section on critical care includes the following language:

> Critical care is the care of the unstable critically ill or unstable critically injured patient who requires constant physician attendance (the physician need not be constantly at bedside per se but is engaged in physician work directly related to the individual patient's care). Critical care services are provided to but not limited to, patients with central nervous system failure, circulatory failure, shock-like conditions, renal, hepatic or respiratory failure, post-operative complications, or overwhelming infection. Critical care is usually, but not always, given in a critical care area, such as the coronary care unit, intensive care unit, respiratory care unit or the emergency care facility.
>
> Services for a patient who is not critically ill but happens to be in a critical care unit are reported using subsequent hospital care codes (see 99231-99233) or hospital consultation codes (see 99251-99263) as appropriate.

Procedures that can be coded in addition to critical care include:

31500 Endotracheal intubation
32020 Tube thoracostomy
36010 Introduction of catheter, superior or inferior vena cava
36011 Central lines (not peripheral lines)
92950 Cardiopulmonary resuscitation

Documentation of critical care services is difficult to standardize because this service encompasses such a wide range of situations. As a general rule, documentation should contain the amount of *time* the physician spent providing critical care services. The fact that the patient is unstable, requires immediate attention, displays abnormal vital signs, and receives immediate management should also be documented in the medical record.

Examples of critical care services (CPT code 99291) include:

- First hour of critical care of a 65-year-old with septic shock
- First hour of critical care of a 15-year-old with acute respiratory failure from asthma
- First hour of critical care of a 6-month-old child with hypovolemic shock secondary to diarrhea and dehydration

The 1994 edition of CPT has also revised the descriptors to allow use of the critical care service code 99291 for 30 to 74 minutes of critical care services. Critical care of less than 30 minutes total duration on a given date would be reported by using the appropriate evaluation and management (E/M) code.

Surgical Procedures. Many surgical and diagnostic procedures are performed by emergency physicians. These procedures are identified with the procedure code applicable to the type of service performed. Payors may reimburse these procedures by set fees for each procedure or by a percentage of the total charge.

Emergency physicians provide numerous surgical services to patients. These services are, for coding purposes, separate and distinct from the evaluation and management services identified with codes 99281 to 99292. Procedures are identified as either major procedures, defined as "global" surgery through the surgical package concept, or "minor" surgery, designated with star or asterisk (*) in CPT. It is important to understand the basis for distinguishing between these two procedure types to ensure that the services provided are coded accurately.

SURGICAL PACKAGE CONCEPT. Many procedures include preoperative, operative and postoperative components associated with the procedure. These components are generally identifiable as a consistent part of the surgical service and, as such, are bundled into the surgical package. Thus these "packaged" procedures are considered to include the three components unless otherwise modified.

It is important to note that these procedures include all *related* preoperative, operative, and postoperative services. Thus any services in excess of those normally included in the procedure would be identified separately with the appropriate evaluation and management or procedure code. For example, a patient sustains a complex laceration as the result of a fall. In addition to suturing the laceration, the emergency physician must determine if the fall was due to underlying medical problems and if, during the fall, the patient sustained other injuries in addition to the laceration. In this case, the complex laceration repair code would include only the preoperative examination and preparation of the wound, the actual suturing, and the wound reexamination and suture removal. An additional code would be used to identify the examination of other parts of the body to determine whether underlying medical problems contributed to the fall or if any additional injuries were sustained.

MINOR ("STARRED") SURGICAL PROCEDURES. Certain minor procedures whose preoperative and postoperative components are variable but whose surgical component is generally well defined are identified with a star (*) in CPT. Certain coding rules apply to use of additional evaluation and management and surgical codes when a starred procedure is performed during an emergency department visit. According to CPT guidelines, when the starred procedure is provided during an initial visit or during a visit that involves a significant evaluation and management service, an evaluation and management code (99281 to 99291) is listed in addition to the starred (*) procedure. However, when the starred procedure is the major service provided during the visit, the code 99025 is used to identify the visit component of the service. Because most payors do not recognize the 99025 code, emergency medicine coding generally requires the addition of an evaluation and management code (99281 to 99292) to identify the visit component of the service.

The starred procedure used to identify the service does not include the postoperative wound check, suture removal, etc. Therefore revisits to the emergency physician would be identified with the evaluation and management code that describes the level of care provided.

Payors may interpret the CPT surgical coding guidelines differently, and the knowledgeable coder will need to determine where payor rules differ from the CPT guidelines and code accordingly. One such example is the Medicare program's guidelines governing minor starred (*) procedures. According to Medicare, all related preoperative, operative, and postoperative services are included in the minor starred (*) surgery package. Medicare assigns a 0 to 10-day postoperative follow-up period for minor procedures and a 90-day follow-up period for major surgical procedures. Further, Medicare does not recognize the 99025 visit code in its fee schedule. Therefore before an additional evaluation and management service can be billed with the minor starred procedure, a significant, identifiable E/M service must be performed.

Diagnostic Interpretation Services. According to CPT "the actual performance of diagnostic tests/studies for which specific CPT codes are available is not included in the level of E/M services." Physician performance of diagnostic tests/studies for which specific CPT codes are available should be reported separately, *in addition* to the appropriate E/M code.

Emergency physicians are often required to interpret the diagnostic tests ordered during the patient's emergency department stay. Emergency physicians generally do not provide the equipment and supplies associated with each test. The interpretative component of the diagnostic study, however, can be identified by adding a −26 modifier to those diagnostic tests that include both the technical and interpretative component. The −26 modifier indicates that the emergency physician provided the interpretative or "professional" component of the test. Whether or not the payor distinguishes the emergency physician's service from the technical component or from the separate interpretation provided by another practitioner (often referred to as an "overread") depends on the payor's own payment guidelines. Thus the emergency physician must understand each payor's methodology for recognizing the emergency physician's professional component of the service for payment to ensure that the coding is accurate. In essence, the requirements for emergency physician's coding for interpretative services can vary among payors.

Modifiers. The use of modifiers is necessary when the service provided differs from the written code description. The modifiers used for services listed in the various sections of CPT are listed in the front of each chapter. In addition to the CPT modifiers, payors may assign unique modifiers for use in coding services according to their own criteria. Therefore it is necessary to understand when modifiers are necessary either to modify the description of a service and/or to adjust the charge or payment for a specific service. Modifiers are necessary to ensure that appropriate payment is made for combination of services according to Medicare RBRVS guidelines. The modifiers most commonly used in the emergency medicine practice are:

−25 Significant, Separately Identifiable Evaluation and Management Service by the Same Physician on the Same Day of a Procedure or Other Service.

This modifier is applied to the appropriate emergency department service (99281-85, 99291-92) when E/M services are reported in addition to the usual services included in operative procedures. Medicare policy specifies that no payment will be made for E/M services in addition to procedures unless the E/M services are significant and separately identifiable. Therefore without the −25 modifier, Medicare reimbursement for these services may be denied.

When a history and physical examination, interpretations, system review, and/or management actions are necessary or when these components are expanded past the stated problem area at the time a procedure is performed, the addition of an E/M code with modifier −25 is appropriate. The diagnosis should state the additional condition(s) that required the evaluation and management service(s) in addition to the procedure.

−54 Surgical Care Only

Certain procedures are considered to be part of "Global Surgery" packages for Medicare and as such include preoperative, operative and postoperative services related to the operative procedure. When the emergency physician provides the preoperative examination and the operative service, but refers the patient to another physician for follow-up, the modifier −54 may be required by the third party payor for accurate billing of the procedure as an indication of the modification in the surgery "package."

The omission of this modifier could result in one or more of the following:

- Nonpayment of follow-up services provided by other physician
- During the claims review process, a payor may determine that the absence of the −54 modifier constitutes a billing error if the patient is referred to another physician for follow-up.

Use of this modifier demands that the coder identify if and where the patient is referred for follow-up. Documentation provided by emergency physicians and/or nurses in the emergency department often omits the "where" from the discharge instructions, thus creating a problem for a coder trying to determine how to identify the provider of the follow-up care.

−57 Decision for Surgery

When an evaluation and management service is performed and results in the decision to perform surgery, the −57 modifier is reported. Use of this modifier differentiates the E/M service from the normal preoperative service and is often used with E/M services billed in addition to global surgery procedures.

Hospital Observation Services. In 1993 three new codes (99218, 99219, and 99220) were assigned for evaluation and management services provided to patients designated and/or admitted to "observation status" in a hospital. The patient does not have to be physically located in the observation area designated by the hospital, he or she can be in an observation area in the emergency department. Typical time ranges have not yet been established for the observation category of service.

The observation codes can be used by the "supervising physician" for the initiation of observation status, supervision of the patient during the observation period, and the performance of periodic assessments by the physician. Evaluation and management services provided by the supervising physician on the same date as the observation service should not be reported separately. Therefore the emergency physician would bill for either the observation or the evaluation and management service, but not for both. For observation encounters by other physicians, these physicians should use office or other outpatient consultation codes (99241 to 99245).

Discharge from observation on a day other than the initial date of observation status is identified with CPT code 99217, Observation Care Discharge, day management.

Other Services. Because of their availability and expertise, emergency physicians are often involved in directing or participating in the resuscitation of hospital inpatients. Determining the most appropriate method of describing the service provided depends on the specific services that the emergency physician performs. For example, when the emergency physician directs the resuscitation team but does not perform any procedures, the cognitive services provided may be described by using critical care codes 99291 and 99292. CPR code 92950 is *not* considered a cognitive service and can be billed separately. In addition, the direction by a physician of CPR performed by another individual would be more appropriately reported using critical care or the appropriate E/M code. When surgical procedures are performed, they may be listed separately. Listing the specific procedures is the preferred method because it offers a better itemization and description of the services rendered.

INTERNATIONAL CLASSIFICATION OF DISEASES, 9TH EDITION, CLINICAL MODIFICATION (ICD-9-CM)

ICD-9-CM precisely delineates, through diagnosis coding policy, the clinical picture of each patient seeking care from a physician or other healthcare provider. It provides precise information, beyond that needed for statistical or healthcare trends analysis, to third-party payors about the reason for the patient's "visit" to the healthcare provider. ICD-9-CM consists of a tabular list of diseases (Volume 1), an alphabetical index to diseases (Volume 2), and a tabular and alphabetical listing of hospital inpatient procedures (Volume 3).

Dating back to seventeenth century England, diagnosis coding was originally used for gathering statistical information through a system known as the London Bills of Mortality. Around 1937, this mechanism for tracking clinical information had evolved into the International List of Causes of Death. In 1948 the World Health Organization published a statistical listing that was used in tracking both morbidity and mortality information. This listing, known as the International Classification of Diseases, became the model for the internationally accepted text in use today—the International Classification of Diseases, 9th Revision.

In 1977 the U.S. National Center for Health Statistics modified this statistical study with clinical information. The clinical modifications provided users with a way to classify morbidity data for indexing of medical records, medical case reviews, ambulatory and other medical care programs, and for basic health statistics. This modification resulted in the development of the International Classification of Diseases, 9th Revision, Clinical Modification (ICD-9-CM).

Congress enacted the Medicare Catastrophic Coverage Act in 1988, which required the reporting of ICD-9 codes on Medicare Part A and Part B claims. This mandate became effective on April 1, 1989, even though the remainder of the Medicare Catastrophic Coverage Act was later repealed. The Health Care Financing Administration published guidelines about the use of ICD-9 codes, which were to be followed by each state. Failure to use or correctly use ICD-9 codes on Medicare claims now carries substantial penalties.

Many healthcare providers and coders are presently awaiting the release of ICD-10. The World Health Organization recently began making available Volume 1 of the International Statistical Classification of Diseases and Related Health Problems, Tenth Revision. Volume 1, which is the tabular list of diseases, has yet to be modified for clinical use in the United States. A second volume, containing guidelines and instructions for the use of the entire reference, is not yet available. In addition, the alphabetical index to ICD-10, contained in a third volume, is reportedly still under development by the World Health Organization. The National Center for Health Statistics, the agency in charge of preparing Volumes 1 and 2 for end users, has conservatively estimated that ICD-10 will not be implemented in the United States before 1998. The Health Care Financing Administration has indicated that implementation of ICD-10 will not occur before the year 2000.

Although introduction of ICD-10 to U.S. healthcare providers is still several years away, it will be a major watershed event in the development of diagnostic coding. Early reports indicate that the chapters in ICD-10 have been significantly expanded, the coding conventions have moved toward an alpha-numeric terminology, and many listings have been reclassified.

Application of ICD-9 in the Emergency Department Setting

The "Official Coding Guidelines" published by the American Hospital Association in its Coding Clinic publication stresses the importance of coding "the diagnosis, condition, problem or other reason for the encounter to be chiefly responsible for the services provided," as well as listing any additional codes that describe coexisting conditions. Coders must assign the highest level of specificity to the codes selected but code only the conditions that are established. "Rule-out, probable, and possible" conditions are not to be coded as though established through the assessment process. Coding should identify conditions to the highest degree of certainty for the encounter event though those conditions are symptoms, signs, abnormal test results, or other reasons for the visit.

For patients receiving only ancillary diagnostic services during an encounter, the V code that most appropriately describes the examination is sequenced first, followed by the diagnosis or problem for which the services are being performed. When surgical services are provided, the diagnosis for which the surgery is performed is sequenced first. All documented conditions that coexist at the time of the encounter or visit that require or affect patient care, treatment, or management should be coded.

It is not uncommon to find payors that reduce payment levels or deny claims when the emergency department treatment is rendered for a nonemergency condition according to the payors' own unique definition of emergency. A subjective approach to defining "emergency" will often result in payment problems. Thus a definition of what constitutes an emergency must be understood by the coder and communicated to the payor to ensure that emergency patient visits are reimbursed.

Coding for emergency services has always presented unique challenges to coders. Payors may deny claims for services provided in the emergency setting that do not appear to be for "true" emergencies. Therefore unless payor policy instructs otherwise, it is often necessary to list symptoms and complaints in addition to the diagnosis for those conditions that appear to be emergencies before clinical assessment. For example, it is not uncommon for an elderly patient to present to the emergency department with "severe" chest pain. This patient would be considered emergent and receive immediate care to determine whether the chest pain is cardiac in nature. This patient may have severe gastritis, a significantly less acute condition; however, the patient is given the benefit of stabilization and treatment until a possible cardiac condition can be ruled out. The discharge diagnosis of gastritis would probably be considered a nonemergency. Payment might be reduced from the standard payment rate for the level of service billed, payment for the emergency treatment might be denied by the payor, or the patient might be held responsible for the nonemergency service that does not meet the insurer's payment criteria. Therefore the emergency coder must consider not just the condition but the payor criteria governing payment for the condition to ensure that the diagnosis information is complete to establish the need for the emergency treatment.

Because coding for emergency services is not a new problem, emergency physicians have attempted to adequately define *emergency* over the years. Most recently, the ACEP has adopted a formal definition of emergency services as follows:

> Emergency Services are those health care services provided in a hospital emergency department to treat medical conditions of acute onset and sufficient severity that would lead a prudent layperson, possessing an average knowledge of medicine and health, to believe that urgent medical care is required to reduce the level of pain, prevent the deterioration of one's condition, prevent disability and/or death.

In essence, patients who demonstrate conditions requiring urgent and/or unscheduled medical care should qualify for immediate treatment. Examples of these types of services would include the following:

Evaluation and management of:

- Acute or significant pain
- Any trauma less than 72 hours from time of incident
- Complications of trauma
- Acute infection or sepsis
- Shock or impending shock
- Obstetric crises and/or labor
- Bleeding or threat of hemorrhage
- Any condition resulting in admission of the patient to a hospital or nursing home within 24 hours
- Suspected abuse or neglect of any person that could result in temporary or permanent physical or psychologic harm
- Any illness or injury that would cause loss or impairment of the following systems: integumentary, musculoskeletal, HEENT, respiratory, gastrointestinal, genitourinary, nervous, or cardiovascular
- Congenital defects or abnormalities in an infant
- A patient suspected to be suffering from a mental illness and/or posing an apparent danger to the safety of himself/herself or others.
- Conditions that pose a threat to public health
- Any acute or significant symptom(s) that might indicate a condition that constitutes a threat to the patient's or family's physical or psychologic well-being requiring prompt medical attention to prevent possible deterioration, disability, or death

Use of this criteria may be helpful in negotiations with area payors to generate appropriate reimbursement levels for emergency services.

DOCUMENTATION REQUIREMENTS FOR EFFECTIVE AND ACCURATE CPT CODING

Complete, legible documentation is the cornerstone of reimbursement and medicolegal requirements. The Joint Commission on Accreditation of Health Care Organizations (JCAHO) standards require that the following key components must exist on the emergency department medical record:

- Incorporation of the emergency department medical record into the patient's permanent hospital record
- Availability of all prior pertinent inpatient and ambulatory care patient medical record documentation, including previous visits to the emergency department
- Entry of the following information for each emergency department visit:
  - Pertinent history of illness or injury and physical findings, including the patient's vital signs
  - Emergency care provided to the patient before arrival
  - Diagnostic and therapeutic orders
  - Clinical observations, including results of treatment
  - Reports of procedures, tests and results
  - Diagnostic impression
  - Conclusion at the termination of evaluation/treatment including final disposition of the patient's condition on discharge or transfer.

Medical record documentation serves three basic functions:

- To minimize the high medical liability risk of emergency physicians
- To support the charges billed to the patient by clearly substantiating the services rendered
- To provide a detailed record of conditions and actions to be referenced by other providers involved in the patient's care.

Increased emphasis on the importance of documentation has resulted in publication of documentation standards by a joint committee of the AMA and the Health Care Financing Administration. Making the transition to these new standards will be difficult for many emergency physicians, as many emergency department medical records provide inadequate room to provide the level of detail that will be required. For those emergency departments with access to transcription services, transition will be less difficult.

For emergency physicians, it is important to remember that all documentation requirements must be met unless a notation is made with regard to the condition or circumstance that prohibited the physician from obtaining the necessary information. Under coding guidelines published by the AMA in its CPT manual, the following should be documented when the related services are provided to the patient during the course of emergency department treatment:

Chief Complaint/Presenting Problem

- Reason for visit (Why did the patient come to the emergency department?)
- Mode of arrival (How did the patient arrive?)
- Triage status (Condition upon arrival?)

History of Presenting Illness

- Illness associated with the chief complaint; includes at least all pertinent negative findings
- Source of history

Past Medical History

- Must be documented relevant to the patient's condition

Family History/Social History

- Must be documented relevant to the patient's condition

Review of Systems

- Cardiovascular
- Endocrine
- Gastrointestinal
- Genitourinary
- Integumentary
- Immunologic/Hematologic
- Musculoskeletal
- Neurologic
- Psychiatric
- Respiratory

(For minor cases, the Review of Systems may be included with the History of Present Illness)

Physical Examination

- Orientation and mental status
- Vital signs (comment on abnormal vital signs)
- Specific body area examined and related area(s):
  - Head and neck: eyes, ears, nose and throat
  - Lungs
  - Heart
  - Abdomen (may include rectal); pelvic; extremities
  - Neurologic
  - Skin

Diagnostics

- Laboratory and radiographic studies (list studies performed, specific results)

Surgical/Medical Procedure Note

- Listing of all procedures, complications, and details about the technique used in performing each

Clinical Impression

- Diagnosis or symptom that is the most likely cause of the patient's major problem(s)

Emergency Department Course

- Laboratory and radiographic studies
- Surgical/medical procedure notes
- Repeat evaluation
- Time of examination
- Vital signs
- Interventions (O_2, medications, IVs)

Differential Diagnosis

- Stated considerations for other possible causes of patient's symptoms

Physicians Contacted for Coordination of Care

- Name of physician(s)
- Comments of physician(s) contacted

Disposition Plan

- Disposition (admit, transfer, home)
- Recommended treatments (medications prescribed, splints, etc.)
- Physician responsible for follow-up
- Specific patient instructions and/or counseling provided to family (activity level, follow-up appointment, risks, etc)

Emergency departments should strive for a uniformity among physicians in their approach to documentation. In addition, routine reviews of compliance with established standards should be conducted to ensure that all physicians meet the standards. It is expected that the documentation guidelines associated with the CPT evaluation and management codes will evolve over time. During this evolution, payors will use these and their own internal guidelines to evaluate whether the documentation supports the services that were billed. This process will require close attention to payor requirements relating to documentation of the services that are billed.

The following checklist may assist physicians in ensuring that all elements of the medical record are reviewed and completed:

- Read and acknowledge nurses' notes.
- Address any conflicting nurse assessments.
- Make sure the entire record is consistent with final diagnosis and disposition.
- Address normal/abnormal vital signs.
- Document complete physician history: Symptoms, past medical history, assessment of risk factors, and past medications and treatments. Never use "As above" when referring to nurses' notes.
- Address chief complaint with patient's perception of the problem.
- Convey positive and negative objective findings.
- Document complete examination and severity of patient's condition.
- Clearly document all initial interpretations, tests ordered, and positive or negative results.
- Avoid the term *Rule out* unless you plan to rule out that diagnosis before discharge from your care.
- Document all procedures performed, medications ordered, consultations and discussions with other healthcare providers, work releases, and disposition.
- Include detailed information on procedure site, length, depth, complicating factors, corrective actions, and follow-up instructions, as applicable.
- Ensure diagnosis and disposition are consistent with history, physical examination, and progress.
- Know what reimbursement problems might result from continued inadequate documentation.
- Recognize your inability to bill accurately for services rendered when they are not clearly documented.
- Provide enough detailed documentation to facilitate the selection of the appropriate procedure code(s).
- Specify diagnosis to permit selection of reimbursable ICD-9 diagnosis code.

CODING ACCOUNTABILITY

Although numerous changes have been made during the last several years in the codes appearing in CPT and in the payor guidelines delineating how these codes are to be used, one rule has remained constant: *The physician in whose name a claim is submitted is ultimately responsible for all information contained on the claim.* Particularly with respect to the Medicare program, where fraud and abuse penalties are extremely severe, physicians who mistakenly believe that their coding responsibility is assumed by another party (e.g., a billing or coding company) can quickly find themselves in an indefensible position when third-party payors begin to question their coding or billing practices. Physicians must be knowledgeable about the processes used to select particular CPT and ICD-9 codes that appear on their claims. This responsibility is assumed by understanding the essential components of procedure and diagnosis coding, taking an active role in monitoring coding personnel and third-party payor guidelines, and regularly reviewing the quality of the coding work being performed.

Ensuring quality coding involves appropriately identifying the applicable responsibilities of physicians and coders in today's reimbursement environment. These responsibilities include ensuring that coding is performed according to established guidelines for each payor, ensuring that available documentation meets the criteria for correctly reporting, through a coding mechanism, each service rendered, ensuring that all billable services are identified with the correct CPT and ICD-9 codes, and reporting physician services in a consistent manner. In addition, physicians and coders have a responsibility to communicate regularly throughout the coding process to refine it into a system that ensures accurate coding and well-documented records.

Although many physicians have codes assigned by others (e.g., billing company, hospital, coding company, group employee, etc.), the responsibility for quality coding ultimately belongs to the physician. Therefore all physicians should concentrate on learning the objective components of documenting the services they rendered, routinely reviewing or auditing the coding performed on their behalf, and proactively working with third-party payors to identify and solve coding problems or concerns. Every emergency physician has a responsibility to help educate third-party payors about coding issues unique to emergency medicine.

RELATIVE VALUE SCALES

A brief discussion of relative value scales/studies (RVS) is included here because some third-party payors use these scales (e.g., the physicians' *Medicare Fee Schedule*) as a tool for modifying CPT coding rules through a reimbursement mechanism. With few exceptions, these older scales/studies are no longer relevant to today's dynamic coding environment. Advances in medical technology, revisions to code numbers and descriptors, and legal challenges have limited the usefulness of most of these relative value scales.

Relative value scales were used initially as early as the 1950s to describe and assign values to the medical services provided by physicians. They were to be used not as fee schedules, but as an *aid* in determining physicians' individual fees. Area physicians were often surveyed to obtain input on assigning values to their services. The RVS was then developed as a coded listing of physician procedures with relative values attached to indicate the relativity within each individual section of median charges. A base procedure was selected for each section of the RVS and was used to calculate an index for all other procedures within that section.

Two primary types of relative value scales exist. In the first, a charge-based relative value scale, a unit value is assigned to each procedure based on historical charges submitted for a given procedure throughout a particular geographic area. In the second, a resource-based relative value scale, values are assigned to each service by measuring the resources expended (e.g., work, practice costs, malpractice costs, etc) in providing the medical service.

Perhaps the best-known example of a resource-based relative value scale in use today in the physicians' *Medicare Fee Schedule (MFS)*. Because of widespread concerns that Medicare's reasonable charge payment system led to imbalances in relative payments between procedural services (such as surgery) and evaluation and management services (such as visits and consultations), Congress enacted reforms in 1989 that led to the creation of the *MFS*. Effective January 1, 1992, the *MFS* resulted from a study funded by the Health Care Financing Administration and conducted by researchers at Harvard University. Phases I and II of the project generated relative work values for more than 2700 unique *CPT* codes. Phase III of the project created relative work values for CPT codes that were not valued during the first two phases, or were valued by extrapolation.

The *California Relative Value Studies (CRVS)*, a charge-based RVS, was the companion to the 1974 revision of the AMA's *CPT*. It was one of the most widely used coding systems adopted by payors in its time. Because many of the codes and services included in the CRVS have not been updated since 1974, however, most physicians and third-party payors have abandoned its use. The CRVS system provided a value for each service based on historical charge data generated by all specialties up to 1974.

The *Florida Relative Value Study (FRVS)*, another charge-based RVS, was based on the AMA *Physicians' Current Procedural Terminology*, Fourth Edition, 1989. The database used in the study consisted of all charge data submitted to Blue Cross/Blue Shield of Florida in 1988 by all physicians. More than 40 million charges were in the database used to develop the *FRVS*. The relative values were established by arraying all charges for each procedure and then calculating the mean value for each procedure. A base procedure was established for each section of the RVS, which was then used to calculate an index for all other procedures within that section. The resulting relative value for each procedure was reviewed by statistical consultants for consistency and statistical validity. Much like the *CRVS*, the FRVS is rarely used today by payors or by physicians.

The *McGraw-Hill/Systemetrics Relative Value Studies* is a comprehensive relative value system still in use today. The research and data used to produce this particular RVS began in 1980, when a research group of medical and legal professionals incorporated as Relative Value Studies, Inc. In 1984 the first edition of *Relative Values for Physicians* was published. A resource-based relative value scale, *Relative Values for Physicians* uses time, skill, severity of illness, risk to patient, and risk to physician (medicolegal) criteria to value a procedure. Physicians across the country are asked to review all procedures they frequently perform and to assign relative values to these procedures. This physician input is then analyzed statistically for validity and for normal distribution. Results are then presented to a cross-specialty comparison group for adjustment, and recommendations are presented to an editorial panel for a final decision.

SUMMARY

Procedure (CPT) and diagnosis (ICD-9) codes describe the services rendered to patients, the reason for the patient's visit to the emergency department, and the medical necessity of the care delivered by the physician. These codes also become the basis for determining payment for the services rendered. Because most coding systems are general in nature and do not effectively translate the acute nature of services rendered in the emergency department, coding for emergency physician services presents many specialized problems. Most third-party payors have a limited knowledge of the practice of emergency medicine, which results in extraordinary pressure being placed on coders to develop a coding process that pertains to emergency medicine without straying too far from accepted coding practices.

The complex nature of today's ever-changing reimbursement system makes it imperative for physicians, administrators, nurses, Emergency Medical Services personnel, and coding, billing, and medical record professionals to work together to ensure that appropriate payment is made for medical services provided to patients. By working effectively with third-party payors, this emergency medicine "team" can develop a better understanding of their respective roles within the healthcare coding and reimbursement environment.

REFERENCES

1. Anzinger RK, editor: *Procedure coding for emergency medicine: an educational manual,* ed 2, Dallas, 1993, American College of Emergency Physicians.
2. Brouch K: *Diagnosis coding for emergency medicine,* errata edition, Dallas, 1989, American College of Emergency Physicians.
3. Bishop M, editor: *Optimizing revenues through effective reimbursement strategies,* ed 2, Dallas, 1991, American College of Emergency Physicians.
4. Drexler JY, editor: *Procedure coding for emergency medicine: an educational manual,* Dallas, 1989, American College of Emergency Physicians.
5. *Physicians' Current Procedural Terminology,* Chicago, 1996, American Medical Association.
6. *Physicians' Medicare Fee Schedule,* 42 CFR Parts 405 and 414, Baltimore, 1993, Health Care Financing Administration.
7. Seare S: *International classification of diseases,* 9th revision, Clinical modification, ed 4, Salt Lake City, 1993, Med-Index Publications.
8. *Relative values for physicians, 1993-1994,* New York, 1993, McGraw-Hill.

ADDITIONAL READINGS

- Commerce Clearing House (CCH) Medicare & Medicaid Guide
  Commerce Clearing House, Inc
  4205 West Peterson Avenue
  Chicago, IL 60646
- Health Legislation and Regulation
  Faulkner & Gray's Healthcare Information Center
  1133 Fifteenth Street, NW, Suite 450
  Washington, DC 20005
- Medical Economics
  Box 55
  Oradell, NJ 07649
- Medicine & Health
  Faulkner & Gray's Healthcare Information Center
  1133 Fifteenth Street, NW, Suite 450
  Washington, DC 20005

- Physician Payment Review Commission Annual Report
  2120 L Street, NW, Suite 510
  Washington, DC 20037
- Medicare Compliance Alert
  United Communications Group
  4550 Montgomery Avenue, Suite 700N
  Bethesda, MD 20814
- Physician's Payment Advisory
  American Health Consultants, Inc
  60 Peachtree Park Drive, NE
  Atlanta, GA 30309
- ACEP News
  American College of Emergency Physicians
  PO Box 619911
  Dallas, TX 75261-9911
- Modern Healthcare
  Crain Communications, Inc
  740 Rush Street
  Chicago, IL 60611-2590
- CPT Assistant
  American Medical Association
  515 North State Street
  Chicago, IL 60610
- American Medical News
  American Medical Association
  515 North State Street
  Chicago, IL 60610
- Reimbursement Report
  Medical Management Resources, Inc
  9550 Regency Square Blvd, Suite 1200
  Jacksonville, FL 32225
- HCPCS Report
  St. Anthony Publishing, Inc
  11410 Isaac Newton Square
  Reston, VA 22090
- Coding Clinic for ICD-9-CM
  American Hospital Association
  Central Office on ICD-9-CM
  840 N Lakeshore Drive
  Chicago, IL 60611

51 Billing

Robert Burleigh

OUTLINE

THE BILLING PROCESS

Administrative Workflows and Costs

At its most basic, the process of accounts receivable and information management is composed of three major elements: (1) accurate and timely gathering of required data, (2) storage and manipulation of required data, and (3) retrieval of stored data in various document formats. This simplification, however, belies the complexity and management requirements of the process. The data gathering activity is complicated by multiple sources of information available in multiple formats, some desirable and some cumbersome. Storage and manipulation of data require the ability to match and move masses of various types of data for many individuals. Information must be retrieved in differing modes to meet requirements of various third-party billing programs and to meet the reporting needs of the involved medical service team.

When considering the administrative workflows and involved procedures, one must also consider the type of healthcare services provider and the variances required of each. In the field of physician practice, there are three basic types (Box 51-1).

With the movement of patients toward the outpatient or private office environment, practice definition lines are not finely drawn. For example, approximately 65% of radiologists perform services at a site other than or in addition to the primary hospital service site (private imaging centers, multispecialty clinics, or industrial sites). Many anesthesiologists serve outside the hospital walls in pain service clinics. Cardiologists often operate diagnostic cardiology and/or catheter laboratorie as part of traditional hospital inpatient activity.

For the purpose of this and future discussions, and because of the common ground and peculiarities of the information processing systems, we will consider all "hospital-based" specialties together, primary care in all facets together (including multispecialty clinic practice), and referral specialities (including private office radiology and anesthesia) together.

Hospital-Based Physicians. The hospital-based physician marketplace differs significantly from private offices of all types. Major differences that affect the billing and receivables process are these:

1. Physicians or physician groups in the hospital setting often have no nonphysician employees, making them prime candidates for outsourcing. In fact, many physician groups actively manage the practice to have no employees other than physicians. This gives the physicians less administrative responsibility and enables them to maximize fringe benefits without having to match required benefits for lower paid employees.
2. These physician groups are dependent on the hospital for demographic information. They are in fact dependent on the hospital for all information required to perform billing activities.
3. Hospital-based physicians may have multiple sources of income (Tables 51-1 and 51-2). Although billing separately for the professional portion of procedural activity provides the majority of their income, hospital-based physicians may also be paid by the hospital for ***A***dministration, ***S***upervision, and ***T***eaching in the hospital department. Physicians in university hospital settings may be reimbursed for additional teaching and/or research and publication activity.
4. Hospital-based physicians have multiple potential reimbursement possibilities. Although most bill separately for their service, they may also be paid on a salary or retainer basis, an annual contract for a fixed sum, or on a piecework basis for services rendered, all paid by the hospital. If the hospital pays the physician group, the hospital must bill separately to the Entitlement programs (Medicare and Medicaid) for the physician service. This still allows opportunity for professional billing on behalf of the hospital.
5. Hospital-based physician billing is for the professional (physician-performed patient care) component only, and not the technical component (use of hospital or clinic facilities not "owned" by the practice) of medical services. Because the hospital is responsible for the technical component of service (all nonphysician costs including equipment, space, technicians, medical disposables, administration, registration, medical records, etc), billings and reimbursements are less than in the private office setting because of the lower overhead costs incurred by hospital-based physicians. Medicare payments range between 30% and 50% of office-based reimbursements for the same procedure.

These differences make billing for hospital-based physicians variant from private office billing. The billing process

BOX 51-1

TYPES OF HEALTHCARE SERVICE PROVIDERS

Primary care practice:

General practitioners
Family practice physicians
Internal medicine
Pediatrics
Obstetrics/gynecology

Referral specialties:

Cardiology
Urology
Neurology
Surgery (in various modes)
Psychiatry/psychology
Physiatry
Dermatology
Gastroenterology
Ophthalmology
Oncology/hematology
Pulmonology
Private Office Diagnostics
Others

Hospital-based physicians:

Radiology
  Diagnostic
  Computed tomography scanning
  Nuclear medicine
  Therapeutic
  Sonography
Pathology
  Anatomic
  Clinical
Anesthesiology
Emergency medicine

Table 51-1 Ranges of Income by Source—Nonteaching

	A,S & T	Professional patient care
Radiology	0%-10%	90%-100%
Anesthesia	0%-20%	80%-100%
Pathology	40%-60%	40%-60%
Emergency	0%-30%	70%-100%

for hospital-based physicians is encompassed in the following 10 activities:

Step 1. Patient demographic and insurance information is gathered at hospital inpatient and outpatient registration areas. This is often on-line directly to the hospital's computer system.

Step 2. Procedural and diagnosis data are gathered in departmental areas and entered into hospital systems.

Step 3. Hospital verifies insurance information and corrects data.

Step 4. Demographic and procedure data are passed to physician billing on separate files with common identification.

Table 51-2 Ranges of Income by Source—Teaching

	A,S & T	Professional patient care
Radiology	20%-40%	60%-80%
Anesthesia	20%-45%	55%-80%
Pathology	50%-75%	25%-50%
Emergency	15%-40%	60%-85%

There are a number of data elements that are critical for billing for the physician services (Box 51-2).

Step 5. Demographic data are held in a suspense data file for retrieval, as needed. Full hospital demographic files, including insurance and personal information for all newly registered inpatients and outpatients, are often transferred without determining which patients have received billable professional services and without knowing if a particular type of physician service was or will be performed. This gross approach is used to avoid the manual steps that would otherwise be necessary to select only those patients who received a billable professional service and because more than 70% of all patients receive at least one type of billable professional service. In addition, the hospital should provide discharge date information, so that demographic files can be effectively purged on a time-sensitive basis.

Step 6. As procedural data are received and entered into the physician system, a search is made for matching demographics. If the patient is an outpatient, a daily bill should be produced. If the patient is an inpatient, billing should be held until a reasonable time after discharge to ensure that all procedures for an entire stay (normally less than 6 days) can be placed on one billing episode.

Step 7. Rebilling for services not paid is optimally done automatically in 28 to 30 days from the initial bill. It is important not to require manual intervention for the performance of rebilling. Particular third parties may be put on alternative (45 or 60 day) schedules if appropriate.

Step 8. Cash is received and posted to patient accounts. This system posts allowances and bills the patient or secondary insurance for balances due, again without requiring manual intervention.

Step 9. After 2 (or 3) detail billings to patients are unpaid, the look of correspondence must change. Normally the system produces a letter format that may have wording indicating the possibility of stronger action in the future.

Step 10. Procedures not paid after the completion of all (four or five) billings are considered for collection activity. Usually fixed parameters guide the system, with exceptions reviewed by senior management or the physicians involved.

There is significant opportunity for cost savings in these processes through accuracy, automation, and assessment. Accuracy and automation help the practice or billing company operate with less personnel. Even in the era of automation, personnel costs can account for 35% to 65% of billing operational expense. Without reducing the personnel hours involved, it is practically impossible to effectively reduce the cost of billing. Assessment of operational and accuracy-related aspects of the practice's particular data capture and data flow can keep the system running smoothly and can

BOX 51-2

REQUIRED DATA ELEMENTS FOR BASIC BILLING

1. Patient's name (last name first)
2. Primary care physician (practice) unique provider identification number (UPIN)
3. Patient's date of birth
4. Patient's gender
5. Patient's relationship to insured
6. Patient's social security number
7. Insured's name (last name first)
8. Insured's address
9. Insured's social security number
10. Insured's date of birth
11. Insured's employer
12. Insured's policy number, group number
13. Procedure code(s)
14. Procedure modifier(s)
15. Diagnosis Code(s)
16. Date of service
17. Type of service
18. Place of service
19. Facility identification
20. Referring physician name
21. Referring physician UPIN
22. Performing physician (Aetna identification)
23. Date of injury/accident
24. Work related (yes/no)
25. Submitting group name
26. Submitting group number

identify needed procedural enhancements at all operational levels.

STEP 1 DRIVER(S)—ACCURACY/AUTOMATION. The most important factor is accuracy. If patient demographic and insurance information is not accurate, a tremendous amount of manual intervention will be required later to search for new information and resubmit billings. Hospitals often verify patient insurance information through on-line systems to major third parties on admission and may revise information several times during a patient stay. The value of accuracy (and the cost of inaccuracy) suggests that it is appropriate to wait until the hospital completes information verification (second or third pass information) before assimilating data for physician billing. The few days lost in this process are insignificant when compared to the positive value of more accurate information; however, this assumes that the verification and research process does occur (a not-always reliable assumption). Necessity has caused some practices to perform their own verification/reverification procedures, trading higher front-end operating costs for reduced back-end remedial and repair costs. The timing of verification for outpatient and inpatient services can also complicate this step.

Automation is also important at this step, but it is secondary to accuracy. Automated inaccurate information is worthless. Passing demographics through computer media when they are verifiably accurate will save significant data entry personnel cost. This alone can reduce personnel by 2 to 3 cost percentage points.

STEP 2 DRIVER(S)—ACCURACY/AUTOMATION. Again, upfront accuracy is most important. Accurate procedural information and CPT coding ensures appropriate reimbursement. Accurate diagnosis coding helps ensure third-party payment approval. All information should be assigned by physician or hospital personnel *after* treatment or procedure. Automation of accurate data through transfer by computer media can save the billings system 2 to 3 cost percentage points.

STEPS 3 & 4 DRIVER(S)—ASSESSMENT. Just as the hospital verifies insurance information, the billing system must constantly evaluate the accuracy and timeliness of information received. Verification of data completeness is extremely important because incomplete information will nearly always cause a claim submission to fail. A system to check physician billings against hospital departmental logs on a daily or weekly basis is critical to ensure that all procedures performed were actually billed. This step can be performed by accessing hospital departmental scheduling and service performance records/systems through direct link or electronic format transfer—or simply by manual checks of written patient presentation or sequentially numbered service logs.

STEP 5 DRIVER(S)—ASSESSMENT/AUTOMATION. A constant evaluation process will ensure that patient demographics are adequate for billing purposes. The system should allow for an automatic match and merge of procedural and demographic information, rather than using the data as a massive database.

STEP 6 DRIVER(S)—ASSESSMENT/AUTOMATION. Bills to third parties and patients should generate without human intervention once all necessary information is present. Sending bills electronically rather than on paper HCFA 1500 forms will speed payment tremendously. In fact, Medicare must, by regulation, hold billings submitted on paper for up to 6 weeks. Verification (assessment) that billings have been received is part of the process that is often not quality controlled.

STEP 7 DRIVER(S)—AUTOMATION/ASSESSMENT. Automatic rebilling is an essential element of any effective billing system. Manual intervention cannot be relied upon, nor is it affordable, except in the smallest of practices. The system must have set parameters to issue new billings for outstanding charges within 35 days for self-pay balances, 35 to 40 days for insurance receivables, and immediately upon receipt of a partial payment. The liquidation of receivables at the end of various billing cycles must be reviewed. By looking at how payments "step through the system," by billing cycle, it is often possible to identify which cycle is ineffective in the collection of outstanding claims and self-pay debts. The elimination or reduction of these cycles can be accomplished, with a positive effect on actual collections and cost savings.

STEP 8 DRIVER(S)—ACCURACY/AUTOMATION. Accurate and timely posting of claims is needed for public relations. If patients are allowed to fall into another billing cycle after they have been notified by insurance that a claim has been paid, it reflects poorly on the practice and may reduce referrals. At the very least, it will result in phone calls and increases the need for personnel.

STEP 9 & 10 DRIVER(S)—ASSESSMENT/AUTOMATION. Automatic entry into deeper phases of the collection process will generally both reduce cost and increase collections. Collection accounts must be reviewed to ensure that collection agencies are not collecting easy dollars. An in-house phone collection system may be well advised for high dollar (>$50) amounts.

Physician Needs Adjunctive to Billing, Collections, and MIS

Traditional Needs (Apart from Basic Practice Billing)

CPT-4 CODING. Submission of claims using the Current Procedure Terminology (CPT-4) system developed and maintained by the American Medical Association and/or the HCPCS system (***H***CFA ***C***ommon ***P***rocedure ***C***oding ***S***ystem) is universally required in order to be paid by third parties. Many systems require that the physician supply the service and procedure codes. This approach is normally fairly accurate and puts the responsibility and the reward in the same hands.

Billing companies who assume coding responsibility may charge an additional 0.5 to 1.5 percentage point (assuming their fee is a percent of collected funds) for the additional service, or an additional $.50 to $1.50 per case, if a flat fee is charged. Some billers expect to provide coding as part of their regular service, and a few **require** that they perform the coding (a potentially dangerous relationship because the biller's motives and provider's risk may be at cross purposes).

Experienced coders regularly command salaries in excess of $30,000 per annum. Physicians must realize that even if they delegate the activity, they cannot escape the responsibility and the liability of prosecution under Medicare's Fraud and Abuse and/or the False Claims Act. The physician is *always* responsible for correct coding.

ICD-9 CM CODING. The ICD-9 CM system for diagnosis coding is also universally required. This coding is normally performed by practice or hospital nonphysician personnel. Without correct codes, payment for services may be denied. Caution must be used to provide a proximate clinical diagnosis rather than accepting and using admitting diagnosis.

AUTOMATED REGISTRATION. Automated reregistration of returning patients presumes there is a database retention of patient demographics on a majority of patients seen. Although this may be feasible for most general practitioners, hospital-based physicians generally see so many different patients (up to 60,000 a year for a typical radiology practice, and as many as 120,000 or more) that information storage can become prohibitive for "small" systems.

An atypical patient numbering system can enhance the data retention and reregistration process. The typical method is to use the hospital's numbering system, which routinely assigns a new number for each encounter; the alternate method is to use a permanent numbering system such as Social Security Number as the basis for storage of long-term database information on each patient. Systems able to hold large files of patient demographics allow billing on a rolling charge and credit basis and even enhance collection efforts at the time of new visit scheduling or registration by affording the registrar the opportunity to ask for past due and bad debt balances.

ON LINE INSURANCE VERIFICATION. On line insurance verification is often offered through a link to insurance company data banks. As government programs move more toward managed care, they will offer similar programs.

LINE ITEM POSTING. Line item posting allows individual payments to be posted in association with individual procedure codes, by line item. This approach allows verification of individual third party allowances and payments and identifies denials by service type. It also allows multispecialty systems to allocate income by specialty group.

INSURANCE CARRIER INTERFACE. Insurance carrier interface will enable the practice to determine eligibility and required deductibles and co-pays upon patient presentation. Any system will need to interface with already existent third-party programs.

Newer Needs (Relating to Risk Assumption and Integration)

PREVENTIVE CARE ASSESSMENT. As groups assume financial and medical responsibility for groups of patients, systems will need to assist in the process of initial patient medical assessments and identification of problem pathologies. Groups will need to schedule proactive visits to prevent more serious episodes of care.

CHART ARCHIVING AND RETRIEVAL. In order for groups to perform quality assurance functions and medical reviews in capitated systems, there will need to be on-line access to detail charts.

CLINICAL PROTOCOLS. Specialty physician organizations are moving toward diagnostic-based clinical protocols. The systems will be designed to suggest an evaluation and treatment pathway that is both medically correct and cost effective. The systems will be used proactively to suggest patterns of care and retrospectively to judge the treatment patterns of individual physicians in aggregated groups. For example, 95% of consultations with a urology specialist require that the urologist have in hand some type of specialized study (i.e., a urogram). Often a patient is referred to the physician specialist, the specialist orders the needed study, and the patient must return for a second consultation after study reports are available. A clinical (critical) pathway system will require or encourage performance of needed studies before any consultation, eliminating the need for a second specialist visit and the associated cost.

CAPITATION MODULES. Within the next 5 years, it is likely that 30% to 40% percent of patient care will be paid through capitated programs. Unlike traditional fee for service, capitated programs pay a fixed fee for a certain menu of services to a certain population segment without regard to the actual number or intensity of services rendered. In essence, the physician accepting capitation is becoming an insurance company. Physician billing systems in all physician segments will need to report utilization by diagnosis, plan physician, insurance plan segment, and multiple other variations on request. They must be able to obtain data from multiple referral screens (i.e., ordering physician to primary physician to gatekeeper) and provide on line patient and procedural program eligibility standards.

PATIENT COMPLIANCE MODULE. Patient compliance with proscribed medical service will be essential to efficient patient care delivery. When a diagnostic test is ordered, how does primary care know whether the test was actually performed? How can primary care track compliance with medication directions to keep patients healthy and out of the acute care setting? Automated systems that are interactive with ancillary service providers will be required.

Overall Systems Considerations. All systems, whether new or traditional, will need to provide for high level database retrieval and user-defined report writing. Systems will need to network both locally and over wide areas dictated by insurance regions. Moving toward more sophisticated information processing systems will not be less expensive; it will be more expensive. ***The goal is not to reduce outlays for the information and processing system, but rather to use a more extensive and flexible system to manage and reduce the cost of medical care delivery.***

Ancillary Business Needs. To provide product differentiation and a more seamless approach to the business side of medicine, many information processing companies will provide adjunctive business services. These services not only enhance the relationship with the physician customer, but also may instill some element of control over reimbursement rates, which ultimately affect the dollars that can be charged for information services. The listing of administrative services in Box 51-3 is included for consideration.

Key Drivers of Performance by Physician Segment

Certain key elements affect the income-generating ability of healthcare organizations, including physician groups, universally. In the physician segment these are geographic environs, practice employed personnel, charges per billable encounter, and service contracts entered.

BOX 51-3

ADMINISTRATIVE SERVICES

1. **Management, Bookkeeping, and Financial Reporting**
   - -Payroll/Bonuses
   - -Accounts Payable Management
   - -General Ledger Management
   - -Checkbook Management
   - -Purchasing
   - -Cash Management
   - -Budgeting/Revenue and Expense
   - -Financial Reporting & Monthly Statements
   - -Year-End Close Out
   - -Tax Returns/Quarterly Payroll, Other (except income tax)
   - -Withholding Depositories
   - -Banking/Lines of Credit
   - -Pension Funding/Calculations/Reporting
2. **Organization and Governance**
   - -Employment Agreements, Restrictive Covenants
   - -Independent Contractor Agreements
   - -Pension Documents
   - -Review of Corporate Meetings/Minutes
   - -Determination of Practice Structure
   - -Professional Corporations (S-Corp, C-Corp)
   - -Partnerships/Nonprofits
   - -Entity Start Up
   - -Equity and Voting Control Agreements (Shareholder Agreements)
   - -Capitalization
   - -Buy/Sell Agreements
   - -Selection of Advisors (Legal, Accounting, Insurance, Pension)
   - -Real Estate Partnerships
   - -Practice Valuation
   - -Officers/Compliance Requirements
3. **Staffing and Compensation**
   - -Physician Compensation/Income Distribution
   - -Pension Structure/Top Heavy Testing
   - -Workload Trends, Forecasts
   - -Physician Training Seminars
   - -Physician Staffing Analysis and Design
4. **Benefits Planning & Operation**
   - -Health Benefits
   - -Life and Disability Benefits
   - -Worker's Compensation
   - -General Liability
   - -Property and Casualty
   - -Professional Liability/Malpractice and Excess Coverage
   - -Trustee Insurance
   - -Medical Education
   - -Support Staff Benefits
   - -Salary Continuation Plans
   - -Travel, Dues, and Journals
   - -Cafeteria Plans
   - -Medical Education Reimbursement Plan (MERP)
   - -Professional Education Reimbursement Plan (PERP)
   - -Voluntary Employee Benefits Association
5. **Revenue Management/Enhancement**
   - -A/R Analysis
   - -Cash Flow Analysis
   - -Coding/Reimbursement Review and Training
   - -Fee Schedule Analysis/Development
   - -Collection Services Selection
   - -Data Collection (lost charges)/Count Controls
   - -Assignment Accounts
   - -Par/Nonpar Decisions
   - -Monthly/Quarterly Reporting
   - -Public Relations
6. **Hospital and Other Contractual Relationships**
   - -Hospital Contract Development/Review and Negotiation
   - -Hospital Support Funding (A, S & T)
   - -Service Contract Development/Review and Negotiation
   - -Review of Hospital Medical Staff By-Laws
   - -Review/Development of Managed Care Contracts
   - -Rental Agreements
7. **Strategic Planning**
   - -Referral Source Analysis
   - -Procedure Mix Analysis
   - -Competitive Positioning
   - -Feasibility Studies/New Ventures
   - -Medicare Fraud and Abuse Compliance Audit/Support
   - -HCFA/Third Party Dispute(s)
   - -Joint Ventures
   - -PHO Integration
   - -MSO Integration
   - -Practice Mergers/Acquisitions

HCFA, Health care financing administration; *PHO*, physician-hospital organization; *MSO*, management services organization.

Geographic Environs. The most important income parameter is location. Location dictates the third-party mix and therefore average payments per activity. It is not unusual to have similar practice groups performing the same service at different locations in the same city with as much as a 100% difference in net physician income. Service providers aiming to maximize income look toward middle class locales with high private insurance penetration. Large, dominant health maintenance organizations (HMOs) or even indemnity plans tend to push down potential earnings through fee controls.

Traditionally, practices have steered away from areas of high Medicaid concentration. Although this still may be true, Medicaid reimbursements in many areas now can approach HMO and Medicare payments. Medicaid-insured patients also may be more desirable than self-pay populations.

Practice Employed Personnel. Practices that employ their own personnel are less often a target for provision of outside business services. Many business functions are performed incident to other services. The infusion of another element of business service generally cannot provide offsetting cost reductions. The billing service provider must concentrate on tools for practice staff to use, rather than on systems designed to eliminate staffing.

On the other hand, practices that employ no personnel will resist systems that require them to take on the cost and administrative burdens associated with large contingents of nonphysician personnel. The exception to this case is the physician or group highly motivated by control over minute aspects of billing function.

Various types of employed personnel can cause variances in provider payments for services rendered. As primary care groups begin to depend more on nurse practitioners and/or physician assistants overall practice income will be enhanced while the income per billable encounter decreases. In the anesthesiology marketplace, various third-party programs will reimburse differently depending on whether the physician or the hospital employs nurse anesthetists.

Charges Per Billable Encounter. Charges per billable encounter depend mostly on the mix of service offerings of the medical provider. Surgical subspecialties provide the highest income per billable unit (mostly in the thousands), whereas diagnostic services, some of which may not even require hands-on physician intervention, will provide the lowest. Although the high dollar per encounter would provide a billing company with the highest potential margin per billing expenditure, there is less need to outsource the function or even computerize data manipulation because of the much lower volume of services (one appendectomy versus ten pathology slides), which allows the practice to handle some billing activities at no increased marginal cost because staff are in-house for other functions and often have time available.

Service Contracts Entered. Service contracts will not only determine the procedural reimbursement pattern of the practice, but also serve to define billing methodology. Many practices accept deep discounts and capitated programs to attract or retain a patient base. Many contract programs are settling toward "percentage of Medicare" payment schemes at between 80% and 120% of Medicare payment levels. With contracted capitation programs, the billing function becomes information management rather than billing and receivables management.

Impact on Billing Service Providers (Table 51-3). We believe that the highest potential net revenue for billing services is outsource operations oriented toward outpatient/ambulatory and office-based referral specialties with a middle income clientelle. Those practices with per physician volumes high enough to make in-house (rather than outsourced) solutions less desirable, but with volumes that are low enough to maintain high income per encounter, will have the best potential for (biller) profitability. These specialties include radiology, radiation oncology, hospital-based anesthesia, and anatomic pathology.

Although these referral specialties may provide the highest return in the near term, consideration also must be given to the future progress of healthcare. Solutions and services need to be offered to larger, control-oriented organizations as part of their vertical integration efforts. These will either be **p**hysician **h**ospital **o**rganizations or **p**hysician **o**rganizations controlled by primary care specialists. Those billing organizations that adapt to the needs of new entities will have the greatest growth and profit potential and will have the greatest likelihood of long-term success.

BILLING SERVICE INDUSTRY DEFINITION

Operational Workflows and Processes

Overview. Commercial* billing organizations can be divided into six size categories. The size of each company is a function of the number of employees and clients and the annual company revenue, as shown in Table 51-4.

*Billers who charge a fee for their services and invoice their unrelated, unaffiliated customers. This *excludes* "internal" billers who provide services for their "owners," such as multisite practices and some hospitals. A few hybrids offer both internal and legitimate retail services, such as MedBill, owned by Coastal; MedTrust (Dallas, Tx) a subsidiary of Metroplex Emergency Services; and VoiçeBillStat, a subsidiary of InPhyNet.

Table 51-3 Typical Medical Practice Billing Performance Inhouse Billing Versus Outsourced Billing

	Emergency medicine		
	Inhouse	Typical	Biller
Average charge	125	105	140
Average adjustment	28	23	35
Average payment	78	72	80
Services/day/doctor	40	35	40
A/R days	75	90	80
Bad debt %	9-12	12-15	10-13
Bad debt rec. %	20	15	18
Bad debt collection cost	30%	25-30%	28%
Billing costs			
% of payments	9	10	11
Per encounter	7	7	9
Per procedure	6	6	8
% Practice cost	9	10	11
% Labor	35	0-40	-0-
% Non-labor	65	0-60	100

Reprinted with permission from: Brandywine Healthcare Services, Inc., 1994.

Table 51-4 Billing Organizations Sample

	Est.#	Revenue	Clients	Employees
Mom and Pop	1000	<$300 K	1-9	3-8
Mom and Pop	350	$300-750 K	6-18	8-15
Company	200	$750 K-$1.2 M	12-24	15-30
Company	110	$1-3 M	18-30	25-60
Corp.	30	$3-12 M	24-48	75-200
Public Corp.	10	>$12 M	>48	>200
Totals	1700	$2.1 B	>15,000	>15,800

Billing companies serve both hospital-based (Radiology, Pathology, Anesthesiology and Emergency Medicine) and office-based practices (e.g., family medicine, internal medicine, pediatrics, obstetrics/gynecology), as well as a variety of other healthcare providers, including ambulance companies, durable medical equipment (DME) companies, home healthcare and home infusion therapy, chiropractors, dentists, and physical therapists. Generally, billers charge in one of two ways: a percentage of **collected** funds, or a flat fee per unit (visit, bill, claim, etc.). Medicare regulations require that billers deposit all federally paid funds into the provider's account and prohibit the biller from having any control over the account into which funds are deposited. Billers typically invoice for their services, in contrast to the collection agency industry, which typically controls the client's funds and deducts related fees from the collected payments.

Although there are both generalists and specialists among billers, the majority of companies specialize in certain medical disciplines. Between 70% and 80% of all billers currently bill for hospital-based practices, although there is now a clear trend to greater use of billers for office-based practices. This trend is dually driven by the billers' interest in expanding their businesses and the market's need for a more capable source of billing performance, particularly among practices owned by institutions and practice corporations. The latter (PhyCor, CareMark, Genesis) is a fairly new phenomenon, and while the predisposition is to provide all services internally, it is likely that a business niche will emerge for a commercial provider to support a rapidly growing or geographically divided practice corporation.

The economics of the billing industry have been relatively predictable in the past, although the level of detail to which (and therefore the amount of potential variability) the economic measurements are/can be made is quite extensive. The recent slowing of medical inflation, downward pressure on physician payments, and managed care growth have all had a significant impact on the factors used to measure medical billing costs and performance.

The general costs billers incur are personnel and management, workspace, technology, supplies, utilities, and postage. Labor and benefits are the largest single cost, representing approximately 50% to 55% of an operations budget. The profitability of a billing company, therefore, has been significantly affected by the management (or lack thereof) of labor and benefit costs. In the future, that success will, in many markets, rely in part or wholly on technology and management expertise related to administration of managed care contracts. Unlike traditional billing arrangements, managed care represents a paradigm shift in the work and processes required to perform "billing" services, which will rely on service reporting (not a claim form), retrospective analysis of fee-for-service equivalent financial results, and prospective contract modeling and analysis.

Workflow. The basis of all professional fee billing is a patient service by a provider, usually defined as a physician, although a physician assistant, certified nurse practitioner, and other paraprofessionals are also considered providers. The basic inputs of professional billing are the following:

- The patient's **identity** and sufficient information to allow the services to be billed to the appropriate party(s);

  Labor: 10% *Nonlabor:* 10%

- Identification of the **service(s)/product(s)** to be billed via a coded [CPT-4] service(s) list;

  Labor: 5% *Nonlabor:* 5%

- The **reason(s)** the service(s)/product(s) were provided via a coded [ICD-9 CM] diagnosis;

  Labor: 2% *Nonlabor:* 5%

- Transmission of the **billing** information to the source(s) responsible for payment;

  Labor: 2% *Nonlabor:* 10%

- Receipt, **posting, and banking** of the payment(s) and claim adjudication outcomes;

  Labor: 10% *Nonlabor:* 10%

- **Resolution of problems** delaying or preventing payment that are identified by the insurer(s) and/or the patient;

  Labor: 10% *Nonlabor:* 10%

- Recording and **reporting** the results of billing to the clients who have hired the biller to provide services;

  Labor: 2% *Nonlabor:* 10%

  TOTAL: 40% TOTAL: 60%

Although simple to list, the seven building blocks further divide and subdivide according to the specialty served, the logistics of the relationship, the quality of the data, the accuracy of the identification of services and diagnosis, and other parameters. Most billers make reasonable efforts to simplify and accelerate the processes without compromising the accuracy and thoroughness of their work. The best billers work daily to master the processes that can be managed and/or modified to produce the quickest, best billing outcome.

Discussed below are the finer increments of activity, the variables that apply to practice types (private office versus hospital based) and some specialties that have material differences in the work or data flow.

DATA COLLECTION. Patient identity and coverage information are collected in a variety of ways, depending on the patient's point of access to the healthcare system.

- For "REAP" (***R***adiology, ***E***mergency Medicine, ***A***nesthesia, ***P***athology) physicians, the hospital registration staff collects the patient's data. Problematic variables include the following:
  - Data supplied on paper, despite the universal ability of hospital systems to permit electronic transfer.
  - Data (electronic or paper) that do not contain the coverage information applicable to the patient's coverage for *physician* services.
  - Barely adequate to extremely poor data completeness and/or accuracy in *most* cases. This is attributable to poor training and/or supervision of the registration staff.
  - Replication/perpetuation of previously recorded information that, although it has changed, is not updated.
  - Rare or ineffective efforts to collect payment (hospital or physician) at the time of service.
- Billers who must overcome the data quality related problems frequently incur additional costs without additional revenue opportunity, as providers are not routinely willing to admit (or resolve even when they *are* willing to admit) that they are responsible for ensuring data quality. Some enterprising billers have turned a problem into an opportunity by offering to **staff** the client's registration activities. Although this does not change the flow, it does improve the quality and further "locks in" the biller's relationship. (Imagine firing the biller and having to start over—from scratch—restaffing the registration function.)

CODING. Assignment of CPT-4 (services-procedures) and ICD-9 CM (diagnosis) codes are a required and critical part of the billing process. The person(s) who assign the codes, their qualifications and expertise, the timing of assignment, and the documentation that supports the codes all play an important part in the generation of a charge, the timeliness of bill submission, the predictability of prompt payment, and the protection of the physician from penalties assessed by federal payers for "overcoding."

- For REAP physicians, the coding of services include the following problematic variables:
  - Coding by hospital personnel routinely diminishes the gross and net income of a practice, as the hospital's employees are not adequately aware of the specialized coding requirements of a medical practice. Even when the coding is "the same" for both providers (hospital and physician) the coding decisions are often necessarily different.
  - In radiology, the service billed by both parties *should* be the same, but it is not in every case.
  - Documentation by emergency physicians is a source of high risk, particularly in view of the newly implemented Documentation Guidelines. Improper coding, ineffective documentation, or both are more likely if the coding is performed by the hospital, although physicians also do not often make good coders.
  - Anesthesiology professional fee coding is unique. It **must** be performed by a qualified coder; substantial income losses are risked if an untrained coder is used.
- Billing companies accrue an income and "benefit" opportunity if they have the ability to offer a solution to these coding problems. They can frequently command a higher fee rate or separately bill for coding and coding-related services. This is particularly true for hospital-based practices, where coding support is often viewed as a part of the standard service. In most cases, coding support allows the addition of $1.00 to 1.50 per case, or the percentage equivalent to a billing fee.

The coding step, if performed by the biller, is either carried out by a biller-employed on-site (in the practice location) staff or coded as the first step on receipt of the chart/medical record to be coded.

DATA TRANSFER. The transfer of data from the collection site to the billing provider is an area of ongoing difficulty, particularly for hospital-based practices, but also for office practices. All hospitals are automated, but their internal ability to accommodate data transfer requests/requirements is inconsistent at best. The hospital's internal dataset (the data element "slots" into which data can be placed) is not a stable and constant structure. There are vendor and hospital maintenance and frequent internally and externally generated changes, such as new fields required by a payor or a clinical department, any of which can corrupt an existing data transfer program/utility, compromising a transfer routine that was working. This is due to the usual approach of "hard-coding" the data transfer software; when the data source has new fields and/or values in it, the transfer program "crashes" on arrival in the biller's system. Although the biller could accommodate the change(s), the hospital or vendor rarely remembers to advise the recipients of the changes they have made.

Many hospitals resist requests for electronic data transfer, explaining "we don't want to" as "we can't" or "our software vendor doesn't support it." In the latter cases, the default solution is to transfer data on paper by courier, express carrier, or mail. This also increases the biller's *costs* by approximately $.70 to $1.20 per case for data entry. More and more billers are taking the position that electronic transfer is part of their pricing, and manual transfer is accommodated as an additional-fee service.

Office practices that use a billing service are frequently manual. In these cases, the data move on paper by courier, courier service, or mail. Those that are automated tend to use the system provided by the billing service. The latter provides the additional benefit to the practice of being able to transact over-the-counter payments and saves the biller the costs of data entry.

DATA ENTRY. Entry of CPT-4 and ICD-9 CM codes is routine for all but some radiology and pathology practices, where the hospital's services are an *exact* match to the physician's. (**Note:** The latter is *never* true of emergency practices.) The entry of the data, which may also include the previously-mentioned manual registration data, should be batched (smaller, less competent billers are not always used to this discipline) as part of the data entry process. In most medium and large billing organizations, the data entry process is a stand-alone function. Smaller billers combine data entry with billing or other functions, usually because their staff is too small to separate this effort.

BILL PRODUCTION AND CLAIM SUBMISSION. This function has evolved rapidly over the last 5 years. A significant portion of all physician claims are now submitted electronically; the paper portion will continue to shrink from the currently estimated 35% to 40% to less than 15% by 1998 (our prediction). Most payers and billing software vendors are making it as easy as possible to submit electronic claims.

Actual bill production normally occurs daily. Some (small) billers schedule bill production 2 or 3 days a week, some only once a week. In the latter case, the limiting factor is usually the biller's software vendor, with only a weekly capability being offered.

Claim production should occur within 3 days of the date of service (+/− an allowance for weekends). The best billers have an established, regular ability to bill within 1 day of the date of service (the "gold" standard). Billers who produce bills more than 3 days from the date of service are performing below acceptable levels unless there is clear evidence of insurmountable mitigating circumstances.

Electronic claim submission is handled by a variety of methods.

- Direct submission by the biller to the payor by modem, tape, or diskette(s). Timing is usually affected by the payor's schedule/requirements; most payors who accept electronic claims pay once a week, with a fixed cut-off day for each week (e.g., claims in by Wednesday will be paid by Monday). The cost of this method is nearly zero, except for media and/or shipping costs of tape(s) or diskette(s).
- Indirect submission by the biller through a clearinghouse (or several). Submission schedules are similar to those described previously. The costs associated with clearinghouse services vary, but are currently $.15 to $.50; some large billers have leveraged lower rates, including free.
- Direct data entry. Some payors accept electronic claims, which are in reality manually input claims entered through an online terminal in the biller's office. The advantage of this alternative is faster payment; the biller incurs all of the payor's data entry costs that the payor would incur if the claim were submitted on paper. This method is used only by small, inexperienced billing companies. It adds to the biller's data entry costs and can amount to $.60 to $.80 per claim or more, plus equipment and line charges.

The average cost of this step has been falling steadily over the last 5 years. Managed care will not eliminate this step, as it is replaced by the "report of service" (a no-charge bill); in fact, the timing and cost of the latter may actually increase this cost component to a higher number in the short term (3 to 6 years).

CLAIM TRACKING AND FOLLOW-UP. Billers are typically fairly diligent in their management of unpaid insurance claims. The timing of their efforts varies; some are more aggressive and focused, whereas others are more passive and generalized. Surprisingly, both strategies can be appropriately defended, depending on the specialty, region, and software system used by the biller.

Claim tracking is primarily a software feature that allows the user to recognize, by payor, the aged and unpaid claims owed (an expectation that may ultimately prove false) by a particular payor. This might be used for example to recognize the atypical drop in claim resolution by a certain Blue Shield plan, suggesting that an entire batch of claims has been lost or sidetracked in the adjudication process.

In all cases, follow-up is driven by the biller's computer system. Follow-up is the active pursuit of the problem by telephone and/or correspondence. Some of the more aggressive billers even resort to in-person follow-up with large payment sources where significant amounts of receivable are affected by a single payor. In the latter case, billers who represent providers with an aggregate receivable of $1M++ can easily cost justify in-person follow-up, even if it involves air travel. This step is often preemptive; an initial visit diminishes the likelihood that future visits will be needed because the payor is made aware of the extremes to which the biller will go to ensure prompt payment. In addition, the visit establishes a level of communication with the individuals involved in claim processing, allows the biller to identify and prevent internal problems that interfere with the payor's prompt payment, and heightens the vigilance of each organization to problems and payment delays.

The timing of the follow-up process is typically between 28 and 45 days from the date of billing. (Some systems track both service and billing dates. For those that do not, service date is the default, with a soft adjustment made to allow for the time between service and billing.)

Larger billers assign follow-up to specialists who develop successful relationships with payor staff and who have a demonstrated talent for high productivity and resourcefulness in resolving unpaid claims. Smaller billers and most office practices expect the billing personnel to perform both tasks; this approach usually proves to be suboptimal for follow-up results.

PAYMENT POSTING. The workflow process for payment posting is fairly straightforward. Payments are received by the biller's office, routed to a post office box, or received by a bank lockbox, with copies forwarded to the biller's office. In the latter case, the lockbox fees are a negotiated item; some billers absorb the cost, but many require the client to pay the fees. Large billers have been somewhat successful in eliminating fees in exchange for a large flow of cash through a single bank. (Remember that it is illegal for a biller to deposit funds into its own escrow account.)

Electronic claims are now mirrored by electronic remittance capabilities from a limited number of payors. Payment posting is thereby automated, allowing the biller to reduce its labor costs. Nevertheless, only a small number of billers (approximately 10% to 12%) have mastered the complex task of electronic remittance, which is far more challenging than electronic billing. This will grow in the future and should become synonymous with electronic submission, for at least 70% to 80% of all electronic claims.

A constant problem that may worsen in the future is the misrouting of payments owed to physicians to the hospital's business office. This is particularly problematic for practices owned by the hospital, ownership of which requires the biller to use the hospital's tax ID number on the physician's claim(s). Because most insurers index their check issuing to a tax ID number, *all* payments end up at the hospital, thus delaying the timely posting of payments and creating follow-up efforts for claims that have already been paid without the biller's knowledge. Hospital business offices are typically unresponsive in facilitating an ongoing solution to this problem.

To be optimally effective, payment posting also should provide for the comparison of the payment received to the expected or contracted payment. Billers who do not have the systems capability (or who have it and do not use it) compromise their effectiveness for their clients or perform the function manually. In the latter case, although it may not disrupt the efficient flow of work, it adds an operational cost that can be avoided.

Finally, many members of the billing industry have not effectively dealt with the issue of internal controls and separation of duties. Although lockboxes provide a major protection from embezzlement, many billers do not adequately control the workflow and duties to sufficiently protect themselves and their client from dishonest employees. In our experience, virtually all billers are eventually victimized by a dishonest employee, but many companies do not carry fidelity bond coverage.

CLAIMS APPEAL AND REBILLING. Adjudication errors are a way of life in healthcare billing. The number and type of "errors" suggest that, in many cases, adverse determinations are a deliberate tactic to avoid, or at least delay, payment. Although error rates vary considerably among payors, payment errors of 10% to 20% are fairly common. Paper claims produce more errors because of data entry errors in the payor's shop, manual handling of claims, and a "lost claim" factor that is markedly reduced (but not eliminated) by electronic submission. Electronic submission does not eliminate payment errors, but it can reduce them by half. Diligent billers build into their system a process to catch erroneous payments and to challenge denials. These steps are triggered by the payment receipt, the receipt of a claim denial, or the expiration of a predetermined time limit (no reply to a submitted claim for XX days).

As discussed earlier, short payments are detected, leading to a resubmission of the claim with a request for full payment. This process can be automated, although few billers have accomplished this. The billing industry has not acknowledged that the personnel who post payments are not actually capable of remembering the details of each payor's *proper* payment for each CPT-4 code. In addition, many billers, especially the smaller and medium sized ones, do not have the software capable of tracking payments for each payor. Many commercial billing software packages still do not have this capability, despite years of evidence that payment tracking is useful and cost effective. We have also observed billers who have software capability for payment surveillance, but do not use it.

In the case of denials, review of the adjudication notice and the decision about what to do is, by necessity, a manual effort. Generation of the rebilling is often automated. However, the process also requires an extra step to match the rebill with the correspondence (from the payor and the biller's reply).

The most frequently automated step is the scheduled rebilling of unanswered claims. The most sophisticated billers tailor the timing of this step *by payor,* but most take a more crude approach and simply rebill everything at a single interval, typically 30 days. The former approach is far more effective (and cost effective) and is based on research and recordkeeping on the payment patterns of each payor. Rebilling too soon wastes effort and money because the payment may already be en route; rebilling too late creates opportunity costs if the rebilling is the cause of the payment.

PATIENT STATEMENTS. As deductibles and coinsurance amounts continue to rise, and as more first dollar payors impose deductibles and co-payments, billing of patients has become a crucial part of the successful biller's activity. Not only does it produce cash flow and information flow (patients will call to offer information instead of payment), statements also identify wrong addresses and indirectly measure the quality of the registration process.

The scheduling and production of statements vary among billers, but fall into several patterns:

- A rolling anniversary method, in which the first statement establishes a date from which all future statements are triggered. Statements are usually produced daily or, at most, weekly.
- A "grouping/batch" method, in which the statements are aggregated by alphabetic groups (A-G, H-O, P-Z) or payor types (Medicare, commercial insurance, self-pay), and statements are issued semiweekly or weekly.
- A monthly date. This is the least efficient and the most disruptive to client cash flow and the workflow in the billing office because of the timing delays built into the system. The billers using this method are either extremely unsophisticated or are using a weak system that only supports this approach.

The interval timing of statements also varies. The less creative billers/systems extend the statement process to 30-day intervals for as long as the account has a balance, despite ample evidence that statements beyond the first three to four produce no marginal value to the client or the biller. Better management of the statement process includes variable statement interval timing (e.g., the first one after 21 days, the second after 15 days, etc.), variable schedules by payor type (Medicare, self-pay, commercial, etc.), and/or Zip Code. In addition, astute billers pay attention to the local community being billed; if the local economy is based on employers who pay biweekly, weekly, or semimonthly, statement production is targeted to the predominant pay-day cycles.

Patient statements often have messages added to them as part of the printing process. The most sophisticated systems allow for variable messages, by payor and event (partial payment, denial, missed installment payment, etc.) and for individualized messages that are input by a billing employee. Other systems force the user to be more crude; statements that are advanced in urgency/aggressiveness based on the statement number (first, second, third), with frequent unintended consequences.

Most systems and billers are now using Zip Code sorting to reduce postage expense; better still are those that use nine digit zip (added, if not supplied by the practice) and bar coding. Some billers now use an outside production service vendor who can provide the more sophisticated levels of mail handling.

SELF-PAY FOLLOW-UP. True self-pay follow-up is largely a myth in the billing industry. The economies of the billing industry do not often allow for the provision of a high-cost, low-return service. Most collectors can only generate six to eight completed follow-up calls an hour, or about 40 to 50 a day. Assuming that 25% of those contacted actually pay **in full** (an optimistic expectation), a collector will only generate about a dozen payments a day. If the collector's salary and overhead costs are viewed as a collection fee, those costs must not exceed 20% of the payments produced; otherwise the return on investment is too low for the biller to support.

Because self-pay balances are frequently small—$20 to $100—the marginal opportunity for the biller is routinely not worth the cost. The customers, on the other hand, are not impressed by the business problem facing the biller and expect that the biller is performing the service. Most billers perpetuate this perception, but few actually live up to it.

Large scale billers are able to consider investment in predictive dialing systems or other collection agency-oriented systems. These collection tools allow for larger billers to be more competitive because the price of entry is greater than $100,000 provided they have the volume to keep the system busy. In cases where the biller is part of a collection agency, or the reverse, the billing efforts may be further leveraged by the technical and skill assets of the collection organization.

In the latter case, there is an inherent conflict of interest because most collectors charge a higher percentage of collections. Common ownership creates the conflict. Some organizations have addressed this issue by offering a blended rate that includes both services for a single price. This approach has been satisfactory to some, but not all, billing clients.

Billers who devise a way to apply carefully selected collection efforts to accounts with a high probability of recovery are often rewarded with increased customer loyalty and higher profits because the client's perception is that the biller has a collection department. This cherry-picking method is less often found than expected, primarily because of the lack of insight in the billing industry with regard to the science of collections.

CONTRACT COMPLIANCE MONITORING. Conceptually, billers are viewed as responsible for monitoring and managing payor-related contractual relationships for their clients. This is a highly fragmented and poorly focused aspect of the service offering for many billers, primarily because of their lack of experience in an area of rapidly changing requirements and newly emerging relationships.

Monitoring a managed care contract requires many elements:

- Preauthorization. Identification of which services must be preauthorized, ensuring that the preauthorization is secured and submitted, and that the payment was not deferred or delayed inappropriately because of a preauthorization issue.
- Included and covered services. Many capitated plans itemize the services covered by a capitation payment, allowing for fee-for-service billing of non-cap services. Unless all services are tracked, many billable services may go unbilled, forfeiting income and undervaluing the cash contribution of a contract.
- Some services are capped at a time-related frequency or threshold. Unless the services provided are tracked, a provider may continue to provide a service that is either billable (exceeding the cap) or free (included in the cap, which was predicated on a typical frequency level).
- Some services are covered by a provision in the provider's independent stop-loss insurance policy. In this instance, the biller must be aware of the policy, know which services may be subject to stop-loss, know when to trigger a claim to the stop-loss carrier, and be sure that the loss is covered.
- Some services are governed by a step-down (or step-up) provision, which increases or decreases the payments for services based on threshold volumes. The biller must know which services are so governed and when the triggering level has been achieved.
- Each managed care contract is unique. Unless the biller receives a copy, the biller is unable to properly format its contract management efforts. It is common, not only for the biller not to have a copy of the agreement, but also for the provider not to have a copy!

Less than 5% of all billers have software that provides an automated means of monitoring and/or managing contract compliance. We believe that this will be a pivotal need for all providers and their billers before the end of the century nationwide. Some markets will evolve more rapidly and reach a higher level of managed care penetration, whereas others will be slower and/or less penetrated. However, this capability is already needed but missing, and the need will increase in the next few years.

Billers who provide some support for this need currently provide it for no additional charge or provide it on a project-related basis for a consulting fee. This will become a significant new or replacement revenue source for billing companies. As managed care becomes a significant share of the claims processed, billers will develop a variety of methods for charging: a percent of the capitation payment; a per-transaction fee; a PM/PM (per member, per month) charge, just as the payor pays the provider; a monthly retainer/flat fee; or some combination. When coupled with the cash and strategic value of contract monitoring, billers may be able to improve their own net revenue because the cost of providing some of these new services will actually require less staff resources, albeit more technology resources.

PERFORMANCE REPORTING. Billers typically provide some level of reporting for their clients. The frequency is most often monthly, with some companies supplying daily or weekly status reports of bank deposits. Ideally, the monthly reports should be completed and delivered within 5 business days of month-end. Acceptable timing is within 10 business days of month-end; a report delivered later than 10 days indicates that the biller is poorly organized, overextended, understaffed, or is assembling the data by hand (copying information from their system reports, by hand, into a spreadsheet or database program for production of readable monthly reports).

The quality and content of billing company reports are weak industry-wide. The average biller, with or without a capable system, does not fully appreciate or respect the information needs of the client. Too often, billing companies approach monthly reporting as delivery of a variety of system-generated "green bar" printouts without any summaries or a digest of the relevant performance ratios and statistics by which the practice can manage itself.

ADMINISTRATIVE SERVICES. Physician enrollment (completion of the required paperwork to register with and be eligible to receive payment from contractually based payors) applications for medical staff privileges is one of the administrative services that billers often provide. In most cases, these additional services are included at no additional fee, although some billers charge a per hour or project-based fee for the additional services. In competitive markets, the number and variety of included services can be extensive because they allow the competitor to tie in additional-cost services that will be difficult to give up or pay for if a change is made in billers.

BOX 51-4

GLOSSARY OF TERMS

Average Charge—total charges ÷ volume/frequency (visits or procedures)

Average Adjustment—total contractual adjustments (Medicare, Medicaid, Blue Shield, HMO) ÷ volume/frequency (visits or procedures)

Average Payment—total cash payments ÷ volume/frequency (visits or procedures)

Services/Day/Doctor—[total physician services (visits + procedures) ÷ total FTE physicians] ÷ days in period measured

A/R Days—1. [gross charges for past three months ÷ # days in those months] = Average Daily Charges
2. Total Accounts Receivable (net of credit balances) ÷ Average Daily Charges = Days Revenue in A/R

Bad Debt %—bad debt write-offs ÷ Gross charges for the same period

Bad Debt Recovery %—bad debt collections (recoveries) ÷ bad debt write-offs for the same period

Bad Debt Collection Cost—collection agency fees ÷ bad debt collections for the same period

% of Payments—billing costs (billing service or total inhouse costs) as a percent of $ collected

Per Encounter Cost—billing costs (billing service or total inhouse costs) ÷ total encounters/visits for the same period

Per Procedure—billing costs (billing service or total inhouse costs) ÷ total *services* or procedures

% Practice Cost—approximate % of practice *income* expended for billing services, whether inhouse or outsourced

% Labor Cost—percent of billing-related costs spent on labor related items, including salaries, benefits, etc

% Non-Labor Cost—percent of billing-related costs spent on *non*-labor expenditures

Typical Emergency Medicine Practice—the national average performance and cost factors associated with the specialty, without regard to the nature of the billing provider, which also includes hospital staff providing billing services

Reprinted with permission from: Brandywine Healthcare Services, Inc., 1994.

In MSO markets, the administrative services (Box 51-3) become a value-added service and can include an extensive variety of programs and services. These are typically billed on an a la carte basis by the service, by the hour, or on a project basis.

This area of the billing industry represents a relatively new and uncontested area of opportunity and add-on revenue. We believe it can produce as much as 40% growth in company revenue, with a fully developed program of services in a mature market.

Service Performance Drivers

The organizational structure of a billing company plays an important role in the quality of the services it provides, the profitability of the company, and its capacity to accept more business without adding more staff on a 1 : 1 basis. The three primary organizational models are (1) functional, (2) client centered, and (3) hybrids.

Each of the models has its advocates. At Independent Billers Association (IBA) meetings, there are passionate debates about the merits and disadvantages of each approach. We do not believe that there is a perfect answer; situationally, each has its place in a billing organization.

Functional Model. This organizational model uses the assembly line approach to the performance of the component steps of the billing processes. Data entry is a staff function using personnel whose primary skill and cost are directly related to the entry of data. Coding, billing, claim follow-up, payment posting, collections, filing, customer service calls (inbound), and all other functions are divided among staff whose skill and compensation are directly related to the specific functions to which they are assigned.

The functional model recognizes that some activities can be assigned to entry level staff with few or no skills whose cost to the biller is low, whereas other skilled positions, such as coding and collections, are more difficult to acquire and retain, and therefore justify higher compensation, as supported by the value their skills adds to the process. It is generally viewed that the functional model is the less costly and potentially most profitable organizational approach, although not necessarily the one that produces the *highest* results for the client.

Provided all staff are productive and the number of personnel assigned to a given function is appropriate to the volume of work, the functional model intends to match the skill and cost to the requirements and volume. The "mix and match" and management of staff skills required to operate a highly efficient functional model is more difficult than those using it appreciate. The most frequent problems are the underutilization of highly skilled (higher expense) staff by having them perform menial tasks (a coder used for filing) and the overextension of underqualified staff. Although the use of full-time staff can create marginal contributions while ensuring employee loyalty and retention, this approach is challenging to manage on a daily basis. Good managers must also pay attention to cross training and back-up staff to allow for volume variations, vacations, new clients, turnover, and other variables.

Operationally, the functional model relies on task accountability, making task performance measurement necessary for good control. Managing results becomes more difficult. Poorly managed, the functional model creates vulnerability to turnover in key positions, which cannot be quickly or economically replaced. If the position is a vital part of the workflow or quality, backlogs can be created in critical parts of the process, breaking down the entire flow of work, and funds and/or the quality of the clients' work can become compromised.

Although the functional model is common, few billers have proved to be good industrial engineers who micormanage all tasks and functions with an eye toward achieving the ultimate "faster, better, cheaper, more" results. Billers whose clients vary in their billing requirements (a different mix or intensity of services than the average client) often complicate the workflow for a functionally organized model. Although customized services are not impossible, they are more complicated to organize and provide. Greater use of automation and mechanization is an advantage in a functional model because "people" costs can be eliminated more easily.

Competitively, the functional model reduces and/or concentrates the risk of a single employee sabotaging a client or leaving and luring the client away. This appears to be significant to small billing owners, who fear the departure of an employee and the consequent elopement of a client with an employee who "knew too much" and had established a close working relationship with the client(s).

Client-Centered Model. The client-centered model creates teams or units who are responsible for performing all of the tasks needed to support one or a small number of clients. The amount of work provided by each client determines the number of staff allocated to a team, although there are rarely less than two.

Some of the advantages of the client-centered model are (1) greater attention to details, which produce higher levels of results; (2) more flexibility for work distribution among team members during periods of overload; (3) the client's perception that there is an employee who is his or her private representative with valuable knowledge of the work and a heightened interest in the client's results; (4) concentration of expertise that is unique to a client or specialty; (5) staff elasticity based on the arrival or departure of clients; (6) the ability to develop performance incentives based on measured results attributable to specific employees; and (7) increased job satisfaction for the employees often because of direct contact with the client(s).

The disadvantages of the client-centered model include (1) a perception that the operating costs are higher because of task inefficiency and poor concentration/distribution of expertise; (2) small units are vulnerable to turnover which may jeopardize a client's performance and/or the relationship; (3) risk of team members developing a relationship with the client, which may lead to the client and/or the employee(s) "going off together"; (4) friction among team members that can be extremely damaging to the process, often before it can be detected and resolved; (5) competitiveness and/or unwillingness of different teams to help each other; and (6) Parkinson's law, which can overtake a team's perception that it can take on another client or more work.

It is generally believed that the client-centered model is more costly to operate, but it often produces better results for the client. The billing company owner(s) must decide whether the additional results, if achieved, are supported by marginally higher fees, or whether the team model spends profits on unfunded higher performance. In some cases, the company makes an informed decision to continue to retain the client, particularly in highly competitive markets.

Hybrid Models. A variety of hybrid organizational models can be found. The most common is the combination of the functional and client-centered models, with some duties organized functionally and others concentrated within a team. For example, many companies "functional-ize" the data collection, data entry, billing, and payment posting processes, while assigning the follow-up, collection, and customer service/patient representative tasks to a client team. This approach provides closer attention to the most patient and client sensitive processes, while reducing the operating costs of the more mechanical tasks.

Another hybrid arrangement is one in which the client provides some of the work, such as with office practices who outsource their billing, but who must continue to register patients, collect payments at the time of service, and perform coding of the charts. The remaining duties may be functional or client-team or combined. In another scenario, nearly all of the processes are automated, such as for **clinical** (not anatomic) pathology billing, wherein all of the data collection, data transfer, charge identification and entry, billing, follow-up statements, and payment posting are fully automated. In the latter example, a client representative may be all that is needed to provide service acceptable to the client.

A number of circumstantial differences also affect the services and performance of a billing organization when working for a given client. These factors may or may not be controllable by either the client and/or the biller. In many cases, however, accommodations can be made for factors that will allow the relationship to operate on a fair and equitable basis, without compromising the biller's ability to provide an appropriate service at a reasonable profit. Discussed below are several of the more important factors that can drive the viability of a billing arrangement.

Specialty Segmentation. Although some billing companies are generalists and serve any and all specialties, most billers become specialized in one or a limited number of medical specialties. As the organizations grow, those who specialize often cannot sustain their growth solely within their own geographic area. In other cases, billers have a more focused desire to be expert in billing for a specialty and seek out opportunities to become a regional or national market leader in that specialty.

As a result of this specialty focus, billers who are not local may be the best qualified candidates to propose to provide billing to a practice that nearly always has local alternatives. This circumstance brings into focus the choice between local service that *may* not be expertly qualified and the expert provider who is not local.

The practice must carefully weigh the distance (miles, time zones, culture, regional accents at either or both ends, rural versus urban, etc.) and its potential impact on cost and/or speed of service. A biller based in Florida serving a client in Oregon would have to deal with accents and time zone differences, as well as the direct costs associated with transporting the work (charts, registration forms, diskettes), which are usually transported by express carrier. Payments are delayed by the time required for mail to be delivered across the United States, although some billers will address this issue by using a post office box in the practice's area and having a forwarding service send it by overnight carrier. Dealing with distance usually involves costs; whether or not the client pays for those costs directly, they do pay the costs.

In this example, the biller would argue that the additional costs and potential delays are more than compensated for by their expertise, which will produce a greater net result to the client. This argument may or may not be true.

Price Competition. In virtually all specialties, fees for billing services have fallen over the last 5 years, primarily because of three main reasons:

- Most, but not all, physicians' fees and payments have risen as a result of resource based/relative valve scale (RB/RVS) changes in Medicare. Physicians incomes have risen faster than the biller's costs, allowing billers to reduce their fees in competitive situations without compromising the company's revenue per visit.

- Operating costs have declined or been stable in most markets because of
  - Greater use of electronic data transfer between providers and the billing organization.
  - Greater use of electronic claims processing.
  - Greater use of electronic remittance processing.
  - Commercial real estate rental rates that have softened in most markets.
  - Salary rates that have risen more slowly in the absence of rapid inflation.
  - Systems capabilities that have allowed some companies to avoid staff additions when new clients were signed.
- Competition from new, small billers, some of whom do not know how to price profitably, and some of whom have lower profitability expectations than older, more traditional billers.

As the billing industry has evolved, a variety of factors affecting price (as defined by a percent of collected dollars or as a flat fee "per account") have developed. As some billers become substantially larger, they are able to take advantage of economies of scale that permit lower prices and/or more services for the market price. In some cases, larger billers continue to exploit their incumbency without modifying their price, allowing their sometimes smaller competitors to underbid them. This is particularly true in cases where incumbents/competitors are less diligent in adopting use of electronic claim submission and electronic remittance posting.

Examples of economies-of-scale opportunities include predictive dialers ($50 to 100 thousand) for use in data collection and follow-up activities (patient contact) for which a minimum of eight collectors would be in need of support; a collection agency system ($80 to 300 thousand) for dedicated collection efforts for which a minimum of twelve collectors would be required to justify the expense; and scanning and document imaging systems ($40 to 200 thousand) for mass storage of client documents, including medical records, an expenditure that would only be justified by encounter volumes in excess of 20,000 to 30,000 a month. Small billers cannot begin to justify these costs, whereas those who can are able to offer a broader array of services, can increase results and performance, and can also reduce costs.

A biller's expertise in a specialty may allow them to *thoroughly* regiment the billing process to the advantage of lower operating costs than those who only bill a portion of their business base in the given specialty. In some markets, outright price competition occurs, particularly when a company perceives that they have a significant competitive disadvantage (the drive to "catch up") or advantage (the drive to "bury" their competitors).

In some billing markets, competition and/or clients have driven prices down by competitively bidding/rebidding their work. Faced with the possibility of losing a client, billers will often succumb to downward price pressures. They recognize that a long-term, referenceable client has the multiple value of ongoing income, margin contribution, marketing advantage, depriving a competitor of a client (maintenance of market share), and the long-term value of a client retention ratio that increases the potential sale value of the company. Highly competitive markets include all of Florida, metropolitan areas of California, the "Metroliner Corridor" (Boston, New York, Philadelphia, Baltimore, and Washington), St. Louis, Dallas, and Seattle.

We believe that in the long term, prices could rise and/or return to higher levels in response to the complex obligations imposed on providers and their billers by managed care programs. Alternatively, billers may "unbundle" their services (some already have begun) for managed care support, depending on the level of sophistication required. In some cases, billers will charge a per-service fee calibrated to the type and amount of work required.

Competence. Billers are significantly different in their level of competence, both by medical specialty and in general. There is a wide range of skill levels among billing organizations. Some apparently successful, long-established companies are not particularly talented or exceptionally competent. They are merely beneficiaries of clients with low expectations (a standard the biller may have set years ago) and/or a noncompetitive market.

Conversely, highly competent billers may be less profitable, although their client retention and/or competitive abilities may be strong. A dilemma facing the company owner is balancing the work, intensity, and skill/competence level and their associated costs, so as to avoid spending the profits on marginal (for the company) services.

In some specialties, such as infusion therapy, interventional radiology, and emergency medicine, competence is a vital part of the profitability and competitiveness of the business. These specialties, among others, rely heavily on the skills of the CPT-4 coders who usually work for the biller. True competence is vital because the risks to the practice and the biller are overcoding and/or misrepresentation of the practice's services, which can lead to exposure to fraud and abuse, false claims, and other sanctions by the Medicare and Medicaid programs. Alternatively, poor coding skills may "cost" the practice lost income because of undercoding or failure to charge and bill for all of the services provided.

Locale. A recognized strategy in the billing industry is the location of the billing office in a low cost labor and/or overhead market. Locating in a rural or low income area is a common method of lowering overhead. When working at its best, this strategy also places a premium on employees with an extraordinarily high work ethic, low salary and benefit expectations, and few alternatives for other employment. Also important is access to transportation for the employees, whether public transportation or strategically near all of the roads leading through the area.

In some markets, "curb appeal" makes a difference to customers, although too much of a good thing can have the opposite effect. A biller in a large city has offices on the top floor of a tall downtown office building, with panoramic views. Visiting prospective customers are concerned that they will be paying a premium for high profile offices, at the expense of high performance results.

There are numerous examples of billers successfully managing all costs, even in challenging high-cost markets such as New York City and Los Angeles. It requires relentless micromanagement to achieve control of costs in these areas, in contrast to rural locations where proximity to the client is not a primary consideration, but work ethic, labor supply, and cost control are important.

Technology. Employees are almost always more expensive than computers. Few of a biller's activities are less costly when performed by employees. To the extent that billers are able to automate, mechanize, or leverage technology in different ways, they are able to be more cost-effective, profitable, and competitive (even when costs are about equal because time can be a competitive advantage). Because of the cost of entry, many small billers are unable or unwilling to make the investment in costly technology. We have observed that these habits often live on after a biller becomes larger and more economically able to use more technology.

Examples of higher-level technology include predictive dialers ($50,000 to $100,000), document imaging ($40,000 to 100,000+), document scanners/OCR ($200,000+), and higher cost billing software from "high-end" vendors. Some billers also consider mail handling equipment such as folder/inserters and automated mail openers as "high-tech," although it is more mechanization than technologic. Potential savings can be expected to range from 10% to 15% overall, although individual circumstances may allow for even greater savings, where the "old" method is mostly manual.

Electronic claim and remittance processing or electronic data interchange (EDI) should also be mentioned here, although we have discussed it in earlier sections. Its importance in this context is that it can be secured through a clearinghouse, even if the biller's inhouse or shared system cannot/does not support two-way EDI.

From a service and performance perspective, leverage of technology is a hallmark of an effective, competitive, and profitable billing company. Those who fail to vigorously pursue greater use of technology in the present and future will be casualties to those who do. Companies who can afford to buy and/or create and master technologies capable of very high volumes, or who can automate/mechanize activities that others can only perform manually will have a critical strategic and competitive advantage.

Payor Mix. There is often little a provider can do to limit or influence the payor mix of the patients. This is especially true of the hospital-based specialties. In a given geographic area, only a limited amount of influence can be applied to the mix of patients seen, particularly in areas where managed care is growing.

Billers are acutely aware of the impact of payor mix will have on their success and the work that will be required to support a new client. For this reason, fees charged will vary from the norm. In most cases, fees are increased for poor payor mixes (high indigent and uninsured and/or payors whose billing requirements are burdensome, such as some managed care and workers' compensation programs), but seldom are rates lowered for superior payor mixes.

As payor mixes evolve, billers may endeavor to renegotiate their rates. This phenomenon is particularly common in areas where managed care and capitation programs are becoming a greater portion of the population for whom billers must process services. Billers who are naive of the impact of managed care and the paperwork and data management requirements on their obligations to their clients will suffer income and/or client losses as a result.

In a larger context, the services and performance levels of a biller are constrained by what is possible to achieve with a particular payor mix. Some clients who have practiced elsewhere may have unrealistic expectations of performance levels, based on their prior experience. In other cases, the payor mix is never stable long enough to allow for a period-to-period comparison.

Finally, hospital-based specialties are vulnerable to another aspect of the payor mix issue; hospital registration staff are notoriously poor at accurate and consistent data capture. Patients who have coverage and/or new data to provide are often not obliged to provide it or to prove it. Simple steps such as requiring positive proof of ID (driver's license or other photo ID), recording the identity of the registrar who recorded the data and holding them accountable for their errors and omissions, and maintaining statistical data on the error rates (using indicators such as returned/undeliverable mail, disconnected telephones, and bad debts). Hospitals, like the physician providers, are unable to affect the mix of patients who use the institution. Their recourse is to assertively and diligently work at preventing losses through data collection.

A few billers have successfully used outside database companies to refresh and improve the addresses and telephone numbers of patients at relatively low cost with sometimes substantial benefit.

Operational Cost Components

What Affects the Cost and/or Necessity of Each Element?

PERSONNEL EXPENSES*. The area labor pool for medical billing, local (un)employment, local customs for fringe benefits, and area wage scales are the primary driving factors in personnel costs. This is not particularly different from all other businesses that are primarily in the skilled-clerical category.

For a billing company, certain key technical skills are so important that a biller will grudgingly pay a premium to secure and protect the ability to provide those key services. These include several already discussed earlier, such as coding, regulatory compliance, contract analysis/negotiation, and systems coordination (particularly important if a commercial software package is used), programming, and integration.

Some labor markets have a ready supply of medically experienced clerical workers. Others, even in major metropolitan markets, have a severe shortage. In the latter case, the biller is forced to consider relocation and/or a "build your own" programming of staff training, taking the risk of becoming the source of supply for his own competitors if compensation, benefits, working conditions, or job security become concerns.

Billers who are major local employers, with 50 or more employees in a small community, often become a sought-after place to work, particularly if the aforementioned conditions are favorable. If local conditions favor unionized clerical workers, most billers will flee, as much to diminish the hassles as to avoid the additional labor costs. Fringe benefits are occasionally an issue, such as in California, where the State mandates an insurance benefits package that is optional in 49 other states.

Local unemployment rates may provide a billing organization with a lower cost labor supply. However, unless the community has chronic unemployment, the advantage will eventually reverse itself. It is believed that areas with chronic

*Salaries, Benefits, and Payroll Taxes 45% of Gross Income.

unemployment dilute the work ethic over time, as motivated workers leave for broader opportunities elsewhere.

OPERATING OVERHEAD*. Proximity to the customer is of dual value to the biller and the client. The latter prefers it in a billing relationship, and the former would rather be close than not. Billers vary in their approach to proximity; in some cases larger billers open branch offices, such as Medaphis. In others a single central facility is used exclusively, such as Emergency Physician Billing Services in Oklahoma City.

A variety of techniques can be used to overcome higher-than-normal rental rates, including use of shifts for activities that do not require business hours contacts (payment posting, data entry, charge posting, evening collection calls, etc.); use of "flex-time" hours; use of "10-4" schedules (10 hour days × 4 days), which has the effect of creating 20% more capacity without the burdens and costs of shift supervision; and subdividing the work among several facilities, some of which are much less costly because of their lack of "cosmetic" appeal to potential client visitors (the "billing factory" approach).

Postage can be managed by use of zip sorting and bar coding; aggressive management of mail returns (why continue to send mail to a bad address?); precise selection of billing cycles to optimize returns on the costs; use of mailing services who perform printing, sorting, stuffing, and mailing at lower cost than may be possible in-house; and maximum use of electronic claims submission.

In the future, we envision actual capture and use of personal (home) e-mail addresses as part of medical registrations, allowing postage-free mailing of digital statements via Internet. Not only will delivery be confirmable, but replies will be more likely and equally well documented, all at higher speed and lower cost.

Cost/Payment/Contract Administration

Management of practice costs has never been more necessary or more challenging. Managed care contracting has placed the practitioner, often for the first time, in the difficult position of making cost-driven decisions about patient care. Not only are some practices now financially responsible for payment, such as in a subcapitation arrangement, but practices are becoming involved in highly structured, complex payment arrangements. Some of these arrangements include specific, limited payments for high-cost and/or single source products, placing the provider in financial jeopardy if costs are not managed to the amounts to be paid.

Selection of an effective and economic billing company is crucial to managing an emergency department. Some additional terms you may encounter are listed in Box 51-4. In making this decision it is important to thoroughly understand the process and to research the prospective companies.

*Rent, Depreciation/Amortization, Telephone, Postage, Technology, Maintenance and Repairs, Insurance 13% of Gross Income.

PART FIVE
Quality

52 Theory of Continuous Quality Improvement

Thom A. Mayer and Richard Salluzzo

OUTLINE

In the late 1980s and early 1990s a revolution swept through American business and industry, constituting a radical reformation of management theory and structure. Continuous quality improvement (CQI) represents a significant departure from traditional management philosophy and practice and has been applied widely in both manufacturing and service industries across the country. In addition, a rich literature has developed regarding the implementation of CQI principles in healthcare settings, including their application to the emergency department.[1-4] The Joint Commission on Accreditation of Healthcare Organizations (JCAHO) has embraced the principles of CQI as a major tool to be used by hospitals in their performance improvement efforts.[5] Continuous quality improvement applications have been particularly relevant to the emergency department given the process focus of quality improvement and the fact that *the emergency department is a process-rich environment* (Figure 52-1). Perhaps the most telling evidence of the application of quality improvement principles in the emergency department is the fact that the game used to teach process management principles is known as "Friday night at the ER." This game examines typical processes in an emergency department to illustrate basic concepts of process management and their application.

The goals of this chapter are to address the following:
1. The philosophic and practical tenets of CQI
2. The origins of CQI and the study of traditional management
3. Similarities between CQI and the scientific method
4. The role of statistical process control
5. The importance of staff empowerment
6. Criticisms of CQI
7. The relationship of CQI to reengineering, redesign, and patient-focused care

PHILOSOPHIC AND PRACTICAL TENETS OF CONTINUOUS QUALITY IMPROVEMENT

Continuous quality improvement arose out of the careful and disciplined study of traditional management approaches by a group of separate but extraordinarily similar thinkers, including Shewhart,[6] Deming,[7,8] Juran,[9-11] and Ishikawa.[12] As their values began to be applied in a practical fashion, it became clear that certain key features were inherent to any CQI approach regardless of the specific formulation:
1. Customer focus
2. Statistical application of knowledge of variation
3. Focus on process
4. Design and redesign (Kaizen)
5. A redefinition of leadership

Customer Focus

For many healthcare providers, the transition of the "patient" to "customer" is the most difficult transition in CQI. The healing professions have a rich tradition of commitment to the patient and the virtues of care, compassion, and concern for the well-being and healing of the patient and family.[13,14] However, this paradigm casts the professional caregiver in a dominant role with regard to the patient, who has traditionally had little input in healthcare management.

Recently, the concept of the patient as passive recipient of the healthcare team's beneficence has changed radically. This change is not primarily the result of CQI, but rather relates to several factors. First, patients have an increasingly high level of understanding and sophistication with regard to the mechanisms of disease and available healthcare options. Second, the development of more customer-focused concepts in society has extended to healthcare. Third, the concept of healthcare as an essential right of the American people has also had an impact.

Because CQI arose from the detailed, statistical study of traditional manufacturing management principles, it is not surprising that the central focus of the philosophy is on the thorough and statistical understanding of customers. Thus CQI has not caused the difficult transition from patient to customer, but rather simply chronicles the elements of that transition, recognizing that a thorough and statistical understanding of customer needs is essential to implementing a successful healthcare system. Chapter 8 addresses the concept of customer service in some detail, but the basic principles are presented here.

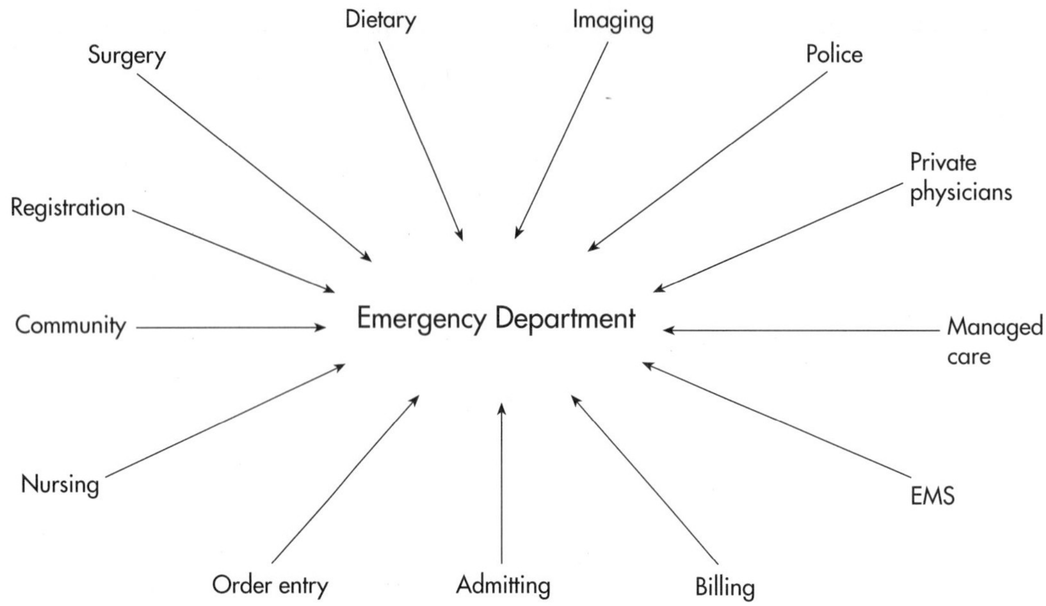

FIGURE 52-1 The emergency department is a process-rich environment. Regardless of size or volume, all emergency departments have multiple, cross-functional processes at work on each patient. Success requires careful, sequential coordination of these processes.

BOX 52-1

INTERNAL AND EXTERNAL EMERGENCY DEPARTMENT CUSTOMERS

- Internal customers
  - Emergency physicians
  - Emergency nurses
  - Emergency department technicians
  - Registrars
  - Core secretaries
- External customers
  - Patient
  - Family
  - Payors
  - Emergency medical services
  - Police
  - Referring hospitals
  - Medical staff
  - Administration

In simplest terms, a customer is any person who is affected by a process or product. This definition includes "external customers" such as patients and their families and "internal customers" such as emergency physicians, emergency nurses, medical staff members, and administration. Box 52-1 contains a more complete delineation of potential customers in the emergency department setting.

Continuous quality improvement defines quality as meeting or exceeding the customer's expectations. An infrastructure that allows customer feedback on an ongoing basis is critical to measuring performance in this regard. It is also important to understand that customer needs are by nature a moving target, subject to change and refinement over the course of time. The idea of continuous improvement in meeting these changing needs is a central tenet of this management approach.

Statistical Application of Knowledge of Variation

Just as DNA is considered the "building block" of life, statistical process control (SPC) should be considered the building block of continuous quality improvement. In the late 1920s and early 1930s Walter Shewhart and his colleagues at Western Electric Laboratories began a detailed analysis of U.S. industry through a series of extraordinarily sophisticated and detailed experiments.[6] The essence of their work became the science that has since been recognized as SPC. Shewhart's early writings and subsequent commentary thereon offer rich detail in the concepts of statistical process control, which can only be dealt with somewhat superficially here. Nonetheless, reduction of variation through statistical means is an essential component of CQI and derives directly from the science of SPC.

To a large extent, healthcare planners have previously considered the end results of their work to be largely unmeasurable. The patient's journey from illness to wellness, although subject to numerous measurements, had been considered to be a largely unmeasurable process, particularly with regard to customer satisfaction, cost, outcome, measurement, and so forth. This is an odd paradox in a field whose very essence concerns the nature of being able to measure quantifiable differences between patients, as well as within the patient, as the course of the disease progresses or improves. Nonetheless, a rich literature has developed that indicates that statistical process control can be applied not only to healthcare processes overall, but to the patient encounter itself.

Understanding the implications of variation in process is a critical skill for the healthcare manager. Common cause variation refers to naturally occurring, statistically predictable

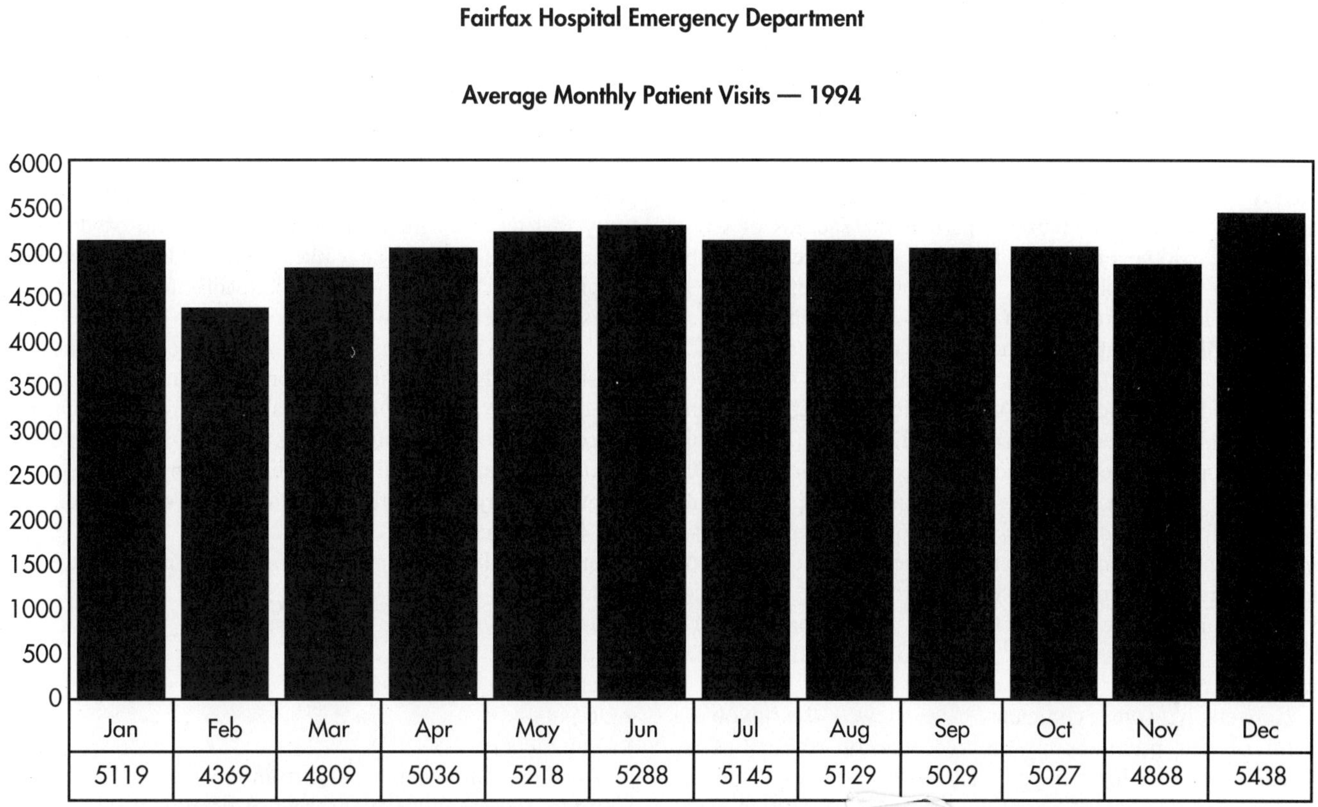

FIGURE 52-2 Emergency department run chart. A run chart is a statistical tool that looks at variations in a process over time. Careful interpretation is required because "tampering," or type I errors, can result. For example, the lower volumes in the nonsummer months do not represent failures of marketing or public relations; they reflect the influx of a large number of patients into the service area of the hospital during the summer months and an increase in injuries during this time. (Courtesy Fairfax Hospital Department of Emergency Medicine, Falls Church, Va.)

variations that are inherent in all processes. For example, emergency department volume can vary widely, depending on the day of the week, season of the year, and other multitudinous factors. Figure 52-2 illustrates this concept through a run chart on emergency department volumes. By applying statistical principles one can determine the variations that are common cause in nature, which helps guide appropriate interventions to improve the system. There are classically a number of problems involving an understanding of common cause variation. These include a lack of understanding of the basic principles of common cause variation and therefore a strong tendency to overinterpret the fluctuations within the system. For example, in interpreting Figure 52-2 this sharp downturn of emergency department volume in the fall months could lead to interventions in the system that fail to take into account the application of statistical principles that show that such variation is predictable. More detailed analysis in this particular case indicates that the high volume in the summer months is due to an influx of population, and therefore patients, during the course of such months. Similar variations may be seen in tropical climates in the winter months, as tourists and seasonal residents increase. Because of the lack of understanding of the basic principles of common cause variation, one of the most common problems is tampering with the system as a result of overinterpretation of data. These errors were originally described as type I errors.[10]

Special cause variation is a natural variation caused by events or circumstances that are nontypical and therefore not inherent in the process. Such special causes are often operator dependent (caused by variation in individuals providing service within the system). This is particularly true in cases in which different operators provide the service through a process that is inherently different from that of other providers. In the emergency department setting, the example of specific emergency physician–nursing team combinations slowing emergency department flow is a pertinent example. Box 52-2 lists other examples of common cause versus special cause variation.

Perhaps the greatest obstacle to successful implementation of CQI in healthcare is the paradox of control of variation (and its short circuit to fear) and the dilemma of empowerment. One of the essential features of CQI is to reduce variation through statistical means. Although certain protocols have always existed within the field of medicine, there has nonetheless been a substantial degree of freedom on the part of the individual practitioner to diagnose and treat patients according to the preferences of the individual practitioner. For example, outpatient management of new-onset hypertension has been shown to have extraordinarily wide variation among the physicians responsible for the patient's care. The development of general hypertensive treatment guidelines have more clearly delineated that any of four initial drug therapies may be effective, when combined with diet and exercise.[15] However, the choice of drugs itself still varies widely, according to the individual practice patterns of the practitioner, the patient's clinical presentation, and the experience that either the patient or the practitioner has had with certain drug therapies. The movement toward more clearly defined clinical pathways in emergency medicine and other specialties represents part of the success of CQI principles. However, there is some resistance to such guidelines in that physicians often view these efforts as a reduction in their freedom to practice in an unencumbered fashion. Bluntly stated, physicians do not want to be told how to practice medicine, nor in general do they want to be constrained in their choice of therapeutic options for a given patient. This represents the "short circuit to fear" in control of variation that medicine faces in the application of CQI principles. However, there are many examples of successful control of special cause variation through accepted treatment protocols including the use of the principles outlined in the Advanced Trauma Life Support Course,[16] the Advanced Cardiac Life Support Course,[17] the Advanced Pediatric Life Support Course,[18] and, more recently, asthma treatment protocols.[19]

Conversely, some clinicians have viewed the involvement of the providers in the redesign of service as a freedom to "do whatever you want." These two elements—viewing the control of variation as a short circuit to fear and viewing empowerment as the freedom to do whatever one wants—form an essential paradox that can arise from the misapplication of CQI principles. It is important for physicians to realize that reasoned and data-supported development of practice guidelines, clinical pathways, and process improvements represent the best CQI has to offer.

Most important, at its essence, statistical process control involves the intelligent design and interpretation of tests that help us understand our fundamental processes. In the case of clinical processes, these "tests" are often analyses of the ways in which we approach and care for patients with certain clinical entities. The commitment to using statistical process control ensures that any such tests are guided by statistical analysis of results, as opposed to more subjective opinions. The application of SPC to emergency medicine is at the heart of CQI principles and harkens back to a reapplication of the scientific method to the processes in which we work on a daily basis.

Focus on Process

In addition to a customer focus and a reliance on statistical process control, a focus on process is the third element present in all CQI formulations. A process is simply any activity that takes an input, adds value to it, and produces an output (Figure 52-3). The value that is added may involve people, materials, energy, equipment, information, or procedures, each element of which is designed to add value. Thus CQI defines a process as a series of supplier-customer relationships in which various macroprocesses in the overall system can be broken down into smaller subprocesses, each of which has a set of supplier-customer relationships involved. Figures 52-4 and 52-5 illustrate the differences between application macroflowcharting and microflowcharting on process improvements.

Juran's analysis of process components includes the following:

- Supplier
- Input
- Action
- Output
- Customers

Any process can thus be analyzed in this manner. By way of example, let us look at the process of obtaining a radiograph in the emergency department (Box 52-3). This process begins with a *supplier,* the emergency physician, who determines the need for a radiograph based on clinical examination. In systems in which advanced triage is used, the supplier may be an appropriately trained triage nurse. The supplier (emergency physician or triage nurse) provides *input,* the x-ray request, which results in a series of *actions:* an emergency department clerk enters the order into the computer; the x-ray technician reviews the order and processes it; the patient then returns to the emergency department, at which time the emergency department clerk or physician is

BOX 52-2

COMMON CAUSE VERSUS SPECIAL CAUSE VARIATION

Common cause variation
- Physical layout
- Staffing policies
- Existing process

Special cause variation
- High volume
- Specific physician–nurse combinations
- New personnel
- New processes (capitation)

BOX 52-3

PROCESS COMPONENTS—EMERGENCY DEPARTMENT RADIOGRAPH

Component	Entity
1. Supplier	Emergency physicians
2. Input	X-ray request
3. Actions	Clerk enters orders
	X-ray technician processes orders, retrieves patient, obtains x-ray, develops x-ray, returns patient to room, informs clerk and physician
4. Output	Radiograph
5. Customers	Physician interpretation
	External customer—patient
	Internal customers—emergency department personnel, x-ray technician, clerk, radiologist, nursing staff

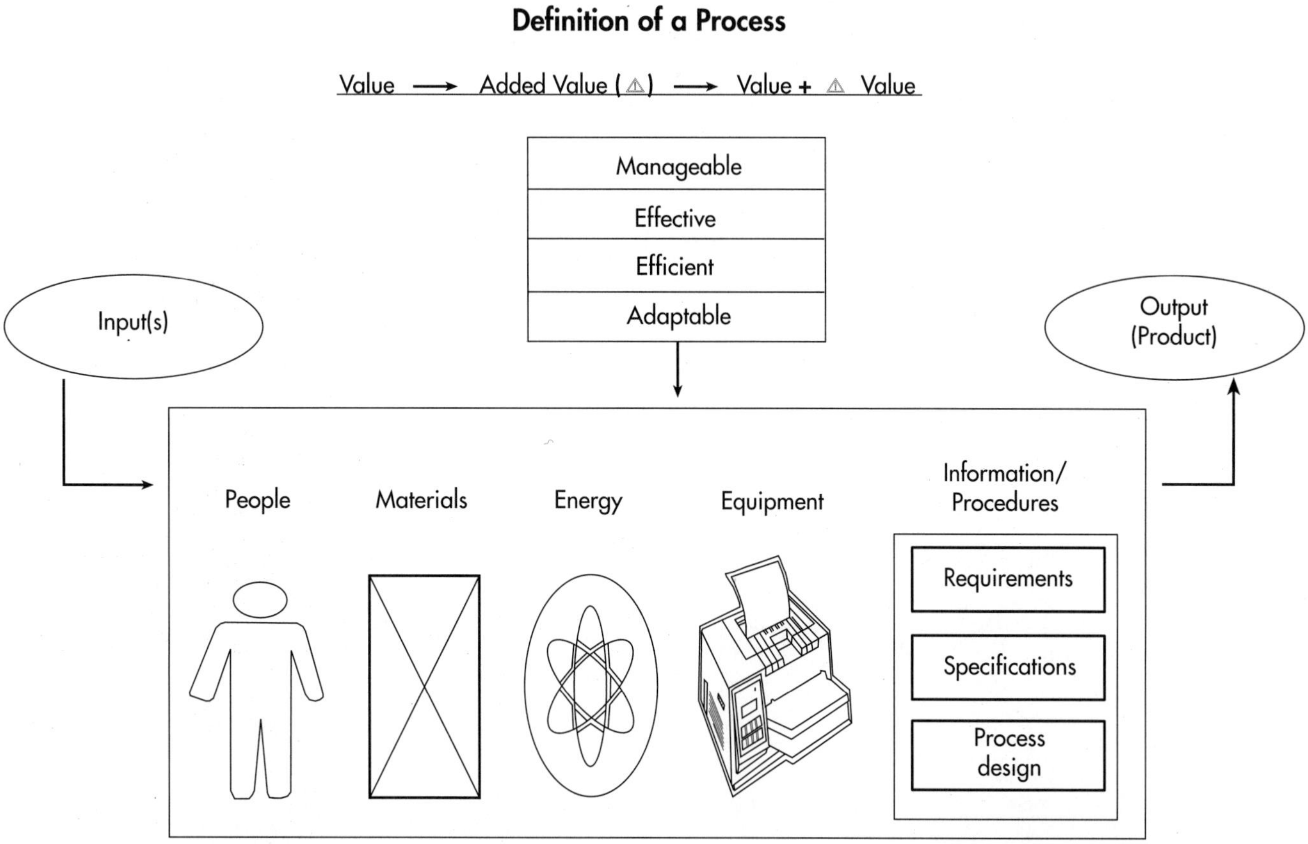

FIGURE 52-3 Definition of a process. A process consists of any activity that takes an input, adds value to it, and produces an output. The value that is added may include people, materials, energy, equipment, information, or procedures. Effective processes must be manageable, effective, efficient, and adaptable to ensure that they are responsive to customer and supplier needs.

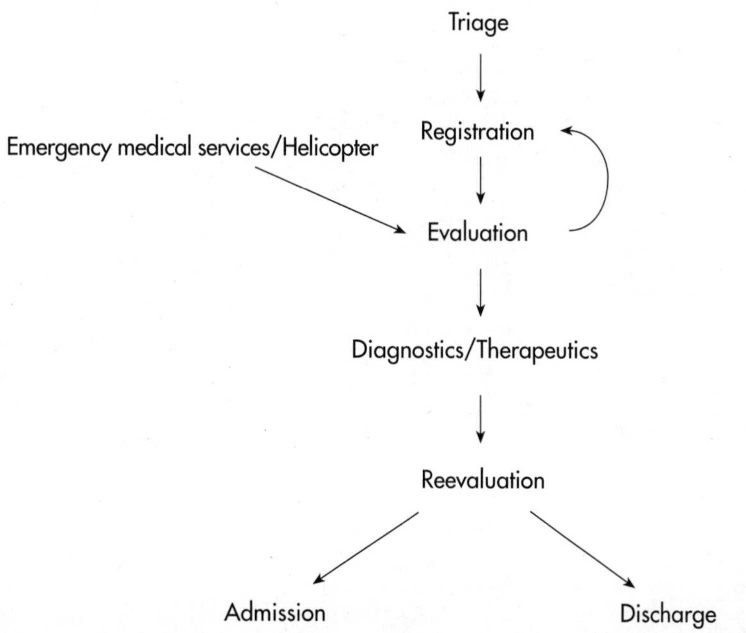

FIGURE 52-4 Macroflowchart of emergency department operations. A macroflowchart is intended to show the major elements of a process, within which multiple subprocesses can be further delineated through microflowcharting. Macroflowcharting is intended to give a general, overall view of a system's processes.

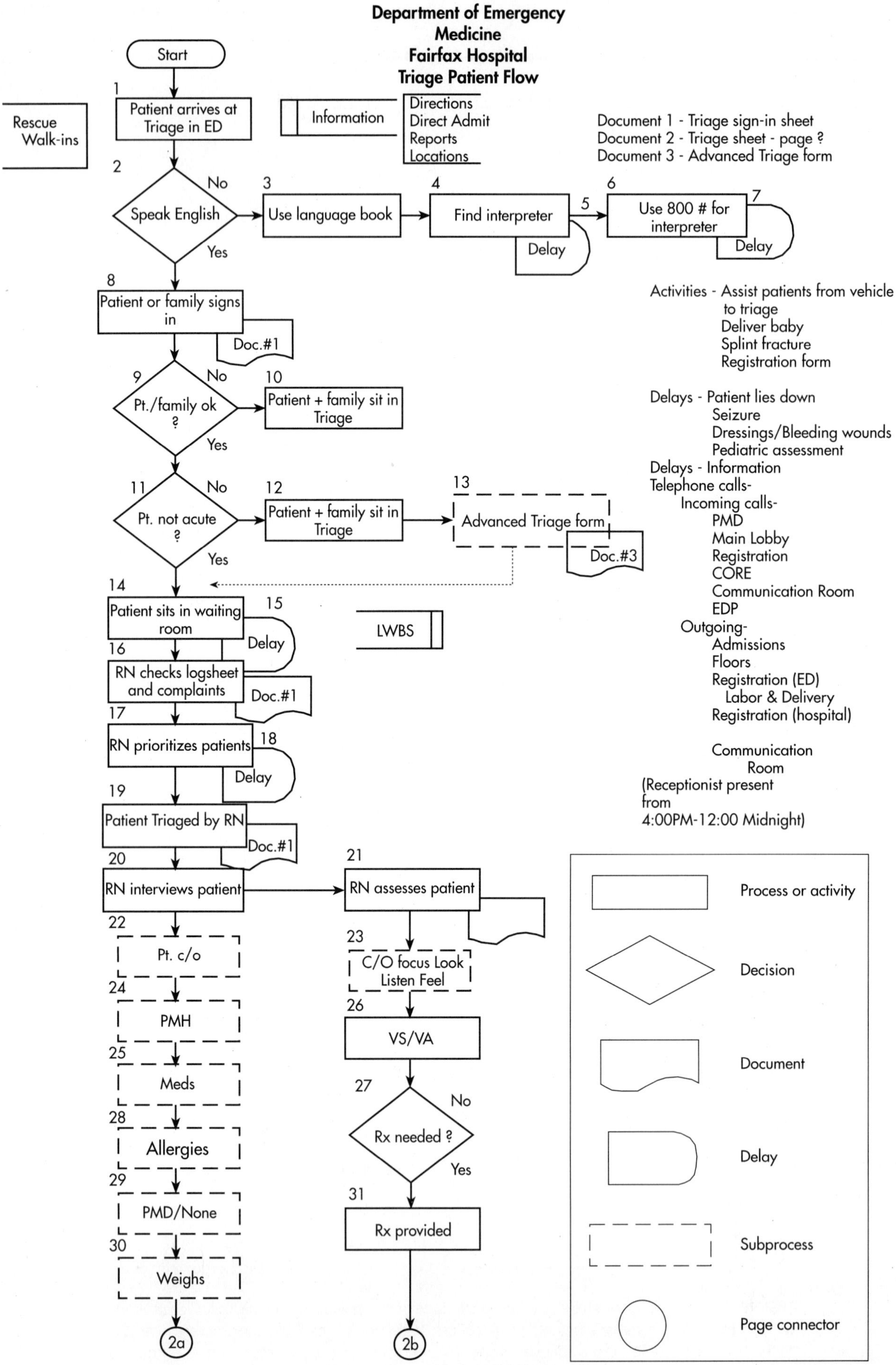

FIGURE 52-5 For legend see opposite page.

informed that the x-ray is completed. It is clear that this process consists of a series of subprocesses that can also be analyzed and improved.

All of these actions result in an *output,* which in this case is both the radiograph itself and the physician interpretation of that radiograph. Each of these outputs has an effect on the *customers,* both external and internal. Viewed in this fashion, the simple process of obtaining an emergency department radiograph constitutes a series of supplier-customer relationships, which are linked in an interdependent fashion to result in a quality outcome.

It is critical to recognize that the emergency department is a process-rich environment. Virtually all interactions in the emergency department involve interdependent, cross-functional processes for their successful conclusion. It is precisely because the emergency department is a process-rich environment that the precepts of CQI hold so much promise for improvement of service. As Deming first noted, 85% of bad outcomes arise from the process itself, whereas only 15% arise from faulty performance by the individual provider.[7,8] Given this fact, CQI attempts to improve processes and systems rather than focus on individual performance, as was the primary purpose of traditional management and quality assurance (QA) programs.

Emphasis on Design and Redesign—Kaizen

Another of the key concepts in CQI is the emphasis on design and redesign. As Donald Berwick has noted, "Every process provides information by which that process can be improved."[20] This focus on process improvement is a dramatic change from the prior emphasis on outlier activity. In traditional QA, quality improvement is attempted by routing out "bad apples" rather than by improving processes and systems.[21] However, quality is more than the absence of adverse events; elimination of outliers in a system may have minimal impact on mean performance. Quality exists to the extent that value is added in the course of the process itself.

The design and redesign concept in CQI is illustrated in Figures 52-6 and 52-7, in which the focus is on analyzing the system in such a way that the entire curve can be shifted to the right, so that "average performance" improves rather than placing emphasis primarily on the outliers with bad outcome. Such shifts of the curve can occur only when there is a team approach to improving customer service, statistical application of knowledge of variation, the understanding of process, and the application of design and redesign for improvement.

A key concept of Kaizen is that the redesign of process is not primarily a management function but a function of the caregivers (providers) themselves. In traditional management systems a central role of the leader is to redesign the system and exhort personnel to follow the process. In the CQI model the process of redesign includes management, but it also involves the staff members responsible for care in an essential fashion. Thus the distinction between "those who do" and "those who think" is fundamentally altered in the CQI system. As Berwick noted, in a CQI system the provider is expected to improve the process in an ongoing fashion.[20]

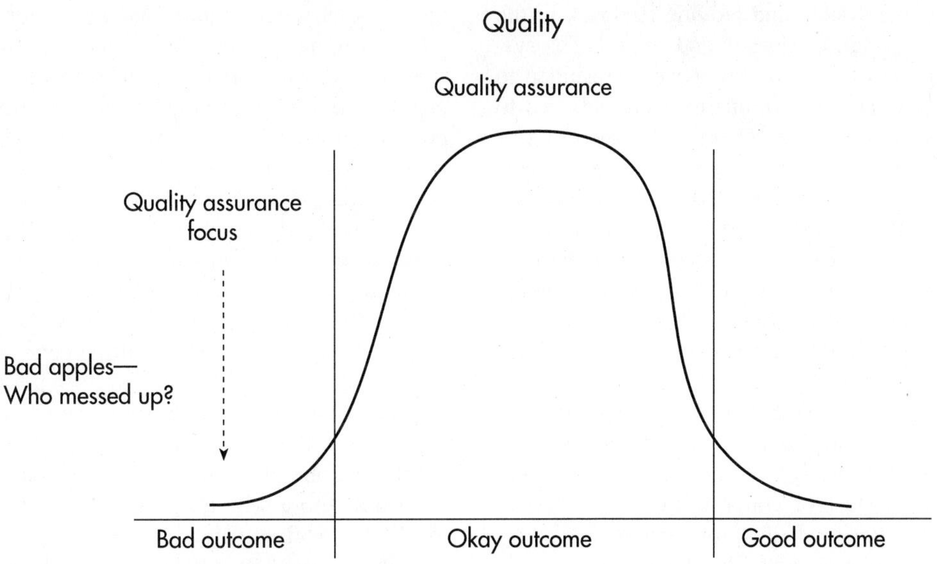

FIGURE 52-6 Quality assurance versus quality improvement. In quality assurance systems, the focus is almost inevitably on the bad outcomes, "bad apples," with specific attention to negative outliers. Little focus is on acceptable outcome, and even less on good outcome.

FIGURE 52-5 Microflowchart. Microflowcharting is a detailed, careful delineation of a process or series of processes. It is intended to give providers a detailed understanding of the numerous steps within a process. Common flowcharting symbols are used to delineate areas in which decisions are made, documents are generated, and so forth.

(Courtesy Fairfax Hospital Department of Emergency Medicine, Falls Church, Va.)

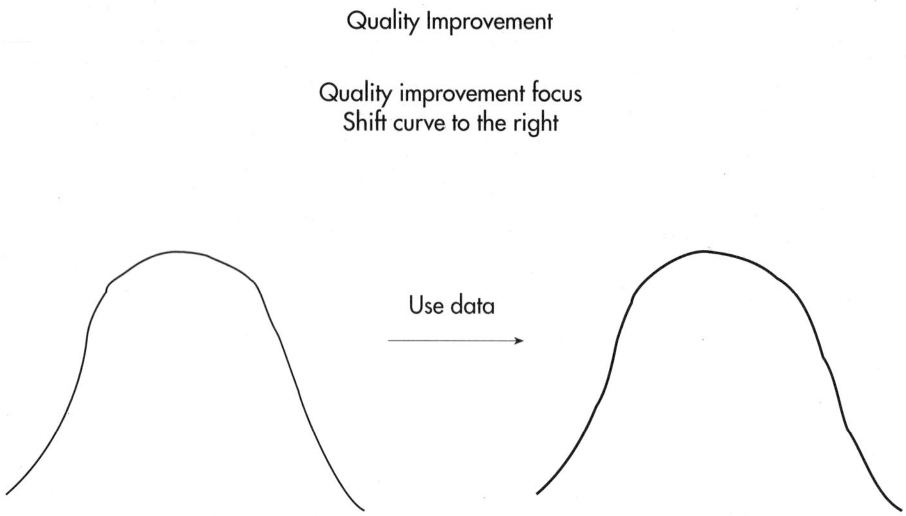

FIGURE 52-7 Quality assurance versus quality improvement. Whereas quality assurance focuses on bad outcomes, quality improvement attempts to move the entire curve further to the right, improving all outcomes in the system.

Leadership Redefined and Empowerment of the Workers

The scions of continuous quality improvement—Deming, Juran, Shewhart, and others—began their development of the CQI philosophy with a detailed, statistical study of traditional management principles that had been applied since the dawn of the industrial revolution. The role of the traditional manager was to observe the system and provide feedback to the staff in the form of exhortation, reward, and control. The system itself and the processes composing it were presumed to be well designed, and variations in quality were believed to be a result of workers who were not properly motivated or skilled. The traditional manager made systems improvements in a unilateral fashion and then inspected the work, seeking outlier performance. By necessity, under such a system personnel problems predominate over process problems. Further, the alterations that are made in process are usually at the hands of middle or senior management. The basic theory of traditional management is that accountability restores will and intention, thereby improving performance and quality.

The founders of CQI proved that such a traditional management approach had certain subtle, inherent, unavoidable, and predictable consequences.[7-12,20,21] For instance, although systems managed in this fashion could result in small, incremental improvements, they could not provide dramatic breakthroughs in quality, as demonstrated by the Japanese in the growth of their auto industry. A second consequence of this traditional approach is the loss of creative redesign input of the providers themselves. Continuous quality improvement recognizes that the continuous redesign of the system must of necessity include the input of those responsible for providing service to the patient or customer. Without input from the provider, management is faced with a sterile and unrewarding task of designing a system in which they are not involved on a day-to-day, minute-to-minute basis. There is an abundant history in manufacturing, service, and healthcare environments to indicate that this active role of the provider in redesigning the system is essential for continuous improvement to occur.[7-12,20-23]

A third consequence of traditional management systems is the development of what Paul Batalden referred to as "functional silos."[24] This concept refers to the fact that in a traditional management system providers tend to narrow the area of their involvement to extremely well-defined and circumscribed areas over which they can be held accountable. Further, as this specialization and narrowing of interest occur, the dissemination and fertilization of information is not shared across the organization, or even across parts of the organization. In effect, this creates functional silos in which processes that are fundamentally horizontal in nature become stratified in vertical silos. As this functional, vertical siloing occurs, the processes of necessity become unlinked, which is usually readily apparent to the customer (Figure 52-8).

All of these elements result in a system in which people are held accountable for systems over which they have limited control, which clearly leads to a tremendous amount of frustration and stress. The redifinement of leadership in the CQI model involves a number of difficult transitions for leaders and managers. Among these transitions is moving from more external models of leadership to more collaborative and facilitative models. Whereas leaders traditionally have been viewed as those who are instrumental in systems redesigns, the CQI model envisions the leader more as a coach, consultant, and facilitator, who ensures that the providers have the appropriate tools and techniques to redesign the processes in which they participate on an ongoing basis. Chapter 1 delineates further the relationship between leaders, managers, and motivation. It is important to understand just how radical this redefinition of leadership is. In many ways, the concepts of traditional management have been mirrored in our educational processes, extending from grade school all the way through residency training programs. Clearly, much of education (and a good bit of child rearing) focuses heavily on an authoritarian, hierarchical structure that still pervades much of the healthcare industry. The concept of having the

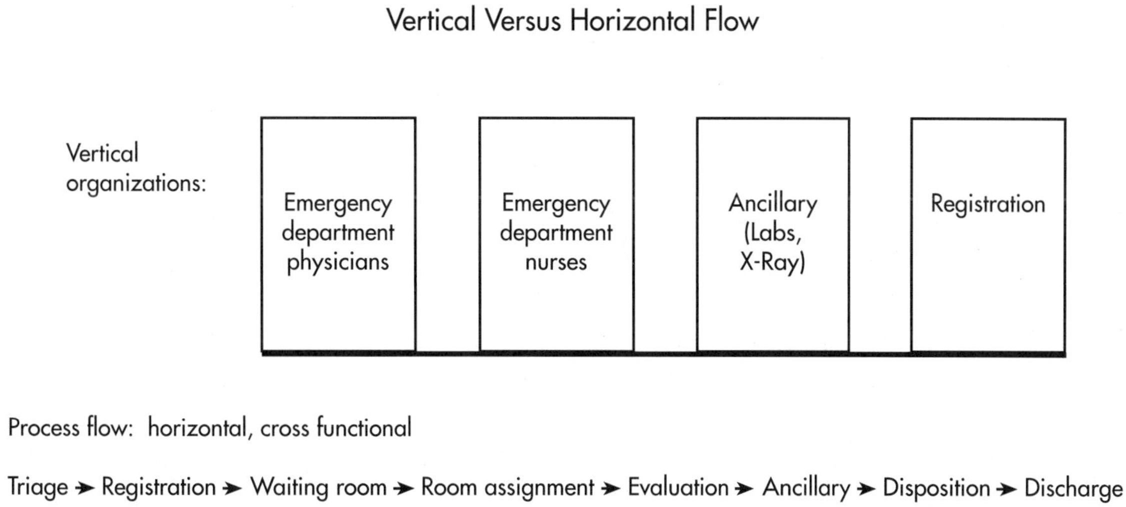

FIGURE 52-8 Vertical versus horizontal flow. Most emergency departments are organized in at least four vertical silos: emergency department nursing, physicians, ancillary services, and registration. However, the patient moves through the system in a horizontal, cross-functional fashion, crossing the vertical silos, in which communication and process may become important issues.

providers of healthcare redesign the ways in which that healthcare is delivered is thus in many ways at cross-purposes to this hierarchical structure. However, medicine has strong roots in the scientific method and is characterized by a deep spirit of intellectual curiosity. For this reason, healthcare providers should make an effective transition to collaborative management philosophy in which governance is shared, workers are empowered, and quality is a function of customer satisfaction.

CONTINUOUS QUALITY IMPROVEMENT AND THE ENHANCED SCIENTIFIC METHOD

At its essence, CQI is in many respects the simple application of the scientific method to cross-functional processes that result in a deeper and more fundamental understanding of the ways in which healthcare delivery can be designed and implemented to meet customer needs. As Box 52-4 illustrates, there are strong similarities between the scientific method and the concepts of quality planning, quality improvement, and quality control, which make up the foundation of total quality management or continuous quality improvement systems. In the scientific method one isolates areas of study, postulates causes, designs experiments and measurements that focus on the area of study, collects data, develops conclusions, and continues to design more focused experiments to help delineate the biologic or physical phenomena under study. This is similar to quality planning's features as outlined by Juran: determine customers, determine customer needs, develop services responsive to those needs, develop processes producing those features, transfer plants to operations, and continue studying data to document success.[9-11] When the close similarity between CQI and the scientific method is highlighted, many healthcare providers find the transition to be somewhat easier.

However, it is important to recognize that, although medicine has been vigorous in its application of the scientific method to the development of new therapies, we have been far less willing to apply those same principles to the everyday processes in which we are involved that deliver those therapies. Thus, although we are careful to study the literature to determine the best methods of handling congestive heart failure by vasodilator therapy, we have been far less rigorous in ensuring that clinical pathways are devised for such patients and that the systems in which such care is delivered are organized around precise customer needs. Yet even in the clinical areas there are substantial applications of CQI that could be of benefit. For example, how carefully have we applied the scientific method to the types of therapy that we offer and to measuring the response to such therapy? How clear are we in the understanding of second- and third-line therapies for patients who fail initial vasodilator or diuretic therapy? Do we have specific criteria under which we use Bi-PAP therapy, or is that simply a "judgment call"?

BOX 52-4

CONTINUOUS QUALITY IMPROVEMENT AND THE ENHANCED SCIENTIFIC METHOD

Quality planning
- Determine customers
- Determine customer needs
- Develop services responsive to those needs
- Develop processes producing those features
- Transfer plans to operations
- Study data to document success

Scientific method
- Isolate area of study
- Postulate causes
- Design parameters of study
- Collect data
- Develop conclusions
- Continue study

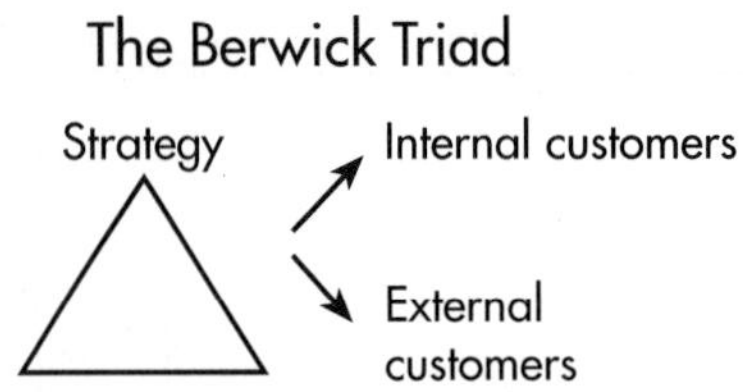

Culture	Techniques	Tools
Leadership	Quality planning	Pareto analysis
Learning organizations	Quality control	Flowcharts
Teams	Quality improvement	Cause & effect diagram
	Process management	Data collection
	Benchmarking	Hoshin planning
		Affinity diagrams
		Forcefield analysis

FIGURE 52-9 The Berwick triad consists of a strategy, which focuses on the customer, enhanced by a culture, in which leadership is deeply committed to quality, and tools and techniques, which form the practical basis of implementation of such programs.

When patients with similar clinical presentations and acuity come to the emergency department, how likely are they to be cared for in identical ways by the emergency physician–nursing teams assigned to them?

In many respects the application of CQI involves the enhancement of the scientific method and applying it to our clinical and management practices in the emergency department. Because this is, in essence, rediscovering our roots in scientific processes, physicians and nurses have often found adoption of the CQI tools and techniques to be far less onerous than has been the case in other businesses and industries.

The Structure of Continuous Quality Improvement—The Berwick Triad

Dr. Donald Berwick has been one of the earliest, most consistent, and most fervent interpreters of the integration of continuous quality improvement principles into the healthcare setting. His description of the so-called Berwick triad is a clear and concise representation of the precepts of quality improvement.[20,21] The Berwick triad (Figure 52-9) consists of a strategy, a culture, and a group of techniques (augmented by specific tools) that constitute the foundation of quality improvement. The strategy begins with, maintains focus on, and ends with a commitment to the customers of the process, including both internal and external customers. Understanding customers is a lifelong commitment that is bolstered by statistical understanding of the changing needs of the customers on an ongoing basis.

The second portion of the Berwick triad is the culture, which is defined by the leadership of the organization. Berwick notes that the leader must define the dimensions of quality for the organization, simply because no one else can. Without the clear commitment of the senior leadership of an organization, quality improvement programs cannot hope to be successful on a long-term basis. The leadership must be committed to ensuring that appropriate learning strategies are in place for the organization and that the organization is appropriately organized into teams that allow for defined ways by which progress can be attained.

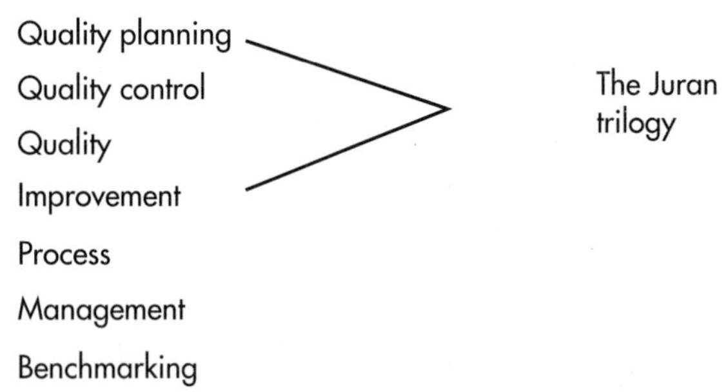

FIGURE 52-10 Building blocks of continuous quality improvement.

The third aspect of the Berwick triad is a series of techniques and tools designed to form the infrastructural quality within the organization. The techniques of quality improvement (Figure 52-10) include the traditional aspects of quality planning, quality control, and quality improvement, to which have been added more recently developed concepts of process management and benchmarking. Quality planning, quality control, and quality improvement have long been recognized as important foundations for quality improvement systems and are often collectively referred to as the Juran trilogy.[25]

Quality Planning

Although there are various means of referring to or defining quality planning, the formulation by the Juran Institute is a concise and accurate description of the process, which

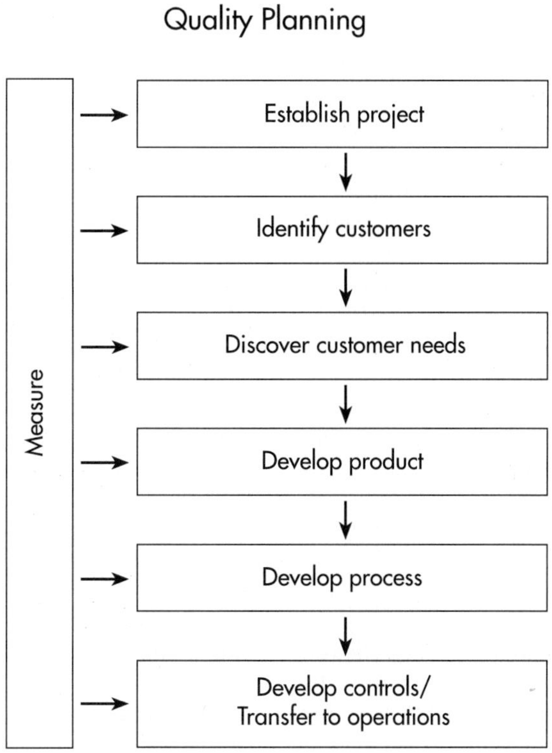

FIGURE 52-11 Quality planning.

involves several steps (Figure 52-11). The first of these steps is to identify the customers of the process, which are defined as all persons or entities that are affected by the processes and products of the provider or manufacturer. After defining internal and external customers, the next step is determine the needs of these customers in a statistical fashion. Once the customers and their needs have been determined, management should develop product features that are responsive to the needs of these customers, particularly in a service environment such as emergency medicine. Too often in emergency medicine, we make the erroneous assumption that our processes and products are in fact responsive to customer needs without having carefully surveyed these customers to determine how closely our concept of quality matches that of the customer.

The fourth aspect of quality planning in the Juran formulation is to develop processes that produce those previously identified features constituting quality for the customer. Finally, it is important to transfer these resulting plans to the operating forces, who will be responsible for ensuring that there is appropriate process capability. In summary, the quality planning process may be referred to in a number of different ways, whether in the formulation of Juran, Hoshin, planning, quality function deployment, and so on. However, the essentials of the quality planning process, regardless of semantics, comprise the activity of developing the products and processes required to meet customer needs and developing processes that will produce those features when deployed by the operational units.

Quality Control

The second element of the Juran trilogy is quality control, which involves the evaluation of actual clinical or management performance, comparison of that performance with goals set in the quality planning process, and identification of actions needed on any differences between the actual performance and preestablished goals. Figure 52-12 shows the elements of the quality control process, which are in many respects similar to more traditional quality assurance in that quality control refers to the actual measurement of performance and is therefore similar to the classic indicators used in quality assurance. Elements of statistical process control are therefore at the heart of quality control programs. The application of run charts, control charts, and other sophisticated statistical techniques forms the basis of the data-driven approach to a meaningful quality improvement program.

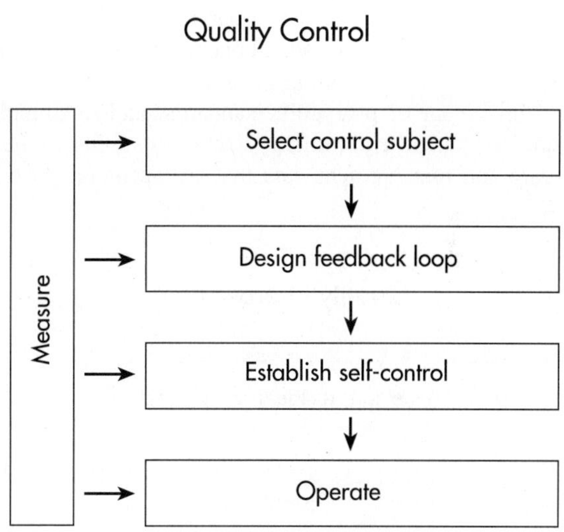

FIGURE 52-12 Quality control.

Quality Improvement

The third component of the Juran trilogy is quality improvement, which is the process of raising quality performance to ever increasing levels. Figure 52-13 delineates Juran's sequence of quality improvement activities, which is the basis for providing an infrastructure for teams focused on specific areas for targeted improvements. As indicated previously, the most important elements in the quality improvement process are ensuring that there are infrastructure in place for the quality improvement team to function and commitment from senior management to ensure its success. Specific needs for quality improvement projects are identified, usually on the basis of previously identified data from quality control mechanisms. A project team is established with clearly delineated responsibilities and appropriate team members to ensure that all aspects of the process are addressed. Finally, the team must be provided the appropriate resources, motivation, and training to diagnose problems, propose remedies, and establish controls to hold quality improvement gains.

When Juran introduced quality planning, quality control, and quality improvement, he compared them with basic financial planning and business processes.[20] Quality planning most closely approximates the budgeting process, and the statistical methods of quality control are similar to cost and expense control processes. The quality improvement process has some parallels with efforts at cost reduction and profit improvement. Box 52-5 illustrates parallels between the quality improvement trilogy, financial planning, and medical process models. Quality planning is similar in some respects to the establishment of protocols, standards, and treatment algorithms for patient care; quality control is similar to the patient care and management data that are accumulated on an ongoing basis. For example, clinical data such as pulse oximetry, pulse and blood pressure monitoring, and clinical laboratory data are all aspects of "clinical quality control" data that we follow on a patient on an ongoing basis. Similarly, turnaround times, cycle times, and data on patients leaving without being seen are all quality control elements affecting management processes within the emergency department. Quality improvement activities are similar to bench and clinical research, in which teams are organized to help solve certain clinical or management problems on an ongoing basis.

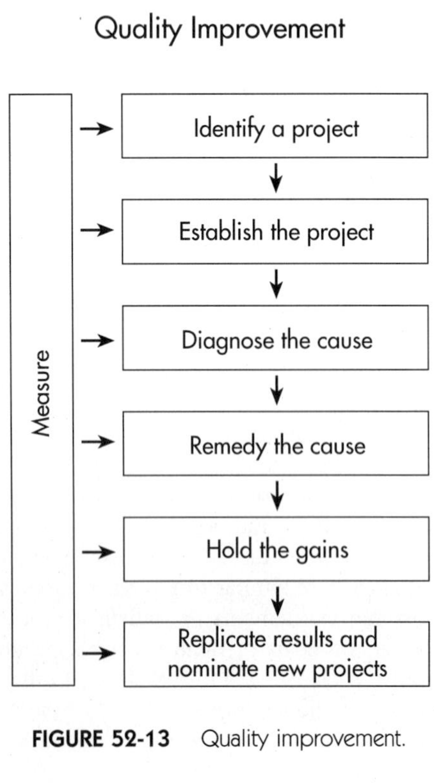

FIGURE 52-13 Quality improvement.

Process Management

Although not originally a part of the Juran trilogy, two additional aspects have been recognized as essential techniques in continuous quality improvement or total quality management: process management and benchmarking. Process management involves the application of specific tools and techniques to examine key cross-functional processes to meet the changing needs of customers. Because the emergency department is such a process-rich environment, utilization of process management tools holds substantial promise for the future of emergency medicine. The quality improvement literature defines a process as an activity that takes inputs, adds value (through a series of subprocesses, activities, and tasks), and produces an output (see Figure 52-2). An essential feature of understanding processes is to see the activities of the emergency department as a series of customer-supplier-processor interactions. Each process comprises several components: people, material, energy, equipment, information, and procedures. Each of these processes, in which an input has valued added to it before production of an output, has several features that are desired. First, the process should be manageable, in that it should be easily communicated to those who are responsible for it and should produce well-defined, discrete output. Second, the process should be effective—it should produce the features that the customers, suppliers, and processors desire. Third, it should be efficient, both from a cost and personnel standpoint. Finally, in the changing world of healthcare, the process should be adaptable to the changing needs of its customers and the environment in which it operates.

Triage is an excellent example of a process operating within the emergency department setting. It meets the classic definition of having an input, value added, and a defined output. There is a combination of people, material, energy,

BOX 52-5

CONTINUOUS QUALITY IMPROVEMENT AND MEDICAL MODELS

Juran trilogy
- Quality planning
- Quality control
- Quality improvement

Medicine
- Protocols and clinical pathways
- Data measurement
- Clinical advances

equipment, and information involved in triage itself. However, the analogy of triage as a process in emergency medicine is instructive in that many emergency departments have failed to recognize the critical aspects involved in the triage process. For example, how many emergency departments are aware of the percentage of patients who come through triage? Is there a clearly understood and widely agreed-to definition of the purpose of triage? Is triage intended to merely classify patients, or is there a substantial customer service aspect also involved in this process? Are we aware of the extent to which we are able to meet customer needs in the course of the triage process? By focusing on key cross-functional processes such as triage, process management in essence offers a structured approach to improving processes on an ongoing basis.

The advantages of process management (Box 52-6) begin with the ability of the organization to focus on the customer as a changing target and to help predict and control change through an understanding of the process functions that constitute the business of the organization. Process management also helps improve the use of available resources by the use of statistical means, promotes a fundamental understanding of inherently complex activities, encourages learning, and manages across boundaries, stakeholders, and interrelationships. As a part of the overall continuous quality improvement or total quality management approach, it also helps accelerate the use of statistical process control and the understanding of variation.

Process management by its nature is inherently more complex and requires a longer-term commitment than quality improvement, quality planning, or quality control (Figure 52-14). In essence, a commitment to a process management team is usually for the life of the organization or the process itself. The work is ongoing because the process continues to be improved by the refinements, redefinition, and reengineering that the process management team undertakes.

Although the overall structure of process management varies from organization to organization, all share features of planning, implementation, and operational management. Because emergency departments are by their nature process-rich environments, process management offers an important and valuable tool to emergency department managers. (See Appendix A for one approach to process management.)

Benchmarking

Benchmarking is the fifth component technique for organizations dedicated to quality improvement. First conceptualized and implemented by Robert Camp at Xerox, benchmarking is formally defined as "the continuous process of measuring products, services, and practices against the company's toughest competitors or those companies renowned as industry leaders."[26] However, a more practical, operational definition is simply "the search for an implementation of best practices." The primary objective of benchmarking is to help further the direction-setting process of an organization and to discover the best practices needed to move in that direction. It differs sharply from traditional management approaches in that the more traditional approach is to establish targets based on the extrapolation of internal past practices and trends. For example, a common goal for an emergency department may be to reduce patient complaints and turnaround times by a certain amount. This goal is set from internal past practices and involves a somewhat arbitrary determination of a target reduction. Benchmarking, on the other hand, seeks to understand what the best practices in regional or national emergency departments are with regard to patient complaint levels and turnaround times. More important, benchmarking involves a rigorous and thorough understanding of the organization's practices, as well as those of industry leaders.[27,28]

There are four basic types of benchmarking: internal, competitive, functional, and generic process benchmarking.[29] Internal benchmarking views similar internal functions that can serve as the baseline to begin to understand processes. For example, laboratory turnaround times may be compared between the emergency department and other critical care areas for an internal benchmarking comparison. However, internal benchmarking in emergency medicine has limited usefulness because of the unique challenges and processes involved in emergency medicine. Competitive benchmarking compares a work process with that of a best competitor in the industry. In emergency medicine this usually involves benchmarking with local or regional competitors, although national competitors can certainly be used as well. An example of competitive benchmarking is comparison of emergency department marketing programs, flight programs, or trauma centers. Looking at best processes and practices within these institutions can lead to improvement for other organizations.

BOX 52-6

ADVANTAGES OF PROCESS MANAGEMENT

- Enables organizations to focus on customer as a changing target
- Enables organizations to predict and control change
- Improves use of available resources by statistical means
- Permits fundamental understanding of complex activities
- Manages boundaries, stakeholders, and interrelationships
- Encourages learning

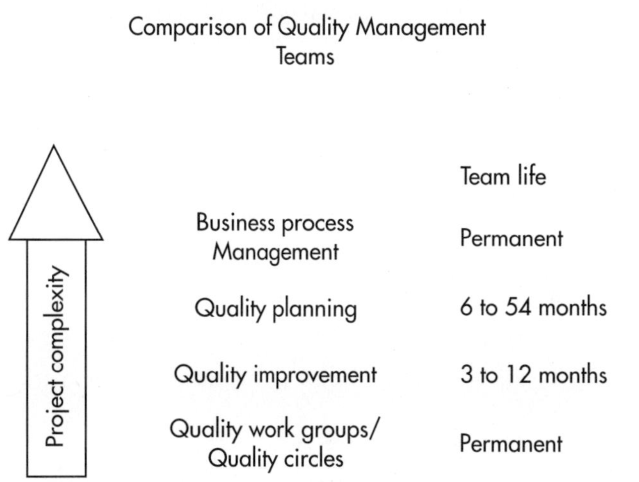

FIGURE 52-14 Comparison of the length of commitment among quality management teams.

Functional benchmarking is the process of comparing a work function to that of a functional leader, often in a different industry. For example, one of the most common functions in an emergency department is entry of physician or nurse orders. Functional benchmarking might look at another industry that also uses order entry as a key functional process. In a similar fashion, generic process benchmarking begins with the identification classification of key business processes, as well as their application in other industrial settings. For example, the process of assigning beds to admitted patients in the hospital might be compared with the assignment of hotel rooms for large hotel chains. Hotel chains are almost uniformly successful in their assignment of beds, but experience has shown that the process of obtaining beds for patients admitted through the emergency department can be long, cumbersome, and subject to extreme variation. The specific steps in benchmarking are perhaps best delineated by the Xerox Corporation itself. Their 10-step benchmarking process is listed in Figure 52-15, which summarizes the detailed nature of the process and the need for careful integration of existing practices with industry standards. Like process management, benchmarking involves a long and detailed commitment to the resources, training, and data measurement necessary to thoroughly understand the process in question and to analyze best practices from other institutions. However, benchmarking shows substantial promise in the healthcare environment and in emergency medicine in particular. As business processes are examined ever more closely, learning from the lessons of other industry leaders can be extremely important in improving the day-to-day clinical and management functions performed in a busy emergency department.

CRITICISMS OF QUALITY IMPROVEMENT

Despite the adoption of quality improvement principles by JCAHO and their acceptance in the healthcare industry in general, there have been several criticisms leveled at continu-

Xerox Ten-Step Benchmarking Process

PHASE I — PLANNING

Step 1: Select a subject to benchmark

- Determine the purpose
- Recruit the team
- Determine the measurements
- Determine the scope and constraints
- Obtain support of all major stakeholders

Step 2: Identify the best practitioner(s)

- Prepare a list
- Select the benchmarking partner(s)

Step 3: Determine the data-collection method and collect the data

- Prepare a list of questions
- Answer the questions for your own operation
- Search for data in existing studies
- Review processes for collecting new data
- Select process(es) and develop guidelines
- Determine who will conduct data gathering
- Review legal, ethical, and protocol requirements
- Collect data using process guidelines

PHASE II — ANALYSIS

Step 4: Determine the current gap

- Tabulate the data
- Analyze data against the purpose of the study
- Determine the benchmark
- Determine the gap
- Determine the general reasons
- Determine specific drivers and practices

Step 5: Project future performance

- Identify assumptions used in the projection
- Project the gap

PHASE III — INTEGRATION

Step 6: Communicate the results of analysis

- Understand your audience
- Determine method of communication
- Organize your analysis
- Obtain acceptance from stakeholders

Step 7: Establish functional goals

- Identify current goals
- Determine what changes could and should be made
- Revise your gap projection
- Obtain commitment to changes
- Revise functional goals

PHASE IV — ACTION

Step 8: Develop action plans

- Prepare action plans
- Organize your plan
- Obtain functional buy-in

Step 9: Implement plan and monitor results

- Implement action plans
- Monitor results

Step 10: Recalibrate benchmark

- Identify appropriate time frame
- Repeat steps 1 to 9

FIGURE 52-15 Xerox benchmarking model. The model contains four major phases: planning, analysis, integration, and action. This model has been widely used and tested in both the manufacturing and healthcare industries.

(Adapted from Camp RC, Tweet AG: *Jt Comm J Qual Improv* 20:229-238, 1994.)

ous quality improvement. Box 52-7 summarizes these general criticisms and the response that quality improvement proponents have made to them. The first and most important criticism of continuous quality improvement is that emergency departments are typically structured with at least three and often four reporting structures. Many emergency departments have a physician structure, a nursing staff structure, a business office structure to accommodate registration, and ancillary services (laboratory and x-ray), which report through a different mechanism. This creates a vertically oriented organization, which can produce fragmentation in terms of the overall purpose of the emergency department's commitment (Figure 52-8). If there is not a clearly agreed to and delineated constancy of purpose among all of the components of the emergency department team, any quality improvement program will have difficulty at best and is doomed to failure at worst. To address this, each of the components of the emergency department team must ensure that there is a clearly delineated and mutually agreed-to sense of purpose in the provision of emergency services and in the importance of the quality improvement program.

The second criticism of quality improvement is that it purports to be a "magic bullet" that will solve the problems of the department in a rapid and sweeping fashion. In fact, CQI is a difficult fundamental change from traditional management, as has been discussed previously. It requires not only a constancy of purpose on the part of the leadership of the emergency department, but a commitment of substantial training and effort toward transition from a traditional management approach to the fundamental changes that are involved in quality improvement. An additional myth is that quality improvement can be somehow delegated to a "quality person" or "quality department." In some emergency departments, a committee is empowered to handle quality improvement activities, but the leadership of the emergency department is not involved in those committees. Similarly, business and industry, as well as healthcare, have often attempted to delegate quality to a single department. The reality of quality improvement is that there must be top level commitment, dedication, and courage to ensure that the senior management of the facility remains committed to the quality improvement initiative on an ongoing basis.

One of the most common criticisms of CQI is that managers somehow lose power in the course of the implementation of such a program. It is presumed that the empowerment of quality improvement and process management teams somehow detracts from a manager's ability to obtain and maintain power and control in the organization. In fact, because of the focus on process and the interrelationships among providers, continuous quality improvement can empower managers further by ensuring that they are armed with statistically derived data to make the difficult management decisions that face healthcare leaders in the 1990s and beyond. A related complaint is that accountability suffers under programs in which the providers of service are empowered to design solutions to existing process problems. However, all of the literature in continuous quality improvement verifies that between 80% and 85% of the sources of rework or complaints regarding industrial inservice models are due to poor design of the system and the processes that make up that system. In 15% to 20% of cases, individual provider problems account for the "defects in service."[7-12] Thus accountability is maintained under a quality improvement system, but the focus is placed more heavily on redesigning the process and maintaining accountability under circumstances in which individual providers are at fault.

One of the most frequently heard complaints of CQI is that it is the latest "management style *du jour*" or "intellectual MTV." The presumption in this criticism is that this is simply the latest management trend, which is sure to pass away as quickly as most such fads do. However, there is substantial reason to believe that CQI as a management philosophy serves as bridge between the rational/scientific management schools and human relations/social science theories of management that have traditionally been taught by business schools. The acceptance of quality improvement as a model for healthcare delivery by JCAHO is an indication of the likely permanence of this philosophy in the medical profession.

Finally, one of the most pervasive myths concerning quality improvement is that it simply "takes too much time." In fact, quality improvement does require a substantial amount of commitment to learning a new approach to management. The majority of continuous quality improvement programs take 3 to 5 years to pay substantial dividends, particularly

BOX 52-7

CRITICISMS OF CONTINUOUS QUALITY IMPROVEMENT

Myth	Reality
CQI is a magic bullet	CQI is a difficult, fundamental change from traditional management
Has been abandoned	Some have "chosen" to abandon CQI
CQI can be delegated	Must have top level commitment and courage
Create quality departments	Quality as a way of life
No focus on profits	Profitability is an outcome of statistical understanding of variation
Managers lose power	CQI is a source of hope
Accountability suffers	Accountability assumes its proper place (80-20 rule)
CQI is intellectual MTV	Bridge between rational/scientific management and human relations/social science theories of management
CQI takes too much time	Realistic option for process change

because the processes themselves must be reengineered to allow for maximum profitability as a legitimate outcome of the statistical understanding of variation that quality improvement entails.

THE RELATIONSHIP OF CONTINUOUS QUALITY IMPROVEMENT TO REDESIGN, REENGINEERING, AND PATIENT-FOCUSED CARE

As quality improvement programs have developed, the concept of radically reassessing processes previously thought to be sacrosanct has become more widely accepted. There have also been a number of different additions to the improvement literature, each purporting to represent radical departures from the essential concepts of quality improvement. Whether these formulations are radical or not depends greatly on the judgment of those who use these processes. Concepts such as redesign, reengineering, and patient-focused care are among the approaches that have been applied in the healthcare setting with good results.[30-32] The simplest concept is redesign, which refers simply to the concept of reorganizing work along process lines, as opposed to along organizational lines. In most cases, focusing on customer outcomes becomes the prime driver of redesigning job descriptions and processes, as opposed to more traditional hierarchical structures. A simple example of redesign is having emergency department technicians draw blood, perform electrocardiograms, apply splints, and so on. This represents a redesign of the way in which work is done in the emergency department, allowing more highly trained and highly compensated individuals to focus on bedside patient care.

The concepts of reengineering have been outlined in detail by Michael Hammer in his innovative books *Reengineering the Corporation* and *The Reengineering Revolution: A Handbook*.[32,33] Hammer defines reengineering as "the fundamental rethinking and radical redesign of business processes to achieve dramatic improvements in critical measures of performance (cost, quality, capital, service, and speed)."[32] The concepts of reengineering differ from those of CQI not so much in philosophy as in the radical nature in which the process is redesigned and the speed in which these redesign efforts are undertaken.[34,35] Both CQI and reengineering are customer focused, are centered on cross-functional processes, and seek improvements of the system. However, reengineering proponents state that quality improvement programs are more incremental in nature, focusing on changes in existing processes.[36,37] Reengineering does not involve changes within a system, but rather makes changes of a system.

Nonetheless, many elements of quality improvement and reengineering are closely aligned, including the need for change, the focus on core processes, and the input of customer and provider. Interested readers are referred to the increasingly rich literature on this subject; however, it may be easiest to envision reengineering as "quality improvement at the speed of light."

A related concept currently being used in many healthcare settings is patient-focused care. Patient-focused care involves redesigning the system to provide seamless care delivery with consolidation of services in the proximity of the patient. Although the original experience with this concept arose in the inpatient setting,[38-40] it has since been extended to the emergency department setting as well.[41,42] Common themes in healthcare redesign include mechanisms for designing the healthcare system that meets patients needs as perceived by the patient rather than by the provider, redesigning patient care processes with the focus on both customer needs and how the work actually gets done, and organizing diagnostic processes and therapeutic protocols around individual patient needs, as opposed to traditional hospital hierarchical structures. How does this differ from CQI? Again, there are far more similarities than differences between redesign, reengineering, and patient-focused care and continuous quality improvement. Although redesign, reengineering, and patient-focused care are not necessarily inherently implied from the initial precepts of CQI, these concepts represent extensions and further refinement of the principles of customer focus, statistical process control, process focus, design and redesign, and redefinition of leadership. In the continuing search for improvement of processes in services, familiarity with the literature of these and other aspects of improvement will be essential. Similarly, concepts such as the learning organization,[43] systems thinking,[44] and idealized design[45] will also be of assistance.

SUMMARY

Continuous quality improvement represents a radical transition from the traditional management philosophy that has been used in medicine for many years to one that focuses more heavily on customer focus, statistical application of the knowledge of variation, understanding of process, the importance of design and redesign, and a redefinition of the role of the leader in the organization. Quality improvement thus entails an unfreezing of our mental models, mindsets, and patterns of reaction that have been learned through decades of training, education, and experience. Rigorous application of the principles of process redesign and a redefinition of our fundamental roles as caregivers and leaders form a substantial amount of the attractiveness of the application of quality improvement to emergency medicine. Most of us have labored under the strong suspicion that the processes in which we were entrapped were fundamentally flawed, in effect preventing us from offering as high a level of service to our customers as we would prefer. Quality improvement principles, particularly combined with elements of change management, boundary management, reengineering, and transformational leadership, may illuminate a path that can truly liberate us to devise strategies that allow us to provide better patient care at lower fixed costs while continuing to enjoy our practices on an ongoing basis.

REFERENCES

1. Mayer TA: Industrial models of continuous quality improvement, *Emerg Med Clin North Am* 10:523-547, 1993.
2. Mayer TA: Quality improvement in emergency medicine. In Schwartz G, Cayten G, Mangelsen M et al, editors: *Principles and practice of emergency medicine,* ed 3, Philadelphia, 1993, Lea & Febiger.
3. Berwick DM: Peer review in quality management: are they compatible? *QRB* 16:246-251, 1990.
4. Dubnicki C, Williams JB: The people's side of TQM, *Healthc Forum J* 35:55-61, 1992.

5. Joint Commission on Accreditation of Healthcare Organizations: *Accreditation manual for hospitals,* 1996, Chicago, JCAHO.
6. Shewhart WA: *Economic control of quality of manufactured products,* New York, 1931, Van Nostrand.
7. Deming WE: *Out of the crisis,* Cambridge, Mass, 1989, Massachusetts Institute of Technology Press, Center for Advanced Engineering Study.
8. Deming WE: *Quality, productivity, and competitive position,* Cambridge, Mass, 1982, Massachusetts Institute of Technology Press, Center for Advanced Engineering Study.
9. Juran JM: *Leadership for quality: executive handbook,* New York, 1989, The Free Press.
10. Juran JM: *Juran on planning for quality,* New York, 1988, The Free Press.
11. Juran JM: *Quality control handbook,* New York, 1988, McGraw-Hill.
12. Ishikawa K: *What is total quality control? The Japanese way,* Englewood Cliffs, NJ, 1985, Prentice Hall.
13. Pellegrino ED, Thomasma DC: *The virtues in medical practice,* New York, 1993, Oxford University Press.
14. Pellegrino ED, Thomasma DC: *For the patient's good: the restoration of beneficence in healthcare,* New York, 1988, Oxford University Press.
15. 1988 Joint National Committee of the National High Blood Pressure Education Program: The 1988 report on detection, evaluation, and treatment of high blood pressure, *Arch Intern Med* 148:1023-1038, 1988.
16. Committee on Trauma, American College of Surgeons: *Advanced trauma life support course,* Chicago, 1994, American College of Surgeons.
17. American Heart Association: *Advanced cardiac life support course,* Dallas, 1994, American Heart Association.
18. American Academy of Pediatrics/American College of Emergency Physicians: *Advanced pediatric life support course,* Dallas, 1995, American College of Emergency Physicians.
19. National Asthma Education Program: *Guidelines for the diagnosis and management of asthma,* Bethesda, Md, 1991, National Institutes of Health.
20. Berwick DM, Godfrey AB, Roessner J: *Curing healthcare: new strategies for quality improvement,* San Francisco, 1990, Jossey-Bass.
21. Berwick DM: Continuous improvement as an ideal in healthcare, *N Engl J Med* 320:53-56, 1989.
22. Berwick DM: Quality convictions: beyond the beginning. Presentation at the Quality Improvement Network Meeting, April 21, 1993, The Healthcare Forum, San Francisco, Calif.
23. Sahney VK, Warden GL: The role of CQI and the strategic planning process, *Qual Manage Healthcare* 1:1-11, 1993.
24. Batalden PB, Buchanan ED: Industrial models of quality improvement. In Goldfield N, Nash DB, editors: *Providing quality care: the challenge to clinicians,* Philadelphia, 1989, American College of Physicians.
25. Juran JM: The quality trilogy: a universal approach for managing for quality, *Quality Progress* 4:19-24, 1986.
26. Camp RC: *Benchmarking: the search for industry best practices that lead to superior performance,* Milwaukee, Wis, 1989, American Society for Quality Control, Quality Press.
27. Spendolini MJ: *The benchmarking book,* 1992, New York, American Management Association.
28. Patrick P, Alba T: Healthcare benchmarking: a team approach, *Qual Manage Healthcare* 2:38-47, 1994.
29. Camp RC, Tweet AG: Benchmarking applied to healthcare, *Jt Comm J Qual Improv* 20:229-238, 1994.
30. Hall G, Rosenthal J, Wade J: How to make reengineering really work, *Harvard Business Review* 71:119-131, 1993.
31. Kennedy M: Reengineering and healthcare, *Qual Lett Healthcare Leaders* 2-10, 1994.
32. Hammer M, Champy J: *Reengineering the corporation,* New York, 1993, HarperCollins.
33. Hammer M, Stanton SA: *The reengineering revolution: a handbook,* New York, 1995, HarperCollins.
34. Drucker PF: The new productivity challenge, *Harvard Business Review* 69-79, 1991.
35. Fralic MF: Creating new practice models and designing new roles: Reflections and recommendations, *JONA* 22:7-20, 1992.
36. Kovner AR: The case of the unhealthy hospital, *Harvard Business Review* 69:12-25, 1991.
37. Morris D, Brandon J: *Reengineering your business,* New York, 1993, McGraw-Hill.
38. Zimmerman D, Skalko J: *Reengineering healthcare: a vision for the future,* Franklin, Wis, 1994, Eagle Press and Zimmerman & Associates.
39. Lowenthal JN: *Reengineering the organization: a step by step approach to corporate revitalization,* Milwaukee, 1994, ASCQ Press.
40. Reeves M, Tory E, editors: *Beyond the basics of reengineering: survival tactics for the 90's,* White Plains, NY, 1994, Quality Resources, Institute of Industrial Engineers.
41. Wakefield DS, Cyphert ST, Murray JF et al: Understanding patient centered care in the context of total quality management and continuous quality improvement, *Jt Comm J Qual Improv* 20:152-161, 1994.
42. Lathrop J: The patient focused hospital, *Healthcare Forum J* 34:76-78, 1991.
43. Garvin DA: Building a learning organization, *Harvard Business Review* 71:78-91, 1993.
44. Senge PM: *The fifth discipline: the art and practice of the learning organization,* New York, 1990, Doubleday.
45. Ackoff RL: *Creating the corporate future,* New York, 1981, Wiley & Sons.

APPENDIX A

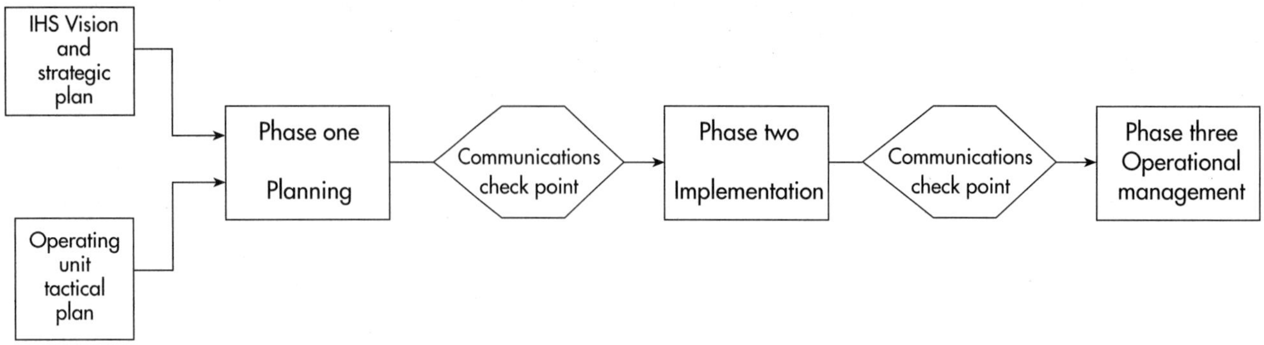

INOVA process management. Roadmap for process management.

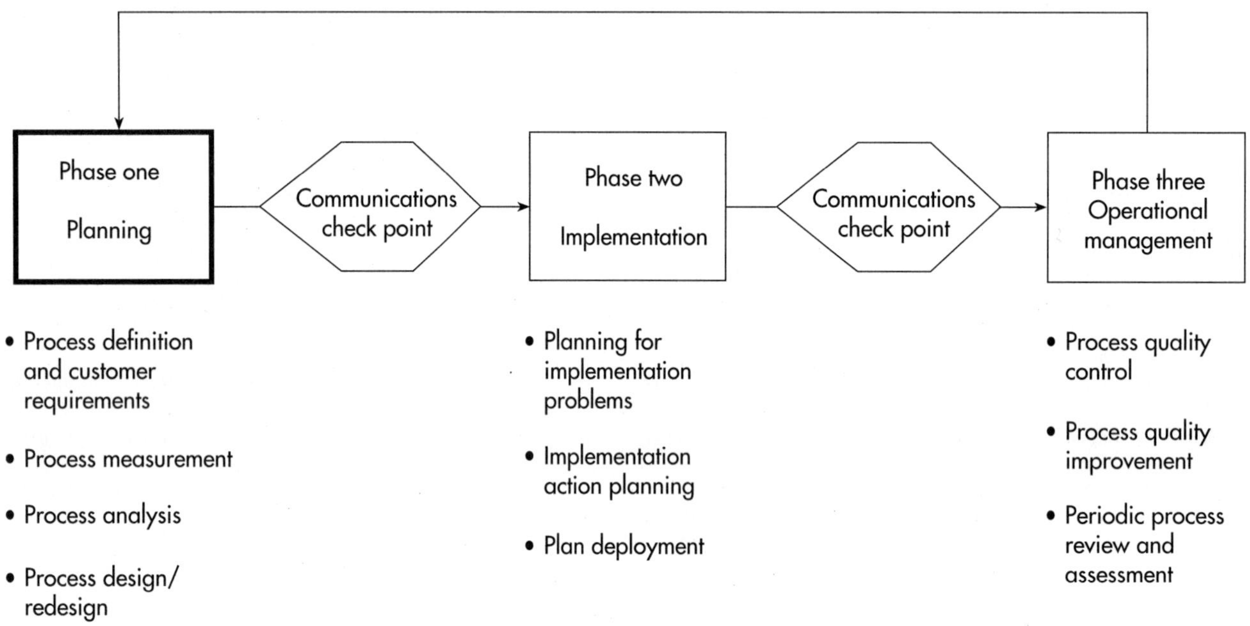

INOVA process management. Roadmap for process management.

Courtesy Inova Health Services, Springfield, Il.

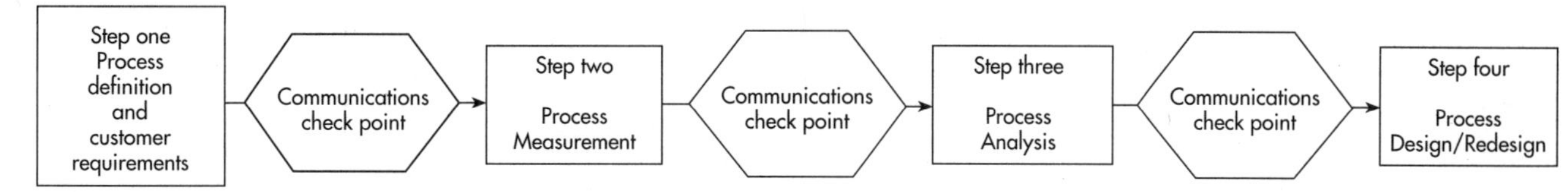

Step one

Establish the process flow
- Macro flow process
- Micro flow process (as required)

Identify key customers and their requirements
- Brainstorm customers of the process
- Select key customers of the process
- Survey key customers to establish customer requirements
- Prioritize and select key customer requirements

Correlate and Prioritize Customer Requirements
- Complete QFD grid
- Develop customer requirement statements (guiding principles)

Step two

Develop initial process performance indicators (based on "current state" measurements):

- Process improvement (i.e., cycle time, reduction in steps, decrease in rework, reduced variation)
- Financial improvement
- Customer satisfaction

Consider customer requirements in measurements

Step three

- Review the macro level flow chart
- Perform value analysis of key activities
- Do value versus cost versus time analysis
- Perform fragmentation analysis
- Perform flexibility analysis complexity analysis
- Micro flow (as required)
- Charter appropriate QI, QP, Reengineering teams

Develop Measurable Targets (future state):
- Process improvement
- Financial improvement
- Customer satisfaction

Review customer requirements

Step four

- Redesign/improve the suspect-value activities within the process
- Additional development of relevant process performance indicators

Incorporate customer requirements

INOVA process management. Phase 1: planning phase.

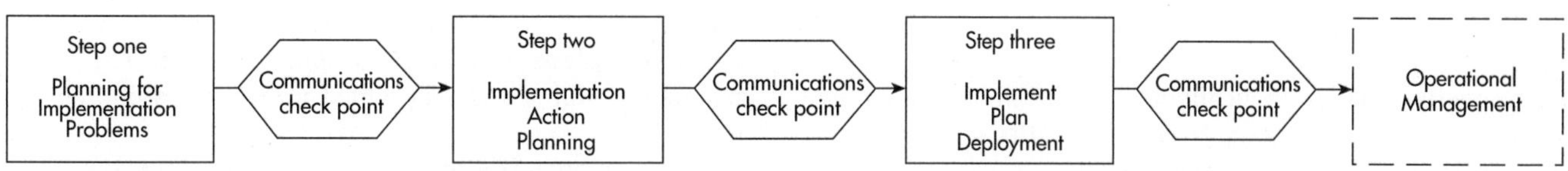

Step one

- Force field analysis
- Plan for contingencies
- Catch ball

Step two

- Documentation of plan
- Action plan template
- Audit
  - Measurement of indicators
  - Holding the gains

Step three

- Allocate resource
- Implement plan
  - Responsibility chart
  - Authority/responsibility/accountability delineated

INOVA process management. Phase 2: implementation phase.

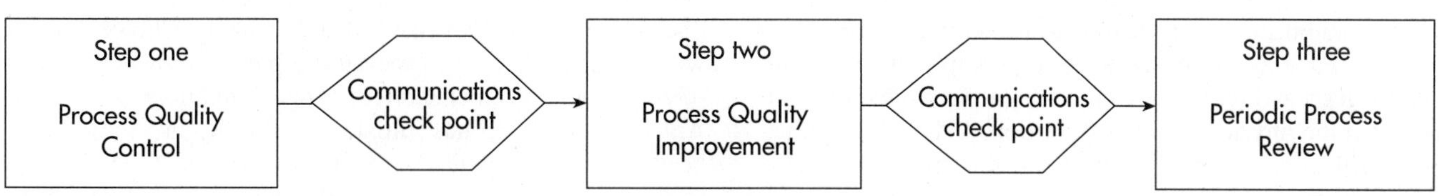

Step one

- Continuous monitoring of process
- Measurement of relevant process performance indicators

Step two

- Act on quality opportunities
- Charter appropriate quality team

  + QI
  + QP
  + QC
  + QB

Step three

- Measurement/trending of indicators
- Holding the gains

INOVA process management. Phase 3: operational management.

53 Service Is a Quality Standard in the Emergency Department

Laura R. Seff

OUTLINE

Traditionally, quality in healthcare has been measured by clinical indicators. Today, however, healthcare providers are expected to evaluate service quality as well. Changes in the healthcare industry are well documented in the medical business literature. Increased competition, rising consumerism, growing public demand for accountability, skyrocketing malpractice claims, and increased awareness of the cost inefficiency of healthcare delivery in this country are among the trends that have drawn attention to the customer's perspective on quality. Because patients are rarely able to evaluate the validity and efficacy of the technical care they receive, the focus of their quality assessment is more often on the affective aspects of how the care is delivered.

As part of the healthcare transformation, traditional roles of patients and physicians have been changing. For much of medicine's long history, physicians practiced medicine as the absolute authorities over the diagnosis and treatment of their patients. Patients were expected to comply with recommended tests and regimens and to accept the professional authority of the physician without question. Although many patients still interact with physicians in this manner, increasingly patients are demanding to be part of the decision-making process in terms of evaluation and treatment. The paternalistic physician is no longer seen as kindly and caring, but rather as arrogant and outdated.

The relationships between physicians and other members of the healthcare delivery system have also changed. New types of care providers such as physician assistants (PAs) and nurse practitioners (NPs) have entered the industry. These providers tend to see the physician as a member of the care delivery team with particular, but not necessarily superior, expertise. More traditional care providers, such as the registered nurse (RN), are increasingly less likely to accept the absolute authority of the physician as well. Growing pressure to control the costs of providing medical care and shortages of these important care providers (PAs, NPs, and RNs) have increased their power and have supported a shift toward democratization and collaboration in the care delivery process.

Pressure for change from patients and ancillary staff is also applied by external agencies that provide accreditation to healthcare organizations. The Joint Commission on Accreditation of Healthcare Organizations (JCAHO) has adopted an "agenda for change," moving their accreditation review emphasis away from retrospective quality assurance systems to more prospective and comprehensive continuous quality improvement processes. In addition, the most recently issued JCAHO standards require accredited healthcare organizations to maintain systems for assessing patient satisfaction with services provided in every hospital department.

Consumer organizations and business coalitions are also pressing for change with patients' rights initiatives and for legislation that requires healthcare organizations to publish patient satisfaction data and other quality of care indicators. For example, Peoples' Medical Society has developed a questionnaire for its members to fill out and send in regarding the "caring" aspects of the healthcare they receive. The American Association for Retired Persons has issued a set of guidelines for healthcare delivery, which includes some indicators of functional quality (reliability, responsiveness, assurance, empathy), and the Group Health Association of America has developed a patient satisfaction instrument for use by payors. The Washington Consumer Checkbook has published ratings of every major hospital in the Washington, D.C., metropolitan area. Hospitals in Cleveland, Ohio, developed the Greater Cleveland Health Quality Choice Project with the specific goal of measuring patient satisfaction with physician and hospital services. The Aluminum Company of America (ALCOA) has initiated a "Buy-Right" strategy for healthcare and requires hospitals with which it contracts to monitor patient satisfaction. Furthermore, ALCOA mandates which hospitals are used based on the satisfaction data results.

To survive in such an environment, physicians must arm themselves with data that will help them better understand what their patients expect from the healthcare delivery system and how patients feel about the medical services they receive. Valid and reliable data are important tools that will enable physicians to take a leadership role in initiating needed improvements. This chapter describes how emergency department medical directors can establish a quality measurement program for their practices.

BUILDING A CUSTOMER SATISFACTION ASSESSMENT PROGRAM

Standards of Care

The foundation of a quality measurement program is a fundamental commitment to providing quality service. To function properly, service systems must create a service culture that conveys an organization's commitment to providing quality services to current and prospective consumers. In the absence of such a foundation, it is difficult to effectively utilize data to change behavior. Data collection and reporting are likely to become meaningless exercises while poor performance continues to plague the organization.

Healthcare organizations can begin to create a quality culture by articulating what behaviors are considered to be exemplary of the desired standard. Although a mission statement is useful as a broad affirmation of commitment, physicians and other providers of healthcare services also need more specific guidelines. Box 53-1 shows a sample "standards of care" document. Five categories of caring behaviors are identified, and specific standards are described within each category.

BOX 53-1

STANDARDS OF CARE

Five caring behavior categories

Timely care
Responsive care
Understandable care
Humane care
Professional care

Responsive care—specific standards

- Patients should be made comfortable from the onset of contact (within 15 minutes of their arrival in the emergency department). Find out if they need a blanket, food, or a place to lie down, and ask a member of the emergency staff to respond to identified needs. If you can't, ask someone else to do this. Be specific when asking the emergency staff to assist; for example, "Please bring Ms. Smith a blanket" or "Please give Mr. Miller directions to the cafeteria."
- Patients in the waiting or examination areas should be checked at regular intervals by a nurse or physician, even if it is only to tell them there will still be a wait. It is the physician's responsibility to ensure that patients have frequent contact with a member of the emergency staff.
- If the patient is in pain, DEAL WITH THE PATIENT'S PAIN. If you cannot alleviate the pain immediately, explain why to the patient. Make sure they understand your explanation and give them a conservative estimate of how soon you will be able to administer medication or when they can expect to feel some relief. Remember that helping patients set realistic expectations about their emergency department experience will make the visit more pleasant and will enable you to give more effective medical care.

Adapted from Sterling Healthcare Group: *Standards of Care*, 1992, Coral Gables, Fla.

Patient Expectations

A number of studies have focused on the link between customer expectations and customer satisfaction, with mixed results. Although the data may be inconclusive, it is appropriate for healthcare providers to attempt to achieve some level of understanding about the expectations of the recipients of healthcare services (i.e., patients).

The work of Zeithaml, Parasuraman, and Berry examines the relationship between customer expectations and satisfaction. They theorize that consumers evaluate service quality along five dimensions (Box 53-2). Consumers enter a service system with expectations in each of these dimensions, and after receiving the service they evaluate to what degree their expectations were met.

Figure 53-1 represents the relationship among the five dimensions of service quality, the expectations that consumers bring to the service delivery system, and the gap between expected and perceived service. This model suggests that consumers form expectations about the five dimensions of service quality based on word of mouth, personal needs, and past experiences. When the service is received, consumers form perceptions of the service along the same five dimensions. Any gap between the expected service and perceived service forms the basis of the consumer's perception of service quality.

Figure 53-2, the gap model of service quality, presents a framework for examining specific points of potential mismatch in a service delivery system that may result in dissatisfied customers. Gap 1 represents the potential for management (in this case, emergency department heads) to make inaccurate assumptions about what customers (i.e., patients) really value and expect from the service system. If management does not understand customer expectations, they are unable to develop appropriate services or to deliver the services in a way that will meet customers' expectations. Gap 2 is the potential discrepancy between management's perceptions of customer expectations and service quality specifications. It is not unusual for service systems to miss the mark on stated goals, and, even if management understands customer expec-

BOX 53-2

FIVE DIMENSIONS OF REFINED SERVICE QUALITY SCALE

Tangibles: the appearance of physical facilities, equipment, personnel, and communication materials
Reliability: ability to perform the promised service dependably and accurately
Responsiveness: willingness to help customers and provide prompt service
Assurance: knowledge and courtesy of staff and their ability to inspire trust and confidence
Empathy: caring, individualized attention the organization provides its customers

Adapted from Zeithaml VA, Parasuraman A, Berry LL: *Delivering quality service: balancing customer perceptions and expectations*, New York, 1990, The Free Press.

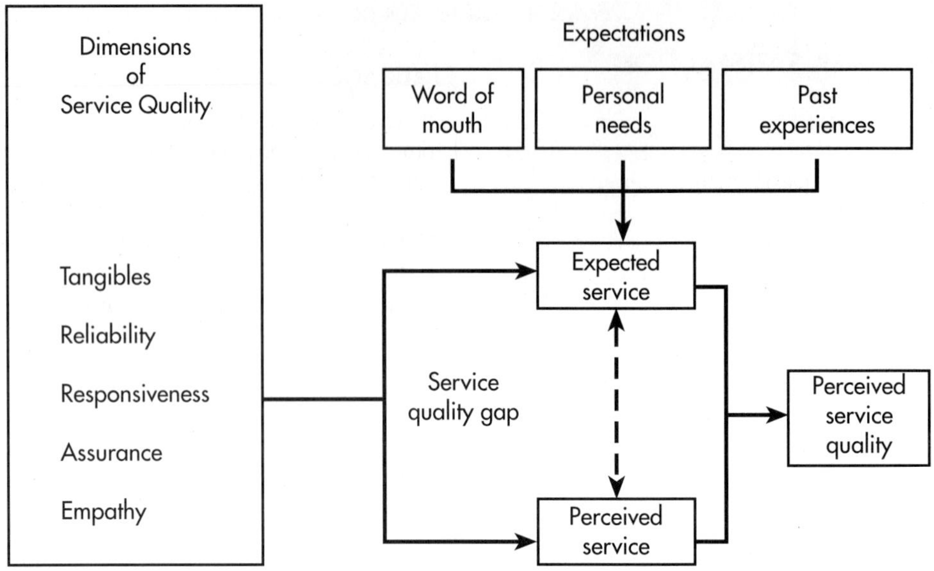

FIGURE 53-1 Determinants of perceived service quality.

(Adapted from Zeithaml VA, Parasuraman A, Berry LL: ***Delivering quality service: balancing customer perceptions and expectations***, New York, 1990, The Free Press.)

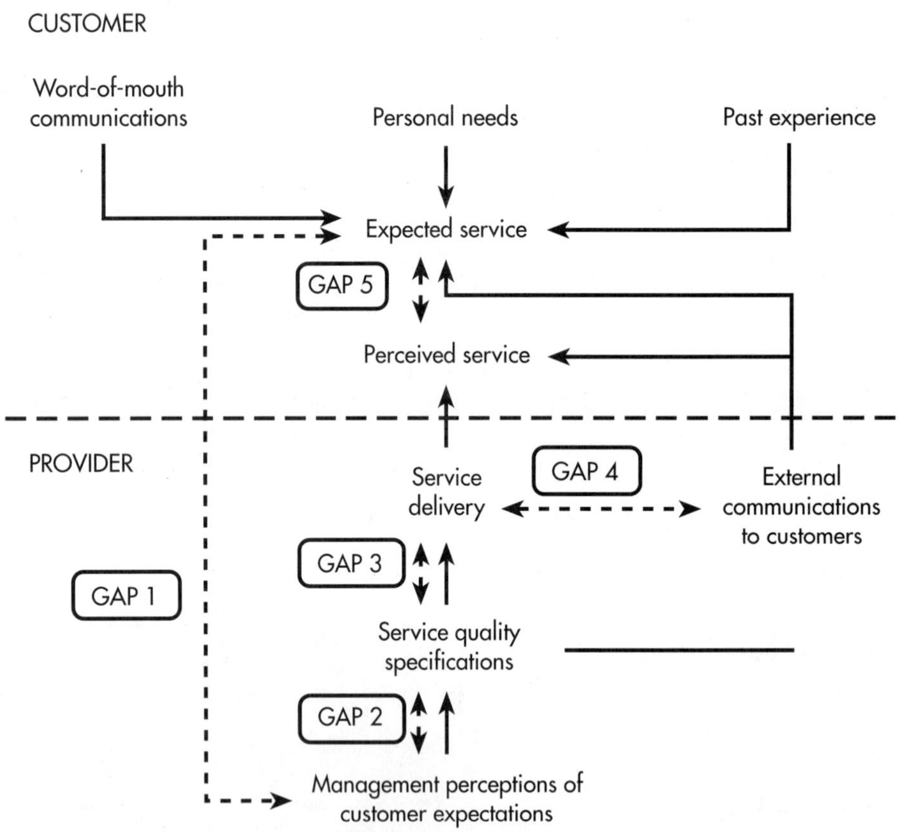

GAP 1: Consumer expectation-management perception.
GAP 2: Management perception-service quality specification.
GAP 3: Service quality specification-service delivery.
GAP 4: Service delivery-external communications.
GAP 5: Expected service-perceived service.

FIGURE 53-2 Conceptual model of service quality.

(Adapted from Parasuraman A, Zeithaml VA, Berry LL: A conceptual model of service quality and its implications for future research, ***J Marketing*** 3:41-50, 1985.)

tations perfectly, the design of the service system may not appropriately address those expectations. If management's perceptions are not accurate, it is easy to see the cumulative effect of problems in both areas. Gap 3 highlights the potential for service to be delivered in a way that does not meet quality specifications. This gap can be especially large when the people who are responsible for service delivery are not involved in development of service quality specifications. Good training for service providers with regard to quality standards will help minimize this gap. Any difference between what the service provider communicates to customers about the service they will receive and the actual service delivered is represented by gap 4. Promotional materials and marketing campaigns sometimes make promises that are difficult for service providers to deliver on. Finally, gap 5 shows the difference between what customers perceive about the service received and what they expected when they arrived for service.

The model suggests that if expectations are confirmed by the provided service, the consumer will be relatively satisfied; if expectations are disconfirmed, the consumer will be relatively dissatisfied. Note that gap 5 is a function of the other four gaps and therefore cannot be acted on directly. To reduce the size of gap 5, gaps 1 through 4 must be remedied. Although there is some controversy regarding the disconfirmation theory, the gap model offers healthcare service providers an interesting and useful way to visualize and articulate where systems run amok, leading to dissatisfied patients. One appealing aspect of using the gap model is its clear focus on systems versus individual performance. This is consistent with continuous quality improvement principles. Continuous quality improvement tools such as the cause and effect diagram, flowcharts, frequency tables, histograms, and Pareto diagrams are useful in identifying opportunities for improvement in each of the five gaps.

Patient Satisfaction

Although it may seem that emphasis on monitoring patient satisfaction with service quality is a recent phenomenon, medical literature dating back to ancient Rome contains references to this timeless issue. In Plato's *The Statesman,* a speaker proposed that because the doctor "cuts us up, and orders us to bring him money . . . as if he were exacting tribute . . . he should be put under rigid control." This could be accomplished by calling an assembly of all the people and inviting opinions about "disease and how drugs and surgical instruments should be applied to patients." The speaker also proposed that the people "elect our physicians from among our number for one year terms, and severely penalize them if they fail to carry out the letter of the law."

Collecting data about patient satisfaction is an important component of any initiative to create a service quality culture. Rhetoric and philosophy may be debated or subjected to semantic dissection, but data provide definitive indicators of actual performance of the service delivery system and the individuals who participate in that system. There are a number of methodologies for collecting information about patient satisfaction. These include complaint tracking, telephone surveys, mail surveys, and focus groups. Each methodology has advantages and disadvantages; a comprehensive data collection program will include more than one approach.

BOX 53-3

COMPLAINT CODE DEFINITIONS

Example of categories

100	Charges
200	Physician
300	Other emergency department issues
400	Billing

Example of definitions within categories

200 Physician	
201 Physician—quality of care	Patient is unhappy with quality of clinical care from physician.
202 Physician—examination	Patient states that he or she was not seen or was not examined by emergency physician.
203 Physician—procedure	Patient states that emergency physician did not perform a particular procedure reflected on the bill.
204 Physician—diagnosis	Patient states that physician's diagnosis is incorrect.
205 Physician—professionalism	Patient states that physician was impatient, unprofessional, rude, poorly groomed, etc.
206 Physician—information	Patient states that he or she was misinformed or received inadequate information from emergency physician re: discharge instructions, billing/charges, referral.

Complaint Tracking. Patient complaints should be tracked as part of every service quality measurement program. Complaint categories should be clearly defined, and each complaint should be coded to reflect all issues addressed by the person filing the complaint. Specific complaint issues should be tracked, rather than complaint incidents, because any one complaint incident may represent more than one complaint issue. For example, a patient may call or write to complain about the bill and may also mention that the nurse was rude and the physician never examined the patient. The bill, the rude nurse, and the invisible physician are three distinct complaint issues generated by one complaint incident. Patients may complain directly to emergency department staff, to hospital administration, to the physician, or to the billing office. Because complaints may be filed in a number of different places, a uniform reporting procedure should be developed as well. Box 53-3 presents a sample patient complaint coding system. Figure 53-3 shows an example of a patient complaint data collection form. Figures 53-4, 53-5, and 53-6 represent the kind of reports that are useful in analyzing patient complaint information.

Tracking complaints is not a substitute for collecting information about patient satisfaction or dissatisfaction using other methodologies. Patient complaint reporting represents an extremely skewed source of satisfaction data and must be supplemented by data collected in a more random fashion.

Attach copy of patient chart

PATIENT COMPLAINTS

Hospital: ____________________

Physician UPIN # ____________________ Medical Record # ____________________

1. Patient Name: ____________________ (Last / First / MI)

Date of E.D. visit: ____________________

Date of complaint: ____________________

Patient admitted: ☐ Yes ☐ No

2. Source of complaint: (CHECK ONE)

☐ Patient ☐ Family

☐ Other ____________

3. What was the primary complaint? (CHECK ONLY ONE)

Charges:
- ☐ Charges high for services patient received from physician
- ☐ Charges in general excessive/unreasonable
- ☐ Other ____________

Physician:
- ☐ Physician quality of clinical care
- ☐ Physician did not see/examine the patient
- ☐ Physician diagnosis incorrect
- ☐ Physician demeanor/attitude/professionalism
- ☐ Physician gave inappropriate referral/ no referral
- ☐ Other ____________

ED Staff:
- ☐ ED staff quality of clinical care
- ☐ ED staff demeanor/attitude/ professionalism
- ☐ Other ____________

Facility:
- ☐ ED wait/delay in care
- ☐ Ancillary services
- ☐ Environment (e.g. equipment, bathrooms, waiting area)
- ☐ Other ____________

4. What else did the patient complaint involve? (CHECK ALL THAT APPLY)

Charges:
- ☐ Charges high for services patient received from physician
- ☐ Charges in general excessive/unreasonable
- ☐ Other ____________

Physician:
- ☐ Physician quality of clinical care
- ☐ Physician did not see/examine the patient
- ☐ Physician diagnosis incorrect
- ☐ Physician demeanor/attitude/professionalism
- ☐ Physician gave inappropriate referral/ no referral
- ☐ Other ____________

ED Staff:
- ☐ ED staff quality of clinical care
- ☐ ED staff demeanor/attitude/ professionalism
- ☐ Other ____________

Facility:
- ☐ ED wait/delay in care
- ☐ Ancillary services
- ☐ Environment (e.g. equipment, bathrooms, waiting area)
- ☐ Other ____________

5. Action Taken. Check all that apply and describe response for each action. Include mode (letter, memo, meeting, call, referral), who made the contact <u>and</u> who was contacted.

☐ With patient	Date: ________	Response: ____________
☐ With ED staff	Date: ________	Response: ____________
☐ With billing co.	Date: ________	Response: ____________
☐ With physician	Date: ________	Response: ____________

6. Perceived status of initiator (CHECK ONE): ☐ fully satisfied ☐ satisfied, not in agreement ☐ dissatisfied

Comments: ____________________

Reviewed By: ____________________ Date: ________

FIGURE 53-3 Sample patient complaint form.

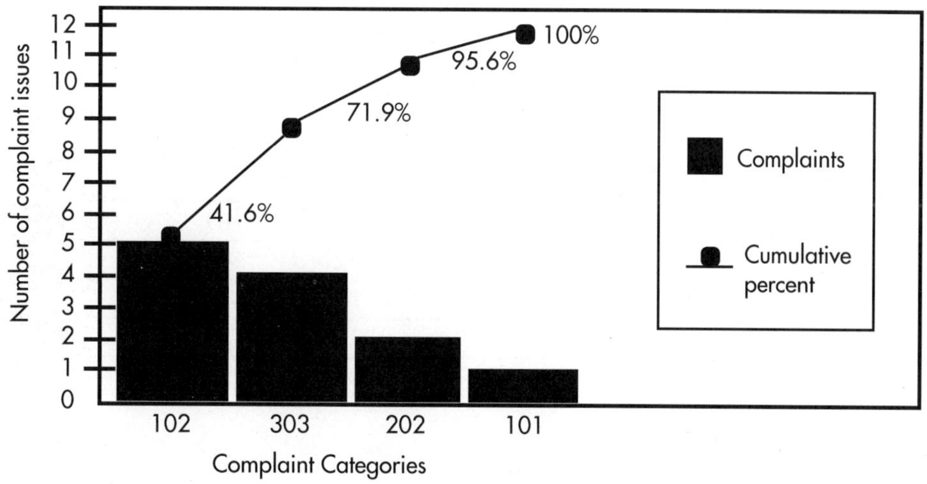

Note: This graph represents the number of complaint issues for one emergency department for a sample month.

FIGURE 53-4 Emergency department complaint issues, Pareto diagram—sample month.

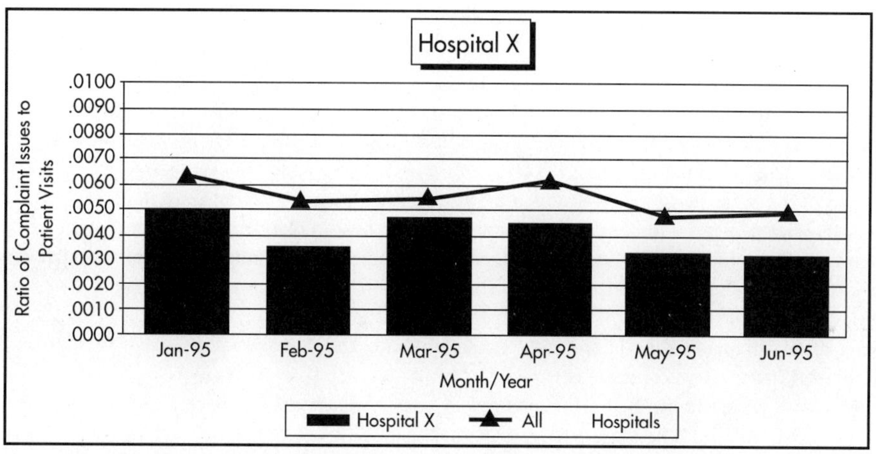

Note: This graph shows the trended ratio (number of complaint issues divided by the number of patients seen) for the practice. An average representation from a reference data base is also provided.

FIGURE 53-5 Trended ratio of complaint issue to patient visits.

Telephone Surveys. Telephone surveys represent an opportunity to pursue a randomly selected sample and to maximize the information gathered by using a mix of specific, open-ended, and clarifying questions. A telephone survey may represent one of the most statistically valid and reliable sources of data regarding how patients feel about the services they receive if the sampling methodology is statistically sound, the survey is developed with statistical rigor, and the surveyors are trained to ensure interrater reliability. However, telephone surveys are expensive, and, for many hospitals or physician practices, telephone surveys will be cost prohibitive.

Mail Surveys. A mail survey offers the advantage of lower cost than a telephone survey and also provides survey respondents with anonymity not offered in the telephone survey method. Mail surveys may be done using a randomly selected sample or may be sent to all patients. Distributing a survey at patient discharge is a variation of the mail survey. Mailing surveys or distributing them at discharge creates some sampling errors, and therefore collected data lack statistical rigor. Nevertheless, data may be used to demonstrate trends in either satisfaction or dissatisfaction with certain aspects of the healthcare delivery system. Mail surveys are generally less expensive than telephone surveys. Distributing surveys at discharge is even more economic. It is important, however, that the survey reply process be facilitated by offering respondents preaddressed, postage-paid reply cards or envelopes. Box 53-4 indicates the steps that should be taken to prepare a survey. Figure 53-7 is a sample of a patient satisfaction survey.

Survey frequency will be a function of economic constraints and the amount of data required. A survey distrib-

HOSPITAL X

Physician UPIN #	Number of Complaint Issues per Month Jan-95	Feb-95	Mar-95	Apr-95	May-95	Jun-95	Year-to-Date Total
A11111	1	0	1	0	1	2	5
B22222	0	1	1	0	0	0	2
C33333	0	0	0	1	0	0	1
D44444	1	2	1	0	1	0	5
E55555	0	0	0	0	0	0	0

Note: This graph shows the number of physician related complaint issues for each physician in the emergency department practice.

FIGURE 53-6 Trended physician-related complaint issues, by physician UPIN number.

BOX 53-4

PREPARING A PATIENT SATISFACTION SURVEY

Step 1: Determine issues or areas that the survey should focus on. For example, the survey in Figure 53-3 looks at seven performance areas, based on the flow of a patient's emergency visit. It is helpful if discrete categories are identified.

Step 2: Select a response scale. Options include a Likert scale, which offers respondents a range over which to identify the *level or degree* of a certain item. Likert scales are often presented as 1 to 5 but may include as many degrees as the surveyor wishes. Define which end of the scale represents the best performance and which represents the worst. Phrases such as "very satisfied" and "very dissatisfied" are helpful in defining the range. Another commonly used response scale is "yes" or "no." It is helpful to add the option of "not applicable" when using a yes/no response scale. On some questionnaires it is also important to have a "don't know" option. Include at least one or two open-ended questions that offer respondents the opportunity to elaborate on any coded responses and to address issues that may not have been covered in the survey questions.

Step 3: Develop questions for each focus area. Make sure each question addresses a discrete issue. One survey pitfall is to ask about more than one thing in a single question. Questions should be stated simply and should be written at no higher than a sixth-grade reading level. Qualifying words, such as all, every, and never, should be avoided. Attention should be paid to whether the question is stated positively or negatively. Survey theory suggests there is value in mixing this; however, mixing positive and negative wording may result in a survey that is difficult for respondents to understand.

Step 4: Test the survey before finalizing it. Start with getting feedback from employees, and then test with a sample patient group. Make modifications as needed.

Step 5: Select a presentation format. Determine how the survey should look. Appearance is important in terms of maximizing response. Patients are much more likely to respond to an attractive, printed survey than to one that comes from a copy machine.

Step 6: Establish a reporting format, and determine how data will be disseminated and used to improve the emergency department practice.

uted at patient discharge will produce a relatively low response rate. It is best to offer a survey distributed in this way to every patient to maximize the response and to minimize distribution bias. Nurses, physicians, and any other staff who might have responsibility for distributing the survey must be trained to ensure that every patient receives a survey and to encourage patients to complete and return the information. The response rate will improve if patients get a clear message that the staff members care about the patients' point of view. With a mail survey, and certainly with a telephone survey, reaching every patient may be cost prohibitive. If every patient will not be surveyed, the sampling strategy and a survey schedule should be predetermined to ensure that data are collected consistently and at regular intervals.

Focus Groups. Focus groups bring together a randomly selected or targeted group of consumers to discuss certain aspects of the service delivery system. Focus groups are used to identify causes of satisfaction and dissatisfaction, to collect information from consumers about how to improve service delivery, to clarify consumer expectations, and to anticipate consumer response to planned product or system innovations. The success of a focus group depends on the skill

PATIENT SATISFACTION SURVEY

We want to continuously improve the services we provide in our emergency department. We pride ourselves on providing quality medical care and on our kindness to the patients we see, their families and friends. Your comments, both good and bad, help us continue to improve.

Directions: Please answer the following questions. Use "N/A" to indicate that a question does not apply to your situation. If you were not the patient, please answer questions about "you" from your point of view.

	Yes	No	N/A
1. Were you the patient?	❑	❑	❑
2. If you were not the patient, the patient is your... (please check one) ❑ parent ❑ child ❑ husband/wife ❑ other relative ❑ friend ❑ employee			
WHEN YOU ARRIVED...			
3. Were you greeted right away when you first came to the emergency department?	❑	❑	❑
4. Did the clerk or nurse who greeted you tell you how long you would have to wait to see the doctor?	❑	❑	❑
5. Do you feel your wait to see the doctor was reasonable?	❑	❑	❑
WHEN YOU REGISTERED...			
6. Did the registration process take a reasonable amount of time?	❑	❑	❑
7. Was the registration staff nice to you?	❑	❑	❑
8. Did the registration staff give you information about the billing process?	❑	❑	❑
WHEN YOU SAW THE DOCTOR...			
9. Did the doctor let you fully explain what the problems were that brought you to the emergency department?	❑	❑	❑
10. Did the doctor let you ask all your questions?	❑	❑	❑
11. Did the doctor clearly answer all your questions?			
12. Was the doctor nice to you?	❑	❑	❑
IF YOU NEEDED TESTS...			
13. Were you satisfied with the care you received from:			
a. Lab technician (person who drew blood)	❑	❑	❑
b. X-ray technician (includes regular, CT-scan, ultrasound)	❑	❑	❑
c. Heart test technician (EEG, EKG)	❑	❑	❑
d. Other (specify) ______ (If N/A, please skip to question #17.)	❑	❑	❑
14. Do you feel the amount of time you waited for the tests, listed above, to be performed was reasonable?	❑	❑	❑
15. Do you feel the amount of time you waited for test results was reasonable?	❑	❑	❑
16. Did the doctor clearly explain the results of all the tests?	❑	❑	❑
DURING YOUR VISIT...			
17. Were the nurses and staff nice to you?	❑	❑	❑
18. Were you kept informed about the progress of the evaluation and treatment during your visit?	❑	❑	❑
19. Do you feel your privacy was respected during your visit?	❑	❑	❑
AT THE END OF YOUR VISIT...			
20. Were you (the patient) admitted to the hospital? (If yes, please skip to question #24)	❑	❑	❑
21. When you left the emergency department did you understand what was wrong?	❑	❑	❑
22. When you left the emergency department did you know how to take care of the illness or injury?	❑	❑	❑
23. Do you feel the amount of time you waited to be released from the emergency department was reasonable?	❑	❑	❑
IN GENERAL...			
24. If you are sick or hurt again, will you come back to this emergency department? Why? ______	❑	❑	❑
25. Please indicate about how long you spent in the emergency department, from the time you arrived to the time you left: ❑ less than 1 hour ❑ 1-2 hours ❑ 2-3 hours ❑ 3-4 hours ❑ more than 4 hours	❑	❑	❑
26. Please check the box which best shows how satisfied you were, overall, with your experience in our emergency department: ❑ very satisfied ❑ satisfied ❑ dissatisfied ❑ very dissatisfied	❑	❑	❑

27. Age of the patient?
❑ 0-12 ❑ 13-20 ❑ 21-30 ❑ 31-40 ❑ 41-50
❑ 51-60 ❑ 61-70 ❑ 71-80 ❑ 81+

28. Patient gender? ❑ female ❑ male

29. Date of the patient's visit to the emergency department? ______

30. Suggestions for improvement:
______
______
______
______

(Additional comments on reverse side)

31. Would you like to talk with someone about your visit to the emergency department? ❑ Yes ❑ No If yes, please indicate:

Patient's name: ______
Your name: ______ Day-time phone: ( ) ______
Address: ______ Night-time phone: ( ) ______
______

FIGURE 53-7 Sample patient satisfaction survey.
(Copyright 1993, Sterling Healthcare Group. Used with permission.)

of the facilitator, the composition of the group, and the degree to which questions are skillfully framed and responses carefully documented.

Some hospitals and physician practices have developed variations on the focus group idea. These include establishing a consumer group that meets periodically to provide input and establishing a regular forum, such as a monthly lunch with the administrator, where interested consumers have an opportunity to discuss issues of importance to them with representatives from the hospital or the practice.

USING DATA TO IMPROVE PATIENT SATISFACTION

Collecting data about patient satisfaction is less than half the battle. The more challenging task is to effectively use the data to modify systems or individual behavior patterns that result in dissatisfied patients.

Data Analysis

Collected data should be entered into databases, with a separate database for each of the data collection programs. With survey data, data entry is straightforward. Responses to open-ended questions should be subjected to some coding scheme so that results can be reviewed in an organized fashion. The coding method suggested for patient complaints in Box 53-3 is an example of how text responses can be categorized for analysis. Data from focus groups may be coded in a similar way. It is extremely important to create well-defined, discrete coding categories and to train coders extensively to ensure reliability.

Data collected with statistically valid survey instruments using statistically sound sampling methodology may be subjected to rigorous analysis. Unless the hospital or emergency staff includes an experienced statistician, it will be necessary to locate someone with expertise in statistical analysis to assist with this process. Data collected in a less rigorous fashion do not need to be statistically analyzed and can be looked at using basic continuous quality improvement tools such as frequency tables, histograms, Pareto diagrams, scattergrams, and control charts. Figure 53-4 is an example of complaint data analysis using a Pareto diagram.

Reports

Special attention must be paid to how data are presented and who sees the reports. Often there is a tendency to keep data "confidential" and control access to reports. However, wide dissemination is essential to the effectiveness of service quality data collection and improvement programs.

Reports should be attractive to look at and easy to interpret. Complicated graphs or charts should be avoided. Some people have an inclination to pack a lot of information into a single data presentation. This approach may save time and paper, but the results will be less than satisfactory because the report will be difficult to interpret. The rule of thumb is that the report reader should be able to look at the graph or chart and, without any explanation other than what is printed on the page, determine exactly what the data indicate. Just as surveys are tested, report formats should be tested to ensure that all readers can gain maximum benefit by reviewing them.

Data from more than one data collection program may be incorporated into a single report. For example, a report might include graphs on patient complaints, graphs on patient satisfaction survey results, and a presentation summarizing a recent focus group. This is a beneficial approach to patient satisfaction data because there may be simultaneous data collection efforts focusing on different aspects of patient satisfaction and service quality that when looked at together provide a comprehensive snapshot. There is a strong argument for including patient satisfaction and service quality data in clinical performance improvement reports. This practice affirms the belief that customer satisfaction and service quality are integrally linked to the delivery of clinical service and are important measures of the effectiveness of any healthcare delivery system. Satisfaction data should also be used in conjunction with the gap analysis (see Figure 53-2) to help identify areas where the service system is not working effectively.

Presentation of the data, however, may not be sufficient to bring about needed change. Therefore wide dissemination of data is highly desirable. Furthermore, the emergency medical director and other hospital leaders must implement organizational structures which ensure that collected data are looked at, discussed, and acted on. These structures may include routine and ad hoc committees, regular departmental meetings, and periodic educational conferences. Successful introduction of these structures is, perhaps, the most challenging aspect of any program to improve service quality. As with all continuous quality improvement endeavors, the ability of the leadership to both inspire and control groups so that they effectively use data to initiate and monitor change is critical.

Separating Systems Problems from Personality Aberrations

Traditionally, customer satisfaction and other service quality issues have been linked to individual performance. Even with the proliferation of continuous quality improvement theory there is a tendency to point a finger at one person when problems are identified. Clearly an individual healthcare provider's personality aberrations or skill deficits may lead directly to a dissatisfied patient. However, it is extremely important, even in what appear to be clear cut situations, to look deeper and determine if there are systems that need to be modified to completely ameliorate the concern. Continuous quality improvement techniques, such as cause-and-effect and Pareto analysis, are effective tools for separating the issues and identifying opportunities for improvement that focus on systems rather than individuals. When systems problems have been ruled out or addressed but dissatisfaction persists, it is then appropriate to focus on an individual whose performance is below standard.

Use of data in one-on-one counseling sessions can be powerful and is often a persuasive motivator for behavior change. Most individuals are not happy to learn that their performance falls below that of their colleagues on well-defined criteria and will work to improve their relative standing.

INTERNAL CUSTOMERS

For any external customer-focused service quality program to succeed, organizations must initiate comprehensive standards for internal customer service quality and measure actual performance against those standards. This falls under the continuous quality improvement concept of "walking the talk." In other words, it is difficult to gain commitment from physician and nonphysician staff for a service quality measurement and improvement system if there is no internal corollary. Furthermore, if the internal environment is characterized by noticeable factionalism, inappropriate competition, and a general sense of disharmony, it will be difficult to make effective use of external customer satisfaction data.

For the emergency medical director, internal customers include hospital administration, emergency medical services, nursing staff, ancillary departments, and the medical staff. All the components of an external service quality measurement system described in this chapter apply to internal customers, and the steps described in the section on building a customer satisfaction assessment program should be followed as the program is developed.

Setting standards of behavior toward internal customers is often overlooked, even when clear standards are established for external customers.

Understanding expectations of internal customers is extremely important. Each type of internal customer may have a different set of expectations about the service delivery system and different ideas about how service quality is defined. Therefore a separate analysis should be undertaken for each customer category. Again, the gap analysis model shown in Figure 53-2 provides a useful framework for examining expectations and understanding points in the system that may lead to dissatisfaction.

The same methodologies described earlier—complaint tracking, telephone and mail surveys, and focus groups—are appropriate for data collection regarding internal customer satisfaction. Likewise, the same principles for data analysis, reporting, dissemination, and improvement implementation should be followed. As with expectations, the satisfaction of each internal customer constituency should be assessed and analyzed separately.

SUMMARY

The emergency physician has an important leadership role to play in setting performance standards, recognizing the need to understand and accommodate internal and external customers' expectations, and placing emphasis on improving customer satisfaction. Clearly, regular collection and review of satisfaction data as part of an ongoing quality assessment and performance improvement program are essential in today's healthcare environment.

Development of comprehensive programs as described in this chapter may seem daunting. The best way to get past that hurdle is to take the process one step at a time. Begin with modest goals and build on successes. Although there is great power in putting all the kinds of information described in this chapter together, each piece is valuable in its own right.

BIBLIOGRAPHY

Lanning JA, O'Connor SJ: The health care quality quagmire: some signposts, *Hosp Health Serv Admin* 35(1):39-43, 1990.

O'Connor SJ, Shewchuk RM, Carney LW: The great gap: physicians' perception of patient services quality expectations fall short of reality, *J Health Care Marketing* 14(2):32-37, 1994.

Nelson CW, Nierderberger J: Patient satisfaction surveys: an opportunity for total quality management, *Hosp Health Serv Admin* 35(3):409-414, 1990.

Yenney SL: Practice management: how to survey patients and staff to improve your practice, *Consultant* 29(12):41-49, 1989.

Press I, Ganey RF, Malone MP: Satisfied patients can spell financial well-being, *Healthcare Financial Manage* 45(2):34-39, 1991.

France KR, Grover R: What is the health care product? *Health Care Marketing* 12(2):31, 1992.

Emanuel EJ, Emanuel LL: Four models of the physician-patient relationship, *JAMA* 267(16):2221-2226, 1992.

Schwartz LR, Overton DT: The management of patient complaints and dissatisfaction, *Emerg Med Clin North Am* 10(3):557-572, 1992.

Jones WS: *Hippocrates*, vol 2 (English translation), London, 1923, William Heinemann.

54 Selecting and Defining Quality Improvement Projects

Linda Greenberg

OUTLINE

Emergency department monitoring data and staff behavior
Benefits of a multidisciplinary approach to problem solving
Creating quality improvement teams
Selecting quality improvement projects
Evaluating continuous improvement
Summary

Quality service will differentiate emergency departments in the future. Departments that provide cost-effective, efficient, and excellent service will be the choice of consumers. The traditional management choice to provide either quality service or cost-effective service is no longer an option; consumers now demand both quality and cost-effectiveness. The department's success will be directly related to the effectiveness of its quality improvement (QI) monitoring.

Quality improvement monitoring can have many benefits for an emergency department. First, a well-organized monitoring plan that focuses on enhancing patient outcomes will meet Joint Commission on Accreditation of Healthcare Organizations (JCAHO) requirements. Quality improvement is also an excellent methodology to assess the efficacy of care delivered, as well as the efficiency and cost-effectiveness of care delivery systems.

This chapter will explain the relationship between emergency department monitoring data and emergency staff behavior change strategies; discuss the benefits of a multidisciplinary approach to emergency department problems; describe how a QI team is created; illustrate how QI projects are selected; and discuss the evaluation of continuous improvement.

EMERGENCY DEPARTMENT MONITORING DATA AND STAFF BEHAVIOR

Implementing changes in staff behaviors can be a complicated and time-consuming process. The QI process can be used as an effective process or tool to assist in implementing such changes. The JCAHO 10-step process (Box 54-1) uses a problem identification model.[1] Once a problem is identified, an assessment of the scope and details of the problem is done, data are collected, a plan of action is recommended and implemented, and the outcomes are evaluated to see if the action taken improved or resolved the problem.

This process focuses on identifying the root causes of the problem, along with changing the systems that are contributing to or causing the problem. Traditional quality improvement models focus on individuals, as opposed to systems.[2] In most cases, the individual did not make a mistake; the system in which the individual was functioning failed. Many systems cause waste, rework, and duplication of services.

Once the root cause is identified, there are three categories in which problems, and the resulting solutions, may be grouped. The first area is systems problems. Systems issues explore how care is delivered, who delivers that care, and how the persons delivering care interact with each other and the patient.[3] Examples of systems problems include communication channels, changes in organizational structure, adjustments to staffing, revising or adding policies and procedures, and changes in equipment.

The second area of problems and solutions addresses deficiencies in staff knowledge. Examples include changing orientation programs, providing inservice education programs, and providing additional reference material. The third area is behavior problems. In these instances, counseling or disciplinary action may be required; however, educational efforts or modifications to systems issues will usually bring about the desired change.

BENEFITS OF A MULTIDISCIPLINARY APPROACH TO PROBLEM SOLVING

The emergency care setting is a dynamic environment with a host of constantly changing personnel and resource needs. All of the various systems interact to yield a final product, and change in one area will affect many others. Because patient care is provided via those intricate relationships with multiple ancillary services from both within and outside of the main facility, improvements in care cannot be done independently by the emergency staff.

One of the tenets of continuous quality improvement (CQI) is ensuring that the right people are present or involved to solve a problem. If the right people are not involved, time may be wasted in the group meeting by not having the authority or resources to solve the problem. Once the root cause of a problem is identified, the group should ask if the right people are present. This step can save time and help maintain the motivation of the team because they feel that their efforts are not wasted.

Another benefit of multidisciplinary teams is the increase in cooperation and teamwork that occurs among departments. Another component of many QI philosophies is empowering the employee with the ability to problem solve. Quality improvement teams create bonds that form a foundation for future problem solving. Instead of waiting for the supervisor or manager to fix a problem, staff can resolve issues imme-

BOX 54-1

JCAHO 10-STEP QUALITY IMPROVEMENT PROCESS

Step 1	Assign responsibility
Step 2	Delineate scope of care and service
Step 3	Identify important aspects of care and service
Step 4	Identify indicators
Step 5	Establish thresholds for evaluation
Step 6	Collect and organize data
Step 7	Initiate evaluation
Step 8	Take actions to improve care and service
Step 9	Assess the effectiveness of actions and maintain the gain
Step 10	Communicate results to affected individuals and groups

From Joint Commission on Accreditation of Healthcare Organizations: *Using QA to CQI. Using CQI approaches to monitor, evaluate, and improve quality,* Oakbrook Terrace, Ill, 1991, JCAHO.

diately, avoiding unnecessary delays and wasted resources. Management's role becomes that of facilitator, assisting the staff to have the tools to solve the problem.

CREATING QUALITY IMPROVEMENT TEAMS

For a QI team to be effective, there should be three key components. The first is the team sponsor. The second is the facilitator. The third is the team members, including a team leader. The facilitator and sponsor roles vary slightly based on the scope of the project.

The team sponsor is the person who provides administrative support and helps ensure that the team has the resources it needs to accomplish the goals of the group. The sponsor runs interference for the team with the rest of administration to ensure that administration understands and supports the project. If the scope of the project is limited (i.e., involves only one or two departments or requires limited resources to resolve) a team sponsor may not be needed. There is also a team leader, whose role is to be the content expert and ensure that the group accomplishes the task. There should always be a team leader.

The facilitator is a person who has special training in the QI process and the tools of CQI. This person is the process expert. The process expert assists the team in using the CQI tools to assess and solve the problem. Process experts are often chosen for their lack of content knowledge and expertise. Their role on the team is only to assist in the process, and they are deliberately not involved with the affected departments.

The team members should involve staff from all levels, both staff and managers or supervisors should be involved. There should be representation from the core department, as well as from customers and suppliers. The core department should contribute 50% of the team members. The remaining 50% should be split equally among the customers and suppliers. If the group is addressing problems with x-ray turnaround time, the core group would be emergency staff. The supplier group would be radiology and possibly the transport department. The customer group may be attending physicians and patients. The optimal number of team members is usually 8 to 10 people.

The team leader and team sponsor meet to identify the initial draft of a problem statement and team charter. The problem statement addresses the current issue, the impact of the current problem, and what the desired state would be if the problem was resolved. This team charter lists the team members, available resources and constraints, and time allotted to address the issue, as well as the problem statement (Box 54-2). Once the team members meet and complete their brain-

BOX 54-2

TEAM CHARTER

Improvement opportunity:
Expressed dissatisfaction from internal and external customers regarding the patient length of stay in the emergency department. There are multiple encounter points during the length of stay with potential delays at each point. The impact of these delays is widespread, affecting multiple internal and external customers. Additional impact includes duplication of efforts, unnecessary work, wasted supply and personnel resources, lost customers, and lost revenue.

The action team will be assigned to assess the various service encounter points and areas of potential delays and choose one area to concentrate on decreasing the length of time to complete that portion of the encounter.

Results expected:
Development and implementation of a plan to decrease turnaround time for an encounter point in the emergency department.

Completion date:
Four months from the date of the first meeting.

Resources provided:
Up to 3 hours per week of administrative secretarial support; 4 to 6 hours per week of facilitation/consultation services.

The action team may ask administration to *consider* physical plant changes that might be incorporated into the emergency department remodel plan.

Constraints:
Changes must be implemented with existing staff or via a reorganization; no new staff can be added as a result of the solution unless additional patient volume is recognized.

Team sponsor:
Mary Jones

Team leader:
Linda Smith

Facilitator:
Jim Frankle

Team members:
Representation from radiology, laboratory, nursing service, and admitting; core team members from the emergency department include an assistant nurse manager, a secretary, a registered nurse, and the emergency medical director. This group will define the problem and then invite other participants based on the problem identified. Additional participants may include pharmacy, patients (e.g., former patient who complained), attending MDs, and other emergency staff.

storming, they rewrite the problem statement, covering the areas mentioned earlier. It is at this point that the group asks the question, "Do we have the right persons to solve the problem?" Adjustments are made to include additional members if needed.

The problem solving can occur on an informal or formal level. The formal process involves a team charter and may or may not have a team sponsor and facilitator. If more than one department is affected, more resources will be required to solve the problem, and a more formal approach may be needed. Informal problem solving can still use QI tools to address issues but may involve smaller groups that meet to brainstorm solutions to a given problem and then implement a solution. The key to either approach is to involve all of the players who have a stake in the issue at hand in the process, at least to obtain their input as to how they and their department are affected by the problem and the proposed solution.

SELECTING QUALITY IMPROVEMENT PROJECTS

There are numerous methods to determine QI projects in the emergency department setting. The more traditional approach is to define high-volume and high-risk topics.[4] These topics are then prioritized and teams formed to address those issues. Another approach is to identify projects after setting goals for the department. Once goals are set and the scope of services is delineated, areas for improvement are noted and form the basis for project teams. The last approach is to assess areas that affect patient flow through the department, using areas with patient flow problems as a basis for the teams.[5]

An example of a problem that would benefit from a multidisciplinary team approach is the coordination of ancillary services. When diagnostic tests are ordered on a patient, the orders are usually put in the computer all at the same time. The typical result is that all of those ancillary departments show up at the same time and try to perform their tests. Because in most cases only one provider can work on the patient at a time, the other providers waste time waiting their turn. If the patient goes to x-ray before labs are drawn, the patient can have an increased length of stay resulting from increased turnaround time waiting for lab results. Increased turnaround time can also lead to delays in interventions; delays in disposition; increased or continued patient discomfort; patient, family, or attending physician dissatisfaction; decrease in bed turnover in the emergency department; potential diversion of incoming patients; and potential increase in waiting time for other patients.

A multidisciplinary team composed of lab, radiology, electrocardiograph, transport services, emergency secretarial staff, and emergency nursing and physician staff can brainstorm problems and solutions. A flowchart of the work process can help point out root causes of delay. The group focuses its energies on solutions that will decrease turnaround time by increasing the efficiency of completing diagnostic tests. The ultimate beneficiary is the patient. Enhanced patient outcomes can be seen when one, some, or all of the problems are resolved.

EVALUATING CONTINUOUS IMPROVEMENT

Evaluation of continuous improvement should be done on an ongoing basis. Regular evaluations should be scheduled to assess specific changes, as well as to continually reassess the needs of the department. The results of monitoring should be used to alter action plans and to revise systems as needed.

In a more structured QI process, the teams identify reporting points at the beginning of the process. Examples of reporting points include after the problem statement is written, after the data collection plan is formulated, after a solution is proposed, and after an implementation plan is developed. Once the plan is implemented, the team should monitor progress quarterly for the first year, and then semiannually during the second year.

Measurement criteria should be developed that reflect the original goals of the team to measure progress at achieving the desired state. Criteria should include monetary and nonmonetary components. The monetary components should include the cost of implementing the solution, in terms of personnel, supply, and capital equipment resources. A comparison between expenses and savings in dollars and time should be noted. The institution and the department should address the need to measure the incremental cost of team time in meetings and in preparing for the meetings.

Nonmonetary issues can address a wide variety of factors. Customer satisfaction should be measured initially and on an ongoing basis. It is important to specify which customers are affected by the problem. It is also important to reevaluate the impact of proposed solutions and solutions on other customer groups. Clinical outcomes are another important measure. Additionally, an impact analysis of the problem and the proposed solution as they affect the values and mission statement of the facility can provide valuable information regarding the success of the project. The team should also note any unintended outcomes that arise. Lastly, the process and the team dynamics should be evaluated.

SUMMARY

The emergency department is an excellent forum for implementing QI. The use of multidisciplinary teams can have many benefits for staff and patients. A structured and efficient process that can be used to solve problems and improve services will enhance patient care and patient outcomes. Satisfaction of all the emergency customers, staff, physicians, other departments, and patients will also be enhanced.

REFERENCES

1. Joint Commission on Accreditation of Healthcare Organizations: *Transitions: from QA to CQI. Using CQI approaches to monitor, evaluate, and improve quality,* Oakbrook Terrace, Il, 1991, JCAHO.
2. McAllister RL: Quality management. In *The hospital emergency department: a guide to operational excellence,* Chicago, 1992, American Hospital Publishing.
3. Greenberg L, Markin D: *Enhancing patient flow in the emergency* department, Chicago, 1993, Emergency Nurses Association Leadership and Management Monograph Series.
4. Emergency Nurse Association: *Emergency nursing core curriculum,* ed 4, Philadelphia, 1994, Saunders.
5. Hellstern RA: *Managing the emergency department,* Dallas, 1992, American College of Emergency Physicians.

55 Implementing and Evaluating the Effectiveness of a Quality Improvement Program

Richard F. Salluzzo, Joel M. Bartfield, and Vincent P. Verdile

OUTLINE

OVERVIEW

One of our greatest challenges as healthcare providers is to ensure that the care we provide is of "high quality." For an organization to successfully implement a new approach to quality, the members within the organization must believe that the new approach will work. One of the major stumbling blocks in acceptance of quality management programs in the emergency department in past years has been a concern by professional staff that such programs generate extra work and really do not improve the quality of patient care. As we are now solidly in the era of continuous quality improvement (CQI), the importance of implementing an effective quality program and the ability to evaluate the effectiveness of this program become essential.

Continuous quality improvement focuses on the overall effectiveness and efficiency of an organization and is therefore systems based. It also attempts to be data driven and places the responsibility for improvement on everyone in the organization rather than a select few. To illustrate the difference in philosophy between traditional quality assurance (QA) and CQI, let us contrast two hypothetical emergency departments: emergency department A, which employs traditional QA techniques, and emergency department B, which has adopted CQI. The emergency departments differ in what they study. In emergency department A, the caregiver is the primary object of review. In emergency department B, the systems of patient care in all of their complexity are the main focus of evaluation. Emergency department A tends to ask the question, Who does what here? Emergency department B asks, How is the work accomplished?[1]

Emergency department A tends to focus primarily on clinical issues; emergency department B examines all aspects of patient care, clinical and nonclinical. Emergency department A is interested in behavioral outliers. Emergency department B also cares about outliers, but places much more emphasis on the average care delivered and how to improve it. Emergency department A is content when the care delivered meets local or national standards. Emergency department B attempts to improve its delivery of patient care even if that care already falls within existing norms. Although many emergency managers are now familiar with the concepts and terminology of CQI, a large number of quality programs still use traditional approaches to performance improvement.

As a point of illustration, suppose that the philosophy of CQI is applied to the issue of patient throughput in the emergency department. Assume initially that the mean turnaround time from patient arrival to discharge is 135 minutes. A preliminary examination of this process may detect two or three major issues affecting this time. Suppose, for instance, that a delay in obtaining vital signs on the part of the nursing staff and a delay during registration are major reasons for delays in this process. By redesigning systems these two problems can be resolved and turnaround times improved to 120 minutes. Further review of the issue may reveal inadequate physician or nurse staffing at peak hours and a delay in discharging patients. Subsequent resolution of these two problems may then result in throughput times of 110 minutes. Other functions that may require review include delays associated with laboratory, x-ray, pharmacy, and so forth.

By examining the individual steps in a process with a view to the bottom line of that process, continual improvement will occur. Contrast this approach with one (traditional QA) in which an arbitrary throughput time (e.g., 120 minutes) is considered acceptable and no further attempts at improvement are made.

An important consideration in the philosophy of CQI involves customer input. For example, if patients perceive that they are being rushed through the system, the improvement in throughput times may not result in improved customer satisfaction. Quality is not a number but rather a function of positive patient perceptions.

Most emergency managers have at least a rudimentary understanding of the principles of quality improvement (QI) and understand the contrast with traditional QA as outlined in the overview. Many emergency managers, however, are not as certain about the steps needed to effectively implement a QI program. The following discussion will attempt to highlight how to accomplish this important task.

MANAGEMENT AND STAFF EDUCATION

The emergency department team should themselves go through a standardized educational program to learn the important elements of a QI program. Several of the managers can then become trainers and begin educating the staff in small group sessions. Certain staff members can learn to be trainers as well, which creates a healthy staff-to-staff interaction. These educational programs should include at least 8 hours of material, which can be taught over two or three sessions. These sessions should be comprehensive with an emphasis on practical examples and the use of the tools of CQI for the statistical evaluation of process. The importance of this educational process can not be overemphasized; an effective QI program cannot be created without staff education.

CHOOSING QUALITY IMPROVEMENT PROJECTS

Many emergency managers have difficulty choosing which processes of patient care are most in need of improvement. In addition, when several such processes have been identified there must be a method to prioritize which of these require the most immediate intervention.

Understanding which processes of patient care require modification is to a large extent determined by reference to the department's quality statement. In QI parlance, quality is defined as meeting or exceeding the customer's expectations, and accordingly those processes that have the most impact on meeting customer expectations should have the highest priority for improvement.

Processes that require improvement may be identified in a number of ways. For instance, patient satisfaction surveys may suggest an unmet customer need in terms of facility cleanliness, patient throughput, staff attitude, or other issues. The emergency staff and the hospital medical staff may also give valuable input about processes that require improvement. Perhaps the most important source of this kind of information comes from the management team itself, which has the broadest overview of emergency care.

Once a specific process has been identified and given priority status, a multidisciplinary team should be chosen to evaluate and improve this process. Team members should be selected on the basis of expertise with the process. For example, if the process of ordering and obtaining a radiograph is in need of improvement, staff members who participate in this process ought to be part of the performance improvement team. In this case, physicians, ward clerks, nurses, radiology technicians, and transporters should all be represented on a performance improvement team. This group must designate a leader and a facilitator, and it is a management responsibility to ensure appropriate oversight and facilitation for the team. The team should start with an opportunity statement defining the team's objective. Typically the team will go through the stages of brainstorming, discord, and ultimate consensus as its members grapple with how best to modify a given process.

Once a team has created a modified process, it is imperative that it also define indicators by which the process can be evaluated on an ongoing basis. This approach will ensure that the "new" process is effectively monitored and functions as designed. Monitoring of this nature is necessary to prevent "evolutionary drift" of the process as various staff members alter the process in unauthorized and idiosyncratic fashion.[1]

Indicators

An indicator, or monitor, is a tool by which a process can be surveilled. Indicators may monitor direct patient care or review processes supportive of patient care. For example, a monitor of direct patient care may involve the workup of females of childbearing age who are admitted to the emergency department with abdominal pain. The indicator criteria might be that such patients require at a minimum a pregnancy test and a pelvic exam. The quality of care as defined by these criteria can then be quantified for this group of patients.

The monitoring of a support process such as ordering a radiograph uses indicators that do not involve direct patient care. These types of indicators often use criteria concerning timeliness, error rate, or patient satisfaction. Although quality improvement teams work on the direct and indirect processes of patient care that most affect customer satisfaction, it is clear that only a few such teams can operate at any given time. Despite the fact that only a few processes can be modified at any one time, it is important to develop indicators and monitor all significant processes of patient care in the emergency department. Such data collection will allow management and staff to have an understanding of how well their processes and systems of care are working. The use of comprehensive monitoring is an essential aid in identifying processes in need of improvement.

Box 55-1 lists some useful indicators for the emergency department. Data from various indicators may show little variations or may provide useful information by which performance can be changed. When this situation exists, the monitor in question should be performed on a "focused" basis rather than as an ongoing monitor because it is only providing "maintenance" data.

BOX 55-1

SOME SAMPLE QUALITY INDICATORS FOR THE EMERGENCY DEPARTMENT

Throughput times
Number of complaints
Patient satisfaction
Physician, nurse documentation
Ancillary performance
Deaths in the department
Unscheduled returns
Invasive procedures
Consultant performance
Cleanliness of the facility
Materials management
Equipment function
Appropriate respiratory isolation
Triage: timeliness, accuracy
Registration: timeliness, error rate
Discharge: timeliness, appropriateness
Patients who leave against medical advice
Patients in the department for longer than 180 minutes
Specific practice guidelines by diagnosis-related group (chest pain, seizure, asthma, febrile infant, trauma, etc.)

Outcome Versus Process Indicators

An indicator may be used to assess an outcome or a process of care. An outcome indicator measures what happens or does not happen as a result of a process. A process indicator measures a discrete activity carried out either directly or indirectly to care for patients.[1] One of the greatest difficulties in emergency medicine has been defining outcome monitors that effectively assess the performance of caregivers. There are many reasons for this difficulty, of which the following are the most important:

1. Generally, patients do not seek follow-up in the emergency department. Therefore it is difficult to know the ultimate outcome of the disease process.
2. Emergency medicine is not a procedure-based subspecialty, and many of the outcomes are a reflection of progression of the natural disease process. It therefore becomes extremely difficult to separate "good care" from "bad care" based on outcome alone.
3. Continuous quality improvement programs in the emergency department are not well integrated into quality assurance programs of the hospital, and the quality programs in the emergency department and hospital are at different stages of maturation, making sharing of information a difficult task. Consequently, an integrated view of a patient's entire experience from emergency department to hospital discharge is generally unobtainable.

For these reasons, indicators for emergency medicine are for the most part process related and to be effective should monitor those processes that are integrally related to outcome. For instance, monitoring how quickly a patient receives thrombolytic therapy in the emergency department is presumably directly related to the outcome of that patient's disease and therefore should prove to be a useful monitor of quality.

For the purposes of our discussion, we can consider indicators to be of two broad types: rate-based indicators and sentinel-event indicators. A rate-based indicator is an indicator that monitors an event for which a certain proportion of the events that occur are expected when state-of-the-art care is provided; further evaluation is required when the rate at which the event occurs crosses a threshold or data pattern analysis suggests opportunities for improvement. For example, to monitor how quickly patients receive thrombolytic therapy in the department we first determine what an acceptable time delay would be considering national benchmarks and the constraints under which we work. If this threshold has been consistently exceeded, a "team" review of how thrombolytic therapy is given in the department would be initiated. Through this review process we would attempt to identify process changes that could be implemented to expedite the use of thrombolytic therapy.[2]

A sentinel-event indicator is an indicator that monitors a serious patient care event that requires further investigation each time it occurs. An example of a sentinel event indicator might be all unscheduled patient returns to the emergency department. In this situation, each case would be reviewed to ensure that care and disposition were appropriate on the initial visit.

Both types of indicators should identify data that provide opportunity for improvement.

EVALUATING THE EFFECTIVENESS OF A QUALITY IMPROVEMENT PROGRAM

The success of CQI is not measured by the number of teams functioning or the amount of paperwork created. The only real parameter of success is the demonstration of measurable improvement in the processes and systems of patient care. Box 55-2 lists examples of processes that might be evaluated by a QI team. Some of these processes are support functions, and others, such as use of thrombolytics and the treatment of febrile infants, involve the development of practice guidelines and clinical pathways. (See Chapter 58 and 59.)

Improvement in the process of care should lead to a measurable enhancement of quality. For instance, a change in the triage process that improves care or efficiency should be reflected directly in enhanced patient satisfaction and other quantitative parameters. For example, creating a clinical pathway for thrombolytic therapy ensuring that it is routinely given within 30 minutes allows compliance with national benchmarks and should satisfy both patients and internal customers (i.e., the physicians who care for these patients).

SUMMARY

This chapter has discussed the importance of process review, the role of QI teams in process change, and some of the important steps that are necessary to create an effective QI program. If a program is effectively identifying, prioritizing, and modifying processes in need of change, it likely possesses certain characteristics.

For one, commitment will be pervasive in the department; both managers and staff will embrace CQI philosophy, which defines quality as exceeding patient expectations and advocates shared governance with an empowered staff. There will be adequate resources for management and staff training, as well as for teams working on specific projects. The projects chosen will be those that have real impact in terms of the department mission and quality statements. The teams chosen to work on these projects will be multidisciplinary and involve staff who are experts in the process under review. Management will act as facilitators for the process improve-

BOX 55-2

EXAMPLES OF IMPORTANT PROCESSES OF CARE IN THE EMERGENCY DEPARTMENT

Triage
Obtaining a radiograph
Obtaining laboratory tests
Practice guidelines for specific drugs
Registration
Discharge
Obtaining an electrocardiogram
Obtaining pharmacologic agents
Physician-nurse interface
Use of thrombolytic agents
Treatment of febrile infants

ment teams, not as design engineers. A series of indicators will be developed by the teams that will monitor the modified process so that variation over time is minimized.

There will be a mission statement clearly defining organization commitment to quality. The scope of the program will be workable and proportionate to the complexity of the services offered. The emergency department CQI program should be integrated whenever possible with hospital quality activities, and the missions of the department and institution should be aligned.

Continuous quality improvement seeks an answer to the following question: Is a given emergency department optimizing the efficiency and effectiveness of patient care and service given its level of resources and its patient mix? If the answer is no and a CQI program is working well, continual improvement in key processes of care should occur, providing evidence of the effectiveness of the program.

REFERENCES

1. Koska MT: New JCAHO standards emphasize continuous quality improvement, *Mod Healthc* 65:41-44, 1991.
2. Joint Commission on Accreditation of Healthcare Organizations: *Development and application of indicators in emergency care,* Oakbrook Terrace, Ill, 1991, JCAHO.

ADDITIONAL READINGS

Berwick M: The clinical process and the quality process, *Qual Manage Health Care* 1:1-9, 1992.

Joint Commission on Accreditation of Healthcare Organizations: *Primer on indicator development and application: measuring quality in health care,* Oakbrook Terrace, Ill, 1990, JCAHO.

Kritchevsy SB, Simmons BP: Continuous quality improvement concepts—applications for physician care, *JAMA* 266:1817-1823, 1991.

Niven D: When times get tough, what happens to TQM? *Harvard Business Review* 11(3):20-22, 1993.

Relman A: Assessment and accountability: the third revolution in medical care, *N Engl J Med* 319:1220-1222, 1988.

56 Preparation for Trauma Survey

Colleen H. Swartz

OUTLINE

Care of the injured patient has become increasingly sophisticated during the last decade. Trauma systems have evolved in terms of scope (e.g., inclusive versus exclusive systems), systems assessment (levels I, II, III, and IV; regional/community facilities), development, implementation, and evaluation. The principles of trauma systems development and evaluation have been firmly established, specifically through the Trauma Care Systems Planning and Development Act of 1990. This Act founded the Model Trauma Care System Plan. Guidelines for systems evaluation have been set forth by the American College of Surgeons Committee on Trauma and the American College of Emergency Physicians. Despite this progress, however, implementation of trauma systems has been difficult.

Traditionally, trauma systems have tended to focus on the major, multiply injured patient in the major level I trauma center cared for by a traumatologist. A shift in focus is occurring, which redirects the focus of trauma systems to a more inclusive approach. This approach addresses the interface of all trauma patients, regardless of injury severity, with *all* facilities that actually render care. The approach of an inclusive trauma system considers the capabilities and resources of all facilities, ranging from the community clinic to the major level I referral center. The patient management rendered by each facility must be evaluated based on the facility's resources and capabilities. All facilities rendering care to the injured patient play an integral role in the continuing vitality of a trauma system.

TRAUMA SYSTEMS: INCLUSIVE VERSUS EXCLUSIVE

The inclusive trauma system provides a model of care in which all injured patients' needs are addressed, not just the major trauma patient who requires the services of a level 1 or 2 facility. Historically, trauma systems focused on the most severely injured patients evaluated in the major trauma center (level I or regional facilities). In reality, only about 10% to 15% of all injured patients require the resources provided by the major trauma center. Thus resources relative to treatment of the majority of patients who had sustained relatively minor injuries were ignored or received little attention. The intent of the concept of the inclusive trauma system is to address the resources, staff, and equipment necessary to care for all patients who have been injured, regardless of severity of injury or facility type. Optimal care must be rendered to all patients, and a match must occur between needs of the injured patient and hospital capabilities, with care rendered in a fiscally responsible environment.

The resuscitative phase of trauma care is critical. In this phase the patient makes the transition from the prehospital arena to the receiving hospital. Timeliness of definitive care, organization of personnel and resources, and early recognition of patients who may require transfer to another level of care are critical issues during this transitional phase. Resuscitation has traditionally occurred in the emergency department; however, some hospitals across the country, specifically level 1 and 2 facilities who can provide immediate access to the operating room, are transitioning patients immediately from the prehospital phase into the operating room based on predetermined criteria.

Thus the capabilities and resources of each trauma center vary depending on the facility's size and commitment. In keeping with the inclusive trauma system focus, however, all facilities rendering care, regardless of size and commitment, must be evaluated to determine their capability. The site survey process is one mechanism for evaluation and should be viewed as a constructive process. The intent of the reviewers is to facilitate development of the facility and provide an objective evaluation of the center's responsiveness, strengths, and weaknesses.

TRAUMA SITE SURVEY

The intent of the site survey process is to review an institution's capabilities and commitment to providing optimal care to the trauma patient care. The site survey process should be conducted as a constructive process to commend the institution being surveyed for its commitment to the injured patient, as well as to facilitate ongoing improvement of care rendered. Site survey is typically performed in the context of verification or designation, usually depending on the level of sophistication of trauma systems within the state. Designation of trauma facilities is a political process in which a standard review process has been legislated by government. Participation in the process is usually mandatory to provide an inclusive trauma system. Verification, on the other hand, is usually performed when the state has no trauma system in place or has not legislated the designation process. Verification is usually pursued on a voluntary basis by facilities.

The site survey process involves evaluation of a facility's capabilities in providing care to the injured patient based on predetermined standards. Standards of care may be generated by (1) a state- or regional-specific regulating agency, as is the case with most states or regions with designation firmly established or (2) another group with expertise in care of the injured patient, such as the American College of Surgeons Committee on Trauma or the American College of Emergency Physicians. In pursuing the site survey process, the facility must be familiar with the standards that will be used during the review process to anticipate potential areas of focus during the review.

Emergency Department Issues

Regardless of the guidelines/standards adopted by the surveying agency or state appointed team, many of the issues addressed during the site survey process specific to the emergency department are consistent. Typically, the survey covers issues about evaluation of the organization, personnel, and resources critical in the emergency department where time is of the essence. One other core component of the survey process is the facility's commitment to ongoing quality improvement in trauma care.

Organization in the Emergency Department

Organization of resources during the resuscitative phase of trauma care is a crucial aspect, which will most certainly be reviewed during the site survey. The resuscitative or receiving area for the trauma patient must be arranged geographically so that it can easily address the priorities of airway, breathing, circulation, and neurologic stability. Equipment necessary to address life-threatening injuries must be readily available to the caregiver. An outline of Trauma Resuscitation Equipment and Supplies can be found in both Resources for Optimal Care of the Injured Patient: 1993, published by the Committee on Trauma-American College of Surgeons and in The Resource Document For Nursing Care of the Injured Patient (1992) published by The Trauma Nursing Coalition.

As part of the survey, protocols, policies, and procedures relative to the resuscitation of the injured patient are reviewed. Each person involved on the trauma team during resuscitation should be familiar with role expectations of themselves and others. Protocols for care of the patient should be firmly established and evidence of protocol adherence should be available to the site survey team. Trauma team responsiveness is a critical component for evaluation in the emergency department. Trauma alert guidelines are available in most level 1 and 2 hospitals to ensure timeliness of trauma team response, usually to a major trauma patient with a complex injury pattern and/or hemodynamic instability. In keeping with the concept of the inclusive trauma system, guidelines should be available for team activation, marshalling the necessary resources in level 3 and 4 hospitals as well. Level 3 and 4 hospitals play a vital role in resuscitation, especially in a rural system of trauma care. Resource availability is crucial in a smaller facility where an abundance of personnel is unlikely. The role of the level 3 and 4 facility is integral, however, in the functioning of the inclusive trauma system. It is not unusual for the survey team to request a team notification during the review process to gauge responsiveness of team members, review roles and responsibilities of team members during a trauma alert, detail frequently used clinical protocols, and generally review system responsiveness to the acutely injured patient.

Other organizational issues are important for the emergency department related to the survey process depending on the level of designation/verification the facility is seeking. For level 1 hospitals, issues related to education and research will certainly be addressed. Clinical care of patients is comparable in level 1 and 2 hospitals. However, patients with complex injury patterns who may require more advanced and extended critical care may require transfer from level 2 to level 1 facilities. Education requirements for level 1 and 2 facilities are similar. Research, on the other hand, is not essential for the level 2 center. The differentiation is based on the level 1 hospital's commitment to education and research. Level 1 hospitals are usually university based with residency programs. Thus during the review process of a level 1 facility, there will be investigation or review of academic endeavors of clinicians. Also of importance in the level 1 facility is the evidence of ongoing education of the community, healthcare providers, and a commitment to injury prevention. All hospitals in the inclusive trauma system, however, must demonstrate commitment to meeting the needs of the community they service. Vigilance in addressing the everchanging focus of the populations serviced must be documented.

Level 1 and 2 Facilities/Regional Hospitals. Clinical organization of the level 1 and 2 facilities is comparable. Clinical concerns that may be addressed during the site survey of level 1 and 2 facilities include the following:

1. Operating room access and availability for the patient requiring immediate surgical intervention. The emergency department must play an aggressive role in notification and transport to the operating room. If an operating suite is not designated and held open for the potential trauma patient, quality monitoring must be available to show the operating room schedule is maintained to provide immediate accessibility for the patient.
2. Monitoring the acutely injured patient while outside the emergency department for diagnostic studies such as computed tomography (CT) scanning or aortography. The provision of a comparable level of care for the patient while he or she is outside the department for diagnostic studies must be demonstrated.
3. Implementation of a bypass/diversion policy. The frequency of implementation and contributing factors should be available to the site surveyor.
4. Advanced resuscitative techniques used in these areas should be documented. Techniques such as the use of open/resuscitative thoracotomy, ventriculostomy, invasive hemodynamic monitoring, and diagnostic peritoneal lavage should be monitored for clinical criteria in application of the procedure, clinical competency in the procedure, and evaluation of patient response to the procedure.

Level 3 and 4 Facilities/Community Hospitals. The inclusive trauma system implies each facility's role is important in rendering care to the acutely injured patient so the most optimal care can be provided under any set of circumstances. Issues relative to level 3 and 4 hospitals include the following:

1. Timeliness of triage/transfer to a higher level of care and rate of overtriage and undertriage.
2. Utilization of aeromedical versus ground transport modes for transfer of patients.
3. Availability and adherence to treatment protocols for the injured patient.

The site survey team will determine the focus of the site review depending on the level of designation/verification sought by the facility.

Emergency Department Personnel

A second general area reviewed during the survey process is the area of personnel. Acuity systems vary widely across the country. Any system to measure patient acuity at the facility should be available to the review team. Staffing patterns and emergency department patient flow patterns must be available to the surveyors to facilitate their vision about how patients move in the system. Reviewers will typically look at the staffing patterns of the emergency department and attempt to ascertain how the needs of the trauma patient are met.

Typical questions include: How many nurses are usually assigned to the trauma resuscitation? What is the availability of a physician to the emergency department? What is the role of the advanced practice nurse in the emergency department for trauma resuscitation when a physician is not immediately available? How are multiple patients handled? Is there an on-call pool of nurses to address multiple patients, and how or when does activation of the on-call staff occur? What inhouse resources can be marshalled when patient needs surpass available resources?

Emergency Department Resources

A third area of interest during the site survey process is the issue of resource availability. Resource application should be delineated in the protocols, policies, and procedures at the facility. Care of the acutely injured patient brings together multiple specialty services (e.g., blood bank, radiology, clinical laboratory) that are crucial to resuscitation. Many of the specialty services are crucial to the patient during the resuscitative phase of care because of their contribution to the diagnostic evaluation of the patient. Radiology is one of the most important areas of evaluation because of its contribution to the timeliness of diagnostic differentiation. The interaction of the radiologist and radiology technologist with the emergency department is worthy of investigation during the survey process. Specifically, in a hospital that services a population of injured patients who have been involved in blunt versus penetrating injury, the diagnostic function of radiology is of utmost importance in determining a differential diagnosis and, ultimately, the plan of care for the patient.

Clinical laboratory and blood bank are frequently investigated by the survey team. Their role in the optimal resuscitation of the injured patient must be clearly defined, with firm expectations in terms of laboratory turnaround time, blood availability and utilization, and other diagnostic studies. The application and utilization of respiratory therapists, social services, communications specialists, physician/nurse extenders, anesthesiologists, and a myriad of other healthcare providers in the context of trauma resuscitation will be reviewed by the survey team. Again, the critical component of organization and cost-effective application of the resources necessary to care for the injured patient is the crux of the review of the resuscitative phase of care. Questions related to fiscal responsibility may include these:

- Is a complete Trauma Laboratory Panel necessary on all patients?
- Which patients would benefit from type-and-hold versus crossmatching?
- How can we minimize extraneous supply utilization during the resuscitation?
- How can we obtain adequate radiographic evaluation of the patient with one attempt by the technologist?
- When do we draw the line between overamplification of resuscitative efforts and futile care?

These questions must be asked in the context of maintaining constant quality clinical outcomes in a fiscally responsible environment.

The resuscitative phase of care that occurs in the emergency department has traditionally been viewed as a short-term piece of the trauma patient's interaction with the acute phase of the hospitalization. However, a national trend has been noted in which emergency department length of stay has been increasing for patients who require critical care resources. As the use of critical care beds continues to be scrutinized and patients admitted to the critical care unit are more acutely ill and utilizing the resource to its fullest, the emergency department is faced with the challenge of providing critical care in the context of the emergency department environment while the patient awaits admission. Regardless of the timeliness of the patient's disposition to another area in the facility, effectiveness of care and outcome measurement in the emergency department are being more critically appraised by survey teams. The facility must demonstrate ongoing quality improvement. The resuscitative phase of patient care offers many opportunities to measure the effect of care rendered during this phase on both short- and long-term patient outcomes. Examples of potential clinical indicators include volume resuscitation/overresuscitation and pulmonary status, blood products availability and administration, backboard times and pressure sore development, trauma team responsiveness/delays, and appropriateness of team notification.

Quality Improvement

More emphasis is being placed on the facility's efforts toward quality management during the site review process. Any facility providing care to the injured patient must demonstrate ongoing evaluation of clinical outcomes, with attention given to the cost effectiveness of care to achieve those outcomes. Quality management, as it relates to trauma populations, has historically presented unique problems. Trauma care systems are complex and difficult to pigeonhole in terms of cause and effect. A smooth running resuscitation involving many professionals all rendering care simultaneously presents a unique set of problems when the processes surrounding patient care are evaluated. Documentation of the individuals and processes during resuscitation is crucial and is addressed later.

The philosophy of quality improvement attempts to afford the individual techniques to analyze processes surrounding the care of patients versus the traditional approach of quality assurance, which focuses on individuals rendering care to the patient.

Clinical indicators should be developed, with a mechanism firmly established to monitor the indicators, such as a monitoring calendar. Several indicator sets are developed or are being developed and tested by organizations such as Joint Commission on Accreditation of Healthcare Organizations (JCAHO) and the American College of Surgeons Committee on Trauma. The clinical yield of the indicators may be marginal or quite substantial, depending on the facility, and for many facilities serve as a gross filter to identify cases for further review. The site survey team, however, may be interested in the emergency department's commitment to recognition of facility-specific issues related to care of the injured patient. Thus facilities should critically appraise their own patient care delivery system and demonstrate ongoing evaluation of processes surrounding care of the injured patient in their facility. Examples of hospital-specific indicators are backboard times and the relationship to pressure sore formation, fluid resuscitation in the pediatric or geriatric populations, ventriculostomy management in the emergency department, and timeliness of transfer for the most acutely injured patients.

The trauma site survey process should be a positive process that allows the facility to demonstrate its commitment to optimal care of the injured patient and allows an objective reviewer to evaluate the system and recommend potential areas of improvement. Typically, the review process invokes anxiety among those responsible for preparation of the facility and those involved the day or the week of review. However, the potential for growth and systems improvement to enhance patient outcomes should override this anxiety.

EMERGENCY DEPARTMENT PREPARATION

Many of the critical areas for review have been discussed in the preceding sections. Departmental preparation is an ongoing process. Reassessment of individuals and processes is integral to continual improvement in care. To prepare the emergency department for survey, much of the energy must be directed toward anticipating education of staff members about potential questions the reviewers may pose. Many of the questions relate to clinical care of the patients. Typical questions address mechanism of trauma team notification, application of clinical protocols, and roles and responsibilities. Site reviewers may often ask staff about their impressions of trauma evaluation and resuscitation and what they identify as problem areas.

Evaluation of care in the emergency department is typically conducted through chart review. Charts are usually requested for review before the survey day. Potential categories of charts are presented in Box 56-1. Each reviewer has specific areas of interest and may require charts with a different clinical focus. Usually, the chart review list can be obtained through a query to the Trauma Registry or through the Medical Records Department.

Documentation of care in the emergency department is *critical.* A typical problem area is physician responsiveness for evaluation of the injured patient. Documentation should include the time physician was notified, the time the physician returned the call, and physician arrival time. The physician's name also should be recorded. For trauma alert patients, all team responders' arrival times and names should be documented. Procedural information also should be recorded, with time and result of procedure, as well as patient's toleration and response to procedure or other interventions (Figure 56-1).

Ongoing evaluation of the patient must be demonstrated in the nursing documentation. The nurse's notes provide the reviewer insight into the patient's condition, response to interventions, and plan of care. Preparing the department for survey often involves months of chart review, documentation, education, and follow-up.

Other areas for departmental evaluation include review of a divert or bypass log, which documents data elements found in Box 56-2, review of emergency department log and/or tracking system, timeliness/documentation of decision to

BOX 56-1

POTENTIAL CHART REVIEW CATEGORIES

Preventable deaths
Potentially preventable deaths
Emergency department length of stay >2 hours with systolic blood pressure <90
Liver injuries
Spleen injuries
Subdural hematomas
Epidural hematomas
Pelvic fractures requiring >5 units of blood
Pediatric patients
Charts that reflect excellence in care
Charts that demonstrate how the quality improvement process works in the facility
Resuscitative thoracotomy performed
Emergency department length of stay >4 hours

BOX 56-2

DATA ELEMENTS FOR DIVERSION/BYPASS LOG

Date
Time of prehospital report
Individual receiving report
Prehospital unit
Prehospital report/injury
Time of charge nurse/emergency department faculty notification
Time of charge nurse/emergency department department faculty response
Orders given, decisions to divert/accept
Reason for diversion
Facility diverted to

CLASSIFICATION I II III IV V	TIME OF ARRIVAL	DATE	AGE	SEX	WEIGHT	MODE OF ARRIVAL ☐ Aeromed ______ ☐ Ambulance ______ ☐ Lex. Fire Dept. EC#______ ☐ Ambulatory ☐ Private Auto

RECORDING NURSE	PRIMARY NURSE	CIRCULATING NURSE	PHYSICIAN

CHIEF COMPLAINT/PRE-HOSPITAL REPORT

Injury time: ______________ ☐ Scene flight

PAST MEDICAL HISTORY ☐ DM ☐ COPD ☐ PSYCH ☐ CARDIAC
☐ Other: ______________ ☐ HPT ☐ CVA ☐ SEIZURES ☐ NONE

Allergies: ______________________________

Medications: ______________________________

Last Tetanus: ______________________________

☐ Trauma Alert Red ☐ Trauma Alert ☐ Trauma Consult	Trauma Surgeon	Anesthes.	Trauma Resident	Neuro-surgeon	Consult	Consult	Blood available	X-Ray	Respiratory Care
Time Called / Time Arrived									
Name									

INITIAL ASSESSMENT

TIME: | NURSING DIAGNOSIS

OXYGENATION

AIRWAY/BREATHING: Ventilator: ☐ N/A TV______ Mode______ Rate______ PEEP______ FiO2______
☐ Patient ☐ Spontaneous ☐ Assisted O2 per______ SpO2______% Trachea: ☐ midline ☐ deviated (R/L)

CIRCULATION: Capillary refill ______ seconds EKG Rhythm: ______

CHEST/LUNGS: Chest expansion: ☐ Symmetrical Other:______ Breath sounds: ☐ clear ☐ equal Other:______
Heart sounds: ☐ S1 S2 ☐ Muffled Other:______ Pain:______

EXTREMITIES/PULSES: ☐ MAE x 4 ☐ Pedal pulses x 4: ☐ palpated ☐ dopplered Splints: Pain:______

ELIMINATION

ABDOMEN: Bowel sounds: ______ Appearance: ______ Pain: ______ Rectal exam: ______

PELVIS: ☐ Stable ☐ Unstable Pain:

COMMUNICATION/SENSATION

Neurologic/Musculoskeletal: ROM: Sensation:

HEAD: ☐ Head blocks ☐ Tape

NECK: ☐ Cervical collar Pain:

BACK/SPINE: ☐ Long spine board ☐ Straps ☐ Scoop Pain:

NUTRITION

☐ NAP
LAST MEAL ______
DIET ______
WT. CHANGES ______

SUBSTANCE ABUSE
☐ ETOH ______
☐ TOBACCO ______
☐ OTHER ______

*PUPILS

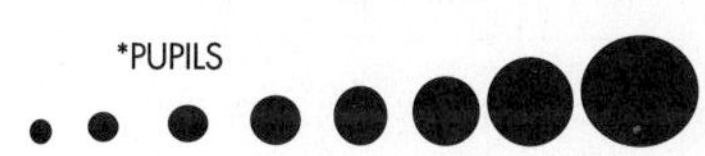

1 2 3 4 5 6 7 8

Right	Size
	Reaction
Left	Size
	Reaction

ACTIVITY/REST

☐ NAP

SAFETY/SECURITY

☐ NAP
☐ RESTRAINTS ______
☐ SIDE RAILS
LEVEL OF PAIN
1 2 3 4 5

SEXUALITY

☐ NAP
LMP ______
GRAVIDA ______ PARA ______ Ab. ______

SELF ESTEEM

☐ NAP
☐ Decreased coping abilities secondary to illness

GLASGOW COMA SCALE			
EYES			
Spontaneously	4		
To verbal command	3		
To pain	2		
No response	1		
MOTOR			
Obeys	6		
Localizes pain	5		
Flexion/Withdrawal	4		
Flexion abnormal	3		
Extension	2		
No response	1		
VERBAL			
Oriented & Converses	5		
Disoriented & Converses	4		
Inappropiate words	3		
Incomprehensible sounds	2		
No response	1		
TOTAL			
		Arrival	D/C

TRAUMA SCORE				
Resp. Effort	10-24	4		
	25-35	3		
	>35	2		
	<10	1		
	0	0		
Resp. Effort	Normal	1		
	Shallow	0		
	Retractive or absent	0		
Systolic Blood Pressure	>90	4		
	70-90	3		
	50-69	2		
	<50	1		
	0	0		
Capillary Refill	Normal	2		
	Delayed	1		
	None	0		
Glasgow Coma Scale	14-15	5		
	11-13	4		
	8-10	3		
	5-7	2		
	3-4	1		
			Arrival	D/C

FIGURE 56-1 University of Kentucky Hospital Trauma/Critical Care Nursing Record for documentation of care during trauma resuscitation.

Continued.

SHADE INJURY AREAS (see legend below)

TIME	pH	pO2	pCO2	BE	HCO3	FiO2/TV/Rate

TIME	TEMP	VITAL SIGNS BP	PULSE	RHYTHM	RR	BS ®/Ⓛ	E	M	V	PUPILS ®/Ⓛ	ICP	SpO2	OTHER	OUTPUT URINE	OUTPUT NG	CHEST RIGHT	CHEST LEFT	DRIPS CONC.	DOSAGE
		Manual L_____ R_____												PTA:					

INTERVENTION

TIME	PROCEDURE
	ET __________ NT __________
	Ventriculostomy opening pressure __________
	CENTRAL SITE
	CHEST (R) TUBES (L) Size
	FOLEY SIZE__________
	NG SIZE__________
	DPL
	12 LEAD EKG
	ARTERIAL LINE SITE:
	Backboard removed
	Cervical collar removed
	OTHER

IV FLUIDS/BLOOD PRODUCTS ☐ Warmer

PTA Crystalloids:

PTA Colloids:

PTA Total:

TIME	AMOUNT	SOLUTION	SITE	TOTAL INFUSED
Crystalloids				
Colloids:				

TIME	LABS/TESTS
	Trauma labs drawn by: Site:
	Urine dipstick:
	Stool guiac ☐+ ☐-
	Serum ETOH/Beradine prep by:
	DRUU
	Other:

INTAKE/OUTPUT TOTALS

Intake	Output
PTA: __________	PTA: __________
Crystalloids __________	Urine: __________
PTA: __________	PTA: __________
Colloids __________	Chest: __________
CT Contrast __________	NG __________
	EBL __________
Total __________	Total __________

LEGEND: A = Abrasion; B = Burn; L = Laceration; EN-W = Entrance; D = Deformity; BS = Breath sounds; E = Eyes; M = Motor; N = Normal; V = Verbal; A = Absent; ↓ = Diminished.

FIGURE 56-1, cont'd. For legend see p. 503.

University of Kentucky Hospital Emergency Department **Trauma/Critical Care Nursing Record**

RHYTHM STRIP

Addressograph

MEDICATIONS

TIME	MED	DOSE	ORDERED BY	ROUTE	BY

TRANSPORT

DEPART TIME	DESTINATION	ARRIVAL	RETURN	ACCOMPANIED BY

ADMITTING SERVICE: VALUABLES CHECKLIST COMPLETED: ☐ Yes

TRANSFER FORMS COMPLETED BY: ______________ R.N.

NOTIFICATIONS

☐ SOCAL SERVICES ______________ ☐ CHAPLAIN ______________

☐ FAMILY PRESENT ☐ FAMILY NOTIFIED ______________

☐ FAMILY ENROUTE

NAME OF RELATIVE ______________ PHONE ______________

☐ POLICE NOTIFIED (TIME) ______________ ☐ N/A

DISPOSITION ☐ MICU ☐ SICU CLASSIFICATION

Report called to: ☐ CCU ☐ Morgue I II III IV V

______________ ☐ CT ☐ OR

☐ NSICU ☐ Floor______________ D/C Time ______________

Time: ______________ ☐ TICU

☐ PICU ☐ Other______________

NURSING EVALUATION

TIME		INITIAL

INITIALS	SIGNATURE	INITIALS	SIGNATURE

FIGURE 56-1, cont'd. For legend see p. 503.

transfer patient from one level of care to another (e.g., from level 3 or 4 facilities to level 1 or 2 facilities), credentialing of emergency physicians (e.g., Advanced Cardiac Life Support, Advanced Trauma Life Support, Board Certification) emergency nurses (e.g., Trauma Nursing Core Course Completion, Advanced Trauma Nursing Course Completion, Advanced Cardiac Life Support, Certified Emergency Nurse) and roles and responsibilities in trauma evaluation and resuscitation, and timeliness of trauma service consultation. Adequate documentation of these areas, as well as any other specific documents requested, must be available to the reviewer.

The site review process involves evaluation of the trauma program in its entirety. A complete discussion of the evaluation of other departmental pieces is beyond the scope of this chapter. In short, the review process looks at the functional status of the entire facility, prehospital care, rehabilitation, and prevention along a continuum.

The emergency department plays a crucial role in the facility's trauma care model and an essential role in the oversight of the inclusive trauma care system concept, as the injured patient, regardless of injury severity, generally interfaces with one or more emergency departments during the course of evaluation. The same cannot be said for any other department in the facility. Thus the emergency department is a focal point along the continuum of patient interaction with the inclusive trauma system. Site survey of the emergency department involves evaluation of preparedness, organization, resource application, and quality improvement. The image of the hospital in the community with regard to optimal care of the injured patient often may be attributed to the care rendered in the emergency department.

57 Case Management in the Emergency Department Setting

Tener Goodwin Veenema

OUTLINE

Public outcry for healthcare reform has mandated that healthcare providers identify new approaches to patient care delivery that achieve and maintain quality, improve efficiency, and are cost effective. The widespread acceptance of managed care and the clinical guidelines/outcomes movement has driven emergency department medical directors and nurse managers to reconsider their present model of unit organization. Case management, a clinical system for the strategic management of cost and quality patient outcomes, has achieved tremendous popularity over the last 5 years. It was originally conceived to address the needs of the acute inpatient population. Work redesign using the concepts of case management can be applied to select emergency department settings to improve care delivery, enhance patient and provider satisfaction, and simultaneously control costs. Case management focuses on the reengineering of care delivery systems through the use of care maps or clinical guidelines, enhanced collaboration and care coordination, and clearly defined time frames for care.

Case management, which has been strongly influenced by total quality management (TQM) and patient-centered care, provides a framework for monitoring and managing clinical processes. In the emergency department setting, case management can decrease emergency department patient length of stays, avoid duplication of expensive healthcare resources, and identify systems strengths and weaknesses. Emergency care is by nature challenging because of its variability in volume and patient acuities. The emergency patient population presents with complaints rather than clearly defined diagnoses. The problem for which the patient is seeking care is often unexpected and episodic. Acuity levels vary among patients presenting with similar complaints. High patient acuities and sudden and frequent changes in the patient's condition make compartmentalization of care into a progression of predictable events more difficult. Traditionally, the "planned care" approach (patients present to the emergency department, and care is rendered based on their presenting complaint) has been used in the emergency department setting. Case management empowers administrators and providers to develop an approach to patient care based on preestablished guidelines. This transition moves providers from a reactive mode to a more proactive mode and establishes a gold standard for the delivery of emergency services. Case management embraces the organization's standard of care and brings it to the bedside, improving the overall quality of patient care.

OVERVIEW OF CASE MANAGEMENT AND MANAGED CARE

The concept of case management emerged in healthcare nearly a decade ago as a nursing initiative at Boston's New England Medical Center, which borrowed the term from engineering project management.[1,2] The model evolved from a 13-year history of primary nursing and an in-depth investigation of nursing and physician practice patterns as they related to outcomes of care.

The goals of this model were to (1) Increase nurse-physician collaboration in patient care, (2) Increase provider and patient satisfaction, and (3) Achieve acceptable patient outcomes, within an effective time line and with appropriate use of resources.

Case management is a method of rethinking patient care needs and clinician roles. The focus of change is the provider and the focus of evaluation is the patient. Restructuring patient care delivery systems using case management assumes that quality is not an elusive goal in healthcare and requires that emergency department medical directors, nurse managers, and administrators ask the following questions:

- What is required by each healthcare discipline to achieve realistic outcomes for patients with similar diagnoses/complaints?
- What is the best way to produce these outcomes?
- Who should be held accountable for these outcomes?
- How can care be restructured so that these outcomes are consistently achieved?

The answers to these questions are found in the key components of the case management model: care maps (or clinical guidelines that are detailed standards of care), care coordination, and time framed clinical outcomes. The evaluation component of the model lies in variance analysis. Case management provides an effective means to target specific patient populations (based on volume, and/or acuity) and operationalizes continuous quality improvement programs where they matter most, at the patient care level. When used effectively, it is a direct and powerful methodology to organize and coordinate services within a complex department or larger healthcare organization.

Yet case management will not work in every emergency department setting, nor will every emergency department benefit from case management. Before investing considerable resources in terms of time and personnel, the emergency department manager must first carefully evaluate the goals of their individual department and how best to achieve them. Is case management the right model for our department? Do we have the resources to support the development of this model? Is the department ready for such widespread change? Will our hospital administration support the implementation of this model? Case management requires a substantial investment in terms of unit resources the first year and can be difficult to implement in a setting as volatile as the emergency department. It requires commitment by staff and all levels of management. At the same time, case management is a model flexible enough to address the unique characteristics of emergency departments and emergency patient populations. Case management can also take into account the chaotic nature of the work environment and the existence of multiple providers and rotating medical staff. Design and development of an emergency department case management project requires the identification of key participants early on in project design, administrative commitment, provider support, and realistic estimations of project development needs in terms of time and resources. It requires the development of a "shared vision" for what the project will look like once implemented. This chapter introduces a framework for applying the key concepts of case management to the emergency department setting.

DEVELOPING A SHARED VISION

The formulation of a clearly defined statement of the purpose for redesigning emergency department patient care delivery that is consistent with the overall goals of the organization is imperative to ensure the success of the project. For example, case management in the emergency department will:

- Improve patient care
- Improve patient satisfaction
- Decrease patient waiting times and length of stay in the emergency department
- Improve staff satisfaction and retention
- Improve resource use and achieve cost containment

Once implemented, case management will function as follows:

- *All* patients will be placed on care maps based on their presenting complaint that will be identified at triage. Some of these care maps will be complaint specific (e.g., thrombolytics, cardioversion), and some care maps will be more generic in origin (e.g., overdose, chest pain, abdominal pain, fever).
- *Select* patients will be under case management plans in which their care is driven by interdisciplinary case management work groups that will design a care plan that encompasses entire episodes of care. These care maps will be located in the emergency department and will be updated on a regular basis.

A clearly defined vision will ensure that all project participants are working toward the same idea.

CARE MAPS

Care maps (or clinical pathways) bring the standard of care to the point of practice at the patient's bedside. A care map is an outcome-based tool that shows the standards of care and establishes a timed-sequenced relationship between these standards and a given patient case type. They describe the clinical responsibility of each professional discipline in terms of clearly measurable outcomes. The care map may include the following:

- Guidelines for assessment
- Diagnostic studies
- Treatments and medications
- Patient activities
- Consultations
- Patient/family teaching
- Discharge planning

Care maps also serve as educational tools for resident house staff and new nursing staff. In emergency departments staffed by multiple medical providers on a contractual basis or who frequently use the services of traveling nursing agencies, the care map conveys the organization's standard of care. For healthcare providers working in the emergency department whose education and training are in a specialty other than emergency medicine the care map can be an invaluable reference tool. For these reasons, many organizations use multidisciplinary teams to drive the development process. Participation by all members of the healthcare team improves communication between providers and provides consensus about patient care management. This reduces the amount of conflict between healthcare providers about the patient's plan of care by proactively determining what the ideal standard of care for that type of patient should be before the patient's arrival. Care maps operationalize the organization's quality improvement program, ensuring the right thing is done for the right patient, the first time and every time.

Emergency department clinical pathways may be in a variety of formats (Figures 57-1 to 57-3). Most do not and should not look like inpatient care maps. Emergency department clinical pathways are more than a new system for organizing and documenting care. Flexible in design, clinical pathways should be an accurate reflection of actual practice rendered and will serve to drive patient care. For emergency department use, the standard columnar format for day 1, day 2, etc that is used on inpatient units will not work. In most cases, attempting to structure patient care on an hourly basis also will not work well. The emergency department care map must recognize that time is played out differently in the emergency department.

THE ISSUE OF TIME IN THE EMERGENCY DEPARTMENT

Successful clinical pathways consider that most emergency care is often rendered within the first hour. Frequently, more

Text continued on pg. 57-58.

University of Rochester
Strong Memorial Hospital
Emergency Department
SMH 133 MR
Isolated Closed Head Injury
Page 1 of 2

Date/Time NOW: ______________________

Date/Time OF INJURY: ______________________

☐ Inpatient ☐ Outpatient ☒ ED

HISTORY:

Sex ☐ Male ☐ Female

Injury Type: ☐ MVA Restrained? ☐ No ☐ Yes Ejection? ☐ No ☐ Yes
Roll-over? ☐ No ☐ Yes Airbag? ☐ No ☐ Yes ☐ Steering Column Intact ☐ No ☐ Yes
Location of patient ☐ Driver ☐ Front seat passenger ☐ Back seat passenger
Location car struck ☐ Front ☐ Rear ☐ Driver side ☐ Passenger side
speed ☐ 0 - 20 mph ☐ 20 - 40 mph ☐ 40 - 60 mph ☐ >60 mph

☐ Motorcycle/Bicycle (circle) speed ☐ 0 - 20 mph ☐ 20 - 40 mph ☐ 40 - 60 mph ☐ >60 mph
helmet ☐ No ☐ Yes
thrown ☐ No ☐ Yes distance __________ feet

☐ Pedestrian Struck Speed of vehicle ______________________

☐ Fall height __________ feet surface ______________________

☐ Sport ______________________

☐ Assault object ______________________

☐ Projectile object ______________________

☐ Other ______________________

Loss of Consciousness ☐ No ☐ Yes Duration: ☐ 0 - 10 min. ☐ 10 - 20 min. ☐ >20 min.

Amnesia Retrograde ☐ No ☐ Yes ______________________
Anterograde ☐ No ☐ Yes Duration: ☐ 0 - 10 min. ☐ 10 - 20 min. ☐ >20 min.

Neck Pain ☐ No ☐ Yes Nausea ☐ No ☐ Yes Emesis ☐ No ☐ Yes

Drug or alcohol use within the last 12 hours? ☐ No ☐ Yes What type: ______________________

PAST MEDICAL HISTORY:

Past history of head injury? ☐ No ☐ Yes when ______________ injury ______________

Past medical history? ☐ No ☐ Yes If yes, ______________________

Medications? ☐ No ☐ Yes If yes, ______________________

Past psychiatric history? ☐ No ☐ Yes If yes, ______________________

History of alcohol abuse? ☐ No ☐ Yes

History of drug abuse? ☐ No ☐ Yes

Coagulopathy (liver/renal failure, coumadin, etc.) ☐ No ☐ Yes ______________________

PHYSICAL EXAM:

Abnormal vital signs? ☐ No ☐ Yes BP ________ P ________ RR ________ T ________

Glasgow Coma Scale on presentation? * ☐ 15 ☐ 14 ☐ 13 ☐ <13

Where was skull struck? ☐ Frontal ☐ Parietal/Temporal ☐ Occipital ☐ Crown ☐ Face

Laceration? ☐ No ☐ Yes

Scalp hematoma? ☐ No ☐ Yes

Possible skull fracture? ☐ No ☐ Yes ☐ Step-off ☐ Battle signs ☐ Hemotympanum ☐ CSF Rhinnorhea

Pupils equal and reactive? ☐ No ☐ Yes

Neuro exam nonfocal? ☐ No ☐ Yes

Normal mental status? ☐ No ☐ Yes If no, ______________________

Cervical-spine tenderness? ☐ No ☐ Yes

Evidence of dementia? ☐ No ☐ Yes

Concomittant injuries? ☐ No ☐ Yes If yes, ______________________

____

FOCAL NEURO EXAM: Neuro Evaluation Q 15" x 2 then
Q 30" x 2
Q 1° x 2
Q 2° x 2 if needed.

* See back for Glascow Coma Scale and Indications for Studies/Labs.

Rev. 10/95

FIGURE 57-1 Sample care map for isolated closed head injury.

Continued.

GLASCOW COMA SCALE FINDING	SCORE	MODIFIED GLASCOW SCALE FOR CHILDREN FINDING	SCORE
Eye Opening		Eye Opening	
Spontaneous	4	Spontaneous	4
To voice	3	To voice	3
To pain	2	To pain	2
None	1	None	1
Best Verbal Response		Best Verbal Response	
Oriented	5	Coos, Babbles	5
Confused	4	Irritable cries	4
Inappropriate words	3	Cries to pain	3
Incomprehensible sounds	2	Moans to pain	2
None	1	None	1
Best Verbal Response		Best Verbal Response	
Obeys commands	6	Normal spontaneous movements	6
Purposeful movement (pain)	5	Withdraws to touch	5
Withdraw (pain)	4	Withdraws to pain	4
Flexion (pain)	3	Abnormal flexion	3
Extension (pain)	2	Abnormal extension	2
None	1	None	1

A Glascow Coma Score is equal to the sum of the scores in each of the three categories.

INDICATIONS FOR RADIOGRAPHIC STUDIES

Cervical Spine X-Rays Recommended for: Neck pain, neck tenderness, altered mental status (e.g., intoxication, head injury) or mechanism of injury suggestive of cervical-spine injury.

Cervical Spine X-Rays NOT Recommended for: The awake and alert non-intoxicated adult patient with a normal neuro exam and gait who has no neck pain or tenderness on examination.

CT Scan Loss of consciousness > 20 min., seizure, altered mental status, Glasgow Coma Score of < 15, neuro deficit, penetrating trauma, structural injury, hemotympanum or other evidence of skull fracture on physical exam.

Skull Series: Penetrating wounds, suspected depressed skull fractures.

INDICATIONS FOR OBSERVATION

Glascow Coma Score < 15 when known to be previously normal.
Loss of Consciousness > 15 minutes.
Persistent vomiting.
Potential closed head injury but no reliable adult to observe patient.

HIGH RISK INDICATORS FOR CHILD/DOMESTIC/ELDER ABUSE

1. History of injury not consistent with physical findings.
2. Other injuries (bruising, lacerations, fractures) at various stages of healing.
3. Retinal hemorrhages.
4. Delay in seeking health care.
5. Signs of physical confinement, e.g., rope burns, decubiti.
6. Malnutrition +/or dehydration, e.g., dry skin, sunken eyes, loss of weight, poor growth.
7. Unexplained venereal disease or other unexplained genital defects.
8. Abnormal interaction between patient and caregiver -- indifference, fear, anger
9. Signs of excessive drugging or lack of medication.
10. Unexplained paranoia of patient.
11. Significant other: answering questions when patient able to do so; unwilling to leave room; suspicious of health care providers.

If any indicators present, notify social worker, ED Attending, and ED RN immediately. DO NOT discharge patient until further evaluation has occurred.

FIGURE 57-1, cont'd. For legend see p. 509.

University of Rochester
Strong Memorial Hospital
Emergency Department
SMH 133 MR
Isolated Closed Head Injury
Page 2 of 2

☐ Inpatient ☐ Outpatient ☒ ED

VITAL SIGN RECORD

INITIALS	TIME	T	P	R	BP	OXIMETRY	GLASCOW COMA SCALE	NURSE NOTES	SIGNATURE
					/				
					/				
					/				
					/				
					/				
					/				
					/				
					/				

Tolerating liquids: ☐ Yes ☐ No

IMAGING/LABS:

Head Cat Scan? ✳ ☐ No ☐ Yes Results ______
Cervical-spine films? ✳ ☐ No ☐ Yes Results ______
Skull films? ✳ ☐ No ☐ Yes Results ______
Ethanol level? ☐ No ☐ Yes Results ______
Tox screen? ☐ No ☐ Yes Results ______
Other studies: ______

ASSESSMENT: ☐ No CHI ☐ Mild CHI (concussion) ☐ Brain contusion ☐ Subdural ☐ Epidural ☐ Intracerebral bleed

MD/NP NOTE: ______

______ Signature

RN NOTE: ______

______ Signature

DISPOSITION: ☐ Neurosurgical consult ☐ Trauma Consult
☐ Discharged ☐ Admitted for observation ☐ Admitted for other reasons
Glascow Coma Scale at end of ED evaluation ✳ ☐ 15 ☐ 14 ☐ 13 ☐ <13

DISCHARGE PLAN:
☐ Closed head injury sheet reviewed with patient
☐ Leaving with a responsible adult who can observe patient for next 24 hours
☐ If no, Social Work Involvement ______ notified ______ time
CHN Involvement ______ notified ______ time
☐ Acetominophen or ibuprofen prescribed
☐ Follow-up with ______

FIGURE 57-1, cont'd. For legend see p. 509.

UNIVERSITY OF ROCHESTER
STRONG MEMORIAL HOSPITAL
SMH 689 MR
EMERGENCY DEPARTMENT CLINIC
OUTCOME BASED CARE MAP
FOR: DENTAL/ORAL AND MAXILLOFACIAL SURGERY

TRIAGE

Date: ______ Time of arrival: ______

Arrival: ☐ Emergency Medical Services ☐ Family member ☐ Self

Primary Dentist: ______ Location: ______

Patient sent in by Dentist: ☐ yes ☐ no ☐ other

Age ______ If under 18, page Eastman Dental Center Pediatric Resident after paging General Practice Dental Resident

VS T ____ P ____ R ____ BP ____ Hx of: ☐ Heart Murmur ☐ Prosthetic Heart Valve ☐ Prosthetic Joint Replacement

Weight (if < 18 years old) ______ ☐ Accompanied by Parent or Guardian

OUTCOME

Time Resident Paged ______

Time of arrival ______

CHIEF COMPLAINT

Toothache ☐ yes ☐ no

Location ______

Onset ______

Duration ______

Post Procedural Complication ☐ yes ☐ no

Date of procedure ______

Type of procedure ______

☐ Bleeding ☐ Persistent Pain ☐ Fever ☐ Swelling

Patient Triaged to Dental Clinic ☐ Yes ☐ No

Time: ______

Patient Taken to Dental Clinic by: ______

If female, last menstrual period ______

TRAUMA

Have the teeth or jaws been traumatized? ☐ yes ☐ no

Time of occurrence ______

Type of trauma ______

Mechanism of trauma ______

Teeth brought to ED ☐ yes ☐ no

Facial lacerations ☐ yes ☐ no

Last tetanus ______

AVULSED TOOTH KEPT CLEAN, PLACED IN SALINE AND GIVEN TO DENTIST UPON HIS/HER ARRIVAL TO ED

☐ **YES** ☐ **NO** ☐ **N/A**

TETANUS GIVEN ☐ **YES** ☐ **NO** **TIME** ______

MANUFACTURER ______ **LOT #** ______

TRIAGE RN ______

HISTORY (to be completed by Provider)

History of Present Illness Time ______

Past Medical History

☐ Heart murmur ☐ CVA ☐ Rheumatic Fever ☐ Angina ☐ Hypertension
☐ Prosthetic heart valve ☐ Sickle cell anemia ☐ Hemophilia
☐ Other clotting factor syndromes ☐ Hx of prolonged bleeding
☐ Jaundice ☐ Hepatitis ☐ Other Liver Disease
☐ Hx of MI ☐ Pregnancy

☐ STD ☐ HIV ☐ AIDS ☐ TB ☐ Seizure Disorder
☐ Psychiatric Treatment ☐ Asthma ☐ Bronchitis
☐ Pneumonia ☐ Emphysema ☐ Cancer
☐ Radiation therapy ☐ Ulcers ☐ Other GI/GU
☐ Med Allergies ☐ Developmentally Disable ☐ Diabetes

Comments ______

Past Surgical History & Hospitalizations ______

Complications of Surgery or Adverse Drug Reactions ______

Current Medications ______

Rev. 4/94

FIGURE 57-2 Sample care map for dental/oral and maxillofacial surgery.

Allergies: ____________________

____

Type of Reaction: ____________________

____

____

☒ ED

ASSESSMENT 1

☐ Informed Consent Obtained
☐ Surgical ☐ Sedation ☐ Pediatric ☐ Other

PHYSICAL EXAM

Extra Oral Exam: ☐ Swelling ☐ Large ☐ fluctuant ☐ airway compromised
☐ Moderate ☐ indurated ☐ multiple spaces
☐ Slight ☐ extended past midline

Location of swelling: ____________

Rate of Onset ____________

☐ Erythema Location: ____________

☐ Sensitivity to Palpation Site: ____________

☐ Extraoral Lesion/Laceration Location: ____________

Approximate size: ____________

Comment: ____________

Intra Oral Exam: ☐ Swelling ☐ Large ☐ fluctuant ☐ airway compromised
☐ Moderate ☐ indurated ☐ uvula deviated
☐ Slight ☐ tongue/floor of mouth elevated

Location of swelling: ____________

Traumatized Teeth ☐ Fracture ☐ Tooth# _____ ☐ Class _____
☐ Avulsion ☐ Tooth# _____

Toothache: Aera/Tooth# ____________

Sensitive to: ☐ Hot ☐ Cold ☐ Percussion ☐ Palpation

Radiographic Survey ____________

Assessment ____________

☐ Oral Surgery Consult Called ☐ Attending Consult Called

Diagnosis ____________

Consent obtained ☐ Surgical procedure ☐ Sedation ☐ Pediatric ☐ other

Type Local Anesthetic ____________

Amount _______ Type of Injection ____________

Assessment: ____________

____

____

____

Plan: ____________

____

____

Treatment Rendered: Antibiotic Prophylaxis begun ☐ Yes ☐ No

____

____

____

____

____

Dentist Signature: ____________

DISPOSITION

☐ Admit to Floor ____________

Report Called ☐ Yes Time ____________

Transfer Time ____________

Admitting Attending ____________

☐ OR ☐ OR Sheet Completed

Transfer Time ____________

Clothing and Valuables

☐ Family ☐ Security ☐ Cashier ☐ Clothing Room

☐ Discharge Home:

Accompanied by: ____________

Transporation: ____________

Time: ____________

Ambulatory: ☐ Yes ☐ No

T _______ P _______ R _______ BP _______

OUTCOME

☐ Patient's pain controlled

☐ Patient discharge instruction sheet complete

Patient/Guardian demonstrates knowledge of:

Discharge Medications ☐ Yes ☐ No ☐ N/A

Activity Restrictions ☐ Yes ☐ No ☐ N/A

Dietary Restrictions ☐ Yes ☐ No ☐ N/A

Need for follow-up ☐ Yes ☐ No ☐ N/A

Follow-Up:

☐ Private Dentist ☐ SMH Dental Clinic

☐ Eastman Dental Center ☐ Other ____________

Appointment Scheduled ☐ Yes ☐ No

Date ____________ Time ____________

Dentist Signature ____________

FIGURE 57-2, cont'd. For legend see opposite page.

UNIVERSITY OF ROCHESTER
STRONG MEMORIAL HOSPITAL
SMH35MR
Emergency Department
Asthma Clinical Pathway
Page 1 of 3

[X] ED

Drug allergies/reaction: ☐ Yes ☐ No

Time: ____________

PMH	Medications	Significant Other ☐ Present ☐ Notified ☐ Yes ☐ No
		Clothing ☐ with patient ☐ with family ☐ locked Valuables ☐ with patient ☐ wiith family ☐ locked

HISTORY

INITIAL EVALUATION BY RN AND MD/NP SHOULD TAKE NO MORE THAN 10–15 MINUTES EACH

Duration of symptoms: ____________

Circle any of the following symptoms that are currently present: wheezing chest pain fever
Cough Shortness of breath URI Symptoms other: ____________

Symptoms precipitated by:
URI cold/heat exposure smoke dust/allergens missed meds other: ____________

Current smoker? Y N If no, does someone in home environment? Y N

Currently on steroids? Y N If yes, when was last dose? ____________

When was last exacerbation? ____________

When was last admission? ____________

Has the patient ever been intubated/admitted to ICU? Y N If yes, when? ____________

Severity of symptoms at this time: ____________

Treatment at home for this exacerbation: ____________

EMS treatment for this exacerbation: ____________

Other history: ____________

INITIAL PHYSICAL EXAM

Vitals: Temp ______ RR ______ BP ______ HR ______ Pulse ox ______

PEFR (best of 3 tries) ______ Predicted ______ Time ______ Initials ______

NOTIFY ATTENDING IMMEDIATELY FOR PEFR OF <25% PREDICTED! (See back of page 2)

Degree of respiratory distress:	None	Mild	Moderate	Severe
Use of accessory muscles:	None	Mild	Moderate	Severe
Cyanosis:	None	Mild	Moderate	Severe

HEENT:

Cardiac:

Lungs: Wheezes: None Mild Moderate Severe

Where? ____________

Expiratory phase: Normal Prolonged
Breath sounds: Normal Decreased
Crackles/Rales: Yes No If yes, where? ____________
Rhonchi: Yes No If yes, where? ____________

Mental Status: ____________

Other physical exam ____________

RN ____________ MD/NP ____________ Initials: ____________

FIGURE 57-3 Sample care map for asthma.

Response to Treatment

1. <u>POOR RESPONSE</u>
   PEFR not improving
   OR
   PEFR < 40% of predicted
   OR
   persistent symtoms

→ ADMIT/CONSIDER ICU
1. Continuous to q 30 minute albuterol treatments
2. Add ipratropium 0.5 mg to each treatment
3. Consider parental therapy (equinephrine or terbutaline) magnesium, theophylline.
4. Antibiotics only if indicated

2. <u>INCOMPLETE RESPONSE</u>
   PEFR > 40% or < 70% of predicted
   OR
   not doubled
   AND
   with mild moderate symptoms

→ OBSERVATION/ADMIT
1. Continue hourly albuterol treatment
2. Add ipratropium if appropriate
3. Upon completion of 5 albuterol treatments if not good responder → Admit to Hospital
4. Consider subcutaneous epinephrine, terbutaline, magnesium, or theophylline.
5. Antibiotics only if indicated

3. <u>GOOD RESPONSE</u>
   Double initial PEFR
   AND
   PEFR > 70% of predicted
   OR
   patient without symtoms

→ DISCHARGE
1. Arrange for medical follow-up within 5-10 days/or while on steriods.
2. Discharge Medications:
   Steriods
   Adult: Prednisone 30–50mg po qd x 5 d (longer if appropriate)
   Pediatric: Prednisone 1mg/kg po qd x 5d (longer if appropriate)
3. Antibiotics only if clearly indicated.
4. Inhaled $beta_2$ – agonist prn.
5. Consider inhaled steriods

<u>FUNCTIONAL PATIENT</u>
Outcomes for Discharge:

Patient able to speak in full sentences,
Feels back to baseline

RR at baseline,
no FiO_2 requirements.
O_2 Sat > 95% with mild or no wheezing

Ambulatory in department without clinical deterioration.

FIGURE 57-3, cont'd. For legend see opposite page.

Continued.

UNIVERSITY OF ROCHESTER
STRONG MEMORIAL HOSPITAL
SMH35MR
Emergency Department
Treatment Sheet
Page 2 of 3

Drug allergies/reaction: ☐ No ☐ Yes

☒ ED

TREATMENT

☐ START O_2 2-4 1 via NC for: ☐ SaO_2 <94% ☐ SaO_2 <90% and history of COPD ☐ all pregnant patients

☐ BEGIN albuterol nebulization (2.5 mg) with O_2 x 3 q20-30 min each (over 90 minutes total)
After 3rd treatment, consult with medical provider for nebulization schedule (see assessment guidelines back of page 1)
CHECK PEFR after each treatment

☐ START steroids if patient requires > 1 albuterol treatment (Relative contraindications: known varicella exposure within 3 weeks, or active herpes)
ADULT: Methylprednisolone 125 - 1000 mg IV **OR** ☐ Prednisone 60-80 mg PO
PEDIATRIC: Methylprednisolone 2 mg/kg IV **OR** ☐ Prednisone 2 mg/kg PO
☐ For pts > 50 or with history of COPD add Ipratropium 0.5 mg to every Albuterol treatment

☐ CXR if high suspicion for pneumonia, foreign body, CHF; localized wheezing after therapy; first time wheezing.
CBC if temperature >38.2°C
ABG, Electrolytes, Theophylline level NOT ROUTINELY INDICATED

SECOND ASSESSMENT of patient should occur:
☐ For initial PEFR >40% predicted, after 3rd albuterol treatment
☐ For initial PEFR <40% predicted, after 1st albuterol treatment
AND notify attending MD Time _______ RN/NP/MD _______________

REPEAT ASSESSMENT Time _____
Degree of respiratory distress None Mild Moderate Severe
Use of accessory muscles: None Mild Moderate Severe
Cyanosis: None Mild Moderate Severe
Lungs: Wheezes: None Mild Moderate Severe Where? _______________
Expiratory Phase: Normal Prolonged
Breath sounds: Normal Decreased
Crackles/Rales: Yes No If yes, where? _______________
Rhonchi: Yes No If yes, where? _______________
Other physical exam:
RN _______________ MD/NP _______________

REPEAT ASSESSMENT Time _____
Degree of respiratory distress None Mild Moderate Severe
Use of accessory muscles: None Mild Moderate Severe
Cyanosis: None Mild Moderate Severe
Lungs: Wheezes: None Mild Moderate Severe Where? _______________
Expiratory Phase: Normal Prolonged
Breath sounds: Normal Decreased
Crackles/Rales: Yes No If yes, where? _______________
Rhonchi: Yes No If yes, where? _______________
Other physical exam:
RN _______________ MD/NP _______________

PRIVATE MD/TIME NOTIFIED

Lab Results
_______ Segs
_______ Bands
_______ Lymphocytes
_______ Monocytes

plt PT _______
PTT _______

Total Bill _______
AST _______
ETOH _______
Amylase _______
Lipase _______
CK-MB _______
Other _______

ABG pH _______
pCO_2 _______
PO_2 _______
SaO_2 _______

U/A Dip _______
Micro _______

Urine Pregnancy _______
EKG _______

X-Rays _______

FIGURE 57-3, cont'd. For legend see pg. 514.

UNIVERSITY OF ROCHESTER
STRONG MEMORIAL HOSPITAL
SMH35MR
Emergency Department
Vital Sign Record
Page 3 of 3

[X] ED

RESPONSE TO THERAPY — Time ____________

☐ GOOD — ☐ Plan to discharge patient to home
☐ INCOMPLETE — ☐ Observe (planned duration)
☐ Admit
☐ POOR — Admit ☐ Floor ☐ ICU

PRCEDURE NOTE Time ____________

ATTENDING NOTE — Time ____________

Critical Care Time ____________

MD ____________

VITAL SIGN RECORD

Initials	Time	Temp	Pulse	RR	B/P	Pulse ox	PEFR	comments
					/			
					/			
					/			
					/			
					/			

INTAKE RECORD

Start time	Amount	Initials	IV gauge	End time	Amount

MEDICATION ADMINISTRATION RECORD

Albuterol nebulization dose: ____________

#1	Time:	RN	#4	Time:	RN	#7	Time:	RN
#2	Time:	RN	#5	Time:	RN	#8	Time:	RN
#3	Time:	RN	#6	Time:	RN	#9	Time:	RN

Steroids Medication ____________ dose: ____________ Route: ____________
Time: ____________ RN ____________

Other Medications ____________ dose: ____________ Route: ____________
Time: ____________ RN ____________

DISCHARGE PLAN COORDINATION

Patient/family teaching

Assess patient's knowledge of asthma management and teach where needed.

Patient/family will demonstrate understanding of:

☐ proper use of medication
☐ precipitants of attack
☐ knowledge of symptom progression
☐ knowledge of ACTION PLAN for increased severity of disease
☐ proper use of (if appropriate):
  ☐ inhaler and spacer device
  ☐ peak flow meter

patient discharged with peak flow meter ☐ YES ☐ NO ☐ N/A

RN ____________

Care coordination

Ensuring appropriate and adequate outpatient plan

☐ Patient knows source of primary care and phone number
☐ Patient aware of need for follow-up visit within 5-10 days
☐ Assessment made for need for community health referral:
  ☐ Noncompliance with medical regimen
  ☐ lack of social support system
  ☐ poor coping skills
  ☐ frequent ED visits or admissions
  ☐ history of missed follow-up appointments

If any indicator yes, make referral

MD/NP ____________

FIGURE 57-3, cont'd. For legend see pg. 514.

than 75% of the clinical pathway content will address assessments and interventions that take place within the first 60 minutes of the patient's arrival.

Therefore a care map that is locked into a rigid chronologic time frame results in a document that is cumbersome, unbalanced, and rarely an accurate report of the emergency care rendered. A flexible time frame that provides reasonable ranges for care to be delivered (e.g., within 15 to 30 minutes certain interventions must be done for the patient) or time framing care maps based on the achievement of desired patient outcomes (perform intervention A until patient outcome A is achieved) will ideally function more effectively. This approach to time framing care based on the patient's response accommodates the uniqueness of each individual patient.

Emergency department clinical pathway construction requires the development of several formats based on the needs of patient populations seen and the types of services each emergency department renders. Short, one page formats can easily address the needs of the nonacute patient, as well as many procedures, such as suture placement, foreign-body removal and cardioversion. The needs of the more acutely ill patient can be met by designing a longer format that takes into account repeated assessments and multiple interventions. Care maps also must be designed to accommodate patient complications and co-morbidities. Clinical pathways based on the patient's presenting complaint at triage (e.g., chest pain, abdominal pain, overdose) allow for the most flexibility in addressing clinical findings later. Clinical pathways may also be symptom based (e.g., fever of unknown origin, pain, shortness of breath). The format of the care map should reflect the algorithmic approach that is inherent to the practice of emergency medicine and nursing, such as including current pediatric advanced life support (PALS) guidelines in the care map for pediatric major trauma. Care maps that are diagnosis-related group (DRG) driven, as on inpatient units, are too narrowly focused to function in the emergency department. For example, the care map designed to address DRG #198 Total Cholecystectomy is of little value in the emergency department. Patients presenting to the emergency department with abdominal pain require a care map with broad enough scope to entertain a wide differential of possible diagnoses.

RESEARCH

Clinical pathways are also excellent data collection tools for emergency care research. Historically, emergency medicine or nursing research required lengthy chart reviews or additional documentation on separate study forms. Clinical pathways facilitate departmental research by building the data pieces of interest directly into the body of the care map, allowing for more accurate data collection and a larger sample size. Simultaneously, they provide a management tool for conveying current research findings as providers strive for clinical application to improve patient outcomes.

DOCUMENTATION

An important decision to make early in the design process is whether the care map will be a documentation tool or strictly a project management tool. Care maps that are interdisciplinary documentation tools are more time consuming and challenging to write; however they ultimately function more effectively. The decision to make the care map the sole documentation tool for the emergency department visit will also ensure compliance. Busy emergency care providers will rarely use documents that they do not have to write on. Care maps are an invaluable tool for streamlining documentation while increasing documentation accuracy. Patient care situations such as a resuscitation, which previously required the completion of many forms by medicine and nursing, can be reduced to one comprehensive care map. Care maps blend easily into the hospital's clinical information system. Once implemented, care maps are reviewed annually by the development team to ensure that the content meets Joint Commission on Accreditation of Healthcare Organizations (JCAHO) standards and reflects the most current treatment modalities available.

Finally, each care map can be coded so that billing can be done directly off the care map, avoiding lengthy chart reviews or additional paperwork. Procedures such as lumbar puncture, electrocardiographic interpretation, and radiographic interpretation are sources of income to the emergency department that are frequently missed. By designing care maps in conjunction with the hospital's billing department, all appropriate charges will be captured and lost revenue resulting from inadequate or insufficient documentation will be avoided.

COMMUNICATION

Clinical pathways articulate with the following:

- Inpatient units
- Ambulatory clinics
- Private physicians
- Other healthcare facilities
- Community agencies

For example, an emergency department care map designed to address the needs of the patient with sickle cell anemia should ideally "link up" with the care map where the patient receives his or her primary care. Individual patient health histories about treatment modalities and pain management can be captured on the care map. The care map should also link directly to the inpatient care map for patients requiring admission. This facilitates better communication across units and consistency of care for the patient. It also avoids expensive and unnecessary duplication of diagnostic tests performed in the emergency department.

COLLABORATION

The case management model states that collaborative care will become the primary model for professional practice. An interdisciplinary patient care management team will oversee the ongoing management of this project, comprised of nursing leadership, physicians, social workers, and community health nurses.

Conceptually, the emergency department is an ideal clinical location for implementing case management. Attending physicians are on site 24 hours a day and a collaborative model is already in place. Healthcare providers render patient care side by side, and communication about patient status is ongoing. Physicians and nurses are already accustomed to an algorithmic approach to patient care by virtue of Advanced Cardiac Life Support, Advanced Trauma Life Support (ATLS), and Pediatric Advanced Life Support (PALS) guidelines. These guidelines parallel the development of time-framed standards of care for specific patient populations that is the hallmark of the case management model.

The design and development of a case management model for the emergency department should be a collaborative project from inception through implementation. Emergency providers are greatly concerned with the issues presented by expanding fiscal constraints, increased state and federal regulation, and increased consumer demand for high quality, cost effective care. Societal factors such as lack of health insurance, increase in random and domestic violence, and substance abuse have contributed to emergency department overcrowding and patient acuity. An outcome-based model for patient care delivery such as case management provides emergency nurses and emergency physicians a common ground to enhance provider satisfaction while improving patient care. Initially, the physician/nurse practitioner determines the medical management of each patient case type and establishes priorities for care. Collaboratively, intermediate and discharge outcomes are identified and transposed onto a clinical pathway. Case management focuses providers on achieving clinical and financial outcomes by improving trust and communication between providers through the use of clinical pathways and shared decision making. This model encourages shared responsibility and shared recognition, enhancing provider satisfaction and facilitating collegial relationships between physicians and nurses, as well as other healthcare disciplines.

Potentially, collaboration could be further defined along patient service lines. For example, because of the disparity in daily emergency department patient volumes and acuity, care will be rendered by physician-nurse teams in their area of expertise. Area of expertise may be defined beyond the present team divisions of medicine, surgery, pediatrics, obstetrics/gynecology, triage, and trauma team. These team partners will participate in inpatient case management team meetings to define standards of care, organize and oversee care of select patient populations, establish clinical outcomes, and identify system variances that are barriers to care.

OUTCOMES MEASUREMENT/VARIANCE ANALYSIS

The use of care maps to guide care allows for accurate measurement of the quality of care rendered through the identification of variation in outcomes. Variances in outcome may be analyzed to identify sources of variation. Traditional variance analysis categorizes emergency department variances into three main sources.

- *System:* This variance occurs when something in the system has not provided the expected support. An example would be a test such as an cytomegalovirus (CMV) titer that is needed emergently but cannot be completed because the laboratory is closed. Another example is a patient requiring radiologic procedures that are not available at the institution 24 hours a day.
- *Provider:* This variance occurs when the clinician has not completed an expected activity based on a generally accepted standard for care.
- *Patient:* This variance occurs when the patient does or experiences something unexpected that results in a prolonged length of stay. Examples might include untoward responses to care or social situations with the patient's family that prolong the emergency department length of stay.

Ideally, variance data should be collected on all patients seen in the emergency department, and variance analysis should take the place of all existing quality assurance activities. Aggregate variance analysis is performed weekly or monthly as needed and can be reviewed at regular staff meetings or morbidity and mortality rounds. Variance analysis should not be part of the permanent medical record.

This process facilitates identification of the sources of variances and offers opportunities to improve systems and ultimately improve patient outcomes. Information learned about patient care through care maps may be aggregated to identify patterns and trends. For example, persistant delays in patient admissions may be tracked to their source (e.g., lack of transport personnel, housekeeping, communication problems). Use of variance analysis also offers opportunities for research to validate the effectiveness of current approaches to patient care and identify opportunities for improvements in patient care.

TROUBLESHOOTING CASE MANAGEMENT

As with the implementation of any project that entails major restructuring of the work environment, problems are bound to arise. With solid planning and continuous vigilance over project development, however, many problems can be easily resolved or avoided entirely. Some of the more common problems associated with case management in the emergency department are presented in the next sections.

Ambiguity in Project Leadership

Because of the scope and nature of the case management project, a project manager must be identified who is both knowledgeable and enthusiastic and has sufficent time to devote to project development. In most cases, the project manager is a nurse who also may be a clinical nurse specialist in emergency services. It is unrealistic in most busy emergency departments, to assume that the nurse manager will also be able to function as the project manager. As with other administrative activities, the role of the nurse manager is to create and maintain an environment conducive to the development of case management. Leadership and guidance from the nurse manager is imperative to the success of the project; however, the daily management of the project requires the time and talents of an individual dedicated to case management.

Inconsistent Use of Care Maps

It is not uncommon for project managers to experience some difficulty in intially gaining widespread acceptance of the care map concept. Part of the problem often lies in the care map development process. Each care map development team must be interdisciplinary, and each discipline must be represented that would normally be involved in the management of that patient. For example, the care map development work group for hip/femur fracture might include nursing, emergency medicine, orthopedics, radiology, and physical therapy. Representation from the inpatient orthopedic unit and the outpatient department will further enhance communication across units.

Select care map authors based on their clinical expertise and enthusiasm for the concept. Content validity of each care map is ensured through a comprehensive review of the literature. Retrospective chart review can help determine organizational practice patterns for review by the group. Inclusion of the "key players" in care map development ensures that everyone who has an interest in the patient is involved, but protects the group from becoming so large that consensus becomes impossible.

VISION FOR THE FUTURE

Case management is designed to ensure continuity of care for patients across all areas of the healthcare system. Emergency department care coordinators and project managers should meet regularly with inpatient units and other critical care areas to ensure the emergency department care maps "link up" with their respective pathways and that they are clear and easily understood. Emergency department personnel should work with their Emergency Medical Services (EMS) providers to design care maps for implementation in the field. Ideally, case management should begin in the prehospital setting.

Case management can address the problem of "emergency department abuse" by targeting patients who repeatedly elect to bypass their primary care provider and go to the emergency department for management of routine complaints. Emergency department providers working together with primary care providers can design care maps to ensure that the care the patient receives during an emergency department visit is consistent with the overall healthcare plan designed by the patient's primary provider. At the same visit, the emergency department care coordinator can review and encourage the patient to use appropriate access of the healthcare system.

"Patient friendly" care maps can be written that would be shared with the patient and the family to allay their fears, establish patient/family healthcare goals, and to help them better understand their emergency department visit.

Case management provides emergency care personnel with a model for outcome-based care that enhances the achievement of clinical outcomes while conserving valuable resources. Case management cannot extinguish the chaos that characterizes many of today's urban and community emergency departments; however, it can reinvest a sense of control for providers through its proactive design.

REFERENCES

1. Zander K: Nursing case management: resolving the DRG paradox, *Nurs Clin North Am* 23:503-520, 1988.
2. Zander K: Nursing case management: strategic management of cost and quality outcomes, *J Nurs Admin* 18:23-30, 1988.

ADDITIONAL READINGS

Ethridge P, Lamb GS: Professional nursing case management improves quality, access and costs, *Nurs Manage* 20:30-35, 1989.

Ison A: Nursing case management: an innovative approach to care in the emergency department, *Top Emerg Med* 13:35-46, 1991.

Mayer G, Madden MJ, Lawrenz E: *Patient care delivery systems,* Rockville, Md, 1990, Aspen.

Veenema TG: The ten most frequently asked questions about case management in the emergency department, *J Emerg Nurs* 20(4):289-292, 1994.

Zander K, Physicians, care maps, and collaboration, *New Definition* 7:(1) 1992.

58 Practice Guidelines For Physicians

Richard F. Salluzzo

OUTLINE

Practice guidelines in emergency medicine
Practice guidelines versus clinical pathways
The use of outcome data
Summary

Emergency medicine, like other medical specialties, is being scrutinized by several interested parties in terms of its ability to deliver cost-effective care. Managed care organizations, the government, and the public are concerned that our country is not getting its money's worth in terms of healthcare expenditures and are particularly concerned about high emergency department costs. Several studies have shown tremendous geographic variability in resource use for the diagnosis and treatment of various diseases. For instance, two adjacent counties in Maine showed significant differences in cholecystectomy and hysterectomy rates per capita, which was clearly not due to discernible differences in demographic factors.[1] The number of catheterizations per unit of population also demonstrates wide geographic variability.[1] Given such data, many regulatory and governmental agencies have promoted the concept of clinical standards—sets of standardized criteria that will drive medical decision making and consequently resource utilization.

Many physicians are apprehensive when confronted with the concept of clinical standards or practice guidelines. They argue that every patient is unique and requires individually tailored care. In addition, they believe that practice guidelines create a "cookbook medicine" style of practice, which is overly simplistic and may expose physicians to additional medical legal liability. Despite these concerns, there has been tremendous interest in the creation of clinical standards or practice guidelines, and there are now more than 2000 such guidelines across the various medical and surgical specialties.[2]

PRACTICE GUIDELINES IN EMERGENCY MEDICINE

Many emergency physicians promoting the use of standards believe they will help create a threshold of acceptable care in the specialty. These physicians argue they have a basic obligation to patients to define and deliver appropriate care. Another important consideration in the development of standards is their impact on quality management. With the development of such standards, quality is no longer defined completely on the local level. As in other specialties, several external forces come to bear on the creation of clinical standards. For instance, both the Agency for Health Care Policy and Research, and the Joint Commission on Accreditation of Healthcare Organizations (JCAHO) have sponsored several panels and task forces to promote the development of clinical standards for specific medical problems such as back pain and trauma care.

There are presently several practice guidelines for emergency medicine. The American College of Emergency Physicians (ACEP) has developed clinical policies for chest pain, abdominal pain, acute blunt trauma extremity trauma, pediatric fever, and seizures. ACEP policies are meant to be flexible and are not intended to replace physician judgment; they may not be appropriate in all clinical situations (Box 58-1).

For practice guidelines to be effective, certain issues should be addressed. A practice guideline should be "user friendly," but not unusually complicated. Such policies should also be flexible enough to allow for individual practice patterns and to some extent varying clinical circumstances.

In creating such guidelines for the emergency physician several considerations should be kept in mind. The development of clinical guidelines will surely fail if the task is oversimplified, lacks institutional support, or is attempted with inadequate data management tools.

The elaboration of effective clinical guidelines is a complex task, which may require significant financial and human resources. The American Medical Association underscores both the importance and the difficulty of creating practice guidelines and has developed a list of desirable attributes for such standards.[3] These suggestions are summarized as follows:

1. Practice guidelines should be sponsored by physician organizations.
2. Appropriate "experts" should sit on task forces creating these standards.
3. There should be a scientific basis to the standard based on appropriate research.
4. They should be comprehensive and flexible.
5. They should be constantly reviewed and upgraded.
6. They should be widely promoted and disseminated.

Some emergency physicians across the country have created their own "tailored" practice guideline so that care is provided in a more uniform way among the group members. The creation of such guidelines has been greatly facilitated by computerized dictation systems, which provide "templates" of documentation and care via the use of valuable "cues" to the emergency physician. For instance, given a specific presenting complaint, the computer might request certain historical detail or "suggest" particular diagnostic interventions.

In the late 1980s, emergency physicians in Massachusetts created practice guidelines for specific high-risk clinical pre-

BOX 58-1

CLINICAL POLICY FOR THE INITIAL APPROACH TO PATIENTS PRESENTING WITH PENETRATING EXTREMITY TRAUMA

Preface

One of the most common presenting conditions in emergency medical practice involves penetrating extremity trauma. The American College of Emergency Physicians (ACEP) has developed this clinical policy to promote consistency of practice and quality of care in patients presenting with penetrating extremity trauma.

This policy concentrates on penetrating extremity wounds during the first 24 hours after injury. ACEP's development of this policy included review by wound care experts and field testing of the policy. The reasons for developing clinical policies and the approaches used in their development have been enumerated.* The experts often were divided on whether a recommendation should be a rule or a guideline, and final decisions were made by ACEP's Clinical Policies Committee. Experts and field testers were derived from a wide geographic area and a wide variety of clinical settings.

ACEP hopes that this policy will help improve and provide consistency in the care of penetrating wounds of the extemities, and will help improve the documentation of these cases. The ultimate evaluation of this clinical policy will occur when emergency physicians use it, evaluate it, and provide feedback to the Clinical Policies Committee.

Inclusion criteria

This policy is intended for use with patients of all ages with any of the following penetrating extremity injuries: lacerations, mammalian bites, gunshot wounds, or other puncture wounds to the extremities.

Exclusion criteria

This policy is *not* intended for use in patients with nonmammalian bites, stings, or envenomations; needle sticks; wounds more than 24 hours old; abrasions; burns; or infected wounds.

Stabilization

This policy assumes that life-threatening emergencies have been treated or stabilized and is not meant to apply to the unstable patient. If a patient presents in an unstable condition, initial resuscitation and stabilization must take precedence over any action in this policy.

Rationale

Wound care represents a significant part of emergency medicine practice. This policy provides rational guidelines for the evaluation and treatment of penetrating wounds of the extremities but does not make definitive recommendations dealing with the prophylaxis or treatment of rabies, tetanus, HIV exposure, or hepatitis exposure. Recommendations in these areas are undergoing rapid evolution, and are currently being addressed by ACEP and other agencies and organizations. Many of the "guidelines" outlined in this policy reflect a consensus opinion of experts in the field.

Penetrating extremity wounds may have numerous complications, including foreign bodies, missed fractures, the development of a compartment syndrome, the development of infection, and associated damage to nerves, blood vessels, or tendons. Special consideration also should be given to crush injuries and to the potential for the development of compartment syndromes, although this policy does not further address these issues.

The scientific evidence concerning wound care is also evolving, and many acceptable techniques for wound management are widely used. For these reasons, ACEP does not advocate any specific wound closure materials or management techniques other than the establishment of early hemostasis, decontamination, the provision of adequate pain relief for the patient, and the removal of jewelry and other potential constricting bands. ACEP does not recommend prolonged soaking of wounds, particularly using cytotoxic agents.

The decision of how and when to close a wound may be complex. Factors to consider include age of the wound, potential contamination, care of the wound before arrival in the emergency department, mechanism of injury and extent of concomitant soft tissue or bone injury, cosmetic and functional considerations, and the potential for wound infection. In addition, consideration must be given to associated conditions and diseases such as advanced age, severe alcoholism, uremia, diabetes mellitus, peripheral vascular disease, malnutrition, and immunosuppression.

The initial evaluation and stabilization of penetrating extremity wounds require complete exposure of the wound, removal of any jewelry or potentially constricting bands in the anatomic area, and adequate hemostasis. Hemostasis usually can be achieved by direct pressure. Blind clamping of vessels in the extremities may be associated with inadvertent damage to other structures. Patients who are anticoagulated or have a bleeding disorder are at higher risk of continued bleeding and may require special interventions to achieve and maintain hemostasis.

Evaluation of some wounds may require the use of imaging techniques to identify foreign bodies, bone or joint damage, or vascular or other soft tissue injury. These imaging modalities may include plain radiographs, ultrasound, fluoroscopy, xeroradiography, computed axial tomography, magnetic resonance imaging, and others. The choice of imaging techniques should be based on availability and the clinician's judgment. The decision to identify a potential foreign body by imaging techniques needs to address the potential benefit of such identification. Some foreign bodies do not need to be identified and may be left in the soft tissues without significant sequelae.

Adequate pain control is an important component of patient care, both during and after the evaluation and treatment in the ED. Immobilization may be indicated to prevent further injury, to minimize pain, and to promote wound healing.

Decontamination should be undertaken for the prevention of infection to penetrating wounds of the extremities, but infections sometimes develop even with the best of care. Decontamination methods involve the removal of foreign material from the wound and debridement of devitalized tissue. Syringe irrigation with saline will remove most debris, although direct visualization of the debris and removal are sometimes required.

American College of Emergency Physicians: Clinical policy for the initial approach to patients presenting with penetrating extremity trauma. *Ann Emerg Med* 23:1147-1156, 1994.

*Schringer DL, Cantrill SV, Greene CS: *Ann Emerg Med* 22:597-602, 1993.

BOX 58-1

CLINICAL POLICY FOR THE INITIAL APPROACH TO PATIENTS PRESENTING WITH PENETRATING EXTREMITY TRAUMA—cont'd

The use of antiseptic solutions has not been proven to be superior to the use of saline alone, and some agents may be cytotoxic or gas forming even when diluted.

Even though there is an absence of sound scientific evidence supporting the use of antibiotics for wounds, clinicians frequently consider and often use them empirically for wounds with certain characteristics. The use of antibiotics, however, must be individualized and is a matter of clinical judgment. Characteristics of extremity wounds that may profit from antibiotic therapy include wounds more than 12 hours old, especially of the hands and the lower extremities; crush wounds with devitalized tissue; significantly contaminated wounds; wounds involving joint spaces, tendons, or bones; mammalian bites; contaminated wounds in patients with preexisting valvular heart disease; and wounds in immunosuppressed patients or in those with other impairment of host defenses.

The need for tetanus prophylaxis should be addressed for all wounds.

Implementing the policy

The rules and guidelines for patient management emphasize those findings with the potential for high risk to the patient. It is important that no single finding be considered independently. Some actions are separated by a slash mark (/), meaning that either action may be appropriate in a given clinical situation; the action is at the discretion of the clinician. The order in which items appear in the rules and guidelines is arbitrary and not meant to imply the order in which they should be performed. In using this clinical policy, it may be helpful to think of the ***rules*** as broad categories that should be recorded as pertinent positives or negatives, whereas *guidelines* are detailed or expanded lists that are meant to prompt the physician to consider many possibilities. Documentation should be sufficient to reflect the clinical decision-making process. It is unrealistic for a physician to perform or document every item in the guidelines.

Rule*	Guideline†
Solicit and record a history that includes:	**Consider these aspects of the history:**
Mechanism of injury	Potential contaminants and foreign bodies, associated crush injury, species of animal if bite or scratch, description of wounding agent, high-pressure injection injuries Circumstances (e.g., self-infliction, assault, domestic violence, or work related)
Approximate age of wound Tetanus immunization status Allergies	**Associated symptoms**: Pain, paresthesia, anesthesia, weakness, loss of function Treatment before arrival in the emergency department **Social history**: Handedness, vocations/avocations **Prior medical history**: Prior injury, prior disability, prior deficits, immunosuppression, diabetes mellitus, valvular heart disease, keloid formation, asplenia, peripheral vascular disease, bleeding disorders, internal prosthetic devices, current medications
Conduct and record a physical examination that includes:	**Consider these aspects of the physical examination:**
	Vital signs: Blood pressure, pulse, respirations, temperature; weight of child
Inspection of the area of injury	Location, length, estimated depth and shape of the wound, nerve function, tendon function, vascular integrity, entrance, exit, hematoma, hemorrhage, evidence of foreign body or contamination, evidence of fracture, palpation, range of motion (active, passive, functional), exploration throughout range of motion when anatomically feasible

*An action reflecting principles of good practice in most situations. There may be circumstances when a rule need not or cannot be followed; in these situations, it is advisable that deviation from the rule be justified in writing. Inability to comply with rules should be incorporated in institutional policies.

Guideline: An action that should be considered but may or may not be performed, depending on the patient, the circumstances, or other factors. Thus, guidelines are not always followed, and there is no implication that failure to follow a guideline is improper.

BOX 58-1

CLINICAL POLICY FOR THE INITIAL APPROACH TO PATIENTS PRESENTING WITH PENETRATING EXTREMITY TRAUMA—cont'd

Implement ACTIONS Based on the FINDINGS for the Following VARIABLES:

Variable	Finding	Action: Rule	Action: Guideline
History			
Mechanism of injury	Potential for foreign body in wound	Explore when anatomically feasible	Imaging
	Potential for underlying injury	Explore when anatomically feasible	Imaging
	High potential for infection due to contamination	Attempt decontamination	Antibiotic administration
	Mammalian bite		Rabies risk assessment Antibiotic administration appropriate for biting species
	Human bite		Assess for joint penetration when proximate to joint Possible delayed closure Antibiotic administration
	Dog bite to asplenic or immunosuppressed patient		Antibiotic administration to prevent infection with *Capnocytophagia canimorsus* (DF-2) Consult
	High-pressure injection injury	Consult	
Age of wound	Delayed presentation		Possible delayed closure Antibiotic adminstration
Comorbidity	Valvular heart disease, immunosuppression, diabetes mellitus, internal prosthetic device		Antibiotic administration
	Keloid formation		Consult/Referral
	Inadequate tetanus prophylaxis	Provide tetanus prophylaxis	Refer to ACEP information paper on tetanus immunization
Physical examination			
Location of wound	Over metacarpophalangeal joint or other joints	Assess potential for joint penetration	Assess potential for human bite Immobilization Consult
	Palmar puncture wound		Imaging Antibiotic administration Immobilization Consult
	Plantar puncture wound		Imaging Consult No weight bearing
Inspection, palpation, exploration, neurovascular examination, range of motion	Nerve injury		Immobilization Consult
	Suspicion of significant vascular injury	Control bleeding	IV access Immobilization Consult
	Tendon injury		Immobilization Repair or consult
	Deformity suggestive of underlying fracture	Image	Immobilization
	Open fracture	Image	Antibiotic administration Immobilization Consult

BOX 58-1

CLINICAL POLICY FOR THE INITIAL APPROACH TO PATIENTS PRESENTING WITH PENETRATING EXTREMITY TRAUMA—cont'd

Implement ACTIONS Based on the Findings for the Following VARIABLES—cont'd

Variable	Finding	Action: Rule	Action: Guideline
Physical Examination		**Rule**	**Guideline**
	Suspicion of joint violation		Imaging Wound exploration Antibiotic administration Immobilzation Consult
	Joint violation	Joint irrigation or consult	Imaging Antibiotic administration Immobilization
	Visible wound contamination	Attempt decontamination	Wound irrigation and cleansing Debridement Antibiotic administration Consult
	Foreign body in wound		Imaging Removal of foreign body
	Significant avulsion injury		Grafting Consult

Implement ACTIONS for the Following VARIABLES:

Variable	Action: Rule	Action: Guideline
Disposition	**Rule**	**Guideline**
Admission	Transfer care to accepting physician	
Transfer	Follow ACEP and other applicable transfer principles‡	
Discharge	Provide referral for follow-up care Provide instructions regarding treatment and circumstances that require return to emergency department	Advise patient about wound care, signs and symptoms of infection, signs and symptoms of compartment syndrome, the possibility of retained foreign body, methods for relieving pain, signs and symptoms suggestive of occult bone or tendon injury, follow-up, suture removal, care of the immobilized extremity/splint

‡American College of Emergency Physicians: *Ann Emerg Med* 22:766-767, 1993.

sentations (e.g., chest pain, abdominal pain) and were able to obtain a reduction in malpractice premiums if these guidelines were followed.[4] Guidelines such as these should not have geographic bias and should create practice standards of both national and regional scope. They should not be so oversimplified for ease of use they are not applicable to the many levels of clinical complexity that define emergency practice.

Perhaps the most important factor in effective practice guidelines is the composition of the task force charged with their creation. The group should be multidisciplinary, with all the significant stake holders involved in the discussion. The group should choose those diagnoses that are high risk for adverse patient outcomes. Guidelines should not be created in those situations where treatment is highly controversial, but should concentrate instead on diagnosis for which standards of care exist and are generally accepted.

Practice Guidelines Versus Clinical Pathways

Some physicians use the terms *practice guidelines* and *clinical pathways* interchangeably. In fact, they are quite different. Practice guidelines refer to suggested interventions a professional (e.g., physician, nurse) ought to make in his/her specialty when confronted with specific clinical situations. For example, the American Academy of Pediatrics suggests a certain approach when a physician is confronted with a febrile

Text continued on p. 531.

Care of Febrile Infants < 90 Days in the Emergency Department

PROBLEM

Great variability in care of the febrile infant < 90 days.

MISSION

To standardize care for the febrile infant.

Team Members

Leader	Physician
Member	Nurse Manager
Member	Nurse
Member	Resident
Member	Pediatrician
Member	Ward Clerk Manager
Facilitator	ED Director

MEASURE OF SUCCESS

Compliance with 'clinical pathway' created by the group.

CONSTRAINTS

Improve compliance with existing resources.

EXPECTATIONS AND SUPPORT

Progress reports every two weeks to emergency department management group.
Project completed in six months.

FIGURE 58-1 Clinical pathway for the febrile infant.

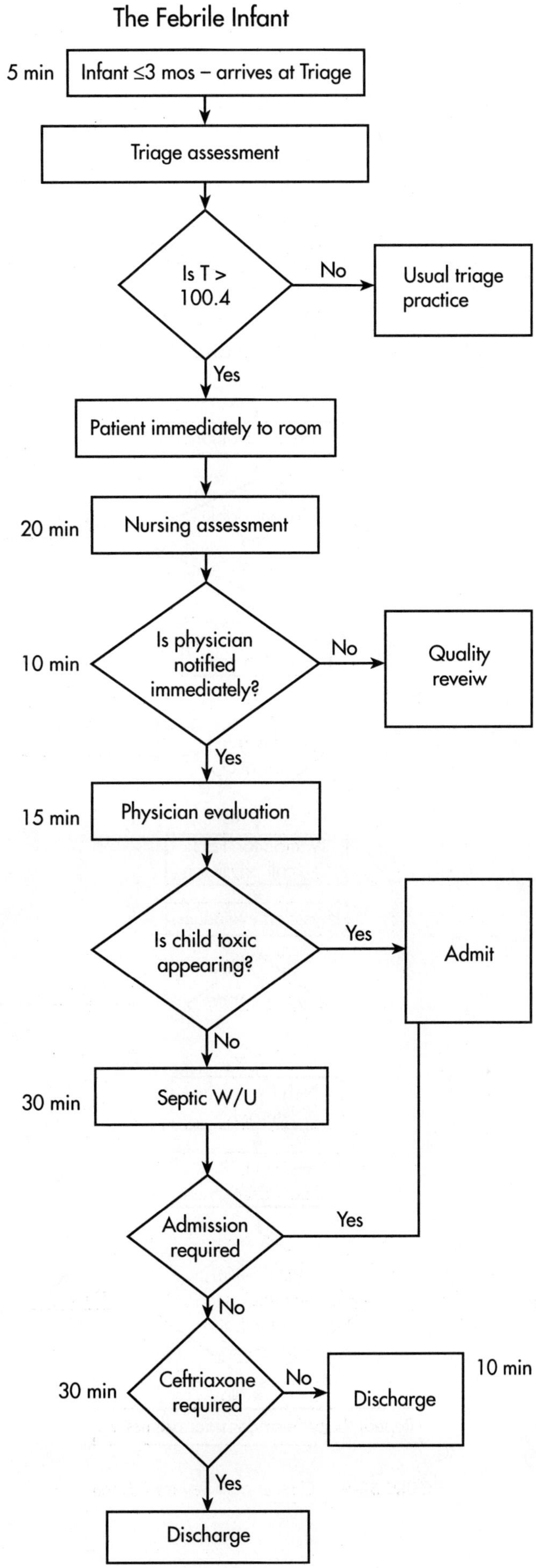

FIGURE 58-1, cont'd. For legend see opposite page.

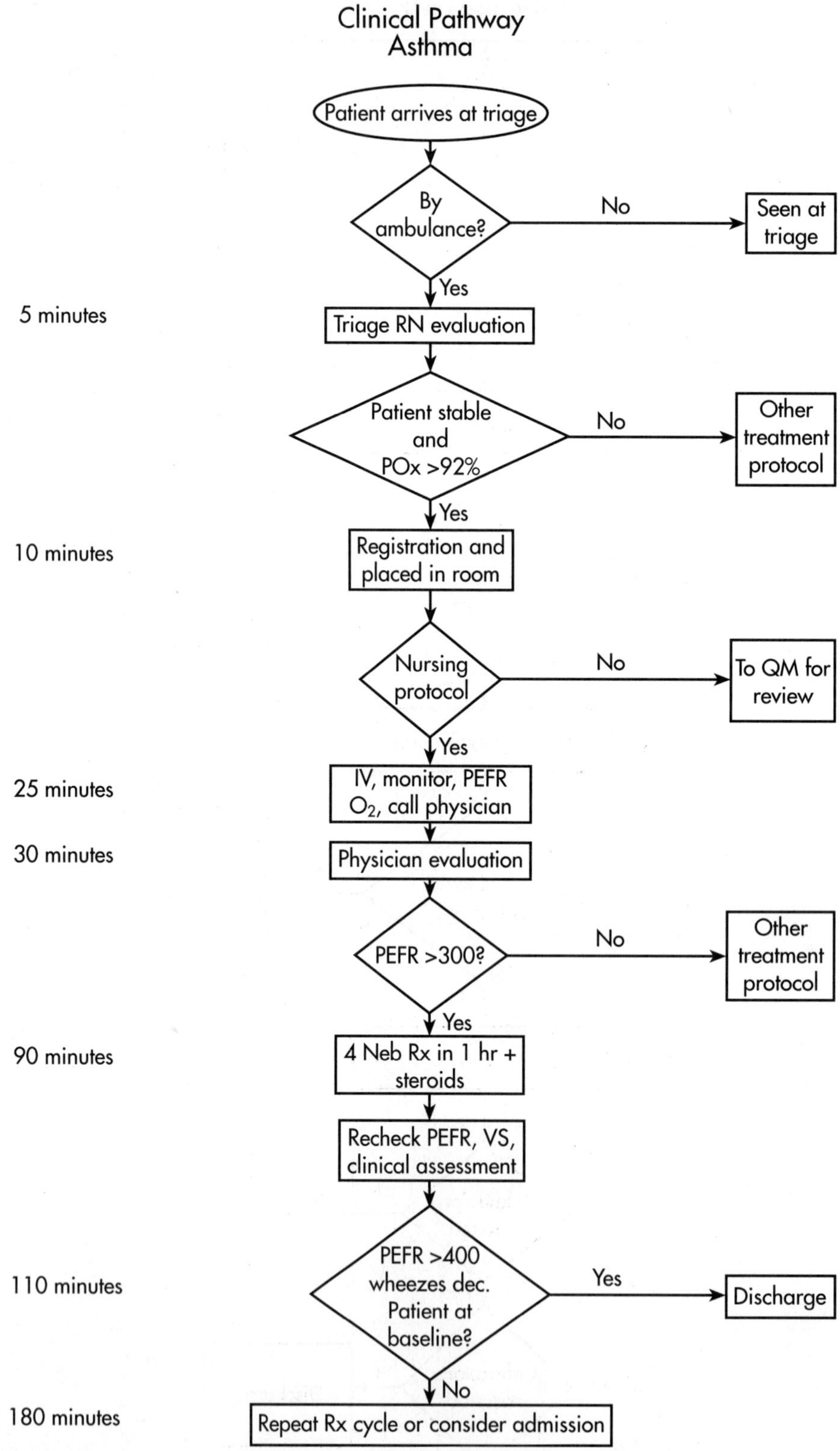

FIGURE 58-2 Clinical pathway for asthma.

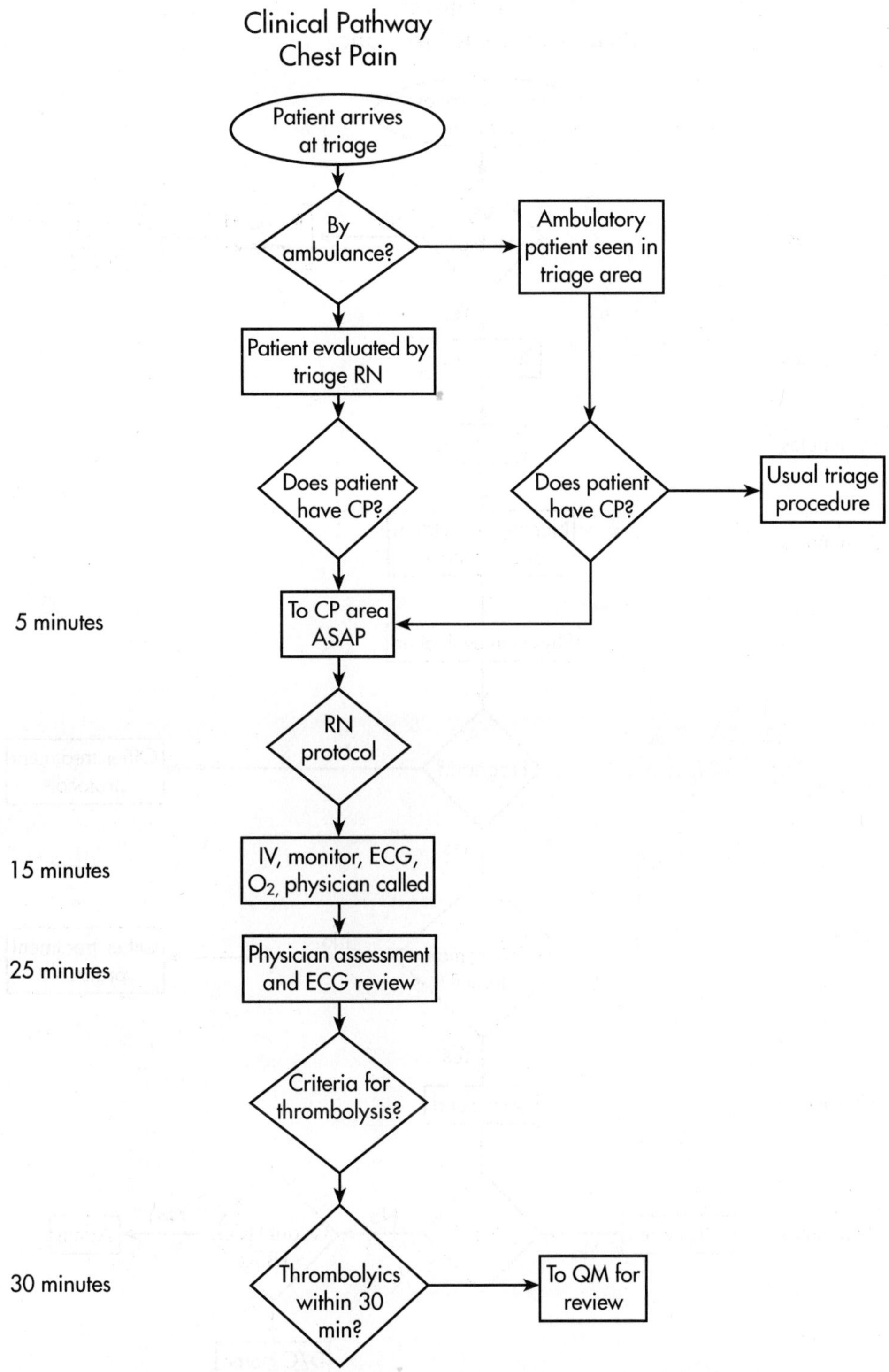

FIGURE 58-3 Clinical pathway for chest pain.

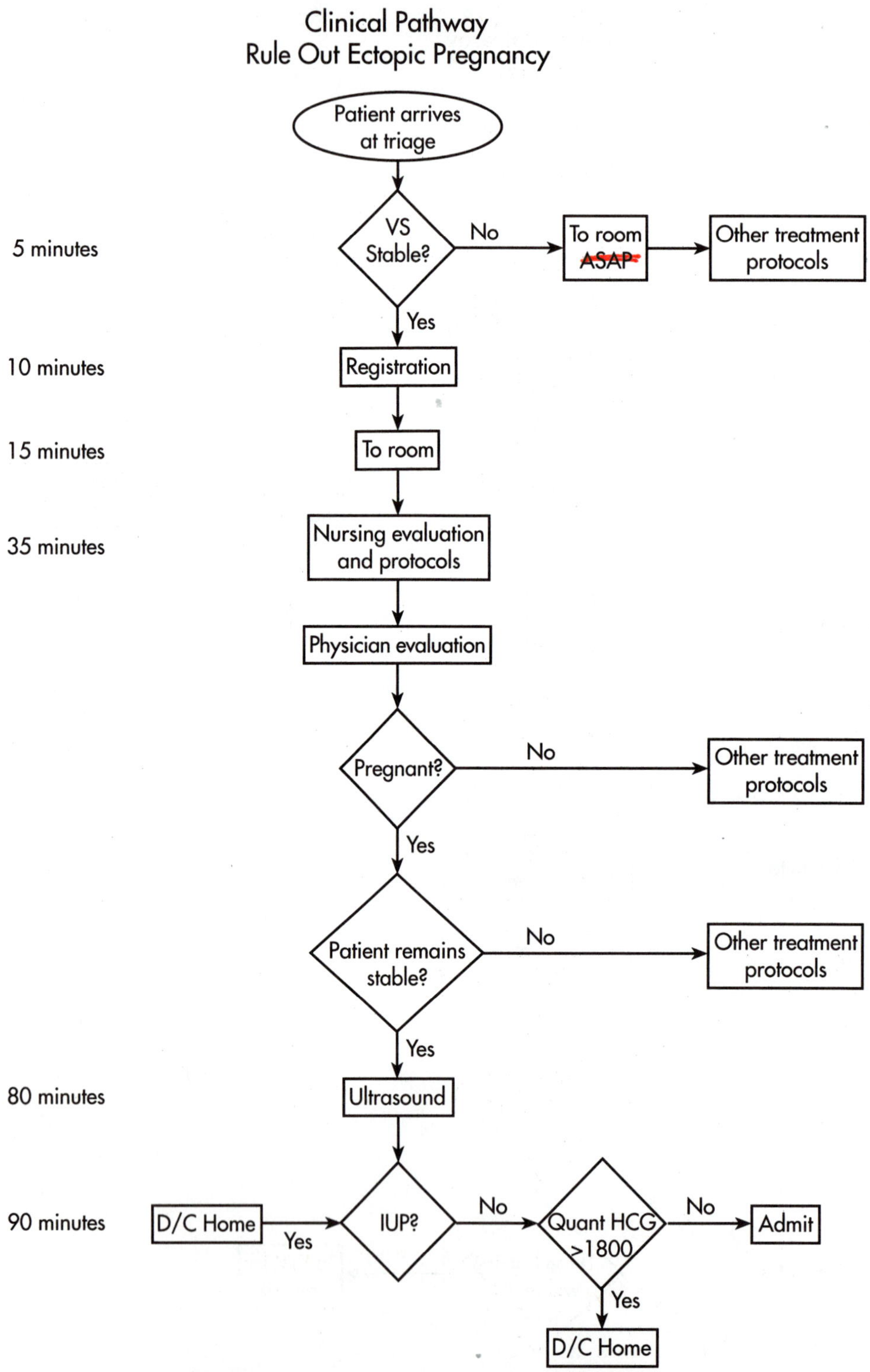

FIGURE 58-4 Clinical pathway to rule out ectopic pregnancy.

infant less than 3 months old[5] (Figure 58-1). In this situation the child should receive immediate treatment if toxic appearing and then a "septic workup" including complete blood count, BC, urine analysis, and lumbar puncture. In nontoxic appearing infants, the results of this workup greatly influence the disposition decision. The physician component of the infant's emergency department course is facilitated by the practice guidelines. However, the care rendered by a physician is only part of the series of Emergency Department processes that a febrile infant experiences from arrival to admission or discharge.

A clinical pathway defines a given patient's "journey" through a healthcare system in a way that optimizes clinical outcomes and is most cost effective.

For example, if a potentially ill febrile 1 month old sat in the waiting room for 2 hours before seeing a physician, the fact that an appropriate workup was performed by the physician does not mean that this child received good care. A clinical pathway defines appropriate "door to door" sequencing of patient care with timelines so that the care given is both of high quality and timely. Representative clinical pathways are demonstrated in Figures 58-2 to 58-4.

THE USE OF OUTCOMES DATA

As noted earlier in the chapter, the healthcare industry in the United States has been unable to deliver consistently high-quality, cost-effective care despite a variety of control mechanisms including market forces, regulatory sanctions, liability risks, peer review, and most recently the creation of practice guidelines. One reason that all of these measures have been ineffective to some extent is the inability of healthcare organizations to understand the link between patient outcomes and medical care practice. Managed care organizations, on the other hand, clearly understand the relationship between medical practice and one important outcome, cost, and have used physician incentives to achieve lower cost care.

It is difficult to understand the potential value and importance of practice guidelines unless patient outcomes are also considered. If physicians do not see a "value" to behavioral change in a practice guideline, they are unlikely to support and promulgate such algorithms. Such value can be defined if appropriate outcomes data are available and used. It may well be that to date practice guidelines have not lived up to their potential, at least in part, because of the absence of relevant outcome data.

Ideally, practices leading to improved patient outcomes for a particular condition would be formulated as a set of guidelines. Providers would model their decisions and behaviors on these guidelines and deliver cost-effective care. Instead, reports indicate that guidelines have had minimal impact on provider behaviors.[6] Implementation has not been easy, and guidelines, even when implemented, have not always produced sustained benefits. There is concern that guidelines do not consider patient preferences, as well as a perception that they are designed for the "average" patient. Both of these issues may reduce the motivation of providers to use guidelines in treatment decisions.

SUMMARY

This chapter has discussed reasons for creating practice guidelines, as well as some of the physician issues concerning their use. Contrasted practice guidelines were compared with clinical pathways, and examples given of each. Finally, the role of outcomes data in legitimizing the use of practice guidelines has been emphasized.

REFERENCES

1. Wolff SH: Practice guidelines—a reality in medicine. I. Recent developments, *Arch Intern Med* 150:1811-1818, 1990.
2. Ellrodt AG et al: Measuring and improving physician compliance with clinical practice guidelines, *Ann Intern Med* 22:277-282, 1995.
3. Hayward RSA et al: User's guide to the medical literature. VIII: How to use clinical practice guidelines. Are the recommendations valid? *JAMA* 274:570-574, 1995.
4. Schriger DL, Cantrill SV, Greene CS: The origins, benefits, harms, and implications of emergency medicine clinical policies, *Ann Emerg Med* 22:597-602, 1993.
5. American Academy of Pediatrics: Guidelines for pediatric emergency care facilities, *Pediatrics* 96:526-537, 1995.
6. Garnick DW, Hendricks AM, Brennan TA: Can practice guidelines reduce the number and costs of malpractice claims? *JAMA* 266:2856-2860, 1991.

59 Practice Guidelines for Nurses

Eleanore R. Kirsch

OUTLINE

Perhaps the most common terms heard today in reference to healthcare are quality, appropriateness, and effectiveness. Is the quality of care that patients receive the best it can be? Is the care they receive necessary, comprehensive, and available to everyone? Is the care effective, that is, the outcome of care is successful or at least what the patient expected?

There are initiatives under way to address these questions. These initiatives are being implemented by nursing, medicine, federal and regulatory agencies, third-party payors, and the public. They address many issues, including formulation of professional standards, database development related to nursing contributions to patient care, funding of healthcare and reimbursement policy development, and the development and implementation of practice guidelines.

Changes are rapidly occurring that affect emergency nursing, and the implications for emergency nurse managers are multiple.

- The guidelines being developed can be useful to emergency nursing practice. Mechanisms must be implemented to disseminate the information.
- Nursing must collect information to demonstrate nursing participation in care. Forms must be developed to assist in this data collection.
- Staff must receive continuing education to keep up with the numerous changes that are occurring.
- Nursing must participate in a collaborative manner with other disciplines to accomplish patient care and develop ongoing patient care guidelines.
- Ongoing quality management must occur to demonstrate that the outcomes of patient care are positive.

This chapter will address these initiatives from a nursing perspective. Nursing's initiatives toward practice guideline development will be a specific focus of the chapter.

HISTORICAL PERSPECTIVE

For the past 20 years, descriptive research has revealed treatment variations of specific health problems. Many variations are unrelated to patient need or preference. Although healthcare is individualized and not expected to be identical from patient to patient, in some instances treatments were not effective and were harmful. Healthcare dollars were being spent on inappropriate, unnecessary, and ineffective care.[1]

There is no consensus among healthcare providers regarding effective treatment for specific health problems. If the research literature is contradictory regarding what constitutes appropriate care, healthcare providers often rely on their own professional judgment, the judgment of their peers, or personal experience in making practice decisions.[1]

Federal Initiatives

Because of escalating healthcare costs and wide variations in clinical practice, the federal government, private insurers, specialty organizations, and other public and private entities have become involved in effectiveness and outcome research. (See Box 59-1 for a list of the organizations involved.) Research findings will eventually influence new ideas regarding the implementation of healthcare, market share for healthcare providers, clinical practice, medical liability, insurance coverage decisions, and reimbursement policies.[2] For example, future research may demonstrate that the most appropriate healthcare provider for certain disease entities may be a nurse practitioner in an ambulatory care setting rather than a physician in a hospital setting.

The federal government's focal point for healthcare effectiveness and services research is the Public Health Service's newest agency, the Agency for Health Care Policy and Research (AHCPR). The purpose of AHCPR is to enhance the quality, appropriateness, and effectiveness of healthcare services so that a greater majority of people may receive health services. Created in December 1989, AHCPR expands on the work of its predecessor, the National Center for Health Services Research (NCHSR) and Health Care Technology Assessment. See Figure 59-1 for an explanation of where AHCPR is situated in the U.S. Department of Health and Human Services (DHHS) and Figure 59-2 for a breakdown of AHCPR components.

The AHCPR commissions expert panels of healthcare providers to develop clinical practice guidelines that address selected conditions. The purpose of these guidelines is to direct practice by providing links between diagnosis, treatments, and outcomes and by describing the alternatives available for each patient. Guidelines provide the basis for evaluation of care and allocation of resources.[3]

The AHCPR bases its clinical guidelines on a comprehensive review of scientific literature, valid evidence presented at open meetings, and professional judgment of panel members and other experts. The panels are multidisciplinary and include representatives from medicine, nursing, psychology, allied healthcare providers, consumer groups, and ethicists.[1]

BOX 59-1

ORGANIZATIONS INVOLVED IN HEALTHCARE EFFECTIVENESS INITIATIVES

Public

Public Health Service
Agency for Health Care Policy and Research (AHCPR)
Health Resources and Services Administration (HRSA)
Division of Nursing
Commission on National Nursing Shortage
National Institutes of Health (NIH)
National Institute for Nursing Research (NINR)
Veterans Administration
Department of Defense (DOD)
Health Care Financing Administration (HCFA)
National Library of Medicine
Prospective Payment Assessment Commission
Physician Payment Review Commission
World Health Organization (WHO)

Private

Joint Commission on Accreditation of Healthcare Organizations (JCAHO)
Institute of Medicine (IOM)
American Hospital Association (AHA)

Organized medicine

American Medical Association (AMA)
Individual researchers
Vendors

Organized nursing

American Nurses Association (ANA)
Nursing Organization Liaison Forum (NOLF)
Sigma Theta Tau International
North American Nursing Diagnosis Association (NANDA)
International Council Of Nurses (ICN)
National Commission on Nursing Implementation Project

From American Nurses Association: *Consultation development workshop on the quality, appropriateness and effectiveness of health care services.* Kansas City, November 4-5, 1991.

The first seven clinical conditions addressed by AHCPR were the following:

- Management of functional impairment caused by cataracts in the adult
- Acute pain management: operative or medical procedures and trauma
- Diagnosis and treatment of benign prostatic hyperplasia
- Diagnosis and treatment of depressed outpatients in primary care settings
- Sickle cell disease
- Prediction, prevention, and early treatment of pressure ulcers in adults
- Urinary incontinence in adults

Additional panels have since been developed to address otitis media in children, the diagnosis and treatment of heart failure secondary to coronary vascular disease, poststroke rehabilitation, evaluation of and early intervention for HIV-positive asymptomatic patients, management of cancer-related pain, treatment of stage 2 and greater pressure ulcers, low back problems, screening for Alzheimer's and related dementias, and quality determinants of mammography.

The intent of AHCPR is to widely disseminate its guidelines for the following purposes:

- Changing the behavior of healthcare providers in the workplace by providing them with science-based knowledge and respected professional judgment for making practice decisions, especially under conditions of uncertainty.[4]
- Enabling consumers to make informed treatment choices and work as partners with their healthcare providers.
- Eliminating or greatly reducing unnecessary and inappropriate healthcare practices.
- Improving the quality of healthcare by enhancing treatment consistency among healthcare providers.
- Decreasing healthcare costs by eliminating less beneficial and costly treatment variations.

To date, nursing has been involved in most of the AHCPR panels, as nursing representatives, chairs, or cochairs of the multidisciplinary panels that set guidelines. Additionally, AHCPR convened an ad hoc advisory panel of nurses on January 31 to February 1, 1990, to provide the nursing profession perspective on its role in the overall initiative. Panel membership comprised 45 nursing leaders with recognized expertise as clinicians, researchers, educators, administrators, and representatives of professional nursing organizations. This panel proposed a definition of "guideline," defined "clinical condition," recommended guideline topics, and recommended formulation of a nursing research agenda on outcomes and effectiveness.[5]

Nursing Initiatives

Through the leadership of the American Nurses Association (ANA) and with the participation of specialty organizations, including the Emergency Nurses Association (ENA), three major initiatives are under way to address the quality, effectiveness, and appropriateness of healthcare services: quality improvement, a database of nursing contributions to healthcare to support clinical nursing practice, and payment reform.

Quality Improvement. The goals of quality improvement are to guide nursing practice through the development of standards and guidelines, to strengthen the evaluation of nursing care by developing criteria to measure compliance with standards, and to promote nursing research aimed at the outcomes of nursing interventions.[6]

Recently, the American Nurses Association (ANA), along with representatives from the National Federation of Nursing Specialty Organizations (NFNSO), developed the standards of Clinical Nursing Practice. These generic standards apply to the practice of all professional nurses, regardless of clinical specialty, practice setting, or educational preparation. These standards were acknowledged by the ENA board of directors in September 1991 and have been incorporated into the third edition of the *ENA Standards of Emergency Nursing Practice*.

The generic standards of clinical nursing practice include both standards of care and standards of professional performance. (See Box 59-2.) Standards of care are authoritative statements that describe a competent level of clinical nursing practice demonstrated through assessment, diagnosis, out-

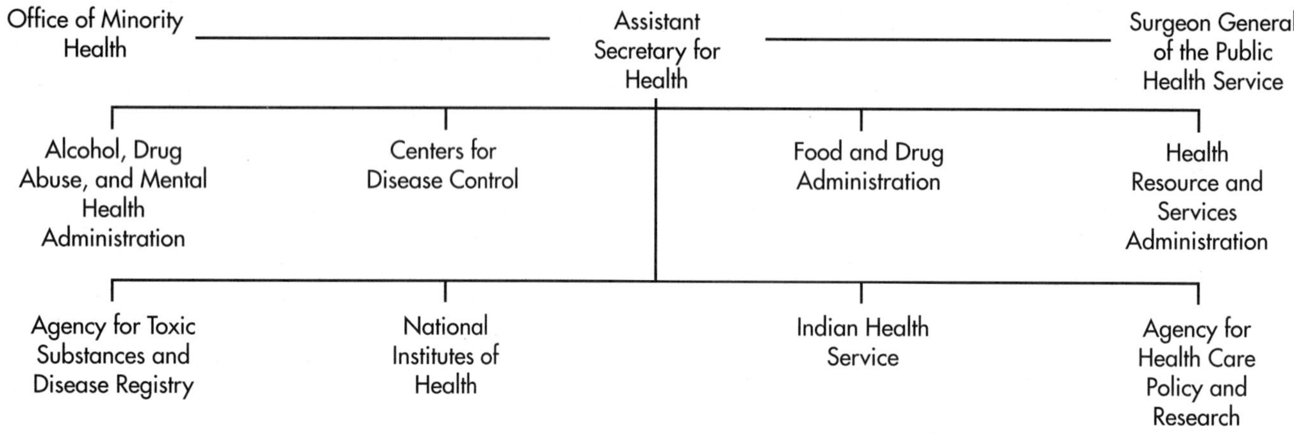

FIGURE 59-1 U.S. Department of Health and Human Services, Public Health Service.

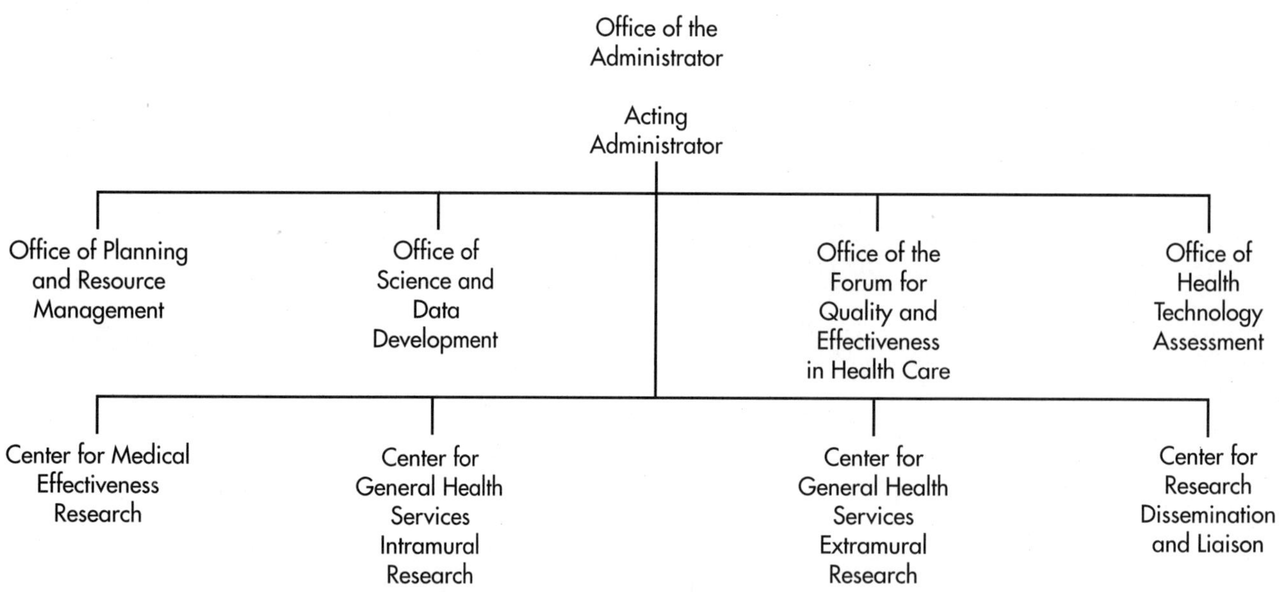

FIGURE 59-2 Agency for Health Care Policy Research.

come identification, planning, implementation, and evaluation.[7]

Standards of professional performance are authoritative statements that describe a competent level of behavior in the professional role, including activities related to quality of care, performance appraisal, education, collegiality, ethics, collaboration, research, and resource utilization.[7] The ENA incorporates both standards of care and standards of professional performance within its standards of emergency nursing practice.

The terms *standards of care* and *standards of practice* have different meanings for different groups. Table 59-1 clarifies these definitions.

Standards and guidelines differ primarily in their scope and intent. The intent of standards of nursing practice is to describe an acceptable level of client care (standard of care) or behavior in the professional nurse's role (standard of professional performance). Guidelines further the intent of standards of nursing practice by defining specific recommendations for care to be provided in various clinical situations or for individuals or groups of client populations.[6]

BOX 59-2

STANDARDS OF CLINICAL NURSING PRACTICE

Standards of care

- Assessment
- Diagnosis
- Outcome identification
- Planning
- Implementation
- Evaluation

Standards of professional performance

- Quality of care
- Performance appraisal
- Education
- Collegiality
- Ethics
- Collaboration
- Research
- Resource utilization

Table 59-1 ENA, ANA, and JCAHO Terminology

	Nurse	Client Outcome
ENA	Standards of practice	Guidelines
ANA	Standards of care	Guidelines
JCAHO	Standards of practice	Standards of care

ENA, Emergency Nurses Association; *ANA,* American Nurses Association; *JCAHO,* Joint Commission on Accreditation of Healthcare Organizations.

BOX 59-3

ELEMENTS OF THE NURSING MINIMUM DATA SET

Nursing care elements

- Nursing diagnosis
- Nursing intervention
- Nursing outcome
- Intensity of nursing care

Patient or client demographic elements

- Personal identification*
- Date of birth*
- Gender*
- Race and ethnicity*
- Residence*

Service elements

- Unique facility or service agency number
- Unique health record number of patient or client
- Unique number of principal registered nurse provider
- Episode admission or encounter date*
- Discharge or termination date*
- Disposition of patient or client*
- Expected payor for most of this bill (anticipated financial guarantor for services)*

*Indicates data already collected in existing systems.

The scope of standards is broader than that of guidelines. Standards of nursing practice apply to the care that is provided to *all* clients and the professional behavior of *all* nurses. Guidelines have a more narrow scope than standards. They are developed for particular clinical conditions or diagnoses addressed by nursing. These clinical conditions may be patient problems manifested as a nursing diagnosis, a medical diagnosis, or a diagnosis made and treated by another healthcare provider, such as a social worker, dietitian, or by multiple healthcare providers.

Nursing guidelines are embedded in standards of practice, standardized care plans, protocols, critical paths, and the core curricula and statements of various specialty organizations and interdisciplinary groups. However, many of these guidelines are not fully developed or are not accessible to many nurses. Therefore a centralized database of existing nursing guidelines needs to be developed.[6]

Database Development. Standards and guidelines for nursing practice provide the unified database for clinical nursing practice. The goals included in a database to support clinical nursing practice are establishing a national nursing database that includes assessment, diagnosis and patient problem, and interventions and services and developing nurse-sensitive patient outcomes and evaluation of nursing care.

The first goal will be accomplished by developing a unified language system that will link and classify assessment, diagnosis, and interventions. The second goal will be addressed by developing guidelines for nursing information systems. These guidelines will address standardized nursing data elements through identifying nursing data elements in existing federal and private databases and conducting secondary analyses.[6]

Unfortunately, clinical nursing is essentially invisible in current hospital, institutional, federal, private-payor, and public policy databases. Nursing's contribution to patient outcomes is largely documented, but it is not retrievable data because it is not a part of the present databases. If a national database for clinical nursing practice cannot be established, nursing will be excluded from the major healthcare policy decisions within the coming years. Additionally, there will be no information available to demonstrate how nursing should be reimbursed for services because no documentation of nursing outcomes can be elicited from the present databases.

Databases are essentially used to monitor patient care, evaluate the quality of care delivered, project personnel needs, authorize payment for services, and conduct research on the effectiveness of care. Sources of healthcare data include the patient record, federal databases, private databases, and bibliographic retrieval systems. Numerous data systems are available that collect information related to healthcare. However, none of them collects information specific to nursing.

A Nursing Minimum Data Set (NMDS) was developed by nurses. It names the minimum data elements to be included in any data set or patient record.[8] Box 59-3 lists the elements of the NMDS. Additional examples of information sources include the following:

- Nursing diagnosis/problem list
  - Nursing Minimum Data Set (NMDS)
  - North American Nursing Diagnosis Association (NANDA)
  - Omaha Visiting Nurses Association (VNA)
  - Saba's Home Care Classification
  - International Classification of Diseases (ICD)
  - Diagnostic and Statistical Manual III (DSM-III)
- Nursing intervention
  - NMDS
  - Bulachek and McCloskey Classification of Nursing Interventions
  - Omaha VNA
  - Common Procedural Terminology (CPT)
- Nursing outcome
  - NMDS
  - Omaha VNA

Examples of large databases in use by the federal government, state and private agencies, and medicine include the following:

- Uniform Clinical Data Set (UCDS)
- Professional Review Organizations (PRO) Quality Screens
- Assessment of needs for continuing care
- Nursing Facility Resident Assessment and Care Screening

Claims data are found in the following:

- Medicare part A
- Medicare part B
- Other federal programs, including Civilian Health Medical Program of Uniformed Services (CHAMPUS) and Federal Employee Health Benefit Program (FEHBP)
- Medicaid
- Private insurance

Recognizing the growing need for a uniform method of documenting and collecting emergency care data, the ENA appointed a task force in 1994 to develop an Emergency Nursing Uniform Data Set (ENUDS). The implementation of ENUDS, along with the movement toward a computerized patient record, will facilitate access to important emergency care data that will complement and supplement other health data. The ENUDS is a set of essential and desirable data elements with uniform definitions and categories concerning the specific dimensions of emergency nursing. These elements will meet the needs of multiple data users in healthcare systems.

The purpose of ENUDS is to do the following:

1. Standardize the collection, storage, and retrieval of core emergency nursing data.
2. Examine patient outcomes influenced by emergency nursing care.
3. Provide national guidelines for data collection.
4. Improve resource allocation.
5. Provide the ability to trend data and to link with existing data systems.
6. Enhance the knowledge base of practitioners by discovering information useful for modifying practice.
7. Identify information useful for workforce redesign.
8. Encourage the analysis of data being collected currently.
9. Identify essential versus desirable (or a more detailed continuum of) data elements.

The NMDS was used as the primary foundation for the ENUDS. The nursing care element for triage acuity classification was added to the NMDS nursing elements because this element is uniquely relevant to emergency patient care. Emergency nurses frequently make triage decisions that require judgments about the immediacy of treatment based on the risk of the patient to lose life or limb. Therefore this information is integral to evaluating emergency department operations. The Nursing Care Elements for the Emergency Nursing Uniform Data Set consist of the following:

1. Triage classification
2. Nursing diagnosis
3. Nursing intervention
4. Nursing outcome
5. Nursing intensity

The ENA supports and promotes the need for standardized nursing data to be included in healthcare system databases and continues to work with other groups (nursing organizations, Centers for Disease Control and Prevention [CDC], American Society for Testing and Materials) that are developing uniform data sets to ensure that emergency nursing data elements are recognized and included. The ENUDS, along with other healthcare elements, patient demographic elements, and service elements, will be a part of the CDC Emergency Department Data Set that was refined at the CDC National Workshop in January 1996 and will be disseminated in 1997.

A manual for the nursing elements has been developed by the ENUDS Task Force. This manual will be used in conjunction with the Emergency Department Uniform Data Set manual from the CDC National Workshop. The ENUDS manual will include topics such as the definition and format of the essential and desirable nursing elements; how to implement ENUDS (computer and paper systems); how to use the data; barriers and problem solving; the CDC Data Set; research priorities for data set development and evaluation; and a bibliography. The manual will be ready for distribution in 1997.

The ENUDS Task Force also identified several areas of research that are needed to further delineate individual ENUDS data elements or to identify the most appropriate classification system for emergency nursing care elements.

Payment Reform. The goals of nursing toward payment reform are to design payment systems to support new practice models and to demonstrate the cost-effectiveness of quality, appropriate, and health-effective nursing care. The first goal will be accomplished by promoting emerging nursing practice models, such as community nursing organizations, and determining methods that clarify the value of nursing diagnosis, interventions, and services. An additional strategy includes lobbying for payment of nursing services for advanced practice.

The second goal will be accomplished by analyzing all nursing literature related to nursing cost-effectiveness and comparisons with physicians, promoting cost-effective nursing services to legislators and the business community, and developing strategies to influence future payment systems.[6]

DEVELOPMENT OF NURSING PRACTICE GUIDELINES

The ANA has been the moving force in nursing's involvement in the development of clinical practice guidelines. The ANA Committee on Nursing Practice Standards and Guidelines has representation from many specialty groups and reports regularly to both NFNSO and the Nursing Organization Liaison Forum (NOLF). The development and dissemination of practice guidelines is based on several assumptions.[9]

- It is in the best interest of the profession and the public health for nurses to be involved and influential in the development and dissemination of national practice guidelines.
- The current status of nursing research and professional consensus justifies guideline development for many clinical conditions and nursing diagnoses.
- If the nursing profession does not actively seize its appropriate role in practice guideline development, others will claim these activities.
- Organized nursing (which includes emergency nursing) is committed to collaborating in the development and dissemination of practice guidelines.

Development of guidelines can be initiated by nursing in at least three ways.[9]

- Nursing participation in the AHCPR initiatives of guideline development
- Nursing participation in the guideline development by other professional groups
- Initiation of guidelines by nursing that could be developed with multidisciplinary participation

The development of guidelines by nursing should follow the process being used by other disciplines to allow collaboration and integration of nursing guidelines with those being developed by others. This entails a different process than that previously used to develop standardized care plans or other nursing documents.

Guidelines must have the following attributes.[9]

- They must be valid—"derived from the synthesis of the best scientific evidence and expert opinion and lead to desired outcomes."
- They must possess reliability and reproducibility—given the same evidence and methods for guideline development, another set of experts would produce essentially the same document.
- They must be clinically applicable—practitioners would consistently apply them to practice in the same manner.
- They should contain clinical flexibility—exceptions to recommendations are identified.
- They should contain clarity—the language should be clear and terms defined precisely.

The ANA and the specialty organizations have developed a format for guideline development. It is consistent with the work of AHCPR and other disciplines. (See Appendix A.) Additionally, ANA has developed criteria for nominating individuals to AHCPR guideline panels. (See Appendix B.)

Legality of Guidelines

Standards and guidelines are used throughout society as the measure of client outcomes, nurse performance, and competency. A standard is a clearly defined legal expectation to which nurses can be held accountable. According to the ANA, practice guidelines reflect only recommended options for care.[9] Although a set of guidelines may be developed to address the typical clinical conditions of a particular client population, not every guideline may be appropriate for or applicable to each individual client and would not be selected for that plan of care. In addition, not all interventions within a particular guideline may be applicable or indicated. The evaluation of nursing practice using practice guidelines therefore requires nursing clinical judgment to evaluate the appropriateness of the guidelines to meet the needs of each individual client. Not using a guideline does not mean that the nurse is providing inappropriate care.

Guidelines, however, can be used as malpractice defense. According to the American Hospital Association,[10] "compliance with clinical practice guidelines can be used as an affirmative defense in professional liability lawsuits." An example of this is the development of parameters for basic intraoperative monitoring in 1986 by the American Society of Anesthesiologists. This guideline development led to a joint underwriting arrangement to offer insurance premium discounts for physicians who agreed to follow the guideline. There have been no hypoxic injury lawsuits among physicians who followed the guideline.[10]

Linkage of Guidelines to Quality Improvement

Quality improvement activities are meant to enhance the quality of patient care. This is usually accomplished by focusing on both the process and outcomes of patient care through data collection and analysis. Clinical patient guidelines can be useful to healthcare providers and institutions in improving patient care. This can be accomplished in the following manner:

- Healthcare providers can introduce completed guidelines into the work environment.
- Quality managers (persons specifically responsible for developing quality improvement mechanisms) can stress the educational value of clinical guidelines documenting the process of care.
- Mechanisms can be established to evaluate practice patterns relative to the guidelines.
- Quality management can support guideline implementation by ensuring that there are adequate systems in place to collect, analyze, and use information related to the guideline.
- Guidelines can be translated into review criteria, standards of quality, and performance measures.

The implementation of guidelines into a quality improvement program can enhance the quality of patient care, facilitate collaboration between disciplines, provide malpractice defense, enhance educational programs, support outcome research, and assist in the development of databases or computerized patient records.

SUMMARY

Nursing must continue its participation in and independent development of clinical practice guidelines. This includes the identification of specific areas for guideline development, the utilization of a consistent process for guideline development, and the development of useful guidelines for both nursing and the public. Specialty groups should continue or begin development of guidelines to address specialty conditions. Because guideline development is expensive, this can occur in collaboration with other nursing or multidisciplinary groups. This is especially appropriate with more universal clinical conditions or nursing diagnoses.

Nursing organizations should also be responsible for educating their members on the process of guideline development and disseminating completed guidelines. Additionally, organizations should budget for the development of guidelines. The ANA has developed a manual to assist in writing guidelines.[11] Organized nursing must continue to work with the nursing research community in the evaluation of newly developed and existing guidelines.

Guideline development is a process that will continue into the next decade. It will take the energies of many organizations and will be an evolutionary process in an ever changing healthcare environment. Nursing can take advantage of this opportunity to position itself in the new reality of healthcare and demonstrate that nursing can make a difference.

REFERENCES

1. AHCPR: *AHCPR commissioned clinical practice guidelines in AHCPR fact sheet,* Rockville, Md, 1992, AHCPR.
2. Bocchino CA: An interview with Jarrett Clinton, *Nurs Econ* 9(4):221-231, 1991.
3. AHCPR: *AHCPR program note: clinical guideline development,* Rockville, Md, US Department of Health and Human Services, Public Health Services.
4. AHCPR: *Purpose and programs,* Rockville, Md, 1990, US Department of Health and Human Services.
5. AHCPR: *AHCPR program note, nursing advisory panel for guideline development: summary,* Rockville, Md, 1990, US Department of Health and Human Services, Public Health Services.
6. ANA: American Nurses Association Consultation Workshop on the Quality, Appropriateness and Effectiveness of Health Care. Kansas City, November 4-5, 1991.
7. ANA: *Standards of clinical nursing practice,* Washington, DC, 1991, ANA.
8. Werley HH, Lang NM, editors: *Identification of the nursing minimum data set,* New York, 1988, Springer.
9. ANA: *Second working paper of the ANA committee on nursing practice standards and guidelines,* Washington, DC, 1993, ANA.
10. AHA: *Clinical practice guidelines: an awareness paper for hospitals,* Chicago, 1992, AHA.
11. Marek KD: *Manual to develop guidelines,* Washington, DC, 1995, ANA.

APPENDIX

A Format for Clinical Practice Guideline Document

I. Introduction
  A. Description of the nursing diagnosis/clinical condition* (hereafter known as the condition)—includes all terms by which the condition is known
  B. Statement of the scope of the condition in nursing practice
    1. Prevalence of the problem and potential impact
    2. Definition of the population affected; precise delineation of the population (e.g., age, symptoms, past history, etiologies)
    3. Settings in which condition is most commonly treated by nursing
  C. Discussion of the significance of the condition
    1. Variations in outcomes affected by nursing practice
    2. Variations in cost of care affected by nursing practice
    3. Degree of independence, interdependence/collaboration, and dependence affecting client outcomes

II. Clinical practice guideline
  A. Identification of decisions that must be based on client preference
  B. Description of the assessment criteria
    1. Identification of assessment criteria that represent the presence of the condition
    2. Description of assessment criteria within context of evidence
    3. Discussion of assessment criteria that are appropriate, inappropriate, or of intermediate or uncertain appropriateness in specific clinical situations
    4. Identification of and rationale for major foreseeable exceptions and alternative assessment strategies
  C. Description of interventions
    1. Description of interventions within the context of the evidence
    2. Discussion of interventions that are appropriate, inappropriate, or of intermediate or uncertain appropriateness in specific clinical situations
    3. Identification of and rationale for major foreseeable exceptions and alternative intervention strategies
  D. Description of expected client outcomes within context of evidence
  E. Identification of and rationale for major foreseeable exceptions and alternative management of strategies
  F. Discussion of the utilization of guidelines across the continuum of care
  G. Development of a model that shows linkages (relationships) between assessment, interventions, and outcomes
  H. Discussion of recommendations for documentation

III. Documentation of guideline development
  A. Identification of organizations involved in the development of the guideline
  B. Description of process used to develop guidelines including but not limited to
    1. Selection criteria for panel members
    2. Review and critique of evidence
    3. Peer review/open hearings
    4. Field testing
    5. Method for arriving at consensus about the guideline
  C. Review of the evidence used in the development of the guideline
    1. Methods used for the selection, analysis, and data extraction of the literature
    2. Processes used to review and synthesize scientific evidence
      a. Metaanalysis
      b. Best evidence synthesis
      c. Confidence interval analysis
    3. Process of expert opinion/clinical consensus evidence
    4. Process to assess the clinical risks and benefits associated with various interventions after review of the scientific evidence and expert opinion

IV. Plan for dissemination and review
  A. Assessment of practice feasibility
    1. Identification of concerns of clients, practitioners, and payors
    2. Identification of limitations of healthcare system
    3. Identification of ethical and societal issues affecting implementation
  B. Description of methods for dissemination
  C. Discussion of implications for professionals and consumers (e.g., client education, professional education, quality of care, credentialing)
  D. Recommendations for future research
  E. Recommendations for periodic review of guidelines
    1. Mechanisms for update and revision
    2. Time table of review

V. Disclaimers/medical-legal statement

VI. Glossary

VII. References

Consider as appendices
1. Samples of assessment tools
2. Samples of documentation tools/systems
3. Client version of the guideline
4. Results of statistical summaries
5. Algorithm
6. Abstract of guidelines for healthcare personnel

*A condition may be a human response, a nursing diagnosis, or a phenomenon of concern.

APPENDIX

B Criteria for Nominating Individuals to AHCPR Guideline Panels

A. AHCPR guideline panel chair
   1. Research experience
   2. Communication ability
   3. Management capability
   4. Previous author of publications or a literature review
   5. Familiarity with statistical methods
   6. Availability to attend all meetings
   7. Knowledge of a large group of experts in the area
   8. Geographic distribution
   9. Clinical experience

B. AHCPR guideline panel members
   1. Research experience
   2. Has published on the topic
   3. Has worked in multidisciplinary groups and can arrive at consensus
   4. Availability to attend all meetings
   5. Geographic distribution
   6. Clinical experience

Optional special skills

   7. Can serve as database coordinator (computer skills)
   8. Can organize an open hearing (organizational skills)
   9. Can serve as panel's methodologist
   10. Can serve as panel's biostatistician
   11. Can serve as panel's consumer
   12. Can translate guideline to patient education documents

PART SIX
Risk Management/Legal Issues

60 Principles of Risk Management

Gregory L. Henry

OUTLINE

The term *risk management* has become one of the buzzwords of the 1990s corporate communities. Practitioners of the healing arts should never forget that the only real risk is to the life and well-being of the patient and that risk management should really mean controlling the variables with regard to medical practice so as to maximize the patient's chances of a satisfactory outcome. To view risk management as any more or any less is to remove it from the traditional duties placed on physicians from the time of Galen. Doing what is in the true best interest of the patient is generally in the short-term and long-term best interests of the healthcare professionals and the institutions they represent.

Traditionally, risk managers have used incident reports, patient complaints, and reported poor outcomes as the impetus for them to begin to "manage risk." In its more traditional form, risk management is reactive and not proactive. Up to this time, it has been the division of the hospital where "bad outcomes" or "bad practice" were mitigated, if not repaired, on an after-the-fact basis. The risk was always viewed as the risk to the assets of the institution and not to the life of the patient. In the past, it was the rare institution that combined its risk management and quality assurance functions in such a way that true changes were triggered in the systematic care of patients. It was also a rare occurrence to see that the risk management personnel had significant input into and influence on creating the quality assurance standards that would prevent poor outcomes.

The newer trends in risk management take a different view of risk. The intelligent risk manager knows that his or her job is proactive, not reactive. The circle of policy formation should include input from risk management on a regular basis. Risk managers are now analyzing the actual causes of adverse outcomes and employing system thinking to help solve the problem.

Before risk can be approached in any meaningful way, several concepts must be internalized. The number one plank in the platform of risk management is that good things happen only when they are planned and bad things can happen all by themselves. Institutions have spent too much time providing the latest bit of equipment and not enough time actually analyzing the physical journey of the patient through the maze found in the usual healthcare institution of the 1990s. Studying this sojourn through the medical system from the patient's perspective is key to understanding where things go wrong.

The second major principle of risk management is taken from the quality assurance literature: that is, to emphasize the fact that 85% of the problems are system based and not based on the incompetent or malevolent actions of workers themselves. Few healthcare workers want anything for the patient but the patient's rapid return to health. But our systems fail to properly inform us of outcomes. Precious little time is spent in coordinating the activities of the various departments through which a patient must pass. Miscommunications between the emergency department and radiology, poor follow-up by on-call physicians, failure to properly relay information between the nurses and physicians—these are the types of system failures that frequently characterize risk management disasters in the healthcare system of the 1990s.

The reasons for such system failures are multiple. Through superspecialization, seemingly every technical aspect of healthcare is performed by a different individual. Such individuals frequently perform their task well but out of context to the overall needs of the patient. The headlong race for technologic superiority and efficiency frequently leave the only person who matters—the patient—in a bewildering haze. Everyone feels that it is someone else's job to oversee, coordinate, and justify his or her role as the patient is pushed along through the healthcare system. The lack of any type of coordinated U.S. primary care policy continues to increase the chances that patients will never have any type of in-depth discussion of why certain healthcare procedures are being performed or what their role is in ensuring that they have received maximum benefit from the system.

Relating the issues of start-to-finish planning of each aspect of a healthcare encounter along with system recognition allows for a conceptual model to analyze both the system's successes and failures. Too much time is spent looking for the "bad apple" employee related to a specific poor outcome. Where time really needs to be spent is in analyzing our successes, our good outcomes, to see what we did right and then duplicating such good behavior. The final reason why the risk management department should exist is to serve as the early-warning radar system for the hospital's policies, procedures, and actual outcomes. Risk management should be picking out those problem areas where the system has not yet succeeded in securing a seamless thread of integrated medical care. It should be considered risk management's duty to bring such problems to the attention of the highest levels of the institution. The intelligent and humane provision of healthcare as viewed by our patients is our only reason for our existence. If U.S. healthcare, which is now the largest and most expensive industry in the world, cannot provide such humane and integrated care, its reason for existence is in doubt. The only way we can know that we are indeed providing such care is through the feedback loop provided by risk management.

A valid test of an institution's commitment to improving its system is the resource base that is allocated to the project. It takes both time and effort to study our systems and improve them. It takes a serious intellectual and financial commitment for a healthcare provider to come to the reality that almost all systems can and should be both monitored and continuously improved. Last, it takes the human touch. It is a willingness to not merely study averages and percentages, but to look at each and every human being who enters the system as our final test and to recognize the outcome, no matter how great or small the problem, as a reflection on the level at which we have performed our functions. The concept of zero defects, which has become the watchword in all manufacturing industries, must now become the credo of healthcare institutions. We must move to the point where unhappiness on the part of the patient with regard to our service should be considered unacceptable.

Understanding the variability in all human systems, each healthcare worker must be trained to handle on-line complaints about the system. Often, the most satisfied patients are those who have had some type of minor problem in the system that, once brought to the attention of the healthcare personnel, has been properly and satisfactorily resolved.

No one method or system avoids risk in all emergency departments. But the principal elements of a risk management format can be summarized in the following manner:

1. Patients come to healthcare institutions anxious, afraid, and in a somewhat diminished capacity to understand what is happening to them. It should be expected that healthcare workers will "go the extra mile" in understanding and in providing explanations to reassure the patients.
2. Every healthcare worker is a risk manager. He or she manages the risk by doing what is necessary to see that the patient's needs are met.
3. When it is apparent that a patient's needs have not been met, any member of the healthcare team has not only the right but the obligation to bring such concerns to the manager in charge of that area to let the manager know that there is a potential risk situation requiring intervention.
4. Continuous communication with the patient, no matter what the outcome or the circumstances, is the best way to show concern on the part of the healthcare team. Whenever conflict is identified, rapid action on the part of both the healthcare worker and the institution to correct the situation is always in the best interests of the patient and the healthcare providers.
5. Whenever conflicts between the patient and the healthcare providers cannot be resolved on line, what is needed to prevent future such episodes is a structured, organized system that will not only respond to the particular patient's problem but will analyze the system reasons for that problem.

HIGH-RISK BEHAVIORS AND ISSUES

Although any interaction between a patient and the healthcare system may result in litigation, it is clear that certain situations lend themselves to system failures. In 3% to 5% of malpractice cases, there is no easily definable pattern. There is an outcome that could not be predicted or mitigated against before the fact. Disease is infinitely variable, and there will be those cases that in the best of hands will have a poor outcome. However, in approximately 95% of cases, the failure in either medical decision making or system logic is evident. Such cases can be and should have been avoided by proper communications and actions in advance. Such system failures are common to most emergency departments and constitute the vast majority of risk situations.

Change of Shift

The troublesome time period when one physician is coming on shift and another is going off is often regarded by experienced observers as an extremely dangerous time for both the healthcare providers and the patient. A casual passing of the baton from one physician or group of nurses to the next can allow the patient to "fall between the cracks." The oncoming physician often feels confident that the patient has been properly worked up, and the patient is frequently given a diagnosis before the oncoming physician's assumption of the case. The patient is frequently not properly reevaluated before a decision is made. Change of shift should be viewed as starting anew, and such times should not result in a lower standard of care for the patient. If, for any reason, a physician cannot properly complete the workup of a patient and such responsibility must be transferred to another physician, a proper and orderly transfer of responsibility and liability must take place. It is important that the physician leaving shift notes the patient's condition at the time of leaving and the fact that the responsibility has be transferred to a specific physician. Similarly, the physician coming on must write his or her own note discussing the condition of the patient and the program that will be followed. The physician discharging the patient should be considered the physician of record and should be considered the physician responsible for the discharge program.

Nursing has, within its role, the same responsibilities as physicians. Nurses who are going off shift or are leaving for break should ensure that the patient's care has been properly transferred to another nurse who will ensure that the observation program and any treatments or studies will be completed. The litigation history of emergency medicine is littered with the stories of patients forgotten in rooms, lost in radiology, or left in the waiting room because of an inadequate transfer of responsibilities. The transfer of responsibility at the change of shift should be a formal and orderly process among not only healthcare personnel but the patient as well. The patient and family should never have any doubt as to who is in charge of the patient's care and who will direct further therapy and plan the discharge program.

Return Visits and Transfers

Patients who return to the emergency department with unscheduled visits, instead of being viewed as potential risk situations, are often treated as medical criminals. Interrogation by medical and clerical staff often sounds more like a police roundup than a medical reevaluation. There is a tendency on the part of healthcare personnel to view such return patients as "doctor shopping" or having some underlying psychologic problem, when in fact nothing could be farther from the truth. Careful studies have been done looking at return visits, and it is clear that at least 75% of the time the patients were poorly instructed, the disease process has taken an unexpected turn, or the initial diagnosis was wrong. This, combined with the fact that getting into the healthcare "nonsystem," which is often through private physicians' offices, can be extremely difficult for many patients. Such inability to access the regular healthcare system should be viewed as a legitimate reason for returning to the emergency department.

Transfers from other institutions have in common with second visits the one thing that gives a false sense of security to the healthcare team and can represent a true impediment to rapid resolution of their problems. Such patients already have a diagnosis. Once a diagnosis is made in medicine, frequently all intelligent thought stops. There is a tendency on the part of healthcare personnel to assume that the original diagnosis for which the patient was seen on the first visits or the original problems identified at the first hospital before transfer are correct. But experienced emergency personnel realize that transfers from another institution must be viewed as totally new patients. It is the conservative course of action for the emergency physician to work up transferred and second-visit patients as if they were new. It is perfectly proper for a physician to refer to previous histories and physical examinations performed and to be aware of previous diagnoses. It is important for the physician to realize that an independent history and physical at that moment in time should form the basis of a current clinical impression.

A rule that more and more emergency physicians are beginning to follow is that when a patient appears for the third time, admission should be strongly considered. It is always troublesome when a patient comes repeatedly to an emergency department. Such patients may have an ongoing medical problem that may not be clear. The fact that the patient has come to the emergency department three times should indicate that somewhere along the line either the patient's true diagnosis has not been recognized or the patient does not understand the nature of the illness and the course of the disease. In any event, such multiple interactions without progress toward a successful resolution should make the concerned healthcare professional anxious to properly resolve the problem.

Private Patients in the Emergency Department

An important concept in both philosophy and law is that regarding patient ownership. It must be understood by all that doctors do not "own" patients. The opposite is true: patients own doctors. The doctor, and indeed the entire healthcare team, is the retained agent and servant of the patient. Patients can change healthcare institutions and physicians anytime they so choose. Whenever patients come to the emergency department, they become, by the very act of their appearing, patients of the emergency physician for at least that visit. The emergency physician has more than a duty; he or she has an absolute obligation to be aware of any and all patients who are in the department and their status at any time. The emergency nursing personnel have a similar duty to evaluate patients expeditiously and to keep the emergency physician informed of patients who are waiting to be seen, particularly those whose situations may be critical. The COBRA law clearly states that each patient must be evaluated to see if an emergency exists. There is no exemption in the law that says patients do not have to be seen if they have "their own doctor" coming to see them.

The usual sticking point in all of these problems is who gets to charge for services. This should be the least important aspect in analyzing such cases. The hospital must go on record—and this must be conveyed to the medical staff at all levels—that patients entering the emergency department will be evaluated, and, if necessary, intervention will take place before the arrival of private physicians. The private attending physician has no right to place in jeopardy the healthcare institution and the emergency department personnel and the patient because of ego issues.

Private patients in the emergency department should be viewed as any other patients. They should be properly triaged and examined, and therapy should be started if they are in an urgent or emergent condition. There is no problem with properly transferring care to a private physician when he or she arrives.

It should be the policy of the emergency department and the institution that patients waiting in the department for their personal physician will be evaluated to determine whether an emergency condition exists. Should the hospital, for the sake of convenience or political purposes, wish to provide an area where private attending physicians may meet their patients for nonemergent conditions, such an area should be provided. It should be away from the emergency department and should not be governed or included in those areas covered by the federal COBRA statutes.

On-Call Physicians

The Joint Commission on Accreditation of Healthcare Organizations (JCAHO) has classified emergency departments into four levels of care. Hospitals functioning at levels I and II are required to have on-call lists for physician specialists. Hospitals are essentially required to enter patients, for at least their immediate problem, into the healthcare system. The hospital and, by extension, the medical staff have a direct duty and obligation to care for emergent patients who have come to the emergency department. A physician who appears on the on-call panel in a hospital emergency department plays an essential role in the functioning of the healthcare system. When such physicians do not respond to calls to the emergency department or refuse to carry out follow-up care on patients seen in the emergency department, and the hospital and the emergency physician are forced to send the patient to another institution, potential violations of COBRA abound. The issue of transferring and economic screening of patients is one of which the federal government is well aware. The

COBRA laws are an attempt to channel hospital and medical staff energies in the direction that would provide greatest protection for the patients and yet leave the private practice of medicine intact. As physicians fail to live up to their obligations with regard to the on-call process, it should come as no great surprise to them that the federal government will move to mandate such care. If such systems cannot be organized in a cooperative venture between the hospital and the administration, there is no question that further federal action will move to secure such benefits for the citizens of the United States.

Several key points of the on-call panel must be emphasized. First, the on-call list is the responsibility of the hospital, not the emergency department. It is incumbent on hospital administrations to secure the services of physicians and to ensure proper entry of patients into the healthcare system. Second, care delayed is care denied. When on-call physicians are not available within a reasonable period of time and patients suffer harm secondary to such lack of care, the institution and the system are equally culpable. Third, the practice of having consultant physicians screen potential patients by inquiring about their financial status or ability to pay should be considered not only ethically immoral but legally prohibited under the federal COBRA and OBRA laws. Last, continuity of care and outpatient follow-up of emergency patients are paramount issues. Healthcare facility on-call panels must serve not only to come to the hospital to see patients, but should accept patients for outpatient management of care for at least the acute illness for which they are referred.

Against Medical Advice

Patients who refuse to follow carefully considered medical advice should be considered high risk. Such patients have essentially announced that they do not respect or trust the professional judgments of the emergency personnel involved. Such actions on the part of the patient frequently provoke less than empathetic responses from the medical staff, who take such patient responses as insults. Against medical advice situations call into play two divergently opposed concepts in law: the concept of a patient's freedom versus the healthcare worker's duty to protect.

The patient's rights to self-determination are unquestioned. A patient of adult years and sound mind has the right to refuse any medical care offered. This virtually always runs counter to the entire question of communication and informed decision making. The patient can always claim that he or she did not understand what was being presented by the healthcare personnel and therefore was prevented from making a proper decision. It is therefore essential that the charting on such cases recognize the major pitfalls in advance. First, a patient or the family may claim that the refusal was uninformed because of diminished mental capacity. The first duty of the emergency staff is to properly document the mental capacity of the patient to make the decision to refuse care. A patient who is encephalopathic clearly lacks capacity; therefore the substitute judgment of the healthcare professionals involved or family members may be appropriate. If, however, the patient is awake and alert, can carry on reasonable conversation and discuss the problems at hand, and has the mental ability to act in his or her own self-interest, the test for competency to exercise judgments on the patient's own behalf is usually met.

Second, in informed refusal cases, it is often claimed that the hospital personnel did not inform the patient in a manner that they could understand. It is important to inform and document that the patient was told in no uncertain terms of the desire of the healthcare professionals and the fact that such discussion was held in terms that the patient could easily understand. Euphemisms should not be used. If the medical staff is afraid of sudden death, the term *death* should be used. If they are afraid that injury to a limb might result in amputation, use of terms that clearly indicate that the limb may need to be removed should be used and recorded on the chart.

A third question in refusal of care revolves around alternative forms of treatment. Patients must be properly informed if there are alternative modes of treatment that would solve the problem, and they should be given opportunities to use such modes of therapy. When acceptable alternatives are not available, this should also be documented.

Fourth, involvement of family is crucial. Should the patient die as a result of noncooperation with the healthcare system, it is the patient's relatives who will bring action against the medical professionals involved. Family or friends who are with the patient must be aware of the patient's refusal. The hard-driving executive who may wish to deny his own chest pain is usually brought into more realistic thinking when he must deny care in front of his wife and children. Should the patient expressly forbid the medical staff from speaking to family or friend, such forbiddance must also be carefully documented. It is perfectly reasonable to inform the family that you have been denied the option to speak to them by the patient. This allows the family to understand that the patient, not the physician, is refusing to discuss the problems.

Last, and least important, is the patient's signature. The signature line on the chart is no replacement for a properly documented record. Many times patients who leave against medical advice do so in a hostile atmosphere and refuse to sign. The fact that the patient refused to sign should also be noted. The myth has long been advanced that as long as a signature is present the patient has waived his or her rights and has relieved the healthcare personnel of legal responsibility. This is not the case. Documentation of against medical advice requires the previously listed four parts of the process. A signature is not a substitute for a legal process, and the signature and the legal process must be accompanied by proper documentation if such situations are to be adjudicated in favor of the healthcare team.

The attitude with which a physician approaches a patient in an against medical advice mode is critical to success. A "take it or leave it" attitude combined with a "my way or the highway" ultimatum frequently makes for noncompliance on the part of the patient. Such situations should not be confrontational.

Left Before Examination

The patient who leaves before examination (LBE) or leaves without being seen (LWBS) constitutes a much different medicolegal problem than the patient who leaves against medical advice. Patients who leave against medical advice virtually always represent a doctor-patient communication problem. In the LBE situation, the doctor was not even given the opportunity to form a doctor-patient bond. Large numbers of LBE patients are system problems and usually represent prolonged waiting time. Analysis of lawsuits regarding emergency medicine find that suit rates go up almost exponentially after a patient has been waiting more than 2 hours. Hostility grows, and hostility is the basis of miscommunication and lawsuits. Substantial or rising LBEs should prompt a systems review to determine exactly why the patient flow is less than adequate. Long waits for labs and x-rays, difficulty in freeing beds because of inadequate or poor admissions procedures, or delays in obtaining needed consultations should all be reviewed to determine why patient flow is inadequate to meet the patient demands.

In-House Emergencies

The emergency physician in smaller institutions is occasionally involved with patients who are doing poorly on the medical and surgical floors. These in-house emergencies vary from cardiopulmonary arrest situations to assessing patients who have fallen out of bed to pronouncing patients dead. All such situations, however, have the potential for liability problems. Whenever the emergency physician is called out of the emergency department, he or she is no longer able to provide immediate care to those who may came through the doors. To the child with an airway obstruction, to the patient in cardiac arrest, to the patient with a tension pneumothorax, the absence of the emergency physician may spell disaster. Therefore leaving the emergency department should be an infrequent event and one that is prompted by true medical necessity. It is wise for the emergency physician to not guarantee in any contract to answer in-house emergencies. The physician is by such action guaranteeing to be two places at once. It is advisable for the emergency physician to agree to respond to in-house emergencies as would any other physician in the hospital when hearing the stat call for a physician. Part of the test of a Good Samaritan action is that it is performed outside the usual practice setting of the physician and that the physician has no established duty to provide such services. A contractual link might obviate a physician's eventual Good Samaritan defense. It is also wise for the emergency physician not to be paid per patient for responding in such events. Direct payment for medical services on a prearranged basis may also obviate a Good Samaritan defense.

It is not the role of emergency physicians to solve all problems of the hospital merely because they are available 24 hours per day. Should a patient become ill on the floor, hospital rules and regulations should clearly delineate the responsibility for the primary attending physician to evaluate his or her patient. If indeed the primary physician cannot attend the patient for some reason, such patients can be brought to the emergency department, where the emergency physician has proper facilities and equipment and is not forced to leave the site of primary obligation.

House Staff in the Emergency Department

House staff in the emergency department are often treated under two erroneous concepts: (1) young doctors learn from their mistakes; and (2) if young doctors are not ready now to see patients on their own, how can they be "graduated" from the program? The premise of learning by mistakes is unsound educationally and morally. I know of no one who wants pilots to learn by their mistakes as they land their 747 without supervision. Educational theory would dictate that the only thing learned from mistakes is how to make mistakes. The great advantage of emergency medicine is that each patient can be supervised in an on-line, real time manner by an attending physician who can help the resident work through the decision process and intervene when the situation requires. No hospitals give a "training discount" reduction to patients because they have been seen by a resident in an unsupervised manner. The resident is a physician in training. Overall responsibility for every patient in the emergency department is borne by the attending physician. It is a cowardly act for an attending physician to blame the outcome of a case on the resident that he or she is supervising. Residents should be concurrently monitored and actively supervised while in the department.

A resident rotating through the emergency department from a specialty other than emergency medicine should be supervised in the same manner as an emergency medicine resident and should be considered to be less familiar with emergency department policies and procedures. Retrospective review of charts, although useful as a teaching tool, is no substitute for on-line, hands-on evaluation of patients and the care being given by residents. Billing for residents' services that are not directly supervised by the physician doing the billing should be considered an extremely high-risk activity. The attestation statements signed by physicians who sign up with various insurance companies generally state that they will charge for only those services that they personally render or supervise. Supervision from a distance is considered no supervision at all. The federal government and many states actively pursue physicians under a doctrine of fraud when they have rendered bills for services in which they have not been directly involved.

Residents frequently feel that because their malpractice coverage is paid for by the institution and they are covered under a doctrine of *respondeat superior,* they are immune from the ravages of lawsuits. This misapprehension should be corrected in all house staff in that they may be sued individually, may be forced to participate in any trial situation that arises, and are not exempt from being reported to the National Practitioner Databank.

An extremely touchy and often volatile situation involves off-service residents who are called down from the floors to evaluate patients in the emergency department. These physicians are still residents and are responsible to the physician in charge. It is often said by attending physicians on medicine and surgery services that their residents can function without reference to the emergency physicians and that they are essentially functioning "as their agents." Such physicians are rarely willing, however, to sign statements that they will assume all responsibility, pay all costs, and have all reported losses against their name in the databank. The emergency physician bears the liability of all patients in the department until they have been properly transferred to another attending physician. The resident, no matter how advanced or from what service, cannot relieve the emergency physician from his or her responsibility to act in the best interests of the patient. Disputes on how a patient should be handled should not be conducted between the emergency physician and the off-service resident, but between the emergency physician and the physician in charge of that resident. All dispute resolutions should be between parties of equal power who will bear equal responsibility. The resident should be considered a nonentity in such discussions.

Telephone Orders from Private Physicians

Outside physicians frequently do not appreciate the extent of liability that the hospital and emergency physicians may incur when a patient is treated without being examined by the emergency physician. Physicians may see patients in their office and wish them to have a medication or treatment that is not conveniently available in their outpatient setting. As a result, such patients are frequently sent to emergency departments, and telephone orders are given to emergency personnel. This practice should be discouraged and eliminated whenever possible. There is no section of the hospital as tightly regulated by federal law as the emergency department. There is no exemption in the COBRA or OBRA statutes for patients being sent from outside physicians' offices. Although this practice is common, it is anachronistic and dangerous. Federal law requires that every patient who enters the emergency department receive a medical examination. Nowhere does it indicate that patients may be seen without such an evaluation. Should the hospital wish to run an outpatient clinic for the convenience of its own physicians, such a clinic should be set up separately from the emergency department, and strict criteria should be laid out as to what can and cannot be done without concomitant physician evaluation.

Similar situations exist with regard to requests for medical staff, particularly screeners and gatekeepers from health maintenance organizations (HMOs), for the emergency physician to just take a "quick look" at a patient. Medicolegally, there is no such thing. When the emergency physician has agreed to see anyone to determine whether an emergency exists, a doctor-patient relationship is established. Such a visit must be memorialized with correct charts and records. Again, there is no exemption in the OBRA or COBRA statutes that says that if a patient is being looked at for an HMO or a preferred provider organization (PPO) the usual duties incumbent on the emergency physician are waived.

Telephone Advice

Many healthcare personnel are not aware that a doctor-patient relationship can be established with the telephone. It is not necessary that a patient physically enter the emergency department for such a relationship to exist. As soon as the patient requests medical advice and the healthcare professional is willing to give that advice, a doctor-patient relationship is established. The rule for the emergency department should be, *We do not give telephone advice*. Numerous studies have documented the poor quality of telephone advice, and common sense would dictate that with a patient not present, the most important clues to correct diagnosis and treatment are gone. It is both acceptable and advised that in a polite and caring manner patients are told that the emergency department is open 24 hours per day and will properly evaluate them for an illness. No patient asks a casual question. People seek advice from emergency departments hoping to do something with that information. It is always better to actually have seen the patient before entering into such discussions.

In no circumstance should advice be given that does not directly state that the patient must be seen and evaluated before any type of medical diagnosis or specific treatment can be given. Telephone advice reiterates the adage that you get exactly what you pay for.

PRACTICAL TIPS ON MANAGING EMERGENCY MEDICINE RISK

Having dealt with some of the larger philosophic issues involved with emergency medicine risk management, it is worthwhile to turn to a more micro level and recognize that risk is either created or avoided one patient at a time. It is an intensely personal decision on the part of each patient and the patient's family to bring action against a healthcare professional and a healthcare organization. The simple fact that "they like you" can mean the difference between a lawsuit and a patient who is still your friend despite the outcome. Emergency medicine is, by its very nature, in the bad outcome business. We tend to see people not at their best, but at their worst. Emergency departments are the place where families receive the news of their child's death, a family member's permanent paralysis, or other incurable lifetime disabilities. No patient in the emergency department is truly prepared for the news that we are to bring, and the old concept of slaying the messenger is still alive and well.

In this, the last half of the twentieth century, the maxim is that no one is truly responsible for anything. Should any evil befall a person or a family, someone must be to blame, and someone must pay. These factors, along with the general impersonalization and technologic isolation of modern medicine, have made it an ideal target for all failings. The corridors of the great healthcare institutions—like our schools, our prisons, and our gigantic workplaces—have become sterile and devoid of perceptible caring. Healthcare is never delivered in the aggregate; it is delivered one patient at a time. The degree to which the physician and healthcare team can individualize and personalize healthcare will determine its ability to prophylactically manage risk. Showing the patient and the family that the healthcare providers are truly the advocates of the patient's well-being will go further than anything else to prevent the hostility and disappointment that frequently are dissipated through legal channels.

It is often said that perception is the only reality. The patient's perception of the care he or she received is influenced by each aspect of the surroundings. The healthcare institution that wishes to reduce risk should begin by sampling the product. Physical access into the system—parking, moving sick patients into the emergency department, and general surroundings—should all be user-friendly. It should be considered the height of embarrassment for a family member to be struggling to get a sick patient out of a vehicle and hospital personnel not available to lend a hand. Such an introductory attitude sets the tone for a relationship that is adversarial as opposed to therapeutic. Hospital emergency departments that have all the charm and aroma of a 1950s bus depot also convey an atmosphere of institutional mediocrity.

It is well documented that patients are strongly influenced by how the health professionals appear. Clean uniforms with proper name tags and other markers of identification are essential. The usual rules of human interaction and polite social discourse often seem to be suspended in emergency departments. Physicians no longer shake hands with their patients and identify themselves. Some physicians treat other family members who are present as invisible instead of recognizing their presence and understanding their role in the system. It is the wise physician who makes friends with the patient and the family.

The patient's first impression of the healthcare provider is formed much like the impression of the institution itself. Patients of all socioeconomic ranks have an amazingly similar view of how physicians and nurses should be dressed. This so-called doctor camouflage is an important element in setting the tone for the doctor-patient interaction. Patients are willing to expose the most intimate details of their lives not because of who we are personally but because we represent a profession with a code of ethics and an oath of devotion to the patient's problems. It is mandatory that the patient believe in the provider. Any hint that information obtained would be used for purposes other than the advancement of the patient would certainly shut down all communications.

The two most prevalent complaints of patients who have been to an emergency department are that they waited too long and that the doctor never "told them anything." Both of these factors lead to frustration, which creates an atmosphere in which hostility can exist. It is perfectly appropriate for a physician and other members of the healthcare team to apologize to a patient for any delay in being seen. Most healthcare professionals would like to see every patient immediately. It is this recognition that no one wants to wait and the recognition that the patient's time is just as valuable as the physician's that tends to reduce hostility. It is the recognition of the situation more than any specific corrective action that is important in changing patient perception.

With regard to the second major complaint—"the physician never told me anything"—the corrective actions are obvious. The moment of discharge for a patient is indeed the moment of truth for the entire healthcare system. It is incumbent on the emergency physician and other healthcare personnel to make certain that the patient understands the discharge instructions and the diagnosis. Any other problems or situations should be sought at that time. Practical matters, such as where the patient is to go, what the patient is to eat, where the patient can obtain medication, and whether the patient needs a note for work, are the real-life nuts and bolts issues with which the patient must deal when being discharged from the emergency department. It is inadequate for the emergency physician to believe that patients innately understand how they are to function outside the walls of the institution. Directly asking patients and their families how these everyday matters will be taken care of not only shows human concern, but on a practical level allows the physician to analyze the therapeutic milieu that the patient must enter. Last, it is important for the physician to ask the patient if there are any other specific issues requiring assistance. All patients enter an emergency department with a specific program in mind. They have specific ideas of what will or will not be accomplished and set notions of desired outcomes. It is impossible to serve the wants and needs of the patient without specifically asking what he or she would like. There is no better risk management strategy than at the time of discharge to make sure that the patient and the family are comfortable with the diagnosis and the healthcare program advocated and have the ability to carry out such a program in their daily lives.

It is estimated that one half the lawsuits in emergency medicine are related in some way to either the discharge program or the inability to enter the patient into a coordinated healthcare system. Virtually all cases of meningitis, missed fractures, abdominal pain, and wounds have to do with how patients are instructed and how they view their own role in the follow-up care.

The principal weapon that any physician has in the risk management wars is attitude. The physician who is secure and happy in his or her work tends to convey that attitude to the patients and the staff. Attitude, like anything of importance, begins at the top. Nurses and ancillary healthcare personnel, as well as clerical personnel, often pick up the tone in the behavior from the physician on duty. Physicians who go out of their way to be kind to the staff and the patients often find such attitudes infectious. This attitude should be expressed not only to patients but to all members of the healthcare team. The attitude of the professional should be one that extends toward the entire patient. Merely going through technical hoops and making certain that the process has taken place is no substitute for outcome, and the physician who can judge outcomes separate from process will be well equipped to manage risk.

61 Interhospital Transfers: THE EMTALA PROVISIONS OF COBRA AS AMENDED BY OBRA 89 AND OBRA 90

Kenneth L. DeHart

OUTLINE

Few circumstances prove to be as difficult as those requiring the safe transfer of patients from one health facility to another. Nevertheless incidents inevitably occur in the daily practice of emergency medicine in which the benefits of interhospital transfer outweigh the risks to the patient. In this chapter, information will be provided regarding the application of the Emergency Medical Treatment and Active Labor Act in the daily practice of emergency medicine. In addition, the implications of the Interim Final Rules, published by the Health Care Financing Administration, June 22, 1994, will be addressed.

EMERGENCY MEDICAL TREATMENT AND ACTIVE LABOR ACT OF 1986

The Emergency Medical Treatment and Active Labor Act of 1986 (EMTALA) was incorporated into the Consolidated Omnibus Budget Reconciliation Act (COBRA) passed by the United States Congress in April of 1986 as Public Law 99-272. The relevant components addressing the interhospital transfer of patients appear under "Miscellaneous Provisions," Section 9121 of this legislation. In addition, the United States Congress further amended components of EMTALA in the Omnibus Budget Reconciliation Act of 1989 and 1990, 42U.S.C. 1395DD:1395cc(a)1(I). The provisions of EMTALA require that a hospital must provide a screening examination, a stabilization process, and an appropriate patient transfer process. The provisions of EMTALA apply to hospitals that historically receive Medicare funds and are applicable to all patients, including U.S. citizens, noncitizens, and illegal aliens that arrive at a hospital seeking care. The provisions do not apply to hospitals without an emergency service, facilities that are not deemed to be hospitals, free-standing emergency facilities that are not owned or formally affiliated with a hospital, physicians' offices, or health maintenance organizations. In addition, it does not apply to hospitals that do not receive Medicare funding such as those of the U.S. Veterans Association.

Provisions of EMTALA

There are three principle components of EMTALA addressing the patient screening, stabilization, and transfer processes. Each of these activities incorporates common terminology, but specific legal definitions have been applied to them in the legislation. In the paragraphs that follow, all references to EMTALA will incorporate the most recent components of the legislation to include COBRA 1986, OBRA 1989, and OBRA 1990 and the Final Interim Regulations of 1986 and 1994.

Patient Screening Requirements

Every hospital with an emergency department is required by EMTALA to provide a medical screening examination within the capability of the hospital's emergency department, including ancillary services routinely available to the department for all individuals requesting medical examination or treatment. The purpose of the medical screening examination is to determine if an emergency medical condition or active labor exists to include psychiatric disturbances, symptoms of substance abuse, and situations with respect to pregnant women having contractions.

The definition of an emergency medical condition, in EMTALA, is "a medical condition manifesting itself by acute symptoms of sufficient variety (including severe pain) such that the absence of immediate medical attention could reasonably be expected to result in:

1. Placing the health of the individual (or, with respect to pregnant women, the health of her unborn child) in serious jeopardy;
2. Serious impairment to bodily functions or;
3. Serious disfunction of any bodily organ or part" [Section (e)(1)(A)].

It should be noted for the purposes of EMTALA that the Health Care Financing Administration, in its published Interim Final Rules of 1994, defined labor as "a process of child birth beginning with a latent or early phase of labor and continuing through the delivery of the placenta." Therefore all women experiencing contractions should be considered in true labor until a physician or appropriate designee certifies that after a reasonable period of time of observation and examination, the individual is experiencing false labor.

The law and the subsequent regulations do not define in greater detail any other parameters of a medical screening examination. It should be sufficiently detailed, however, to address medically indicated diagnostic tests and mental status evaluations. For obstetric patients, the screening process should include the evaluation of fetal heart tones, the regularity and duration of uterine contractions, and the status of fetal position, station, and cervical dilation. For individuals suffering from substance abuse or psychiatric illness, the medical screening examination should include documentation regarding relative suicide risk and threats to self or society.

The 1994 Interim Final Regulations do not require a physician to perform a medical screening examination. They do require, however, that the hospital specify in its bylaws, rules, or policies what type of healthcare provider constitutes a "qualified medical person" for the purpose of providing an appropriate medical screening examination. It is incumbent on the institution to comply with its own methodology. In the event that a physician is not physically present in the emergency department 24 hours a day, the screening examination should be performed by trained ancillary personnel according to written policies, procedures, and algorithms that are consistent with state medical practice and nursing practice acts. It is imperative, however, that providers recognize that although the hospital may determine under what circumstances a physician is required to perform an appropriate medical screening examination, the Health and Human Services Secretary may, in accordance with the 1994 Final Interim Rules, not necessarily accept the hospital's determination of what circumstances require that a screening examination be performed by a physician. The Health Care Financing Administration reserves the right to determine, retrospectively, in certain circumstances that an individual did not receive an appropriate medical screening examination because the condition of the individual required the expertise of a physician to determine whether an emergency medical condition existed at the time of presentation. It should therefore be concluded that it is the position of the Health Care Financing Administration that one cannot assume, unequivocally, that an examination by a nurse or other nonphysician medical personnel will be deemed appropriate in all circumstances.

Clearly, the medical screening examination process is required on all patients who arrive at the hospital. The 1994 federal regulations clearly indicate that the law applies to all individuals who attempt to gain access to hospital property for emergency care. An individual may not be denied services simply because the individual failed to enter the facility's emergency department. Furthermore, "hospital property" is interpreted to include the ambulances owned and operated by the hospital, even if the ambulances are not on hospital grounds at the time of the patient encounter. It is therefore incumbent on hospital-owned ambulance services to recognize the Interim Final Rules published by the federal government in 1994, which necessitates the application of EMTALA considerations to all patients once they have entered the ambulance.

The screening provisions of EMTALA also apply to all patients regardless of payor status. This applies to patients participating in managed care organizations seeking preauthorization for care. Providers should deem this process as "authorization for payment" but must not confuse it with the legal requirements in providing the screening examination process regardless of the patient's payor status. No preexisting health maintenance organization or managed care agreement, protocol, or contract can circumvent the legal requirements of a hospital in providing a screening examination to all patients who arrive at or on hospital property.

Stabilization Requirements

EMTALA requires, in individuals who are suffering from an emergency medical condition, a medical stabilization process to occur. The term *to stabilize* means "with respect to an emergency medical condition to provide such medical treatment of the condition as may be necessary to assure, within medical probability, that no material deterioration of the condition is likely to result from or during the transfer" [Section e(3)]. In the case of a pregnant woman who is having contractions the term *to stabilize* is interpreted to mean the delivery of the child, including the placenta. In individuals suffering from an emergency medical condition, the stabilization process should include documentation of competent and traditional healthcare to include but not be limited to the following:

1. Establishing and securing an adequate airway and optimal ventilation.
2. Initiating control and management of hemorrhage.
3. Stabilizing and splinting any fractured extremities.
4. Maintaining adequate access routes for fluid or drug administration.
5. Maintaining and intervening when indicated by abnormalities of the patient's vital signs.
6. In cases of active labor, delivery of the infant and placenta.

It is important to note that the stabilization process should use the appropriate ancillary services routinely available to the emergency department. Therefore if computed tomography scans of the abdomen are a diagnostic modality typically available to the emergency department, when medically indicated, this and other similar resources should be available and incorporated into the stabilization process.

TRANSFER PROCESS

The term *transfer* means "the movement including the discharge of an individual outside the hospital facility at the direction of any person employed or affiliated directly or indirectly with the hospital."* It is important to recognize the specificity of the language of the definition of the transfer process to include the routine discharge of any patient from the hospital.

EMTALA specifies that patients who have not been stabilized may not be transferred or discharged unless one of the two following conditions exists:

1. The patient or legal guardian, acting on behalf of the patient, requests after informed consent a transfer or discharge in writing after the hospital has educated the patient of its obligations.
2. A physician, after providing an appropriate screening and stabilization process, signs a certification of transfer stating that, based on the information available at the time of

*From Frew SA: *Am Coll Emerg Med* 1991.

the transfer, the medical benefits of the transfer outweigh the risks.

It should be pointed out that individuals who are deemed to not have an emergency medical condition, or who have been stabilized, may be transferred or discharged at any time.

In those individuals in whom a transfer decision is made, EMTALA and federal regulations have addressed three important considerations in the process. These relate to the accompanying medical records and certification of the transportation process itself [Section 489.24(d)(2)(iii)].

EMTALA clearly states that hospitals transferring patients must provide the receiving facility with all medical records or copies of them related to the individual's emergency condition at the time of transfer, including available records related to the individual's emergency medical condition, observations of signs or symptoms, preliminary diagnoses, and results of diagnostic studies. In addition, other records to include test results not available at the time of transfer must be sent as soon as practical.

In those instances in which an on-call physician has refused or failed to appear within a "reasonable period of time" for backup physician availability to provide the necessary stabilization treatment, the name and address of that physician must also accompany the patient at the time of transfer. EMTALA does not legally require providers to report EMTALA violations. It does, however, provide physicians with a "whistle-blower" provision that allows physicians to be protected from civil penalties for transferring patients because of the unavailability of on-call subspecialty care.

EMTALA and the subsequent regulations do not clearly define "a reasonable period of time" for the purpose of enforcement of this legislation. It should be concluded, however, that any institutional bylaws or staff regulations regarding the timeliness of response will be an initial reference consideration. It is therefore incumbent on providers to be compliant with the hospital's own bylaws regarding the timeliness of their response. Given these provisions, prudent healthcare providers should consider developing preprinted forms such as certificate of transfer documents on which informed consent can be documented. In instances of unstabilized patients the benefits, as compared with the risks, should be identified. In addition, a pretransfer checklist identifying all data, such as history and physical examination documents and laboratory and radiology results, should be delineated so that the transferring hospital can document the completeness of the medical record information transferred with the patient.

EMTALA addresses the transfer methodology to be used in interhospital transfers and requires that a transfer be effected by "qualified personnel and appropriate transportation equipment" as required, including the use of necessary medically indicated life support measures during the transfer. The 1994 final rules do not unequivocally state that emergency medical technicians are "qualified" personnel for these purposes. It should be concluded therefore that, depending on the individual's condition, there may be situations in which a physician's presence or some other specialist's may be mandatory for EMTALA compliance. Clearly, individuals requiring advanced life support interventions should not be transported by basic life support services. Similarly, there may be instances in which the presence of nurses or physicians will be indicated to comply with the "qualified personnel" of EMTALA provisions.

Receiving Hospital Issues

In addition to being compliant with the aforementioned provisions, EMTALA requires that a receiving hospital have available space and qualified personnel for the treatment of the patient and that appropriate hospital representatives have agreed to accept the patient in transfer. It is therefore important for all prudent practitioners to identify not only the agreement of the receiving hospital to care for the patient, but also to identify the individual contacted and a recognition of their willingness to accept the patient.

In addition, EMTALA also addresses specialized services provided by receiving hospitals. Hospitals with specialized capabilities, such as burn units and neonatal intensive care units, may not refuse to accept an appropriate transfer of an individual who requires such services if the hospital has the capacity and human resources to treat the individual at the time of request. Failure to comply with these provisions, or so-called reversed dumping, is an important amendment to EMTALA.

Other EMTALA amendments include the whistle-blower protection afforded by Section 489.24(d)(3). In these provisions, the Health Care Finance Administration prohibits hospitals from penalizing or taking adverse action against a physician or qualified medical personnel who refuses to authorize a transfer of an individual with an emergency condition that has not been stabilized or against any hospital employee or associate because the individual reports a violation of this regulation. In addition, the whistle-blower provision protects the transferring physician from civil penalties that could otherwise be imposed for transferring an unstabilized patient if the treating physician is unable to obtain an adequate intervention from an on-call physician for the purpose of effecting the completion of the stabilization process. In those instances, the practicing physician must identify the physician who fails to comply with the on-call provisions of EMTALA by documenting the name and address of the physician. When the clinical benefits outweigh the risks to the patient, this rationale should be documented and the patient transferred in compliance with other relevant EMTALA provisions. The 1994 regulations clearly reaffirm the whistle-blower protection of Section 489.24. They do not, however, explicitly protect physicians from reprisals that could result from circumstances in which the treating physician reports that he or she was forced to transfer a patient to another facility because an on-call physician did not respond in a reasonable amount of time to a request for care. The potential for civil actions between physicians exists; however, as of the date of this writing, none have been reported.

Penalties under the Emergency Medical Treatment and Active Labor Act

EMTALA incorporates a number of provisions backed by significant financial penalties and exposure to lawsuits for individuals or hospitals that are found to be in violation of its components. EMTALA includes civil monetary penalties of up to $50,000 per violation for hospitals or physicians found to be in noncompliance. It is important to note that a single patient encounter may precipitate multiple violations as they relate to the screening, stabilization, and transfer process. As an example, multiple hospitals, as of this date, have been fined in excess of $100,000 from single-patient encounters. It should also be noted that this action is typically initiated by the Inspector General's office or state agencies delegated by the Inspector General for the purpose of enforcing the provisions of EMTALA.

In addition, the law also allows private individuals suffering personal harm as a direct result of a hospital's violation to recover damages from the offending hospital. EMTALA presently limits these damages, however, to those available under the personal injury law of the state of jurisdiction in which the services were provided. In addition, any medical facility that suffers financial loss as a result of an EMTALA violation can also obtain damages to the limit of the law of the state of jurisdiction. Examples of institutional damages may include the total health care cost involved in caring for a patient transferred in violation of EMTALA.

A recent Florida court decision *(Dearmars v. AV/MED)* upheld that EMTALA allows lawsuits only against hospitals and physicians. In addition, it ruled that health maintenance organizations were covered by the Employee Retirement Security Act (ERISA), which protects health maintenance organizations from EMTALA lawsuits. EMTALA-based liability suits initiated by private individuals and medical facilities are limited to no more than 2 years after the date of violation. It is important to note that private individuals may not initiate civil suits against physicians separate from medical malpractice for seeking relief under the provisions of personal injury. EMTALA is clear in its scope to limit these actions to those against hospitals. In addition to the civil monetary penalties for hospitals and physicians found negligent under the law, there are instances when either party may have its Medicare participation agreements terminated. In instances when a physician's violation is gross, flagrant, and repeated, the Health Care Financing Administration may elect to exclude the practitioner from all Medicare and Medicaid programs. In addition, hospitals that flagrantly and recurrently fail to meet the requirements of EMTALA may also be subject to termination of their Medicare Provider agreements. As of this writing, termination of Medicare agreements have occurred but have numbered less than five throughout the United States. Clearly, enforcement of this provision can prove to be economically catastrophic to providers and hospitals alike.

Judicial Review

Although the federal regulations for EMTALA were published in 1988 and 1994, a number of vagarities in the application of EMTALA will ultimately be decided by judicial review. The essence of a multitude of court rulings would support the following consensus of opinion in the implementation of EMTALA. A number of cases have suggested that the demonstration of economic discrimination is not necessary to violate EMTALA. Although the law was written to address concerns regarding care for the indigent patient, EMTALA's coverage clearly extends to any individual entering hospital property.

Economic Discrimination Implications

The following cases throughout the United States have addressed the issue of economic discrimination and are consistent with the opinion that it is not necessary or incumbent on the Health Care Financing Administration to demonstrate economic discrimination for the purpose of enforcement of EMTALA:

1. *Brooker v. Desert Hospital Corp.,* 947 Fed. 2d 412 (9th Cir. 1991)
2. *Delaney v. Cade,* 756 F.Supp.1476 (D.Kan. 1991)
3. *Burrows v. Turner Memorial Hospital, Inc.,* 762 F.Supp. 848 (W.D. Ark. 1991)
4. *Foster v. Lawrence Memorial Hospital,* No. 91-1151-C (D.Kan. 1992, W.L. 24099)
5. *Jones v. Wake County Hospital System, Inc.,* No. 90-523-CIV-5 (E.D.N.C. Nov. 4, 1991) WL 325271
6. *Urban v. King,* 783 F.Supp. 560 (D.Kan. 1992)
7. *Lee v. Alleghany Regional Hospital Corporation,* 778 F.Supp.900 (W.D. VA 1991)
8. *Gatewood v. Washington Health Care Corp.,* 933 R. 2d 1037 (D.C.Cir. 1991)
9. *Cleland v. Bronson Health Care Group, Inc.,* 917 F. 2d at 269, 270 (6th.Cir. 1990)

Misdiagnosis Implications

A number of court decisions have recently affirmed that misdiagnosis in and of itself does not necessarily constitute an EMTALA violation. Although early court decisions were inconsistent, a growing number of decisions have supported the contention that a misdiagnosis alone does not necessarily constitute an inadequate screening or stabilization process. Clearly, the preponderance of recent interpretations would support the contention that an appropriate screening examination for the purposes of EMTALA may be effected in individuals who are ultimately determined to be misdiagnosed. A number of recent cases have supported this contention and include the following:

1. *Petrovics v. Prince William Hospital Corporation,* 764 F.Supp.415 (E.D. VA 1991)
2. *Jones v. Wake County Hospital System, Inc.,* No. 90-523-CIV-5 (E.D. N.C. Nov.4, 1991 WL 325271)
3. *Gatewood v. Washington Healthcare Corp.,* 933 Fed. 2d 1037 (D.C. Cir. 1991)
4. *Coleman v. McCurtain Memorial Medical Management Inc.,* 771 F.Supp.343 (E.D. OK 1991)

Managed Care Implications

Compliance with the provision of EMTALA has proven to be challenging in patients participating in managed care organizations. Recent court decisions have found that health maintenance organizations cannot be found culpable under EMTALA provisions. Health maintenance organizations are not typically hospital entities receiving Medicare funds. In addition, recent rulings such as *Wickline v. State of California,* 192CALCAL.APP 3d 1630, 239Cal.RPTR.810 (1986) have upheld the opinion that third-party payor reimbursement methodologies do not absolve participating physicians in hospitals from their obligation to exercise appropriate and independent professional judgment and compliance with the screening, stabilization, and transfer provisions of EMTALA. Most managed care networks are requesting emergency departments to provide first contact physician screening assistance. Historically, physician service descriptors such as CPT-4 did not recognize a specific and unique screening examination. In 1996, however, specific screening language was included in the descriptor of services relating to all evaluation and management services provided in any emergency department setting. The provision of the screening services required by EMTALA can now be accurately reported by the amended coding nomenclature.

In addition a number of legislative initiatives at the state and national level have been initiated to develop a consistent "prudent, lay person" definition of emergency services consistent with EMTALA. These initiatives in some states are also requiring a 30 minute response time for payment information and in a limited number of states mandatory payments for required screening services provided to a managed care network. Regardless of the outcomes of these legislative initiatives, the fundamental requirements of EMTALA will remain preeminent to the healthcare provider.

It can be expected that more aggressive efforts by managed care networks will be exerted to redirect patients from emergency department settings. As an example, in 1993 the American Hospital Association data identified 357 emergency department visits per 1000 population. In that same year, utilization rates in competitive managed care environments were as low as 75 per thousand.* Clearly, the managed care environment will prove to be challenging in the years ahead for prudent and conscientious providers in emergency department settings.

SUMMARY

The Emergency Medical Treatment and Active Labor Act, as amended by the Omnibus Budget Reconciliation Act of 1989 and 1990 and as further refined in the 1988 and 1994 Interim Final Regulations disseminated by the U.S. federal government, incorporates issues that affect the daily practice of emergency healthcare. In the aggregate, the provisions require three important services to all patients who come to a Medicare-participating hospital: a screening process by qualified medical personnel; a stabilization process incorporating the usual and customary ancillary services provided by the hospital; and, when indicated and necessary, a transfer process consistent with the requirements of law. In spite of the 1988 and 1994 Final Interim Regulations, a number of uncertainties exist in the compliance with this law. Therefore the Emergency Medical Treatment and Active Labor Act of 1986 and ongoing judicial review will significantly affect the practitioner's approach to patient care in the years ahead.

*Greene J: *Modern Healthcare* 26(5):37-40, 1996.

BIBLIOGRAPHY

Ansell PA: Patient dumping in emergency rooms, *McNeil Lehrer News Hour,* NBC TV, August 1, 1987 (recorded interview).

Berliner HS: Patient dumping: no one wins and we all lose, *AJPH* 78(10):1279-1280, 1988.

Birmingham Baptist Hospital v. Crews, 229ALA 398, 157-224, 1934.

Committee of Government Operations: *Equal access to health care: patient dumping,* report no. 100-131, Washington, DC, 1988, US Government Printing Office.

Cushing M: In case of emergency, *Am J Nurs* 90:1175-1178, 1988.

Enfield LM, Sklar DP: Patient dumping in the hospital emergency department: renewed interest in an old problem, *Am J Law Med* 13(4):561-594, 1988.

Emergency Nurses Association: *Standards of emergency nursing practices,* St Louis, 1983, Mosby.

Frew SA: HMO's and COBRA liability, *Patient Transfer News* 1(3):1-8, 1993.

Frew SA: Patient transfers: how to comply with the law, *Am Coll Emerg Med* 1991.

Frew SA: Power: A risky appeal, *Patient Transfer News* 1(2):1-3, 1993.

Frew SA, Roush WR, LaGreca K: COBRA: implications of emergency medicine, *Ann Emerg Med* 17(8):835-837, 1988.

George JE, Qualtrone MS: New federal law governs patient transfers: "anti-dumping" legislation enacted, *J Emerg Nurs* 12(5):318-319, 1986.

Greene J: ERs adapt to era of HMOs, *Modern Healthcare* 26(5):37-40, 1996.

Krentz M: Working with COBRA to ensure access to care, *Ann Emerg Med* 17(8):859-860, 1988.

Lebow M, Rodney WM: Patient transfer to a public hospital, *J Emerg Med* 6:447-450, 1988.

Maxwell B, Miller B: Smooth the way for safe emergency transfers, *RN* 51(6):34-47, 1988.

Perkins A: The effects of health care cost containment on the poor: an overview, *Clearinghouse Review* 19:831, 1985.

Roper WL: From the health care financing administration, *JAMA* 260(12):1681, 1988.

Rosen P: Patient dumping or work aversion? *J Emerg Med* 6:429-431, 1988.

Schiff RL, Ansell DA, Schlooser JE, et al: Transfer to public hospital: a prospective study of 467 patients, *N Engl J Med* 314:552-557, 1986.

Scott V: "Dumping": interhospital patient transfers, *J Emerg Nurs* 12(5):256-257, 1986.

Stark FP: Patient dumping, *Congressional Record* PE 265-267, 2 Feb 1989.

Sullivan D J: *Yearbook of law and emergency medicine,* Oak Brook, Ill, 1993, Sullivan.

Tammelleo AD, editor: Uninsured patient bled to death: Nursing dilemma, *Regan Rep Nurs Law* 27(9):1, 1987.

Wilmington General Hospital v. Manlove, 54 Del at 20, 174 A.2d at 140 (1961).

62 Medical Record Documentation

Daniel J. Sullivan

OUTLINE

The rationale for effective documentation
- Patient care
- The regulatory environment
- Forensic evidence
- Medical malpractice litigation
- Reimbursement

Essential elements of effective documentation
- History
- Physical examination
- Emergency department management
- Laboratory and diagnostic evaluation
- The diagnosis
- Discharge instructions

Documentation issues and problems
- General charting issues
- Errors, alterations, and late entries
- Consent
- Resuscitation
- Against medical advice
- Other patients who leave before evaluation and treatment
- Federal transfer legislation
- Telephone follow-up
- Shift change
- On-call physician or consultant delays
- Problems and incidents

Medical record documentation methodologies
- The handwritten record
- The transcribed record
- Structured, complaint-specific encounter forms
- The future of medical record documentation

Summary

The ability to perform a high-quality history and physical examination, make a diagnosis, and manage the critically ill patient represents only half the battle in the practice of emergency medicine. The are several other critical elements to a successful practice of emergency medicine, such as communication skills, time management, organization, and leadership. In addition, it is essential that the emergency physician create a medical record that reflects the many requirements of proper documentation.

To understand what to write or dictate, the emergency care provider should understand how the emergency medical record is used by subsequent care providers and reviewers, including researchers, attorneys in legal actions, billing companies, third-party payors and managed care organizations, national accrediting organizations, and a myriad of others. Armed with that understanding it is possible to address the patients' needs, practice good risk management, code for appropriate reimbursement, meet national quality standards, and address other important issues as they arise.

Although the essential elements of a proper history and physical examination have not changed in many years, the requirements of documentation have changed rapidly and dramatically. One example was seen when emergency care providers altered their documentation habits in response to the implementation of COBRA transfer legislation. Another example occurred when the Health Care Financing Administration changed the Medicare reimbursement formulas and the associated documentation requirements.

Emergency care providers and hospital administration should familiarize themselves with the choices in documentation technology. Armed with quality comparisons, turnaround times, cost estimates,and other factors, they can then make informed decisions about the best documentation methodology for a particular site. Handwritten records may be appropriate in certain settings, but other departments with high volume and acuity may require one of the dictation technologies.

Staying abreast of documentation requirements is difficult but necessary. Emergency medicine training programs should teach residents the essentials of record keeping and the methods of acquiring additional information after graduation. Practicing emergency care providers can attain this information through specialty newsletters, the quality improvement process, peer review, and continuing medical education. Whatever the source, this information will be a continuing asset to the practicing emergency care provider.

THE RATIONALE FOR EFFECTIVE DOCUMENTATION

Patient Care

Documentation can be critically important during a patient's visit to the emergency department. Documentation of medications, allergies, and recent and past medical history can guide the healthcare providers in the patient's acute management. A review of the trend in vital signs can herald a change in the patient's condition. Serial Glasgow Coma Scale scores provide useful information about a patient's changing neurologic condition.

Thorough documentation of a patient's presentation and management during the emergency department visit will assist the subsequent providers in giving the highest quality of care. Careful documentation of the critically ill patient's presentation and management helps the admitting team understand the patient's presentation and clinical course, which is essential for ongoing care.

The patient's record is certainly helpful in disposition and follow-up. Accurate and complete documentation will assist the subsequent provider in the appropriate management of patients discharged from the emergency department. This is true whether follow-up is accomplished in the private physician's office or the patient makes a return visit to the emergency department. Eventually, the patient's transcribed, computerized record will be available on-line for subsequent caregivers.

The Regulatory Environment

Joint Commission on Accreditation of Healthcare Organizations. The Joint Commission on Accreditation of Healthcare Organizations (JCAHO) is a voluntary national accrediting body. Its mission is "to enhance the quality of healthcare provided to the public."[1] Failure to pass a JCAHO review can result in sanctions against the hospital. The JCAHO guidelines contain a laundry list of requirements addressing medical record documentation. In 1995 the JCAHO dramatically revised the manual as it pertains to emergency departments. In the past, the manual contained a long list of requirements specific to the emergency department documentation. The list has been significantly shortened, and now includes only the following:

IM.8.1.6.1 A continuously maintained control register for emergency and outpatient services includes at least the following information for every individual seeking care: identification, such as name, age, and sex; date, time, and means of arrival; nature of complaint; disposition; and time of departure.

IM.7.6.1.1 Time and means of arrival.

IM.7.6.1.2 The patient's leaving against medical advice.

IM.7.6.1.3 Conclusions at termination of treatment, including final disposition, condition at discharge, and any instructions for follow-up care.

IM.7.6.2 When authorized by the patient or his or her legally authorized representative, a copy of the record of emergency services is available to the practitioner or medical organization responsible for follow-up care.[1]

The section relating to emergency medical records includes a list of items that all medical records are required to contain. Specifically, evidence of the following must be included in the medical record:

IM.7.2.3 Emergency care provided to the patient before arrival, if any.

IM.7.2.5 A statement of the conclusions or impressions drawn from the medical history and physical examination.

IM.7.2.6 The diagnosis or diagnostic impression.

IM.7.2.7 The reason(s) for admission or treatment.

IM.7.2.9 Evidence of known advance directives.

IM.7.2.10 Evidence of informed consent for procedures and treatments for which informed consent is required by organizational policy.

IM.7.2.11 Diagnostic and therapeutic orders, if any.

IM.7.2.12 All diagnostic and therapeutic procedures and tests performed and the results.

IM.7.7.13 All operative and other invasive procedures performed, using acceptable disease and operative terminology that includes etiology, as appropriate.

IM.7.2.14 Progress notes made by the medical staff and other authorized individuals.

IM.7.2.15 All reassessments, when necessary.

IM.7.2.16 Clinical observations.

IM.7.2.17 The response to the care provided.

IM.7.7.18 Consultation reports.

IM.7.2.20 Every dose of medication administered and any adverse drug reaction.

IM.7.2.21 Every medication dispensed to or prescribed for an ambulatory patient.

IM.7.21.22 All relevant diagnoses established during the course of care.

IM.7.2.23 Any referrals and communications made to external or internal care providers and to community agencies.[1]

Some items on this list pertain specifically to the inpatient component of the medical record. For example, the hospital must review advance directive status with every patient admitted to the hospital. Thus the emergency department would not be obligated to provide this documentation to pass JCAHO scrutiny. There are several other items commonly identified as important on emergency medical records:

- Presence of allergies to medications or chemicals
- Routine and current medications
- Pregnancy, if germane
- Tetanus immunization history, if germane
- Name of the personal physician
- Patient's signature acknowledging receipt and understanding of the follow-up instructions[2]

Emergency department compliance with JCAHO standards, including those relating to the medical record, is generally not difficult and is essential for the hospital. Failure to comply with JCAHO standards can result in loss of accreditation and significant financial sanctions. If a hospital loses JCAHO accreditation it can no longer contract with the federal government for Medicare reimbursement. Furthermore, residents must be trained in a JCAHO-accredited institution. Emergency department leadership should work closely with the administration to ensure compliance.

Peer Review Organizations. Titles XI and XVIII of the Social Security Act provide statutory authority for the creation of peer review organizations (PROs). The PROs were created to monitor the quality and appropriateness of medical care for recipients of federally funded programs such as Medicare. In general, PRO examiners begin their review with inpatient records. While reviewing these records, examiners may review the entire medical record for appropriateness of care, including emergency department documents. In certain instances, the PRO will specifically request emergency department records and focus its review on the documentation of care rendered there.

Intervening care. If a Medicare patient has two hospitalizations within a 31-day period, the PRO reviews all "intervening care." Intervening care includes outpatient and emergency care.

Inappropriate transfer cases. (See the section on federal transfer legislation later in this chapter). Cases of alleged violations of the federal antidumping laws may result in a PRO review. These cases are initially referred to the state office of the Health Care Financing Administration (or designated state agency). When questions of inappropriate care or transfer arise, the case is then referred to the PRO for review of potential COBRA violations.

Beneficiary hotline. Anyone receiving benefits under Medicare may call the beneficiary hotline to complain about perceived problems with medical care. The PRO may then review the care provided. The review will begin with an assessment of the care as described in the documented medical record. Although most cases are resolved without sanctions, the review process is tedious, time consuming, and stressful.

Sources at the Illinois PRO indicate that 60% to 70% of the "problem" cases are related to documentation issues. Therefore appropriate documentation would have led to rapid and favorable conclusions in the majority of PRO reviews.

Only 30% to 40% of cases involve substantive issues. If substantive problems are identified, sanctions may be applied against the medical practitioner. The examiner's questions about emergency medical care should be answered by thorough documentation on the medical record, so more intense scrutiny can be avoided.

State Law Requirements. Several states have enacted some form of legislation or regulation that mandates the provision of emergency medical care to an individual regardless of the individual's ability to pay.[3] Other states regulate the content of the emergency department medical record. For example, the New Jersey Administrative Code contains specific requirements for the emergency department medical record and the emergency department registration log.[4] The scope of services and specific medical records requirements vary from state to state.

Forensic Evidence

Several types of forensic medical events require careful emergency department record keeping so that justice may be served. These events include, but are not limited to, sexual assault, domestic violence, child abuse, intoxicated motorists, and injury from guns, knives, razors, ice picks, and other potentially lethal implements.

Emergency care providers can provide tremendous assistance to the coroner, medical examiner, or criminal investigator by providing well-documented information about the patient's presentation and certain physical findings. For example, gunpowder around a wound may be washed away during resuscitation, but documentation of its presence provides valuable information about the distance from the gun to the victim. Gunpowder on the hand of a gunshot victim may suggest suicide. Documentation of these facts on the medical record is extremely helpful. This is particularly so when patients expire after admission to the hospital and there is a substantial delay between the injury and presentation to the medical examiner.

Emergency providers should also carefully document procedures and interventions. For example, careful documentation will help the medical examiner distinguish between knife wounds to the chest and thoracostomy tube sites once the tubes have been removed. Victims of car accidents, particularly hit-and-run victims, often have foreign matter in wounds. Documentation of the presence of metal or paint fragments may be helpful in the subsequent investigation.

Emergency care providers should be familiar with the pertinent statutory reporting requirements of the state and federal jurisdiction in which they practice. Emergency department leaders and hospital administrators should develop protocols to clarify what forensic evidence should be documented and how the event should be reported.

Medical Malpractice Litigation

Emergency providers must also keep in mind that the well-documented medical record provides the strongest defense in the event of medical malpractice litigation. Well-documented, high-quality emergency practice is hard to beat in a malpractice contest. One single document, the emergency department record, is the primary documentation of the patient-physician or patient-nurse encounter. It is considered the central piece of evidence in a malpractice proceeding.

The maxim "If you didn't document it, you didn't do it" obviously is not technically correct. On medical records, particularly those that are handwritten, there are many things that are done but never documented. In a malpractice scenario, a critical omission will be scrutinized, though many other elements of a physical examination may be recorded. For example, a poorly documented neck and neurologic exam on a 2-year-old who later developed meningitis will be emphasized. The physician will claim that the neck and neurologic examinations were done, because this is the routine on every febrile child. The problem is apparent. The physician's claims will seem self-serving, and the plaintiff's attorney will underscore this point with the jury. The maxim should be, "If you don't document it, you have a really difficult time proving it."

Also consider that in many jurisdictions, the medical malpractice action will not be tried until 3 to 5 years after filing. In many cases, caregivers in medical malpractice cases do not have an independent recollection of the event and must rely completely on the medical record for factual information. It is imperative that the record reflect what was actually done for the patient—that is, all history taking, the complete examination, reevaluations, involvement of consultants, procedures, and all other aspects of care. New chart writing technology allows documentation far superior to handwritten records and is a giant step in emergency care risk management.

Reimbursement

Medicare. Several third-party payors scrutinize the emergency department record to form a basis for reimbursement. For example, Medicare reimbursement is contingent on documentation of the level of service, or care, provided. When performing chart audits, the Medicare reviewers use three key components to assign the level of care: the history, examination, and medical decision making.

Auditors evaluate documentation of historical information, including the presence and complexity of the history of present illness, review of systems, past medical history,and social and family history. Appropriate documentation of physical examination includes a review of relevant body areas (e.g., neck, abdomen) and organ systems (e.g., cardiovascular, respiratory). The auditor also looks at the complexity of the physical exam performed, ranging from the problem-focused exam, which is limited to an affected body part, through the comprehensive multisystem examination. Complexity of medical decision making is the third component used by auditors when assigning of level of service. There are four levels, ranging from "straightforward" to "high complexity."

Although the specific formula for Medicare reimbursement

has changed, reimbursement is clearly based on the level of documentation. For the hospital or medical group to receive appropriate reimbursement, close attention must be paid to the Medicare requirements for documentation.

Medicaid. In several states, physicians working with state regulatory agencies review Medicaid charts retrospectively to determine if a "true emergency" existed. Whether a case is deemed an emergency often turns on the level of documentation. A retrospective review revealing inadequate documentation and nonemergency cases can lead to reduced reimbursement, or "payback," to the state government based on Medicaid "overpayments."

Other Third-Party Payors. Insurance companies and managed care organizations do not dictate a medical record formula for reimbursement. However, third-party payors are increasingly denying full reimbursement based on usual and customary charges. Careful documentation of the examination and medical decision making will result in appropriate reimbursement for services rendered.

ESSENTIAL ELEMENTS OF EFFECTIVE DOCUMENTATION

History

The medical history provides the emergency physician with an overview of why the patient is in the emergency department. Several people write historical information on the chart. This may include registration personnel, the triage nurse, the primary nurse, technicians, social workers, and multiple physicians. It is important that the author be clearly identified on the record.

Inconsistency between the nursing and physician history should be recognized and addressed. Resolution of the conflicting information often results in important fact finding. For example, the patient's condition may have changed between the times of triage and physician evaluation. Further, the triage history is only a screening examination and is less thorough than the physician evaluation. As a result, the triage examination may be insufficient to draw a conclusion regarding the nature of the problem or may simply be in error. Inconsistencies should be addressed squarely in the physician's history. For example: "The triage nurse noted that the patient has substernal chest pain. However, the patient does not have substernal pain, it is an epigastric and left upper quadrant pain. The patient very clearly points out that her chest is not painful now, nor was it painful at any time since the epigastric pain began."

Using phrases that refer to the nursing notes, such as "See above" or "Refer to nursing notes," is appropriate if that adds factually to the history. As the exclusive documentation of the physician history, it is inadequate.

A review of systems identifies signs and symptoms related to the patient's present illness that the patient may have experienced. Examples include constitutional symptoms such as fever and weakness and cardiovascular, respiratory, and gastrointestinal symptoms. The length of the system review is dictated by the complexity and acuity of the patient's condition. An ankle injury may require a single system musculoskeletal review. An abdominal pain presentation requires a multiple system review.

That patient's past medical history includes a list of medical conditions or problems and related medications. Surgeries and prior admissions may also be documented. Family history documentation should include a review of relevant family diseases. For example, a family history of cardiac disease, diabetes, or asthma may be critical factors in creating a differential diagnosis. Social history completes the thorough historical examination. Descriptions of living and working conditions, marital status, alcohol or tobacco use, or other substance use may be important factors in reaching a diagnosis and in determining patient disposition.

Historical prompts can be extremely useful. The emergency department document often contains several key items filled in at triage or by the primary nurse. Examples include last normal menstrual period (LNMP), history of smoking, and tetanus status. These "mandatory fill-ins" can improve quality of documentation and help identify critical information in some cases.

Physical Examination

Vital signs are, as the name implies, a critical element of the examination. If abnormal, they should be repeated and documented. Most emergency departments have a policy that directs staff to repeat and document vital signs in some predesignated time period.

A directed physical examination, as indicated by the chief complaint and history, should be documented. Generally, a problem limited to a single area, such as an extremity laceration or a sprained ankle, requires examination and documentation limited to that and the surrounding area. Additional documentation is usually not relevant, not legally protective, and not a good use of physician resources. The complex case or the difficult diagnosis will require a more thorough physical examination with corresponding documentation.

When documenting a complete physical examination, especially when handwriting the record, there is an inclination to abbreviate certain elements of the examination—for example, "Neurologic examination WNL" (within normal limits). This may be appropriate in a patient with cough, fever, and sputum production, but it is not adequate in the patient with a transient ischemic attack, headache, or fever with stiff neck. When an organ system is potentially involved in the patient's chief complaint, it is necessary to document a thorough, textbook physical examination of the relevant system.

In a malpractice action, the healthcare provider always has the opportunity to explain what was meant by "WNL." He or she can then recite the complete evaluation of that system. However, it is far more convincing at deposition or trial to provide testimony based on a documented complete evaluation.

Emergency Department Management

If the patient receives any significant intervention in the emergency department, ongoing management should be recorded. Patients with tonsillitis or urinary tract infection need little or no documentation of emergency department management. However, the ongoing management of patients with chest pain or respiratory distress requires accurate documentation of interventions.

Important interventions and response to treatment should be timed and recorded. Although this may be difficult in a busy emergency department, it is necessary information for subsequent care providers and for proper reimbursement, and further, it may be legally protective. Intervention by a consultant, attending, transfer team, or other care provider should also be documented.

Emergency physicians should feel comfortable using adjectives and adverbs that reflect the speed with which a task was accomplished. For example:

> This 7-year-old child presented with a rash that was strongly suggestive of meningococcal meningitis. After a rapid examination, I immediately ordered antibiotics, started an IV, and set up for lumbar puncture. Antibiotics were given immediately upon initiating intravenous access.

Laboratory and Diagnostic Evaluation

Abnormal labs, x-rays, special imaging, electrocardiograms, and other evaluations should be acknowledged and, when appropriate, acted on. Many emergency departments design their chart with space for documentation of abnormalities. A user-friendly form for this purpose is a great asset in the busy emergency department.

The Diagnosis

The diagnosis, as the name implies, should reflect what is known rather than what is unknown. "Rule out" is not an appropriate prefix for a discharge diagnosis. It may be an appropriate part of the physician's thought process before discharge. At the time of discharge, the emergency physician should either have a clear diagnosis in mind or, at least, indicate what is known about the diagnosis. For example, if the cause of abdominal pain is unknown, the diagnosis might read, "Abdominal pain, etiology unknown."

A diagnosis such as "rule out appendicitis" is problematic. There is no billing code for reimbursement of "rule out appendicitis." Also, the "rule out" diagnosis may increase the emergency physician's risk of liability. A jury may have difficulty determining why a physician would discharge a patient home to rule out appendicitis. Ruling out a potentially life-threatening problem is something that is supposed to occur in the hospital.

The diagnosis should be consistent with the history and physical examination. For example, a child with vomiting but no diarrhea does not have gastroenteritis. The diagnosis might be gastritis, but there is no evidence of enteritis. A child with vomiting and diarrhea may have a routine viral syndrome. The child with vomiting alone requires close attention and follow-up.

Discharge Instructions

The discharge instructions provide the critical link between emergency department management and the remainder of the patient's clinical course. Bad or unexpected outcomes do occur; some patients' clinical conditions do deteriorate. Management does not end when the patient leaves the emergency department. Discharge instructions help bridge the gap between the hospital and the next medical intervention.

In a malpractice action for "failure to diagnose," the discharge instructions can be a strong ally. The standard of care does not require that the healthcare provider always have perfect judgment or always provide a precise diagnosis. The discharge instructions incorporate the patients in the continuing care. Patients who fail to follow clear and adequate instructions assume some responsibility for problems that may result.

Many malpractice suits against emergency care providers hinge on the failure to provide appropriate discharge instructions or failure to provide appropriate follow-up with a consultant or private physician. Evidence presented at trial may clearly demonstrate that the discharge instructions do not instruct the patient when and under what circumstances follow-up care is necessary. The emergency physician's attempt to demonstrate appropriate follow-up care 5 years later during deposition or trial, without supporting documentation, may be all but impossible.

Follow-up Time Frame. Proper discharge instructions provide the time frame for follow-up, which will vary based on the patient's condition. For example, the repair of a dirty wound may need a wound check within 48 hours and suture removal at some later date. A painful snuffbox (i.e., possible wrist fracture) with a negative initial radiograph will need a follow-up in several days for another x-ray. These instructions are fairly straightforward.

Minor medical conditions may need an "as needed" follow-up. A minor viral syndrome with a low-grade temperature may not need any follow-up unless the condition worsens. With this type of follow-up instruction, the caregivers obviously intend some patient judgment. If the condition improves as expected, no follow-up is necessary. However, the instructions must clearly and specifically state that if the condition persists or worsens or some other problem develops, follow-up is necessary. Thus simply writing the words "as needed" or "prn" is inadequate.

The "mandatory" follow-up is common. This instruction indicates that follow-up is necessary and should occur within a certain specified time frame. The mandatory follow-up is particularly valuable when the patient's diagnosis is not known with certainty. For example, an otherwise healthy 25-year-old male has right lower quadrant abdominal pain. Initially there is tenderness, but it resolves over a 2-hour period. The laboratory evaluation is unremarkable. As in many cases of abdominal pain, when the diagnosis is uncertain, the patient does well and is discharged. The time for follow-up should be specified, perhaps within 12 to 48 hours.

Specifying Reasons for Follow-up. The discharge instruction should include a list of possible occurrences for which the patient should return to the emergency department or call his or her private physician immediately. For example, a patient with abdominal pain on presentation may become asymptomatic and be discharged from the emergency department. The discharge instructions should alert the patient to be seen as soon as possible if he or she develops vomiting, fever, or a return or worsening of the pain, heralding a significant change in the condition.

Another example is the patient with vaginal bleeding. Dysfunctional uterine bleeding and threatened abortion may generally be managed on an outpatient basis. However, both conditions can result in life-threatening vaginal bleeding, requiring emergency surgery. Therefore the patient with vaginal bleeding should receive careful instructions about the amount of bleeding that should prompt a call to the private physician or an immediate return to the emergency department.

It is impossible to list all of the contingencies or possible problems that may arise. Therefore it is prudent to tell the patient, and write in the discharge instructions, that he or she should seek care sooner than specified if the condition worsens or a new problem arises.

Follow-up in the Emergency Department. In the event that a patient is referred to another physician for follow-up, and for any reason that physician is unavailable, the emergency department may serve as the backup resource. The private physician may be out of town, or the on-call physician may not be readily available. Follow-up in the emergency department may be particularly useful for patients requiring a mandatory follow-up within a short time frame. For example, a patient with a burn may require reevaluation on a Saturday or Sunday.

Patient Education. Discharge planning provides a good opportunity for patient education. For example, parents of a child with fever may benefit from information on how to take a temperature, when to use antipyretics, and how to bring high fevers down using a tepid bath.

It is a fact of life that a patient's condition may worsen or change or be misdiagnosed. The discharge instruction provides a safety net to deal with that reality. The emergency physician and nurse should ask, "What if the diagnosis is wrong?" The answer should be that the discharge process and instructions have provided enough education to allow the patient to recognize a problem and seek care promptly.

Computerized Discharge Programs. Several companies sell software programs for emergency department discharge instructions. Computerized discharge planners are user-friendly and allow customized instructions. Some allow the inclusion of the name, address, and telephone number of the private or on-call physician. Some programs calculate the proper dosage schedule when the child's weight is entered (e.g., acetaminophen or pediatric ibuprofen). Some software packages print prescriptions. Some print instructions in multiple languages.

Healthcare providers in emergency departments using these software packages generally have a high level of satisfaction. One potential drawback is the tendency to overload patients with information. Critical information may be lost among pages of less useful information. Great care must be taken when organizing the instructions so that patients can understand the critical information for continuing care, follow-up, and intervention in case of deterioration or change in condition.

Several companies sell preprinted discharge instructions for emergency departments. These instructions are useful but are not tailored specifically for a particular patient. If preprinted instruction sheets are given to the patient, that should be indicated on the discharge form that the patient signs.

Both the emergency physician and nurse are responsible for ensuring that appropriate discharge instructions are provided, even when they do not actually give the instructions. In many departments, physician assistants, medical technicians, or other personnel appropriately may be responsible for this task.

Documentation of the Discharge. The patient and the individual providing the instruction should sign the discharge instruction sheet. It is imperative that the patient has a legible instruction sheet. The patient should receive the original copy of the instructions because the second and third copies are often difficult to read. A copy of the instructions should become part of the permanent medical record.

DOCUMENTATION ISSUES AND PROBLEMS

General Charting Issues

Black ink. Black ink is generally used on legal records and is recommended for emergency medical record documentation. Use of black ink facilitates copying, microfilming, and computer processing.

Blank lines. Blank lines and spaces may be interpreted as demonstrating an incomplete note. There should not be any blank lines left between notes. A line should be drawn through blank spaces.

Signatures. The chart should be signed by anyone who participates in the patient's care. The legal signature should include the first initial, last name, and license or certification.

Chronologic order. Charting should be done in chronologic order. This lends credibility to the accuracy of the recording.

Abbreviations. Each hospital has standards for documentation. The records should be in compliance with those hospital standards.

Military time. Use of military time decreases confusion and is recommended.

John/Jane Doe. If the patient cannot be identified, indicate why on the medical record. In addition, document attempts to notify family or next of kin and notification of police or social service personnel who will be assuming responsibility for further attempts to identify the patient.

Ownership. The medical record is the property of the hospital.

Errors, Alterations, and Late Entries

Medical record entry errors are inevitable. The hospital or the emergency department should establish clear procedures for correcting chart entry errors. Generally, the person correcting a charting error should draw a single line through the error, enter the correct information, initial the correction, and enter the time and date the correction was made (if not otherwise shown in the entry). If information is recorded at a time later than the emergency department visit or the time when the chart is initially completed, include a notation of "late entry" with the date and the time of entry.

Mistakes in the chart should not be erased or obliterated. Such erasures and changes will create suspicion in the minds of those subsequently reading the chart, including a jury. A single line through the incorrect entry leaves no doubt as to the original information being corrected. When the correction requires more space than is available near the original entry, the person correcting the record should make reference to an addendum on the record and enter the more lengthy correction in the addendum.

Because of the increasing prevalence of emergency department dictation, it is necessary to address the types of errors that occur with that charting format. If the transcriptionist does not understand the word, there may be a blank line or space left on the chart. Simply fill in the blank line or space and initial and date the addition. No other words need to be added.[5]

A transcriptionist may hear a medical word and transcribe it improperly, perhaps misspelling it or substituting an entirely different word. Misspelled words should be crossed out with a single line. Watch carefully for this because it occurs frequently with medications. Put a single line through the wrong word, write or print the correct word, and then initial and date the change. Document the reason for the change as a "dictation error."

Changing a medical record can be a high-risk activity. However, attention to detail will keep this practice safe. Do not make the mistake of changing a record after the visit date without clearly dating the change.

After an adverse outcome, emergency physicians often go back to the medical record and recognize that the documentation is inadequate or does not properly reflect the clinical evaluation and management. There is a strong inclination to want to add something to the record as a late entry or create another document to fill in the details. This may or may not be advisable. It is critical that the emergency physician speak with hospital risk management or defense counsel before considering such action. It may be extremely helpful or extremely harmful to any subsequent litigation, depending on specific circumstances. Expert counsel is necessary in this situation.

Consent

Obtaining consent is legally required before the provision of medical care and treatment. Typically, the emergency department registration or triage staff request that the patient sign a general consent provision, such as the following:

> I, or my child or ward, have a condition which requires medical treatment and/or admission to the hospital. I request and consent to St. Elsewhere Hospital and its professional and nursing staff as well as the ABC Emergency Group, a group of independent medical practitioners, to perform such medical and surgical procedures that may be necessary for my diagnoses and treatment including, but not limited to, a physical examination, x-rays, drawing/testing blood, or the administration of medications and/or injectable, as the physician may consider necessary and desirable for diagnosis and treatment.

Once signed by the patient, this form represents an express consent to treatment. Such forms explain the relationship between the emergency medical group and the hospital. When the emergency group is independent, this statement may provide some insulation for the hospital against claims that the physician is an agent of the hospital (i.e., vicarious liability) in malpractice actions.

Most emergency department consent forms contain additional consents and acknowledgments that address a wide variety of hospital concerns. In addition to the consent for medical and surgical care, there is usually a statement about release of information concerning the patient. This allows a release to third-party payors and is limited to the information necessary to accomplish payment. Some hospitals request a release of information so that a copy of the record can be sent to the patient's attending or private physician. In many states, the routine sending of a patient's emergency department chart to the private physician is technically a breach of patient confidentiality. This information should not be released without the patient's consent. A simple checkbox (YES__, NO__) on the consent form provides a simple mechanism for this release. Most consent forms also contain an assignment of benefits and a statement regarding personal property.

Although the vast majority of emergency department patients sign the consent form, it is uncommon for patients to take the opportunity to read and understand its contents. However, it is generally held that most patients have a reasonable expectation of what will occur in the emergency department. Therefore lawsuits regarding consent issues in emergency medicine are extremely rare.

There are some situations in which express consent is considered unnecessary. These include patients not functionally competent to consent to treatment, having a life- or limb-threatening condition, or for whom a delay for the purpose of obtaining consent will adversely affect the patient. It is important for the emergency physician to clearly document the basis for both decisions: (1) that the patient is not functionally competent to consent to, or refuse, treatment; and (2) the nature of the emergency medical condition.

Resuscitation

By its nature, a resuscitation is a rapid assessment with immediate therapeutic interventions performed by a multidisciplinary team. A comprehensive and contemporaneous record of the assessment, interventions, responses, and outcome is necessary. An organized and effective approach generally requires the assignment of one person with the responsibility of documentation. To properly document the sequence of events, the team should vocalize essential findings and interventions as they are being performed.

The role of scribe is generally filled by a nurse or emergency technician. The physician typically writes or transcribes a progress or resuscitation note. Also the physician usually signs the resuscitation form, indicating agreement with the comprehensive documentation.

Against Medical Advice

The discharge of a patient against medical advice (AMA) represents a medicolegal risk. Good medical care dictates a certain approach to the patient leaving against medical advice. Documentation of that approach will provide protection against liability for adverse events after the discharge. A retrospective review of the records of patients leaving AMA revealed that physicians documented that patients understood their diagnosis (36%), the proposed treatment (44%), and the clinical consequences of refusal (57%).[6] This does not represent an adequate effort at managing the risk that accompanies patients leaving against medical advice.

After unsuccessfully trying to convince the patient to permit a necessary evaluation or treatment, the caregivers should take certain steps. They should be convinced that the patient has given an informed refusal. The patient's capacity to understand the care being refused and the consequences of the refusal must be determined and documented. Proof of competence necessitates evaluation of the patient's state of consciousness, orientation, and other elements of a mental status examination.

Additionally, the chart should reflect the fact that the patient has received all treatment and management possible within the parameters of the patient's decision. Document efforts to ensure expeditious follow-up, including discussions with the private physician and family members. Sometimes these people, known and trusted by the patient, can alter the patient's decision.

The chart should contain complete documentation of the elements discussed previously. The caregivers should not rely on a brief hospital preprinted form which simply states that the patient is leaving the hospital AMA and has a space for a witness to sign. This minimal documentation will not provide an adequate defense in subsequent litigation. An AMA note should be specific and individualized and may read as follows:

> The patient has decided to leave against medical advice. The patient has a normal mental status and understands his/her condition (be specific) and the risks of leaving, including permanent disability and/or death, and has had an opportunity to ask questions about his/her medical condition. The patient has been informed that he/she may return for care at any time, and follow-up has been arranged.

Legal cases demonstrate that the AMA note can provide significant protection in cases in which patients clearly have a normal mental status, the physician has respected the individual's right to make a decision regarding healthcare, and every effort has been made to provide a continuum of healthcare.

Other Patients Who Leave before Evaluation and Treatment

Emergency caregivers should carefully document the circumstances surrounding the care of a patient who "absconds" or "elopes" from the emergency department. Generally, these are patients who have entered the emergency department treatment area, may or may not have been examined, and then leave the department, usually without informing anyone.

The Incompetent Patient. Functionally incompetent patients who leave the department before completion of the evaluation create a particularly great risk. Problems will arise if one of these patients, after leaving the department, deteriorates or causes an injury to a third party. When a functionally incompetent patient elopes, carefully document all efforts to retrieve the patient. These efforts may include a security search, telephone calls to the patient's residence, or a mailed letter or cable requesting return or follow-up. It may be necessary to include the police in the search.

The Patient Who Leaves without Treatment. Some patients leave the department from the waiting room without receiving any treatment. This group is described as having left without treatment (LWOT). Though these patients may leave at any time, most often they have been triaged and registered and while sitting in the waiting room become impatient and leave. In this instance, the limited documentation should become part of a permanent record. It will be helpful in case there is a claim that treatment was refused or the patient was denied a medical screening examination under the COBRA laws.

Managed Care Patients Who Leave without Treatment. A second group patients who LWOT deserve special consideration. These are patients who have entered the system but decide to leave when they realize that their managed care entity will not authorize reimbursement for the visit. As with all patients, it is imperative that the triage and registration personnel clearly indicate to the patient that medical care is being offered and is not contingent on reimbursement. The staff should carefully explain that nonauthorization for payment does not prevent medical evaluation or treatment. These discussions should be documented clearly.

The hospital and emergency staff may consider having this group of patients sign out against medical advice. The staff member at triage would be an appropriate person to document this informed refusal of care. Some training would be necessary. COBRA provisions indicate that the hospital has met its obligation if it offers medical examination and treatment and informs the individual of the risks and benefits of examination and treatment, but the individual refuses to consent to the examination and treatment. The law further states that the hospital shall take all reasonable steps to secure the individual's written informed consent to refuse such examination and treatment.[7] Therefore a properly secured AMA would be protective when patients refuse to stay for treatment. This record should then become part of the permanent file.

Increasingly, managed care entities will ask that emergency departments provide "medical screening examinations" for patients in the plan who present to the emergency department. In this time of transition, many emergency physicians and hospitals have questions about the nature and propriety of this type of screening examination. At this time there is no guidance found in the COBRA statute or the regulations for such practice, and there is little practical experience in this area. The plain language of COBRA requires an examination within the capacity of the hospital, including history and physical, lab, radiology, and so forth.

Federal Transfer Legislation

Most emergency care providers are now familiar with the federal antidumping legislation, the Consolidated Omnibus Budget Reconciliation Act of 1986, or COBRA.[8] The law is also known as the Emergency Medical Transfer and Active Labor Act, or EMTALA. The law requires hospitals that participate in the Medicare program to provide emergency medical care to patients regardless of the patients' ability to pay. The legislation applies to any physician responsible for the medical evaluation, treatment, denial of treatment, or transfer of a patient. This section will address COBRA issues related to emergency department documentation. For a more complete discussion refer to Chapter 61.

The legal implications of the medical record are significant. The patient's medical record must demonstrate the hospital's compliance with the statute. Failure to maintain a complete and accurate record of the hospital's actions with respect to emergency patients can create substantial exposure for the institution and its medical staff.[9] Documentation must address several issues.

Medical Screening Examination[10]. The act does not specifically define medical screening, nor does it specifically require a medical screening examination record. However, it is clear that the hospital should develop a record for any person requesting emergency medical care at the hospital. It has been generally understood that the nursing and physician notes showing evaluation and management are adequate to establish that the patient received a medical screening examination.

If a hospital has established a formal protocol for a medical screening examination, the circumstances of the evaluation and the patient disposition should be carefully documented on the emergency record. When patients leave before completing evaluation or leave against medical advice, the emergency care provider should carefully document efforts to evaluate and manage the patient. Further, some patients leave without treatment because a third-party payor has not authorized reimbursement. In these circumstances, the hospital's personnel should be carefully trained to offer and document the offer of examination and treatment to those who leave.

Necessary Stabilizing Treatment[11]**.** If the medical screening examination identifies an emergency medical condition[12] or a pregnant woman having contractions[13] the hospital must provide stabilizing treatment or a transfer to another medical facility.[14] Treatment provided by the hospital for the emergency medical condition should be clearly documented in the patient record. The record should include the staff (e.g., on-call physicians) that provided such treatment and the facilities used in evaluation and management.

Transferring an Unstable Individual. In certain circumstances a hospital may transfer an individual with an emergency medical condition to another medical facility. For example, many community hospitals do not have pediatric intensive care units or the capability of treating multiply traumatized patients. Before transfer, the facility must stabilize a critically ill or injured patient within its capabilities. In such cases, transfer is "appropriate"[15] if the following are true:

1. The transferring hospital provides the medical treatment within its capacity to minimize the risk to the individual's health and, in the case of a woman in labor, the risk to the unborn child.
2. The receiving facility has available personnel and space for the treatment of the individual.
3. The receiving facility has agreed to accept the transfer of the individual and provide appropriate medical treatment.
4. The transferring hospital sends to the receiving facility all medical records (or copies thereof) related to the individual's emergency medical condition.
5. The transfer is effected through qualified personnel and equipment.

The law also requires that a physician prepare a certified statement that the benefits of transfer outweigh the risks of transfer, before the transfer.[16] The federal courts have given us some guidance in filling out the certificate in Burditt v. U.S. Department of Health and Human Services.[17] In Burditt, the court said that COBRA "requires more than a signature; it requires a signed certification." The court indicated that it would be a violation if (1) the signer has not actually deliberated and weighed the medical risks and the medical benefits of transfer before executing the certification; (2) the signer makes an improper consideration a significant factor in the certification decision; and (3) the signer concludes in the weighing process that the medical risks outweigh the medical benefits of transfer, yet signs a certification that the opposite is true.

The medical record must document that the requirements of COBRA have been met. Optimally, the emergency department or hospital transfer form contains preprinted information that allows the staff to address each of these issues. Many emergency departments use a transfer form that contains check boxes and a section for certifying that the benefits of transfer outweigh the risks of transfer. Use of the form is strongly recommended because it can greatly facilitate compliance with the legal requirements.

Telephone Follow-Up

A telephone follow-up system can be a great aid in patient management and reduction of medicolegal risk. Telephone follow-up procedures can be used when new or additional information is obtained, such as amended x-rays, amended electrocardiograms, and lab abnormalities. This procedure can also be used to check on patients discharged with a high-risk diagnosis (e.g., headache, abdominal pain).

The results of follow-up should be included in the patient's permanent medical record. It is useful to have a single form that addresses each of the four areas described previously. This form could also be used for callbacks initiated by the patient for problems or concerns. All of these calls are an important part of patient management and demonstrate professionalism, care, and concern for the patient's condition.

Shift Change

Shift change is well known as a high-risk period in emergency medical practice. Emergency physicians should take great care in the transfer of patient care to an incoming physician. It is wise to document and time the transfer of patient responsibility to the incoming physician.

On-Call Physician or Consultant Delays

Problems with contacting on-call or consulting physicians are common. The problem has gotten worse with increasing numbers of patients participating in managed care plans. The emergency physician or staff should carefully document the time a call is placed to a consultant and the time the call is returned. Each institution should have a policy addressing the "reasonable" time for callback. If that time frame is exceeded, additional steps should be taken promptly and documented.

Callback delays should not result in editorials in the patient record. The documented times speak for themselves. If an unnecessary delay results in deterioration or an adverse outcome, the emergency physician may want to specifically address the delay in a progress note or an incident report. If the delay in reaching an on-call physician results in the need to transfer a patient, that must be specifically addressed.

Problems and Incidents

There is a tendency to blame others when a problem occurs. In the heat of a busy shift, anger and emotion can be reflected in the medical record. The emergency physician should carefully avoid this type of documentation. This practice can lead to tremendous hostility among physicians and departments. Further, it may seriously compromise a coordinated defense in a medical malpractice action.

Enter information describing incidents on a hospital or incident reporting form. The internal review process is a confidential forum for problem resolution and may not be discoverable. Even mentioning that an incident report has been on the medical record filed may compromise confidentiality and nondiscoverability.

MEDICAL RECORD DOCUMENTATION METHODOLOGIES

The Handwritten Record

There is clearly a trend toward typed records. However, through 1995 the majority of emergency departments continued to handwrite emergency medical records. Problems with completeness and legibility of documentation make this form of documentation less than optimal.

Limited Documentation. In a study performed in the early 1980s on 20,000 emergency medical records, the average length of the handwritten record was 54 words.[18] Presumably, the written record has increased in length in the heat of the recent malpractice climate. Regardless, even a 50% increase in the number of words leaves the emergency medical record hopelessly inadequate to meet the multitude of requirements for emergency medical documentation.

The importance of appropriate documentation in the reduction of malpractice risk is well established.[19,20] In a study of 15,009 emergency department medical records, handwritten records rendered unsatisfactory documentation 95% of the time.[21] This investigation focused on several high-risk areas of diagnostic failure, including myocardial infarction, meningitis or central nervous system bleed, appendicitis, ectopic pregnancy, epiglottitis, and wounds with occult nerve or tendon injury or occult foreign body in an extremity laceration.

Agency Review. Many agencies, such as state and federal government agencies, insurance companies, and managed care entities, carefully scrutinize emergency medical records. The written record is often inadequate to achieve appropriate reimbursement for services provided, to demonstrate acuity or utilization patterns, or to demonstrate to the regulatory agencies the intensity of services provided.

Retrospective review of Medicare or Medicaid billing may lead to federal investigation under the fraud and abuse rules and regulations. Penalties can be severe.

Coding must adhere to the formulas outlined by the Health Care Financing Administration, which are based largely on documentation. The term *upcoding* refers to the practice of coding medical services at a level of intensity higher than that which was actually performed. Appropriate coding unsupported by adequate documentation may create the appearance of fraudulent billing. For instance, the chart may reveal documentation of a history and physical and not management, procedures, and interventions that actually occurred. However, the billing form may be coded for the high level of care and critical care management that were rendered.

Although there appears to be a laundry list of problems with the handwritten record, this form of emergency department documentation will be with us for some time. Clearly it is important to avoid the problems outlined previously. In busy emergency departments, it may be necessary to hold charts until the end of the shift for completion of entries. Also, emergency caregivers can be provided with the list of critical elements necessary for documentation of high-risk clinical entities. Further, they can be familiarized with the elements of documentation reviewed by Medicare and other third-party payors for appropriate reimbursement.

The Scribe System. A "scribe system" may be a useful alternative. Scribe systems generally result in high-quality handwritten medical records. Generally, the physician is accompanied into the patient examination room by the scribe. As the physician elicits a history, the scribe records it. The physician then articulates the findings on physical examination, which are again recorded by the scribe. Although there may be some initial discomfort, physicians using the scribe system have a high level of satisfaction. Beyond documentation, the scribe often assists with procedures and other aspects of patient care.

An obvious drawback is the cost of the scribe system. Adding several full-time equivalents to the payroll may be prohibitive. Although the scribe system is well liked where it has been implemented, it is not in widespread use.

The Transcribed Record

Adequate documentation of the emergency department encounter is far easier to accomplish with the sophisticated technologies now available to the emergency care provider. Transcription methods include transcriptionists and computer-generated voice-recognition systems. Transcribed charting has become increasingly popular. In one study of over 20,000 transcribed records, the average record contained 156 words.[18] The average time to dictate a record was less than 2 minutes. Given the salary and benefits of the transcriptionist and the average time of transcription, the average cost of a transcribed record is probably about $1.75 today.

Dictation Using a Transcriptionist. There are several transcription methods. The handheld recording device provides a simple and effective method of transcription. The system uses a microcassette recorder. This system allows the caregiver to include continuing management, addenda, procedure notes, disposition, and discharge information on the dictation. The cassette is left with the chart and reinserted into the handheld recorder whenever a chart update is required. After completion of the recording, the microcassette tape is attached to the chart or sent to the transcriptionist.

The most popular transcription method is dictation over the telephone to an in-house or contracted out-of-hospital service. In-house or in-department transcription provides the most efficient turnaround times, usually ranging from 15 minutes to a few hours. The out-of-hospital services generally take longer to return the transcribed record, from 1 to 24 hours. Out-of-hospital services use modems to print the chart in the department. The cost for out-of-hospital transcription services can range from $2 to $5 per record.

A further enhancement of this system sends the transcribed record back to a computer at the site of origin. Using a word processor, the physician then has the opportunity to review and revise the chart on-line before printing. Also, misspelled words and other transcription errors can be corrected on-line without marking up the chart. The computer may also be programed to perform quality improvement tasks and provide ICD-9 and CPT coding. This type of computer database provides a great opportunity for medical research.

The dictated and transcribed medical record is an excellent vehicle for documentation. It is easy to use, and the emergency care provider may document a lot of information in a short time. However, it is important to point out that the dictation-transcription system does not guarantee quality records. The dictated and transcribed record is inferior to records created by voice-activated systems.[21] Also, a record with a transcribed history and physical may still require handwritten management and discharge notes.

Emergency care providers should consider ways of improving the quality of these documents so that they may optimize risk management, billing, utilization of services, and other important aspects of care. Consider the following:

1. *Cue cards.* There are preprinted plastic cards available that contain the optimal history, review of systems, and physical examination. This information could be available in the dictation area and used in dictation as a prompt to document a complete examination.
2. *Computer macros.* The transcriptionist can work with macros, which can be physician specific. For the most part, the physical examination contains several normal organ systems, with one or two abnormal findings. The normal systems could be disposed of without having to dictate the entire examination. The physician would specifically dictate the abnormal systems and findings. For example, the dictated words "normal cardiac" would prompt the transcriptionist to press the key that would insert the typical cardiac exam for this particular physician. Establishing such a system carries some risks. There may be a tendency to overdocument by dictating a normal exam when a portion of that exam has not been performed.
3. *Prompted exams.* Prompts for the high-risk diagnoses are helpful. The great strength of the voice-recognition systems is *prompting*. In the case of a sore throat, the prompted system may require answers to questions such as "Is there stridor?" or "Is there trismus?" Prompted systems successfully induce emergency care providers to address high-risk and other critical issues. In a transcription system, a series of preprinted prompts or requirements to be used in dictation for abdominal pain, chest pain, and other high-risk cases may significantly improve the quality of documentation.

In those departments using in-house transcriptionists, 24-hour coverage may be cost prohibitive. Cost-saving alternatives exist for quiet periods, such as the graveyard shift (11 PM to 7AM). Dictation can continue during the shift, and transcription can follow in the morning. Alternatively, charts can be handwritten during the night shift, when volumes are usually low and there is more time for writing. Many departments require that a completed chart accompany patients admitted to the hospital and, in particular, patients transferred to other hospitals. In those cases, chart completion cannot wait for subsequent availability of a transcriptionist and must be handwritten.

Computer-Generated Voice-Recognition Systems. Voice-recognition systems for emergency department documentation have been available since the late 1980s. There has been great enthusiasm for the potential of these systems. They use preformatted templates of basic histories, physical examinations, interventions, diagnoses, and discharge instructions. For instance, the operator tells the computer "sore throat" and the computer quickly brings to the screen a predetermined history and physical examination (H&P). The H&P contains multiple prompts specific to the problem or diagnosis. The user creates a patient-specific record by responding to the prompts by voice (usually), keyboard, or mouse.

Prompting is one of the greatest advantages of this system. Using the example of a patient with chest pain, the user is required to include the quality and location of the pain, presence or absence of shortness of breath, diaphoresis, cardiac risk factors, and so on. Consistent and repetitive prompting educates users on the documentation requirements of many clinical entities, including those that are high risk. This results in high-quality, legible, and comprehensive medical records. In addition, the users may edit the prompts and templates to reflect changing standards of care, address quality improvement issues, perform research projects, and so forth.

There are several other advantages:

1. *Cost savings.* These systems cost between $30,000 and $50,000 each. Compared with the cost of several transcriptionists or purchased dictation at $2 to $5 per chart, the voice-activated system rapidly pays for itself.
2. *Ease of use.* These systems usually work off of a popular or easy-to-use word processor. This allows easy manipulation of text and rapid retrieval of charts from the database.
3. *Twenty-four-hour availability.* The system is always available. As long as the computer is functional there is no downtime. If the department has come to depend on use of these units, the loss of a unit is a significant problem. Companies selling this technology typically have user agreements that replace a unit within 24 hours. This may offer substantial advantages over the time required to hire and train a new transcriptionist.
4. *High-quality documentation.* Records created by voice-activated word processors have been found to be superior to handwritten records and dictated and transcribed records.[21]
5. *Vocabulary.* The earlier versions of these systems had limited vocabularies, and much of what was dictated in free text mode could not be recognized. However, product upgrades have increased the vocabularies to 50,000 or more words. This allows the computer to recognize almost any words the user might dictate.

There are several disadvantages to the use of the voice-recognition technology.

1. *Slow speech.* It is slower to use than standard dictation. Dictation in free text is much slower than normal speech. For the computer to understand the speech the user must speak as follows: "This—is—a—fifty—year—old—male—who—was—in—an—MVA."
2. *Flexibility.* Some users consider the prefabricated H&Ps to be inflexible. Changes can be made through dictation of free text mode or typing. Many users are not proficient typists.
3. *One user at a time.* The user typically generates a voice profile, which must be loaded into the memory before use. The voice profile is individualized and supports a single user. It has not proven practical to switch back and forth between users because of the length of time for loading the profiles and the fact that two caregivers may need to dictate at the same time. Product updates and faster computers have decreased the loading time to approximately 1 minute. Departments using this technology usually re-

quire the same number of computer systems on-line as caregivers on duty actively using the system. Thus if there is double coverage and a triage module, the department may require three units.

4. *Learning curve.* A substantial commitment of time and effort is necessary to get a department up and running on voice-activated equipment. In some departments, the equipment has been purchased and then mothballed.
5. *Overdocumentation.* Use of the prefabricated text may result in overdocumentation. As described in the discussion of computer macros, there is a significant potential to document an exam that exceeds what was actually performed. The user must be intellectually honest and diligent in revising those aspects of the history and physical exam that are different from the predetermined text.

In summary, the computer-generated voice-recognition systems offer many advantages over the handwritten record. With continuing technologic advances, this documentation methodology may become the most popular form of charting in the future.

Structured, Complaint-Specific Encounter Forms

Structured, complaint-specific encounter forms are designed to simplify and expedite chart documentation. The caregivers use complaint-specific preprinted encounter forms that include the key items necessary to address the particular patient complaint. Guidelines for the use of laboratory tests and radiographs may also be incorporated. A check-off system is then used with minimal use of free text.

The development of this format follows the national trend for establishing clinical guidelines and standards, and it conforms to the need for consistent high-quality documentation in emergency medicine. A study performed comparing the preprinted encounter form to handwritten records revealed that the structured problem-specific forms improve documentation, resource utilization, and clinical practice.[22] In a second study, the use of programed charts with complaint-specific entry criteria resulted in improved documentation of history, physical examination, and laboratory studies but did not show any correlation with improved patient outcome or patient satisfaction with the quality of medical care.[23]

The preprinted forms contain check boxes or blanks that prompt the caregiver to fill in the critical data for the specific clinical entity. The forms also contain areas for ongoing assessment. The back of the form contains information important to management of the particular clinical entity. For example, the asthma/COPD flowsheet contains "Guidelines for Management of Asthma/COPD Exacerbations in the ED," and the Closed Head Injury Flowsheet contains a Glasgow Coma Scale for adults and children, indications for radiographic studies, indications for a neurosurgical consult, and other elements.

The forms appear to be user-friendly. This system may be a useful substitute for a handwritten record with certain clinical entities. Because there will not be a form for every clinical entity, handwritten charts will still be necessary. Those using these forms seem satisfied.

The Future of Medical Record Documentation

In the future, emergency departments will access the complete patient files through health information systems. These systems will provide users throughout a healthcare organization information on diagnostic studies, treatments, discharge summaries, operative reports, x-rays, and other stored information. This "point of care" technology will make information available to the user from a variety of sites, which may include the emergency department, freestanding facilities, clinic, and the home. Experts predict the systems will take 10 to 15 years to materialize.[24] This technology will create a virtually paperless system, resulting in improved patient care, increased productivity, and reduced duplication, and it will provide a database for research and outcome management.

Today, bits and pieces of health information technology are making their way into emergency departments. For example, St. Mary's Hospital in Grand Junction, Colorado, has implemented an emergency department document imaging system.[25] The document imaging system dramatically reduces the number of steps in the chart-handling system. With the optical disk–based system, transcription is typed and stored on-line as a data file. The data file includes the laboratory reports and x-rays using a computer output to a laser disk, replacing microfilm. Handwritten documents can also be scanned onto the imaging system.

Users of this system need approximately 2 hours of training. Ultimately, all of the data on disk will be available online in the emergency department. Near-term plans will tie the emergency department with an outpatient, family practice residency center to gain access to ambulatory-patient records.

Emergency department computerized tracking systems have been developed at various centers around the country. These systems allow a real-time snapshot of a patient's relative status within the care process. The emergency department staff has access to information on all patients in the waiting room, their chief complaint, and a date and time stamp. The system tracks all patients currently assigned to beds in the patient care areas, provides the length of time within the department, and can alert staff to retake vital signs or to delays in blood drawing or radiologic studies. The systems are expensive but provide efficient alternatives to present systems.

SUMMARY

Medical record documentation is a significant part of the practice of emergency medicine. In the last several years, there has been an increasing demand for comprehensive documentation placed on emergency caregivers. This trend will continue. New technology is providing an opportunity to improve the quality and legibility of emergency medical records.

Documentation is a learned skill. To develop and maintain the necessary expertise, time and attention must be given during training, quality improvement initiatives, peer review processes, and continuing medical education. Once acquired, this skill empowers the emergency caregiver and creates a new comfort level in clinical practice.

REFERENCES

1. Joint Commision on Accreditation of Health Care Organizations: Accreditation manual for hospitals, Oak Brook Terrace, Ill., 1994 JCACO.

2. Bukata WR: Emergency department medical record. In Henry G, editor: *Emergency medicine risk management,* Dallas, 1991, American College of Emergency Physicians.
3. Hawaii Revised Statutes §221-232 (1990); Illinois Revised Statutes ch. 111 ½, par. 86 (1989); Cal. Health and Safety Code §1317 (West 1991); New York Public Health Law, §2805-b.
4. New Jersey Administrative Code, 8:43G-12.7(O) and 8:43G-12.7(j).
5. Sullivan DJ: Foresight: Ask the experts, *Am Coll Emerg Physicians* 31:6, 1994.
6. Dubnow D: Emergency department discharges against medical advice, *J Emerg Med* 10:513-516, 1992.
7. 42 USC 1395dd(b) (2).
8. 42 USC §1395dd. (West 1983 and Supp. 1991.)
9. Roach WH: Legal review: the medical records implications of state and federal anti-dumping provisions, *Top Health Records Manage* 12(4):83-90, 1992.
10. 42 USC §1395dd(a).
11. 42 USC §1395dd(b).
12. 42 USC §1395dd(e) (1).
13. 42 USC §1395dd(e) (1) (B).
14. 42 USC §1395dd(b) (1) (A) and (B).
15. 42 USC §1395dd(c) (2).
16. 42 USC §1395dd(c) (1) (a) (i) and (ii).
17. *Burditt v. U.S. Department of Health and Human Services,* 934 F.2d 1362, 1371 (5th Cir. 1991).
18. Klimt CR, Becker S, Fox BS, et al: A transcribed emergency record at minimum cost, *Ann Emerg Med* 12(9):556-558, 1983.
19. Dunn JD: Risk management in emergency medicine, *Emerg Med Clin North Am* 5(1):51-69, 1987.
20. Hill MD: Preventing malpractice in emergency medicine: identifying the scope of the problem, *QRC Advisor* 5(12)1-8, 1989.
21. Holbrook J, Aghababian R: A computerized audit of 15,009 emergency room records: an analysis of the quality of handwritten versus dictated records, *Ann Emerg Med* 19(2):139-144, 1990.
22. Wrenn K, Rodewald L: The use of structured, complaint-specific patient encounter forms in the emergency department, *Ann Emerg Med* 22(5):805-812, 1993.
23. Humphreys T, Shofer F: Preformatted charts improve documentation in the emergency department, *Ann Emerg Med* 21(5):534-540, 1992.
24. Harrell A: Building a patient record system, *Health Progress* April 51-54, 1994.
25. Barnett E: CQI and emergency room document imaging, *Healthcare Informatics* April 28-30, 1994.

63 Capacity and Consent

James E. George

OUTLINE

It might seem as if the matter of consent in the emergency department is a simple issue. What patient, after all, would come to the emergency department, but *not* wish to be treated? Certainly, if one does not want to be in the emergency department, there are countless better places to spend an evening.

Unfortunately, not all patients come to the emergency department voluntarily. At one end of this "unwilling patient spectrum" are minor children brought by their parents or guardians. These children often simply refuse to allow the emergency physician to administer medications via the dreaded needle, or may not even submit to the examination at all. At the other end of this spectrum are patients such as prisoners in the custody of law enforcement officials. They may be under arrest for driving while intoxicated and not be apt to cooperate with the nurse or physician who will draw the blood that may furnish the evidence to convict them of the charge. Of course, all manner of unwilling patients are to be found between these extremes.

Patients who are treated without their express consent may have the right to bring battery or other, even more serious, charges against the doctor. On the other hand, patients, even rebellious and obnoxious patients, who are denied treatment may have a cause of action for negligence or, worse, a right to bring a suit under the federal COBRA statute. Understanding the issues of capacity and consent are therefore of utmost importance to the emergency physician.

CAPACITY—AN OVERVIEW

For a physician to legally treat any patient, the patient must have the capacity to consent to that treatment and willingly give informed consent to undergo the procedures, absent any legal exceptions. What is capacity? Simply put, it is the ability to understand and use the information one is presented with to make an informed decision.

One person may have varying levels of capacity at differing times. For instance, an insulin-dependent diabetic may have full command of his faculties and hence full capacity when his blood sugar is within normal limits. However, that same diabetic may have a "diminished capacity" to appreciate the consequences of his decisions when his blood sugar falls. When the patient's capacity to make an informed decision is in doubt, most jurisdictions make provisions for the selection of a surrogate decision maker to make the choice for the patient.

A problem for the emergency physician arises when attempting to determine whether the patient has sufficient capacity to make an informed decision regarding his or her treatment at the time that the decision needs to be made. A good general rule is that if the patient seems to lack capacity, as assessed by objective criteria (Box 63-1), an alternate decision maker should be sought.

If a situation should arise in which the patient's capacity is in doubt, hospital policy or local law will usually provide a hierarchy for choosing an alternate decision maker. A patient's right to make healthcare decisions should not be disregarded. However, where the patient's best interests will be served by appointing a surrogate, one may be chosen from the statutory list (Box 63-2), shown typically in order of preference.

An example of this type of statute, Georgia Code section 31-9-2 (1983), provides that "upon the inability of any adult to consent for himself" the following list of surrogate decision makers should be used:

1. Any adult child may give consent for his or her parents.
2. Any parent may give consent for his or her adult child.
3. Any adult may give consent for his or her brother or sister.
4. Any grandparent may give consent for his or her grandchild.

The statute contemplates that a person who is thus empowered to give consent for another will "act in good faith to consent to surgical or medical treatment or procedures which the patient would have wanted had the patient understood the circumstances under which such treatment or procedures are provided."

Certain classes of persons may be legally presumed to lack capacity to render effective consent. State statutes may appoint a specific official to give consent for these individuals. For example, New Jersey law states: "[The] chief executive officer of a state or county institution for the mentally ill, mentally retarded or of a state or county penal or correctional institution is hereby authorized to give consent for medical, psychiatric, surgical or dental treatment to incompetent patients, or inmates under age 21" (quoting N.J.S.A. 30:4-7.2).

If none of the statutorily authorized persons can be reached, local policy may require the hospital administrator

BOX 63-1

CRITERIA FOR DETERMINING CAPACITY

1. Evidence of intoxication/substance ingestion:
   a. Blood alcohol > 100 mg/dl
   b. Positive urine drug screen
   c. Physiologic signs and symptoms of drug use (constricted pupils, disorientation, diaphoresis, ataxia, etc.)
   d. Positive response to drug antagonists such as naloxone or flumazenil
   e. Reliable reports from emergency medical services, law enforcement, or family members regarding the patient's substance intake
2. Evidence of illness or injury causing diminished capacity:
   a. Head injury, with or without neurologic or motor deficit, with or without syncope
   b. Diabetic history/blood sugar abnormally low or high
   c. Signs of profound shock
   d. Signs of stroke/cerebral bleed with cognitive dysfunction (simple motor deficit alone is not enough)
   e. Signs of developmental disability/retardation
   f. Signs of severe emotional/psychic trauma or mental illness
   g. Alzheimer's disease/organic brain syndrome
   h. Any other condition that might affect the patient's capacity to think or reason
3. Statutorily imposed incapacity:
   a. Minority (the age of majority varies jurisdiction by jurisdiction)
   b. Divorce—a noncustodial parent may not be able to give valid consent for the treatment of a child
   c. Arrest—a prisoner may lack capacity to refuse treatment if law enforcement authorities request that treatment (suturing, blood alcohol/drug levels, etc.)
   d. Any other legally specified situation

BOX 63-2

POSSIBLE PATIENT SURROGATES

1. Spouse (if the patient is currently married)
2. Parent of the adult patient
3. Adult children of the patient
4. Adult siblings of the patient
5. Adult uncle or aunt of the patient
6. Grandparents of the patient

on call to make a decision regarding the care of a legally incompetent patient. A familiar scenario in which so-called administrative consent is usually obtained is when a minor comes to the emergency department without a parent or guardian, the parents cannot be reached, and there is no substitute consent (such as a school medical treatment form) available. When administrative consent is necessary, *all* other attempts to obtain consent should be well documented.

Inevitably, the emergency department will be faced with a situation in which a patient who is incompetent to give informed consent seeks treatment. Although this chapter attempts to give some guidance in the form of the general legal principles that concern competency, the specific statutory and case law will vary from jurisdiction to jurisdiction. Because of the constant change that characterizes the U.S. legal system, it is impossible to give a comprehensive list of rules from which competency may be determined. Therefore it is of vital importance to be familiar with the regulations that govern the particular locality in which you practice.

HYPOTHETICAL CASE 1—"CRAZY DELORIS"

In the middle of the afternoon, an ambulance crew arrives with "Crazy Deloris," the town "eccentric." She is unwashed, covered with loathsome sores, and is harboring several forms of insect life. She also has a large gash on her forehead, which she claims to have gotten from "sticking her head in some place it just didn't belong." She is alternating demands for medical treatment with claims that there is a conspiracy against her at the emergency department.

She is well known in the emergency department and has often left in the middle of assessments or treatment. After a difficult period of questioning, you determine that she is oriented to person, place, and time and that she does desire to be rid of her lice and have her head sutured. Does "Crazy Deloris" have the capacity to consent to treatment?

If your assessment reveals that the patient is oriented and is expressing a desire for treatment, past patterns of conduct probably do not negate demonstrated capacity. If the patient appears to be able to rationally understand the risks and benefits of treatment at the time they are explained, the likelihood that the patient may unjustifiedly fly off the handle after treatment begins does not change the right to make a healthcare decision while rational. It would be wise to document your findings regarding capacity and perhaps have a nurse or other professional witness your assessment.

The Capacity of Minors—A Special Case

A minor is defined as a person whose age falls below a statutorily fixed level. Generally, the common law presumes that all such minors lack the maturity, experience, and judgment necessary to make healthcare decisions. Thus the general rule requires parental consent before performing any healthcare procedure. Unfortunately, as with any rule, the standard does not allow for any deviation for individuals who may not have been considered when the rule was drawn.

In recognition of this shortcoming in the doctrine, the law has evolved to allow limited exceptions for minors who possess the experience and demonstrate the maturity necessary to make healthcare decisions on their own. Such individuals are referred to as emancipated or mature minors. An emancipated minor is considered to have the capacity to consent to medical treatment because he or she is mature enough to understand the full significance of the contemplated treatment. Some minors who are approaching the age of legal majority, some who are married, and those who are self-supporting and living separately from their parents or guardians may be considered competent to consent to medical treatment. The factors to be considered in deciding whether a minor is truly emancipated typically include those shown in Box 63-3.

Most states have enacted procedures for minors who wish

BOX 63-3

DETERMINING FACTORS FOR EMANCIPATED MINORS

1. Age
2. Maturity
3. Marital status
4. Economic self-dependence
5. Ability to understand the nature of the proposed treatment
6. General level of self-sufficiency

BOX 63-4

CALIFORNIA EMANCIPATION CRITERIA

1. The minor is at least 14 years of age.
2. The minor lives apart from his or her parents, with their consent.
3. The minor manages his or her own finances.
4. The source of the minor's income does not depend on criminal activity (Cal.Fam.Code §7120; operative Jan. 1, 1994).
5. The minor has entered into a valid marriage, regardless of whether the marriage has since been dissolved.
6. The minor is on active duty with the armed forces of the United States (Cal.Fam.Code §7002; operative Jan. 1, 1994).

to have a judicial recognition of their independent status. As an example, California law allows minors to petition the court for a declaration of emancipation if they meet the criteria in Box 63-4.

California laws also pragmatically recognize that some minors who are living apart from their parents without their consent (homeless, runaways, etc.) may come to the emergency department seeking care. In the case of such a minor above age 15 who manages his or her own financial affairs (regardless of the source of income), the law recognizes that consent may be validly given (Cal.Fam.Code §6922). The law, ever a realist in California, also allows the treating physician to notify the minor's parents or guardians if the physician has reason to know their whereabouts, without violating patient confidentiality laws.

Aside from the general rules, some state laws grant minors the legal capacity to consent to treatment for certain specified medical conditions. Again, California law makes provisions for this type of consent by minors seeking medical care related to the prevention or treatment of pregnancy (Cal.Fam.Code. §6925), reportable communicable or sexually transmitted diseases (Cal.Fam.Code. §6926), and cases of substance abuse (Cal.Fam.Code. §6929).

A good general rule for the treatment of minors is to attempt to contact the parents before rendering any treatment, unless a specific consent exception is applicable or the patient's condition does not allow the time to do so. (See the discussion of the emergency doctrine in the following section.)

HYPOTHETICAL CASE 2—UNMARRIED WITH CHILDREN

Jane is a 14-year-old who refuses to give a permanent address or the names of her parents or guardians. She comes to the emergency department seeking treatment for a case of gonorrhea. She is dressed in dirty clothing and exhibits poor personal hygiene, suggesting homelessness. At her side is a sleeping 8-month-old infant. Jane claims that this is her daughter, Everlasting Rainbow. Does Jane have the capacity to consent to treatment?

In many jurisdictions, the answer to this question is yes. Often, minors who have children of their own are presumed to have the capacity to offer consent for themselves, as well as their children. The authorities may have to be notified of any reportable disease Jane may have contracted. Additionally, social welfare agencies may be notified of Jane's suspected homelessness or truancy.

In summary, it is important to remember that every decision regarding care should be based on what is best for the patient. If no responsible party can be found to make such a decision for the patient, the emergency physician should exercise his or her best medical judgment. Explaining one's actions in erring on the side of appropriate treatment is infinitely preferable, both ethically and legally, to suffering liability by failing to treat a patient who suffers harm as a result.

CONSENT

Once it has been determined whether the patient possesses the capacity to make a decision regarding care, the next step before treatment is to obtain informed consent. Even if the treatment rendered to a patient meets all the applicable standards of care, the failure to obtain informed consent can still lead to liability for the caregivers. This is because the common law acknowledges that a person has a right to determine what treatment he or she should or should not receive. One of the earliest cases concerning consent to medical treatment recognized that "every human being of adult years and sound mind has a right to determine what shall be done with his own body; and a surgeon who performs an operation without his patient's consent commits an assault, for which he is liable in damages." (*Schloendorff v. Society of the New York Hospital,* 105 N.E. 92 [1914], opinion of Cardozo, J.)

For consent to be considered legally valid, the patient must be informed of all of the attendant risks of the treatment under consideration. Consent given after this type of disclosure is therefore called *informed consent.* Because this is such an important concept, its requirements bear repeating. For consent to be truly informed, the patient must understand all of the following:

- The nature of the proposed treatment
- The risks and benefits of the proposed treatment
- The available alternatives to the proposed treatment and the risks and benefits of those alternatives
- The risks and benefits of no treatment at all

The burden for obtaining this consent falls squarely on the shoulders of the treating physician. However, in the emergency department, it is invariable that emergency nurses will assist the physician with this responsibility. Whoever procures the patient's consent must remember that the patient must be informed of the risks and options available to him or her in a neutral, professionally objective manner. If the information is presented to a patient in a manner calculated to frighten him or her away from a particular procedure and toward another option, the consent may not be considered voluntarily given or may not be deemed fully informed.

Express Consent

The law generally recognizes two types of consent: *express* and *implied.* Express consent is that consent which is directly communicated to the nurse or physician by a competent patient, after the risks of and alternatives to the procedure have been explained. Consent may be expressed in writing, orally, or by nonverbal, nonwritten means.

In the eyes of the law, written consent is best. A typical consent form usually includes a description of the procedure to be performed, a listing of the risks of the treatment, and the available alternatives to the procedure. Other forms simply state that the patient gives his or her consent for "treatment in the emergency department." Any form will contain spaces for the patient's signature, the time and date of the signing, and a space for a witness signature.

Whichever form is used, the fact that the patient has signed it makes it difficult to later deny that consent was in fact given. If the consent is given orally, it should be documented and witnessed in writing. This documentation will have the effect of supporting the validity of the consent if there are any later questions. The following is an example of the statutory significance given to written consent:

Code of Georgia, section 31-9-6(d) (Medical Consent Law): A consent to medical and surgical treatment which discloses in general terms the treatment or course of treatment in connection with which it is given and which is duly evidenced in writing and signed by the patient or other person or persons authorized to consent pursuant to the terms hereof, *shall be conclusively presumed to be a valid consent* in the absence of fraudulent misrepresentations of material facts in obtaining the same. *[emphasis added]*

Implied Consent

Remember that patients who may not be able to write or speak may still wish treatment. For instance, a patient with severe exacerbation of chronic obstructive pulmonary disease (COPD) may be concentrating all of his or her energies on breathing. If this type of patient has the capacity to understand the consequences of a healthcare decision (absent any neurologic deficit or legal disability), he or she can give an informed consent to treatment. Unfortunately, the patient may not be able to express this consent because of the distress or disability.

In such cases the emergency physician does not have many worries about consent issues. This is because consent does not have to be expressly given if it is validly *implied.* If a patient comes voluntarily to the emergency department with a clear medical complaint and submits to treatment without any indications that he or she does not wish to be so treated, his or her actions may imply consent to the treatment.

The key to obtaining implied consent is a reasonable belief that the patient's actions have manifested his or her consent to the treatment. Many times, when a patient complies with any affirmative instruction, such as "open your mouth so I can look in your throat," the lack of a verbalized refusal is the equivalent of implied consent. Of course, as with any type of consent, the patient should understand the risks and alternatives to the treatment.

How far will this implied consent go? Implied consent is a limited doctrine. A patient who limps into the emergency department with a fractured tibia and sits on an examining table has probably given implied consent to stabilization of the fracture, administration of pain medication, and perhaps a radiographic examination. However, later decisions such as the method of fracture reduction would require express informed consent. In any situation where there is doubt about whether the patient has consented or not, it is best to attempt to obtain express, written informed consent.

How Much Consent Is Enough?

The general consent form signed by patients on registering at the emergency department generally provides express consent for an examination. However, when specific procedures are proposed to remedy the patient's condition, other than the prescribing of medications or basic procedures such as suturing, it is wise to obtain additional consent.

For example, parents may sign a general consent form allowing an examination of their febrile child with nuchal tenderness. However, to perform a spinal tap the physician must review the specific risks, benefits, and alternatives to the treatment with the parents and obtain specific consent for the lumbar puncture. Although the parents' silent acquiescence to the tap may be considered implied consent, the far better alternative is to obtain express consent, in writing. Some state laws even make specific provisions for obtaining such additional consent. For instance, Title 31, Chapter 9-6.1 of the Code of Georgia requires such additional consent for the following:

1. Any proposed treatment requiring general anesthesia
2. Any proposed treatment requiring spinal anesthesia
3. Any proposed treatment requiring major regional anesthesia
4. Any proposed treatment involving intravenous or intraductal injection of contrast material
5. Amniocentesis

Other laws require that special types of consent be given for specific procedures. New Jersey Statutes Annotated 45:9-22.2 requires that patients undergoing surgery to explore a breast tumor be offered a specific consent form, allowing one of the following:

1. Consent only for a biopsy of the tumor
2. Consent to any procedure necessary, including mastectomy, if the patient is determined to have a malignancy or "other breast abnormality"
3. Consent for a biopsy and "an additional operation or procedure, if necessary"

Any procedure that goes beyond routine care should be explained to the patient, and express consent should be obtained to limit any potential liability.

The Emergency Doctrine

Courts and legislatures have recognized that the unique, time-intensive nature of emergency medicine sometimes requires relaxation of traditional consent requirements. The patient's clinical presentation may require immediate action by the emergency physician to save or preserve the patient's life. In such a case the patient may be unconscious or otherwise unable to give consent. Therefore a type of implied consent known as the emergency doctrine has evolved. The purpose of this doctrine is twofold. First, it serves to protect emergency medical personnel who act in good faith to preserve life from the traditional liability that would accompany nonconsensual treatment. Second, it encourages those personnel to act decisively in the patient's best interests, without wasting time on unnecessary formalities.

The first requirement for implying consent under this doctrine is that an emergency truly exist. In short, if the patient's life or health is significantly endangered by the medical condition and rapid treatment is necessary to save or preserve the patient's life, an emergency most likely exists. Next, the patient must be unable to give consent on his or her own. Finally, there must be no other surrogate decision maker available, or the time involved in contacting such a surrogate would endanger the patient's life.

If all of these conditions are met, the physician may treat the patient to the extent necessary to preserve the patient's life and health. Be aware that the emergency doctrine will not authorize the performance of elective procedures. Furthermore, if the patient makes an informed refusal before losing consciousness, such refusal may not be negated by the doctrine.

The emergency doctrine is considered so important to the practice of emergency medicine that it has been enacted into law in many states. Although the form varies from jurisdiction to jurisdiction, most statutes conform to the content of the Georgia statute presented as an example.

CODE OF GEORGIA, TITLE 31, CHAPTER 9-3

(a) As used in this Code section, the term "emergency" means a situation wherein (1) according to competent medical judgment, the proposed surgical or medical treatment or procedures are reasonably necessary and (2) a person authorized to consent under (the medical consent law) is not readily available and any delay in treatment could reasonably be expected to jeopardize the life or health of the person affected or could reasonably result in disfigurement or impaired faculties.

(b) In addition to any instances in which a consent is excused or implied at law, a consent to surgical or medical treatment or procedures suggested, recommended, prescribed, or directed by a duly licensed physician will be implied where an emergency exists.

The case law and statutes that have developed to codify the emergency doctrine are invaluable adjuncts to the rendering of emergency care. It is comforting to know that emergency care, provided in good faith and in the light of the practitioner's best medical judgment, will not lead to civil liability for battery or other charges, as long as the requirements of the emergency doctrine are met.

However, the best policy is always to attempt to obtain express consent from the patient or an authorized surrogate decision maker whenever possible. Should one be unable to contact any alternate consent giver, the attempts made to do so should be well documented, witnessed, and made a part of the medical record.

HYPOTHETICAL CASE 3—ADVENTURES IN BABYSITTING

The doors to the emergency department fly open, and a young woman runs in with a blanket-wrapped bundle in her arms. She is not making much sense. You unwrap the bundle and see an approximately 6-month-old infant having a seizure. The child's temperature is 104.9° F.

The young woman is Dawn, the child's babysitter. She states that she is 15 years old and a neighbor of the baby's parents. She moans, "I told them I wasn't ready for this kind of responsibility—I can't even be trusted with a dog yet!"

Dawn tells you that the child's parents will be home in about 2 hours, and that they can't be reached until then. She has the name of the child's pediatrician, but no other information. Can the infant be treated, and, if so, what can be done?

Under the emergency doctrine, the child may be treated for the febrile seizures to the extent necessary to save his life. Blood work, cooling, and the administration of antipyretics and anticonvulsants would be allowed. However, if the parents will be available in 2 hours, it would probably be best to wait until they can be reached before performing a lumbar puncture. If, however, the parents were not expected home for a significant amount of time and the blood work and examination indicate that a spinal tap is necessary, this procedure may be allowed as well.

A Note on Jehovah's Witnesses

Persons of the Jehovah's Witness faith routinely refuse to allow the administration of blood or blood products to themselves or their loved ones, even if such a refusal might have fatal consequences. This practice arises from the biblical proscription in "abstaining . . . from blood" (Acts 15:28,29). Although Jehovah's Witnesses do seek most types of medical care freely, they view this particular biblical passage as prohibiting transfusions of whole blood, packed cells, plasma, white blood cells, and platelets. This prohibition is absolute, and any Jehovah's Witness who receives either a voluntary or involuntary transfusion of blood or blood products believes that they have lost their chance at resurrection and eternal life.

Unfortunately, the patient care benefits provided by the administration of blood or blood products is often not replicable by substitutes such as lactated Ringer's solution. Therefore in certain situations blood or blood products are administered or are sought to be administered to patients who are known to be Jehovah's Witnesses. These cases, in which the emergency physician is acting to save the patient's life, have led to many instances of healthcare litigation. Although a few cases have found liability for the physician in these actions, fortunately, there does seem to be a discernible judicial trend toward the liberalization of the treatment of these individuals.

If the patient makes an informed refusal of blood products and then becomes incompetent to render consent, courts have held harmless physicians who administer blood products in good faith where it was reasonably necessary to save the patient's life. Often, the judicial theory is that the patient may not have been truly aware of the risks of refusing blood products. In other cases, consent was obtained from a family member, or a legal guardian was appointed to consent to the administration of blood.

Every effort should be made to accede to the wishes of these patients. Given the magnitude of their beliefs, it is understandable that they do not wish to violate such an important tenet of their faith. However, this does not mean that the emergency physician's hands are tied when treating such patients, especially because they may arrive at the emergency department without warning and without an opportunity for prior consultation about the risks of and alternatives to refusing administration of blood products. If there are doubts as to whether the patient has indeed given an informed refusal and an emergency exists, the emergency doctrine may imply consent to administer blood products. In any case, if no alternate decision makers are readily available, it may be best to err on the side of treating the patient and preserving life.

Case Studies in Capacity and Consent Law

Miller v. Rhode Island Hospital. In *Miller v. Rhode Island Hospital,* 625 A.2d 778 (R.I. 1993), the plaintiff was involved in a motor vehicle accident on February 12, 1987. At trial, the plaintiff indicated that he had consumed 7 to 12 alcoholic drinks on the day of the accident.

The plaintiff was a passenger in an automobile that was struck by another vehicle. He was not wearing a seat belt. As a result of the accident, the plaintiff sustained lacerations over his right eye, on the bridge of his nose, and on the right side of his forehead. He also incurred a bruise of his ribs.

The plaintiff was transported to the defendant hospital by rescue personnel. At the emergency department, he was evaluated as a "surgical emergency." It was undisputed that his blood alcohol level at this time stood at 0.233.

The plaintiff's fiancée, T.N., was brought into the emergency department, and the emergency physician asked her to consent to treatment on the patient's behalf. Nickerson refused, on the grounds that she was not yet married to the plaintiff. She gave the doctor the name of the patient's sister, who lived nearby. The sister was called, and she arrived within 10 minutes.

The plaintiff heard one physician order him prepped for a diagnostic peritoneal lavage (DPL). He questioned the physician about the procedure, and then stated, "No, I don't want you to do that." The physician allegedly replied that the patient was in no condition to refuse the procedure because he had been drinking so heavily. The DPL was then performed over the patient's objections. The patient sued the hospital, claiming battery. The jury awarded the patient $10,000 in compensatory damages, and $100 in punitive damages.

On appeal, the hospital argued that the patient's intoxication made him incompetent to render an informed refusal. Experts in emergency medicine testified that the hospital's policy of requiring a nonconsensual DPL on any patient who has the required traumatic mechanism of injury and whose mental status is impaired by drugs, alcohol, or head injury met the national standards imposed by the Committee on Trauma of the American College of Surgeons. Both of these issues had been excluded from the jury's deliberations by the trial judge.

The Supreme Court of Rhode Island ruled that "the doctrine of informed consent must, at times, yield to the practical considerations of emergency medical treatment." The damage award was vacated, and the case was remanded for a trial, with the understanding that the patient's intoxication and the nature of the hospital's policy were to be fully explained to the new jury before making their deliberations.

The trial judge attempted to rule that only patients who are legally incompetent to make any sort of decisions for themselves, such as insane persons, may be considered incompetent to give an informed refusal. Fortunately, the Supreme Court of Rhode Island recognized that intoxication can and does affect the ability of patients to make informed decisions regarding their care.

In Re Merrill. Sometimes, a physician or hospital official will seek court-ordered authority to treat a patient who does not have the capacity to consent to such treatment. *In Re Merrill,* 531 N.Y.S.2d 201 (1988), is one such case.

Vera Merrill, a 78-year-old woman, was found wandering near her home, in a state of disorientation. She had not eaten in several days, but she denied having pain or discomfort. She was taken to Binghamton General Hospital and was admitted with a diagnosis of cardiac dysrhythmia. A physician implanted a permanent pacemaker to correct this dysrhythmia, using the implied consent offered by New York State's emergency doctrine.

During the pacer implantation, a suspicious mass was discovered in the patient's breast. The patient's physician had a special guardian appointed for the patient, and then moved in New York Supreme Court (the trial level jurisdiction in New York State) for a court-ordered biopsy and possible further treatment.

The court was presented with testimony which indicated that the patient was "cooperative, coherent, but somewhat illogical." Other testimony tended to show that she was a poor historian, was "hard to understand at times," and was reportedly "disoriented and confused." The special guardian, two evaluating psychiatrists, and the treating physician all concluded that the patient "lack[ed] mental capacity to give her informed consent to the biopsy and subsequent medical treatment." The treating physician did not tell the court that the patient refused the procedures; rather, he indicated that he did not attempt to obtain consent because the patient lacked capacity and could not give valid consent in any case. Additionally, there were no relatives or other surrogate decision makers available.

The court ruled that a court order was not necessary for the treating physician to perform the biopsy or other procedures. Section 2805-d of the New York State Public Health law allows a physician to "take the full responsibility for the course of nonemergency treatment of a person under a disability without judicial authority." The law provides a defense to a battery action if "informed consent is 'not reasonably possible.'"

The court noted that if the patient's physician reasonably felt that the patient was incompetent, such a belief would provide the statutory implied consent necessary to perform the biopsy. On the other hand, if the physician had reason to believe that the patient was competent, the patient's consent should have been sought. In either case, no court intervention was necessary. The New York law does an excellent job of ensuring that physicians may care for incompetent patients with a minimum of unnecessary legal intercession.

Patrich v. Menorah Medical Center. An overwhelming majority of cases find no liability for emergency care providers who use restraints or treat patients against their will when appropriate. *Patrich v. Menorah Medical Center,* 636 S.W.2d 134 (1982), involved claims of assault, battery, and false imprisonment. Mr. Patrich was found unconscious in his apartment by police, who had broken in at the request of a concerned friend. He was admitted to the hospital on August 27, 1976, with the diagnosis of probable self-administered drug overdose.

The emergency physicians and nurses on duty treated Mr.

Patrich immediately for his condition. Over the next 2 days, physicians were able to completely detoxify him. He was also given a Foley catheter and antibiotics to combat partial urinary problems secondary to the overdose. When he regained consciousness, he apparently objected to the continued antibiotic injections, which were nonetheless given with "firmness."

After the patient regained consciousness, it immediately became obvious to the hospital staff that he was mentally ill. As a result of this observation, Mr. Patrich was transferred from the intensive care unit to the mental health treatment area of the medical center. A search of old records indicated he had been treated twice previously for mental illness. His psychiatric diagnosis was given by the defendant as "psychotic depression, schizoid personality severe."

The patient brought a civil suit for assault and battery as a result of the continued antibiotic injections and for false imprisonment in restraining him and transporting him to the mental ward. Mr. Patrich conceded that the actions of the police in breaking into his apartment, the emergency medical services personnel in transporting him to the hospital, and the hospital staff in treating him while he was in a coma were privileged (because of necessity). They were probably authorized as well under an implied consent theory.

The court found that the hospital had a reasonable belief that Mr. Patrich was not competent to refuse the treatment and transfer. They also found that the treatment and transfer were necessary and reasonable to preserve Mr. Patrich's life and health. Therefore the hospital had no liability for assault or battery resulting from the treatment. Finally, the court found that the medical center had legal justification to restrain Mr. Patrich for his own safety, without his consent. Again, this justification was due to his lack of competence to refuse treatment.

The first lesson this case illustrates is the concept of implied consent. We can look at Mr Patrich's unconsciousness as simply another form of incompetence. No one would deny an unconscious patient treatment, if it could be rendered safely. Physicians should be similarly concerned when they are faced with incompetence of a different nature, whether it is substance abuse, mental disease, or hypoglycemia.

This case is also valuable because it shows that, even in the face of a specific refusal of a specific procedure, the hospital was protected because of the patient's incompetence and the demonstrated need for the procedure. Courts look unkindly on plaintiffs whose lives were saved by the administration of necessary care, who then attempt to gain financially from the situation, based on an incompetent refusal.

64 Refusal of Care and AMA

Richard Tobey and Gregory L. Henry

OUTLINE

Common situations of refusal of care
Response to patients refusing care
Informing the patient and AMA documentation
The AMA form
After the patient leaves
Cases

Whenever a patient "refuses" hospital admission, rejects a proposed procedure, or insists on leaving the emergency department before the evaluation is complete, the physician is faced with a dilemma and a myriad of questions. Should the patient be allowed to leave the emergency department, or should the patient be prevented from doing so? If the patient is to be permitted to leave, how may the physician best serve the patient's welfare and also shield himself or herself from the legal consequences of an imprudent patient decision? If the patient is to be restrained in the emergency department or procedures performed against his or her will, how can the physician justify and document such intervention?

Under what circumstances does a patient commonly refuse care? What is the most effective response to a patient's refusing care? How is the patient best informed of the risks and consequences of refusal of care? Just as important, what are the essential elements to document on the emergency department record, and what instructions should be given to the patient at the time of discharge against medical advice (AMA)?

Responding to a patient refusing care requires a good measure of tact, sensitivity, and clinical judgment to arrive at the best possible disposition—one that protects both the patient and the clinician.

COMMON SITUATIONS OF REFUSAL OF CARE

There is no well-defined, extensive profile of patients refusing care or signing out AMA from emergency departments. Only one relevant study is cited in the medical literature.[1] It involves 52 consecutive emergency patients refusing care. Chief complaints in the study were related to chest pain in 41%, trauma in 10%, abdominal pain 6%, headache 4%, orthopedics 4%, genitourinary illnesses 3%, fever 4%, respiratory diseases 2%, and miscellaneous problems in 25% of patients in this series. Fourteen of seventeen patients who could be contacted later stated that they had signed out AMA because they did not agree with the physician's assessment or management plan. Three cited the inconvenience of hospitalization. A study of 107 chest pain patients who left the emergency department against medical advice revealed that these patients' symptoms tended to resemble more a group of patients who received regular discharges rather than a control group of admitted chest pain patients.[2]

One can speculate that patients with milder, less typical symptoms may not share their physicians' perception of risk and may well refuse an admission, especially one intended for the purpose of monitoring or cautious observation and recommended, moreover, by a physician they are seeing for the first time.

Studies of admitted patients who sign out AMA reveal a disproportionate number of young, single, male patients, often with a history of personality disorders, alcoholism, or substance abuse.[3-7] Anecdotally, some patients refuse admission because of concern about inadequate insurance coverage; others are concerned about family responsibilities or the impact an absence might have on their employment status. Refusal of care may be a form of denial or an expression of panic in some patients who, subconsciously perhaps, fear discovery of serious illness. Some individuals become impatient, frustrated, or resentful over long, unexplained waits in the emergency department because they may feel that their illness is not being taken seriously. Finally, a conflict or misunderstanding with a staff member, real or perceived, may precipitate an angry reaction in a patient who is ill, frightened, or in pain.[7-10]

RESPONSE TO PATIENTS REFUSING CARE

Patients who declare their intention to leave the emergency department against medical advice may exasperate the emergency staff. The decision is a rejection of the advice being given and may imply dissatisfaction with the care in the emergency department. An abrupt announcement may also create an unwelcome administrative crisis if staff are actively involved in caring for other, perhaps sicker, patients. In this instance, it may be impossible to respond immediately to the expressed displeasure or demands. In such circumstances it is important to resist having the patient simply "sign the AMA form and go." This is an inadequate disposition and clearly will not protect the patient or the physician should there be an adverse outcome. The patient may later claim not to have understood the risks of leaving. Emergency personnel must understand AMA as a process and not just a signature on a piece of paper. When signing out a patient AMA, the physician should be prepared for a longer and more laborious discharge process rather than the shortcut to departure that might be expected.

An intemperate response is, of course, inappropriate. To threaten denial of future care, to refuse alternative treatments, or to threaten physical restraint (unless fully intended) is self-defeating. Such responses only inflame a volatile situation, inevitably fail to dissuade a patient from leaving, and reduce the likelihood of timely follow-up care.

Although one would hope to be able to persuade all potential AMA patients to change their minds and accept admission or completion of the emergency department evaluation, this will not always be possible. When confronted with a patient threatening to sign out AMA, it is a wise strategy to keep a "second-best" plan in mind. This type of approach accomplishes several positive outcomes even though the patient may ultimately sign out AMA. For instance, the patient might agree to comply fully with alternative treatment and to follow up promptly and might genuinely understand the need to return to the emergency department should the condition worsen. To reach a satisfactory disposition the physician should first mollify the patient sufficiently so that he or she will stay long enough to receive proper discharge instructions. By remaining a friendly advocate for the patient while going through the necessary explanations inherent in the AMA process the patient and the clinician will come to a better understanding of what is at issue. Even if the patient does not change his or her mind, a placated patient will be more disposed to comply with discharge instructions and follow-up referral.

Should the patient be so upset that he or she refuses to stay to receive discharge papers but instead insists on leaving the department immediately, the critical issue is whether or not the patient is "competent." If the patient is competent, then, insofar as possible under the circumstances, he or she should be given verbal explanations of his or her condition and the assumed risks of leaving along with verbal and written discharge and follow-up instructions.

The concepts of competence and consent are beyond the scope of this chapter (see Chapter 63) but are crucial in judging whether a patient is to be allowed to sign out AMA.[9,10] If the patient is unimpaired and able to understand the physician's explanation of the situation and the possible consequences of premature departure, he or she cannot be held against his or her will. One is allowed to restrain patients only if they are, or have the potential to be, a danger to themselves or others based on an evaluation of their mental status.[11]

Often, incompetence, or lack of capacity, is based on a patient's temporary impairment requiring observation (e.g., for alcohol intoxication). Temporarily impaired, intoxicated, or sedated but otherwise healthy patients may be discharged in care of responsible family members, or they must be prevented from leaving until they demonstrate ability to ambulate safely and to care for themselves. The impaired patient with significant illness or injury must wait to be fully cleared of mind-altering drugs before he or she can be allowed to sign out on the same terms as a competent patient. If there is any indication of possible impairment the chart should clearly reflect the patient's mental status and physical capacity at the time of the AMA discharge.

For those patients willing to remain in the emergency department long enough to formally sign out against medical advice the task is less stressful and more clear-cut, provided the patient is indeed competent. The physician should begin by acknowledging the patient's right to make his or her own decisions. The process of going through the AMA form (Figure 64-1) will provide an opportunity to discuss thoughts and feelings that may clarify a particular misunderstanding and perhaps lead to a resolution of the conflict. Frank and full discussion between the patient and the physician, as should occur during an AMA discharge, may be the very communication the patient had previously lacked in a busy emergency department.

INFORMING THE PATIENT AND AMA DOCUMENTATION

Once the physician understands the patient's reason for seeking discharge he or she is in a better position to explain to the patient the tentative diagnosis and the rationale for proposed tests, treatments, procedures, or hospital admission. One should carefully and simply express concern for the patient about not accepting the care proposed. The doctor must explicitly warn the patient of the potential clinical consequences of refusal and specifically include the worst possible outcome. For example, a patient with chest pain who decides to sign out AMA should be warned about heart attack, disability, and sudden death. It is advisable to involve the patient's private physician, family, or friends in the discussion, while simultaneously respecting the patient's rights to confidentiality. The support of family and friends is often effective at calming the patient's fears and may at times be necessary to persuade the patient to follow a prudent course.

Often when patients are discharged AMA, no alternative treatment is provided. This may be a regrettable component of a physician's strategy to coerce the patient into staying. More justifiably the physician may not want the patient to rely on suboptimal therapy or might be concerned about masking a condition with treatment. In most circumstances, however, it is reasonable to be more flexible and provide judicious alternative treatment. For example, oral antibiotics may be prescribed instead of the recommended admission for parenteral antibiotics. This alternative is appropriate if it will not interfere with subsequent assessment or diagnosis, provided the patient has agreed to comply with follow-up arrangements.

The patient should not be ridiculed or made to feel guilty about the decision to leave AMA. The fact that a patient has exercised the right to sign out AMA need not be taken as a personal affront, nor need it be an antagonistic or confrontational matter.

An amicable closure is more likely to lead to a more positive outcome with prompt follow-up and better compliance with discharge instructions. The physician should welcome the patient to return to the emergency department should the patient change his or her mind or should the condition worsen.

THE AMA FORM

The AMA is not a form but a five-part legal process. An AMA chart should look like the physician's formal exam in medical school. Although a "Refusal of Advised Medical Care" form is not required, such a form conveniently incorporates all the recommended elements of documentation, provides a framework for discussion, and thus can serve as a helpful guide.

AMA DOCUMENTATION FORM

(Should have standard number of carbon copies, with a copy being given to the patient)

REFUSAL OF ADVISED MEDICAL CARE

Name ______________________ MR# ____________________
(Person being advised)

Physician ____________________ Date ____________________ Time __________

Care being refused (specify and describe)

____
____
____

Significant risks/complications that may result from refusal of the above care, include but are not limited to the following:

____
____
____

CAPACITY STATEMENT

I, ______________________________, M.D., have personally examined the above named patient and, based upon this examination, it is my opinion that the patient is mentally capable of understanding the risks of refusing care and is capable of making an informed decision.

Signature ____________________________, M.D. Date ________________________

RELEASE

I, ______________________________, acknowledge that on ____________________ (date) ____________________, M.D. advised me of the above-stated risks and/or complications. It is still my desire to refuse the advised medical care stated above. My reasons for refusing advised medical care are:

____
____
____

____________________________ Date ____________________________ am/pm
Signature of patient/parent

____________________________ ____________________________
Signature of witness (family or friend) Signature of witness (staff, not emergency physician)

DISCHARGE INSTRUCTIONS

You are more than welcome to return to this emergency department should you change your mind or should your condition worsen. The discharge instructions that follow are offered as a second-best alternative to the recommended care that you are refusing. (Standard hospital emergency discharge instructions are then appended)

FIGURE 64-1 Against medical advice (AMA) documentation form.

The Five-Part Process of an AMA Discharge

1. Description of recommended care and the risks of refusal
2. Capacity statement
3. Release statement
4. Witnessing the AMA document
5. Discharge instructions

An initial section, completed and signed by the emergency personnel, advises the patient about the specific care or treatment plan being offered and lists the significant risks or complications that may result from the refusal of this care.

There should be a declaration, signed by the physician, stating that the patient has been found to be competent and capable of making an informed decision. The patient is then asked to sign a release acknowledging the stated risks and complications. The patient should be asked to write in his or her own words the reasons for refusing care. This will attest to the patient's understanding of the situation.

The completed form should be read to the patient in the presence of witnesses, including someone accompanying the patient and another member of the emergency staff. The witnesses should then sign the AMA form. When a patient refuses to sign or refuses to even wait for discharge instructions, a witness to the physician's account of the events is particularly important. Although the terminology of the AMA form may seem unduly harsh at times (stern warnings of dire consequences) it is far preferable to sign a patient out AMA than to compromise one's evaluation by allowing a regular discharge. By doing so, the patient may appreciate the importance of the refusal of care. Further, a properly executed AMA form may indicate that the proper legal process has been followed.

A copy of the AMA form is usually not given to the patient. It is generally considered important only for medicolegal purposes. However, it may be advisable to provide the patient with a copy of the AMA form. This form complements the discharge instructions and spells out the issues of disagreement. It also allows the patient a later opportunity to reflect on the potential consequences of his or her decision. Alternatively, the discharging physician should repeat the description of recommended care and the risks of refusal on the discharge form.

It is essential to give the patient standard discharge instructions as well. Include the diagnostic impression, injury or wound care instructions, a list of any prescribed medications, and a referral to the private or service physician. Emphasize and document an invitation to return to the emergency department if the condition worsens or the patient changes his or her mind about accepting advised treatment.

AFTER THE PATIENT LEAVES

The department should consider routine, documented follow-up calls by the emergency department staff. This will ensure that the patient is complying with instructions and will demonstrate the appropriate concern of the staff. All AMA charts should be reviewed by the risk management director of the emergency department.

CASES

The following cases demonstrate the principles introduced in the chapter.

CASE 1—PATIENT WITH UNSTABLE ANGINA

A 52-year-old executive experienced mild central chest tightness with nausea and diaphoresis. He initially resisted leaving work and argued about the need for ambulance transport when the paramedics arrived. The patient finally agreed to go "just to have an ECG." En route, he was placed on oxygen and the symptoms abated.

In the emergency department, the emergency physician took the history and felt that admission was warranted because the nature of the chest pain was suggestive of coronary artery disease. The patient noted that the computer analysis printout on his ECG indicated a "normal ECG." He decided that he should be discharged. When the need for hospital admission was mentioned the patient angrily demanded to sign out of the hospital and began pulling off the monitor leads. The physician acknowledged that the patient had a right to leave and asked for an opportunity to discuss the situation and complete the proper forms. This had a calming effect on the patient.

In the meantime, the patient's family arrived at the bedside and a relaxed discussion of unstable angina, the need for further studies, and the potential complications ensued. The family supported the physician's recommendation. The patient relented only to the point of allowing a cardiologist to provide a consultation in the emergency department. The cardiologist later admitted the patient.

CASE 2—PATIENT WITH HYPOGLYCEMIA

A 28-year-old male patient was brought by police from a local shopping mall where he had been acting in a bizarre and irrational manner. In the emergency department, the patient refused to undress for examination and loudly demanded to be released. He claimed that he was fine and just wanted to go home. The emergency physician was occupied with a multiple trauma case and could not attend the patient.

The initial vital signs were normal, and staff members were unsure how to proceed. The physician told them to complete a screening evaluation, including pulse oximetry and finger-stick glucose. The physician authorized this evaluation "even if the patient objects." The finger-stick glucose was 30, and the patient was treated with intravenous (IV) administration of 5% glucose in distilled water. He became fully coherent, cooperative, and affable and revealed that he was a "brittle" diabetic with frequent bouts of hypoglycemia.

CASE 3—PATIENT DEMANDING PRESCRIPTION

It was a busy day in the emergency department. The nurse informed the emergency physician that a patient was angry at the long wait and was preparing to leave. The chief complaint was "ran out of antibiotics and wants a new prescription." Though other patients had waited longer and seemed to have more urgent problems, the physician attended this patient. The patient told the physician that he had had an argument with his girlfriend and had swallowed a 2-month supply of his isoniazid "just to scare her." He denied having had any intention to harm himself and said he felt fine. He stated that he was now going to leave "with or without the prescription." The patient could not be convinced that this "antibiotic" that he had been taking for several months could possibly be dangerous. He refused IVs, blood work, and gut decontamination procedures. After some deliberation the physician gave the patient access to a bedside telephone and gave him the number of the local poison control center for advice and gave him permission to telephone his girlfriend if he wished. Security staff were posted at the door.

The patient then agreed to be treated. Unfortunately, he had a prolonged seizure before therapy could be started. He was then promptly intubated, lavaged, and given activated charcoal. He required so large a dose of IV pyridoxine that vials had to be pooled from area hospitals.

REFERENCES

1. Dubow D, Propp D, Narasimhan K: Emergency department discharges against medical advice, *J Emerg Med* 10(4):513-516, 1992.
2. Lee T, Short L, Brand D: Patients with acute chest pain who leave emergency departments against medical advice, *J Gen Intern Med* 3:21-24, 1988.
3. Jankowski C, Drum D: Diagnostic correlates of discharge against medical advice, *Arch Gen Psychiatry* 34:153-155, 1977.

4. Long J, Marin A: Profile of patients signing against medical advice, *J Fam Pract* 15:551-556, 1982.
5. Schlauch R, Reich P, Kelly M: Leaving the hospital against medical advice, *N Engl J Med* 300:22-24, 1970.
6. Pennycook A, McNaughton F: Irregular discharge against medical advice from the accident and emergency department—a cause for concern, *Arch Emerg Med* 9:230-238, 1992.
7. Selbst S: Leaving against medical advice, *Pediatr Emerg Care* 2:266-268, 1986.
8. Albert H, Kornfield M: The threat to sign out against medical advice, *Ann Intern Med* 79:888-891, 1971.
9. Griglak MJ, Bucci RL: Medicolegal management of the organically impaired patient in the emergency department, *Ann Emerg Med* 14:685-689, 1985.
10. Mayer D: Refusal of care and discharging "difficult" patients from the emergency department, *Ann Emerg Med* 19(12):1436-1446, 1990.
11. Hill H: Leaving against medical advice. In Henry G, editor: *Emergency medicine risk management,* Dallas, 1991, ACEP.

65 Discharge from the Emergency Department

John D. Dunn

OUTLINE

More than 70% of emergency department patients are discharged from the emergency department, and more than 90% of malpractice cases brought against emergency physicians involve patients discharged from the emergency department.

Emergency healthcare providers have increasingly been burdened with responsibilities for patient education, continuity of care, and follow-up care. We have become the provider of last resort for a portion of the population and, as such, the medical safety net for the society in general. Because a significant portion of the population has no regular healthcare providers other than those in the emergency department, the discharge process must be accomplished with the same attentiveness and consideration as the evaluation and treatment of the patient while present in the emergency department.

CAPACITY TO UNDERSTAND

The courts recognize that patients bear significant responsibility for their own care.[1] Patients are held to have absolute control over their choices of care with a few exceptions, including incompetence, impairment, immaturity, or lack of information. When those exceptions exist, the emergency department and its healthcare providers can be held liable.

If the patient is incompetent or uninformed, that patient's choices and ability to comply with discharge instructions are reduced. For example, if a patient is instructed to take his or her temperature twice a day but has no understanding of why it is important, the discharge instruction might be judged to be inadequate. Discharge instructions might be considered inadequate if the risks and the benefits of a particular instruction are not explained. A failure to assess the patient's ability to understand the instructions because of language difficulties or mental incapacity would also create increased liability for the emergency department staff.

Individuals require special attention and special provisions when they are mentally retarded, intoxicated, or suffering from a condition that might impair their mental capacity even if they are not legally incompetent or declared incompetent. Discharge instructions to an incapacitated or incompetent individual are considered adequate only when a responsible family member or friend can assist and will take responsibility.

In many jurisdictions, minors are considered legally competent to consent for emergency care under certain circumstances. These may include the treatment of sexually transmitted diseases, pregnancy care, and care of mental health or drug and alcohol abuse and chemical dependency problems. Minors may become emancipated in most states by several mechanisms, including parenthood, legal and financial independence, membership in the armed services, or marriage. For example, in most states a 13-year-old with a child can give consent for her own care, as well as the care of the child. The ability of the 13-year-old to understand discharge instructions usually is adequate to allow an emergency department to rely on that individual's competence and capacity.

DISCHARGE PROCESS

The basic principles to be considered in evaluating the adequacy of discharge are that patients should understand their medical condition, their responsibilities, how the illness may progress, and what to do if it does. The patient must be properly warned of the risks and benefits of the proposed treatment. Proper warning includes an evaluation of the patient's or family's ability to understand the instructions, to comply with the instructions, and to consider the risks and benefits of the instructions.

The components of good discharge instructions include the following:

- Issues of understanding
  - Cultural and intellectual capacity of the patient or family
  - Literacy and ability to understand the language of the discharge instructions
  - Ability of the family or patient to comply with the instructions and directions
- Form of instructions—written and verbal
- Follow-up instructions
  - Specificity
  - Home care needs

Language of the Discharge Instructions

The first question that must be answered is, What is the primary language of the patient? There are many circumstances in which English is a second language, and limited knowledge of English prevents adequate understanding of the discharge instructions. This can be resolved by having a translator explain the instructions. The care provider must then document on the record that a translator was used and include the name of the translator. This will demonstrate that a sincere effort was made to enhance the patient's understanding of the instructions. In areas where a language other than English is a commonly spoken primary language, it would be appropriate to have preprinted instruction in that language.

Literacy

It is equally important to present the information in a form understandable to the patient. Healthcare providers often use terms that are not understandable to the lay public. For example, the term *lethargic* is difficult for healthcare workers to define in a consistent manner, so it is probably more appropriate to use terms such as *sleepy* and *hard to wake up* instead. College-educated individuals may know words such as anterior and posterior but be unfamiliar with their use in a medical context. Grade school–educated individuals may have no understanding of technical terminology.

Remember that a significant portion of the adult population is functionally illiterate. The average American functions at the sixth- to eighth-grade level. It is critical to write the discharge instructions in simple, understandable language without using medical terminology. The instructions should then be given verbally with attention to using common words with common meaning to achieve the highest possible level of understanding at the lowest level of education.

Impairment

There are situations in which the medical condition of the patient reduces the likelihood of adequate understanding and compliance with discharge instructions. Some of these situations include the presence of mind-altering drugs or alcohol, underlying dementia, and mental incapacity. Under these circumstances, observation in the hospital or special arrangements for discharge may be necessary.

Provision of subsequent supervision or custodial arrangements may be necessary. Such supervision could be provided by responsible family members or friends who are documented in the chart as being responsible, capable, and willing. Although the absolute determination of custodial care for every impaired patient is not the responsibility of the physicians or nurses of the emergency department, they should adopt an approach that reasonably ensures compliance with discharge instructions. Decisions regarding discharge under the conditions of incapacity and impairment should be documented clearly in the chart.

Written and Verbal Instructions

The instructions should be both verbal and written. The instruction process is the last opportunity for the emergency department staff to evaluate the capabilities of the patient and the family and their understanding of what was done in the emergency department. It is the final opportunity to explain the working diagnosis and the plans for follow-up. Written instructions should be used to reinforce the verbal instructions. Both should provide specific instructions.

Follow-up Instructions

The discharge instructions should include warnings, precautions, monitoring, and specific instructions regarding reevaluation. Loose and unclear follow-up instructions such as "as needed" or "prn" are inappropriate and should be eliminated in favor of specific, relatively rigid criteria for follow-up. Any patient who comes to the emergency department with a potential emergency condition must have a specific instruction and time interval for follow-up. For musculoskeletal disorders, perhaps a few days; infectious diseases may require reevaluation in 24 hours if the patient does not improve; and for other kinds of conditions, a change may require immediate reevaluation. For example, if an infant or child with fever is discharged and the child is expected to improve within the next 24 to 48 hours, the family should be given instructions on the signs and symptoms that would indicate a deterioration of the condition. Other examples include patients with abdominal pain or chest pain who should be reevaluated at specific times under specific circumstances.

Home healthcare follow-up may be an appropriate part of the discharge plan, particularly in extremes of age. The elderly patient with minimal or no home support may require social services and home healthcare follow-up. Again, follow-up requirements should be clear, specific, and relatively rigid.

REFERRAL ISSUES

Referral problems have led to increasing concern among emergency department healthcare providers. This is particularly true for those working on a staff in which the private practitioners begrudgingly accept assignment of emergency department follow-up responsibilities. In these circumstances issues of access, scheduling, and finances may create substantial barriers to adequate and prompt follow-up.

When prompt follow-up is difficult to attain, the emergency department staff should look for reasonable alternatives and instruct the patient on access to those alternatives. One option is to have the patient return to the emergency department as the follow-up resource. Further, the alternatives should be clearly documented on the discharge instructions. This eliminates the possible accusation subsequently that the patient was not provided an adequate follow-up alternative and as a result was unable to obtain appropriate care.

Many cases require specific specialty follow-up, such as casting of a stable fracture. Alternatives should be available even in these situations. For example, a patient referred to an orthopedist may not keep the appointment because of access, a medical complication, misunderstanding of instructions, or a missed appointment. Patients should always be instructed that they may return to the emergency department.

The politics in many medical staffs require that emergency physicians not appear to be encouraging follow-up in the emergency department. However, it is important to give the patient the option because emergency department care is available 24 hours a day. Most other physicians are not able to provide immediate follow-up, particularly for new patients who are not already enrolled in the practice.

These referral problems increase the burden on the emergency department. However, it is critical for emergency department providers to provide their patients with adequate follow-up. The liability issues that arise from a failure to provide a reasonable alternative for follow-up care make this strategy economically a much better choice. One malpractice suit based on an allegation of inadequate follow-up arrangements could consume in defense costs alone the cost of follow-up visits for a year.

TYPES OF DISCHARGE INSTRUCTIONS

Recent concern about appropriate patient discharge from the emergency department has led to an increase in the number of conditions for which departments provide written instructions. For example, it has been customary in the past to provide discharge instructions for such conditions as wound care, head injury, sprains, vomiting and diarrhea, urinary tract infections, and a few other conditions, but other conditions also may warrant written instructions.

Written discharge instructions should be added to include other common and potentially high-risk diagnoses, such as abdominal pain, febrile infants, and chest pain. These may be developed by the staff within the department or purchased from an organization that has instructions printed or available on computer disk. Several companies produce standard sets of discharge instructions, which can be purchased in a variety of forms.[2]

General Instructions to All Patients

Some basic rules about general instructions to all patients include the following.

Limitations of Emergency Care. Patients should understand the limitations of emergency care, and this should be communicated as part of the general instructions on discharge. It should be explained and written that emergency care is episodic and cannot be comprehensive. Complete accuracy cannot be guaranteed because the diagnosis may be difficult to make without a more comprehensive evaluation than is available in the emergency department. Conditions change, and adequate follow-up is necessary.

Diagnosis. Patients should be informed of the initial impression of the emergency care provider. Patients should also be aware of the fact that this is a "working diagnosis" that may be modified by time. The specific discharge instructions attempt to identify potential problems and the need for follow-up.

Referral. Patients must know at the time of discharge that follow-up with a physician or return to the emergency department may be necessary to ensure adequate care for the condition.

Medications. Patients must understand that following instructions with regard to therapy and medications and filling prescriptions is essential to proper management of the case.

Laboratory Tests. Patients should understand that some laboratory tests, such as cultures or special studies, may be delayed. Patients should be instructed that they will be informed of the results but still given a phone contact number. Although some emergency departments instruct patients to call back, this method does not ensure that the results will be appropriately reported to the patient. It is best to call the patient and document the call on the chart.

X-Rays. Patients should be informed that radiologists have special training and skills in reading x-ray studies and that those skills are an absolute necessity in emergency department care. Patients should understand that the radiologist's impression will be the final interpretation of the x-ray and that the emergency physician's initial impression occasionally will be modified by the radiologist's review. Patients should provide a contact number in case it is necessary to inform them of a change in the diagnosis.

Signature. Provide for patient or responsible party signature on the written discharge instruction.

High-Risk Diagnoses

It is easy to develop a list of high-risk situations that create special problems for patients discharged from the emergency department. The list should include nontraumatic chest pain, respiratory distress, changes in mental status, changes in neurologic function (such as sensation, strength, and seizures), febrile illnesses in the extremes of age, abdominal pain, head trauma, headache, pregnancy-related problems, diabetic problems, eye problems, orthopedic injuries, and wounds. Prewritten discharge instructions for common and high-risk problems will ensure consistency and comprehensiveness.

Specific Medications

It is difficult to anticipate and describe all side effects of all discharge medications. Many emergency departments have overcome this issue by using general and prewritten specific instructions. Pharmacies have these instructions available for their patients, and they may be a resource for obtaining these medication instructions. Drug interactions also must be considered.

Specific Follow-up

Follow-up discharge instructions should be specific, with time intervals appropriate for the complaint. Specific complications should be listed with clear instructions, including follow-up intervals, if they occur. As described, it is important to provide patients with reasonable alternatives to remove barriers to reevaluation.

COMPUTER-GENERATED DISCHARGE INSTRUCTIONS

The emergency department with preprinted or computer-generated discharge instructions increases its patients' education and quality of care. Many companies produce standard sets of computerized discharge instructions that can be bought on disk, electronic media, or preprinted booklet. A copy of the instructions signed by the patient and attached to the medical record will demonstrate that the discharge instruction was given. Computer-generated discharge instructions can be signed and then duplicated before being attached to the chart. An additional advantage of computer-generated discharge instructions is that they can be developed and revised as necessary when new information is available.

Standard computer-generated discharge medication instructions may be available from the pharmacy. These can reduce the chance of misunderstanding about medication side effects. It is also an opportunity to limit the likelihood of medication reactions that might otherwise have been overlooked.

AN EXAMPLE DISCHARGE INSTRUCTION

To demonstrate the proper content of a discharge instruction, it is worthwhile to go through the exercise in Figure 65-1. Important things to remember on discharge instructions will be addressed by this example (Figure 65-1).

CASE STUDIES

Ella Crawford sued the Earl K. Long Hospital of Baton Rouge, Louisiana, because of an incident related to emergency care at that hospital's emergency department on August 17, 1975. During an altercation, her son was hit in the head with a baseball bat and stabbed in the shoulder. He was evaluated and treated in the emergency department. He was discharged to the care of his mother, who came to the hospital to pick him up and take him home. Instructions were given to awaken the patient and check him for mental status and comprehension. Mrs. Crawford's son died after being discharged from the emergency department.

Mrs. Crawford brought suit alleging improper and inadequate diagnosis and treatment. Legal issues cited by the Appellate Court in this case were specifically related to the discharge instructions. The court stated in its opinion, "It is proper to release the patient to his home under the supervision of family members or friends." The court also said, "It was also established that oral instructions may be more effective than written, depending on the person to whom the instructions are given. We find no error in the determination of the trial court that the method of giving instruction was adequate." "We are impressed, as was the trial court, with the fact that the nurse insisted that the plaintiff come to the hospital to get her son rather than sending him home in a taxi as was requested by the plaintiff. This insistence conforms with the defendant's contention that the sole reason for having the plaintiff come and get her son was so that home care instructions could be given by the nurse." The Appellate Court therefore upheld the trial court decision in favor of the hospital. [*Crawford v. Earl K. Long Memorial Hospital,* 431 So.2d 40 (La.App. 1 Cir. 1983).]

This situation demonstrates that, even with a bad outcome, appropriate instructions on discharge can support the healthcare providers. In contrast to the Crawford case, each of the following cases demonstrates the converse. In these, large awards were made primarily based on a question in the jury's or judge's mind about the discharge instruction. One should be able to anticipate what discharge instructions might have been provided to reduce the risk. Each should have contained warnings and instructions related to potential complications. Sometimes it is less the diagnosis at the time of discharge than the instructions and expectations that the patient has that are responsible for good and bad outcomes and liability.

A 9-year-old girl was brought to the emergency department at Caledonia Hospital complaining of fever, vomiting, and a loss of appetite. Examination resulted in diagnosis of tonsillitis, and she was discharged with medications. Two days later she began to vomit blood and was taken to another hospital, where severe peritonitis was discovered secondary to ruptured appendix. Plaintiff and her mother brought suit alleging improper diagnosis by the emergency physician. A verdict in excess of 1 million dollars was awarded. [*Hunter v. Caledonia Hospital,* No.1247281 (King's County Sup. Court, April 27, 1982).]

A 17-month-old child was taken to the emergency department with a change of voice, whininess, and shakiness. Examination resulted in diagnosis of pharyngitis, and prescription for antibiotics was given with instructions to see a pediatrician in 10 days. Two and one half hours after being released from the emergency room, the child's crying became hoarse and labored and he suffered a cardiac arrest and was taken to the hospital and diagnosed with epiglottitis. A verdict of 1.3 million dollars was awarded. [*Pitt v. St. Luke's Memorial Hospital,* No.F1-2309 (Wis. Patient's Compensation Panel, Aug. 10, 1985).]

A 5-year-old girl was brought to the emergency department complaining of sore throat, runny nose, and a cough of three weeks' duration. Defendant pediatrician conducted a visual examination of the patient, diagnosed a common cold, and released the patient with a prescription for cough syrup. The patient returned to the hospital 8 days later with a high fever and was diagnosed as having meningitis. The jury in a King's County court awarded 29 million dollars because she had brain damage and a life expectancy of 55 years. [*Marcelin v. St. John's Hospital,* No.24450/80 (King's County Sup. Court, Oct. 1982).]

The legal and medicolegal literature are replete with cases related to emergency department claims of patients who were discharged after evaluation. The discharge process is a critical, medicolegal step in the process of care.

SUMMARY

One indication of an efficient and patient-oriented emergency department is a healthcare team that pays close attention to good discharge instructions. Carefully written and presented discharge instructions provide an opportunity to educate patients, reduce confusion, prevent misunderstandings, and provide quality patient care.

Healthcare changes in the United States require emergency physicians to take increasing responsibility for primary care. It is therefore even more important for emergency department personnel to provide for the safety and continuing care of patients once they are discharged from the emergency department.

Emergency department personnel must understand the following points related to patient discharge and instruct patients accordingly:

1. Emergency care is limited, and a change in condition should prompt further evaluation by a patient's choice of physician or a return to the emergency department of original care.
2. Discharge instructions should include warnings of the complications of the presenting problem. Patients must understand that a condition can get worse. Documented

XYZ HOSPITAL
Instructions for Parents of a Child With Fever

What is a Fever— Temperature above 100° is usually considered a fever. Fever is a normal response to infection. Fever is the body's way to fight infection so do not be afraid when your child has a fever. Fevers can be the sign of minor or more serious infections.

How to Prevent Dehydration— Dehydration occurs when a child does not take in enough fluids. It is important to make sure your child does not develop dehydration. You may reduce the chance of dehydration by having your child drink plenty of fluids. Your child should wear loose light clothing and not be bundled in lots of clothing that may make your child more uncomfortable. Signs of dehydration are weakness, unusually quiet behavior, dry tongue and eye, sunken eyes, soft and loose skin, and a decrease in the amount of urine. A child with dehydration will not have tears when he cries and diapers will be drier than usual.

When a child has a serious infection, there are other changes that you need to watch for. Watch for the following:

* Change in behavior, a loss of energy, development of weakness, and sleepiness.
* No interest in eating of feeding or drinking for hours.
* Poor eye contact or unable to recognize parents and family.
* Crying for long periods or time.
* A high-pitched different sounding cry, jumpiness, or severe fussiness.
* Breathing problems.
* Jerking or a seizure (fit).

Your child has been diagnosed with an infection that can be treated at home. Watch for the problems that are listed above. If your child has any of these problems, have the doctor recheck the child right away. If you are unable to see your doctor, please return to the emergency room.

If your child continues to be sick for more than twenty-four hours and does not improve, then your child should see your doctor right away. Bring along all of the medications that were prescribed.

Medications— Your child was prescribed:

____

____

____

Give all prescribed medicines and complete the prescription. Give Tylenol every four hours in the doses recommended to control the fever. Remember, some fever is okay because it helps the body to fight infection.

Recheck— Your child should be rechecked in ________ hours or _____ days by Dr. ________________. The Telephone number is: _________________. The address is: ____________________________________

Remember, you are welcome to come to the emergency department if you have any problems getting to your doctor.

X-ray and Laboratory Tests— If x-rays were preformed during this visit, the Radiologist will read the x-rays, and we will contact you if there is a change in the official reading. If the results of laboratory tests performed during this visit were not available when you left, we will contact you if there is a change in the diagnosis.

Signature ______________________ Witness ____________________

Date ___ / ____ / ____

Time ___________

FIGURE 65-1 An example discharge instruction.

written and oral discharge instructions that include warnings and precautions are much more defensible for the emergency department.

3. Use simple language with simple instructions. Do not overestimate the ability of people to understand medical terminology and concepts.
4. The nature of uncertainty in emergency medicine requires that intervals for follow-up are short and definite rather than long and vague. Although this does not eliminate patient or healthcare provider responsibility, it does help support the defense of a case in which the patient claims ignorance as the reason for inappropriate follow-up decisions.

These points also emphasize the importance of careful evaluation of unscheduled revisits or repeat visits to the emergency department.

REFERENCES

1. *Kaspar v. Schack,* 237 N.W. 2d 414 (Neb. 1976). Sec State Law on Comparative fault, Texas Rev Civ Stat. art 2212a; N.Y. Civ. Prac. Law Sec 1411-1413; *Hoffman v. Jones,* 280 So. 2d 431 (Fla. 1973), *Crawford v. Earl K. Long Memorial Hospital,* 431 So.2d 40 (La.App. 1 Cir 1983).
2. Aftercare by Micromedix, Denver, Co; Checkout by Logicare Corp., Eau Claire, Wisc; Emergency Patient Instruction Compiler by Epic Software Inc, Ashland, Or.

66 Complaint Management

Robert W. Strauss

OUTLINE

People complain when they are dissatisfied. Add the anxiety, confusion, and potential peril of an emergency and the number and seriousness of complaints increase. For example, a tearful 2-year-old with an earache and fever is brought to the emergency department by his mother. After waiting 3 hours, the child is seen by a hurried nurse and then once (for 2 minutes) by a physician who performs a limited examination and barely speaks to either mother or child. The patient is discharged on a very expensive antibiotic and 2 days later still has a fever and has developed a rash. The private physician states, "I can't believe they put you on that medication for an earache!" Two months later, a very dissatisfied parent receives a bill for $200.00. She is angry and on the phone waiting to speak with you.

Complaint recognition and management are critical components of the successful emergency department manager's armamentarium. When handled properly, a dissatisfied and angry person can achieve satisfaction. Alternatively, the improper management of a complaint can lead to a disgruntled person who seeks retribution.

The benefits of effective complaint management go beyond meeting the perceived needs of the individual complainant. Institutions that recognize the importance of consumer opinion seek opportunities to improve by taking steps to reduce the root cause of dissatisfaction.

To address these issues, this chapter is divided into three sections. The first section describes who complains and why they do. It includes the most common reasons for complaints and methods of prevention. The second section describes a successful method of complaint management. The processes and tools necessary to implement the system are provided. The third section is a supplement that reviews several classic emergency department complaints. Underlying issues and methods of resolution are presented.

EMERGENCY DEPARTMENT COMPLAINTS

All emergency departments receive complaints. Inevitably, some people will voice their dissatisfaction with the quality of care, length of stay, attitude of providers, or cost of care. The approach of the department leadership and the institution toward the receipt and management of these complaints distinguishes the providers seeking improvement and satisfaction from the providers destined to repeat mistakes. To develop an effective approach, it is necessary to first understand why people complain.

We all experience dissatisfaction with some interactions because "reasonable" expectations go unmet. The emergency department is particularly prone to create dissatisfaction among those who use its services. Patients, private physicians, emergency medical services (EMS) providers, and staff all cross the threshold with expectations of rapid, quality care by an attentive and kind staff. Unfortunately, it is impossible to always meet these expectations.

The Complainer

Why do people complain? Generally, people are dissatisfied because their expectations go unmet. When, in addition, they perceive that they have been inconvenienced and treated rudely, they are much more likely to voice their dissatisfaction in the form of a complaint.

Brief Relationship. Although the reasons for patient dissatisfaction are myriad, certain generalizations can be made. The duration of the relationship between the healthcare provider and the patient is positively correlated to patient satisfaction.[1,2] The longer the relationship, the more satisfied the patient. The relationship between an emergency care provider and the patient is measured in minutes rather than years. This brief exposure allows little opportunity to develop the bond that may exist between a patient and a private physician.

Effective Communication. Patient expectations of healthcare providers go beyond that of clinical competence. Patients expect their practitioners to be friendly, kind, and concerned and to take the time to explain the situation and answer questions.[3] In the stressful setting of the emergency department, the ability to develop a rapid rapport with the patient and family will enhance patient satisfaction. The greatest number of complaints lodged against healthcare workers in an emergency department are related to attitude and poor communication.[4]

It follows that those healthcare providers who adequately explain the nature of the problem or procedure are found to score higher on patient satisfaction scales than those who do not.[1,5,6] More complete explanations create a better understanding and more realistic expectations of the course and outcome. An understanding of the likely course allows the patient and family to participate more actively in the continuing care. In addition, those who are encouraged to and actually do ask questions about their illness are more satisfied.[1,3,6]

The Demographics of Complainers. There is substantial literature reviewing the characteristics of the complainer. Considerations of age, sex, and income levels are frequently cited.[2,4]

The relationship between age and complaint behavior is unclear.[2,4] Although it has been suggested that the elderly are less likely to voice a complaint, this has not been substantiated in several studies. The gender of the person registering the complaint is more likely to be female. This may relate to the fact that women are more likely to be involved in family healthcare decisions.

Those with higher incomes voice complaints more often and are more likely to choose another provider.[2] This may result from higher expectations, greater resources, and increased options to obtain alternative providers of care.

Reasons for Concern

Successful delivery of emergency care entails recognizing our responsibility to address the needs of those using our service. There are many ramifications of dissatisfied and complaining patients, peers, and customers. The emergency department census may drop, medicolegal cases may increase, and ultimately the ties between the practitioner and the institution may be severed.

People who are dissatisfied with your service have three choices.[7] They may "voice" a complaint, choose another provider ("exit"), or continue to use the service despite being dissatisfied (remain "loyal"). Interestingly, loyal but dissatisfied consumers are considered passive, seeming to "suffer in silence."

Many dissatisfied people do not complain.[5,8-10] They don't express their dissatisfaction because they believe it is not worth their time and effort, they don't know how or where to complain, or they don't believe it will do any good. In fact, fewer than 25% of patients with dissatisfaction voice a complaint to the service provider.

Many of these "noncomplaining" consumers may have a more subtle impact. Although unwilling to complain to the service provider, they may complain to friends and family, influencing their behavior and creating "negative word of mouth."[11] Further, they may seek satisfaction from third parties, such as governmental agencies or the legal system. Finally, they may choose other providers as suggested by the following passage[12]:

> "You know me, I'm a nice person. When I get lousy service, I never complain. I never kick. I never criticize and I wouldn't dream of making a scene. I'm one of those nice customers. And I'll tell you what else I am. I'm the customer who doesn't come back. I take whatever you hand out because I know I'm not coming back. I could tell you off and feel better, but in the long run, it's better to just leave quietly. You see, a nice customer like me, multiplied by others like me, can bring a business to its knees. There are plenty of us. When we get pushed far enough, we go to one of your competitors."

Census Impact. Exit, or changing providers, once a relationship is well established is difficult and requires substantial effort.[2,13] However, recent literature reveals that up to 63% of patients change physicians when dissatisfied.[10,14] This is much higher than had been previously demonstrated. Those with medical (quality of care) complaints are twice as likely to seek alternative providers as those with nonmedical (administrative, length of wait, attitude) complaints.[2]

As the environment becomes increasingly competitive, patients may find the option of changing providers more attractive. This is particularly true in an emergency department setting because

- The provider-consumer relationship is superficial.
- Interactions occur unpredictably.
- The consumer's absence will go unnoticed.
- Many alternatives are available.

In the emergency department, a contraction of census will decrease the need for service providers, including nurses, physicians, and support staff. For an emergency physician group that exists within a fee-for-service environment, a dwindling census may be devastating. For employed emergency physicians and emergency nurses, fewer patients may obviate the need for their positions.

Medicolegal Implications. Third-party actions are increasingly viewed as an acceptable method of seeking satisfaction. Multiple agencies have created systems to receive and respond to consumer complaints. These include the Office of Consumer Affairs, Better Business Bureau, and state medical societies. There is an increasing tendency to use the legal system to seek redress.

Consumers have a greater tendency to seek third-party actions when they perceive that more direct interaction, such as voicing a complaint, is unlikely to lead to resolution. Consumers perceive healthcare providers to be among the least responsive to complaint resolution among the service industries.[13] Only about one third of the consumers who voiced complaints believed their problems were satisfactorily addressed.[8] As a result of not handling or mishandling complaints, we unwittingly encourage third-party actions.

Contract/Job Security. If there is a perception of ineffective problem management, your relationship with the institution may become tenuous. Effective administrators expect problems to be found and solved. They develop procedures that improve the system. Emergency care providers in management positions must participate in this process of improvement, or, by their avoidance, they allow these problems to continue unabated.

Nonparticipation will be perceived as an "I don't care" attitude, which is often the reason for the complaint in the first place. Hospital administrators, managed care organizations, and others may react decisively against unresponsive individuals and organizations by looking for alternative contractual relationships.

Consumers dissatisfied with the medical care are unlikely to voice their complaints and easily change providers. They are least satisfied with the response to their complaints and most ready to invoke third parties, including the legal system, when dissatisfied with the response. Unfortunately, although third party actions are particularly prevalent in the medical industry, these actions seem to have little impact on the providers.[13]

The Regulatory Imperative. Regulatory agencies look at problems, the systems used to handle those problems, and the methods to prevent their recurrence. The presumption is that if you have an effective system you will recognize and resolve the problem, at least, and preferably prevent it.

The Joint Commission on Accreditation of Healthcare Organizations (JCAHO) looks specifically at the institution's complaint management process. Reviewers often specifically ask for evidence of the system. The JCAHO requires that guidelines regarding complaint management be incorporated into the organization's procedures. The following passage is an excerpt from the 1996 Accreditation Manual for Hospitals[15]:

> The hospital has a formal process for reviewing patient complaints and helping to resolve conflicts. This process includes a plan to inform patients and their families of their right to make complaints and how to go about having them resolved. . . . Those issues that cannot be resolved in this manner are referred to the hospital administration for intervention.

Other regulatory bodies such as the New York State Department of Health further define the process necessary for institutional complaint management. In code 405.7.23, the regulation states[16]:

> The hospital shall afford each patient the right to: . . . express complaints about the care and services provided and to have the hospital investigate such complaints. The hospital shall provide the patient or his/her designee with a written response if requested by the patient indicating the findings of the investigation. The hospital shall notify the patient or his/her designee that if the patient is not satisfied with the hospital's oral or written response, the patient may complain to the New York State Department of Health's Office of Health Systems Management. The hospital shall provide the telephone number of the local area office of the Health Department to the patient.

We are responsible for developing and implementing a mechanism to promptly receive and respond to patients' and families' complaints. The organization must thoroughly analyze the complaint and when indicated take appropriate corrective action. The patient or family member making the complaint must receive a response that substantively addresses the complaint.[13]

Providing Satisfaction

Our job entails providing high-quality care while satisfying the perceived needs of those around us. It is helpful to look at patients, colleagues, staff, and others who use and interact with our service as customers. This business philosophy enables us to look closely at what our patients and others as a group and as individuals want from us. To do this, it is necessary to first define customer satisfaction:

> **Prepurchase expectations of the product or service are met or surpassed.**

We can create satisfaction only by meeting, surpassing, or modifying expectations.

Patient Satisfaction. The ultimate goal is patient satisfaction. And yet, so often, we create dissatisfaction by raising expectations. An emergency physician says, "The nurse will discharge you in *a minute*." An emergency nurse says, "The doctor will be in to see you in a *few seconds*." A private physician says, "Just go to the emergency department and get an x-ray." The inexperienced patient may believe this will be a 10-minute excursion. If it takes an hour and the patient did not plan for it, every little additional delay creates frustration.

Patients are customers and we offer a service. If it is not delivered properly, we will lose our customers. Webster's defines a customer as "a person who purchases a commodity or service." Unfortunately, some practitioners who work in the emergency department reject the concept of patients as customers. This disregard is a form of arrogance that essentially communicates: "I'm in control. If the patients don't like what I say or how I say it, they can go somewhere else."

Are patients fundamentally different from people who buy computers, gas, or food? A person who comes for treatment of a broken toe and the one who orders food in a restaurant both want service delivered quickly, courteously, with quality, and at a fair cost.

PATIENT EXPECTATIONS. Patients want the same things that all customers want—the four *C*s: convenience, caring, care, and cost.

- *Convenience*. When patients have a choice about emergency care, they tend to choose the place that will get them in and out most quickly. Interestingly, healthcare providers rarely have the patience to wait in the waiting room of their own emergency departments when they or their family members are ill.
- *Caring*. We must develop rapport quickly. The success of our treatment approach once the patient is discharged depends on the trust we have developed. Our patients judge us most often based on the level of caring rather than the level of care.[5,10]

  Caring goes beyond giving a high standard of care. The classic response, "I did everything correctly; just look at the chart," just isn't good enough. And, when dealing with people and complaints, the complaint manager initially must focus on how the process did not work for the patient (complainer) rather than trying to provide education while defending the process.
- *Care*. Generally, the lay public cannot judge the quality of care provided. Consider how difficult it is for an unsophisticated consumer to assess whether the examination was complete, the testing was appropriate, or the antibiotic was the best. It is only when the outcome is poor and unexpected that questions arise, perhaps even leading to questions of competence. Therefore it is critical to recognize the patients' expectations and meet, surpass, or modify them. It is often expedient to both say and document: "You should improve with this treatment. If you are not better in __ days or you get worse, I would like you to immediately see your doctor or come back here."
- *Cost*. Value is the important issue for those who use our service. If a patient waited for hours, was treated rudely, or got worse in spite of treatment, the cost of care may seem inappropriate no matter how inexpensive. Alternatively, patients who perceive that they received value—

treated quickly, courteously, and correctly—are much more willing to pay a reasonable bill.

COMPLAINT PREVENTION TECHNIQUES. Though it is not always possible to meet patients' initial expectations, we have many opportunities to modify or reset patients' expectations.

Realistic Triage. Triage provides the first opportunity to recognize and influence the patient's expectations. We know that the most common complaint is related to duration of stay. We also know that patients typically have unrealistic expectations based on a poor understanding of the process. The triage nurse may positively modify the patient's expectations by spending a few extra seconds to explain what will happen to the patient.

For example, to a patient requiring an x-ray, the nurse could explain: "From here you will be registered and then wait in the waiting room until a bed is available. Once you are in the examining room, you will receive a more in-depth evaluation by both the RN and the MD. If an x-ray is necessary, it will be ordered. Once taken, it will be read by the physician who will determine your treatment and follow-up. You will then get discharge instructions from the nurse. Generally, the entire process takes an hour. Do you have any questions?"

It is appropriate to add a few minutes to the estimate of the patient's duration of stay to allow for the interruptions that typically occur in an emergency department. If the evaluation is completed sooner, the patient is thrilled and you have surpassed the now "modified" expectation.

Triage Ordering. Operational protocols that empower the nursing staff to order necessary, ancillary tests and begin treatments on patients can dramatically reduce the duration of stay. An x-ray or lab test that has been completed by the time the patient arrives in the examining room will reduce unnecessary waits.

Resetting Expectations. Once triaged, patients expect rapid care. Often, however, it is not always possible to meet this expectation. There are several appropriate opportunities to modify the patient's expectation during the wait. After a particularly busy time, such as a resuscitation, the nurse or physician may go out to the waiting room with two or three charts in hand. An apology for and explanation of the delay—displaying respect and providing a legitimate reason—are usually very much appreciated. Then bringing two or three people back to the emergency department proper will confirm that the situation is improving.

Once a patient is in an examining room, the same outcome can be achieved on an individual basis. "Hello, Mrs. Jones. I am Dr. Smith. I know you have been waiting a while. I am taking care of a very unstable patient and expect to be back with you in about 20 minutes. In the meantime, I will ask the nurse to make sure we get your evaluation started and keep me informed." The caveat is that if you reset the expectation by providing a specific time, you must be there at that time or send someone in to say it will be a little longer.

Just Say YES. It is often helpful to begin the response to a request or inquiry with a form of "YES!" Consider the following response to a patient asking for something unreasonable: "No, you don't need that." The message is that I am the trained specialist and I know what you need. Once you start with "No" the communication begins to deteriorate and it becomes increasingly difficult to further develop a therapeutic relationship. Alternatively, according to the "Yes" theory, one might respond by saying, "Yes (Sure), I can see that it is bothering you. Let me take a closer look so that we can figure out exactly what is wrong." The communication now is one of acceptance. The practitioner has agreed to work with the patient to further elucidate the problem without actually agreeing to meet the unreasonable request.

The Unnecessary Test. You've examined the patient and believe that he or she does not need an x-ray or a lab test, but the patient is convinced that it is necessary. What do you do? When practical, one usually successful strategy is to involve the trusted private practitioner in the discussion. However, on occasion, it may be appropriate to provide the desired test. The patient will leave satisfied and believing that you cared enough to make sure that he or she is OK. This is not substantially different from the practice of most practitioners who obtain ankle, knee, or cervical spine films that are of questionable necessity.

Closing Questions. It is a good practice for each practitioner who participates in the discharge of the patient to routinely ask, "How else may I help you?" or "Is there anything else I can do for you?" Occasional patients, if given the opportunity, divulge their true concern only at the end of the visit, such as "Can I get a work excuse?" or "Is it cancer?" Without that final opportunity to ask the question, the patient may leave dissatisfied. Other patients may notice or describe an additional complaint, such as "What about my wrist?" that may have been previously overlooked. Most often, the patient will respond with a "No, but thanks." The closing question allows the patient and the practitioner to come to a definitive closure.

Other Customers

ADMINISTRATION. The hospital administration runs a service business. A service business, to be responsive, must listen to its customers. Included among the most influential groups are the patients and their insurers, who use the service and pay the bills; the primary care physicians and orthopedists, who control which of the paying patients will use the hospital's service; and the hospital board of trustees, the institution's governing body, which directly oversees the administrator. Notice that the emergency care providers are not among the most influential groups.

What does the administration typically want from the members of the emergency staff? They want problem solvers who do not generate a lot of complaints and who keep the influential customers—the patients, physicians, and the board—happy.

When an effective emergency complaint management system exists, the process of handling a complaint follows a well-worn path. On receipt of an emergency complaint (written or oral) by the administrator or anyone else in the hospital, it is immediately forwarded to you or your department's complaint manager for resolution. That is because every time it has been forwarded to you in the past, it has been handled immediately with rapid proclamation (in writing) of resolution. The appropriate management of complaints, including trend analysis (which might point out certain deficiencies), cannot be overemphasized as one of the key tasks of the emergency department leader.

EMERGENCY STAFF. The emergency staff requires leadership that solves problems. For instance, if a nurse or physician comes to you as an emergency leader and states that he or she is having a problem with another person or a process, you must make efforts to resolve the problem. These issues generally do not go away and if ignored erode the confidence of the staff toward the department leaders. If you do not at least attempt to find a resolution, you become part of the problem.

The Disney Corporation describes a customer service concept called "on-stage, off-stage."[17] According to the concept, when the service providers (employees or emergency practitioners) are "off-stage" they may be themselves, but when they are "on-stage" they must always be in character. The emergency care practitioners' on-stage role is to make people feel better. Those who believe their only responsibility is to take care of patients may mistreat their colleagues. In other words, "on-stage" does not begin when you walk into the patient cubicle; it begins when you walk into the hospital.

THE COMPLAINT MANAGEMENT SYSTEM

Successful complaint management systems contain consistent components. This section will examine each of the following components in detail:

- Positive approach demonstrating sincerity and concern
- A system to track, investigate, resolve, and document the complaint
- Follow-up and reporting mechanisms
- A compliment tracking system

The Approach to Complaints and Complainers

A positive approach to this sometimes unpleasant task can be the best tool you have for improving others' perceptions of your services. People who complain are looking for something they did not get during their first interaction with your system—satisfaction. By calling you, the complainer is providing you with a challenge and an opportunity to transform the previously dissatisfying interaction into a favorable one. A response that conveys the sentiment, "Oh no, not another complaint!" will confirm the complainer's misgivings. Alternatively, an open and sincere approach that conveys the sentiment, "I want to satisfy your needs" will demonstrate caring and concern.

Real-Time Management. If presented with an opportunity to rectify a situation while it is occurring, try to achieve immediate reconciliation. Five to ten minutes spent now getting a situation back on track may obviate hours of investigation and embarrassment later.

Most practitioners recognize when a patient is frustrated and dissatisfied. Effective responses may take several forms. When certain that the patient is upset, the practitioner may simply observe, "You seem upset, may I help?" Alternatively, send in a colleague to confirm and investigate the perception of an angry or dissatisfied patient. A problem uncovered may be resolved. Left unresolved, the patient will leave dissatisfied. The dissatisfaction may develop into frustration and anger resulting in a complaint voiced directly to someone in the institution or indirectly to friends and acquaintances. Also, unresolved dissatisfaction is likely to result in the patient's seeking alternative providers in the event of subsequent need for services.

Tripping the System. Determining which complaints require a formal process of resolution is individual to each institution. This is one of the reasons that it is difficult to objectively compare the volume of complaints among institutions. Should a comment such as the following be included in a formal complaint process? "My patient Mrs. Smith says that she had to wait to be discharged because your emergency doctor/nurse was on the phone ordering dinner!" Should complaints from a "repeater" patient who comes to the emergency department every Saturday night to get warm and sober be taken seriously? What about the patient who comes to the emergency department two or three times a week for a migraine who says that Dr./Nurse Peterson was rude and wouldn't give the normal dose of Demerol?

What do you do with "bogus" complaints? How do you separate legitimate from groundless complaints? It's like asking what is a true emergency. Is it our definition or is it the patient's? The same is true for complaints: they are all legitimate from the perspective of the complainer.[19] It is my contention that more rather than fewer complaints should be included in the formal system of complaint management.

Handling the Complaint. Unfortunately, the staffs of most organizations react adversely to complaints, ignoring them, leading to denial, which in turn leads to perpetuation of the problem. Complaints are most appropriately viewed as an asset. On one hand, complaints create additional and sometimes difficult work for the complaint manager. On the other hand, the person who calls and lets you know that your system didn't work cares enough to let you know and has the great potential to be satisfied.

The person managing the complaint should demonstrate concern, sincerity, and empathy.[13] The handler must convey the feeling that the issue is important to him or her. In one sense, we are all experts at handling complaints. We do it all the time as part of our routine in the emergency department when we try to figure out how to solve the patient's medical problem. It is simply a matter of putting the same effort into managing the complaint as you do to resolve the medical problem. Even the questions "How may I help you?" and "How did it happen?" are similar. Attempt to make the complainants feel important.

The complaint manager may be able to give the complainer a sense of great value. The message should be some form of: "Thanks for letting me know . . . This is a real concern to me . . . I'm going to investigate this now and get back to you." Complaint managers who are continuously trying to improve their systems may with sincerity say, "Your call comes at an opportune time. We are looking at ways to improve our service. What happened? How is he/she doing now?" This type of attitude displayed to a complainant may actually transform the complainer's self-perception from a slighted, depersonalized object into a valued consultant.

You have taken the first step in resolving the complaint.

Determining the Issue. The second step is to find out what the complainer really wants. This can be accomplished only by hearing it from the complainant's perspective. Allow the person to leave the conversation thinking "I'm glad I called, I've made a difference."

People with complaints want one or a combination of the following:

- *Respect and understanding.* It is necessary for complainers to believe that you sincerely want to hear and resolve the issue—that it is important to you. Empathic listening may itself provide the caring and compassion that were missing from the initial interaction, which in many cases is all the complainer wants.

- *Immediate investigation and follow-up.* You will demonstrate your sincerity to a complainer by agreeing to perform an immediate and thorough investigation and promising rapid follow-up. This approach conveys a powerful message: "Your issues (you) are so important that I will address them immediately and report back to you." A neglected person who has been frustrated by the system is now able to establish some control.
- *Censure.* Some complainers have been so slighted by the process that they believe satisfaction can best be achieved by some form of punishment, reprimand, or censure. These people want to know that the responsible person "will pay the penalty." This most often occurs as the result of uncaring, inattentive, or rude behavior exhibited by caregivers. (See Dr. Jerkyl later in this chapter.)
- *Assurance that the problem will not recur.* It is very satisfying to conclude an interaction knowing "I've made a difference." If the complaint manager is able to transform the complaint into a system or a behavior change, the complainer can walk away with the feeling that he or she has improved the system and the care rendered to others who follow.
- *Reduction of the bill.* Many complaints occur at the time the bill is received. For a variety of reasons the patients may not believe the service rendered justifies the bill received. These patients will want reconsideration of the amount. They may be satisfied with a negotiated reduction of the bill. Some will ask for complete elimination of the bill, and a few may even request compensation. (See Dr. Mercedes later in this chapter.)

The System

To achieve the greatest success in complaint management and effect the greatest system improvements, it is necessary to formalize the complaint management process. This entails the development of the following:

- Complaint manager
- Situation assessment form and process
- Follow-up and reporting mechanism
- Log

The Complaint Manager. It is necessary to identify a single person to assume responsibility for the overall management of complaints. Only in this way can the process be consistent. Further, the development of the position and title encourages all potential recipients of a complaint to immediately direct the complaint to a single place and person. As stated, the complaint manager must be someone who has the authority and the leadership skills to create change.

Preferably, the complaint manager will be the director or associate director of the department—someone with the imprimatur of leadership and authority. Of course, if a complaint is received about the person who typically handles the complaint, it is most appropriate for another person to perform the investigation.

The Situation Assessment Form and Process. An example situation assessment form is provided in Figure 66-1. It is presented as a single page for the convenience of the reader. The situation assessment form is invariably longer, sometimes requiring several pages to thoroughly document the assessment.

IDENTIFYING INFORMATION. Identify the patient by name and medical record number. In addition, the patient should have an identifying number particular to the log system. The practitioners should also be identified by a number, rather than by name, when referring to them in the body of the situation assessment. For instance, in the example that follows, Dr. Smith is referred to as "emergency physician #107", and Nurses Jones and Peters are referred to as "emergency nurses #2214 and #1020", respectively.

DATES. Delineating the dates of service, complaint, and resolution may be helpful in many ways. A complaint expressed immediately after care is rendered implies a problem with the care or caring. A complaint articulated months later may relate more to the receipt of the bill. A review of the average time between date of complaint and date of resolution will measure the efficiency of the system.

In some institutions, particularly those in which the complaint is not immediately forwarded to the emergency complaint manager, it is necessary to have lines for both date of complaint and date complaint received.

TYPE OF COMPLAINT. Differentiating the type of complaint into various types, such as quality, attitude, and length of stay, allows data trending. Simply look at the most common types of complaints received over the previous year to create your list. A single complaint may involve more than one type.

SOURCES (INITIATED BY). Anyone can be the source of a complaint. Entry into the system should be easy—patient (oral or written), physician (directly or by word of mouth), or a staff member. A legal inquiry may uncover a problem of care. Routine chart reviews, such as 72-hour return visits, may identify possible problems of care and become an entry point into the system.

THE ASSESSMENT. The actual assessment contains three components—the issue, investigation, and resolution. As stated, the assessment may require several pages to thoroughly document the information gathered.

Issue. This issue is obtained by discussion with the complainant and review of the records. It should be described from the perspective of the complainant but documented in an objective manner. For instance, a patient might state, "The doctor was a jerk and treated us like animals!" This could be documented as, "The patient was angry and felt emergency physician #107 was rude and uncaring."

The issue section should contain enough detail to understand why the complaint is being lodged and to direct the subsequent investigation. Typically, several issues are elucidated by the complainant. Each should be described in this section and then addressed in the process of investigation and resolution.

Investigation. This section should begin with a description of the sources of the investigation and end with the results of it. For example, "The following sources were used to investigate this case: the patient, the medical record, emergency physician #107, emergency nurses #2214 and #1020, and *ABC Textbook of Emergency Medicine*."

The investigation should be driven by the desire to objectively determine what actually occurred. To be effective, the complaint manager must gather information without precon-

EMERGENCY TREATMENT ASSOCIATES

QUALITY ASSURANCE PROGRAM
SITUATION ASSESSMENT

LOG# ______________________

Patient Name ____________________________________ ID# ______________________

Date of Service ____________
Date of Complaint ____________
Date of Resolution ____________

Type of Complaint
____ Attitude
____ Cost of Care
____ Documentation
____ Follow-Up Instruction
____ Length of Stay
____ Quality of Care
____ Other (Specify)
____

INITIATED BY:	NAME	DATE
____ Chart Review	____________	____________
____ Hospital Administration	____________	____________
____ Nurse	____________	____________
____ Patient	____________	____________
____ Physician	____________	____________
____ Billing Rep	____________	____________
____ Other	____________	____________
____________________		

ISSUE:
____
____
____

INVESTIGATION:
____
____
____

ASSESSMENT:
____
____
____

DISCUSSED WITH:	NAME	DATE
____ Emergency Nurse	____________	____________
____ Emergency Physician	____________	____________
____ Patient (Family)	____________	____________
____ Private Physician	____________	____________
____ Hospital Representative	____________	____________
____ Billing Representive	____________	____________

Investigated By:	____________________	Title: ____________
Print Name:	____________________	Date: ____________
Physician:	____________________	Date: ____________
Print Name:	____________________	Rating: ____________

FIGURE 66-1 Situation assessment form.

ceived notions of right or wrong. This is not an opportunity to assess blame, but rather to clarify and improve perceptions and performance. In other words, when approaching the emergency care provider, the query should be without reproach or criticism: "It was Mrs. Smith's perception that her care was . . . What happened?" Each person implicated or with substantive information to add should get an opportunity to describe the occurrence.

Resolution. The resolution must address each concern raised in the previous sections. The goal is to educate, improve performance, and correct inappropriate behaviors, faulty perceptions, and misinformation. The complaint manager will determine that many complaints, after investigation, do not require any change in the system or individual behavior. These assessments are particularly valuable. The complaint manager not only satisfies the complainer by a thorough investigation and follow-up, but also supports the caregivers by a positive conclusion.

Other complaints require specific actions to effect a change in behavior or fund of knowledge. Complaint-specific resolutions are presented in detail later in the chapter. The following are typical resolutions:

Problem	Resolution
Misread radiograph	Review radiograph. If trend or significant misread, read chapter and spend time with radiologist.
Misunderstood medical process	Perform in-service (by practitioner).
Delay in care	Improve lab reporting system.

SIGNATURE. This final section is completed on a separate page. The complaint manager or person investigating the complaint determines a rating and then signs the form. The involved practitioner reads, signs, and may comment. This process guarantees that the practitioner has knowledge of the conclusions you have drawn. Occasionally, a determination is made with incomplete or erroneous information. In these cases, the review by the practitioner allows appropriate modification.

In any case, this document resides in the practitioner's file. It is inappropriate to hold this information without knowledge of the involved person. Concealing the information limits the opportunity to change and improve. Further, if the information only surfaced subsequently when the practitioner was applying for another position, the complaint manager might be subjected to legal scrutiny.

RATING. The rating system is necessary to determine the significance of final assessment. The rating should incorporate two elements. First, the complaint manager must judge whether the standard of care was met. If not, there must then be a determination of whether an adverse patient outcome (APO) occurred directly as a result of the deficiency. (See Box 66-1 and Table 66-1.) In other words, if the standard of care was met and the patient nonetheless had a poor outcome, the rating will not reflect an adverse outcome. The following examples will be illustrative:

BOX 66-1

STANDARD OF CARE

Symbol	Standard of care
+	Met
+/−	Questionable
−	Deficient

Standard of Care	Adverse Patient Outcome	Rating
1. Deficient	Pneumothorax (related to deficiency)	−/3
2. Met	Death	+/0*
3. Deficient	Death (unrelated to deficiency)	−/0*

The Log. The purpose of the log is to document in a single and consistent manner the essential data and status of all complaints (Figure 66-2). Information entered into the log is derived from the situation assessment form. At minimum, the log should be used as a tracking system to identify the patient, nature of the complaint, and its present status and resolution.

A more sophisticated log can be used to extract a variety of information about the providers and the provision of care in your institution. For instance, a comprehensive log can be used to determine the number of complaints, types of complaints, and outcome data.

NUMBER OF COMPLAINTS. The absolute number of complaints is important. However, when initiating this type of system, there will be a substantial increase in the number of complaints. Complaints that were previously ignored or could not be handled by the system will now be sought, recognized, and documented. Develop a new baseline once the system is functioning smoothly.

The total number of complaints should be broken down by provider. If you use this "per provider" number to *compare* practitioners, it is necessary to consider other individual factors, including the following:

*In these cases there was no APO related to the deficient standard of care.

Table 66-1 Adverse Patient Outcome

Symbol type	Change in patient outcome/management	Examples (management changes that would not have occurred if standard of care had been met)
0	None	
1	Minor-temporary	Additional visit, splint, antibiotics
2	Minor-permanent	Facial scar, decreased function fifth digit
3	Major-temporary	Ruptured appendix, pneumothorax, ICU care
4	Major-permanent	Loss of functional use of limb, cardiac cripple
5	Death	

EMERGENCY TREATMENT ASSOCIATES
COMPLAINT MANAGEMENT LOG

LOG #	NAME	MR#	DOS	DOC	DOR	TYPE	INV BY	MD#	SA COMP	CONCL	COMMENT
025	H Jones	244190	3-1-93	3-3-93	3-7-93	Attitude	RS	16	✓	+/-, 0	Cust Serv Disc
026	R Reagan	362141	2-2-93	3-9-93	3-12-93	Qual	GN	24	✓	-, 1	CME
027	G Bush	371122	1-16-93	3-12-93	3-12-93	Cost	RS	14	✓	+, 0	—
028	S Bono	349725	3-7-93	4-2-93	4-6-93	Qual	GN	16	✓	+, 0	—
029	A Rose	379111	3-9-93			Qual	RS	92			

FIGURE 66-2 Example log.

- Relative number of patients cared for and hours worked by each provider
- Types of shifts worked (days, nights, swing, fast track)
- Complaint type and severity and patient outcome

TYPES OF COMPLAINTS. It is helpful to determine the types of complaints received over time and trend the data. This will over time expose or confirm system and provider problems such as delays, attitude, and cost of care issues.

OUTCOME DATA. A sophisticated log can quickly identify providers whose care is associated with poor outcomes or a particular type of poor outcome. A provider who has several complaints with an APO of 0 may be delivering high-quality care but low-quality caring. Alternatively, a provider who has more than one case with an APO of 2 or greater is likely to have significant quality of care problems. (See Practicioner Follow-up in the following discussion.)

Follow-Up and Reporting

Follow-Up to the Complaining Party. When possible, the complaint manager should contact each complaint source. Not all persons registering a complaint will achieve complete satisfaction. However, it is usually possible to provide them with the gratification of knowing that their issue was addressed quickly and with respect and sincerity.

When the complaining party is the patient or a family member, it may be appropriate to send a letter thanking them for sharing the issue with you. An example of such a letter follows:

Dear Mr. Jones:

Thank you for taking the time to let us know how we can better serve you. Your direct feedback about our services is vital to us. Though we closely monitor the medical care in our department, evaluating the perceptions of the patients and their families is more difficult to assess. Letters (Feedback) such as yours are the best means we have of determining how well we are achieving our goal of providing excellent medical care in a caring manner. I am encouraged that part of your experience was positive. I hope that should you or your family need emergency care in the future that you again consider ________ Hospital.

Sincerely,

Chairman,
Department of Emergency Medicine

Practitioner Follow-Up (Monitoring Performance). Individual performance must be monitored and trended over time. This allows for group, intragroup, and self comparisons. Initially, it may be necessary to compare practitioners with their cohorts to persuade them to change. In the long run, however, it is more important for practitioners to be made aware of their own strengths and weaknesses so that they may recognize areas for improvement. This continuing feedback can also demonstrate progress, providing positive reinforcement.

An effective monitoring system identifies practitioners with particular types of deficiencies. When a trend is noted, the emergency complaint manager should provide direct feedback to the individual practitioner and when appropriate develop a plan of corrective action. This should be communicated in both oral and written form.

Reporting and Maintaining Confidentiality. The complaint management process should be an essential part of the overall quality management program and linked directly to the credentialing and reappointment process. Create practitioner profiles incorporating this data at least yearly.

When discussing, documenting, and reporting these situation assessments, it is imperative to avoid specifically referring to the practitioner. Names should not appear on any circulated data. Many systems use coded numbers to identify staff members. To maintain the tightest security, some emergency departments have their own coding system separate from the hospital's system, which generally can be decoded by anybody in the institution.

As with all continuous quality improvement (CQI) materials, these situation assessments should be circulated on a limited "need-to-know" basis only. If these materials are widely available, they lose the protection of confidentiality usually afforded to peer review activities. In our system, situation assessments are distributed during our departmental CQI meeting and collected at the conclusion of the meeting. Participants in the process, including the support personnel who gather the materials and enter data, must be aware of the significance, sensitivity, and confidential nature of these efforts.

The Compliment Management System

An approach based on responding to complaints is only part of a complete system. Many complaint managers concentrate so heavily on complaints and "what went wrong" that the opportunity to recognize and share "what went right" is squandered. A more comprehensive approach to performance improvement includes the management and promotion of compliments.

The system should look for opportunities to praise success.

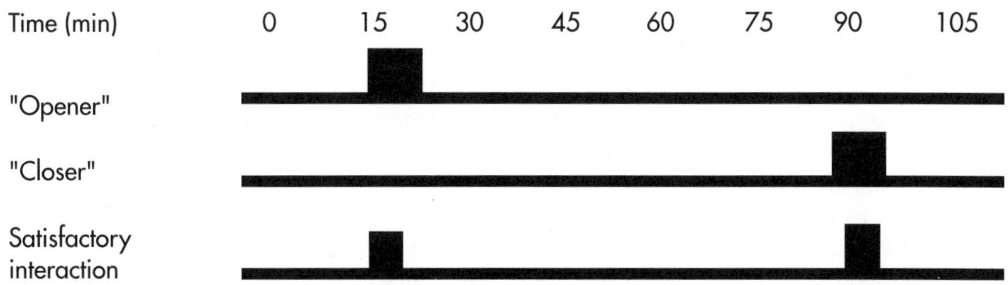

FIGURE 66-3 Dr. Zippy.

A compliment tracking system demonstrates to all who participate in the system—practitioners, administrators, and even regulatory personnel—that the system is balanced. The complaint manager should look for, document, and incorporate compliments in the practitioners' performance appraisals. Further, compliments should be distributed. For example, the following compliment was received in our system:

Dear Dr. _______________

We know that you were instrumental in saving our son Jim's life. We can't even begin to imagine our lives without him and are so grateful that he is healing. You are a very special person and we would like to commend you and your staff for excellence in every area. We have a long road but are progressing. You will never ever be forgotten and we will remember you in our prayers always. Thank God you were there.

God Bless You
Our Love

The _______________'s

This written compliment was sent to the provider with a cover letter of congratulations for a job well done. It was then distributed widely throughout the institution. Consider its effect on the medical director who is often dealing with physician problems, the CEO who expects the vast majority of written material crossing his or her desk to create more work, and all the others who share responsibility for the emergency department. Take credit for the good that you do.

CHANGING PERCEPTION AND BEHAVIOR

In this section I review the most common complaints and describe the basic techniques for resolving these complaints. After defining the issue, the resolutions will be examined from two perspectives. The retrospective solution will deal with the complaint that has already been voiced. This process focuses on damage control and satisfying a dissatisfied person. The prospective solution will describe prevention strategies, specifically examining the behavior or the system that has been identified as a problem.

Necessary Steps

Collect information, when possible, even before talking with the complainer. Responding to a complaint without information is like walking in a minefield. If a secretary answers the phone, have him or her make arrangements for you to call the person back. Get the chart immediately, and critically review the records with an eye for the appropriateness of the medical care.

If it is not possible to prepare for the complaint in advance with a copy of the chart, do the following:

- Take all of the information.
- Empathize: I can understand why you might be upset.
- Promise to call back after an investigation.

Common Complaints

The following is the list of common complaints that will be reviewed in the final section of this chapter. Every complaint manager will confront these issues.

- Dr. Zippy—"He only saw me for thirty seconds."
- Molasses General Hospital—"I waited so long."
- Dr. Mercedes—"Too much money!"
- Dr. Frankenstein—"But he was dead when he got there!"
- Dr. Jerkyl—"The doctor yelled at me!"
- Dr. Vesuvius—"He blew his stack again at the nursing station!"
- Dr. Terry Bradshaw—"The Monday morning quarterback."
- Dr. Helen Keller—"She missed the fracture!"

Dr. Zippy

"He never touched me," or "He only saw me for 30 seconds and my bill was 100 bucks . . . that means he's making $12,000 per hour! No wonder healthcare is so expensive!!"

At Issue. This patient has one of three problems. The patient is concerned about the lack of caring and thoroughness, a possible missed problem, or the expense of the bill. To respond effectively to the actual concern, listen carefully and ask questions to determine the true nature of the patient's complaint. If your review demonstrates a consistent pattern of complaints, you may have a doctor problem.

This doctor appears in a variety of forms. He or she may be lazy, unconcerned, or lack an understanding of what patients want. Some are good "openers"—they evaluate the patient near the beginning of their emergency visit but don't provide closure (Figure 66-3). They do not tell the patient the results of tests, summarize, or provide an opportunity to ask questions. Instead, these physicians send in another professional to act as a designee.

Alternatively, this physician may be a good "closer," only arriving to meet the patient for the first time after the decisions have been made. This doctor may believe the patient has come to the emergency department for a simple answer to a simple question—"Is it broken?" or "Do I need to be admitted?" Patients want more. They want time and touching. They want caring and compassion and consideration.

Retrospective Solution. Listen to find out the specific nature of the complaint. A missed problem may be resolved with a reevaluation or arranging appropriate aftercare. A missed opportunity to demonstrate a caring environment with concerned professionals can often be resolved by demonstrating caring during the discussion and a commitment to follow up. A bill that is perceived by the patient as too expensive should be dealt with as discussed in Dr. Mercedes.

Prospective Solution. This problem can be prevented by retraining the practitioner to provide the patient with early contact and late closure. Without both, the patient may believe that the practitioner has only a fleeting awareness of the patient's presence. Evaluating the patient at the beginning of the visit and providing a conclusion at the end creates in the patient the belief that the practitioner is aware of and concerned about the patient during the entire visit (Figure 66-3).

Molasses General Hospital

"I waited so long," or "Those party animals! I waited so long and nothing was done . . . and the staff was just sitting around laughing and figuring out what they were going to have on their pizza!"

At Issue. The most important issue for patients who have a choice of where they get their emergency care is convenience. The second most important issue is caring. Convenience means easy access and parking, efficient systems, and being evaluated and treated quickly so that they can return to the rest of their lives.

If you are unable to provide convenience, you must provide caring. Most patients lack the sophistication to scrutinize the actual quality of care provided. As a result, we are usually judged more for our level of caring than for our quality of care. Provide patients with what they want—contact and caring.

Retrospective Solution. Demonstrate objectivity by an expression of understanding. "It is frustrating to wait when your child is in pain. How is he doing now?" There is very little to offer other than empathy and a promise that you will investigate the delay and get back to them. But this is usually enough. People who are complaining that they were not taken care of in a timely and caring way when they were first seen are asking to be taken care of in a timely and caring way—now. DO IT!

Prospective Solution. Particularly during the periods of time that your emergency department is unable to provide rapid and efficient care, it is necessary to provide caring care. Methods include the following.

THE SIT DOWN APPROACH. When you have the opportunity to spend time with the patient, sit while you are obtaining the history. Sitting often results in a more efficient communication. Patients may be more trusting and specific when the practitioner demonstrates that he or she is not rushed and is willing to spend the time necessary to complete the evaluation.

THE FREQUENT TOUCH. Some practitioners walk by patients as if they were wearing blinders. Some are worried that if they make eye contact, the patient will be able to pull the practitioner away from the important matters at hand.

In fact, a comment such as "We are waiting for your lab tests to come back; is there anything I can do for you?" or "Are you OK?" will usually result in nothing more than the patient realizing that the practitioner is concerned. Most patients respond with a smile and "No thanks" or a request for something to make them more comfortable. Occasionally, they alert you to a change in their condition. And always they are appreciative. Patient satisfaction is higher when multiple practitioners are checking on them than when they feel ignored and unappreciated.

PROVIDE REALISTIC EXPECTATIONS. When providing care in a busy setting, patients particularly appreciate a realistic appraisal of when they can expect to be evaluated. One effective approach is to introduce yourself, explain the situation, and when possible get initial lab or x-ray studies ordered. When walking by a patient that he or she has not seen yet, the practitioner may simply say, "Mrs. Jones, I'm Dr. Smith. I have two patients to see before I can spend time with you. I should be with you in about 20 minutes. Are you OK?"

Dr. Mercedes: Too Much Money

"I can't believe they charged me this much money, all they did was . . ."

At Issue. For many complaint managers, the majority of the complaints come at the time the patient receives the bill. The recipient of the complaint must look for the underlying concern. The three most common reasons for this complaint are limited ability to pay, inappropriate bill, and dissatisfaction with care. The key to the approach to these complaints is to let reason prevail. And if you decrease or eliminate a bill, always make it clear that you are addressing an issue of patient satisfaction rather than poor-quality care. The appearance of the latter could be perceived as an admission of guilt.

Retrospective Solution

1. *No money.* Some patients may voice dissatisfaction with the care, the lack of care, or the cost of care because of their inability to pay the typically expensive bills generated by a visit to the emergency department. When this issue is recognized, patients may be satisfied to go on a payment plan and to know they will not be placed into collection. You may on occasion write off part or all of a bill. However, be careful to avoid developing a reputation in the community. Usually, patients are willing to pay part or most of the bill, and it is reasonable after the discussion to say, "I understand that it is difficult to pay this bill, would you be able to pay . . .?" or, although somewhat more risky, "What do you think would be fair?"
2. *Inappropriate bill.* Occasionally, the bill is incorrect. Removal of a superficial tick may get mistakenly coded as a removal of a deeply embedded foreign body. When this is recognized, apologize and thank the person for bringing it to your attention so that you can make an immediate change in the billing process. Without this step, some patients will believe that you are trying to gouge the public when you can get away with it.

   When a bill is decreased or eliminated for one of these reasons, it is appropriate to send an explanatory letter to the patient. Avoid any reference to having done anything wrong in the provision of care. Instead, describe the reason for the change as a means of satisfying the patient and maintaining the patient's patronage.

I understand that you are not satisfied with the bill you received as a result of your visit to the Emergency Room. Your satisfaction and patronage are important to us at XYZ Hospital and for that reason we have decreased your bill to $XX.00. Thank you for the opportunity to discuss this matter. I hope that in the event that you require emergency services in the future, you will again give us the opportunity to serve you.

3. *Dissatisfaction with care.* This is a quality issue and should be addressed directly. Find out in what way the patient's expectations weren't met, investigate the situation, and get back to the patient quickly. A different issue arises if the patient unexpectedly deteriorates and concerns exist about the quality of the care provided. Because an expensive bill may be perceived as adding "insult to injury," some practitioners advocate not sending a bill in this situation. However, this is a dangerous practice. If it is discovered that the bill was intentionally eliminated, a plaintiff's attorney will effectively demonstrate your early "admission of guilt."

Prospective Solution. Remember the four *C*s: convenience, caring, care, and cost. An organization that effectively deals with the first three gets fewer significant complaints about the fourth. Nonetheless, it is inevitable that an emergency department will receive some complaints about the cost of care. And with increasing managed care penetration, each facility should review its cost structure to be certain that it remains competitive with other local providers.

Dr. Frankenstein: But He Was Dead When He Got There

"The ambulance arrived and I overheard them say there was no chance . . . but they kept working on him. I'm not sure why. And now I've got this huge bill. Why are you charging me so much?"

At Issue. This is a particularly poignant variation of "too much money" (see Dr. Mercedes). Clearly, the anguish and suffering associated with the grieving process is only compounded by the receipt of the large bill that typically follows a resuscitation. This becomes particularly distressful when the grieving party believes that "there was no chance" or that "you were working on the dead body of my loved one." Arguing with the grieving person or trying to explain how the billing process works will only reinforce the belief that you are uncaring and only interested in the money.

Retrospective Solution. Remember, the grieving person is often distraught and dealing with many unresolved issues. Empathize with complainants and objectively repeat back to them the issue. For example, you might say, "I'm very sorry your husband died. It is difficult to deal with money at a time like this." Then wait and listen. If you are a good and patient listener, by the time the grieving spouse is done, she may be ready to listen to you.

It then may be appropriate to explain the situation in a way that demonstrates compassion and caring. "The resuscitation team was called. We really thought that there was good reason to try our hardest to resuscitate your husband. We performed *x, y,* and *z* just like the American Heart Association recommends and unfortunately he didn't survive. We did the best that we could. However, I understand that what you're going through is difficult and it is a lot of money. Let's work something out."

Prospective Solution. Some emergency departments, by policy, do not bill for care rendered to patients who are dead on arrival (DOA). Though the definition of DOA may vary broadly, the intent is usually the same—to avoid the additional burden of an expensive bill to an already grieving family. In this situation, it may be appropriate to send a letter of condolence describing your concern for the grieving spouse and your resultant willingness to eliminate the bill. This allows the department to give solace and get credit for the good deed.

The process of forgiving a bill should be done in a way that does not imply that something went wrong. (See Dr. Mercedes.)

Dr. Jerkyl

"The doctor yelled at me because I came in last week for the same thing. Well, it wasn't better," or "The doctor said that this is an emergency room and that my case was not an emergency. Well, it was to me and to the surgeon who took me to the operating room the next day!"

At Issue. It is difficult for some practitioners to understand that each individual has his or her own definition of an emergency. Instead these practitioners are often intent on explaining how the emergency room works rather than listening to the patient's issue. This pedantic attitude is, at least, humiliating to the patient. Further, it may be dangerous if, as a result of the lecture, the patient is reticent to seek appropriate care in the future.

The practitioner may believe that he or she is just educating the patient. The patient, on the other hand, may believe that the practitioner is arrogant, lazy, and unwilling to spend the appropriate time with the patient. There is a saying, "Jerks who are right are jerks; jerks who are wrong are defendants." When insulted, the patient may get angry. When things go wrong, the patient may seek retribution.

Retrospective Solution. Once you've determined that the nature of the complaint is rudeness or inappropriate behavior on the part of the practitioner, empathize with the complainant and agree to investigate and get back to him or her soon. Remember, if the person believes that he or she got disrespect instead of caring and compassion, you now have an opportunity to give the patient what he or she wanted. Avoid lengthy explanations about the way the emergency department works. Instead, describe your expectations of respect and courtesy.

You may even admit guilt about caring, but never about care. "It seems like you've been treated rudely and we did not meet either your or our expectations. This type of attitude is unacceptable. Thank you for letting me know. I will investigate it and get back to you on Tuesday." Then, either you or the practitioner, if he or she is caring and capable, should get back to the slighted patient. "He/she is sorry that you perceived him/her as rude. It was not intended; in fact, he/she was very upset that you left dissatisfied. We both appreciate that you brought this to our attention."

Prospective Solution. If this is a consistent problem of a particular practitioner or, worse, among many practitioners within the emergency department, it is necessary to create a behavior change. Changing the behavior of an individual is very difficult. Changing the behavior of a group may require professional consultation.

SCREENING INDIVIDUALS. When possible, look at individuals carefully before hiring them. Ask them, "What is the worst thing I'm going to hear about you?" Extensively check their backgrounds with specific attention to issues of patient relations. Create a probationary period and have the practitioner do some shifts. Then talk to the staff with whom the practitioner works to find out how they get along. It may be much simpler to avoid a problem than to try to change or correct a personality.

OPEN-MINDED INDIVIDUALS. Open-minded practitioners that are responsible for numerous complaints may change their approach if they realize how much discomfort they are causing. It is particularly valuable to incorporate these individuals into the complaint resolution process. Review the complaint management procedure and its desired outcome with them. Then have them respond to and follow up on complaints about other practitioners. This may be enough to create a behavior change. If not, once they have learned the complaint management process, supervise them in the management of complaints directed toward them.

CLOSED-MINDED INDIVIDUALS. Other practitioners may reflect that they do not care what people think about them. "After all, I'm providing good care; just look at my charts!" Such a practitioner does not understand that people want more than appropriate care, they want time and touching, care and compassion. Unfortunately, it is nearly impossible to create caring where none exists.

DYSFUNCTIONAL GROUP BEHAVIOR. When several members of the emergency department or any group are perceived to be rude and uncaring, a serious organizational problem exists. It may be as simple to solve as bringing in new leadership that understands customer service and how to rebuild morale. Usually resolution requires a great deal of time and the same caring and compassion for the practitioners that you would like to see them give.

Dr. Vesuvius

A private physician on staff charges up to the nursing station and blows his stack again, screaming: "I can't stand to have my patients come here! You never get anything right around here!"

At Issue. Everybody is upset and embarrassed, and worse, if it is directed at someone in particular, that person may be humiliated by the outburst.

Many physicians have their only significant emergency department experience during their residency. For some, their memory of the emergency department is a wild, uncaring, chaotic environment with nobody responsible or particularly interested. It was a brief and sometimes distasteful assignment, the purpose of which was to provide exposure or meet a service obligation.

Further, the physician may be used to a supportive office staff that responds immediately to his or her needs. Arriving in this more clamorous and confusing environment may be very stressful. Unfortunately, some people handle high-stress situations by becoming aggressive and blaming.

Retrospective Solution. Success with this physician requires showing respect and then creating the understanding that the emergency department is your office. Make an appointment and go to the physician's office. This demonstrates that you respect the physician's time and are willing to go to him or her with *your* issue. (Remember, it is your issue, not the physician's.) Then do the following:

1. Find out what happened and deal with it. Determine the nature of the problem that caused the outburst. You must listen and try to solve the physician's problem before the physician will listen and consider solving yours. Deal with the predicament that caused the physician's frustration.
2. Describe your complaint management process. Encourage the complaining physician to come to you any and every time that there is a problem with the emergency department or the care being rendered there. Let the practitioner know that it is important to you for the emergency department to be a user-friendly environment and that you take very seriously any concerns that the practitioner may have with the emergency department. Once the physician is convinced that you understand and are willing to try to fix the problem and that you want to deal with any problems that arise in your emergency department, you now have the opportunity to solve the problem.
3. Explain that the emergency department is your office. Describe how, in your practice environment, you assume responsibility for the patients and staff as does the practitioner in his or her office. Relate how important it is for you to create the most positive and caring environment for those who use your facility. If you had a problem with something related to the physician's patients or practice, you would never express your concerns in a public forum with the practitioner's staff or in front of patients. Instead, you would either call or make an appointment and privately discuss your concern.
4. Gain commitment to work directly with you when problems arise.

Prospective Solution. The person expressing his or her discontent may not recognize the inappropriateness of the behavior. If a disruptive situation is occurring at the nursing station and you are uncomfortable with the expression of emotion in this public arena, you may be able to intervene by doing the following:

1. Stand in front of the person and try to gain his or her attention. Establish eye contact.
2. Quietly and firmly say: "I can see you're upset; I want to talk with you about this over here," and move toward a more private space. If you have gained the practitioner's attention and you are in a position of authority, it is likely he or she will follow you.
3. Deal with the issue. Repeat the steps listed in the retrospective solution.

Dr. Terry Bradshaw: The Monday Morning Quarterback

"My doctor said that I had a ruptured appendix . . . and your doctor screwed up!"

At Issue. This patient is angry and wants satisfaction. The patient is perhaps offering you your only opportunity to resolve a high-risk situation. Ignoring the issue at this point is fanning the fire. It is essential to understand what the patient wants. However, in the long run, it may be even more important to ascertain if and why the physician criticized the emergency department care. The private physician may be upset with the care and inadvertently may have planted a seed of discontent; he or she may be angry with the emergency department, an emergency physician, or the hospital; or may be implicating another for his or her own protection.

Retrospective Solution

THE PATIENT. When talking with the patient, demonstrate your concern by listening carefully to the story—now. Seek to understand what the patient wants as a result of this discussion, or even ask: "What would you like to see happen?" Perhaps it is to make sure that this mistake does not happen again. The patient may want the practitioner to be punished ("his head on a platter!"). Agree to look into the situation and get back to the patient quickly. Review the care and determine if it was improper or led to a poor outcome.

If the care rendered was within the acceptable standard, then you must deal with the patient's perception and expectations. At the very least, it is important to empathize with the patient and try to provide a satisfactory answer. One response is the following:

> "Yes, I've talked with your Dr. Smith [private physician] and understand her concern. There are several ways to evaluate and treat abdominal pain. Dr. Jones [emergency physician] was very concerned about you and your pain. He performed the correct tests and encouraged you to see your doctor immediately if the pain got worse. He was very glad to hear you're feeling better . . . How may I be of further help to you?"

Avoid further complicating the situation by criticizing the private physician. This will only lead to a battle that you are likely to lose.

If the care did not meet the standard, you must again deal with the patient's perception and help to meet his or her expectations. Be particularly careful not to make statements to the patient that subsequently may be used against you. In other words, avoid an admission that a staff member or the hospital was guilty of poor care. This is equivalent to becoming the plaintiff's witness.

THE PHYSICIAN. Discuss the situation with the private physician. Again, make an appointment to meet with the physician in his or her own office. It demonstrates a level of deference that may help you while trying to enlist the support of the private physician. Try to figure out if and why the physician denounced the patient's care. This must be done in a nonaccusatory manner, such as, "It was the patient's perception that you were not happy with his care in the emergency department. How might we have done better?"

Usually when faced with this type of situation, the private physician will recognize the gravity and implications of his or her conversation with the patient. You may gain support by asking the physician to participate in the advancement of care in the department. Methods include designing a clinical protocol, giving a lecture, participating in a journal club, selecting upgraded equipment, and so forth.

Prospective Solution. The only prospective solutions to this problem involve techniques of prevention. As soon as you recognize that there are physicians or groups of physicians who are unhappy with the care of their patients in the emergency department, seek them out. Ascertain their issues. Work with them to seek solutions that demonstrate that you are eager to continuously improve the level of care in the department. Incorporate them into the solutions by cooperating in the development of clinical guidelines. Above all, assure them that your greatest interest is providing the best care you can to their (your) patients.

Dr. Helen Keller: Missed X-Ray

"The doctor told me my x-ray was okay and now you tell me that my son has a broken bone!"

At Issue. Patients expect high-quality care and accurate diagnoses. They are sometimes intolerant of what they perceive to be mistakes. As in other complaints, this is a second opportunity to provide the correct care, and caring.

Retrospective Solution. There are two important issues. First, make sure that the patient now gets the appropriate and necessary care for the injury. If appropriate in your setting, demonstrate your concern by bringing the patient back to the emergency department for further care. "How is your child now? Would you like to come in now and I'll take care of him myself?" Otherwise, take the initiative to secure definitive care for the patient by making all the necessary arrangements with the primary care physician or orthopedist.

Second, reassure the patient that the system worked. It is acceptable to admit that the x-ray was not read correctly. That is why you have developed a system in cooperation with the radiologists that ensures that a second expert, a radiologist, reviews every x-ray taken in the emergency department. You must be in a position to say: "I'm pleased that the system works so well." Depending on what the patient expects, such as that it won't happen again, it may also be necessary to add: "Our system also requires that Dr. Jones (emergency physician) review the x-ray to become an even better physician."

Prospective Solution. The prospective solution involves three components.

OVERREAD SYSTEM. Develop an effective protocol for overreading x-rays. Elements include the following:

- Rapid identification of misread radiographs
- Immediate notification of emergency personnel
- Determination of significance, and when appropriate
- Patient or physician notification
- Arrangements for follow-up care
- Documentation
- Physician review of radiograph, preferably with radiologist
- Physician trending, and when appropriate
- Physician education

PATIENT EDUCATION. The patient being discharged should get a thorough and caring explanation of the continued management of the injury. As part of the discharge process, it is appropriate to advise the patient that, "Though I don't see anything wrong with your x-ray, we always have the radiologist review the films in the morning." By informing the patient before discharge, you may prevent subsequent misunderstanding and anger.

PERFORMANCE IMPROVEMENT. The performance improvement system must identify members of the department who misread radiographs, particularly those that lead to a subsequent change in patient management. Depending on the type, frequency, and seriousness of the misread radiographs, it may be appropriate for the practitioner to read a chapter on the topic, spend time with the radiologist, or participate in a course dedicated to emergency department radiology.

REFERENCES

1. Adamson TE, Schann JM, Gullion DS, et al: Physician communication skills and malpractice claims—a complex relationship, *West J Med* 150:356-360, 1989.
2. Solnick S, Hemenway D: Complaints and disenrollment at a health maintenance organization, *J Consumer Affairs* 26:90-103, 1992.
3. Korsch BM, Gozzi BK, Francis V: Gaps in doctor-patient communication, *Pediatrics* 42:855-871, 1968.

4. Schwartz LR, Overton DT: Emergency department complaints: a one-year analysis, *Ann Emerg Med* 16:857-861, 1987.
5. Buller MK, Buller DB: Physicians' communication style and patient satisfaction, *J Health Soc Behav* 28:375-388, 1987.
6. Evans BJ, Kiellerup FD, Stanley RO, et al: A communication skills programme for increasing patients' satisfaction with general practice consultations, *Br J Med Psychol* 60:373-378, 1987.
7. Hirschman AO: *Exit, voice and loyalty: responses to decline in firms, organizations and states,* Cambridge, Mass, 1970, Harvard University Press.
8. Best A, Andreasen AR: Consumer responses to unsatisfactory purchases: a survey of perceiving defects, voicing complaints, and obtaining redress, *Law Society Review* 18:701-742, 1977.
9. Ley P: Complaints made by hospital staff and patients: a review of the literature, *Bull Br Psychol Soc* 25:115-120, 1972.
10. Schneiderman N: Patient complaints. In Henry G, editor: *Emergency medicine risk management,* Dallas, 1991, American College of Emergency Physicians.
11. Day R, Gabricke K, Schaetzle T, et al: The hidden agenda of consumer complaining, *J Retailing* 57:86-106, 1981.
12. *Bits and pieces,* vol 3, Fairfield, NJ, 1991, The Economic Press.
13. Singh H: Industry characteristics and consumer dissatisfaction, *J Consumer Affairs* 25:19-56, 1990.
14. Andreasen AR: Consumer responses to dissatisfaction in loose monopolies, *J Consumer Research* 12:135-141, 1985.
15. Joint Commision on Accreditation of Health Care Organizations: *Accreditation manual for hospitals,* Oak Brook Terrace, Ill, 1996, JCAHCO
16. State of New York: *Official compilation of codes: rules and regulations,* Albany, NY, 1995, Department of State.
17. Peters TJ, Waterman RH: In search of excellence: lessons from America's best run companies, New York, 1983, Warner Books.
18. Truelove A: On handling complaints, *Hosp Health Serv Rev* 229-232, 1985.

67 The Litigation Process: DEPOSITIONS, TESTIMONY, AND OTHER DANGEROUS PRACTICES IN THE EMERGENCY DEPARTMENT

William H. Ginsburg

Deposition and trial testimony are nothing more than methods of communication. Communication between a physician who is a litigant and the judge and jury in a litigated case is as essential as communication between physician and patient in the context of medical treatment. Understanding of the litigation process and the important role of communication in the litigation setting is an essential tool to winning a case. Physicians must be trained in how to act in the context of an adversarial proceeding and what to expect in the way of questioning technique and style. The jury watches the party litigant and bases a significant part of its decision on the jury members' reactions to the way the party handles himself or herself in the litigation process, thus the importance of following prescribed rules of conduct and behavior when giving deposition or trial testimony.

THE IMPORTANCE OF COMMUNICATION IN THE LITIGATION PROCESS

It is fundamental that litigation takes a great deal of time and costs a great deal of money. It is equally fundamental that litigation is to be avoided if possible.

However, if litigation becomes unavoidable, in the context of risk management, effective communication is the single device that makes litigation successful and that makes the gargantuan task of winning manageable.

William H. Ginsburg is a noted trial lawyer who has devoted his career to the defense of medical providers and medical devices and pharmaceuticals. He has tried over 200 jury trials and is a fellow of the American Board of Trial Advocates and a Fellow of the American Society of Law and Medicine. He is Senior Partner in the Los Angeles–based law firm of Ginsburg, Stephan, Oringher & Richman.

Communication is the key to success. Effective communication and the development of rapport, with counsel, judge, and jury, in deposition and trial, are extremely important goals. The purpose of this chapter is to bring the litigation process into focus in such a manner that the importance of communication becomes apparent and the role of communication in winning a trial becomes the standard for all physicians who must undergo a trial.

The litigation management phase of risk management is the process of attempting to define and contain the risks of litigation. During the litigation process, the object of risk management is to win the case. The ability to employ effective communication skills demonstrates a fundamental principle of risk management in the context of the deposition process and courtroom testimony and is the key to winning.

At the outset, the ideal way to prevent claims and lawsuits is to foment good patient relations through communications and to ensure that the delivery of medical care is of the highest quality.

Establishment of a "rational alliance" with a patient is important. Nobody likes to go to the doctor or the dentist because it portends illness and pain. Even in the context of such unpleasantries, the experience of visiting a doctor can be a positive one if the physician or dentist makes it so.

It is just as unpleasant for juries, witnesses, and physicians to be in a courtroom as in a doctor's office because the circumstances are uncomfortable, anxiety producing, and frightening. Thus the "players" in the courtroom drama feel the same way as the litigants about the experience.

Just as it is critical for a physician or dentist to create a rational alliance with the patients, it is equally important for a physician to establish a rational alliance with a judge and jury when a physician is party to a litigation.

Communication is the foundation of risk management. Good communication and patient rapport causes acceptance of less than perfect care and avoidance of a great number of claims by otherwise potential litigants. Many claims are never asserted because of the rapport established between doctor and patient, hospital and patient, and other relevant members of the healthcare team. Patients often feel willing to waive their complaints if they feel their doctor is their "friend" or if they have otherwise gotten to know him or her and have established a mutually respectful communicative relationship. Thus the physician "wins" in that he or she is looked at with the respect and tolerance that allow a margin for error.

In the courtroom, the same factors influence "winning and losing." The ability of a physician litigant to communicate in a manner that breeds respect, persuades, convinces, and molds the opinion of the decision maker (in the courtroom, the jury), is the key to litigation success.

A fundamental rule that must always be remembered by the physician litigant is that the litigation process is different from the practice of medicine. The concepts, the method of preparation, and the result to be achieved do not necessarily have anything to do with the physician's concept of reality, but rather with the reality created by the lawyers and perceived by the jurors and judge.

A Jury of Peers

The concept of being tried by a jury of peers may seem unreal and unattainable in the U.S. system of justice. However, nothing could be further from the truth. Peers, or members of the same community in which a physician is practicing, decide the standard of care after hearing other members of the community, as well as the physician litigant, testify about the subject. Just because the jurors are not doctors does not disqualify them as peers any more than a doctor would be disqualified from a jury trying a case about automobile repair just because he or she is not an auto mechanic.

Some doctors believe that they are not getting a fair deal and that they are better than others because of what they do. Thus, rather than use the system in its intended context and manner, they demand a separate system for their profession. This chapter tries to recognize some of the practical problems that face physicians to ensure the most effective utilization of the process as it presently exists.

THE ESSENCE OF A MEDICAL MALPRACTICE CLAIM AND THE ROLE OF DEPOSITION AND TRIAL IN THE CONTINUUM OF EVENTS

Medical malpractice claims are essentially rooted in the concept of negligence. They are essentially composed of allegations that, when added up, state that the physician and other healthcare providers acted in a manner that was below the standard of care.

The standard of care is defined as the way a similarly trained and qualified physician would have acted under the same or similar circumstances. Once a claim of negligence, replete with damages as a result of the negligence, has been made by a patient, the litigation process has potentially begun. If the claim is not settled or resolved in its early stages, it progresses to a lawsuit or arbitration. Throughout the lawsuit process, communication and rapport with lawyer, judge, and jury become essential.

The Litigation Process

The actual litigation process commences when a complaint is filed in the court. Service of the complaint then takes place, and an answer to the complaint is filed, usually denying that anything wrong was done. The allegations of the complaint allege some deviation from the standard of care, and the answer to the complaint states that the standard of care was met. The complaint also defines that there were damages, and the answer denies the severity as alleged by the plaintiff or claimant.

Discovery of facts begins after the initial filing and serving of the summons and complaint and the filing of a response or answer. Medical records presumably will have been copied or obtained in advance, but if incomplete, additional records are gathered by subpoena and stipulation.

Discovery then proceeds to interpretation of the records and exploration of the history of the plaintiff and the medical services rendered or not rendered. These are usually in the form of "interrogatories," written questions that the physician and others will be required to answer. After the interrogatories and answers, the process turns to deposition, questions asked of the physicians and other parties in person, orally.

At deposition proceedings, lawyers ask questions of parties and witnesses in the presence of shorthand reporters with transcription machines. They attempt to determine what a physician did and did not do and what the physician's reasoning process was in determining a course of action.

The lawyer's purpose in a deposition is threefold: to gather facts; to develop contradictions and ways to impeach the litigant; and to develop premises that will justify the desired conclusion, liability for the plaintiff with no liability for the defense. These purposes can be translated simply as follows: to gather facts is to get a medical education; to develop contradictions is to make the physician litigant look ineffective, uncaring, and unskilled; and to develop premises is to get admissions that one or more of the litigants breached the standard of care.

The deposition process was designed by lawyers to elicit facts and materials deemed necessary to make their case. The making of a case, the gathering of facts, and the information to "win," may be different from what is "right" or "wrong."

It is a fundamental principle that the litigation process has as much to do with "winning and losing" as "right and wrong." The anger that this concept foments in the minds of most physicians can be an advantage to the plaintiff's counsel, and lawyers are trained to use every advantage. It is important to recognize this reality and develop resistance to the anger. This will neutralize the advantage that the opposition believes exists.

Fact Finding

Facts that need to be developed in the pretrial deposition process are as simple as what was the diagnosis; how did the physician arrive at the conclusion he or she did; and what was the course of treatment or care provided by the physician.

Information necessary to develop the case includes the physician's background and current educational status and determining the physician's weak points. The attorney will attempt to use them against the physician in question.

When determining what occurred in the case, peripheral facts and observations about the parties are also discerned, such as how a party presents himself or herself, what might be effective in the questioning process, how the party is likely to appear to a jury, and determination of the party's inherent weaknesses and biases. A physician must remember that the object of trial to an attorney is winning. An attorney is trained to develop facts and create a favorable environment to win a case.

The Jury Must be Persuaded

Juries and arbitrators are often moved by both relevant and irrelvant facts that give them impressions and feelings that influence their vote and therefore the outcome of the case. It is common sense and fact that jurors spend a great deal of their time in a case ultimately trying to develop a "trial story"—what happened and why. Thus it is important for the lawyers to feed them the facts in the most influential way they can conceive and to try to make the physician in question look as good or bad as possible.

The jury gleans images of the litigants as the trial proceeds. It is necessary for the physician to exude a confident demeanor. Juries, who make every good faith effort to decide cases fairly, are not technically adept and thus glean their information from what they see, hear, and otherwise sense.

Consider the following exchange of irrelevant facts that can move a jury. Assume a rural venue with only a small hospital and a few doctors. Assume further that the plaintiff's lawyer has brought in a "big city expert" who has testified in a medically perfect manner in the sense that almost everyone would agree that the doctor being sued did something wrong. The defendant doctor's attorney is trying to rehabilitate the defendant effectively and change the image of the jury about his work, as described by the expert:

Q Doctor [defendant], I notice you have not written any articles or chapters in books, nor have you addressed any major medical colleges or societies over the past 35 years that you have been practicing. Given that plaintiff's expert has coauthored over 75 articles with titles like "Histological Pathogenesis of Blood Borne Infectious Diseases" and a whole bunch of others like that, and has addressed the International Society of Surgeons and the National Health Care Coalition of Physicians, how do you justify not having done all that and still claim you can practice to the standard of care?

A I don't understand how Dr. [expert] could have done all of that and still keep up with his clinical practice. I admit I haven't written anything or made all of those fancy trips; I've just been here in Elmville, treating the folks for everything that's wrong with them. I'm proud of my 35 years of service to this community.

Q Doctor [defendant], do you have any criticism of Dr. [expert's] analysis of the case we are trying here today and in which you are the prime defendant?

A Yes, I do. Dr. [expert] is cloistered in his big city teaching hospital with all of his interns and residents and fellows to assist him. We are just country doctors out here, practicing the medicine we know how to practice and just serving the folks in the community.

The point of this example is that lawyers may manipulate information and facts to pursuade the jury.

The Ability to Persuade Is Critical. Persuasion is not always completely rational or logical or in accord with the thought process of a scientist or doctor. There are elements of human nature, demography, and practicality in persuasion.

A clinically correct physician who is a wonderful professor and marvelous teacher is useless in the courtroom if he or she cannot convey the essence of the point to be made in a coherent and persuasive manner. The converse is also true. A mediocre physician who testifies incorrectly and without foundation, but with sincerity and resolve, and in a professional manner, may be believed. Accuracy of facts should not be confused with results in the context of litigation.

The reality of this lesson must be recognized to properly prepare for deposition and trial. There are aspects to the litigation process that are "not fair," but they are real, so they must be accepted and dealt with on a rational and preparatory basis.

Pretrial discovery proceedings, depositions, and trial must be treated as a type of theater by the physician who faces the event. It becomes crystal clear, then, why the preparatory stages of the conflict, including the deposition, are critical.

The Deposition

The deposition sets the stage and freezes in time and place the physician's image and sense of what was right and wrong at the time of the event that led to the claim and lawsuit.

It is essential then that the deposition be taken seriously. It will be written down or videotaped. Eventually in the trial, the jury will be listening to and watching everything that is presented to them and will seek telltale signs of weakness or patterns of consistency and strength. There is an element of stage presence, rehearsal, and preparation that enters into all cases at both the deposition and trial stages.

It is also important to remember that experts for the opposing side of the case will review the deposition and will comment and draw on statements of the physician to show inaccuracy and inconsistency. The lawyers representing the claimant often lack significant medical knowledge and look to the physician defendant and the experts that they engage to educate them. The deposition then may also educate the plaintiff's counsel. The object is to deal with the questions without educating the plaintiff's counsel or providing the plaintiff's expert fodder from which to predicate a theory against the physician defendant. The deposition should be directed to turning what the plaintiff's attorney is trying to do—get an education and gather material to be used to criticize and eventually defeat the physician—into a positive experience for the defendant physician and a negative effort for the plaintiff's attorney.

The physician who is about to give a deposition in support of his or her actions and in defense of a claim must remember several rules.

The Question is the Enemy. Listen carefully to the question, and do not do more or less than respond to the question asked. An inexperienced physician may mishandle a question as the following illustration demonstrates:

Q Can you tell us what color the sky is today?
A Blue.

As foolish as it sounds the sequence should go as follows:

Q Can you tell us what color the sky is today?
A Yes.
Q Will you tell us what color the sky is today?
A Yes.
Q What color is the sky today?
A Blue.

The difference between the first and second sequence is that in the first sequence the final question was assumed and answered without regard to the fact that the questioner had not asked it.

In the second sequence, the questions were specifically answered as they arose and were not assumed or superimposed on one another. It is common to answer the question that was not asked, particularly when the person answering has additional information. In deposition and courtroom testimony, this can be a fatal flaw.

In medical context the question could well have been, "Can

you tell us what bone was broken here?" The answer could have been, "We have a comminuted compound fracture of the femur that could have confused an average practitioner." How silly to answer assumed questions when the answer to the question is simply "Yes."

It is essential to keep to the point and not volunteer more information than is necessary to answer the question in deposition and trial testimony.

Another form of the same trap—falling prey to the unasked question—is illustrated by the following sequence:

Q Doctor, what procedure do you follow when a person presents with a lacerated finger?

A Well, first we take a complete history. In this case the patient told us he was 38 years old and had considerable experience on his job as a painter using a spray device under pressure. He told us about his history and that he had hurt his finger before with the device. He also told us where he had that injury treated. He showed us the finger and we looked at it. We called for an x-ray and then we discussed the matter. I was not sure if we should call an orthopedic specialist or not, because I felt I could debride the finger successfully myself, and it did not appear too complicated an injury. *[and on and on and on . . .]*

The correct answer to the question should have been something approximating the following:

Q Doctor, what procedure do you follow when a person presents with a lacerated finger?

A We assess the injury and decide whether a specialist needs to be called or whether we can handle the laceration ourselves in the emergency department.

The clarity of the latter statement is obvious. The first response was confused. The physician lost the whole point of the question, began rambling, and volunteered myriad points, creating a potential disaster. Such voluntary "exposés" can only open up whole areas of further questioning that may never have been broached if the physician had maintained control and been aware of what he or she was doing.

The question can be the enemy and the answer can be fatal. Keep the response pointed and focused on the question. Force the plaintiff's attorney to ask the whole series of questions. If counsel is unprepared, the physician will accomplish what he or she set out to do—realize a positive result from the process.

Trust Your Attorney to Give You a Chance to Say All That Must Be Said. There is plenty of time at deposition and trial to "recover." Remember that lawyers are trained to think inductively, and they are always searching for reasons to justify their conclusions. What this means is that the fact-finding mission embodied by discovery is one in which counsel seeks not the truth, but information to justify to a jury a sometimes specious conclusion.

Lawyers can sometimes persuade a jury with seeming irrelevancies. The image of the physician will make a difference.

Physicians are taught to think deductively. They develop premises leading to a logical conclusion. Lawyers are trained to think inductively. They use facts to support their conclusion. Put another way, if the lawyer does not get the facts needed to support the premise, he or she will simply continue the search to secure "facts" that develop the premises sought. The physician, by trying to deductively reason his or her way out of the case, may unwittingly provide facts that can be developed into a persuasive story against the physician. Thus it is essential to remain focused and to the point.

No matter how much information a physician thinks he or she is conveying in support of a position, overly verbose and rambling presentations only bolster the perception that the physician has something to defend. Lawyers are trained to understand which facts and concepts require further explanation. The physician will be given a chance to amplify and clarify responses during the presentation of the case for the defense under "friendly fire" with preplanned questions and considered responses.

Thus there is no need to attempt to explain everything at the time of initial questioning by the plaintiff's lawyer. Simple, direct answers are best with an expression of the need to clarify. If counsel allows it at the time, simple clarification or qualification is acceptable, otherwise the physician's counsel will note the need to clarify. The physician will have a chance to clarify during the presentation of the defense.

The physician should understand the sequence of trial and recognize that he or she will have a chance to say and explain everything necessary to make the case favorable to the jury. The physician defendant should always keep in mind that the defense puts on its case last and the information conveyed during the defense is the last material the jury considers. The jury is more inclined to absorb and remember the most recent material. Be patient and trust that counsel will allow full explanation and clarification at a later time, as the following exchange illustrates.

To set the stage, assume that the plaintiff's counsel asked the defendant physician, who is being sued for medical negligence, if the plaintiff, who was suffering from a possible cervical injury, was intubated at the time of his presentation in the emergency department. The physician litigant answered by saying, "Yes, but I feel I should explain that decision," whereupon counsel for the plaintiff said, "You can clarify later, Doctor, all I asked was whether my client was intubated and you have answered the question."

At a later time, after plaintiff's counsel is finished with his or her questions, the defendant physician's counsel might stand up and ask the following, giving the defendant physician a chance to respond and clarify:

Q Doctor, during plaintiff's examination of you, you were asked several questions about your diagnosis and treatment of plaintiff. In one instance you were asked about your findings regarding the condition of his airway at the time he came into your emergency department. You answered the question, and you wanted to clarify, but counsel suggested you should defer your clarification. Would you please clarify now?

A Yes, thank you, counsel.

Q Please proceed.

A When plaintiff presented he was having difficulty breathing. Both I and my team had to decide if he was suffering from an airway obstruction or a condition that required medical intervention. The decision to intubate a patient with potential cervical spinal injuries is one that must be carefully but quickly assessed, because it is well known that intubation in the presence of severe cervical spinal injury can cause an exacerbation of the injury, and that is not desirable. On the other hand, to withhold intubation in this situation would have almost certainly led to the patient's death.

This exchange, clarifying what counsel for plaintiff would not allow, is now set in the minds of the jury and in a manner that they will remember when it is raised to them again. This illustrates the point that there is time to recover and that counsel will assist the physician defendant in clarifying what is unclear and making all of the necessary points.

Trust Your Attorney to Appropriatly Cross Examine the Plantiffs and Their Experts. The physician must remember that the right of cross-examination is the greatest "engine of justice" available, and the lawyer for the physician will have a chance to lessen much of the impact of the plaintiff's case during that process. Consider the following cross-examination of an expert for the plaintiff after the expert has testified that the physician defendant breached the standard of care:

Q Doctor [plaintiff's expert], do you agree that medicine is as much an art as it is a science?

A Well, there are aspects of "art" to it, but it is mostly science.

Q Doctor, medicine involves judgment, doesn't it? I mean doctors have to exercise clinical judgment all the time, right?

A Right, they do.

Q And to exercise clinical judgment you have to be there to observe, to see, to hear, to feel, to smell, and to use all of your senses as a physician; isn't that right? You can't make a clinical judgment without examination and judgment, can you?

A Not necessarily; you can make clinical judgments from a set of records.

Q True enough, doctor, but the fact is you were not there when Dr. [defendant] examined the patient and you did not have the benefit of seeing, hearing, touching, and smelling; you did not have the benefit of all the things that he had to rely on in making his judgment, correct?

A That's true, I wasn't there.

Q Yet you are prepared to sit here in judgment now as a Monday morning quarterback, aren't you?

A I have analyzed everything Dr. [defendant] did and I have concluded it was below the standard of care and not good practice.

Q Amazing, Dr. [expert]. I wish I had your God-like abilities to make judgments that involve facts that are important that you had no opportunity to observe. I have nothing more, your honor.

Note that the cross-examination has nothing to do with the medical care provided. It is an issue of image with a direct attack on the credibility of the expert. Tremendous headway can be made before a jury with effective cross-examination. There is time for the physician defendant and his or her attorney to recover lost ground on technical points during the presentation of their case.

The physician who quietly follows the lead of the lawyer appears professional. The physician who impulsively interrupts and tries to lead the examination appears to be a "know-it-all" who considers himself or herself better than the other people involved in the process. Trust and confidence in one's lawyer must be developed early and renewed often. Ultimately the physician will have much riding on the attorney's skills.

Watch out for the Ambush and the Negative Pregnant Question. A common tactic is to ask questions with implied negative answers. The correct way to answer the "negatively pregnant" question is to avoid it and dispel the negative:

Q How many times has a patient died while you were performing an intubation, doctor?

A No one has ever died, to my knowledge, as a result of an intubation that I have performed, counsel.

Another example:

Q Is your poor performance in this case, doctor, indicative of your poor training or your lack of continuing education in the field?

A My training was excellent and I am very proud of my continuing education in the field.

The "negatively pregnant" question can be especially disconcerting when it is asked as an ambush in the midst of a comfortable chat. After a pleasant trip down memory lane regarding a physician's medical education, internship, residency, honorary associations, fellowships, hospital staff privileges, and other relatively benign chatter, a question can be quickly laid out as follows:

Q Why did this patient die in your hands, doctor?

The obvious answer is as follows:

A Due to causes beyond my control. We exercise the best judgment we can in circumstances that present themselves but we cannot guarantee results.

Such a question can be an ambush, and the reaction, if not calculated, can be devastating. Be alert and expect the ambush question in many forms.

A Deposition is an Algorithm, and This Should be Remembered at all Times by a Party to a Case. A deposition of a party to a case may be used for myriad purposes at trial. It may be read in whole or in part, to refresh memory, to impeach, or to prove a point. Because defense attorneys can read from party depositions, it is best if there is nothing in the deposition that may be used or manipulated by the opposing party. This is another reason to keep answers short and pointed, with the algorithm concept closely in mind.

Most judges will not allow a lawyer to read only part of an answer or part of a question, but they will allow the reading of selected portions of a deposition. Thus answers to questions should be couched in terms that are sympathetic to the physician's position, are responsive to the question, and demonstrate awareness that the answer can be read back at will to the jury. Consider the following example:

Q Why did you feel comfortable, doctor, ruling out the myocardial infarction?

A Because the patient felt better and wanted to leave. I didn't feel it would be a problem to let him go if he promised to see his private doctor in the morning. He seemed OK to me and I did not feel further workup was justified or necessary. Besides, it's hard to hold patients in the hospital if they don't want to stay. You have to do a shift as a pit doc to understand the problems of our business. No matter what you do, it's never enough. We lose patients all the time because they don't listen and won't comply with what we tell them.

Contrast that with this:

Q Why did you feel comfortable, doctor, ruling out the myocardial infarction?

A All of the tests we did and all of the history taken and physical examination performed at the time the patient presented mitigated, in my judgment, against the diagnosis suggested.

Consider how the testimony could be linked if later in the deposition the following material appeared and was used at the trial:

Q Doctor, did you call a cardiologist to consult on this matter?

A No.

Q Why not?

A Because I didn't think it was necessary.

Q Do you always let patients go just because they feel better, even if you know they are at risk?

A We try to evaluate each person thoroughly and as completely as is indicated by the circumstances.

The first example demonstrates a physician in trouble because the physician has "cornered" himself or herself. The algorithm is broken because the second passage is not consistent with the first passage, and counsel can make the doctor look like he or she is unsure of the diagnosis made or the reasoning behind it. The second passage is consistent with the later deposition answer—obviously if a physician has sincerely ruled out a heart attack, there is not need to call a specialist. The answers are consistent.

The second passage, to put it another way, is scientifically based and is consistent with the judgment not to call a specialist. The first sequence could and probably would be read in the plaintiff's closing argument to the jury in conjunction with the later testimony from the same deposition. The reader need only contrast the effect of the two responses to see the potential impact.

Assess the Demography of Your Jurisdiction and Dress and Act Appropriate for That Venue. Jurors expect physicians to look and act professionally. They expect care, concern, professional behavior, bedside manner, and confidence. They expect surefootedness and the maturity and appearance of one who is capable of dealing with life and death. Because jurors all have medical problems and doctors, they will identify with the patient and will sense poor communication, lack of rapport, insecurity, and poor professional demeanor.

It's OK to wear Hawaiian shirts in Hawaii and cowboy boots in Texas, but it probably is not advisable to do so in New York or Chicago. Clean fingernails, trimmed hair and beards, a modicum of makeup, or other signs of good grooming and personal hygiene are essential. After all, isn't that what physicians would expect when being treated themselves?

Physicians are expected to follow all of the basic rules of hygiene and appearance because they are presumed to know the consequences of not following the rules. Juries are not iconoclastic people. They are the good citizens that respond to their community responsibilities. Although no one can state with clarity what a "good" or "bad" doctor looks like, many people "know one when they see one." The ability to instill confidence is a direct function of appearance and grooming, as well as being a method of expression.

A Physician Must be Aware of How He or She Sounds and What the Physician's Affect is in Every Circumstance in Which Jury Trials are Involved. Failure to be conscious of physiologic traits easily visible to others can be devastating.

Attempt to work out affect and personal physiologic traits that are annoying or that give mixed signals. Bad habits and traits that come out when a physician is nervous can be dangerous. Videotaped sessions with hard questions and critical review after the fact can mitigate large problems.

Along the same lines, use of jargon is to be discouraged because it tends to bore the jury and may make them think that the physician believes he or she is better than them.

Q How did the patient present himself to you?

A He was diaphoretic, febrile, had pain plus 7, with labored respirations and a slight rub. While I had not yet ruled out pericarditis since he had a history of recent URI, I felt he might well be suffering from MI so I ordered a CPK, an EKG, and requested that a team stand by with a crash cart including 02 sat monitors, ET tubes, atropine, sodium bicarb, and other medication. Fortunately his enzyme test was negative, his ST segments were flat, and I did not see any arrhythmias or signs of heart block, so we went on to assess him for triple A and possible ascending dissection because his radiographic studies showed a dilated and tortuous aortic pattern.

Such a manner of expression will be met with boredom, disdain, and a poor outcome. It does not matter whether the answer is incomplete, correct, incorrect, overly verbose, to the point, or otherwise. The jury *is listening,* and they just will not understand. Juries expect the physician to be clear and concise and to explain the facts and circumstances in a clear manner. They are not impressed with jargon or attempts to fool them or "hide the ball." They no more appreciate that kind of conduct in a trial setting than they do in the office setting where they are patients themselves.

A wonderful postulate that all physician defendants should keep in mind when they are testifying is that all jurors have had medical care—some with good result and feeling about the provider and some with bad results and feelings. They will consciously and subconsciously compare the treatment, care, and concern the physician defendant expresses with their own experiences. Jurors do not leave their experiences or their common sense at home.

Accents, affect, and manner of expression must be worked out in advance of deposition and trial. Care, concern, professionalism, sincerity, confidence, and surefootedness are the keys for success before the jury.

Stick to the Chart and Records—Memory Never Serves the Physician Well in the Trial or Deposition Context. No matter how smart a physician is, the physician is well advised to always refer to the chart. It is inconceivable that a physician can recall one patient out of thousands over a long period of time. It is acceptable to remember name, gender, and hospital where an incident may have occurred, but all else should come from the chart and records.

A jury expects a physician to have reviewed the records in close proximity to testimony at deposition or trial. They also expect a physician to be thorough and to refer back to the chart to ensure that the physician has the exact facts, times, medications, dosages, names, and orders stated correctly and in perspective. Having the names of colleagues such as consulting physicians and nurses identified in advance is reassuring to a juror as opposed to stumbling over names and words. If a physician cannot read a note in court, how could the note have been read under the pressure of the moment that preceded the untoward result over which the lawsuit is being litigated?

A physician gets demerits for being unsure, wrong, or for stating facts out of order. *A physician gets no points for good memory.*

Thus there is a need to refer to the records, which the jury expects to be complete and from which they expect the doctor to be able to reconstruct the facts. Pertinent portions of the record may include the presentation, how the physician and the nurse resolved differences in history and physical findings, what the reasoning was for the initial impression, how the "rule out" diagnosis was made and reasoned, the fact that the physician eliminated all of the conditions that were potentially catastrophic first and then moved on to lesser diagnoses, the emergency department course, the informed consent that was given for treatment, medication, and the thoroughness of follow-up and care.

All of these items must be in the chart. If they are not, referring to the chart is not only futile, but the physician will have to justify why the missing elements were not included. That can be devastating because an inference will be raised, and can fairly be raised, that sloppy in charting is sloppy in reasoning and sloppy in care.

Dictated charts with complete histories and physicals, a recitation that informed consent was given for treatment and medications, an explanation of the diagnostic process and the reasoning process used to get to the working diagnosis or impression, the emergency department course, and clear follow-up instructions are the first line of defense. They will also serve the physician well in the courtroom and at deposition. They show care, concern, and professional pride.

Be Convincing and Sincere—Bedside Manner with the Jury is as Important as Patient Rapport. The following question is often asked in trial, and it can make or break the trial depending on the skill of the attorney in asking it, its timing, and the skill of the physician answering it:

Q Doctor, I know you have been concerned about this case for 4 years now. You have contemplated and considered it and wondered if you could have done anything differently. Doctor, if the same patient presented himself today as presented himself 4 years ago, with exactly the same symptoms and circumstances, would you do anything different now than you did then?

A *[after some contemplation—in a sincere and caring manner]* No! What I did 4 years ago was correct medicine and so I would do it again.

Juries can accept human error or untoward results. They cannot and will not accept a lack of surefootedness or insecurity about a physician's decisions. The public image is of surefooted scientific healers who are tired, overworked, wise, and dedicated—the *Marcus Welby affect,* it has been called—and they expect every bit of that affect in trial and out of trial, as well as in deposition.

It is important to recognize the need to be surefooted and to inspire the kind of confidence that makes jurors want the physician on trial to be their doctor at the end of the trial.

Do Not Become an Unwitting Expert Against Your Hospital or Your Colleagues. A frequent source of rancor among healthcare professionals occurs when one professional unwittingly does harm to another. The best intentions can be thwarted by carelessness in the deposition and trial process. Making one defendant doctor an expert against another defendant is a favorite technique often employed by plaintiff attorneys. The typical exchange might go like this:

Q Doctor, do you have any criticism of the staffing provided to you at Community Hospital?

A Yes; I think we are shortchanged on nursing staff as well as technicians, especially in the emergency department. By the way, we could use an ultrasonographer as well on a 24-hour basis.

Obviously, the jury now believes that the testifying physician holds the opinion that the hospital is holding back on necessary care. It only remains for the plaintiff's counsel to link the untoward events to a shortage of personnel for a plaintiff's victory to occur.

The correct answer to any questions about a colleague or an institution, if you wish to avoid becoming an inadvertent expert against that person or entity, is, "I am not an anesthesiologist and I don't really know whether Doctor Jones' performance was within the standard of care for anesthesiologists—I only know he tried darn hard and I respect his efforts."

Another acceptable answer could be, "I am not a hospital administrator and I can't tell you if the hospital is properly staffed. Our emergency department group has always felt comfortable with the hospital and the administration and we are pleased and proud to work with them."

Care must be taken to avoid unintended implications. Remember, a deposition is an algorithm—say only what is necessary and do not volunteer information.

Always address the people who will be making the decision—the jury. It is important to always address the decision maker, because the jury focuses on relevant as well as irrelevant issues during the course of a trial. Frankness, and honesty, and noncondescending earnestness are essential to make the decision maker believe you are sincere. The art of trial is in making the jury believe that the defendant (or the plaintiff) believes in his or her case and decision-making process. Jury studies have repeatedly shown that the jury process is mostly one of assessment of the parties themselves because it is axiomatic that each party will have an expert who will testify favorably for them.

It is then the only other expert left, the defendant, who can speak to the technical issues and who can convince the jury that the case should be decided for the defendant. Sympathy, passion, and emotion have no place in a trial according to the law, but it would be a rare jury, judge, lawyer, or physician who could look at a severely handicapped child, a teenager paralyzed from the neck down, a despondent mother who had lost her child, or a little girl who had lost her dad and not feel sympathy.

To feign a dispassionate affect is foolish. Expressing the tragedy of the human condition as everyone perceives it and then addressing the real issue—can the tragedy of the human condition always be controlled and prevented?—is truly the best way to face a jury. Addressing the jury sincerely and directly can defuse any number of otherwise potentially explosive issues, and it always goes a long way in demonstrating courage of conviction and decisiveness.

The physician must prepare his or her lawyer to examine and cross-examine. The emergency physician should choose lawyers who specialize in emergency medicine from among the available panel of lawyers employed by the institution or the insurance company that provides legal coverage. Lawyers within the malpractice defense field have subspecialties just as physicians do. The physician must identify the person or firm that makes the physician most comfortable and then have an in-depth discussion regarding the case and perhaps even demonstrate the involved procedure. This process will help develop an informed and comfortable relationship between the counsel and the physician. A high comfort level between physician and lawyer will breed mutual trust and enhance the ultimate performance of both at trial.

There is an old adage known by salespeople all over the world: if you don't believe in your product, you cannot sell it to anyone because you will not be able to make them believe in it either.

The physician's attorney must believe in the physician individually. However, even more important, the physician's attorney must understand the clinical and conceptual aspects of what happened and why the conduct of the client was within the standard of care. Every procedure is different, and it is wrong to assume that a lawyer is as conversant with the concept or the clinical aspects of the concept even under the best of circumstances. In addition, to the extent that there is a bibliography of dispositive articles or material in the medical literature, pointing those materials out to the lawyer can only be supportive.

Review prior depositions and trial transcripts to avoid being impeached or contradicted in front of the jury. Whenever a physician is deposed or testifies in a case, whether as an expert, a party, a witness, or a subsequent treating physician, a transcript of the proceedings should be obtained and added to the physician's library. The plaintiff's bar will have "the book" on the physician party or expert witness and will uncover other cases in which the physician has testified and will obtain the transcripts of those prior efforts. It is foolish to be caught in a contradiction because all of these materials are also available to the physician.

Jury reporting services provide names and specialties of experts who have testified, as well as court titles and case descriptions, thus making trial testimony easily available. Additionally, the network of attorneys around the country maintains lists of people who have previously testified and provides those names to colleagues. Thus prior depositions are always available.

It is acceptable to have changed an opinion either because the circumstances are different or because the theory or practice of medicine has changed in the interim between the prior testimony and the present. However, one should be prepared for the apparent contradiction and ready with the explanation rather than be surprised and appear flustered when the issue is raised. Consider the following exchange:

Q Doctor, you have now told us, if I am not mistaken, and you correct me if I am wrong, that a case of meningitis can be definitively diagnosed by observation of a child alone; is that correct?

A Essentially that is true. Observation is the most important aspect of early diagnosis, and early diagnosis is essential to successful treatment.

Q Doctor, do you recall giving your deposition in the case of *Jones versus Smith* in [the adjacent state] 3 years ago in which a similar question was asked of you?

A Not specifically; let me see what you have there.

Q Your honor, I have a certified copy of the deposition of Dr. Smith from the trial here and I would like to read from page 29, lines 1 through 12.

The judge instructs counsel to proceed, and counsel then reads the transcript:

Q Is observation the most important element in the diagnosis of meningitis in a child?

A Absolutely not, counsel; without a lumbar tap and additional tests you can never be sure; observation isn't even close to enough.

Q Thank you, doctor, I have nothing further.

Caught in a major contradiction, the physician has assisted the opposing counsel in making a point about the honesty and integrity of the testimony under consideration by the jury.

How much easier it would have been to be aware that the prior testimony existed and to have been prepared for it. The original answer could have been, "Observation is the most important element in early diagnosis. Lumbar tap and other tests are considered important, but not as important as observation." If the lawyer still tried to use the certified prior deposition, the doctor could have answered the question regarding whether the physician recalled the earlier testimony by stating something like the following: "Yes, I do recall that testimony, but the facts and circumstances of that case were totally different and they must be explained or the answer I gave there will be out of context and misunderstood by the jury." The difference in impact is so dramatic that such a foolhardy attempt to create the appearance of contradiction by plaintiff counsel could be turned into an asset by the defense. Be prepared for such a contingency by reviewing prior testimony, which should be available to the physician directly or through counsel representing the physician.

Never argue or become frustrated in deposition or courtroom testimony. It is extremely unwise to fight or argue in a testimony. Attorneys often attempt to vilify the opposition in the presence of a jury so that the jury will more readily identify with their client's cause and circumstances.

If an attorney can get an opposing physician to perform in an arbitrary or argumentative manner under examination, the attorney becomes the controlling factor. Calmness, competence, and patience are what the jury expects. After all, the jury expects these attributes when they are under the care and treatment of a physician.

Becoming argumentative can work to the benefit of the plaintiff and against the physician under examination. The physician should avoid showing frustration at the lawyer's apparent inability to understand basic anatomy, basic procedure, and the dynamics of the emergency department setting. In fact, a physician with self-control will respond calmly and not answer a question if it is a nonsequitur. Consider the following:

Q Doctor, I understand the pain medication that was most desirable here was supposed to be given parenterally; so my question is, doctor, why did you give the shot in the buttocks?

A I don't understand your question, could you please rephrase it?

Q What don't you understand, doctor?

A I'm terribly sorry, counsel, but your question doesn't make any medical sense and I cannot answer it in its present form. I would like to try, but you will have to rephrase it.

Contrast that with the following:

Q Doctor, I understand that the pain medication that was best in this situation was supposed to be given parenterally; so why did you give the shot in the buttocks?

A Counsel, I am so tired of having to give you a medical lesson on everything you ask that I can't begin to tell you. If you would just do a little preparation you would understand that a shot in the buttocks *is* parenteral administration of medication. I don't know what you have in mind but it would be nice if you could figure it out before you asked it.

The jury is listening! The second answer gives everyone an education from someone who is annoyed, angry, and obviously feels superior to everyone else in the courtroom. "Why am I being subjected to these ignorant people who are not my 'peers?' "

This is an example of the exasperation and frustration that can anger a jury and give a plaintiff an edge. Under no circumstances should a physician express pique or anger at counsel or the plaintiff. The results in the eyes of the jurors can be serious.

Don't become fatigued or tired during the testimonial effort—take time to refresh. The physician does not have to "run a marathon" during testimony. The physician should ask for a break if he or she tires and loses concentration and the ability to keep the facts, rules, and purposes of the effort in mind.

It is acceptable to request a break in the proceedings for water, toilet relief, or just because of fatigue. Attorneys, juries, judges, clerks, court reporters, and bailiffs all have personal needs, and if the physician under examination is fatigued, they probably are too.

The privilege should be exercised when needed, but not abused. In most cases it will be respected.

Avoid the use of slang, and take care not to fall into the trap of familiarity. Respect for the process of law, the court, and the jury are expected. All parties to the process should avoid slang and terms of familiarity. Casual use of the word "yeah" in place of "yes" is in poor taste. Do not refer to patients by first name, even if the previous relationship permitted it. Avoid expressions of familiarity, such as "Look, son . . ."

Also be conscious of and try to avoid familiar colloquialisms such as "Ain't no way," or "You got it Jack," or "Heck no." Other examples of poor taste and expression are "No way, Jose," "Yup," or even more offensively, "He acted like a girl" or "He was as queer as a three-dollar bill." The latter examples are not only politically incorrect phrases but also offensive to large segments of the population. They are demeaning, pejorative, and inappropriate. Avoid their usage.

If you are referring to someone's appearance do so carefully and without any potentially pejorative meaning. For example, if someone is asked to describe a patient after she returned from a vacation in Hawaii, she might be described as "well tanned" as opposed to "dark as a Polynesian princess." Certainly phrases such as "He was as black as the ace of spades" or "He was typically Jewish looking" are absolutely contraindicated. Unlikely as these examples may seem, they are actual examples of expression that are part of some normal (however misguided) conversations, but they have no place in deposition or courtroom parlance.

It is appropriate to be a little more formal than usual in normal social and business intercourse. The legal process has a solemnity about it, and the extra dignity that a physician might be able to bring to it can only be a benefit.

Once again, the recurrent theme: *the jury is listening and watching!*

SUMMARY

The art of communication is extremely important in the practice of any profession. It is especially important in the medicolegal setting. The ability to create an image of surefooted self-confidence without appearing haughty or condescending, the ability to convey care and concern in the face of a catastrophe, and the ability to make all of the listeners relate favorably to the person communicating is the heart of the exercise.

Effective communication is an asset that cannot be overpracticed. It can be learned and always improved on. It is essential that the physician faced with a claim understand the value of effective communication.

68 The Expert Witness—His, Hers, and Mine

William H. Ginsburg

"I don't know the key to success:
I do know the key to failure:
Trying to please everybody all the time!"

Wm. Cosby, Jr.

OUTLINE

The standard of care
It's about winning and losing, not justice
The emergency physician as a unique expert
Selecting an expert
- Make sure expert qualifications are genuine and in order
- The jury is listening and trying to decide who they can trust
- Make sure counsel knows all of the expert's qualifications
- Disclose all prior literature written in the expert's name for review and inspection
- The right experts must be selected

The hypothetical question
Credibility is the ultimate test of an expert
- Convert negative questions into positive answers
- Make the jury see you as an expert
- Never condescend to a jury
- The expert must be prepared
- Rehearsal for trial and deposition
- Use of medical literature

Some practical tips for prospective expert witnesses

The concept of expert testimony is as old as the jury trial system. An expert is defined as a person who can shed light on a topic not generally considered to be within the grasp or understanding of members of the general public who are generally selected to be jurors.

This chapter describes the role of the medical expert in medical negligence litigation. A case alleging medical negligence or a defective medical product cannot proceed without at least one medical expert. It is safe to say that the "art" of forensic medicine has risen to the status of a minor industry for those physicians who want to extend their talents into the forensic arena. Certainly, the role of the expert has expanded in direct proportion to the number of medical negligence cases being brought in the courts of this country.

Although many people consider medicine as much of an art as a science, it is sufficiently alien to a lay jury as a discipline, with concepts and clinical practices unknown to any but those involved with healthcare, and with a language all its own, that it must be explained with care and great detail. This allows the lay jury to apply the principles of medicine to the law as explained to them by the judge. Thus an expert is needed to guide, explain, and translate.

Doctors and their associations have self-generated a "magic of medicine," which is resented by many jurors. The need to unwind (unravel) and reverse the concept is present in most trials. A feeling that physicians are no different from everyone else can go a long way toward the process of persuasion.

It should never be assumed that the lawyer who engaged an expert has any working knowledge about the specific aspects of medicine involved in the case at hand. The lawyer engaging the expert should use the expert as a bellweather to ensure a level of knowledge in the specific areas in question so that it can be understood by the jury. The lawyer is just as uneducated a peer as a juror in most cases of alleged medical negligence.

A good rule of thumb is the following: If the attorney who has engaged an expert is sufficiently conversant with the medicine involved in the case at hand, enabling him or her to discuss it intelligently, replete with analogy and clinical insight, then the expert has successfully reduced the detail and terminology into an acceptable forensic package.

The trained emergency physician who harbors the belief that the concept of a "jury of peers" has anything to do with educational background or knowledge is sadly mistaken and is simply not in touch with the definition of the word *peer* or the very nature of the jury system. A peer is a citizen on an equal footing with the persons to be tried in a civil or criminal matter. Peers are equals under the law, people who have the same background of citizenship and the associated rights. Otherwise, there is no guarantee in the constitution or any document that people who will sit on juries must be specially educated or knowledgeable. Thus the physician, as an expert, must convey the concepts of clinical practice and the general knowledge of medicine to a group of his or her peers in an effective way so that the information can be used and absorbed in a meaningful manner. Whether acting on behalf of the plaintiff or defendant, the medical expert must be convincing while conveying technical information in an interesting and noncondescending manner.

THE STANDARD OF CARE

All of the information with regard to the standard of care must come from the physicians, including the defendant, who testify at trial.

The standard of care is purported to be national in its scope rather than local or regional. In fact this is rather idealistic because it suggests that the care rendered in every setting should be held up to some undefinable and elusive standard. Demography, circumstances, the quality of lawyers representing the parties, and the persuasiveness of the experts engaged to assist in the trial all play a role in the ultimate determination of the width and breadth of the standard of care.

It is clearly evident that "old Dr. Jones," who has delivered and cared for virtually every citizen of "Elmville" over the last 40 years, would be held to a different standard of care in a trial venued in Elmville than in New York, Chicago, or Los Angeles.

To determine what is meant by "standard of care," the jury must determine the credibility of the experts and sort out their opinions to arrive at the baseline question: Was the defendant doctor negligent in the performance of care and treatment of a medical nature?

It is easy to see how the uncrowned poet laureate of the United States, Robert Frost, could issue the cynical statement, "A jury trial is a contest between two people to see who has the better lawyer." The word *expert* could easily be exchanged for the word *lawyer.*

The entirety of a jury trial consists of efforts to persuade the jurors of one's position and dissuade them from the position of the opponent. It is a boxing match of words and wit, knowledge and personality, and ego and will.

IT'S ABOUT WINNING AND LOSING, NOT JUSTICE

Lawyers, who are trained to win, care about truth. They may have little concern, however, with justice as an abstract concept because justice always, by definition, requires his or her client to win. Such an attitude has given rise to folklore personified by the story of the lawyer who was told upon the verdict of a jury having been read that justice was done. The lawyer immediately replied, "Shall we take an appeal?" The experts then are, by definition, a necessary weapon in the arsenal of both sides of a case and must be garnered by plaintiff and defendant to enable them to proceed.

THE EMERGENCY PHYSICIAN AS A UNIQUE EXPERT

With the exception of a few states,* any physician can qualify to testify for either side regardless of training or background because, by theory, all physicians are able to shed light on the science applied by another physician.

As a practical matter, however, the experts sought by both plaintiffs and defendants are those that share the same training and specialty. The reason is obvious—credibility. Thus even in states where an emergency physician is not required to testify in cases involving emergency physicians, it is likely that lawyers will select emergency physicians as experts in their cases. The reason, as stated earlier, is that only such a physician involved in the practice of day-to-day emergency medicine is able to render an appropriate opinion credibly.

SELECTING AN EXPERT

The problems of expert selection to the attorney are evident. Counsel does not want anyone too academic for a nonacademic situation, nor does it want someone too folksy or undercredentialed. Like most phenomena in jury trial work, perceptions, sometimes artificial and irrelevant, are often more important than reality.

Membership in national associations, leading to letters after one's name, is a competitive factor. An expert is considered more qualified if he or she is a FACEP, FAAFP, FACOG, FACP, FACS or some other "alphabet qualified" individual. Much time may be taken to discuss these organizations if a lawyer thinks it is a selling point to a jury. Thus the doctor who can list his or her name with board certification, such as Fellow of the American College of Emergency Physicians (FACEP) and other titles, is to be respected, but no more revered than any other person who has pride in what he or she does. Juries can appreciate that type of approach. However, much diversion from the issues can occur if the importance of these organizations and concepts is not handled with humility and care. The best way to handle the situation when overemphasized by the opposing side is to indicate that the organizations are challenging and great resources to ensure continuing education, but that "letters" do not make someone more qualified. Quality, care, and concern, as well as dedication, are the essentials of the profession. Board certification is important as a personal challenge and as a mechanism of self-testing, but it is not the pinnacle of ability or credential.

Physicians may find themselves in a defensive position by trying to support the importance of their credentials or justifying their nonmembership or participation in organizations and activities. This diverts attention from their position and opinions and makes them vulnerable in their qualifications.

Physicians who are not board certified, although potentially still excellent physicians, are eyed with suspicion, especially when the defendant doctor or the plaintiff expert is board certified. Board certification is not the sine qua non of medical criteria with regard to the qualifications of physicians to practice medicine or surgery, but in the world of the courtroom that simple qualification has become a competitive factor.

One need only use imagination to understand the fodder a lawyer has for examination of a doctor who could not or did not "pass the boards." This problem becomes pronounced if the doctor tries to defend his or her position as opposed to just accepting the reality of the situation and dwelling on the real issue, the standard of care, and the treatment given or received in a particular case.

Make Sure Expert Qualifications are Genuine and in Order

The first principle of being an expert is to make sure that qualifications and credentials are in order and that the limits of their value and importance are understood. The concept of humility and understatement cannot be stressed enough.

*See California Health and Safety Code, for example, where Section 1799.110 states in relevant part, "In any action for damages involving a claim of negligence against a physician and surgeon providing emergency medical coverage for a general acute care hospital emergency department, the court shall admit expert testimony only from physicians and surgeons who have had substantial professional experience within the last 5 years while assigned to provide emergency medical coverage in a general acute care emergency department . . ." California courts have stated that the threshold question as to whether an expert can testify against an emergency physician, is not whether the care rendered was "emergency care", but whether the defendant physician was acting as an emergency physician in an emergency department when the defendant physician did the allegedly negligent acts. (Zavala v. Board of Trustees Stanford University decided July 1, 1993—Sixth Appellate District). This is not the majority view around the country, but is considered the better view.

In this day of specialization, the old time family general practitioner with an internship and no residency is limited to rural and isolated areas. Virtually every major metropolitan community has specialists replete with residencies and fellowships, as well as clinical teaching positions.

The fact that the public thinks that physicians consider themselves "better than others," which has been verified in more than one study and survey,* can only be brought home in failed expert testimony where the expert is haughty or self-righteous about credentials instead of understated and humble. The typical examination regarding qualifications goes something like this:

Q Doctor would you give us a brief rundown of your education after high school?
A Yes. I went to the University of [State] where I majored in biology [zoology] [chemistry] [science]. I graduated with a Bachelor of Science degree. I then went to the University Medical School and graduated in 19_____ with my MD degree.
Q Did you do an internship thereafter?
A Yes. I did a rotating internship at Our Lady of Great Agony Hospital in Anytown, USA (explanation of a rotating internship versus a straight internship).
Q Thereafter did you do a residency?
A Yes. I did a residency at University Medical Center in Othertown, USA for 4 years in emergency medicine, which I completed in 19_____.
Q Did you receive any honors while you were in your residency?
A Yes. I was chief resident for 1½ years. I received the Dr. Ralph Knowitall award for best diagnosis in a New York minute and I was a member of Sigma Sigma medical association, which is the honorary association for academic achievement at the hospital teaching center.
Q Did you then go into practice?
A In a manner of speaking I had been in practice all through my residency; we saw 45,000 patients a year at the hospital and many more in the clinics. In addition, after I completed the residency I did a fellowship, advanced training, at Crosstown University Medical Center.
Q At that point did you go into practice with a private group?
A Yes. I went to work with Emergency, Inc. as a doctor at St. Elsewhere hospital and have been with the group for 12 years now as an emergency physician. I work several shifts a week at St. Elsewhere and see about 200 people a week for various problems and ailments, including people just like the one that is involved in this case.
Q Do you currently do any teaching?
A Yes. I am an associate clinical professor of medicine at Holy-Holy-Children's- Catholic-Jewish-Baptist-Methodist-Lutheran-Presbyterian-County Community Hospital where I teach interns and residents how to practice in the real world.
Q Have you written anything?
A I have participated in the writing of 12 articles, 3 chapters of textbooks, and have presented 12 papers to Medical Societies and Hospitals in my field (explanation of some of papers and articles).
Q Do you belong to any honorary societies?
A Yes. I am a member of the International Academy of Emergency Physicians, the United States Clinical Emergency Medical Physician's Association, and the Phi Phi Phi Medical Fraternity.

This approach can get tedious. Jurors are interested in credentials, but only to a point. Counsel decides how far to take this issue and the expert should be compliant in giving all information requested. Even the area of credentials can subject the expert to cross-examination, a taste of which might be illustrated by the following:

Q Doctor, you do not have to take an examination to get into the American College of Emergency Physicians do you? I mean you make an application, send in your dues, and you are in, right?
A Well, yes, but they do screen every applicant to make sure they are licensed . . .

Another "attack" might be as follows:

Q Doctor, you never did a residency in Emergency Medicine, did you?
A No, I did not.
Q You were grandfathered into eligibility for the boards, weren't you?
A Yes I was.

Note that there is no need to be defensive or explanatory. If the jury perceives the expert is skilled, such ad hominem attacks will be poorly received and probably dismissed as being inappropriate and boorish. The point is that even an issue as simple as credentials can be the source of cross-examination.

The Jury is Listening and Trying to Decide Who They Can Trust

The jury is listening and each side is trying to convince them with as much material as they believe can be absorbed, attempting to find the "button" that gives the expert credibility with each juror.

Lawyers even try to appeal to the charitable side of jurors in their examination. Consider this:

Q Do you give time to the church, Doctor Expert?
A Oh yes, we do a clinic for the poor every week—and by the way I forgot to mention I served 2 years in the United States Marine Corps serving our country.

Only to have defense counsel ask:

Q Where?
A Maui, 1981 to 1983—it was tough work, but someone had to do it.

There is fire and backfire, all at risk of alienating the jury, which may well tire of the incessant games that lawyers sometimes play to win their favor. At the end of the "shelling," the jury should have an impression favorable to one side or the other.

Make Sure Counsel Knows all of the Expert's Qualifications

The second principle is to make sure the counsel who engages you as an expert has all the information necessary to qualify you effectively, including strengths and weaknesses. This avoids problem areas such as disclosure that during a recent military action you were stationed at a beachside hotel in Maui, Hawaii.

*See American Medical Association study and Harris poll of 1991.

Also be sure that the counsel with whom the expert is working understands the implications of all of the organizations and associations listed on the expert's curriculum vitae. Sometimes a preemptive strike, taking the thunder away from the opposing side, is appropriate. In that way the credentials can be laid out, examined, criticized under friendly fire, and thus defused as a nonissue. This can only be accomplished, however, if it is disclosed, digested, and understood by counsel who is orchestrating the trial.

Counsel should be familiar with the subject and content of your papers and chapters if they are at all relevant to the subject at hand.

Disclose all Prior Literature Written in the Expert's Name for Review and Inspection

The third principle is that an expert has given depositions or has testified in court before about a similar matter, the content should be disclosed so that counsel can be prepared to handle it in advance. There is nothing more embarrassing than having opposing counsel armed with your prior testimony when your counsel is not aware.

Experts should demonstrate balance in the cases they review. Lawyers easily attack the doctor who has become a professional witness—who testifies for a living rather than practices medicine. Another easily attacked expert is one who always testifies for one side or is the constant expert of one lawyer.

To say that an expert reviews cases for both plaintiffs and defendants suggests a more unbiased witness. An expert who agrees to take those cases that are meritorious and in fact has taken 60% defense cases and 40% plaintiff's cases (or some other reasonable ratio) is more appealing to a jury. It is also helpful when the physician expert is able to say that income from testifying and reviewing records accounts for only a small percentage of the total income (5% or less).

The Right Experts Must be Selected

Mixing and matching experts also may be necessary. Counsel does not always have the luxury of selecting experts with knowledge of the other side's selections, but when possible, such maneuvering may be important to engineer.

Often members of the same specialty or subspecialty are competitors or friends, and knowing in advance the effect of such a relationship is important to the lawyer, as well as to the physician expert. Interdisciplinary hostility can thus be avoided or exploited and a more effective result can be achieved.

A desire of eviscerating an opponent is not healthy or desirable. Likewise, testifying in opposition to a friend or colleague can be uncomfortable and can potentially destroy the effectiveness of the testimony because of conscious or subconscious considerations.

Once an expert is selected and approved, it may be wise to meet with both counsel and the physician defendant. Some counsel keep the experts away from the defendant for strategic reasons. This allows counsel to say the expert is being purely objective, does not know the defendant physician, and was not influenced with any facts brought to bear by the defendant. Others like to expose the expert to the defendant in controlled circumstances so they can listen and learn and so the expert can say he or she took the defendant's clinical observations and findings into account in arriving at his or her opinion.

The plaintiff's experts are unable to meet with the defendant for ethical reasons. Instead the plaintiff's experts must wait for the deposition of the defendant to factor the findings into their opinion.

THE HYPOTHETICAL QUESTION

The principal method of questioning expert witnesses is the so-called hypothetical question. Counsel can ask experts questions in a hypothetical fashion and then ask them for their opinions. The key to understanding a hypothetical question is that it is not hypothetical at all. It is the facts of the case at hand, and each counsel must ask true and accurate hypotheticals to make them meaningful. If a counsel asks a question in a hypothetical fashion that is inaccurate in some respects, it does not have to be answered.

Counsel monitoring the case on the side of the expert may not realize the problem with and object to a particular hypothetical question. In that situation the expert might signal the counsel by gently protesting that the facts do not comport with actual events in the case at bar.

Counsel is technically allowed to ask any hypothetical question as long as they are willing to represent that they can prove the facts underlying their hypothetical question. Few counsel are willing to go out on a limb to represent to a court and jury that they can prove something that they cannot prove.

It is essential that the expert recognize that hypothetical questions always have substantial flexibility. As a result, the answer can be molded into the opinion that is essential to support the case the expert is trying to present.

The expert can always mold the answer to fit the issue. Consider the following exchange:

Q Doctor I want you to assume a patient who is 54 years old presents in your emergency department with substernal chest pain radiating to his arm. It is early in the morning and he is on his way to work. He has a history of heart disease in his family. His father, who died at age 56 from coronary causes, was a smoker for 15 years before giving it up 3 years before his death. Please assume further that the patient was ashen gray when he presented in the emergency department and had pain of +7 as reported by the nurses. He had some diaphoresis and labored respirations. The doctor gave him a "GI Cocktail" consisting of Xylocaine, Mylanta, and Donnatol and decided he had gastroenteritis. The patient was discharged after 45 minutes in the emergency department with a diagnosis of gastroenteritis and recommended to see his private medical doctor the next day or immediately if the pain recurred. Three hours later the patient died from a myocardial infarction. Do you believe the doctor was in violation of the standard of care?

A Not necessarily, no.

Q Doctor, can you tell us, in your opinion, the proper procedure to follow with a patient diagnosed as having a myocardial infarction?

The problem of being an expert witness is illustrated by the above exchange because the expert now has a choice.

This first answer reflects clearly what a plaintiff's expert would say:

A A complete workup would have been conducted including cardiac enzymes after admission and monitoring of the situation including the administration of analgesics and other essential medications. In essence, the patient would have been cared for instead of released in the community to die.

The defense on the other hand might wish to respond as follows:

A Without further information I cannot state what would have happened next.

Q What further information do you need?

A What did the doctor do upon review of the nurses' notes and the presentation of the patient to him or her?

Q Assume the doctor talked to the patient and otherwise was receptive to the concept of the pain being suffered by the decedent. Assume further that he wanted to do more but the plaintiff did not want to stay. He felt better and wanted to go to work, where he was originally headed.

The plaintiff's expert may go forward with a continued answer as follows:

A Under the circumstances, the physician in charge should have admitted him; if he was reluctant, the physician should have been persuasive and should not have let him go. The risks of heart attack and death were too great.

The defendant's response might again differ as follows:

A What the physician in charge would do very much depends on the circumstances. A physician is in no position to force anyone to stay in a hospital. Persuasive behavior that might well be appropriate here must be judged carefully. Establishment of a patient alliance and engendering sufficient patient confidence may be more important than mere insistence. I cannot fault the physician for not insisting on a stay and an admission because nothing in this life is sure and the physician was no more clairvoyant than the patient. Everything in medicine is a judgment call and a decision. This circumstance is no different.

The difference in approach is obvious. In one case there is certainty and in the other there is room for judgment. Thus the expert who is most persuasive will probably prevail. The jury listens to and watches experts carefully. They write off some and believe others. The difference is always in trust and credibility, which cannot be described, only recognized when seen and felt!

The expert is a key player, and the professionalism manifested by the expert is a key to success in a trial. It may well seem an overstatement to say that an expert must be a salesperson replete with warmth and charm and the ability to convey a sincerity and insight that makes a jury want the expert as their doctor, but that is just what is needed.

CREDIBILITY IS THE ULTIMATE TEST OF AN EXPERT

Experts must be perceived by the jury to be credible, well versed, and in touch with the practical problems experienced by both the patient and the physician in the day-to-day practice of medicine. The 10 things that all counsel look for when examining how to best handle an opposing expert are the following:

1. How will the expert appear physically to the jury—appealing and warm or cold and detached?
2. Can the expert be caused to become emotional and out of control?
3. Does the proposed expert have real credentials or are they assailable? Is he or she board certified, grandfathered into eligibility for the boards, teaching at a reputable institution, properly licensed, previously disciplined, or otherwise in trouble?
4. Can the expert's credentials be attacked by virtue of the "ivory tower" status of the expert, or is the expert in the day-to-day practice of medicine in a facility similar to the defendant being sued?
5. Has the proposed expert significantly favored one lawyer or one side to such an extent that the validity of the expert's testimony can be questioned?
6. Has the expert said or written anything in previous depositions, testimony, or articles that would contradict his or her testimony in the present matter?
7. Does the expert have personal, financial, or other motive for testifying in the manner in which he or she is testifying?
8. Can the expert be turned into becoming an expert for the side against whom he or she is testifying?
9. What will be the jury's impression of the proposed expert at the end of the testimony?
10. Does the proposed expert's testimony really make any difference to the real issue in the case?

Knowing these 10 items enables an expert to prepare to testify by exposing all of his or her potential weaknesses in advance and thus preparing to counter them before they are raised by the other side. Often, knowing the weaknesses that may be raised by the other side can be an asset, and the potential problems can be defused.

An illustration of that concept can be found in the "Aren't you being paid as an expert" line of questions. A related line of questions for some counsel is the following:

Q How much are you receiving for your testimony in this trial, doctor?

A I get $3,000.00 a day for my testimony.

Q How much in addition to that, which I assume you will be paid for today, have you already gotten or at least billed in this matter.

A Let's see . . . I have billed an additional $7000 for reviewing records, depositions, and consultations.

From those questions and answers, counsel will call the expert, "His opponent's well-paid expert" in closing argument or some other choice epithets.

The answers to these questions should be treated like all questions that are negatively pregnant with pejorative implications.

Q How much are you being paid for your testimony here today, doctor?

A I am not paid for my testimony; I am paid for my time including the cost of shutting down my office and having to specially reschedule all of my patients.

Q How much are you being paid for your time?

A To keep my office open and pay my support staff and management people I require $3000 a day.

Q How much in addition to the $3000, which I assume you are getting for today, have you already gotten or at least billed in this matter?

A I do not recall, but I can assure you I have billed for my time at an agreed upon rate of $250.00/hour for all time taken in reviewing records, depositions, and other pertinent material to prepare myself to give a fair and reasonable opinion here today. I want to be fair and thus I did prepare.

The difference in the answers is evident, and a major item has been defused.

Convert Negative Questions into Positive Answers

An expert is not perfect, nor is an expert expected to have all the answers. An expert should not answer a question that is not clearly understood. The question must be understood so that the answer has meaning in the context of the question.

The expert should keep in mind that a lawyer can order partial transcripts on a daily basis and literally read back questions and answers. Thus it is necessary for the expert to concentrate on the question and relay a meaningful answer so that if read back in context, it creates a positive impression for the jury.

Consider the following illustration:

Q Did Dr. [Defendant] act in a manner below the standard of care in rendering the treatment and care to Mr. [Plaintiff] that he rendered or failed to render as we have established thus far in this trial?

A No, he did not.

While that is an acceptable answer that is not subject to criticism from anyone, consider the following answer and decide if it is better:

A No, he did not. He acted with extreme care in a manner that comports with the best training and skills available in emergency medicine today. Mr. [Plaintiff] was a victim of circumstances beyond Dr. [Defendant's] control, and nothing Dr. [Defendant] did caused his problems.

The second answer has reinforcement and is much more effective either if read back intentionally by one party or the other in closing argument or if read back to the jury at their request.

Make the Jury see you as an Expert

If a question is not comprehensible, it should be responded to in a short but meaningful way that does not embarrass the lawyer asking the question. The jury should recognize and identify with the confused expert rather than sympathize with the lawyer who has been deridden by the expert with the superior knowledge.

Contrast the following:

Q In a patient suffering apnea, when they have elevated ST waves could that explain their fever?

A That question is totally incomprehensible counsel and is silly on its face!

The jury will identify with counsel who will then undoubtedly say, "I'm sorry doctor, what is silly to you is not to me . . . I'm just trying to represent Mr. Jones' widow and children and I am sorry to be wasting your time." In a word, the expert fell for the bait and was set up by counsel for the statement that the jury will remember after the expert is gone.

Consider a better way:

Q In a patient suffering from apnea, when they have elevated ST waves could that explain their fever?

A Counsel, I respect your attempt to do your job and I want very much to answer your questions. However, the question you have just posed is a bit confusing to me in its present form. I certainly would appreciate it if you could restate it and perhaps break it down so I am sure we are both on the same track.

The jury will respect that answer. They will not be critical of the doctor who is helping them understand a question that was even more incomprehensible to them than to the doctor on the witness stand. Become a guide, a colleague, and a mentor to the jury rather than an adversary, a boor, and a bore. Make the jury like you as an expert, and you will do your job successfully.

Never Condescend to a Jury

Remember that the jury is listening all the time. They do not want an expert to condescend to them or to dazzle them. They want to learn by listening and understanding.

An idea conveyed in a meaningful manner will allow the jury to feel like experts and colleagues. It will provide them with insight into the medical world replete with its "magic," nomenclature, and taxonomy of unique procedures and treatments.

Convert the "baited question" to a positive approach.

A question that asks whether something is possible can be answered with a wry, "Anything is possible," or it can be answered, "No, I really don't think that what you suggest is at all probable, medically. It is much more likely that the patient would have been suffering from a gastrointestinal disorder than a heart attack under the circumstances that presented themselves to Dr. [Defendant]." If the expert's overall approach to the trial has been perceived as positive up to that point, the jury will be likely to believe the expert now.

The Expert must be Prepared

Counsel who engages an expert must ensure that the expert is prepared. The expert must be presented with readable copies of all medical records and depositions as well as witness statements and other important material necessary for the expert to render an opinion. The more prepared an expert is when rendering their opinion, the more credible their testimony.

Familiarity with the materials and the issues shows care, concern, and credibility. Care must be taken to ensure that the other side does not make the expert appear to be a phoney. Incomprehensible medical records that counsel cannot read generally cannot be read by anyone, including the expert.

Counsel must be certain the materials are translated and that the expert is advised of the content of the unreadable parts. Otherwise an exchange with opposing counsel proving that a whole section of records was not considered by the expert in arriving at his or her opinion will certainly be presented in the trial.

If the expert cannot read the records, the suggestion will be raised that the expert relied on selected parts of the record and obviously was biased to supporting the position of the side that paid him or her. It is easier and more wiser to prepare than to have to explain the circumstances at trial.

Rehearse for Trial and Desposition

Rehearsal is important so that the tough questions can be anticipated and appropriate responses discussed in advance. The concept of rehearsal is just that—a chance for the expert to get into the mood of the proceeding. No lawyer will ever tell any party or expert, or for that matter any witness, what to say. It is appropriate to tell a witness who is properly contacted **how** to say what he or she wants to say as long as no lie or false testimony is being suborned.

The courtroom is an artificial environment to all parties except for lawyers and court personnel who use it all the time. It is neither uncommon nor beyond the comprehension of jurors that a witness would be nervous or "out of his or her element" in presenting the evidence to them. In fact, a perfectly appropriate response by an expert to a question about pretrial preparation with counsel might involve the expert openly stating that the courtroom is a frightening experience and much preparation took place so that the expert could effectively convey an independent and honest opinion. Members of the jury are just as nervous when questioned about their qualifications as jurors as the expert is in testifying. Such identification with the jury is positive and fair game.

Use of Medical Literature

Expert witnesses are frequently concerned with the use of literature from the various medical journals and academic sources. One of the expert's roles is to bring positive and negative literature to the attention of counsel to enlighten them. Supportive literature should be adapted and used. Unsupportive literature should be discussed because it is a reasonable probability that the other side has found the literature and will divulge it.

Experts often fear that literature will be used against them. Generally, however, unless an expert states that he or she is familiar with an article, a book, or a paper and has a working knowledge of it or has relied on it in forming opinions, it will not be admissible on cross-examination.

However, a caveat must be issued in connection with well-known and important literature. A qualified emergency physician is expected to be aware of important recent literature in relevant journals such as the *Annals of Emergency Medicine* and *Journal of Trauma*. The expert's professed ignorance of important well-known literature will negatively influence the jury's perception of the expert's credibility. However, the expert's knowledge and understanding of the literature and his or her ability to distinguish or differentiate it from the case on trial will enhance the credibility of the expert. If the literature comes from an obscure source, it is appropriate not to be familiar with it and to say so openly in court. The same rules apply to basic texts as opposed to obscure and remote publications.

Literature may be used to the advantage of a position that an expert is advocating. Because little is written about the standard of care, the literature often defines it. Reliance on an emerging body of literature and recognition that it is reflective of current thinking in an area are not only logical, but also persuasive to a jury, who will undoubtedly not understand the literature on direct reading.

PRACTICAL TIPS FOR PROSPECTIVE EXPERT WITNESSES

1. *Engagement letter:* Make certain that there is an engagement letter, or agreement, between the expert and counsel hiring or engaging the expert to review the file, chart, or case. Misunderstandings about fees, obligations, and independence can be avoided if such an agreement exists. It can also aid in receiving payment by the other side for depositions and other activities in which the other side may question an expert's fees.
2. *Monetary arrangements:* Do not take an active monetary percentage interest in a case. It is questionable to even be testifying on a lien at an hourly rate. Credibility concerning the independence of the expert is subject to scrutiny under those circumstances. The same is true if an expert has a substantial account balance with the party that hired him or her.
3. *Timing of payment:* Get paid in advance by the other side for deposition time. It is always good to include in the engagement letter the fact that counsel who has engaged the expert guarantees any such funds if counsel requests that you go forward with the deposition without payment. In that regard, get an estimate of the time that counsel for the other side intends to use for deposition and hold counsel to that estimate consistent with money paid for the expert's time. All bills should be paid by the time of the court appearance so that no motive for testimony can be implied by counsel.
4. *Rates:* If an expert is in doubt about what to charge for his or her time, talk to respected colleagues and other lawyers and people who are in tune with the custom and practice in the community where the expert is expected to give testimony. Rates vary around the country, and experts should be aware of the rates, as well as the need to have expenses prenegotiated and prepaid.
5. *Handling records:* Preserve all records and other material entrusted to you until you have written permission to destroy them. If in doubt, send them back to the counsel who forwarded them to you with a cover letter to be preserved in your skeleton file.
6. *Maintaining personal testimonies:* Keep copies of all depositions and transcripts prepared regarding your testimony. If a daily transcript of an expert's testimony at trial is made, the expert should insist that he or she get a copy for the library of materials kept by the expert. Commercial databases exist that keep all the material that is contributed, and the opposite side may have access to all previous transcripts. Having transcripts at the expert's disposal makes the expert that much more ready to act as an expert.
7. *Promoting expertise:* Do not directly advertise your availability as an expert. It creates a bad impression with juries and often impairs credibility. Make your availability known as an impartial expert through your colleagues and members of the bar who you know and trust. There are agencies that act as registries that will list names and cre-

dentials of experts and make them available for forensic work to inquiring lawyers. It is acceptable to become involved with such an agency as long as its reputation for reliability and its reputation in the medical and legal communities are first explored, and as long as its bias toward clientele is understood (i.e., is it a plaintiff agency or a defense agency?). It may be an accident of statistics or some other quirk that defines its bias, but that fact must be determined.

8. *Testify respectfully without lecturing:* Do not "overstep" in the presence of a jury. Juries want to be an expert's colleague, not their student. Remember what it felt like to be an intern on rounds during training. Do not make the jury feel like they are interns on rounds with you. Treat counsel and the court with respect and try sincerely to help, teach, and convey an opinion.

9. *Prepare:* Be prepared to testify at deposition and trial. All records, depositions, and other documents that could make a difference in an expert's opinion must be reviewed carefully. Showing surefooted familiarity with all important documents is persuasive. Always refer to the records and the depositions for specific information. Never rely on memory; a human being, who is, after all, what an expert is in the final analysis, can have a failure of recollection, which can only look bad coming from a scientist whose whole purpose is to persuade.

Experts are essential people who, in the process of trial, deserve to be treated with respect and confidence. The ability to act as an expert in an effective and meaningful fashion is an art, as well as a science. Like all art and science, it must be studied, considered, and honed to a fine edge.

69 National Practitioner Data Bank

Daniel J. Sullivan

OUTLINE

In the mid 1980s Congress became concerned about several aspects of medical care in the United States. In passing the Health Care Quality Improvement Act (HCQIA) of 1986,[1] Congress noted the following:

1. The occurrence of medical malpractice was increasing.
2. The quality of medical care needed improvement.
3. Incompetent physicians should be restricted from moving state to state without disclosing previous damaging or incompetent performance.
4. More effective peer review could remedy the previously mentioned problems.
5. Physicians were discouraged from participating in effective peer review because of potential antitrust and other civil liability.
6. Physicians required an incentive and protection to participate in peer review.

Regulations were published in the *Federal Register* on October 17, 1989. [2]

This law has two basic components. Part A is titled *Promotion of Professional Review.*[3] This section encourages professional peer review and provides protection from exposure to liability for physicians who participate in this process. Part B is titled *Reporting of Information.*[4] This section creates the National Practitioner Data Bank (NPDB), which collects information adverse to physicians.

It is imperative that emergency physicians have a basic understanding of the law. Specifically, the reader should be familiar with the following:

1. The peer review protection and immunities provided by the law
2. The basic operations of the NPDB
3. Physician and hospital reporting requirements
4. The NPDB dispute resolution process

Whether the HCQIA has had its intended effect is an open debate. Arguably, the spirit of peer review has not changed dramatically since 1986, and the NPDB has not been in operation long enough to determine its effect on the quality of healthcare.

ANTITRUST IMMUNITY

Background

Recent triple damage antitrust lawsuits involving physicians in peer review caused a chilling effect on further peer review activities.[5] Congress sought to encourage continued physician participation in peer review activities by enacting the HCQIA. The new law provides protection from federal antitrust and other lawsuits to individuals involved in peer review activities that meet certain standards. The law states that an individual participating in peer review "shall not be liable for damages under any law of the United States or of any State (or political subdivision thereof) with respect to the action."[6]

The Act provides immunity to healthcare entities and to physicians involved in the peer review process as long as the professional review action was:

1. Furthering the quality of healthcare
2. Obtaining the facts of the matter
3. Affording adequate notice and hearing procedures to the involved physician
4. Warranted by the facts known after such reasonable effort to obtain facts[7]

The law and regulations describe specific methods for providing notice and due process, and for conducting peer review proceedings.

Application

HCQIA has now effectively shielded hospitals and physicians from antitrust liability arising out of a professional review action. In *Austin v. McNamara,*[8] a physician sued a hospital and five individual physicians alleging violations of the Sherman Antitrust Act.

Dr. Austin's staff privileges at Santa Barbara Cottage Hospital were summarily suspended 3 days after the HCQIA took effect. Two days later, after a hearing, the medical executive committee recommended revoking his staff privileges. Dr. Austin sued the hospital and physicians alleging an antitrust violation. Dr. Austin alleged that the defendants acted out of personal hostility in seeking his suspension. The Court granted the defendants' motion for summary judgment based on the immunity from federal antitrust liability conferred by the HCQIA. That is, a trial was avoided because the court believed the HCQIA criteria for peer review, listed above, were met. Thus the HCQIA immunities were held to provide an effective protection to conduct that falls within the scope of professional peer review. On November 6, 1992, the U.S. Court of Appeals for the Ninth Circuit affirmed the lower court decision. The court held that pre-HCQIA activities culminating in a post-HCQIA adverse professional review action are necessarily included in the coverage of HCQIA immunity.

This was the first case in which HCQIA immunities were applied in the antitrust setting. Several similar federal court cases are pending. It appears that the law has created some immunity from litigation related to peer review. Although antitrust violation is the most common allegation resulting from peer review, presumably this law also will protect against allegations of slander, libel, interference with contractual relationships, and other allegations resulting from peer review proceedings. The law specifically **excludes** protection from damages relating to an individual's civil rights.[9]

THE NATIONAL PRACTITIONER DATA BANK

Purpose

The HCQIA was also intended to prevent healthcare practitioners from concealing a damaging history by moving to a different state. Toward that end, the HCQIA required the Secretary of Health and Human Services (HHS) to establish a NPDB to which healthcare entities, insurance companies, and State Boards of Medical Examiners would be required to report certain types of information. The NPDB serves as a registry for malpractice and professional misbehavior by physicians and other healthcare practitioners.

Reportable Events

Under the HCQIA, events that must be reported to the NPDB include the following:

1. *Medical malpractice:* This includes any payment under a policy of insurance, self-insurance, or other settlement (or partial settlement) in connection with medical malpractice cases. Any hospital, other healthcare facility, or insurance company that makes a payment or settlement in satisfaction of a judgment in a medical malpractice action must report these data to the NPDB and to the appropriate state licensing board. The rules broadly define a medical malpractice claim as a written complaint or claim demanding payment based on the provision or failure to provide healthcare services. Therefore the traditional formal malpractice complaint initiates the process. In addition, an informal letter to the hospital from a patient making a claim of injury for alleged failure to provide services also would initiate the process. For example, if the hospital pays $1000 to avoid further action on the patient's claim, the payment is reportable.[10]

   Interestingly, under the present rules, if the hospital wrote off a debt of $1000, technically this would not have to be reported under the law.
2. *Disciplinary licensure information:* Actions taken by the State Board of Medical Examiners that revoke, suspend, or otherwise restrict a physician's license for reasons relating to the physician's professional competence or professional conduct must be reported. In addition, the board must report any action that censures, reprimands, or places the physician on probation for reasons relating to the physician's professional competence or professional conduct.[11]
3. *Professional review actions:* A professional review action adversely affecting a physician's clinical privileges for a period longer than 30 days must be reported to the NPDB. "Adversely affecting" includes reducing, restricting, suspending, revoking, denying, or failing to renew clinical privileges or membership in a healthcare entity. Healthcare facilities must also report surrender of clinical privileges by a physician while an investigation related to possible incompetence or improper professional conduct is underway or in return for not conducting an investigation.[12]

Immunity for Good Faith Reporting

Individuals and healthcare entities providing reports to the NPDB have immunity from liability if the reports are made in good faith, without knowledge that the reports are false.[13]

This issue arose in the recent case of *Bearden v. Humana Health Plan, Inc.*[14] In *Bearden,* the plaintiff physician filed suit in federal court seeking damages from the defendant Humana Health Plan (Humana) for termination of his employment as a primary care physician and the resulting injury to his reputation. In addition, the plaintiff sought to enjoin Humana from reporting the circumstances of his termination to the NPDB. Humana moved for summary judgment on the breach of contract count and for dismissal of the damaged reputation claim.

The court determined that Humana was entitled to summary judgment on the breach of contract claim. The court next turned to the plaintiff's damaged reputation claim. Humana argued that it was immune under the HCQIA for any reports to the NPDB. The court agreed with Humana and cited provisions of 42 U.S.C. § 11137(c), which state that "no person . . . shall be held liable in any civil action with respect to any report made under this subchapter. . . without knowledge of the falsity of the information contained in the report."

The court noted that the plaintiff did not allege that defendant health plan knew that any reports to the NPDB were or could be false. Therefore the court ruled that Humana was entitled to the protection of the statute's immunity provision, and the plaintiff's claim was dismissed.

Querying the NPDB

The HCQIA imposes a duty on hospitals to obtain information from the NPDB. Other entities may query the NPDB.

Hospital. All hospitals must query the NPDB every 2 years regarding those on their medical staff or those holding clinical privileges. Hospitals also must query the NPDB when negotiating to bring individuals onto their medical staff or grant them privileges.[15] A hospital may query at other times as it wishes. The intent is to make this request an integral part of the appointment and reappointment process.

State Licensing Board. State licensing boards may query the NPDB regarding an individual when they need information to achieve their mission.[16]

Other Healthcare Entities. Other healthcare entities, including health maintenance organizations (HMOs), may query the NPDB when entering an employment agreement or when a physician applies to the entity for clinical privileges or appointment to the medical staff.[17]

Plaintiff's Attorney. When a lawsuit is filed against a hospital or one of its practitioners, an attorney may access the NPDB regarding that practitioner if the hospital has failed to query the NPDB regarding that particular individual as outlined earlier. This information is discoverable and may be used in a lawsuit against the hospital.

Individual Practitioner. Individuals may query about their own records in the NPDB. Note that physicians will receive from the NPDB a copy of the data being entered into the bank each time a report is received from any source. Also, the individual may obtain his or her own record at no cost, whereas others who query the NPDB must pay a user's fee.

Research. The private company holding a contract for the NPDB (UNISYS) will provide a research service program through which data stripped of identifiers will be available to interested parties.

Failure to Comply

A hospital must comply with the professional review action reporting requirements to obtain the immunity benefits of the HCQIA.[18] The hospital also must comply with the due process requirements in making credentialing decisions to obtain immunity. Civil money penalties may be imposed for failure to make the required reports.[19]

With regard to a medical malpractice action, if a hospital fails to request information about a physician, the hospital will be deemed to have known the information that was available in the NPDB.[20]

Managing Risk Created by the HCQIA

Physicians have expressed several concerns about the NPDB. The issues of foremost concern are incorrect or unwarranted reporting, confidentiality, the use of data by plaintiff's attorneys, and funding.

Reporting Safeguards. Safeguards are in place to shield a healthcare practitioner from unwarranted or incorrect reporting. The physician will receive notice and a duplicate report each time a report is made to the NPDB. Physicians should be certain that the report is accurate.

Physicians have an opportunity to correct any reporting mistakes. If data are inaccurate, the first challenge should be directed to the reporting agency (e.g., hospital, state licensing board). If the response is unsatisfactory, Health and Human Services (HHS) should be contacted to initiate the dispute resolution process. This requires a written request for review directed to the Secretary of HHS.

Also, if HHS reviews the file and decides not to change the report, a physician may have the file permanently marked "disputed" and include a copy of his or her version of the events in the file. However, if a decision is overturned, either by the Secretary or the dispute panel, the record is expunged. The secretary then will send a letter to all parties who might have received the incorrect information.

Given the potential negative effect of unfavorable file data on a physician's professional standing, considerable conflict about the accuracy of file information can be anticipated. For example, in the case of *Melendez v. Hospital for Joint Diseases Orthopedic Institute,*[22] an orthopedic resident disputed the authority of his employer, Bronx Lebanon Hospital, to settle a malpractice claim on his behalf. The resident claimed that the hospital's decision to settle the case without his consent was a breach of the hospital's fiduciary duty to him. The resident acknowledged that he was challenging the settlement to avoid its disclosure to the NPDB, claiming that this blemish on his professional record would cause prospective employers to view him in an unfavorable light.

Bronx Lebanon Hospital contended that the reports were mandatory and further contended that the resident had forgone his opportunity to obtain an administrative review of the settlement and, therefore, had not exhausted his administrative remedies. Moreover, the hospital contended that the NPDB regulations specifically provide that the reports are not to be construed as a presumption that medical malpractice has occurred. The court agreed with the hospital and denied the plaintiff's motion to modify the terms of the settlement.

Failure to Query the NPDB. Hospitals that fail to query the NPDB regarding a practitioner will be deemed to have had knowledge of all information contained in the physician's file. This presumption could increase the hospital's exposure to liability based on the hospital's failure to remove or restrict the privileges of the potentially incompetent physician.

For example, hospital A fails to query the NPDB for a physician's 2-year review. The physician's record would have disclosed that he was sanctioned for practicing under the influence of alcohol at hospital B. The physician then commits malpractice at hospital A, allegedly while under the influence of alcohol. In a subsequent malpractice action against the hospital, the court will presume that hospital A had this information when recredentialling the physician. This may create increased exposure to liability for the hospital.

Failure to Report to the NPDB. Any entity that fails to make a timely report risks penalties. Each failure to report carries a fine. In addition, antitrust immunity provided in Section A of the HCQIA is lost for 3 years. Because antitrust monetary awards carry a treble damage provision, this could be costly for both the hospital and members of the professional review panel. Physicians participating in peer review should verify that the hospital is up to date with the NPDB.

Confidentiality. The list of agencies with the right or duty to query the bank has been discussed. Access by others to NPDB files is a matter of great concern. Reported information is generally confidential under the HCQIA. The hospital's duty to obtain information under the HCQIA "is intended to be used solely with respect to activities in the furtherance of the quality of health care."[22]

After approximately several years of operation, the confidentiality of databank information continues to be a concern for physicians. Professional liability insurers and preferred provider organizations (PPOs) that are not authorized to query the NPDB are increasingly asking physicians to supply their self-queries as a condition of participation.

In addition, Congressional investigators have found NPDB security procedures too lax. Bank reports have ended up in the wrong hands because of incorrect mailing addresses, errors in recording the organization that initially queried the NPDB, and mistakes in identifying practitioners. A Government Accounting Office analysis indicates that during 1991 a monthly average of 250 reports mailed to incorrect addresses were returned to the NPDB. In addition, at least six NPDB users have told officials that they received sensitive information about practitioners to which they were not entitled. The NPDB now provides data from more than 1000 queries weekly. Reportedly, steps have been taken to minimize mailing errors. Officials believe a conversion to a totally electronic system will address security concerns. The NPDB now receives many of its queries electronically.

Miscellaneous Information

Payment Ceiling. The American Medical Association argued that payments of less than $30,000 should be omitted from a physician's NPDB record. The AMA reasoned that settlement of nuisance suits should not affect a doctor's NPDB record.

In the first 2 months of the NPDB's operation, more than 2800 malpractice payments and more than 550 hospital and state medical board sanctions were recorded. Since the inception of the NPDB, the HCQIA has required that all malpractice payments of $1 or more be reported to the NPDB. To date, the NPDB has not accepted the AMA's recommendations.

HMO and PPO Reporting. There is confusion about the reporting requirements and access to the NPDB by HMOs and PPOs under the new law.

REFERENCES

1. 42 U.S.C.S. § 11101 *et seg.*
2. 45 C.F.R. § 60.1—§ 60.14.
3. 42 U.S.C.S. § 11111.
4. 42 U.S.C.S. § 11131.
5. For example see *Patrick v. Burget* (1988) 486 US 94, 100 L Ed 2d 83.
6. 42 U.S.C.S. § 11111 (a)(1).
7. 42 U.S.C.S. § 11112 (a).
8. 731 F. Supp. 934 (C.D. Cal. 1990).
9. 42 U.S.C.S. § 11111 (a).
10. 42 U.S.C.S. § 11131.
11. 42 U.S.C.S. § 11132.
12. 42 U.S.C.S. § 11133.
13. 42 U.S.C.S. 11137 (c).
14. No. 92 C 4019 (N.D. Ill., Sept. 22, 1992).
15. 42 U.S.C.S. § 11135 (a).
16. 42 U.S.C.S. § 11137.
17. 42 U.S.C.S. § 11137.
18. 42 U.S.C.S. § 11133 (c)(1).
19. 42 U.S.C.S. § 11131 (c).
20. 42 U.S.C.S. § 11135 (b).
21. 575 N.Y.S. 636 (N.Y. Sup. Ct. 1991).
22. 42 U.S.C.S. § 11137 (b)(3).

70 Emergency Department Telephone Advice

Vincent P. Verdile and Neal Little

OUTLINE

The telephone is perhaps the most universal tool of contemporary technology. It has become an integral part of our day-to-day lives, both in business and personal endeavors. The newer adaptations of telephones, such as the facsimile machine and the computer modem, have made information access and transmission simple. Application of these technologies has become almost essential to the everyday practice of emergency medicine. Communication by telephone or facsimile machine to obtain patient-related data has become the cornerstone of medical practice. In addition, some emergency departments are using the telephone to enhance patient/customer relations.[1-3]

Patients and their families routinely use the telephone to access the emergency department for medical information.[4-6] Although computerization of the emergency department may reduce the number of outgoing calls necessary to facilitate patient care, there is an irreducible number of incoming telephone calls with which the emergency department staff must contend on a regular basis.

The department manager (physician, nurse, or administrator) rarely determines who answers the telephone and the roles and responsibilities of this individual. In addition, the lay public calling the emergency department can often place unreasonable demands or requests on the staff, distracting them from their immediate duty, which is to care for the patients at hand.

This chapter highlights the importance of providing a medically sound program to address telephone calls for medical advice to the emergency department. The emergency department manager must be aware of the several areas of potential medicolegal risk to which the emergency physician or the hospital may be subjected if carefully designed policies and procedures are not followed when the emergency department staff answers telephone calls for medical advice.

POISON CONTROL CENTERS

Poison Control Centers (PCCs) have a long history of providing telephone advice to just about anyone who calls and asks for it. The services provided by the PCCs routinely involve the telephone triage, management, and disposition of patients, making it analogous to the services provided in the emergency department setting. Several operational aspects of the telephone management offered by PCCs are worth noting. First, since 1978, the American Association of Poison Control Centers has recommended that all regional PCCs develop standardized protocols to manage telephone calls for advice.[7] These protocols should elicit from the caller the patient demographics, the substance to which the patient was exposed, the amount and route of exposure, and any symptoms the patient may have from the exposure.

PCCs use information specialists who undergo 200 or more hours of specialized orientation and training before being allowed to take telephone inquiries. Finally, protocols for patient follow-up are an integral part of their programs, especially for patients exposed to hazardous materials. Protocols, trained personnel, documentation, and follow-up are the mainstays of the telephone advice system for PCCs.[8,9] PCCs provide an excellent model of effective and comprehensive telephone management of patients.

Emergency Medical Dispatchers

Emergency Medical Dispatchers (EMDs) are an example of another successful telephone advice system. EMDs, as described by Clawson and Dernocoeur,[10] not only dispatch emergency medical technician teams, but also provide prearrival medical instructions to the caller based on the information solicited on the telephone. Basic cardiopulmonary resuscitation (CPR) is one example of the type of instruction that can be provided by an EMD to a caller witnessing a patient suffering sudden death.

Training of EMDs includes the use of dispatch priority cards that are complaint specific and prompt the EMD to ask specific questions about the caller's or patient's complaint. These dispatch priority cards help the EMD focus on the type of emergency medical response required. These dispatch/priority cards are similar to protocols used by PCCs and involve a checklist approach. EMDs have proven to be a successful and an integral part of emergency medical services' healthcare delivery.

Other Applications

Other medical disciplines such as pediatrics, family practice, and internal medicine have found it valuable to incorporate telephone advice into office practice.[11-15] Advice is largely given by nurses or nurse practitioners, but in some venues it has been performed by physicians. These telephone advice programs are thought to be successful and account for as many as one fourth of the medical contacts between primary care healthcare providers and their patients.[12,16,17]

Although the American Academy of Pediatrics has developed guidelines for the telephone management of pediatric problems, several studies have demonstrated that telephone assessment of patients by pediatricians is imperfect and errors in diagnosis and management are made.[13,18-22] These errors have been attributed to a lack of formal house staff training in this area. In a survey of 127 pediatric residency programs, only 50% of the programs offered any training in the telephone management of patients.[23] Recently, formalized training programs, although not widespread, are being offered in some pediatric and other primary care residency programs.[24,25]

Wasson et al[14] have demonstrated that telephone care is a reasonable means to reduce the number of routine clinic visits and ultimately results in cost savings. The majority of the telephone calls to patients (83%) lasted 10 minutes or less and for the study period resulted in no untoward outcome for the enrolled patients. The authors concluded that clinician-initiated telephone calls are a reasonable substitute for routine clinic follow-up visits and offer an opportunity for cost savings to patients and hospitals.

The telephone has played a preeminent role in the new healthcare delivery paradigms of managed care organizations (MCOs). The "gatekeeper" system for accessing medical care has become a mainstay feature in an attempt to achieve cost containment. For instance, studies have demonstrated decreased use of emergency departments when a gatekeeper system is in place.[26,27] Often this telephone triage/advice process does not directly involve the emergency department staff if patients call their MCOs before arrival. Nevertheless, some patients first come to the emergency department and then call the MCO gatekeeper from there.

It is unrealistic to assume that an emergency physician will be cognizant of all of the nuances of each MCO's requirements for authorization and payment for emergency department care. There are substantial variations in the emergency physician's responsibility and liability for complying with gatekeeper mandates. Nonetheless, whether or not authorization is obtained, it is clear that emergency physicians must always act in the patient's best interest and deliver quality medical care based on professional medical judgment and the standard of care.[28] If an emergency physician assumes the role of a gatekeeper, the obligations under the federal Emergency Medical Treatment and Active Labor Act of 1986 must always be met first.[29]

EMERGENCY DEPARTMENT TELEPHONE ADVICE

Telephone advice given in the emergency department is an entirely different phenomenon from telephone advice given in PCCs, EMDs, and office practice settings. The emergency department setting is not necessarily amenable to providing telephone advice. It has been demonstrated that the lay public routinely calls emergency departments for medical advice.[4,6] Calling the emergency department for medical advice is convenient, inexpensive, and much quicker than an in-person visit. Emergency department telephone advice may be fast and inexpensive, but much like fast food, it may not be of high quality.

Verdile et al[30] enlisted a research assistant to call 46 emergency departments and present a scenario that could have reasonably been interpreted as myocardial ischemia. The research assistant (caller) asked to speak to a physician but, regardless of who answered the telephone, presented the identical scenario. The caller's father was having "bad indigestion and heartburn" and the caller asked the emergency department what to do. If questions were asked of the caller, further suggestive history was provided.

The caller was allowed to speak to a physician on only two occasions, although each emergency department had a physician on duty at the time of the call. Forty calls were managed by a nurse, and four calls were managed by the secretary or ward clerk. None of the emergency department respondents asked to speak to the patient directly.

Of the emergency department respondents, 26 (56%) failed to ask additional questions of the caller. Although further questioning by 20 of the 46 respondents suggested they were considering the diagnosis of myocardial ischemia, only four instructed the caller to summon an ambulance. Another 24 respondents advised the caller to bring the patient to the emergency department without suggesting ambulance transportation. Of the call takers, 15 instructed the caller to give the patient antacids, several even after eliciting information that supported a possibility that the "indigestion" might be myocardial ischemia. One respondent told the caller to administer one sublingual nitroglycerin tablet every 5 minutes and suggested if the "heartburn" persisted it was not likely to be cardiac in origin.[30]

Isaacman et al[31] performed a similar study but used a pediatric scenario when telephoning emergency departments. The research assistant represented herself as a mother with a febrile child. A total of 61 emergency departments were telephoned, half of which were associated with pediatric residency programs. If the respondents questioned the caller, the patient was described as being 5 weeks old with a fever of 102° F and having signs that were suggestive of meningitis. All of the emergency departments were presented with the same initial information: "My baby has been having a fever all day, and I can't seem to get it down."

A nurse was responsible for providing telephone advice in 42 of 53 emergency departments that offered medical advice. Of the emergency departments, 14 (26%) provided advice without ever asking the age of the child or the degree of the fever. The respondent rarely attempted to elicit any historical information from the caller. Of those emergency departments that asked questions, 4 asked about irritability, 11 asked about fluid intake, 8 asked about urine output, and 6 asked about breathing patterns.[31]

Of the departments, 38 advised the caller to seek medical help for the patient. Of these, 32 suggested a same-day evaluation. Several respondents failed to recommend same-day evaluation despite eliciting information such as the degree of the fever, irritability, and lethargy.[31]

O'Brien and Miller[32] performed a similar study soliciting telephone advice from 100 free-standing Urgent Care Centers (UCCs) in 13 different states. The caller asked what the appropriate dose of acetaminophen was for a 3-month-old child with a fever. If questions were asked of the caller, the patient was described as a 5-kg male infant, with an acute onset of a fever to 103° F, and with a new rash covering the entire body. The authors thought that ideal medical advice would include the suggestion that the child be seen by a physician as soon as possible.

Of the 100 UCCs contacted, advice was provided by a receptionist 45 times and by a nurse 43 times, although a physician was always on duty. Only 22 UCC respondents asked further questions about the patient. Half of the call takers provided the dosage of acetaminophen only, eight of whom supplied the caller with a dosage that exceeded the manufacturer's recommendation. Forty-three UCCs refused to provide any medical advice over the telephone. Only 17 of the 100 UCC respondents suggested that the child be seen at an emergency department or the UCC, and no one suggested ambulance transportation.[32]

These studies suggest that emergency departments and UCCs are currently providing telephone medical advice, and it appears that often no formal policies or procedures exist that govern who manages the calls or the information provided to the public. In fact, some medical advice provided to these researchers could have jeopardized the welfare of the theoretical patient. Successful telephone advice programs should be modeled after that of the PCC or EMD systems. Furthermore, these studies suggest that there may be medicolegal implications to the emergency department staff or hospital for providing inappropriate telephone medical advice.

MEDICOLEGAL CONSIDERATIONS

Studies demonstrate that emergency departments are frequently called for medical advice on a wide variety of issues.[5-7] Hospitals may perceive telephone advice from the emergency department as an important community outreach program.[33] For the caller the advice is inexpensive and convenient. For the emergency department the ability to triage patients away from an already too busy facility can be attractive.

It has been demonstrated that emergency department staff spend a considerable amount of time answering telephone calls for advice.[5] This could have a significant impact on the number of healthcare workers available to care for the patient's already in the department. Furthermore, the studies discussed in this chapter suggest that the telephone advice provided by some emergency departments and UCCs is inconsistent and inadequate to the point of jeopardizing the welfare of the patients for whom medical advice is being sought.

Questioning a caller about a problem is reasonable and acceptable. However, providing medical advice could imply that the staff member or the hospital has developed a provider-patient relationship and assumed a duty and an obligation to the caller for any advice given. Selbst and Korin[34] believe that telephone advice from a pediatric emergency department is a liability risk. They recommend telling parents to bring the child in to be seen. Other authors describe litigation that has arisen out of telephone medical advice provided through clinical settings other than emergency departments.[35,36]

It is easy to provide substandard medical advice over the telephone when relying on an assessment from a nonmedical person, without prior knowledge or experience with the patient or caller, and without the benefit of medical records at the time of the telephone call. Besides offering potentially inadequate or harmful medical advice to unknown patients over the telephone, the nurse or physician providing such advice may be neglecting the patients already under their care. This could expose the physician in the emergency department to increased exposure to litigation should an adverse outcome occur when the physician or nurse is on the telephone.

PROPER IMPLEMENTATION OF EMERGENCY DEPARTMENT TELEPHONE ADVICE

If telephone advice is provided, regardless of the setting, thorough documentation of the exchange between the healthcare worker and the patient is necessary.[20,23,34,37,38] For medicolegal and quality reasons, only trained healthcare professionals should answer telephone calls for medical advice and the advice should be guided by medically sound treatment protocols analogous to PCCs and EMDs.

If telephone advice is an outreach program of the hospital, the emergency department should have policies and programs that promote the dissemination of high quality medical advice to the lay public. These policies and programs should be developed under the guidance of the medical leadership of the emergency department and subjected to regular quality improvement measures. The positioned paper from the American College of Emergency Physicians (Appendix A) can serve as a guide for those emergency physician managers who would like to develop a formalized program for managing emergency department telephone advice inquiries.[39]

Without a formalized program, emergency departments should not be providing telephone medical advice but, instead, should refer all patients to the nearest appropriate healthcare facility. There may be two circumstances when emergency department telephone advice should be encouraged. The first is for the patient who has been recently discharged from the emergency department and requires an explanation of the discharge or follow-up instructions. The second appropriate use of telephone advice is to offer potentially life-saving information, such as the Heimlich maneuver for a choking victim.

SUMMARY

Studies have demonstrated that emergency department telephone medical advice is provided routinely. The studies also suggest that the advice provided is often inconsistent and of poor quality. Emergency departments should have policies and procedures and training programs that ensure a uniform approach to telephone calls for medical advice. Telephone advice activities in the emergency department should be consistent with the overall mission of the hospital and its risk management practices.

Medically sound protocols, documentation, and quality improvement measures must be a part of any telephone medical advice program from an emergency department. If they are not, emergency department physicians, the hospital, and patients may be subjected to unnecessary risks.

REFERENCES

1. Shesser R et al: The effectiveness of an organized emergency department follow-up system, *Ann Emerg Med* 15:911-915, 1986.
2. Shah CP, Egan TJ, Bain HW: An expanded emergency service: role of telephone service in the emergency department, *Ann Emerg Med* 9:617-623, 1980.
3. Kulberg A: Follow-up care by telephone, *Hosp Physician* 7:13-16, 1985.
4. Singh G, Barton D, Bodiwala GG: Accidents in emergency departments response to patients inquiries by telephone, *J R Soc Med* 84:345-346, 1991.
5. Knowles PJ, Cummins RO: ED medical advice telephone calls: who calls and why, *J Emerg Nurs* 10:283-286, 1984.
6. Coates WC, Lucid EJ, Cottington E: Emergency department telephone advice: who's calling (abstract)? *Ann Emerg Med* 22:951, 1993.
7. American Association of Poison Control Centers: Regionalization criteria, *Vet Hum Toxicol* 20:117-118, 1978.
8. Thompson DF, et al: Evaluation of regional and nonregional poison centers, *N Engl J Med* 308:191-194, 1983.
9. Geller RJ et al: American Poison Control Centers: still not all the same? *Ann Emerg Med* 17:599-603, 1988.
10. Clawson JJ, Dernocoeur KB: *Principles of emergency medical dispatch,* Englewood Cliffs, NJ, 1988, Prentice-Hall.
11. Marklund B et al: Evaluation of the telephone advisory activity at Swedish Primary Health Care Centers, *Fam Pract* 7:184-189, 1990.
12. Fischer PM, Smith SR: The nature and management of telephone utilization in a family practice setting, *J Fam Pract* 8:321-327, 1979.
13. Perrin EC, Goodman HC: Telephone management of acute pediatric illness, *N Engl J Med* 298:130-135, 1978.
14. Wasson J et al: Telephone care as a substitute for routine clinic follow-up, *JAMA* 267:1788-1793, 1992.
15. Johnson BE, Johnson CA: Telephone medicine: a general internal medicine experience, *J Gen Intern Med* 5:234-239, 1990.
16. Hessel SJ, Haggerty RJ: General pediatrics: a study of practice in the mid 1960s, *J Pediatr* 73:271-279, 1968.
17. Bergman AB, Dassel SW, Wedgewood RG: Time—motion study of practicing pediatricians, *Pediatrics* 38:254-263, 1966.
18. American Academy of Pediatrics: *Standards of child health care,* ed 2, Elkgrove Village, Ill, 1972, AAP.
19. Nickerson HJ, Biechler L, Whitte F: How dependable is diagnosis and management of earache by telephone? *Clin Pediatr* 14:920-923, 1975.
20. Strasser PH et al: Controlled clinical trial of pediatric telephone protocol, *Pediatrics* 64:553-557, 1979.
21. Greitzer L et al: Telephone assessment of illness by practicing pediatricians, *J Pediatr* 88:880-882, 1976.
22. Brown SB, Eberly BJ: Use of a telephone by pediatric house staff: a technique for pediatric care not taught, *J Pediatr* 84:117-119, 1974.
23. Fosarelli P: The emphasis of telephone medicine in pediatric training programs, *Am J Dis Child* 159:555-557, 1985.
24. Evans S, Curtis P: Using patients-simulators to teach telephone communications skills to health professionals, *J Med Educ* 58:894-898, 1983.
25. Kosower E, Inkelis SH, Seidel JS: Telephone T.A.L.K.: a telephone communication program, *Ped Emerg Care* 7:76-79, 1991.
26. Hurley RE, Gage BG, Fraund DA: Rollover effects in gatekeeping programs: cushioning the impact of restricted choice, *Inquiry* 28:375-384, 1991.
27. Hurley RE, Fraund DA: Gatekeeper effects on patterns of physician use, *J Fam Pract* 32:167-174, 1991.
28. Lydon DR, Hamilton FN, Ross CS: Knocking at the gate: gatekeep system creates liability concerns for ED physicians, *Emerg Legal Brief* 5:73-80, 1994.
29. 42 United States Code 1395dd (1988 and Supp. III 1991).
30. Verdile VP et al: Emergency department telephone advice, *Ann Emerg Med* 18:278-282, 1989.
31. Isaacman DJ et al: Pediatric telephone advice in the emergency department: results of a mock scenario, *Pediatrics* 89:35-39, 1992.
32. O'Brien RP, Miller TL: Urgent care center pediatric telephone advice, *Am J Emerg Med* 8:496-497, 1990.
33. Data watch: Telephone health information services are popular, *Hospitals* 65:14, 1991.
34. Selbst SM, Korin J: The telephone in pediatric emergency medicine, *Pediatr Emerg Care* 1:108-110, 1985.
35. Katz HP, Wick WL: Malpractice, meningitis, and the telephone, *Pediatr Ann* 20:85-89, 1991.
36. George JE: *Law in emergency care,* St Louis, 1980, Mosby.
37. Broome ME: Telephone protocol for pediatric assessment and advice, *J Emerg Nurs* 12:142-146, 1986.
38. Dunn JM: Warning: giving telephone advice is hazardous to your professional health, *Nursing* 8:40-41, 1985.
39. American College of Emergency Physicians: Providing telephone advice from the emergency department, *Ann Emerg Med* 19:600, 1990.

APPENDIX

A ACEP Policy Statement

Providing Telephone Advice from the Emergency Department

Approved by the ACEP Board of Directors August 1995*

The emergency department (ED) often receives telephone calls from recently discharged patients or from the public. Each ED should have a procedure to identify the nature of all calls coming into the department. Calls from an individual concerning life- or limb-threatening medical emergencies should be given information on accessing the emergency medical service (EMS) system. Calls from patients recently discharged from the ED should be managed according to prearranged protocols.

This statement replaces one with the same title approved by the ACEP Board of Directors September 1989; Ann Emerg Med *19:600, 1990.*

Many medical conditions cannot be accurately diagnosed over the telephone; however, individuals often call the ED seeking general medical information or advice. In the interest of good patient care, ACEP recommends that such advice only be given by a designated service or healthcare provider trained in the relevant medical and legal ramifications.

**ACEP,* American College of Emergency Physicians.

71 Confidentiality and Reporting

James E. George

OUTLINE

PATIENT CONFIDENTIALITY

One of the most common causes of patient anger is the violation of the patient's right to confidentiality. A casual comment about the patient's condition may not seem like much to the person who makes it. However, if these words reach the patient's ears from an unexpected source or, worse, in distorted form, the patient may react with unexpected venom. People regard confidentiality in a detached manner until it is *their* confidentiality that is violated. Then they seek revenge.

What issues are confidential? At one extreme, some argue that *all* information imparted by a patient in furtherance of care should be held in the strictest of confidence. Others contend that a more liberal rule, shielding only identifying information, is appropriate. Typically, state laws attempt to draw a balance between these two extremes. Unfortunately, no two states have enacted identical requirements. Therefore some general guidelines are described here, which should be followed when considering confidentiality issues. Bear in mind, however, that it is usually best to err on the side of nondisclosure if such nondisclosure will not harm patient care.

The issue is further clouded by statutes that seemingly require the emergency physician to violate patient confidentiality. Confidentiality statutes provide a penalty for the emergency physician who releases information inappropriately. Reporting laws that cover a multitude of diagnoses and situations provide liability for *failing* to release information. Caught in between is the emergency physician, seeking, as always, to provide the best in patient care while not running afoul of medicolegal statutes.

Finally, remember that confidentiality issues are separate from the physician-patient privilege. Confidentiality statutes govern what types of disclosure may be made on a day-to-day basis. The physician-patient privilege refers to the narrow right of the patient to prevent his or her physician from testifying about healthcare issues during a trial. Many states provide that the privilege is waived if the patient has otherwise revealed the information in another setting or if the law requires that the information be released to prevent the occurrence of a criminal act. Confidentiality covers a much wider territory.

GENERAL PRINCIPLES OF CONFIDENTIALITY

Common law doctrine recognizes that people have a desire to keep their private matters to themselves. When forced by necessity to share this information, patients wish for the most limited disclosure possible. Thus most states have passed laws that protect this right of privacy. Several are presented as an example (Box 71-1).

It is evident from the language of these statutes that several competing interests are considered by the confidentiality doctrine. These interests include (1) the protection of personal privacy, (2) ensuring the free exchange of information necessary to a good physician-patient relationship, (3) the public's interest in developing and maintaining efficient healthcare delivery systems, and (4) the patient's interest in prompt reimbursement of healthcare costs.

Thus confidentiality statutes attempt to weigh each of these interests, as well as others too numerous to list here, to draw an equitable balance between secrecy and disclosure. Unfortunately, this balance is not drawn in the same way in each jurisdiction. In fact, the disclosure of a particular state-required reportable incident in one jurisdiction may be expressly prohibited in another. What is permissible in New Jersey may lead to civil penalties, licensure suspension or revocation, or, in extreme cases, even criminal conviction in neighboring New York. Because of this variability between jurisdictions, physicians must become familiar with the confidentiality provisions applicable to the area(s) in which they practice.

THE DUTY TO REPORT

Many if not all states have decided that the public interest in preventing the spread of certain types of diseases, in preventing some forms of physical and mental abuse, and even in preventing automobile accidents outweighs the rights of some patients to complete confidentiality. Because of the special positions that physicians and other healthcare professionals hold and the access to confidential healthcare information they possess as a result, many states have imposed reporting requirements on them. These reporting requirements may seem to fly in the face of confidentiality and the physician-patient privilege. However, reporting statutes demonstrate the

BOX 71-1

THREE EXAMPLES OF STATE CONFIDENTIALITY LAWS

New Jersey

New Jersey Bill of Rights for Hospital Patients (New Jersey Statutes Annotated 26:2H-12.8): Every person admitted to a general hospital as licensed by the state Department of Health . . . shall have the right: * * *

f. To privacy to the extent consistent with providing adequate medical care to the patient. This shall not preclude discussion of a patient's case or examination of a patient by appropriate health care personnel.

g. To privacy and confidentiality of all records pertaining to his treatment, except as otherwise provided by law or third party payment contract.

New York

Rights of Patients in Certain Medical Facilities (NY Pub. Health L. §2803-c, 3(f)): Every patient shall have the right to have privacy in treatment and in caring for personal needs, confidentiality in the treatment of personal and medical records, and security in storing personal possessions.

California

Disclosure of Medical Information by Providers (West's Ann.Cal.Civ.Code §56.10):

(a) No provider of healthcare shall disclose medical information regarding a patient of the provider without first obtaining an authorization, except as provided [by law]. * * *

(c) A provider of healthcare may disclose medical information as follows:

(1) The information may be disclosed to providers of healthcare or other healthcare professionals or facilities for purposes of diagnosis or treatment of the patient. This includes, in an emergency situation, the communication of patient information by radio transmission between emergency medical personnel at the scene of an emergency, or in an emergency medical transport vehicle . . .

(2) The information may be disclosed to an insurer, employer, healthcare service plan, hospital service plan, employee benefit plan, governmental authority, or any other person or entity responsible for paying for healthcare services rendered to the patient, to the extent necessary to allow responsibility for payment to be determined, and payment to be made.

balancing act at the heart of the body of confidentiality jurisprudence.

Impaired Drivers

One common type of reporting statute requires that physicians inform certain state authorities when they treat a patient who suffers from certain specified conditions that might make it unsafe for the patient to drive an automobile. As an example, details from a relevant Pennsylvania statute are provided (Box 71-2).

This type of reporting statute has engendered much litigation. In fact, in 1991 this Pennsylvania statute was the basis for a lawsuit, which gives the practitioner some idea of the limitations of the liability that can be based on this category of law.

The Crosby Case. In *Crosby v. Sultz,* 592 A.2d 1337 (Pa.Super 1991), the plaintiff and her children were struck by an automobile while crossing the street. The car was driven by James Jackson, a diabetic who was a patient of the defendant, Dr. Sultz.

The plaintiffs argued that Jackson had suffered a syncopal episode while driving, that the syncope was directly related to his diabetes, and that this syncope caused the accident. They sued Dr. Sultz, claiming that he negligently failed to report Jackson's diabetes, in violation of the physician reporting statute. The plaintiffs claimed that Dr. Sultz's failure to report Jackson's diabetes was a proximate cause of their injuries.

The court that heard the case on appeal noted that there was no evidence that the patient had ever suffered a syncopal episode related to his diabetes. Therefore the court concluded that, under Pennsylvania's impaired driver reporting statute, Dr. Sultz had no duty to report his patient's condition to the Department of Transportation.

Furthermore, the court ruled that even if there had been a duty on the part of Dr. Sultz to report his patient's diabetes, "it is not the physician's job to protect all third parties who might come into contact with the affected individual." The reporting statute requires physicians to evaluate the patient's ability to operate a motor vehicle and to make a report if the patient cannot safely be allowed to drive. This type of reporting was held to be different from "imposing upon a treating physician the duty of protecting the entire public from any harm that might result from his or her patient's actions."

The reasoning of the Pennsylvania court supports the importance of confidentiality in physician-patient relationships. When a condition is so serious that the danger to the public outweighs the patient's right to privacy, ethically speaking, it should be reported. Otherwise, the patient's expectation of confidentiality should be held inviolate.

Communicable Diseases

Obviously, the state has an interest in protecting its citizens from the spread of communicable diseases. The type of disclosure required to meet this goal often strikes close to home for the affected patient. One reason is that many of the re-

BOX 71-2

IMPAIRED DRIVER STATUTE EXAMPLE

From Title 67, Chapter 83, Pennsylvania Code Physician Reporting Requirements for Impaired Drivers

When a physician's examination of a patient reveals a condition which may potentially affect the ability to drive safely, the physician is required to report the patient's name, address, date of birth, and the particular condition discovered, within ten days, to Pennsylvania authorities. The conditions that are required to be reported include:

1. Seizure disorder
2. A single seizure
3. Unstable or brittle diabetes or hypoglycemia (unless there has been a continuous 6-month period free from related syncopal episodes)
4. Cerebral vascular insufficiency or cardiovascular disease (if resultant syncope, vertigo, or paralysis has occurred)
5. Periodic episodes of syncope of unknown origin
6. Vision deficiency (combined vision of less than 20/100 with best correction or combined field of vision of less than 140 degrees in the horizontal median)

Confidentiality and enforcement

The statute also provides for the confidentiality of required reports. "[I]nformation regarding the source or content of the report" will not be revealed, even when an inquiry comes from the patient himself or herself.

Title 75, Section 1518(f) of the Pennsylvania Code gives a reporting physician immunity from civil or criminal liability that otherwise might result from providing the information required. The Pennsylvania Department of Transportation has also indicated that physicians who fail to comply with the reporting requirements may be "convicted of a summary criminal offense."

BOX 71-3

COMMUNICABLE DISEASE STATUTE EXAMPLES

New Jersey

New Jersey Statutes Annotated 26:4-15: "[E]very physician shall, within 12 hours after his diagnosis that a person is ill or infected with a communicable disease . . . , report such diagnosis and such related information as may be required by the State Department of Health . . .

California

California Health and Safety Code Section 3125 provides that: "[a]ll physicians, nurses, clergymen, attendants, owners, proprietors, managers, employees, and persons living (sic), or visiting any sick person, in any hotel, lodging house, house, building, office, structure, or other place where any person is ill of any infectious, contagious, or communicable disease, shall promptly report that fact to the health officer, together with the name of the person, if known, that place where he is confined, and the nature of the disease, if known.

Texas

Texas Health and Safety Code 81.042:

(a) A report under Subsection (b), (c), or (d) shall be made to the local health authority, or if there is no local health authority, the regional director.

(b) A dentist or veterinarian licensed to practice in this state or a physician shall report, after the first professional encounter, a patient or animal examined that has or is suspected of having a reportable disease.

portable afflictions are sexually transmitted diseases. Thus it is vitally important to follow the letter of the statute when reporting these cases. Failure to follow the correct procedures can cause the patient emotional distress and lead to the same liability for unauthorized reporting or the failure to report. See Box 71-3 for examples of state requirements for the reporting of communicable diseases.

Note that these exemplar statutes provide varying periods of time for making the required report. The New Jersey law requires reporting "within 12 hours" of the diagnosis. The Texas provision simply requires reporting after the "first professional encounter," and the California statute contains no reference to time requirements at all.

Human Immunodeficiency Virus Testing in the Emergency Department

On the matter of human immunodeficiency virus (HIV) testing in the emergency department, there is a very short answer—**don't.** Because of the prolonged turnaround time and the need for pretest and posttest counseling (whether the test is positive or negative), patients requesting HIV testing in the emergency department should be referred to their private physician or an outpatient clinic.

It is likely that the matter of a patient's HIV status will become known to the healthcare practitioner. Although it is important that staff who treat the patient be aware that the patient is seropositive for HIV, the fact must be guarded jealously from anyone who does not have the right or need to know. In recognition of this fact, the New Jersey legislature passed a series of statutes providing for the reporting of cases of HIV infection, while at the same time protecting the confidentiality of that information (Box 71-4).

One well-known case involving the unauthorized release of such information actually involved an HIV-positive physician. In *Estate of William Behringer, M.D. v. The Medical Center at Princeton,* 592 A.2d 1251 (N.J.Super. 1991), Dr. Behringer was a board-certified otolaryngologist and plastic surgeon. He had been an attending physician at the defendant medical center since 1979.

In mid 1987 Dr. Behringer began to feel ill. On June 16 of that year he was seen at the medical center's emergency department, complaining of respiratory distress. A pulmonary consultation was obtained, and a bronchoscopy was performed. Additionally, blood was drawn for an HIV test. The plaintiff was then admitted to the medical center.

The next day Dr. Behringer's treating physician informed him that his bronchoscopy was positive for *Pneumocystis ca-*

BOX 71-4

EXAMPLE OF HIV REPORTING STATUTE

New Jersey statutes annotated 26:5C-6

All diagnosed cases of AIDS and all diagnosed cases of HIV infection shall be reported to the department [of health] along with the identifying information for the person diagnosed.

New Jersey statutes annotated 26:5C-8

a. The content of a record referred to in section 3 of this act may [only] be disclosed in accordance with the prior written informed consent of the person who is the subject of the record or if the person is legally incompetent or deceased, [but only] in accordance with [the provisions] of this act.

New Jersey statutes annotated 26:5C-11

Any record disclosed under this act shall be held confidential by the recipient of the record and shall not be released by said recipient unless the [confidentiality] conditions of this act are met.

HIV, Human immunodeficiency virus; AIDS, acquired immunodeficiency syndrome.

rinii pneumonia (PCP). Later that day he also notified Dr. Behringer that his HIV test was positive. Dr. Behringer's response was "who else knows?" The treating physician stated that only himself and his wife, both close personal friends of Dr. Behringer, were aware of the test results.

An epidemiologist was consulted, who recommended that Dr. Behringer be hospitalized at a reference facility. The plaintiff was discharged from the hospital the next day, with plans for home care. It was noted that the treating physician, the epidemiologist, and the plaintiff were all aware of the implications that would result from the plaintiff's HIV status becoming public knowledge.

That day Dr. Behringer received calls from various colleagues, expressing concern over the plaintiff's positive HIV test. The next month, when he returned to practice, many patients canceled visits, indicating their knowledge of the plaintiff's HIV status. Several of his office employees resigned, including one who stayed only one day after she learned of his HIV status. Dr. Behringer died on July 2, 1989.

Dr. Behringer's estate sued the medical center, arguing, among other claims, that the medical center breached their duty of confidentiality with regard to his HIV test results. This claim was based on the fact that the HIV test results attached to his chart were not kept reasonably confidential.

The trial court ruled that "the easy accessibility to the charts and the lack of any meaningful medical center policy or procedure to limit access" caused the breach of the duty of confidentiality. Furthermore, the court held that

> [b]ecause the stakes are so high in the case of a physician being treated at his own hospital, it is imperative that the hospital take reasonable steps to ensure the confidentiality of not only an HIV test result, but a diagnosis which is conclusive of AIDS, such as PCP. These precautions may include a securing of the chart, with access only to those HCWs (health care workers) demonstrating to designated record-keepers a bona-fide need to know, or utilizing sequestration procedures for those portions of the record containing such information . . . The court recognizes that in some circumstances, such as rounds at a teaching hospital, exposure to a patient's records must be greater than to solely physicians or students directly involved in the patient's care. It is incumbent upon the hospital to impress upon these physicians or students the significance of maintaining the confidentiality of patient records.

Given the increase in the number of HIV cases treated in the emergency department every year, it is obvious that this issue is not going to go away. Unfortunately, society places a great and unfair stigma on HIV-positive individuals, no matter what the circumstance of their infection. Thus HIV status must be treated with the utmost discretion and confidentiality.

Child Abuse or Neglect

There is perhaps no subject more disturbing than the mistreatment of children. State requirements for the reporting of such abuse or neglect seem almost moot. After all, who would *not* report such incidents to the authorities to prevent them? A problem arises, however, when faced with injuries that *may* indicate abuse but are not *conclusive* evidence of such behavior. In these instances, most required reporting statutes leave the decision to report up to the judgment of the physician. The decision whether to err on the side of caution or to aggressively protect the rights of innocent children is a personal one to be made with the full knowledge of local statutes and the specific facts of each case. The Pennsylvania law provides a good example of this type of discretionary reporting requirement (Box 71-5).

It is important to remember that suspected child abuse is an issue of extreme sensitivity, and that, as in any other confidentiality situation, the letter of the statute must be followed closely. Because an incorrectly filed report can adversely affect parental rights or result in public embarrassment or even ridicule, the penalties for erroneous reporting of such incidents can be severe. One illustrative case regarding the issue of erroneous reporting was decided in 1992.

The Comstock Case. In *Comstock v. Walsh,* 848 S.W.2d 7 (Mo.App.W.D. 1992), the case involves a child who was brought to the emergency department. The child's mother stated that her daughter had a "pain in the bottom," and had been sexually abused. The emergency physician on duty examined the child and questioned her with the aid of anatomically correct dolls. As a result of the examination, the emergency physician developed a suspicion that the child had been sexually abused. She then reported her suspicions to the local police department.

Pursuant to Kansas law, a hearing was held to determine if the noncustodial father's visitation privileges should be altered. The outcome of this proceeding limited the father's visitation rights. As a result of this limitation, the father filed a lawsuit against the defendant physician, claiming that the report of suspected sexual abuse was made negligently.

The reporting statute at issue in this case, Revised Statutes of Missouri, Section 210.115.1, requires "certain persons, including physicians, to report cases of suspected child abuse to the Division of Family Services." There is no pro-

BOX 71-5

CHILD ABUSE/NEGLECT REPORTING STATUTE EXAMPLE

23 Pennsylvania consolidated statutes annotated §6311

(a) General rule.—Persons who, in the course of their employment, occupation or practice of their profession, come into contact with children shall report or cause a report to be made . . . when they have reason to believe, ***on the basis of their medical, professional or other training and experience,*** that a child coming before them in their professional or official capacity is an abused child. The privileged communication between any professional person required to report and the patient or client of that person shall not apply to situations involving child abuse. . . . (emphasis added)

(b) Enumeration of persons required to report.—Persons required to report under subsection (a) include, but are not limited to, any licensed physician, osteopath, medical examiner, coroner, funeral director, dentist, optometrist, chiropractor, podiatrist, intern, registered nurse, licensed practical nurse, hospital personnel engaged in the admission, examination, care or treatment of persons, a Christian Science practitioner, school administrator, school teacher, school nurse, social services worker, day-care center worker or any other child-care or foster-care worker, mental health professional, peace officer or law enforcement official.

vision made for reporting to any other person or agency. Section 210.135 confers immunity for prosecution on persons making the reports required by Section 210.115.1. The trial court held that the defendant physician was protected by the statutory grant of immunity and granted summary judgment in favor of the defendant.

On appeal, the Missouri Court of Appeals examined the reporting and immunity statutes carefully. The court noted that the physician's report was made to the local police department and not, as the statute contemplated, to the Division of Family Services. Because of this technical deficiency, the appellate court ruled that the physician was *not* entitled to the protection of the immunity statute. The case was reversed and remanded to the trial court for a hearing on the merits.

Child abuse reporting statutes are effective mechanisms for detecting and preventing a heinous and reprehensible crime. The information contained within such reports is extremely sensitive, and the consequences of an erroneous report are far reaching. Therefore it is important to be familiar with the exact requirements of the statute in force in your jurisdiction and to make reports compliant with those strictures. If not, even a report made in good faith may lead to liability.

Criminal Offenses

Many states provide that suspected criminal offenses must be reported by physicians who come into contact with perpetrators or, more likely, victims of the crimes. A list of such incidents will typically include gunshot wounds, stab wounds, rape or sexual molestation, and, sometimes, drug abuse. Some states provide for strict reporting of any incident meeting defined criteria (i.e., *all* gunshot wounds must be reported). Others allow the physician to use his or her discretion and experience to evaluate the injury and the accompanying tale. After this assessment, if the physician reasonably concludes that a crime was committed, a report must be made. The Oregon provision is typical of such statutes, which rely on the physician's experience (Box 71-6).

BOX 71-6

CRIMINAL OFFENSE REPORTING STATUTE EXAMPLE

Oregon revised statutes 146.750

Injuries to be reported to the Medical Examiner

(1) . . . [A]ny physician, including any intern and resident, having reasonable cause to suspect that a person brought to the physician or coming before the physician for examination, care or treatment has had injury . . . inflicted upon the person other than by accidental means, shall report or cause reports to be made in accordance with the provisions of subsection (2) of this section.

(2)An oral report shall be made immediately by telephone or otherwise, and followed as soon thereafter as possible by a report in writing, to the appropriate medical examiner.

Oregon revised statutes 146.710

As used in ORS 146.710 to 146.780, "injury" means a physical injury caused by a knife, gun, pistol or other deadly weapon.

Another extremely sensitive topic is rape. Often, the victim is accompanied by law enforcement authorities to the emergency department, thus obviating the need for any reporting. However, a patient may present seeking care for injuries inflicted during a sexual assault, but requesting complete confidentiality. Rape itself is a matter of a legal conclusion arrived at in a court of law. Thus depending on the wording of a local reporting statute, it may be appropriate to provide treatment without making a report to the police. To be sure, it is important to review the applicable statutes in your area. Of course, all such patients should be encouraged to seek counseling and to disclose the details of the incident to the appropriate authorities as soon as possible so that the perpetrator can be apprehended and brought to justice.

One final type of statute that falls into this category is the required reporting of animal bites. These laws exist in all jurisdictions. Typically, they require that the bite be reported to the local health department within a specified number of hours after the injury occurred. Additionally, the type and location of the animal that inflicted the injury should be included, if available.

The goal of such statutes is to aid law enforcement authorities in solving crimes. Therefore penalties for failure to comply are typically criminal in nature. Whether the crime is a misdemeanor or a felony, the condemnation of a criminal conviction should not be taken lightly. Thus it is important to know the requirements of such laws and to follow them with precision.

Release of Records

A typical request for the release of medical records does not involve the emergency department. Usually the patient will send a written authorization form to the hospital's medical records department and will receive the required copies in return. The emergency department is neither consulted nor informed.

A common practice in many emergency departments, however, brings a confidentiality issue to light. Often, patients can be medically cleared for discharge, with the exception of the return of one or two laboratory test results. Previously, these patients had been asked to wait in the emergency department until all of their tests were complete so that they could be advised of the presence and consequences of any abnormal values. Although this practice is safe, it unfortunately causes a backup in the emergency department, where patient care space and personnel are usually at a premium. Patients who are asked to remain in the waiting room until their results are available are often not there when the test comes back.

Because of these problems, many physicians have begun to discharge stable patients who are awaiting the results of noncritical laboratory tests. These patients are instructed to call the emergency department at a predetermined time to be apprised of their test results. Be aware that the transmittal of these values over the telephone *is* a release of confidential medical information.

How can the physician avoid a violation of patient confidentiality in this circumstance? The answer is relatively simple. If the caller can give sufficient identifying information to emergency department personnel, the release of information is authorized by the patient's assent to the procedure when he or she left the department. Name, address, and date of birth should be sufficient to determine the identification of the caller. It is also important to obtain the patient's phone number so that if laboratory values are abnormal, and the patient neglects to call, he or she may be contacted with the information and follow-up instructions.

Media Communication

Few situations can be as frustrating as dealing with the news media. When a news videocamera appears in the emergency department, the disruption in routine and in the process of patient care can be intolerable.

It is important not to reveal any confidential patient information on camera, on audio tape, or "on the record" to print journalists. Even allowing the camera to record on videotape the emergency department status board, where the names of the currently admitted patients are posted, could be a breach of confidentiality. The best advice is to offer "no comment" and refer the media to the hospital's public relations department, or, if the request for information comes after hours, to the administrator on call.

If one chooses to cooperate with the media, it is wise to consult the public relations department anyway. They will be able to caution about the tactics the media may use to obtain information to which they are not entitled. One should always caution against revealing the names or conditions of patients unless they have given their express permission for this disclosure.

Many patients will not mind public exposure, and some, in fact, will even revel in their "15 minutes" of fame. However, patients who do object to the exposure will not want their right to privacy violated. Because of this potential for liability, many hospitals have enacted a "no information" policy, whereas others will only reveal whether the person in question is indeed a patient and a general classification as to their condition (e.g., stable, critical). The best policy is "no comment."

Dead-on-Arrival Patients

Another reportable event of importance to emergency physicians is the presence of a dead-on-arrival (DOA) patient in the emergency department. These cases should be routinely reported to the local medical examiner so that the circumstances of the death can be investigated. As innocent as a death may appear, foul play may still have been a contributing cause, and an autopsy may be indicated. Therefore these patients should be handled as little as possible until the report is made to the medical examiner so that any potential evidence is not disturbed if an investigation is necessary.

SUMMARY

The issue of confidentiality underlies the entire practice of emergency medicine. The patient's expectation of privacy is not to be taken lightly. However, when the rights of the public at large are infringed by that interest in confidentiality, it is the duty of the emergency physician to make the required report. The essence of such reporting is compliance with the letter of the statute that applies to the jurisdiction in which one practices. Subjective good faith may not provide protection from later liability.

PART SEVEN

Human Resource Management

72 General Principles of Human Resource Management

Lloyd E. Greene

OUTLINE

Emergency departments, as with other hospital-based departments, lend themselves to rich and complex applications of human resource philosophies, skills, and practices. Twenty-four hours a day, 7-day a week demands on a highly specialized, professionally diverse team functioning in a truly "open system" environment require consistent and thoughtful attention to human resource issues. Effective human resource management should help create an environment that provides equity, encourages productivity, organizes people to achieve goals and desired results, and meets individual needs for recognition, achievement, and growth. Best practice human resource management is able to accomplish these goals. Human resource management can also be a core competency, which can lead to a competitive advantage. Given that people compose 60% to 70% of a healthcare organization's operating budget and that there is a need to establish effective teams to address the complex issues inherent in providing care to patient populations of ever increasing acuity, there is no question that human resource management skills are critical in today's healthcare delivery environment.

This chapter outlines the functions essential to a human resource management role and includes in this functional description issues of external mandates as well as internal philosophies and needs with respect to staff that should be considered by a leader or manager in a healthcare environment. The fully developed human resource function includes employment, compensation and benefits, policy development and employee relations and training, and development. To add the greatest value, these functions need to be aligned with and directly connected to the business and strategic objectives of an organization, department, or unit. In this sense human resources can take a proactive leadership role in helping organizations accomplish their objectives.

TRENDS IN HOSPITAL HUMAN RESOURCE MANAGEMENT

Trends in human resource management include the evolution from a reactionary personnel department to a more proactive human resource function.[1] As Table 72-1 indicates, the more traditional human resource role included record keeping and technical attention to policies, benefits, and compensation administration. The role tended to be reactive, unaligned with organizational objectives or strategies and tended to function in a closed system model. That is, "personnel" did not need to respond to, nor was it significantly affected by, external forces. As external mandates and demands increased, employee requirements also changed and as organizations, particularly healthcare organizations, began to see the need to more fully partner with stakeholders including employees, the approach to human resource management radically changed. The role evolved to be a strategic business partner in both a programmatic and consultative sense. Predictions about future direction for human resource roles indicate a change of less programmatic to more consultative application of human resource principles. This will be driven, in part, by reengineering of the human resources role to reduce cost and focus on customer needs.

From an internal perspective, the growing complexity of healthcare organizations demanded that environments be created where expertise, skill, and knowledge from all levels of an organization could be tapped and used as a way to improve problem solving, increase productivity, respond to employees as customers, and attempt to accommodate both individual and organizational needs. Because healthcare is in an era of fundamental change, there will be a continued need to reduce costs and to align human resource philosophies, functions, policies, and practices to the strategic objectives of an organization. This will include the need to draw on the richness and value that diversity can and will bring to the work force.

External mandates that are changing the philosophy, strategy, and deployment of the human resource role include increased federal oversight, for example with respect to Occupational Safety and Health Administration (OSHA), Family and Medical Leave Act, "Glass Ceiling" audits, the Americans with Disabilities Act, and the Joint Commission on Accreditation of Healthcare Organizations (JCAHO). Given these internal and external forces on healthcare organizations, it is clear that organizations that can improve quality and productivity, align employees with the goals and objectives of an organization, and effectively help employees cope with system complexity and constant change will have established an important core competency and competitive advantage.

Table 72-1 Hospital Personnel and Human Resource Management Models

Time	Before 1965	About 1965-1975	About 1975-1985	After 1985
Attribute	**Simple personnel model**	**Labor relations model**	**Human resource model**	**Matrix model**
Approach to personnel management	Benign neglect Indifference	Containment of external forces	Human resources perspective (emphasis on people as the most important resource)	Modified human resources perspective
Role	Record keeping	Cope	Intervention (for change)	Intervention (for organizational survival)
Process	Simple functional (not integrated)	Fully functional	Integrative functional	Creative functional
Organizational philosophy about employees	Neutral (employees are just another resource)	Conflict and confrontation	Collaborative-cooperative (organization and employees have mutual interests)	Competitive Participative
Predominant strategy	Inactive compliance	Reactive	Proactive	Innovative
Influence on organizational policy	Minimal	Increasing	Enhanced	Greater
Acceptance by managers and staff	Minimal	Necessary	Enhanced	Greater

Additionally, organizations that can deploy human resource functions in a strategic way so that connections can be made between the human resource functions and organization's goals will be able to achieve a clear advantage. All too often, organizations deploy human resource functions in an unplanned way. Episodic changes to human resource functions such as benefits, compensation, or employee relations can leave staff feeling confused, management having lowered credibility, and contribute to the inefficient use of resources and energy.

The next sections of this chapter deal with basic human resource functions and define their meaning, describe their legal basis where applicable, and discuss practical issues related to application at the department or unit level.

RECRUITMENT AND EMPLOYMENT

The legal basis for most employer-employee relationships is known as *employment at will.* This concept defines the relationship between the employee and employer to exist "at the pleasure" of either. Fundamentally, this can be described as a noncontractual relationship, either implicit or explicit. However, in terminating the employment relationship, most organizations have adopted methods that allow for grievance hearings and progressive discipline for involuntary terminations.

Some organizations have attempted to establish an independent contractor relationship with employees, which specifies length of time for employment and allows for employment outside of normal policy, payroll practice, and the traditional employer-employee relationship. (See Chapter 37 for a more complete discussion of employee versus independent contractor issues.) The use of an independent contractor status for employees is receiving increasingly more scrutiny by the Internal Revenue Service (IRS) as well as other government agencies and should be used only after careful consideration and consultation with human resource professionals or legal counsel. It should be noted that healthcare organizations can maintain an independent contractor relationship with physicians. This is one group of employees or contractors that is generally allowable under IRS and federal regulations.

Over the years employment law has evolved to be complex and encompassing. Examples of federal laws frequently applied to the employment relationship include the National Labor Relations Act, Fair Labor Standards Act (FLSA), Occupational Safety and Health Act, the Civil Rights Act of 1991, Americans with Disabilities Act (ADA), Equal Pay Act, Age Discrimination in Employment Act, Family and Medical Leave Act, the Privacy Act, Immigration and Naturalization Service Policies and Procedures, the Equal Employment Opportunity Act, and various state and local employment practice laws. Although this chapter does not fully explore each of these legal mandates, it is important for line managers to understand that the employment relationship is increasingly complex and, in many cases, externally mandated. It is clear that the federal government intends to take a greater role in advocating and mandating employee rather than employer rights. This role involves job applicants, as well as current employees. Although these legislative mandates are generally intended to have a positive effect on employees and employers with respect to individual rights and the work environment, it is important to understand that these mandates do exist and to consult with human resource professionals with respect to their implementation and implications. In the best practices organizations, an employment climate can be established in anticipation of many of the federal mandates. Best practices organizations are defined as those organizations that have the best methods, processes, and results anywhere in the world.[2] In addition, these mandates can be linked with organizational strategy, for example, in the areas of work force diversity training and development.

BENEFITS AND COMPENSATION

Much of the basis for establishing compensation and benefits practices is dictated by federal, state, or local mandates. One of the overriding external mandates is the federal FLSA and associated Wage and Hour Law. Additional legal issues relative to compensation are found in the Equal Pay Act, which requires equal pay for performance of the same or similar job functions by all who perform those functions. In addition to external mandates, it is incumbent on organizations to have an equitable and consistently applied wage and salary system. This system should include not only establishing objective methods for making hiring offers, but also making internal adjustments to wage and salary levels and having systems and procedures for compensating those individuals who are promoted internally.

There is growing interest at the federal level to narrow the gender gap with respect to wage and salary. Recent information published by the Department of Labor and reported in the *Harvard Business Review* indicates that the gender pay gap is increasing rather than decreasing.[3] Salary systems that look at experience and market data as a way of establishing hiring offers, and as the basis for pay adjustments, are increasingly being scrutinized at the federal level by the Department of Labor, particularly for organizations that are federal contractors. Credit for experience is coming to be defined more broadly, and market as a factor for determining hiring offers and salary adjustments is being reviewed more rigorously for its validity and its effect on the gender gap.

Salary systems and structures are a way to codify and provide equity in delivering pay. Traditional salary systems are intended to look at experience, credentials, market, internal equity, and breadth of responsibility, including decision-making authority in determining where a specific job or job title should be placed. Given the highly specialized environment of most healthcare organizations, the number of job titles relative to other industries is numerous. This presents unique challenges to place jobs in appropriate job grades or groupings. This must be accomplished with careful attention to detail, as well as a thorough understanding of the roles and responsibilities of the job itself. Placing of positions in appropriate grades or slots and reviewing external market conditions must be ongoing, often as frequently as quarterly, but certainly annually.

In addition to the legal and internal equity framework, it is important for organizations to think strategically about establishing compensation philosophies. Does an organization want to pay at the top of its market, at the middle, or within a range relative to the mid-point of its market? It must identify strategically what it is intending to accomplish by its wage and salary system. In addition to making base wage adjustments, is it important for an organization to have merit pay, gain sharing, or bonuses of some kind? These strategies can be connected to organizational objectives such as encouraging teamwork, rewarding productivity, or recognizing individual achievement. As a motivational strategy, however, it might be useful to review an article that synthesized 30 years of research on incentive plans and merit pay. One of the conclusions of this article's author is that reward systems or incentive plans have no effect on productivity or quality outcomes and, in fact, can be counterproductive because of their manipulative character.[4]

Benefits

As with compensation and related pay practice issues, the area of benefits design and administration is to a large extent mandated from the federal level. For example, the Employee Retirement Insurance Security Act (ERISA) mandates who must be offered pension plans, details from a financial perspective an employer's responsibility to fund those plans, and generally contains provisions that help guarantee certain aspects of pension rights for employees. The Consolidated Omnibus Budget Reconciliation Act (COBRA) similarly outlines an employer's responsibility to continue health insurance coverage for employees who are terminated, either voluntarily or involuntarily, from employment with an organization. Generally, minimal provisions of COBRA require that an employer provide, at group rates, continuation of health insurance for a minimum of 18 months. There are conditions around which this time period can be extended for employees as well. Given the current reform movement in healthcare and pending federal legislation regarding access to coverage, as well as who must be covered and for how long, it is likely that COBRA or other legislation will be enacted that could significantly change the current requirements. Additionally, there is benefits legislation that allows claims of discrimination to be made where more highly compensated employees receive substantially different benefits than lower compensated employees. Generally, benefits costs for employers can amount to between 15% and 30% payroll costs on an annual basis. For this reason it is critical for employers to consider the value of benefits and their perceived worth to employees.

Benefits, as in other areas of compensation, can be deployed strategically. For example, if choice and relevance are important, "cafeteria" style benefits plans are often advantageous. These kinds of benefits programs assign a certain dollar value per benefit-eligible employee and allow the employee to spend those dollars on benefits that he or she deems valuable or important. Additionally, providing child care programs, portable pension programs, or early retirement options are other examples of benefit alternatives that can have strategic links.

Benefits typically fall into the categories of health, disability, pension, leave time, life insurance, workers compensation, unemployment insurance, and usually some form of tax deferred annuity. Additional mandated benefits accrue under Social Security. The area of benefits development or design, given its impact on cost and its increasingly complex nature, requires technical expertise and strategic expertise in human resources. From a line manager perspective, it is important to understand the array of benefits available to employees and, at a minimal level, be able to answer basic questions and refer employees to the appropriate resource.

A benefit that is growing in healthcare is the use of employee assistance programs or counselors who generally are not employed by the sponsoring organization but who are available on a referral or direct contact basis to provide assistance with personal counseling to deal with areas of stress, financial counseling, addictive related disorders, and family and social concerns or problems. Typically, these programs are offered for a basic service at no cost to employees and generally become a working part of an organization's benefits package. In addition to employee assistance programs, more organizations are looking at preventive or proactive approaches to maintaining employee health, both physically and psychologically. In this regard, organizations are contracting with wellness centers or health clubs or developing on-site facilities of their own and creating incentives for employees to adjust their life styles to reduce potential disease and illness. For example, incentives that will lower health insurance premium rates or offer bonus payments to employees for adjusting their life styles or being involved in a wellness activity such as aerobics are more and more common. With all that is available and becoming available in the benefits area, it is clear that organizations must have a strategic approach to development, administration, and monitoring of benefits programs and costs.

EMPLOYEE RELATIONS

Establishing effective employee relations can be thought of from at least two perspectives. The legal framework around which employee relations must be managed is a basic perspective and consists of policies and external requirements. Additionally, creating an effective employee relations environment from a programmatic approach is a second perspective.

Legal Framework

As mentioned earlier, many complex federal laws govern the relationship between employee and employer. Laws such as the ADA or the FLSA are intended to ensure that employees are treated fairly and consistently with respect to policies, procedures, and practices that govern day-to-day occurrences in the workplace. It is important for managers to know that these legal mandates exist, at least in title, and to know when to contact human resource professionals when questions arise about their interpretation or applicability. From the standpoint of internal requirements for organizations, human resource policy development should connect directly to business objectives, as well as strategic intent of an organization. For example, policies and procedures that highlight the importance of internal promotions often can be used to show the importance placed on internal candidates for positions, as well as provide ways of recognizing current employees and thereby motivating them. It is critically important for line managers to know the nature of human resource policies and to be sure that they apply these policies when applicable, particularly policies that can impinge on an employee's status or basic working conditions or result in reassignment from his or her current job responsibilities or duties.

Policies and procedures that relate to employee discipline are particularly critical in terms of establishing an effective employee relations environment. These policies must be thoroughly understood and consistently applied. Often disciplinary actions need to be reviewed by human resource professionals. It is generally good practice to have a progressive disciplinary process that affords several steps for employees to go through before or if they are involuntarily terminated. A corollary to a good progressive disciplinary process is a grievance or appellate process that allows for outside or objective third parties to consider both sides of a disciplinary case up to and including termination. This process can either be open to any management action or be more restrictive in scope. It is important for the grievance process to have several steps, which could include a panel of employees hearing the grievance or a chief executive officer or senior level manager independently hearing the grievance process. Grievance processes are not intended to shift accountability and authority for disciplinary actions, but rather provide support to line management in carrying forth their duties relative to employee discipline. Grievance processes and structures that are set up with this approach in mind typically result in an environment that can be owned and supported by both line management and employees.

Strategic Employee Relations

An organization, division, or department that *plans* to create effective employee relations typically has an advantage over those organizations that do not take this approach. Elements of a strategic approach to employee relations include training and development of supervisors and managers, focusing on communication practices and styles, consideration for job content and design, and organizational structure in general. Management development should attempt to connect the role of managers as it relates to creating effective employee relations. Managers who are developed to become leaders typically have a role that could be thought of as designer of their organization or department, teacher, and steward to employees. Manager or leader as designer is a role taken up by careful consideration of job design and its relationship to job satisfaction, as well as the overall design of an organization or department with respect to how the work gets done and how many layers there are. Manager or leader as teacher involves the identification of developmental needs, applying appropriate resources for staff, and the creation of a real learning environment. Manager or leader as steward implies seeing oneself as a servant, both to employees and to other customers. Managers who help create meaningful work, provide opportunities for growth and achievement, believe in recognition, delegate responsibility and authority for vital decision making, and keep employees informed will have taken major steps toward creating effective employee relations.

Communication as a method for establishing effective employee relations comes in many shapes, sizes, and forms. The symbolic nature of communication in the sense that one takes time to meaningfully and frequently communicate to staff is thought of as being critically important to establishing effective employee relations. Communication in this sense also involves effective listening and understanding of employees with respect to needs, issues, ideas, and thoughts. Taking the role as communicator also means taking a leadership position with respect to reflecting the outside environment to staff, as well as communicating staff needs upward to appropriate channels and levels. Communication is often taken for granted in terms of form and content, as well as in its perceived value to maintaining job satisfaction and effective employee relations. It is an aspect of organizational life that must be continually focused on and reviewed from the standpoint of a variety of stakeholders.

A key ingredient in establishing effective employee relations is involving employees in significant decisions that affect their jobs, informing them about the status of their work (i.e., giving them feedback on how they are doing), as well as how the organization in general is doing, and providing them with respect and developing their competencies. Organizations that continually attempt to increase the capacity of their employees tend to establish extremely effective employee relations.

Employee relations is a system of interrelated variables that attempts to balance individual needs with the needs of an organization. In this sense, having an organizational vision is critical. It helps employees know where the organization is going and how they might contribute. In addition, in periods of rapid change, it helps employees and staff in general begin to be more certain about the future, rather than having to make up their own potentially negative fantasies about the future.

Another aspect of the systemic nature of employee relations is the creation of systems to get clear and understandable information about employee needs and expectations. This feedback must be obtained frequently and in a risk-free method for employees. Employee opinion surveys, focus groups, town hall meetings, and other methods are extremely effective and show symbolically the importance that an organization places on communication.

TRAINING AND EDUCATION

As with other human resource functions, training and education have both internal and external requirements. This characteristic is particularly true of healthcare organizations. For example, the JCAHO requires that training and job evaluation be made on age-related skills and criteria needed for specific patient populations. In addition, OSHA requires that employees be trained on such issues as infection control and potential hazards in the workplace. Educational issues that range from fire safety to specific continuing education requirements for licensing are endemic in healthcare organizations.

Training and education can be thought of from at least two perspectives. Training is generally defined as providing job-related skills that can be immediately applied in a given work situation. Education is generally thought of more broadly to include development of skills and capacities that employees could potentially use on their job or in other positions. As pointed out in the employee relations section, keeping both perspectives in mind and implementing programs to address each are vitally important. It is critical for effective managers and leaders to continue to think about developmental needs of employees. This ability requires, in addition to observation and feedback, having a formalized approach for identifying developmental needs. Often it is useful to identify these needs with an employee. For example, it is useful to have employees use an instrument or ranking system to identify what they believe their development needs are while simultaneously having the supervisor or manager similarly identify the employees' development needs. The results then can be pooled to build consensus on training needs and resources.

It is most often useful to identify training and education needs as they relate either to outcomes that are expected from a particular job or needs as identified by the organization. This kind of needs identification tends to become grounded in relevant activities that can be used immediately or sometime in the near future. Training only on the basis of needs assessments of employees often does not have the relevancy that a combination of organizational or departmental needs can identify. The former format, often known as the "menu model" approach, is more akin to an academic setting in which a variety of educational programs and sessions are offered with the hope that some of them will interest employees and be useful to the organization. Although this kind of training can have a positive effect and may be useful, it tends to be less efficient, to consume more resources, and to not always be on target.

In truly creating a learning organization, it is important to create an environment that allows mistakes to be made, assumptions to be tested, openness to others' ideas, and true dialogue and application of inquiry skills. For most people this process requires a fundamental shift in the way they think, feel, and act. Being vulnerable, being willing to take risks and make mistakes, and admitting that one's information may not be the best information or approach are more difficult, particularly for highly trained professionals or as one ascends the organizational hierarchy. In fact the opposite is most likely to be true. We develop what Argyris calls "skilled incompetence."[5] That is, over a period of time we have trained ourselves to be less open to learning or in fact to learn. Senge[6] characterizes several learning disabilities for organizations that must be overcome to create a learning environment. These disabilities are characterized by the following:

1. *Thinking that I am my position.* My identity is consumed by and tied up by my job description and the things I do. This makes it difficult for people to admit that they may have made a mistake or that they are capable of learning more about what it is that they do.
2. *The enemy is out there.* This disability is characterized by assumptions that the problems that are encountered are caused by others or outside forces.
3. *The illusion of taking charge.* This disability is characterized by wanting to immediately solve problems, become the manager as hero, and ride in on a white horse and solve the problem.
4. *The fixation on events.* This disability has the characteristic of looking only at symptoms or episodic activity and reacting to those to solve problems. It does not allow people to look at underlying themes, currents, or structures.
5. *The delusion of learning from experience.* Although it is true that people can learn well and, in many cases, best from experience, in complex organizations or systems it is usually atypical to see a cause-and-effect relationship

from what one does. That is, results of action are often too far distant or too complex to analyze as a cause-and-effect relationship.

Drucker[7] sums this up well when he says that we have to learn to manage in situations where we do not command authority, where we are neither controlled nor controlling, and where the complexity of the job, the information it uses and generates, and the different kinds of relationships needed to do the work define the role, not the numbers of direct reports.

In applying the training and education function to its fullest extent and greatest utility, the issues related to creating a learning environment are endemic. Although training and education can be implemented as human resource functions in "learning disabled organizations," attempts to do so are often less useful and more frustrating and can lead to results that require considerable rework and retraining.

FUTURE DIRECTIONS

Best practice human resource functions must continue to develop the themes of operational connection, proactive strategies, and consultative roles for human resource staff. For example, there is an emerging need to construct connections between human resources programs and practices with total quality management in healthcare. This is an example of how the human resource function can link more closely to the operational and strategic needs of an organization.

REFERENCES

1. Robbins A, Rakich S: Hospital personnel management in the late 1980s: A direction for the future, *Hosp Health Serv Adm* 31(R):18-33, 1986.
2. O'Dell C: Building on received wisdom, *Healthc Forum J* 36(1):17-21, 1993.
3. Perkins G: Wage inequality, implications and explanations, *Harvard Business Review* 71(5):10-11, 1993.
4. Kohn A: Why incentive plans cannot work, *Harvard Business Review* 71(5):54-63, 1993.
5. Argyris C: *Overcoming organizational defenses, facilitating organizational learning,* Boston, 1991, Allyn and Bacon.
6. Senge P: *The fifth discipline: the art and practice of the learning organization,* New York, 1990, Doubleday/Currency.
7. Drucker P: The new society of organizations, *Harvard Business Review* 70(5):95-104, 1992.

73 Physician Recruitment

John H. Wales

OUTLINE

As emergency medicine has evolved as a specialty, so has the need for high quality physician staffing. Recruitment and retention of qualified emergency physicians for staff and administrative positions have become a matter of survival for patients, hospitals, and groups staffing emergency departments. These physicians are the lifeblood of our practice and are essential to compete effectively today. Therefore a thorough understanding of the essentials of effective recruiting is key to success in emergency medicine.

Based on several estimations, there are not enough qualified emergency physicians to staff all emergency departments. Higher levels of patient acuity, rising standards of care required, restrictive hospital bylaws, and state regulations requiring certified providers have created a stronger demand for relatively fewer qualified emergency physicians. An increasing number of residency programs has boosted the production of emergency medicine trained physicians, but numbers still lag behind the necessary supply. Estimates of their rate of emergency physicians attrition range as high as 5% annually (50% within 10 years). This high demand plus low production and high attrition make successful recruitment and retention of primary importance.

Physician recruitment is serious business; that is, it must be viewed as serious and approached like a business. Effective physician recruiting today requires a much more intensive effort than ever before. With many individual and contract groups, in-house recruiters for hospitals and health maintenance organizations (HMOs), and physician search firms, the competition to attract and hire the most qualified physicians has never been so keen. Whether upgrading the quality of the staff, adding additional staffing, or filling vacancies, finding and hiring the right physician require a serious business-like approach to be successful.

Some emergency departments have an easier time filling vacancies than do others. Regardless of the need to find a single physician or multiple physicians, implementing no-nonsense, results-oriented recruiting is like going to war. It must be planned well in advance and prioritized to move forward quickly in a timely fashion to maximize results. Achieving top results takes planning, organization, leadership, priorities, financing, and aggressive action.

UNDERSTANDING THE PHYSICIAN CANDIDATE

Understanding the candidate is crucial for successful recruiting (Box 73-1). All physicians are target candidates; they just don't know it yet. It is important to know what makes each of these emergency physicians tick. What is important to them as they decide where to practice? Emergency medicine is a portable specialty. It is easy to pick up and move with short notice, which is great for individual freedom, but scary for employers. It has been said that emergency physicians vote with their feet.

Every candidate has a "what hurts" list. Find out about it. These are generally factors in their professional or personal life that don't fit well. It could be the busy pace of the emergency department, number of nights and weekends, a disagreeable patient population, the director's style, or the lack of adequate medical staff backup. Personal issues may be a lack of cultural activities, adverse climate, inadequate school systems, high crime rate, or distance from friends or family. Apart from this problem list, it is important to be aware of the candidate's wish list. Spouse and family needs are of primary importance, especially as the aging of emergency physicians brings family concerns. Regardless of the candidate's professional needs, spouse and family are strongly influential and generally wield ultimate veto power despite a physician's wishes.

Geographic location is usually a major concern. In many cases this relates to location of family and friends. With ag-

BOX 73-1

UNDERSTANDING THE PHYSICIAN CANDIDATE

1. "What Hurts" List
2. Spouse and Family Needs
3. Geographic Location
4. Career Pathway
5. Hospital Setting
6. Compensation Requirements

ing grandparents and growing children, proximity to visit becomes important. In other cases, a change in climate after a few years of cold weather and snow may be just the reason for something different.

Career pathway, whether early on, mid-career, or late transitioning is important to many physicians in selecting their next job. It is not unusual for an emergency physician to change jobs every 3 to 5 years, sometimes for location, responsibilities, teaching, or compensation. Physicians with an interest or talent for management may seek positions offering growth opportunities in this area. These opportunities may range from part-time administrative assistant with responsibilities for scheduling, continuous quality improvement (CQI), Emergency Medical Services (EMS), education coordinator, to full-time medical director. With career emergency physicians spending several years in this specialty, the practice of "changing gears" to preserve career longevity is becoming more common.

Emergency physicians practice in many different hospital settings, including academic, teaching, and community. Actual positions usually are staff or administrative at some level. Both hospital type and position play strong roles in a candidate's decision making.

Compensation requirements are less likely to be discussed initially, but are of paramount importance in many physicians' minds. Compensation includes salary and benefits, along with any partnership, bonus, retirement, or other consideration. Indebtedness from college and medical school loans is a bigger issue with recent graduates. Retirement tends to be more important for older physicians.

Steps for Success in the Recruiting Process: Getting Prepared to Recruit

Recruitment Needs Analysis. Serious recruiting starts with a thorough needs analysis. Generally, any recruiting effort should be started at least 12 months in advance. The exact staffing need, whether administrative or staff, and the start date required must be discussed and agreed on. Projected needs for staffing, including program changes (e.g., fast track, occupational health), new contract acquisition, and administrative or academic assignments will help dictate future staffing needs. This type of strategic planning may involve members of the emergency department along with hospital administration, contract managers, and others. Effective planning for the next steps in the recruitment process will be based on these anticipated staffing needs.

Too often, unfortunately, staffing vacancies occur with little notice, creating a disaster situation. Given this all too frequent experience, all emergency department groups should have a recruitment "disaster plan" that is preapproved and can be put into practice on short notice.

Prioritize Search. Once the organization has a demonstrated need for additional physicians, the priority of the search must be understood. In cases in which contract viability is contingent on successful recruitment and staffing, high priority is generally given to recruitment efforts. Previous search efforts, results, expenditures, and time frames should be reviewed.

If results are not crucial and time frame is flexible, search efforts will probably not receive priority. For most groups, however, recruitment results are crucial and search efforts must be made a top priority to be successful. This means that all members must agree to make recruitment efforts a top priority, from funding to allocating their time and efforts whenever recruitment is involved. Too often, emergency department groups recognize the need for recruitment, but fail to commit their time and efforts to its success.

Develop Time Frame and Process for Search. Proper coordination of successful recruiting starts with a careful understanding by all parties involved of the time frame for events. As most recruiting requires 6 to 12 months in the best of cases, it is important to assess your own timetable to organize the steps in the process. Identify specific phases and milestones in each search including sourcing, screening, interviewing, and offers. Each step in the process is quite involved and should be mapped out in advance including who will be participating in the process.

Recruitment Budget. The budget for recruitment should be spelled out, line by line, in advance. Recruiting is rarely inexpensive and can be quite costly. In conjunction with your recruitment needs analysis, prioritization, and recruitment time frame, the estimated costs should be reviewed and approved in advance. Appointing a representative to be responsible for recruitment without the approved budget would be wasting time. Without a budget, there is no serious commitment to success.

The following expenses may be part of a recruitment budget:

1. Staff time—whether physician's time or nonphysician recruiter's salary; organizing and conducting search from startup through hire
2. Office space and overhead for recruiting activities
3. Secretarial costs
4. Telephone costs
5. Advertising
6. Direct mail—materials, mail lists, handling, etc
7. Postage
8. Conference attendance
9. Exhibit fees
10. Interview expenses—travel, lodging, meals for candidates and spouses
11. Attorney's fees
12. Moving expenses
13. Sign-on bonus

Provide Incentives for Search Efforts. Consider offering a "bounty" for anyone bringing forward a qualified new member to the group. There must be proper identification and notification of such candidates within the group to avoid conflicts. A bonus of $1000 to $10,000 can provide a strong incentive to the recruiting efforts and create great enthusiasm among the group. These recruitment incentives can be payable half on signing the new physician and half on starting work. Even though such recruiting by group members can be considered "part of their job," a bonus can be extremely cost effective. To maximize return on the bounty investment, some groups have held the recruiting physician responsible for successful orientation and mentoring of the recruit through the first year.

Market Research or Getting to Know the Competition. It's important to know the competition to get top results from recruiting efforts. Guessing wastes too much time and money. Market research is important to find out how well your offer compares to others. Failure to adequately analyze the competition can lose qualified candidates who will choose to go elsewhere.

For many qualified candidates, competition is regional and perhaps national. By making some inquiries, or even asking the candidates directly, you will discover who your competition is.

Compensation, including salary, benefits, profit sharing, and bonuses, as well as clinical or academic hours required, are important to know as you strategically plan your package.

What really matters is the total value of the package compared to other packages. Furthermore, it is actually only the clinical hours that count in most jobs, not the vacation or sick time that is "paid." It is important to carefully evaluate and maximize the package's value to compete effectively. To make a full comparison, information on patient workload should also be factored in to derive an average compensation figure per patient seen. Table 73-1 shows calculations for two jobs. There are many ways to present the job for sale to a candidate. On quick first impression, without considering the value of benefits, clinical hours worked, or clinical load, hospital A looks attractive. On closer scrutiny, hospital B may be the better job.

Know what your opportunity represents and know the competition. Don't spend a year spinning recruiting wheels only to find out the package wasn't competitive.

Table 73-1 Comparison of two jobs

	Hospital A	Hospital B
Relationship	Independent Contractor	Hospital Employee
Compensation	$110/hr	$160,000/yr
Benefits-Value		
Health Insurance	0	5000
Disability Insurance	0	3000
Life Insurance	0	3000
Malpractice	0	20,000
CME/Dues	0	4000
Moving Expense	0	10,000
Value of Benefits	0	45,000
Package Value	$198,000	$205,000
Annual Hours	1800	2080 (40hr/wk × 52 wk/yr)
Actual clinical hours	1800	1750
Compensation value/clinical hour	$110/hr	$117.14
Annual Patient Volume	25,000	35,000
Physician Coverage	24 hr/day	36 hrs/day
Average Patients/hour/physician	2.85	2.66
Average Compensation/Patient	$38.60	$44.04

Choosing the Team of Key Players

Organization of recruitment efforts is key. Team members who will have the responsibility and authority for recruitment must be identified early and empowered accordingly to act for the group. This is a key position that should be chosen carefully. These individuals should be prepared to coordinate the search process and capable of best representing the group and achieving the recruitment goals.

Participating members in the search process who will help in screening candidates, conducting interviews, and making offers to the right candidates should be selected early. In some cases, it may be wise to choose some members from outside of the emergency department physician group to include nursing, medical staff colleagues, and hospital administration to participate.

Finally, agreeing on the decision maker(s) is important to keep the program on track to completion. If this is a committee, make sure that no more than three to five members make the decisions. Choosing an odd number will eliminate tie votes. Deciding who has the final authority to offer a contract to the candidate should occur well in advance of starting candidate interviews.

For purposes of input in the decision-making process, you might want to consider including the following members:

Emergency Department Administrators. Emergency department administrators include the director and assistant director. These key people should be looked at to provide most of the formal information and to address most of the candidate's questions. As administrators for the department, their involvement will generally ensure that the recruiting process moves along in a timely manner.

Staff Emergency Physicians. An emergency department staff physician will be helpful to add the perspective of "one of the troops." This perspective helps the candidate communicate his or her outlook and provides important feedback to the group on the staff physician's impression of the candidate.

Another useful strategy is to have one of the less administrative physicians keep in touch with the candidate's real concerns (candidate advocate). This relationship usually starts during the interview, when the candidate can freely ask certain questions that normally would not be asked of the director. This same staff member can then be used at a later date, if needed, to get an accurate reading on "where the candidate is coming from".

It is sometimes prudent to have a recently hired emergency physician speak with the candidate. This strategy may be especially helpful if the physician and candidate have similar backgrounds and if the new physician had good reasons for choosing the group. Of course, it is important to choose a physician who is happy with the group and will project a positive image.

Clinical Chiefs, Medical Staff Officers, or Medical Staff Colleagues. In institutions in which emergency medicine is within another department, it may be beneficial to have the clinical chief or representative member of this department involved in the recruiting process. In hospitals with separate emergency medicine department status, there may be reasons to include a medical staff officer or a member of an outside department, especially if that member exerts heavy influence, is viewed as an asset, or has a frequent presence in the emergency department (such as a trauma team). These selected individuals should be supportive of the emergency department program.

Key Hospital Administrators. Most groups usually work with either a hospital medical director or an administrator who oversees the emergency department. If this administrator is an influential player, he or she should be included in the recruiting process. If possible, every interview should include time for the candidate to talk with an administrator. The administrator can help answer questions the candidate might have with regard to the administration's outlook on emergency medicine and the emergency department.

Manager or Nurse Manager. Both of these individuals can be helpful if they are integral to the operation of the department. Because of the close working relationship of emergency physicians and nurses, nurses are likely to give a slightly different but important perspective of the department for the candidate. An invitation for involvement will also give the emergency department manager or head nurse/nurse manager the message that their opinions are valued. Anything that helps build on the emergency department physicians' "collaboration" with nursing or administration is beneficial.

Board of Trustees Member. Having a board of trustee member involved can be helpful for many reasons in some searches. It gives the candidate a feeling of importance and keeps the board involved and supportive of the department's efforts.

Community Representatives. For some smaller communities, it may be prudent to invite a representative from the community to participate. This strategy gives both the candidate and the community representative an opportunity to share some nonmedical information. Community participation also can be helpful in supporting the efforts of the department.

Organize the Team Early. By organizing the team early in the process, each member can prepare his or her presentation to provide the appropriate information as well as questions for the candidate. The emergency department director or recruitment coordinator may wish to address specific areas each member should cover to ensure that important aspects of the job are discussed with prospective candidates.

By making a list of the positive aspects of the emergency department, hospital, and community, this information can be shared with other members of the recruiting team so that the team will collectively present the most positive picture. Emphasize those laudable qualities and accomplishments and be able to project a vision of where the program is headed.

Select only players who will present the best impression. Beware of the disgruntled staff physician who seizes the opportunity to ventilate ill will to a prize candidate.

Invariably, there are questions about the emergency department and the director that cannot always be asked or answered sincerely if the director is in the same room. It is important to provide the candidate with sufficient privacy during an interview. Sometimes the presence of the director can inhibit candid interactions of a candidate with members of the interview team.

The Paper Chase: Getting Ready to Win

Job Description. The job description should be clear and concise. Whether an administrative or staff position, the job description should outline the position's duties and responsibilities. In this way, all involved with the process, including hospital administration and medical staff, will have a clear understanding of the position being recruited for. This description may also include required qualifications including training, board certification, and experience to help reach consensus in advance on the appropriate candidate. Minimal physical requirements for the position, such as the ability to work in a standing position for 12 hours, may be important in avoiding any discrimination issues based on the Americans with Disabilities Act.

Agree on Candidate Qualifications. The group should agree on the qualifications required for the position. Some consideration might be given to MD versus DO degree, board certification, residency training, and international medical graduates. Preference based on gender, age, race, religion, or cultural background is illegal. Clarifying qualifications is important to organize group efforts.

Emergency physicians come in every shape and size with differing clinical abilities, personalities, and interests. With the shortage of qualified emergency physicians in today's increasingly competitive market, it is important to be reasonable, but practical when selecting the "right" physician.

A good emergency medicine group is like an orchestra—individually different instruments that together make the music. Likewise, a wise group selects quality physicians with different personalities, strengths, and interests. In dealing with the wide variety of patients, nurses, administrators, and medical staff, a diverse group of emergency physician bodes well for long-term survival. It is important to keep an open mind when considering qualifications. Unless your contract, state regulations, or hospital bylaws mandate specific background training or board certification, be flexible. Many fine emergency physicians have been hired without formal training or board certification. In many cases, hiring members with different backgrounds can add a healthy diversity to the group.

There is no one perfect emergency physician mold to fit. Preconceived expectations, qualifications, and professional requirements can be helpful in making the selection. These selection criteria should be broad enough, however (given the realities of the emergency physician supply and demand situation), to hire a qualified physician in a reasonable time frame.

Given available compensation, benefits, and practice environment, you should be prepared to work with a given group of qualified candidates in a timely manner. Just as candidates will not get 100% of what they are looking for, the "perfect physician" may not be available in the immediate to near future.

Waiting that extra few weeks or months, just to see who else is "out there" is not an advisable course of action. Be realistic. If the qualified candidate has 75% to 80% of what the group is looking for, he or she will most likely be able to provide quality emergency medicine in the department. A protracted recruitment process prevents the group from carrying out the job of providing quality medical care.

Compensation Package. Consider the following areas when putting together a competitive package:

- Status—Independent Contractor versus Employee
- Salary or Wages
- Board Certification Pay
- Bonus or Profit Sharing
- Partnership

Other Compensation

- Retirement Plans
- Creative Financing
- Home Loans
- Tail Coverage Loan
- Malpractice insurance
- Loan Forgiveness Programs
- Moving Expenses
- Sign-on Bonus
- Incentives
- Administrative Stipends

Benefits

- Malpractice insurance
- Continuing medical education—time and funding
- Vacation
- Disability Insurance
- Life Insurance
- Expense Account

Physician Candidate Contact

INITIAL CANDIDATE CORRESPONDENCE. The initial correspondence to a candidate should be prepared in advance. This first contact letter should sell the highlights of the opportunity, the hospital, and the community. Detailed information profiling highlights of the emergency department as well as the hospital's capabilities can be attractive. Keep in mind that all of this information should be sales oriented.

The information must reach out to build on the candidate's initial interest. This marketing-oriented letter can be easily formatted and stored in a computer system for the next candidate.

PROMOTIONAL PACKAGE. Additional information promoting the employment opportunity can be sent along with the initial correspondence and may include the following:

1. Hospital annual report including a financial statement
2. Hospital public relations-oriented information about the hospital including any hospital newsletters, medical staff newsletters, and so on.
3. Local chamber of commerce, real estate, newcomer's guide, or tourism information promoting the area including information on school systems, recreational facilities, taxes, real estate costs, etc.
4. State tourism information, if applicable
5. Any upbeat articles describing the area that may have appeared in area or regional publications
6. Copy of the local newspaper, especially on a Friday when the "weekenders" section might list the diversity of entertainment possibilities in the area
7. Professionally produced video of the community or hospital

This information should be prepared in advance and on file to be mailed out anytime. The hospital's marketing or public relations department can often provide assistance.

GETTING READY FOR THE OFFER

Actual Offer. The structure of the actual offer, including compensation, clinical or academic commitments, various bonuses, time to partnership, and moving expenses, should be defined in advance. Outlining this offer with some flexibility based on candidate qualifications gives the recruitment coordinator approval to move quickly with the right candidate. Negotiations can be preapproved for several concessions or improvements in the offer to maintain the momentum in the recruitment process.

Letter of Intent. A letter of intent should be drafted to be sent expeditiously to the right candidate to introduce the offer, usually a contract. In cases where a bonafide contract is not part of the employment agreement, a letter of intent can serve to signify intentions to hire and the candidate's intention to join the group.

Without a formal contract, such a letter should outline the actual offer including compensation, benefits, and any bonuses or partnership pathways. In addition, clinical or academic commitment, start date, term of agreement, termination provisions, and any specific duties and responsibilities not covered in a job description should be stated. Agreement to the terms covered in this letter can be signified by the candidate's signature.

Contract. The actual contract should be written in advance. It is strongly suggested that such a document be called and labeled an *employment agreement*. The word *contract* usually sends candidates running to an attorney. In most cases, an attorney is required to help draft the contract to minimize cost and time; it is preferable to avoid participation of a candidate's attorney.

For promising candidates, giving a copy of a sample contract and spending some time reviewing it will expedite the recruitment process and minimize potentially fatal misunderstandings later. Without advance preparation, significant delays in making an offer may jeopardize chances to successfully recruit a qualified candidate. In addition, it should be determined which areas of the contract have flexibility and which are ironclad as written. Even with the best preparation, subsequent negotiations and changes in the contract will likely occur.

Power Sourcing for Physician Candidates

All recruitment starts with sourcing for qualified physician candidates. To conduct a successful search, all methods for candidate contact should be considered. Some methods such as advertising are quite passive; others such as conference attendance and telemarketing can be quite active.

Networking. Networking is the most basic method of generating candidates. A good approach is to organize the group members to make a certain number of contacts among their colleagues from previous jobs, residency, or medical school. Always ask for referrals and help jog their memories. Emergency medicine is a small world and with an effective program, many good candidates can be generated.

Journal Advertising. Journal advertising is probably the most commonly used method to elicit responses from qualified physicians. Although some find their recruiting needs met through journal advertising, others may run ads for several years only to get a handful of underqualified responses. In approaching journal advertising, several important considerations should be made:

1. Circulation of journal: Find out the journal's circulation by total number, numbers by specialty, and mailing list. Certain journals enjoy high circulation among emergency physicians; others have a circulation among all physician specialties. Organizations such as Society for Academic Emergency Medicine (SAEM) and Emergency Medicine Residents Association (EMRA) have their own periodicals and newsletters in which to advertise.
2. Frequency of publication: Some journals are published monthly; others are published weekly. Based on the need to attract attention, this factor should be considered. Some publications are published only annually as a directory; these should be considered if the recruiting need is perennial.
3. Lead time to publication: Some journals require a minimum of 6 weeks notice; others can be much shorter. If the need to advertise is immediate, it is important to determine the journal's lead time.
4. Line ad versus display ad: Line ads can be created quickly and called or faxed into a journal to expedite publication. A display ad is usually one-eighth to one-fourth page or larger in size and usually requires much more thought, preparation, and money. In many cases, outside help from an advertising or graphic design agency may be helpful.
5. Confidentiality: To allow group confidentiality for unannounced or covert searches, a box ad can be run. In these cases, a box number and address are given.

All journal advertising is extremely passive. Responses to the ad is contingent on the candidate reading the ad among a sea of ads and being moved enough to respond.

Direct Marketing. Direct marketing has become an active modality in physician recruitment. The same techniques used to sell catalog clothing, magazine subscriptions, or compact disks can be used in physician recruiting. The goal is to generate a qualified response by carefully targeting the audience with the right message at the right time.

Several key elements must be considered in direct marketing:

1. Target list: Strategically targeting the audience is key to direct mail. Many associations and mail list distributors have mail lists for rent or sale. It is important to know the source of the list of names and its accuracy or deliverability. Accuracy will vary based on how frequently it is updated with change of address information. To enhance cost effectiveness, it might be important to find out if the list can be sorted by multiple criteria such as geographic region or state, physician specialty and/or board certification status, age, MD versus DO, and office- or hospital-based practice. Commonly used lists for emergency physicians include the American College of Emergency Physicians (ACEP), American Medical Association (AMA), EMRA, and SAEM membership lists.
2. Format: Make sure the direct mail piece gets the candidate's attention. Whether the information arrives in an envelope, on a postcard, in a Band-aid box, or in a cylinder, the format must be considered. The initial impact must prompt the addressee to open the mail to receive the message. If the mail doesn't get opened, the message is dead.
3. Graphics and copy: Make sure the piece is graphically pleasing to create interest. The actual copy (written text) must contain enough information to motivate the candidate to take the next step.
4. Response vehicle: The candidate's ability to respond is key to enhancing the number of responses. A toll-free telephone number will greatly enhance the candidate's ability to respond. Consider a postage-paid business reply envelope to eliminate the hunt for a stamp and to maximize candidate confidentiality.

Direct mail experts base their results on cost per response. In today's direct mail for physician recruiting, a 1% response rate is considered acceptable. Delivery factors such as day of week and time of year can also contribute to your outcome. Follow-up mailings or telemarketing dramatically increases response rates and should be considered.

Telemarketing. Telemarketing has been used successfully in physician recruiting. It may include initial calls to a list of physicians or follow-up calls in conjunction with a direct mail campaign. It can also include "cold calls" to other emergency departments in pursuit of qualified candidates. Telemarketing is fairly labor intensive and must be well organized.

Actual connections are less than 30% from initial calls. Messages must be left to elicit return calls from the candidate. A system to log the next call and to schedule call backs is essential. Calls can be performed in-house or, for a fee, can be contracted out to telemarketing or recruitment agencies.

Conference Attendance. Attending major conferences has been one of the most popular methods of active recruitment. Airfare, hotel, entertainment and meal costs, costs of any materials for distribution, and conference tuition are the major expenses involved with this approach. Most conferences allow employers to post notices of their openings with hopes of personally contacting candidates who may be in attendance. There are also opportunities to list openings with an on-site computerized matching service in some cases. Actively "mingling" and working the crowd of attendees has become a predictable activity at many conferences for employers seeking new hires.

Actually setting up a booth and exhibiting is far more aggressive, expensive, and possibly productive. This involves the cost of such an exhibit itself, the booth charges, materials for distribution, and preconference flyers inviting candidates to stop by. Most of the major contracts groups now have booths and private receptions to optimize chances for contacting new candidates.

Residency Programs. Emergency medicine residency programs are prime targets for contacting qualified physicians if hiring recent residency graduates is the goal. Personally contacting each residency director and chief resident by telephone is a great way to begin the process. Persuasion can often produce a list of residents to contact. In addition companies now sell the list of graduating residents for a fee.

Following up initial contacts with a letter along with information that can be posted is helpful. Remember that the information and opening is probably competing with several hundred others. Make sure that yours stands out.

Arranging a didactic presentation is a way of getting a first hand, face-to-face contact with prospective candidates. After wowing them with your knowledge, you can talk to them about a job.

Military Candidates. Physicians who are completing military or public health service commitments are an excellent source of qualified candidates. They generally have smaller educational debts to pay, excellent residency training, and several years of good clinical experience to offer. Contacting the Government Services Chapter of ACEP is a good way to contact such physicians. The AMA also tracks military and public health service candidates.

The Internet. Cruising the World Wide Web is the latest development for candidate power sourcing. Employers can now connect with the world's largest computerized network to explore this virtual dimension for physician recruitment. Healthcare organizations, hospitals, universities, medical journals, professional recruitment firms, and individual physicians are among those who have developed thousands of web sites and home pages to communicate information about available positions or candidates.

Various sites on the Internet offer basic job listings resembling an electronic version of the classified ad pages from newspapers and professional journals. For the more sophisticated recruiter, eyecatching graphics along with actual photographs can be used to highlight a comprehensive narrative describing the opening. A broad array of information applicable to recruitment including immigration, employment status, managed care, and even CV forms can be found along the way. Many educational and CME oriented web sites allow sponsorship or payment to advertise an opening among its readers/web surfers. Response to these listings can be communicated easily through electronic mail. Although relatively new and unproven, the Internet offers new potential for physician recruitment that should be carefully explored.

Screening and Developing Candidate Profile

Initial Contact. Once candidates have responded to your sourcing efforts, you need to move quickly to develop a candidate profile. Most responses come by mail or telephone call. Contact each candidate by telephone within 24 hours to demonstrate your interest in their response. In this first conversation, be able to quickly "size up" the candidate and decide on the next step. After reviewing the candidate's qualifications, share some highlights of your opportunity.

For viable candidates, the next step is to send out a prepared boiler plate computer generated letter reviewing the position and requesting a CV, if needed. The previously described promotional package would be appropriate at this stage. If the candidate cannot be reached within a reasonable time frame, send along an introductory letter advising the candidate of your efforts. Don't ignore the candidate, even if he or she is obviously underqualified. Be courteous at all times. You never know who may turn out to be a real find or have a qualified friend.

Curriculum Vitae. The CV is the only meaningful way to review and sort candidates. Most recruiters want to quickly establish a candidate's board status, background training, and practice experience. Then an employer can quickly triage candidates for further action.

RED FLAGS TO WATCH FOR. Reading between the lines is important when reviewing a candidate's CV. Look carefully and avoid surprises. The following are some red flags that should be considered in carefully evaluating a candidate:

- *Short-term stays:* A candidate who has made several moves within a short time should be questioned further to better understand the reasons. In some cases, this job hopping could be based on a problem clinical performance or personality conflicts, which you may not want to inherit.
- *Gaps in dates:* Carefully review the chronology of each position on a CV. Explanation for gaps should be sought. In some cases, the missing dates may represent time off for personal or professional problems, burnout, or perhaps a substance abuse problem.
- *Multiple residency programs:* Emergency medicine offers several residency pathways to entering the specialty. Be alert, however, for physicians who have recently bounced around in several programs to practice emergency medicine. Do they really know what they want to be when they grow up? Make sure they weren't cut for good reasons from training programs along the way.
- *Other advanced degrees:* Although many emergency physicians are earning advanced degrees such as JD, MBA, MHA, and MPH, the candidate's need for overachievement should be discussed. What are their intentions in joining your organization?
- *Multiple licenses:* The more licenses a physician has, the more suspicious an employer should become. Is this physician a wild rover? Were there problems that contributed to the need to practice in many states?
- *ABEM prepared, but not certified:* By now, practice track American Board of Emergency Medicine prepared candidates should have taken the certification examination. Be concerned about candidates who consider themselves ABEM prepared without having taken the examination.
- *Alternative specialties:* Find out why a generally higher paid specialist (such as surgical specialties) decided to switch to emergency medicine. Traditionally lesser paid specialties such as pediatrics, family practice, and internal medicine have made the transition to emergency medicine careers for good economic sense.

Further Developing Physician Candidate Profile. Information can be gathered during the initial telephone conversations and interview. Personal and professional references help round out your candidate's profile. The AMA offers a physician profile service for a fee to formally verify a candidate's training background. The National Practitioner Data Bank is only accessible by credentialing bodies or the candidates themselves.

Reference Checking. Candidate reference checking should be conducted for most qualified candidates. This time-consuming process usually occurs after the initial conversation with a candidate and review of the CV. For some promising candidates, references can be contacted after the interview. A thorough recruiter will be able to develop an accurate portrait of most candidates through references.

Some candidates are reluctant to provide references early in the recruiting process, especially if their search is highly confidential. A good recruiter will be able to discern the quality of a candidate after the first telephone call and review of the CV. If further information is necessary before an interview, references may be helpful.

Most references volunteered by the candidate are biased in favor of the candidate. Out of courtesy, permission should be obtained before contacting other references. Strongly consider exploring a nursing recommendation to round out an emergency physician's evaluation.

Most written references are only a starting point, neutral at worst, and represent a tacit permission to call to discuss things further. Be aware of current feelings of liability in giving a reference indicating less than satisfactory performance. Confidentiality is not assured, especially in a written document; be prepared to "read between the lines".

Specific candidate reference forms can be used to maximize results and consistently address important areas for evaluation. Participating members of the recruiting team should be briefed in advance on the process and use of this form to get the best information.

When discussing a candidate with a reference, allow an initial monologue following and open-ended question such as: "what can you tell me about Dr. __?" Then unanswered questions can be asked and clarification can be sought. Plan ahead to make reference checking a productive and fail-safe part of the screening process.

Candidate Interview

An interview is a "face-to-face exchange between two or more people communicating via both verbal and nonverbal behaviors." Each individual in the interview plays a specific role and has specific objectives. In the job interview, the basic objective of the interviewee is to get a job offer; the objective of the interviewer is to assess whether the candidate might fit the position.

The goal of an interview from a candidate's point of view is to evaluate whether the job is desirable and if so convince the employer (hospital/group) to hire him or her. The candidate must provide information that is salable and transferable, show an interest in and a knowledge of the hospital/community based on research, and bridge the gap between what he or she has to offer and vice versa.

An interviewer seeks to obtain significant information about the candidate's background, personality characteristics and attitudes. From there, the interviewer attempts to determine if the candidate fills the department's needs and fits in with the hospital/community structure. After determining the candidate as suitable, the recruiter's job is to continue developing the physician's interest.

Essentially, there is a mutual exchange and evaluation of information and ideas between the candidate and the hospital/group to see whether there is a match. View all interview team members as active participants in the process. Effective interviewing is a no-nonsense necessity in deciding whether the candidate is right for the organization.

Meeting with candidates is an expensive and time-consuming process. Appropriate screening, evaluations, and telephone interview will help identify only the most qualified and serious candidates to interview.

Interviews can sometimes be a sure way to make a good hire, or they can be as unpredictable as a Saturday night poker game. Conducted properly, interviews will consistently help select the best people for the job. Done improperly, they waste time, alienate applicants, or place the wrong person in the position.

The subject of interviewing is of paramount importance and is described in Chapter 75. Appropriate planning, organization, and arrangements help in attracting and screening the best candidates for the position. Priority should be given to rapid action, careful planning, prioritizing the candidates schedule of availability, appropriate briefing, and debriefing of interview team members to maximize efforts.

Interview Wrap-Up

After the interview is completed, a "wrap-up" should be conducted. Make sure to offer the candidate the opportunity to ask any questions left unanswered. It may be a good idea to ask about the other jobs the candidate is pursuing. If the candidate is interested in the job, be prepared to answer questions about the competition for the position.

In some cases, the candidate may indicate that the opportunity is a good match for him or her. Others may give no indication. Don't expect a "yeah or nay" on the first interview.

If you are interested in the candidate, you should probably indicate it at this time. Give the candidate a good idea of the timetable for other interviews and when decisions will be made. For a strong candidate, consider giving the physician a copy of a sample employment contract.

It is not necessary to make an actual offer at the time of the first interview. In many cases, the interview team must be debriefed before making such an offer. If referencing has not been accomplished previously and for serious contenders, make sure to obtain a list of three to five references before the candidate leaves.

Interview Follow-up: Thumbs Up or Thumbs Down?

After the interview is completed, the work of a recruiter is far from over. Soon after the interview, everyone who has met the candidate must be carefully debriefed and asked to individually rate the candidate. Invest some time in developing and incorporating an actual interview debrief form to be completed by each participant. By doing so, each participant will be prepared to provide valuable feedback for debriefing. It is sometimes helpful to compare each candidate to others, in case several interviews have been accomplished and offers are to be made.

Physician candidates who do not show promise should be eliminated gently and professionally. They should be contacted soon after this decision is made. Don't forget how much time and energy the unsuccessful candidate may have put into the interview process. Be courteous and respectful. Following the conversation up with a letter demonstrates professionalism and will be well regarded by the candidate. Remember what a small world it is in emergency medicine. This candidate or a colleague may come your way in the future with more promise. In addition, changes in staffing needs and qualifications may prompt a need to recontact this candidate.

Debriefing the Physician Candidate

If the evaluation is complete and you are interested in the candidate, follow the plan to contact the candidate to move toward presenting the offer. Before the actual presentation, however, any outstanding candidate questions or concerns should be addressed and discussed. If significant issues remain, work on a plan to address these.

It is critical to be aware of the candidate's time frame as it relates to the position being offered. There may be several other interviews ahead or counteroffers at home. In some cases, the candidate may need to arrange a second visit. You must have complete understanding of the candidate's agenda to make an effective offer. Timing is critical. There is no sense in making an offer when the candidate is not receptive.

Even if issues still await clarification, send off a quick letter summarizing the discussions and encouraging the candidate's continued interest. Thank the candidate for his or her time and interest, reiterate the position's high points, and advise the candidate of your intended actions and time frame. This approach keeps a strong line of communication open between you and the future employee. Demonstrating a sense of organization and recognition of the candidate's priorities will favorably impress him or her.

Time for an Offer

A Serious Offer must be in Writing. An offer should be made only when both sides are ready. An offer usually is not considered to be serious by a candidate unless it is in writing through a letter of intent with or without an employment contract. In either case, express mail the offer to the candidate.

Limit Time for Offer or Contract. Each contract offered should be a limited time offer. Unless there are outstanding reasons, allow only 10 days to 2 weeks for the candidate to act on the offer. Without such a time limitation, the candidate may be inclined to procrastinate to play one offer against another or to see if another offer comes along. The longer an offer sits on the table, the less likely it will come through.

Contract Negotiations

Contract negotiations are reviewed in detail in Chapter 34. This is the final frontier on your quest for recruitment success; a make or break, do or die point on your road to results.

Avoid overnegotiating a contract. Get what you need and move along. A contract is only a beginning. It is the people and intentions on either side of a contract that make or break the relationship over time.

It is surprising how many well-suited matches go sour because of impasses in contract issues. Be reasonable. Both you and the newly recruited physician will benefit from a fair "win-win" outcome that becomes the basis for a lasting relationship.

HIRING AN IN-HOUSE RECRUITER

In-house recruiters are rapidly becoming key players in organizations committed to success in physician recruitment. Competition for qualified physicians is keen and the stakes are high. Many larger groups and hospitals are hiring individuals to direct their recruiting efforts to maximize results. The costs of salary, benefits, office space, and support staff can be substantial. The cost effectiveness for some organizations who need to hire several physicians annually, however, can be justified.

The physician recruiter's position and support must be a priority and funded accordingly. From an organizational effectiveness viewpoint, this position should report to top management and not be buried beneath several layers of reporting structure. From staffing needs assessment, physician sourcing, screening, to interviews, offers and follow-up, this position carries a great deal of responsibility. In some organizations, these recruiters may also be given related responsibilities for retention and ongoing rapport with existing staff members.

Be careful to hire the best recruiter for this position, not a disenchanted physician or nurse who is burned out and ineffective. Few experienced physician recruiters are available; suitable candidates for this position may come from backgrounds in sales, marketing, hospitality services, or healthcare.

Good verbal and written communication skills, computer literacy, enthusiasm, ability to take rejection, and great organizational skills are essential for top performance. Performance expectations from sourcing candidates through to placement should be discussed and understood. Developing and administering a recruitment budget are important. The recruiter should report to the physician group on a regular basis.

Compensation for this position should be incentive based. Base salary plus bonus appears to work well. Whether the candidate comes from their contacts, a member of the group, or through an outside search firm, the in-house physician recruiter should receive a bonus to encourage strong efforts.

COST CONSIDERATIONS

Cost of Recruiting

When the total time and resources expended by all members participating in the recruitment process are considered, recruiting physicians is usually expensive. Estimates range from several thousand dollars to more than $50,000 for each physician recruited. Costs are quite variable and may include compensation and support for in-house recruiters, advertising, direct mail, telephone, interview expenses, attorneys fees, conference attendance and exhibits, and outside search firms. Each participating member's time has a cost and should also be considered. Additional costs for new physicians including moving expenses and sign-on bonuses or other incentives must also be considered. With recruiting so costly, retention becomes a key to survival.

Cost of not Recruiting

The financial impact of recruitment should be viewed as a cost of doing business—an occupational hazard. Not recruiting, in many cases, can be even more costly. Consider the repercussions. Fewer staff are generally requested to work more shifts. Adding moonlighters (if you can get them) on the schedule tends to add stress to full-time double coverage physicians and nursing staff and often decreases the quality of care rendered and the group's reputation. Posting the schedule in advance becomes problematic and adversely affects full-time staff.

Locum tenens physician coverage (if you can find it) is a costly alternative to staffing shortages in most cases. Overall stress on the core group increases and burnout may occur. Paying bonuses may buy time while your disgruntled physicians shop for new jobs. After the first staff member leaves, the line forms quickly to abandon ship. Ultimately, administration hears about "problems" in the emergency department, the reputation of the group suffers, and it loses its contract with the hospital.

UNDERSTANDING SEARCH FIRMS

Demystifying Search Firms

With the increasing demand for qualified physicians, many search firms are engaged in physician recruiting. Today's physician search firms have worked hard to learn about the industry, and most stand by a strong code of ethics subscribed to by members of the National Association of Physician Recruiters.

Most search firms provide two basic services:

1. Recruiting: They start with a job opportunity and a list of qualifications and then locate the most qualified candidate for the job.
2. Candidate Job Targeting: They start with the physician candidate and find the best career opportunity that meets the candidate's preferences.

In free labor markets, recruiters fill an important need for the client. In emergency medicine, in particular, the emergency department is open 24 hours a day. It is imperative to have a fully staffed department of high qualified professionals.

Physician recruiters are not only filling positions, but are keeping hospitals and groups alive (as well as their patients). Positions can certainly be filled without using search firms; however, groups and hospitals that are serious about providing the best care are pulling out all the stops to find the most qualified emergency physician as soon as possible.

When to Use A Search Firm

Search firms can be a valuable asset to a physician recruitment program. Whether or not they are used, you should be aware of what they have to offer. In addition to a traditional full-service recruitment program, many firms are now offering unbundled services including physician sourcing, telemarketing, database systems, and consulting.

A search firm should be considered in the following circumstances:

- When a qualified physician is needed immediately.
- When multiple physicians are needed over time or on a regular basis.
- When the current recruitment program is not yielding results.
- When the physician sought is in short supply and more difficult to recruit.
- When a larger variety and quantity of candidates are desired.
- When the group does not have the experience or personnel to conduct an effective search.

Retainer versus Contingency

Although most firms offer a variety of services, there are two main types of arrangements.

Retained Search. With this type of search arrangement, the firm is usually paid an up-front fee to start the search, with the remainder of the fee paid over time or at completion of the search. Some firms bill actual "out of pocket" costs including telephone, postage, direct mail, advertising, and search consultants' time and travel expenses. Other firms charge a monthly administrative fee or break up the remainder of the search fee to be paid over time. With some firms, the cost arrangements can vary, with incentives provided for expeditious or multiple placements.

With a retainer search, the *firm represents the client,* not the candidate. Because of financial commitment by the client, there is a greater sense of obligation by the firm to produce results. Search firms believe this commitment also creates a much closer and responsive working relationship.

Retainer firms tend to have fewer searches and can focus their attention to their paying clients. This attention is especially helpful in harder to fill or more urgent searches or when multiple placements are necessary. Retainer firms are more likely to make a site visit to best represent a first-hand view of the opportunity. These strategies generally develop a close working relationship, which produces better results in physician recruitment. With retainer search, you are really paying for the whole process of recruitment using the search firm as consultants and as an extension of your office.

Contingency Search. With this arrangement, the search firm gets paid contingent on filling the position. No placement, no fee. This fee is usually agreed on in advance and is usually paid on signing and start date. Generally, this arrangement does not require any up front fees and is usually nonexclusive.

Contingency firms tend to be candidate driven; that is, they *work on behalf of their candidates.* They are likely to have more active searches; each individual search gets less focused attention. Search firms know that most contingency searches are relative long shots for placement and work less for each contingency client than for retainer clients. Without the financial commitment of a retainer, the working relationship with their contingency clients can be suboptimal; therefore, successful placement less likely. Contingency firms tend to do less candidate screening and are less likely to make a site visit. With contingency search, you are really paying for the results—the placement, more than the process.

Exclusive versus Nonexclusive

There are two search relationships apart from retainer or contingency: exclusive and nonexclusive.

In an *exclusive* arrangement, all candidate leads must be channeled through the search firm, which allows for qualifying, and reference checking, and are significant parts of the recruiter's job. Generally candidates who may have come forward through other means, such as the group's own networking contacts, are included. An exclusive arrangement protects the firm's right to be paid if their recruiting efforts produce a candidate who may have indirectly heard of the position and is hired. Exceptions to exclusivity are sometimes made by excluding a certain small pretargeted list of candidates who the client may pursue on his or her own.

A *nonexclusive* arrangement allows the group to conduct its own search efforts simultaneously, as well as use other nonexclusive search firms. In this arrangement, whoever establishes the initial contact with the physician candidate has the responsibility of representing that candidate and the group and moving forward through the recruiting process.

How a Search Firm Gets Paid

Search firms can get paid in a variety of ways. In all cases of physician recruiting, these fees are paid by the client (the group or hospital that does the hiring), *not* the candidate.

In a retainer arrangement, there is usually a nonrefundable up-front preliminary fee ranging from $1000 to $10,000 per opening. Ongoing monthly fees may vary from a fixed amount, a share of the remaining fee paid over several months, or "out of pocket" expenses. Some firms bill a final completion fee on candidate acceptance.

In a contingency arrangement, the total placement fee is commonly paid half on candidate acceptance and half on start date. In either case, lower fees for multiple placements often can be negotiated.

Unbundled Services

Many search firms are now offering unbundled recruitment services. In addition to the traditional full-service search, separate services are now available such as the following:

1. Targeted Lists: In-house database lists of candidates can be purchased with or without software to help with physician candidate sourcing. Some firms even offer training sessions to accompany this information.
2. Direct Mail: Firms offer full direct mail production or consulting.
3. Telemarketing: Clients can contract out telemarketing to physician candidates with exact scripts to obtain helpful candidate information. Consulting to help a client perform this function in-house is also available.
4. Reference or Background Checking: Clients can contract out these services to some firms.
5. Consulting: Many firms now offer consulting on an hourly basis to include site visit, review of current systems, planning, organization, recruitment modalities, etc.
6. *Locum Tenens:* Many search firms and others offer *locum tenens* coverage in emergency medicine. Based on a client's required qualifications, the firm brings forward available physicians to work an assigned schedule of shifts. Some firms offer to contract blocks of shifts; others assign individual physicians.

Locum tenens fees vary from a fixed percentage of the hourly wage to a specific hourly cost paid directly to the firm. Some *locum tenens* providers supply malpractice coverage; in other cases, it is provided by the client. Travel costs to and from the assignment, housing, and local transportation are usually covered by the client, although this arrangement can vary.

Most arrangements offer an option (and separate fee) for permanent placement if the *locum tenens* physician is hired by the client.

Advantages of Using A Search Firm

The following are common advantages in using a search firm:

- Overall experience with recruiting
- Large selection—qualified candidates from in-house database
- Prescreening of candidates—thorough references/candidate profiles
- Perspective on the opportunity and offer from an outsider
- Assistance with educating the team and developing the process
- Assessing the competitiveness
- Avoiding discrimination problems
- Quiet searches—unadvertised
- Exploring the competitor's physicians as candidates
- Constant presence—availability
- Active sourcing of candidates not actively looking for job
- Coordinating interview arrangements
- Debriefing interviews and offers
- Going after the hot candidates
- Dispositioning the not-so-hot
- Coordinating communications with candidates
- Contact with residents and military
- Conference attendance and exhibits
- Direct mail/Advertising/Marketing experience
- Ongoing objective feedback through process
- Assistance in preparing letters of intent, offers, contracts
- Reviewing contract with candidates
- Third-party negotiating
- Ongoing consultations
- Confidentiality

Choosing a Search Firm

Carefully select a search firm that will work best with the group. Colleagues may offer advice about firms they have used. In addition, the National Association of Physician Recruiters* is a great place to obtain a list of member search firms. Such member firms subscribe to a common code of ethics and allow an arbitration route with any member firms if the need arises.

During the initial contact with a search firm, find out about their services and their fees. Ask about their experience in emergency medicine searches and their knowledge of the specialty. What has been the time to search completion and rates of completion on similar searches? Find out about staffing and resources to conduct the search. What will they do for you in conducting your search? How many searches does each recruiter have ongoing? What does the recruiter do for candidate screening and reference checking? Will the candidate be sent to other jobs that they represent? Request marketing information and a sample contract along with a list of client references.

Search Firm Contracts

Search firms usually have an agreement that is used to set forth the understanding between client and search firm in undertaking a search. This agreement can range from a one page letter of agreement to several pages of legalese. Included in many of the contracts are the following sections:

- Client and Search Firm Responsibilities
- Search Assignment: specialty, position, and number
- Term—usually 1 year, mechanism for extension or termination
- Payment and Terms
- Other expenses that client is responsible for—"out of pocket"
- Guarantee—if present, in case physician leaves (varies from 60 to 360 days with half to full refund or replacement)

Other Contract Clauses:

- Previous candidate contact based on time limitations—ownership issue
- Confidentiality of contract terms—not to be shared with candidates

*Phone (800) 726-5613.

- Confidentiality of candidates—not to be shared with others potential employers
- Subsequent hiring of candidates presented—usually with time limitation
- Exclusivity—may be for full term or only first 90 days

When working with a search firm, it is important to be realistic with time frames. It takes commitment and great communication to develop effective teamwork to coordinate all efforts to be successful. Be careful when working with multiple search firms to separately identify dates and firms that notified you about specific candidates. Make sure to be candid with search firms to make them aware of your progress and agenda so that they can communicate effectively with candidates on your behalf.

WORDS OF WISDOM

Read these "pearls" for successful recruitment and review them often:

- Successful recruiting is a sales job. You may want to tell it like it is, but you need to "sell" it like it is. To spark initial interest in a candidate, talk up the highlights and advantages of the opportunity and community. Brutal honesty can wait.
- Recruiting starts with relationship building. Take time to get to know the candidate and family early on. With spouses, talk early and often. Listen to them to find out their personal and professional needs and then present the opportunity with this information in mind. Spouse and family needs are of primary importance in effective recruiting. Whether it be cultural, educational, religious, or spouse career needs, find out how the opportunity will meet these needs.
- Recruit in parallel, not in series. Keep several balls in the air until you're sure you have a viable hire. Be cautious not to stake your hopes on one candidate, no matter how promising. Having competition for your job will also make it more attractive to the candidate and give you an advantage in negotiations. Some candidates are good poker players and may be playing more than one good hand. Have some backup in case things fall through. In recruiting, "it ain't over 'til it's over". Don't slow down until the candidate has signed and started.
- Seasonality plays a role in recruiting. Job moves usually occur in predictable periods, such as during the summer coinciding with residency graduations and school vacations. It is usually harder to recruit for a December opening than for a July opening. Be flexible. Even though the candidate can't start for 3 months, think twice before turning down the candidate.
- Time kills deals. Forward momentum in the search process is important. Respond quickly to inquiries and move expeditiously with the recruitment plan with each candidate. Many qualified emergency physicians operate their job search within a limited time frame and have only a limited "window of interest." Lack of action sends a message of lack of interest. Reliable follow-up is crucial. Communicate your time frames for action and then stick to your plan.
- Prioritize search efforts and make sure all are in agreement. Work schedules around the candidate's schedule. Be candidate friendly to get results.
- Nothing is forever; keep things in perspective. You're hiring for a here and now need, not for life. Don't be looking for a lifelong commitment to the job.
- Sell the personal and family aspects of the job. These aspects contribute 60% of the reasons a candidate accepts a job.
- Don't assume anyone sees the job the way you do. Take an objective view.
- When the candidate has only "one more job to hear from," your job is at best number 2 on his or her list.
- If the candidate hasn't talked things over with his or her spouse, the candidate isn't really serious.
- Not recruiting can cost more than the cost of recruiting. Finding good physicians is an occupational hazard that can't be underestimated.
- Respect candidate confidentiality. Most candidates prefer that job hunting efforts remain confidential. Unless otherwise permitted, keep conversations about candidates within the recruiting team. Contact references only with the candidate's permission.
- An offer is not an offer until it is in writing. A verbal offer is only tentative. Don't string along one candidate waiting to see if a better one comes along.
- You have only one chance to make a great first impression. Plan to make the best first impression you can. Whether during the first telephone call or arranging the interview, put your best foot forward.
- Physicians prefer dealing with other physicians. Although a nonphysician can be involved in the recruiting process, early on during the process, it is important to have a physician remain in contact with candidates. This will maintain the candidate's feeling that you are interested in him or her.
- Be prepared to make an offer for the right person regardless of the point in the process. You may have planned to look at several candidates before making any decisions. Agree that if the right candidate comes along, you can move forward with an offer, out of sequence if needed.
- Be honest with candidates. There may be potentially negative issues about your community or job that a candidate should know. Be fair and inform the candidate of these issues. In addition, don't string along a candidate who is not being seriously considered.
- Effective recruiting takes thorough planning. Commit now to take the time to organize recruitment efforts following the steps in the recruitment process outlined in this chapter. Good preparation shows through from start to finish.

BIBLIOGRAPHY

Barnett AA: New recruits. The IRS is changing the rules for hiring doctors. Hospitals & Health Networks Sep 20;69(18):41-42,44, 1995

Berger J, Boyle R: How to avoid the high costs of physician turnover, *JAMA* 270:1993.

Bonds RG: Recruiting with southern charm, *South Hosp* 58:24-25, 1992.

Bonds RG: Some inside information on recruiting physicians, *Mod Healthcare* 22(4):33, 1992.

Bonds RG: Aggressive physician recruiting: why and how, *Healthspan* 8:10-12, 1991.

Bonds RG: *Physician recruitment and retention: practical techniques for exceptional results,* Pulliam, KS, 1991, American Hospital Publishing.

Burda D: Physician pay, perks vary by employer, *Mod Healthc* 1992.

Dismuke BJ: The hospital's lifeline: recruiting well-qualified physicians, *Healthc Exec* 4:27-9, 1989.

Cejka SA: Hospital-physician relations: the recruitment perspective, *Top Health Care Financ* 20(4):55-62, 1994.

Connor RA, Hillson SD, Kralewski JE: An analysis of physician recruitment strategies in rural hospitals, *Health Care Manage Rev* 20(1):7-18, 1995.

Dismuke BJ: Physician recruitment in a competitive market, *Healthc Exec Curr* 32:1-4, 1988.

Murray D: Emergency physicians: they're racking up big gains, *Med Econ* 69(5):153-163, 1992.

Grayson MA: Physician recruitment under way at most of nation's hospitals, *Trustee* 42:18-19, 1989.

Hawkins J: Recruiting physicians within IRS and HHS Guidelines, *Health Care Strateg Manage* 10:13-14, 1992.

Halen TN: How a Hospital Attracts MDs, *Hosp Prog* 60:53-55, 1979.

Incentive packages key part of physician recruiting, *AMA News* 20, 1994.

Ingram D: Hospital can avoid costly, frustrating searches for physicians by focusing on three key factors, *Mod Healthcare* 22(21):32, 1992.

Internet gives job hunters a powerful tool, *New Orleans City Business* 20-21, 1996.

Johnsson J: The best approach to recruiting women MDs, *Hospitals* 65:58, 1991.

Koska MT: Physician recruiting 101: avoid the classic mistakes, *Hospitals* 64:46-50, 1990.

Koska MT: Survey: hospital abandoning search for solo practitioners, *Hospitals* 64:42-43, 1990.

O'Leary J: Physician recruitment: a three-step strategy, *Hospitals* 66:84, 1992.

Physician recruiting: do you know where your dollars go? *Healthc Financ Manage* 45:52, 54, 56, 1991.

McCormick B: Physician recruitment strategies, *Trustee* 42:12-13, 1989.

Poggio FL: Physician recruitment: the role of the hospital information system, *Healthc Financ Manage* 46:56,58,60, 1992.

Prabhu SS: A generalizable framework for information systems for physician recruitment/referral, *Manage Med* 9(4);24-30, 1995.

Reaves CF: IRS proposed "physician recruitment" revenue ruling offers few kernels in search for, *Physician Executive* 21(7):50-2, 1995.

Rourke JT: Politics of rural health care: recruitment and retention of physicians (editorial) Comment in: *Can Med Assoc J* 149(5):531, 1993 (discussion) *Can Med Assoc J* 148(8):1281-4, 1993.

Stanton J: In-house recruiters: new role needs clear direction to benefit, *Health Care Strateg Manage* 10:14-15, 1992.

Strategic recruitment need executive leadership, *Healthc Exec* 8:25, 1993.

Wales JH: *All the right moves: the insider's guide to successfully choosing the best emergency medicine opportunity for you,* Albany, NY, John Wales & Associates.

Walker R: Recruiting must adapt to MD payment changes, *Hospitals* 64:64, 1990.

Zuckerman A: Medical staff development: manpower or strategic plan? *Health Care Strateg Manage* 11:10-11, 1993.

74 Nurse Recruitment

Walter Page Young, Ford N. Kyes, and Barbara A. Kyes

OUTLINE

The success or failure of an emergency department is based largely on patient satisfaction with its services. Consumers make judgments primarily on the basis of their interactions with staff during their emergency department visit. The human interaction between staff and patients is clearly the greatest determinant of patient satisfaction.

Balancing staffing demands with patient care needs is the challenge of every emergency department manager. Often wide fluctuations in patient acuity and census add another dimension to the challenge of maintaining appropriate staffing levels. Nationwide, emergency department managers stretch staffing resources to cover the day-to-day schedule while expending time and effort on recruitment and retention of staff. The cycle continues: a new nurse begins orientation; an experienced nurse leaves. The emergency department manager, through the use of ingenuity, commitment, and proactive planning, can minimize the effect of this cycle on the delivery of safe care to the patient.

This chapter reviews several emergency nurse recruitment strategies, illustrates the relationship between recruitment and retention, explains how recruitment strategies are evaluated, and provides a guide for the development of a recruitment plan after conducting an appraisal of the specific emergency department setting.

BACKGROUND

Before discussion of emergency department nurse recruitment strategies, it is important to understand some of the issues that have affected the nursing profession in general, as well as the emergency department nurse specifically. The nursing shortage has waxed and waned since the early 1980s. Although a chronic shortage has existed nationwide, registered nurses (RN) have actually been plentiful in one region while severe shortages have existed in another. Historically, the emergency department has largely escaped the effects of the nursing shortage because emergency nursing has been viewed as an advancement opportunity for many nurses. However, the demand for experienced emergency department nurses has become critical in many parts of the country. Hospitals have also been exploring the use of nurse substitutes to aid in covering shortages, as well as to reduce costs in the emergency department staffing budget.

Urban hospitals located in large population centers with all the perceived amenities of life have a larger applicant pool from which to draw than that available to rural emergency departments. Lower salaries, limited opportunities for professional development and continuing education, and the stigma of rural healthcare all contribute to the shortage in rural areas.[1] Emergency departments with air medical units have a greater attraction for nurses who aspire to become members of the flight team. Increased opportunities for education and professional advancement attract nurses to university hospitals, with their reputation as teaching centers. Whatever the type of hospital (rural or urban, university or community, or with or without air medical services), the hospital emergency department often has vacancies.

Movement of nurses in and out of the emergency department is a common occurrence. Depending on the source consulted, the hospital turnover rate for nurses ranges from 15% to 20%.[2-4] Historically, nurses who made frequent job changes were avoided by managers. However, many managers welcome nurses who possess a variety of experiences and nursing expertise. The negative stigma of frequent job changes has been replaced with a belief that nurses who have made frequent job changes tend to be flexible and bring valuable experience to the department.

Although turnover is accepted and considered normal in the emergency department, it is important that managers do not become complacent and stop questioning turnover. The danger is that managers may view turnover as beyond their control and inevitable. High turnover can quickly result in a dysfunctional department. Valuable information for recruitment can be gained by a thorough evaluation of frequent job changes. Five of the most common causes for a nurse to leave a position are time-off policy, scheduling practices, fairness in dealing with staff, wages and benefits, and inappropriate match between position and employee.[5]

Nursing shortages can impact the emergency department in a myriad of ways. The first problem encountered is filling "the holes in the schedule." Next is the potential inability to meet patient needs followed by the potential for increased costs to the emergency department for premium staffing resources (overtime, internal pool, agency, and incentive pay), recruitment, and training. The use of premium staff and the lack of adequate staff can have further negative effects on retention of the remaining staff, as well as the hospital's image and medical staff relationships. In its most elemental form, a staffing shortage in the emergency department must be defined in the context of patient care and the mission of the institution: It is an inability to meet the needs of patients at a specific time, on a specific day, or during a specific shift.

Table 74-1 Cost of Registered Nurse Turnover

Direct costs	Indirect costs
Advertising and recruitment	Orientation and training costs
Unfilled position (premium pay to cover for vacancy)	Termination costs
Hiring procedure (cost of human resources personnel and recruiters)	Decreased productivity of new registered nurse and impact on existing staff

From Jones C: *J Nurs Admin* 20:30, 1990.
The total cost was estimated in 1990 to average $10,200 per registered nurse turnover ($6650 for direct costs and $3550 for indirect costs).[6]
The cost of registered nurse turnover can be calculated by combining the estimated direct and indirect costs.

Emergency departments are experiencing an increase in patient acuity. Driven primarily by changes in medical insurance reimbursement, more patients are receiving outpatient treatment for less serious complaints and hospital length of stay is decreasing. With fewer nurses to care for higher-acuity patients, patient flow can easily be disrupted. As the manager attempts to meet patient needs through staffing resource management, the emergency department budget can be negatively affected. The estimated cost of filling a vacant RN position is about $10,198[3] (Table 74-1).[6] In this context the nurse manager is challenged to develop a plan for recruiting, training, and retaining appropriate staff.

DEVELOPING A RECRUITMENT PLAN

Recruitment is the act of finding and hiring the most qualified and appropriate applicant for an available position. To maximize success, a balanced approach to recruitment, involving both selling and marketing, should be implemented.[7] The primary focus of selling is placed on the needs of the hospital. The hospital advertises its need and expects the applicant to respond to that need. Recruitment that focuses heavily on selling (advertising) is short-sighted and will not be successful in recruiting the highest quality applicant or in retaining quality staff. Marketing, on the other hand, focuses on the need or self-interest of the applicant, believing that if the needs of the applicant are met, the need of the organization will be met. When demand is great and supply is limited, marketing is the most advantageous and productive approach to recruitment. The department or institution must project a powerful, dynamic, and attractive image. Emergency department managers must have a full understanding of the mission of their institution, the goals and objectives of their department, and the specific aims to be accomplished through recruitment. Often it is difficult to balance the goal of acquiring the *best* candidate with the competing goal of recruiting *quickly* to maintain staffing levels for quality nursing care. For most managers, recruitment is a daily activity.

For the proactive emergency department manager, the *quality* of the staff far outweighs the quantity of staff. The ability of the emergency department to meet its goals and objectives and to fulfill the mission of the institution is directly related to the quality of the employees recruited. Recruitment of staff with ability, promise, and motivation rather than employees seeking minimal commitment should be the primary recruitment goal of managers.

Recruitment and retention coexist. Recruitment is ineffective and impotent without retention. The manager may commit time and financial and personnel resources to recruitment but accomplish little if retention of that registered nurse (RN) is not a priority after recruitment. Retention strategies and planning are addressed elsewhere in the text, but, in general, recruitment may be thought of as an offensive tactic and retention as a defensive tactic.

The development of an effective and productive recruitment plan requires the emergency department manager to conduct a comprehensive appraisal of the department. A useful tool for the manager in appraisal is the Strengths, Weaknesses, Opportunities, and Threats (SWOT) analysis.[2] Originally a marketing and strategic planning tool, SWOT analysis can easily be applied to healthcare and recruitment. Identifying strengths, weaknesses, opportunities, and threats is the goal of this helpful planning tool.[2] Best results are obtained from a brainstorming session with a group of knowledgeable nursing staff and emergency physicians. During the planning session the group is guided to identify and list departmental strengths, weaknesses, opportunities for improvement and factors that may pose a threat, such as higher salaries at a competitive hospital (Box 74-1). Once completed, a SWOT analysis should allow the manager to capture the essence and character of the department and to use this knowledge to formulate recruitment strategies. The objective is to build on the department's strengths and correct or minimize weaknesses through identification of meaningful opportunities to reduce threats.

On completion of the SWOT analysis, specific goals and objectives should be established. For example, a goal in recruitment might be to establish an effective and productive recruitment committee with nursing and physician representation. Objectives should be specific, measurable, and time limited. One objective in support of that goal might be to identify recruitment members and conduct five meetings in the next 6 months. Through the planning process, realistic but meaningful goals and objectives for recruitment should be established and modified periodically (at least annually).

One of the most difficult duties of the emergency department manager is to assess and project potential staffing needs based on patient care demands and anticipated turnover. Specific recruitment objectives should be based on the projections of needs and anticipated turnover. Assumptions for all variables (work demand, census, and organization design) must be specified and validated when possible so that forecasts can be made for recruitment needs for a specified period of time such as the fiscal year. Box 74-2 illustrates a forecasting methodology.

BOX 74-1

THE STRENGTHS, WEAKNESSES, OPPORTUNITIES, AND THREATS (SWOT) ANALYSIS

A SWOT analysis identifies the key strategic issues that must be addressed during the planning period.

- Strengths and weaknesses are controllable (to some degree) by the organization.
  - *Strengths* - These are internal factors that enhance the organization's ability to effectively deal with recruitment in the environment.
  - *Weaknesses* - These are internal factors that could be improved to lead to more effective recruitment in the environment.
- Opportunities and threats are external factors that generally are not subject to the control of the organization.
  - *Opportunities* - These are external factors that provide opportunities for the organization to improve its recruitment effectiveness or its competitive position in the marketplace with regard to recruitment.
  - *Threats* - These are external factors that may have a negative effect on the organization's ability to recruit qualified candidates.

Data from Dubuque S, Neathawk R: *J Home Health Care Pract* 5:1-8, 1993.

BOX 74-2

PROCESS STEPS FOR PROJECTING RECRUITMENT NEEDS

1. Determine historic annual average daily census (ADC) and identify range of low and high volumes for the previous year. Set projected ADC at the midpoint of the range. (It is important to review the distribution to determine variations based on seasons, hours of the day, and days of the week.)
2. Review factors that may result in future changes in ADC.
   - Environmental factors may include volume shifts to ambulatory care areas, increased competition, socioeconomic changes, crime rates, mission changes, marketing changes, insurance (managed care), and corporate contracts.
   - Operational factors may include changes in scope of practice, facilities, and skill mix of staff.
3. Based on review of factors above (step 2), adjust projected average ADC.
4. Develop staffing plan based on projected average ADC including determination of total staff (expressed as full time equivalents) required to meet plan.
5. Using full time equivalents (FTEs), compare current actual staffing to staff required at projected average ADC:
   R_c = FTE requirements − current actual FTEs
   R_c represents recruitment needs (FTEs) as a result of the adjusted ADC.
6. Calculate turnover rate (based on historical trend):
   % Turnover Rate (TR) =
   $$\frac{\text{Terminated registered nurse FTEs}}{\text{Average registered nurse FTEs employed}} \times 100$$
7. Determine amount of staff required as a result of turnover:
   R_t = Total FTE requirements (for staffing plan) × %TR
   R_t represents FTE requirements as a result of turnover
8. Determine total recruitment needs:
   Total recruitment needs = $R_c + R_t$

EXAMPLE

9. ADC = 125
10. Adjusted ADC = 135
11. FTEs required per plan = 60
12. Current FTEs per plan = 55
13. $R_c = 60 - 55 = 5$
14. $TR = \frac{7}{53} \times 100 = 13\%$
    (Example assumes 7 employees terminated and unit averaged 53 FTEs employed during last year.)
15. $R_t = 60 \times 0.13 = 7.8$
16. Total recruitment needs = 5 (R_c) + 7.8 (R_t) = 12.8

Recruitment Strategies and Tactics

Recruitment strategies should focus on what can be done to attract qualified applicants to apply for vacancies. Tactics are specific steps taken in support of the strategy. For example, a recruitment strategy might be to enhance the knowledge of senior nursing students at Main University with regard to career opportunities in the emergency department after a minimum of 2 years' experience in the ICU setting. The tactics to support that strategy might include attendance at Main University's nursing career day, distribution of hospital brochures including emergency department information, and selection of a Main University graduate from the emergency department staff to attend and answer questions. It is of primary importance to focus recruitment resources in tactics that have the greatest opportunity for success in meeting the objectives established in the recruitment plan. The SWOT analysis can also be used to appraise recruitment strategies. The manager should function as the facilitator in marketing the department to optimize communication with the potential applicant, but staff at all levels of the department must also be involved if the plan is to succeed.

The position of nurse recruiter, common in large hospitals, requires a clear and direct line of communication between the recruiter and the manager. Making initial contact with prospective applicants and establishing a relationship are the responsibilities of the recruiter. The emergency department manager must effectively and clearly communicate and provide the recruiter with information about vacancies, qualifications required of prospective applicants, and the manager's expectations of potential staff. During the initial interview, the recruiter can use the information as a guideline with which to screen out those unsuited for the position before scheduling the secondary interview with the manager. Information about vacancies, qualifications, departmental organization, and culture must be accurate when provided to the recruiter. The nurse recruiter is responsible for clearly communicating the applicant's interests and needs, as well as the recruiter's impression of the prospective applicant. A circular exchange of information is essential in promoting a viable and healthy relationship between the nurse recruiter and the manager.

Establishing a positive and accurate emergency department identity influences recruiting. Image building influences both applicants and currently employed nurses. Current nursing staff feel special knowing they accepted a position in a dynamic environment that is well perceived by the community. By building a unique identity and a positive image for the emergency department and the institution, the applicant pool will increase as individuals view the institution and department as a desirable place to work. Careful attention to patient satisfaction, development of comprehensive quality improvement programs, and establishment of an active liaison with local media sources are just a few of the opportunities that should be explored in building and sustaining a positive image for the department.

Selection of Recruitment Tools

The three most important reasons cited by nurses for accepting a position were location, available shifts, and the reputation of the hospital.[5] Additionally, RNs have identified the following recruitment issues as being of importance to them: benefits, salary and shift differential, flexible scheduling, advancement and promotion opportunities, work environment, staffing, and management support relationships.[2] Recruitment communications by the emergency department manager can capitalize on these reasons and the other strengths of the department identified in the SWOT analysis. The recruitment tools should also stress the value of the potential employee to the department. Departmental needs and position qualifications must be communicated clearly and concisely to the applicant. When new nurses find recruitment information accurate, their positive perceptions of working in that particular hospital are reinforced, thus enhancing retention. Equally important is the follow-through by the nurse recruiter in response to employment inquiries of applicants. The response should be prompt and courteous because the applicant's first impression is most important. The emergency department manager should regularly evaluate the human resources department response to prospective applicants and aggressively correct any problems quickly.

The emergency department manager should capitalize on as many recruitment resources as possible. Familiarity of the marketing tools both inside and outside the department is important. The "4 Ps" of marketing can be found in Box 74-3.[1] Advertising in a competitive market demands creativity, as well as recognized logos, slogans, or abbreviated mission statements. Successful recruitment uses multiple tools, including newspapers, professional journals, nursing conventions, schools of nursing, state board bulletins, career fairs, direct mailing, recruitment brochures, employee referrals, inducements, and walk ins.

Newspapers. In addition to internal communication vehicles, local and out-of-area newspapers are the most common tool used in recruitment. When placing the advertisement, the information should be employee-centered, deal with specifics, and highlight advantages for the prospective employee. When recruitment advertisements provide a specific salary range rather than generic terms such as *salary commensurate with experience* or *competitive salaries,* the applicant is far more likely to respond to the advertisement.[7] A distinctive look and message are essential so that the advertisement will not be lost among the others.

BOX 74-3

THE 4Ps OF RECRUITMENT MARKETING

Product	With regard to recruitment, product is the nature of the position that is vacant, including educational and advancement opportunities, expectations for quality, and opportunities for respect and fulfillment.
Place	Geographic locality and working conditions should be considered: availability of flexible scheduling, parking, child care, and reputation of the facility.
Price	Salaries and benefits (both starting and growth potential), differentials, bonuses, merit programs, and career ladders.
Promotion	Various strategies and tactics used to communicate to potential applicants that a position that meets their specific needs is available. Included may be sales promotions, advertising, personal selling, and publicity.

Data from Dubuque S, Neathawk R: *J Home Health Care Pract* 5:1-8, 1993.

Professional and Specialty Journals. Advertising in professional and specialty journals is expensive but can be directed toward specific target audiences. Journals are especially helpful if the applicant pool is small because of qualification limitations such as those for manager or director positions. Because a postsubmission delay of the advertisement can be expected, the use of reply coupons may enhance the return of applicant information. When determining the appropriate journal to target, the emergency department manager can request a demographic breakdown of subscribers to the journal.

State Board Bulletins. State board bulletins reach a wide group of potential nurses, but application information may be slow because of the monthly publication dates.

Nursing Conventions. Nursing conventions, notably specialty conventions, also can be a source of possible applicants. Because of the expense, it is not feasible for most hospitals to conduct on-site recruitment unless the convention is held locally.

Schools of Nursing. Although most emergency department managers do not hire new graduates, schools of nursing are a long range source for the proactive manager. Regrettably, few nursing schools provide clinical experience in the emergency department as part of the curriculum. Managers should encourage student participation and provide a learning atmosphere whenever possible. By serving as a clinical site for nursing students or nursing internship programs, the emergency department will attract interested students after completion of their educational program. Familiarity with the emergency department allows for a smoother transition and faster orientation of employees, promoting productivity.

Career Fairs. Career fairs can be an inexpensive tool for long-term recruitment. Contacts can be made with new graduates who may not be initially eligible but who may want to transfer to the emergency department later, when eligible. It is important to send a graduate of the specific institution as the emergency department representative whenever possible to create a natural link to the potential employer.

Recruitment Brochures. Recruitment brochures are a convenient advertising tool. The brochure should list salary ranges, benefits, the philosophy of the organization, and something about the community in which the hospital is located.

Direct Mailing. By obtaining member lists from professional organizations or other direct mailing businesses, advertisements can be sent to selected target audiences. These advertisements should be designed for ease in mailing and should include reply materials with return postage guaranteed.

Inducements. Promises of inducements such as cruises and large sign-on bonuses may attract some nurses for a critical shortage in the emergency department, but these tools usually do not result in meaningful retention for nurses and may be detrimental to the morale of the presently employed staff.

Walk Ins. Applicants who are either unfamiliar with the human resources department or assertive enough to bypass it may telephone or walk in to the emergency department. In the authors' experience, the odds of recruiting a suitable candidate through this source are about the same as with advertising.

Employee Referral. Of all the recruitment resources, employee referral is the most reliable and preferable. The applicants from this source usually have been fully informed about the department and come with expectations based on fact. The retention rate for employee referrals is much higher than from any other sources.[6]

Publicity. Positive publicity can be an excellent recruitment tool. Active liaison with the local news media can promote feature stories, local news documentaries, and appearances on television and radio shows, which will enhance the department's image. Management and staff should be encouraged to publish articles in professional journals that publicize departmental achievements and advances.

Ethical Recruitment. Recruitment must be ethical. If it is not, the hospital or department is in danger of losing its credibility. Offering recruitment incentives designed to target and attract staff at the expense of other local hospitals is considered by many to be unprofessional. Results at best are usually short term because nurses recruited by this method are likely to move on, lured by the next more attractive incentive.

Internal and External Recruitment. Most emergency department managers must recruit externally to meet the needs of their departments. External recruiting, however, is expensive, and individuals hired from outside the institution take longer to be productive. Internal recruitment is less expensive, shortens the learning curve of the individual, and tends to produce a more productive employee in less time. Although external recruitment brings in fresh personnel and new perspectives, excessive reliance on external recruitment can result in inconsistent values, role expectations, and difficulty in building loyalty and common values. Even though internal recruitment only shifts the RN vacancy from one department to another in the hospital, it does provide an outlet for recognition, advancement, and learning desires of hospital employees. Internal recruitment, if used judiciously, may actually enhance overall hospital retention. Heavy reliance on internal recruitment, however, can result in an inbreeding of values, a strong resistance to change, and resentment from other areas in the hospital.

Evaluation of Recruitment Strategies. When evaluating the efficacy of recruitment strategies, the results usually speak for themselves. If recruitment needs have decreased as the result of obtaining productive employees, the immediate recruitment objectives and goals have been met. If recruitment objectives are measurable, the success or failure of the recruitment objective should be apparent. No studies identify the best recruitment tool. The recruitment tools used most commonly are newspaper advertising and internal posting of positions. With frequent evaluation of recruitment strategies, the emergency department manager can assess which tools produce the best results for their particular department. The manager should evaluate the recruitment response frequently and adjust the mix of strategies and tactics accordingly. Studies have demonstrated a significant correlation between recruitment source and subsequent employee performance.[8] In a nonclinical study, absenteeism of employees recruited by newspaper advertisement was twice the rate of those employees recruited from other sources.[8] When evaluating employee performance the manager should correlate the performance with the recruitment source to evaluate which tool or strategy obtains the highest quality employee for the department. The emergency department manager will want to continue to use what works best but should not be afraid to try new strategies and tactics based on the available information and a regularly updated SWOT analysis.

SUMMARY

Nursing shortages, increased acuity of patients, complex technology and specialization of nurses, with expansion of employment for nurses outside the traditional hospital setting, have all affected nurse recruitment in the emergency department. Recruitment is the act of locating and hiring the most qualified and appropriate applicant for the position. Marketing a positive but accurate image of the emergency department is an ongoing process that is essential in building a successful recruitment program. The manager should involve staff at all levels in the recruitment process. Developing a specific recruitment plan starting with a SWOT analysis and concluding with an ongoing evaluation of the plan provides an objective means to guide the team's efforts.

REFERENCES

1. Stratton T et al: Recruiting and retaining registered nurses in rural community hospitals, *J Nurs Adm* 21:30-34, 1991.
2. Dubuque S, Neathawk R: Applying a marketing framework to staff recruitment and retention, *J Home Health Care Pract* 5:1-8, 1993.
3. Jones C: Staff nurse turnover costs: part 2, measurement and results, *J Nurs Adm* 20:30-34, 1990.
4. Shannon M: A comparative analysis of recruitment and retention of health care professionals, *Health Care Manage Rev* 18:41-51, 1993.
5. Birkenstock M: Recruitment and retention, *AORN J* 53:110-118, 1991.
6. Florida Hospital Association: *1993 Fact Sheet: (1993) Supply of Nurses,* Orlando, Fl, 1993, FHA.

7. Pattan J: Developing a nurse recruitment plan, *J Nurs Adm* 22:33-39, 1992.
8. Breaugh J: Relationship between recruitment sources and employee performance, absenteeism, and work attitudes, *Acad Manag J* 24:142-150, 1981.

ADDITIONAL READINGS

Blackshaw D: Recruit, retain, return, *Nurs Stand* 5:54-55, 1991.

Brady D et al: Unification of critical care nurses: an approach to recruitment and retention, *Nurs Adm Q* 14:61-65, 1990.

Henderson C, Wiggins S: Proactive versus reactive recruitment and retention strategies, *J Nurs Staff Dev* 9:193-195, 1993.

Huston C, Marquis B: *Retention and productivity strategies for nurse managers,* Philadelphia, 1989, JB Lippincott.

Klemm R, Schreiber E: Paid and unpaid benefits, *J Nurs Adm* 22:52-56, 1992.

Krizek M: Emergency nursing recruitment and retention, *Emerg Nurs Reports* 2:1-6, 1987.

McAndrew T: Nurses: to have and hold, *Pa Nurse* 47:5-6, 1990.

Pattan J: Nurse recruitment: from selling to marketing, *J Nurs Adm* 21:16-20, 1991.

Smeltzer C, Tseng S, Harty L: Implementing a strategic recruitment and retention plan, *J Nurs Adm* 21:20-28, 1991.

Spitzer-Lehmann R: Recruitment and retention of our greatest asset, *Nurs Adm Q* 14:66-69, 1990.

75 The Interview Process

Jan Rich

OUTLINE

Interview preparation
Beginning the interview
Types of questions
Crucial questions to ask
Hiring recovering nurses
Group interviews
Critical indicators
Closing the interview
Exit interview
Preparing to be interviewed
Summary

Few decisions are as crucial to the success of a department as the selection of its team members. One decision made without adequate preparation, careful consideration, thoughtful reflection, from trained interviewers, can result in endless conflict and frustration when the wrong candidate is chosen. The right candidate can enhance collaboration, provide clinical or managerial expertise, instill enthusiasm, inspire co-workers, and become a welcome and valuable team member.

INTERVIEW PREPARATION

The professionally qualified applicant may not always be the right person for the department. It is imperative in the interview process not only to establish clinical or managerial competence, but also to identify job candidates who share organizational values and who will fit in with the culture of the department. Important characteristics to consider include the candidate's values, temperament, decision-making processes, conflict resolution style, service orientation, beliefs, and personality.[1]

Well-conducted interviews improve the probability of selecting candidates who are most likely to succeed.[2] Three main skills to master in interviewing job candidates include the following: regulating what you do and do not say, asking the right type of questions, and listening well.[3] It is essential to identify clues about the applicant's abilities to process information, make judgments, provide leadership, delegate, appreciate cultural diversity, and other important traits.

Application review provides an early opportunity to avoid interviews with unqualified or inappropriate candidates. The manager should carefully examine education, employment, credentials, references, and the care with which the application is completed. The applicant may be asked to complete the application in person. In reviewing the application, the following should be noted: misspelled words, illegibility, nonsequential dates of employment, past job-related injuries if indicated, and evidence of progression in job responsibilities.

Resumes can be both valuable and deceptive. Some are prepared personally by the candidate, whereas others are professionally prepared. Avoid placing an inordinate amount of importance on the resume itself. The candidate is the one hired . . . not the resume.

Whenever possible the manager should personally check the candidate's references. Many hospitals have established policies prohibiting comments about former employees. Many managers, however, listed on employment applications will provide enough feedback to prevent a catastrophic decision. Historically, if candidates had attitude, attendance, or performance problems at a former institution, the risk is high that this behavior will recur. One strategy is to ask the candidate, "What will your former supervisor tell me about you?" If the responses of the two differ significantly, one should assume there has been a definite difference of perception about the candidate's attitude or performance.

The interviewer should ask for evidence of licensing, certification, and any other qualifications necessary for the position. Ideally, the candidate will have an opportunity to review the job description before the interview. If the department has a mission statement or a list of written expectations for employees, that too should be shared.

BEGINNING THE INTERVIEW

If possible, job candidates should be greeted in the reception area or outer office rather than from behind a desk. Any interview should be conducted without a desk as a barrier and with both participants seated at the same level. The candidate should be seated in a comfortable chair and out of the direct sunlight. Eye to eye contact should be ensured.

The interview should be timed so that a private meeting can be held without interruptions. All phone calls should be held and beeper responsibility delegated. The interview should be arranged at the interviewer's best time of day. For example, Friday afternoon at 3 PM is probably not the fairest time for interviewing. It is unwise to schedule multiple interviews consecutively. An hour or two between interviews allows time to make notes, stretch, and refocus for the next candidate. If a group interview is scheduled, the candidate should be told who will be in the group (e.g., management, immediate supervisor, a peer).

The applicant should be greeted with a handshake and an introduction. A beverage may be offered, and the candidate should be asked to be seated. The applicant should be informed about the interview process and duration. This sets the agenda for the interview and may help the candidate relax.

TYPES OF QUESTIONS

The applicant should talk 90% of the time. This is the hardest part for most interviewers, but one technique is to stick a note on a clipboard with the word "listen" written on it.[3] The most important information the employer communicates is a sense of the mission of the institution, job responsibilities, and expectations. It should be remembered that both parties are conducting an interview. Box 75-1 lists typical questions asked in an interview.

It is important to understand clearly what candidates mean when responding to questions. If answers sound vague or confusing, they should be paraphrased to clarify the candidate's response. For example, "What I heard you say is that you do not support the concept of shared governance?" The candidate is allowed the opportunity to reply so that both interviewer and candidate have the same understanding.

Closed questions can generally be answered in fewer than five words. Closed questions are used to provide specific information, for example, dates of employment, licensure information, and questions with "yes" or "no" replies.

Open questions force the candidate to provide more than yes or no answers. For example, instead of asking "Did you enjoy your last job?" rephrase it in an open ended format, "What are three things you particularly appreciated about your most recent employment?" Because many candidates do not like to admit weaknesses, it is preferable to ask, "What are the most significant challenges you faced in your last position?" Open questions are useful in determining attitudes, feelings, and opinions.

Leading questions will likely provide misleading, unreliable, or false answers and should be avoided. For example, avoid statements such as, "I expect with your past experience that you are comfortable caring for pediatric patients."

Providing candidates with hypothetical situations is a way of obtaining valuable information about the candidate's critical thinking abilities. For example, this situation could be described: "The emergency department is very busy and you have just received a phone call that a bus crash has occurred. You will be receiving several dozen patients with varying injuries. How would you proceed?" One way to incorporate staff into the interview process is to ask employees to provide the interviewer with actual problems they have encountered with co-workers, physicians, and outside agencies. These problems can be developed into hypothetical questions.

Providing the candidate with several situations in which priorities have to be set will help identify clinical expertise and decision-making abilities. These situations may relate to assignment of staff, triage of patient conditions, directing physician or ancillary resources, involvement of supporting staff, or consideration of outside agency referrals.

CRUCIAL QUESTIONS TO ASK

The most important component in successful relationships is effective communication. The candidate should be asked to describe strategies he or she has used with peers to overcome barriers to effective communication.

The candidate can be asked to relate several difficult situations for which they have successfully used troubleshooting skills. The purpose of this question is to establish each candidate's perception of how problems should be solved on the unit. This is an ideal opportunity to establish whether a candidate always sees problems as "other" related and provides the interviewer the opportunity to identify each candidate's particular coping skills when confronted with problems. It is important to realize that stress reactions can be as different as withdrawal, anger, attack, and acquiescence. Identifying how the candidate responds in adverse circumstances is helpful. Clinical skills can be taught; however, relationship skills are for the most part ingrained in the candidate. Of management problems, 80% will probably be generated by 20% of employees.

Each candidate should be asked to describe collaboration strategies for use with members of the health team. By asking the candidate to list members of the team with whom collaboration is important,[4] one can determine who the candidate perceives is fully vested in the team.

There are several ways to elicit clinical experience. Information about clinical experience can be obtained by asking these questions: With what types of patients do you particularly enjoy working? With what clinical populations do you find it difficult to work? Describe your short and long-term clinical or management career goals. Describe your involvement, to date, in continuing education.[4]

BOX 75-1

COMMON QUESTIONS ASKED AT AN INTERVIEW

What knowledge and experience will you bring to this position?
What are your greatest assets?
What are the greatest challenges you face in the emergency department?
How do you create a positive environment?
What are your expectations for your emergency department management team?
How do you deal with conflict with other team members?
What continuing education have you completed in the last year?
Why should we choose you for this position?
When I contact your references, what will they say about you?

HIRING RECOVERING NURSES

With the recent changes in healthcare reform, including mergers, declining patient census, and layoffs, the need to hire less than the cream of the crop has diminished. When faced with the option of considering a recovering nurse, the interviewer has a special responsibility. The applicant's previous choice of drugs and details about past and current treatment should be elicited in the interview. Information relating to types of treatment (inpatient and outpatient), length of time spent in treatment, and method of intervention assist in assessing a recovering nurse's readiness to reenter the work setting. Other factors to assess are physical appearance, attitude, and identification of current support persons. Does the recovering nurse appear well groomed and healthy? Does the nurse make positive statements about self and others? Has a significant other been identified as a source of strong support? The interviewer should review the hospital's contract for recovering nurses.[5] The interviewee should receive information during the interview about procedures for obtaining random urine samples. As additional precautions, previous employers, references, and a case worker should be contacted. The validity of the license and any pending action against the license should be evaluated.

GROUP INTERVIEWS

Increasingly, management practices include working with and through individuals and groups to accomplish organizational goals. Group interviews can be conducted in several ways. Several persons can individually interview the prospective employee at different times. One group may conduct the job interview at the same time. A simple definition of group interviews is the process of using a committee to interview all acceptable applicants for a particular position, each committee member asking applicants the same set of questions and serving on the committee until the position is filled.[6]

The sharing of employment responsibility is an opportunity that can strengthen teamwork and augment unit effectiveness. After all, staff nurses who provide bedside care around the clock are the ones who best understand the specific skills and knowledge that their working group needs to provide care successfully.[7] It is extremely valuable for several individuals to hear a candidate's answers. Each may perceive the answer from a different point of view. When the committee discusses these various perceptions, someone may recognize a benefit or a problem area that someone else completely missed or interpreted another way.

Inviting clinical staff members to interview candidates for peer positions is a natural way to acknowledge their professional interest in working with competent colleagues and in participating in the management of their practice environment. Having the opportunity to influence hiring can motivate more willingness to undertake charge nurse responsibilities and to precept new staff members.[7] The commitment required by interview team members includes time for interviews and decision-making sessions, completion of interview training, and willingness to accept the empowerment for decision making.[8]

In group interviews the nurse manager acts as educator, facilitator, and coordinator. As educator, the nurse manager teaches the staff the federal, state, and local mandates and constraints that condition terms of employment. Managers must specifically educate staff about how to comply with regulations governing employment and rehearse effective interviewing techniques.[7]

The manager has the responsibility to eliminate unqualified applicants and set up interviews when all team members are available. The manager should verify references, licensing, and certifications and share resumes or applications with all team members before the interview.

Barriers to team interviewing may include inability of team members to get away from their work, lack of commitment from management to support the process, lack of training, and resistance of staff members to the process. Reaching group consensus can be a problem. A decision should be made in advance about how the group will proceed if there is not consensus.

At the conclusion of a group interview, each interviewer summarizes information about the candidate. Assessment of the candidate's suitability can be determined according to each of seven dimensions: (1) education and training, (2) clinical experience and expertise, (3) professional goals, (4) sense of teamwork, (5) interpersonal skills and self presentation, (6) willingness to learn and teach, and (7) match between competencies and unit needs.[7]

In short, assessment of a candidate's capabilities, experience, adaptability, and other qualities may be more accurate when derived from a group than from a single interviewer. Furthermore, asking preset questions ensures that the interview process is complete, consistent, and fair to all concerned.[6]

CRITICAL INDICATORS

Several indicators should be critically analyzed before an applicant is hired. Have there been unexplained gaps in employment? Has the applicant moved from job to job frequently? Is there a reluctance to answer any questions during the interview process? Does the applicant refuse permission to call a present employer? Has the candidate worked under a restricted license?

Emergency department managers may hire staff knowing that the new employee's stated preference is to work in another specialty area. The manager may believe that the staff member will become attached to the new unit. However, study results suggest that staff do maintain clinical preferences and eventually transfer to the desired unit.[2] The significant time and effort committed to orientation and development of a competent emergency nurse warrant careful consideration of any candidate who is uncertain about his or her short- or long-term commitment to emergency services.

The interviewer should determine whether the candidate is truthful. Body language changes when people lie. Their eyes tend to shift and their voices drop. If an answer seems suspicious, the applicant can be asked to explain further. Most people will stumble on details about events they are making up.[3]

During the interview, the interviewer must be careful not to be overpowered by halo effects. This includes judgment bias that occurs when the interviewer develops a positive impression of the interviewee, which may be contradicted by subsequent interview data. This halo effect can occur when the interviewer is reminded of an admired colleague, a reliable staff member, or a similarity to the interviewer. Halo effects can be stimulated by a sense of comfort in the interviewer's presence, ease in communication, or the interviewee's background such as graduation from a respected educational facility. Once the halo effect is established, it is usually entrenched; interviewers are unlikely to be sensitive to subsequent information that suggests a candidate's possible inability to meet job requirements.[4]

Federal law prohibits employers from discriminating against people because of gender, age, race, national origin, or religion (Box 75-2).

The Americans with Disabilities Act prohibits employer discrimination in all hiring, firing, promoting, awarding ben-

BOX 75-2

QUESTIONS ILLEGAL TO ASK DURING AN INTERVIEW

1. Age or date of birth (you may ask if applicant is over 18)
2. Length of time at present/past address
3. Whether dwelling is owned or rented
4. Religion/church preference
5. Father's surname
6. Mother's maiden name
7. Marital status
8. Room/apartment/housemates
9. Residence of spouse or children
10. Number and age of children
11. How child care will be provided while applicant works
12. How the applicant will get to work
13. Name of bank
14. Information about outstanding loans
15. Whether wages were ever garnished or whether applicant has declared bankruptcy
16. Whether applicant has ever been arrested or convicted of a crime
17. Hobbies, clubs
18. Foreign language fluency (unless a job requirement)

efits, and managing of employees and applicants with disabilities. Because of ongoing legislative changes, it is wise to remain updated on federal and state laws that protect people who fall into these categories. Because of the demands of emergency services, however, most hospitals have policies on an employee's ability to lift, bend, and tolerate long periods of standing.

Certain questions are illegal to ask during an interview. Legal issues usually hinge on whether the questions asked have any bearing on the applicant's qualifications to perform the job. Some information can be gathered simply by rewording questions. For example, an applicant may not be asked about national origin, parentage, ancestry, naturalization, or the status of parents, spouse, or children. However, the applicant may be asked if he or she is a U.S. citizen or a resident alien with the right to work in the United States. Questions may not be asked about the applicant's religion, church, synagogue or parish, or the religious holidays he or she observes. Because the company operates 7 days a week, 24 hours a day, the applicant may be asked if there is a problem with working this schedule.

CLOSING THE INTERVIEW

The applicant should be informed when 10 minutes remain in the interview. This time is used to elicit questions or to let the applicant mention anything not yet covered. The interview should end at the predetermined time. Standing and shaking the person's hand make it clear that the interview is over. The applicant is walked back to the initial greeting place. The candidate is thanked for his or her interest and is provided with a time frame for hearing about an employment decision. The interviewer, on returning to the office, writes down any last-minute impressions.

Criteria for choosing the right candidate should be objective and consistent for all candidates. Follow-up should be conducted as promised. If the candidate is not selected and is a current employee in the department, feedback should be offered. The employee deserves to know what issues were considered, how the employee may have interviewed more successfully, and what the employee needs to do in preparation for future promotion.

EXIT INTERVIEW

The purpose of the exit interview is to learn why some employees are leaving in an effort to consider ways of reducing the number of departures. Finding out why people leave sometimes helps correct conditions that cause them to leave. The exit interview is a rational attempt to learn what, if anything, the department employee feels is undesirable about working for the organization.[10]

As in any effort to solicit feedback, there is little point in conducting exit interviews unless some mechanism is in place to address legitimate issues identified in the process. Many managers name three critical elements for obtaining useful information in an exit interview:

1. Ensure confidentiality.
2. Make sure the feedback correlates with other available information such as employee surveys or peer and supervisor performance reviews.
3. Take action. At companies with a history of responding to exemployees' perspectives, people believe their comments may have an impact.[11]

Ideally an exit interview will be held informally with the employee's supervisor (this could be any member of the emergency department management team) followed by an interview in the human resources department. The exit interview should be timed to occur during the employee's final week, but preferably not on the last day of work. The last day should be reserved for closing out records, changing status of benefits, turning in keys, and saying goodbye to others.[10] Phone interviews or surveys mailed to former employees at home 6 months to 1 year later may generate more candor.

The exit interview is an information-gathering review, not a gripe session, witch hunt, or problem-solving meeting. It should occur in private and be unhurried and uninterrupted. Both participants must be aware that the purpose of the interview is to determine whether anything can be learned that can help make the organization a better place to work.

A detailed study of several organizations revealed that the same or similar exit interview topics tend to be used in all organizations. The following common exit interview topics are listed in order of frequency:

1. Reason for leaving
2. Opinion of job
3. Opinion of supervisor
4. Opinion of pay
5. Appeal of new job or pursuit
6. Perception of advancement opportunity
7. Suggestions (e.g., for improvement)
8. What was liked best about employment

BOX 75-3

REASONS FOR LEAVING EMPLOYMENT

1. Lack of recognition or appreciation and the feeling that one is not making a difference
2. Lack of advancement or lack of opportunity for promotion
3. Money or the feeling that one is undercompensated
4. Too many bosses, hazy lines of authority, or feeling of being pulled in too many directions
5. Personality conflicts
6. Underqualification or "in-over-my-head" feeling
7. Overqualification or lack of challenge or interest in work

BOX 75-4

PREPARATION FOR INTERVIEW: THE CANDIDATE CHECKLIST

1. Create a professional image in appearance and attitude.
2. Identify the reasons for making a job change. What can the job offer you? What can you offer the job?
3. Review the job description.
4. Learn as much about the organization as possible before the interview.
5. Ask who will be included in the interview process.

9. What was liked least about employment
10. Opinion of working conditions
11. Likelihood of returning
12. Whether organization could have prevented resignation
13. Assessment of training received

No supervisor should wish to curtail all turnover. Not everyone who leaves is a loss. New employees can bring new perspectives, fresh ideas, and renewed enthusiasm to the department.

People quit their jobs for many reasons. A study by the Administrative Management Society more than 20 years ago and revalidated periodically identified the seven most frequently cited reasons for leaving a job (Box 75-3).[10] When examining reasons for leaving, it is important to evaluate how much of the reason is employer controlled or influenced.

PREPARING TO BE INTERVIEWED

At some point the manager will likely be on the other end of the interview process. Healthcare is a competitive environment, even for managers. Positioning oneself to obtain a desirable position requires a professional approach. Resumes should state accomplishments and achievements clearly and concisely, be no longer than 2 pages, and reflect the type of position being sought.[12]

A person who projects a professional appearance has an edge even before the interview begins. Starting an interview on the wrong foot occurs when a candidate wears inappropriate attire, demonstrates poor grooming and hygiene, reflects adverse body language, uses slang grammar or jargon, has poor posture and expressions, chews gum, or smokes.[13]

It is important to communicate enthusiasm and interest. Negativism, arrogance, cockiness, egotism or overconfidence, abrasiveness, rudeness, a "know-it-all" attitude, lack of self-confidence, extreme nervousness, and inflexibility should be avoided.

Within several moments of the beginning of the interview process, much of the potential for future employment has already been decided. Tardiness is inexcusable. If the interviewee is unfamiliar with the location of the interview site, it is important that he or she make a trial run before the interview date. An informal visit before an interview can provide the opportunity to explore the environment and meet people informally. Unforeseen circumstances such as traffic or weather problems should be anticipated and planned for. An interviewee who cannot arrive on time should always call the interviewer. Making poor eye contact; making racist, prejudiced, or sexist remarks; falsifying resume information; or being more interested in what the company can do for the interviewee than what the interviewee can do for the company are fatal mistakes.

The applicant should request and review a job description before the interview appointment. Box 75-4 lists preparation strategies.

If certain issues are particularly important and the answers could affect the decision to accept employment, it is crucial to ask them in the interview process. This is especially true in relationship to the ethical issues surrounding abortion, euthanasia, decision making for incompetent patients, religious matters, living wills, organ procurement, and do not resuscitate situations.

The applicant should ask the following crucial questions:

- How much job security does this position have?
- What previous experience does this job require?
- What are the requirements for working weekends? Rotating shifts? On-call?
- What are the opportunities for promotion?
- What are staffing policies?[14]

An ill-prepared candidate will be an unemployed candidate. The candidate should be prepared to outline qualifications before the interview and to talk about his or her current position and the reason for leaving. Questions to ask the interviewer should be written down. Unnecessary rambling and failing to answer questions directly should be avoided. Honesty when answering questions, especially with regard to knowledge or competence issues or a former employer, is always the best policy.

The candidate should enter the interview with a smile, a firm hand shake, good eye contact, and clear thought and communication. The key to a successful interview lies in preparation and salesmanship. A candidate will never market a more important product and should never leave anything to chance.[15] If the candidate is familiar with other candidates and a future employer asks who he or she believes is the best person for the position, the answer given could well determine who gets the job. The candidate should always believe he or she is the best candidate.

SUMMARY

Interviewing is a complex and demanding responsibility. The more knowledge brought to the process, the greater the likelihood of correctly predicting effective performance. To interview on the basis of intuition alone, or "gut reaction," is no longer acceptable in the face of all that is known about effective interviewing techniques.[16]

REFERENCES

1. Eubanks P: Hospitals probe job candidates' values for organizational "fit," *Hospitals* 65(20):36-38, 1991.
2. Heslin K, Faux S: The staff nurse employment interview selection process: judgment and decision errors and how to avoid them, Part I, *Can J Nurs Adm* 4(4):25-28, 1991.
3. Hallas G: Hiring top-notch employees, *J Emerg Med Serv* 17(2):54-56, 1992.
4. Heslin K, Faux S: The staff nurse employment interview: predicting performance outcomes, Part II, *Can J Nurs Adm* 4(4):30-36, 1991.
5. Ebener K: Hiring recovering nurses, *Fl Nurse* 39(2):11, 1991.
6. Garcia L: The why and how of the group interview, *Medical Laboratory Observer* 20(1):45-48, 1988.
7. Ott J et al: Peer interviews: sharing the hiring process, *Nurs Manage* 21(11):32-33, 1990.
8. Mills J, Oie M: Autonomous staff selection teams, *JONA* 22(12):57-63, 1992.
9. Swansburg R: *Management and leadership for nurse managers,* Boston, 1990, Jones and Bartlett.
10. McConnell C: The exit interview: locking the barn door, *Health Care Supervision* 11(2):1-10, 1992.
11. Pearl J: Exit interviews: getting the truth, *Working Woman* 18(6):16-17, 1993.
12. Houlihan R: Interviewing tips for the 90's nurse, *Mass Nurse* 61(8):4, 1991.
13. Rodriguez K: Avoid interview turn-offs to ensure success, *Am Nurse* 24(8):18-19, 1992.
14. Black J: Interviewing, *Plast Surg Nurs* 12:41-42, 1992.
15. Flores D: Marketing yourself in an interview, *Nursing 92* 22(8):100-102.
16. Loretto V: Recruitment: effective interviewing is based on more than intuition, *Pers J* 65(12):101-107, 1986.

ADDITIONAL READINGS

Fish J: Preparing for an interview, *Br J Nurs* 1(4):201-204, 1992.

Fish J: How to respond at interview, *Br J Nurs* 1(5):252-255, 1992.

Fish J: How to respond at interview: 2, *Br J Nurs* 1(6):307-309, 1992.

Fish J: How to choose the right applicant, *Br J Nurs* 1(7):352-355, 1992.

Fish J: How to choose the right applicant: 2, *Br J Nurs* 1(8):409-411, 1992.

Husted G: Ethical questions nurses can ask potential employers, *AORN J* 53(3):791-792, 1991.

Netherton H: Tips on successful interviewing, *NSNA/IMPRINT* 39(1):27,29, 1992.

76 Physician Credentialing

Dighton Packard

OUTLINE

The credentialing process
 Hospital and medical staff responsibilities
 Staff membership versus privileges
Special issues
 National practitioner data bank
 Change in the delineation of privileges
 Recredentialing and quality assurance
Summary

Concepts and practices surrounding professional staff credentialing in hospitals have undergone a fundamental shift in the last 25 years. Before 1965 the hospital and its medical staff were considered separate entities with distinct missions. Patient care was the primary domain of the physician members of the medical staff, and the ultimate responsibility for guaranteeing this quality of care rested within the medical staff. This structure had been derived originally under the principles of the American College of Surgeons Hospital Standardization Program, which dates from the early 1900s. In the 1950s the Joint Commission on Accreditation of Healthcare Organizations (JCAHO) was developed and added to this program. Then in 1965 the judicial system became involved in the credentialing process with the now famous Darling Decision. Under this decision hospitals were made to serve a much greater role than the mere provision of facilities for treatment. The hospital, through its board of trustees, is now charged with the overall responsibility for the quality of healthcare delivered to patients, including those elements delivered by physicians practicing as members of the medical staff. Although this shift of responsibility for medical care was a truly landmark decision, the courts have never wavered from this first judicial opinion. Through the years other court cases have taken place that seek only to affirm and expand the responsibility for the hospital and its board of trustees.

Therefore the medical staff is now considered part of the hospital. Peer review is delegated to this staff, but ultimate responsibility is retained by the board of trustees through a quality assurance reporting system and retention of the authority to grant staff membership and clinical privileges. The hospital is now held to a "standard of care" in selecting all staff members and recredentialing these same staff members. Throughout these judicial rulings the JCAHO has remained steadfastly a certifying agency for the hospital and its medical staff. JCAHO now certifies that the hospital not only has the facilities to treat the patients, but also has the necessary organization in place to grant privileges to physicians and to recredential these same physicians. In addition to judicial rulings and organizations such as the JCAHO, hospitals and their medical staffs are also being spurred onward in the area of credentialing and recredentialing by health agencies such as health maintenance organizations, the National Center for Quality Assurance, and similar organizations, which are now demanding that hospitals perform to a certain standard in the area of credentialing and recredentialing for them to obtain contracts with such healthcare entities. These external elements have been the major forces driving the increased need for effective systematic credentialing.

In addition to these external forces, internal forces are also driving us to the same conclusion. The first has to deal with the myriad of medical and legal issues surrounding the interaction between the medical staff and the hospital. The hospital is now seen as being responsible for the quality of medicine practiced by its physicians within its walls, and it is often brought into malpractice suits along with the physician. A major question in these suits is whether the physician was properly credentialed or, in some cases, recredentialed. The matter of peer review documents, which once were sacrosanct and absolutely protected by law, are no longer as well protected. In many states, rulings are being delivered that will allow these records to be reviewed in a court of law when the question of proper credentialing or recredentialing has been raised.

At the other end of the spectrum, hospitals are now being sued by physicians when credentials are not granted, recredentialing is not carried out in a proper manner, or a punitive process is carried out against the physician. The physician's basis of the suit often is on matters of antitrust and center around whether the hospital followed its procedures precisely and whether its procedures were correct under law in the area of credentialing and recredentialing. As a result, the hospital and its medical staff are being pressured from all sides to ensure that their credentialing process is thorough and systematic. In addition, emergency medicine also continues to maintain a high emphasis on quality patient care. This is usually referred to in some type of peer review process, whether quality assurance or continued quality improvement (CQI). These processes are still ongoing. Individual physicians, even in this day of CQI, are still being reviewed individually and their individual care and use of services scrutinized.

Another major internal force now driving credentialing and recredentialing has to do with matching the physician's and hospital's needs. The hospital has a right to have a medical staff plan in place that spells out the number and types of physicians it needs to adequately perform its mission. In addition, it has the right to set credential requirements as it sees fit, as long as they are set uniformly across the board and across the medical staff. This can allow a hospital to restrict, or even not to offer, applications to certain physicians.

Thus a series of external and internal forces has changed the accreditation process over the last 25 years. Through a series of court precedents and rulings, changes in accreditation processes and certain internal forces, combined with the overpowering costs and quality pressures in the development of clinical information systems have set the stage for more rigorous hospital medical staff credentialing processes than would have been dreamed of 25 years ago.

THE CREDENTIALING PROCESS

Hospital and Medical Staff Responsibilities

Each hospital has its own corporate bylaws. These bylaws describe the overall responsibility of the ruling boards in the area of credentialing and recredentialing. The medical staff bylaws and their attended policies and the policy on appointment, reappointment, and clinical privileges outline the role of the medical staff in the hospital and in the credentialing process. It is important that these documents be internally consistent. It is also important that physicians are familiar with those sections of the bylaws that deal with the medical staff.

As stated earlier, hospitals have the right, and even the responsibility, to have a medical staff plan. This staff plan can follow many routes. It can allow the free market to satisfy the needs of the hospital and the medical staff, or it can completely close the medical staff by ceasing to accept any application for appointment. In most cases hospitals and their medical staff follow a third route; they periodically review their needs and may close or open applications as needed in certain areas of the medical staff (i.e., recruit for one specialty, but another specialty may be closed). These staff plans and the ability to cease the acceptance of new applications for one specialty or another are fraught with some hazards. The plans must be followed meticulously and without bias to avoid antitrust- or antitrade-type allegations.

The hospital and its medical staff have the responsibility to set out all criteria for applicants to their medical staff. These criteria should be uniform, but they should clearly delineate the amount of formal training, clinical experience, and ongoing training needed to obtain and to maintain staff credentials.

The physician applicant also has certain responsibilities. The applicant has the responsibility to fill out all forms completely and truthfully. The applicant must see that all documents required are properly obtained and delivered on time to the medical staff office. The applicant should be available at the times necessary for interviews or review by hospital committees. This process takes 60 to 90 days and should not be rushed; proper credentialing takes time and energy. The documentation required for credentialing and recredentialing varies among hospitals and organizations. Some hospitals use a preapplication, which is used to screen out all applicants who are not eligible by bylaws for appointment to the medical staff. Preapplications also can be used to screen out allied health professionals who are not appointed to the specific staff. A separate application form and credentialing process are often used for these mid-level practitioners. Preapplication is, in essence, a letter that outlines the basic criteria for appointment, explains the review process, and requests the applicant to provide proof that he or she meets these criteria. In addition to identifying those individuals who do not meet the preapplication criteria, the preapplication also has the additional advantage of possibly discouraging applicants who do not intend to make a substantial commitment to the hospital in question. After the preapplication has been returned and it is decided that the applicant does meet the basic criteria, the applicant is usually sent an application form and is often sent a copy of hospital and medical staff bylaws and a letter outlining the procedures the applicant must go through to finish the application process. In many areas there is also a dollar cost to the applications. These nonrefundable fees serve two basic purposes. First, they defray the increasing costs of processing an application because they are becoming more intricate. Second, they discourage applicants who do not have the necessary commitment to the hospital.

A preapplication form may include basic demographic data, such as the applicant's address, office address, and practice specialty. In addition, it may ask for the amount of practice the applicant anticipates pursuing at the facility in question, where the applicant currently holds privileges, the applicant's current license number and DEA registration number, proof of liability coverage, proof of residency training, and postgraduate training as necessary.

The application itself will include all information given on the preapplication and will probably include other items such as curriculum vitae, evidence of board certification as applicable, more specific personal identification data, citizenship data as applicable, and a series of questions that have to do with disciplinary actions taken against the applicant by other hospitals, state boards, or entities. Questions will be asked about health or disability, whether the applicant has been convicted of a criminal or civil offense, and any malpractice history. They will require in-depth educational data, listing people who will provide references from each level of education, teaching appointments, postgraduate education, if any, institutional affiliations, professional associations, board certification data, and in-depth professional liability data. In addition, the applicant is usually asked to sign a consent and release form that releases anyone the hospital may contact to give information about the applicant's professional and personal attributes. These releases often read differently, and it is advisable to read a release before signing it. The applicant also may be asked to grant immunity to the hospital or its medical staff for all matters relating to appointment or reappointment of clinical privileges. Because this process is so in depth and often so costly, many hospitals and geographic areas are banding together to form one centralized application process (i.e., all information is forwarded to one group who then credentials physicians for many hospitals). This approach reduces the cost of each individual application. However, because there now appears to be a separate entity credentialing all physicians for those hospitals, it is difficult to put any type of pressure on this system to increase the speed. Therefore applications tend to take longer to process than in the past.

The next phase of the process usually takes several months. All the data provided by the applicant must be verified by the hospital's committees and personnel. In general, the hospital requires original certifications or reference letters, which can easily take 2 to 3 months or longer to obtain. The application process does not proceed until the application is complete and all references and information have been returned. To ensure that the application is processed in a timely fashion, the applicant should put as much pressure as possible on those individuals and organizations responsible for delivering their recommendations and documents to the hospital in question.

After the application is complete, it then enters the committee and hospital credentialing process. The application is generally screened by a credentials committee with input from the prospective department chairman and with possible input from other staff members. The committee's report generally goes to the hospital executive committee, then to the hospital medical board for its review, and then to the board of trustees for the ultimate delivery of staff membership. The credentials committee usually has a variety of alternatives. They can ask for approval of provisional privileges or, in some cases, for approval of temporary privileges. Provisional privileges are generally the starting point in most hospitals. This allows the hospital and the applicant to review each other over time before having a permanent membership attachment. In addition, some hospitals use *locum tenens* privileging, which can be an entirely different process covered under a different area of the medical staff bylaws. *Locum tenens* is usually seen as a short-cut for certain medical staff appointments. However, a *locum tenens* membership often does not imply full rank and privileges with other members of the medical staff. The hospital bylaws should spell out these differences.

The provisional appointment is usually used in the self-evaluation system and may be as simple as a perfunctory to an in-depth perusal of all charts and documentations before obtaining full staff membership. The committee process itself may be finished within a month, or it may take 6 to 8 weeks, depending on the efficiency and the timing of the committees. Once membership credentialization has occurred, it is important to understand other elements of staff membership.

Staff Membership versus Privileges

It is important to differentiate privileges granted to a physician from the granting of staff membership. Staff membership is obtained through the process previously outlined. Staff membership does not state what the physician might be privileged to do within the confines of that hospital. The delineation of clinical privileges is a process by which the hospital determines the specific procedures that may be performed by each medical staff applicant and appointee in the hospital. Staff membership title may be courtesy, provisional, assistant staff, or full staff. At the same time, the same privileges throughout all categories of membership may be obtained. They are separate entities.

In general, the criteria for obtaining each specific privilege are set out in print long before an applicant applies to the hospital. That is, to obtain a specific privilege, the applicant must have a certain amount of formal training, on-the-job experience, or education that can be substantiated. The JCAHO mandates that every individual who is permitted by law and by the hospital to provide patient care in the hospital have delineated clinical privileges. According to the JCAHO, it is the responsibility of the department chairperson to recommend to the medical staff the criteria for clinical privileges in the department. The criteria for appointment to the medical staff are general requirements that are met by all applicants, whereas certain criteria for the delineation of privileges specify the certification or specific training or experience required for eligibility for specific clinical privileges in a specific specialty. Therefore two members of the medical staff may be practicing side by side in the same department but have different privileges. Also, two members of the medical staff may be credentialed by different departments practicing the same privilege. Furthermore, these same two physicians may have obtained the privileges by satisfying different requirements. It is the credentials committee's job and responsibility to see that these different requirements are both justified.

The privileges are usually granted by a simple form on which a check-off list of those privileges requested by the applicant is delineated. The request is then compared with a preset delineation of education, training, and experiences necessary for each privilege. This comparison is usually made by the medical chairperson of the department. He or she then recommends to the credentials committee the privileges that shall be granted; those privileges are then granted by the committee and follow the same line as the applicant's general application up through the medical board and the board of trustees. Individual privileges may be restricted without affecting the medical staff membership.

In the specific area of emergency medicine, the delineation of privileges is perhaps simpler than in some other specialties. In general, anyone capable of practicing general emergency medicine must have privileges for almost all procedures performed within the emergency department. However, in larger departments that have a division of care, such as in a major trauma or medicine unit, an observation unit, or a fast track, it is possible to have privileges to practice in only one area of the emergency department (Appendix A).

In summary, obtaining privileges is a completely different process than obtaining hospital membership. It is necessary for the hospital bylaws to treat membership and privileges separately. They can be taken together, but most often they need to be looked at as separate components. This is particularly true if there are questions about one's individual privileges. If questions arise about certain privileges or staff membership, an area within the bylaws of every hospital and medical staff should pertain to investigations, hearings, and appeals. These areas of the bylaws must meet all standards of applicable state and federal law to protect the individuals who must sit on these committees to hear the investigations or appeals. The policies should include when a hearing may be requested, a step-by-step procedure pending a favorable or unfavorable recommendation, a statement of grounds and reasons, the notice of hearing, the place of hearing, who shall attend the hearing, whether attorneys may be attending, the discovery process, whether witnesses are allowed, the burden of proof, the admission of certain evidence, and appeals. All of this must be set out carefully in the hospital's bylaws or regulations attending these bylaws. A physician may have one or more privileges denied or taken away without affecting that physician's staff membership. It is important, therefore, for the physician applicant to maintain this separate identity (i.e., that staff membership does not equate to complete and universal privilege). Membership gives the applicant the right to request certain privileges; the granting of those privileges is a separate action.

In the general area of credentialing and privileging, certain questions arise with regard to special and separate issues. The next section describes some of these special issues in the area of physician credentialing.

SPECIAL ISSUES

National Practitioner Data Bank

The Health Care Quality Improvement Act of 1986 was passed by Congress in October and signed by President Reagan on November 14, 1986. The critical underlying assumption of that law is that malpractice is increasing and that professional review can remedy the problem. Another less critical underlying assumption is that physicians are more likely to be candid and aggressive in the performance of peer review if the threat of antitrust exposure is removed. The act provides two different immunities. One is for individuals who provide information to healthcare entities such as a hospital. The other is for individuals and entities who take professional review action against a physician. The act states that any person who provides information to a professional review body about the competence or professional conduct of a physician shall be immune from liability and damages under any federal or state law, unless the information provided is false and the person providing it knew it was false.

For individuals who participate in professional review, it spells out that these persons are protected from damage suits as long as the professional review was taken (1) in a reasonable belief that the action was in the furtherance of quality healthcare, (2) after a reasonable effort to obtain the facts of the matter, (3) after adequate notice and hearing procedures are forwarded to the physician involved, and (4) in the reasonable belief that the action was warranted by the facts known. As long as these standards are met, the healthcare entities and those persons involved in its professional review activities will be immune from damage. This immunity does not apply to actions brought under the federal Civil Rights Law, injunction or declaratory judgment actions, actions by governmental agencies such as the Federal Trade Commission, or criminal proceedings. The immunity also does not apply to actions brought by nonphysician practitioners such as podiatrists and chiropractors. Immunity also could be lost if the action was based on improper motive, such as actions based on the patient's affiliation with any professional organization, fee structure, advertising or business solicitation methods, or affiliation with any health maintenance organization (HMO).

The Health Care Quality Improvement Act of 1986 also mandated the establishment of what is called the National Practitioner Data Bank for Adverse Information on Physicians and Other Health Care Practitioners. The purpose of the databank is to serve as a central repository for information related to the professional competence or conduct of physicians, dentists, and other healthcare practitioners, specifically, information about malpractice payments, adverse licensure actions, and adverse actions pertaining to clinical privileges. The Health Resources and Services Administration, a division of the Department of Health and Human Services, is responsible for the databank's implementation. The databank contains reports about actions taken against malpractice payments, disciplinary actions taken against physicians by hospitals or medical societies, and actions taken against physicians' licenses by state medical licensing boards. A hospital is required to query the databank of all physicians at least every 2 years, and all physician applicants for new medical staff appointment.

Certain actions do not have to be reported. The actions that do not adversely affect a physician's clinical privileges such as censure, reprimand, or admonishments do not have to be reported. Actions that are not based on a physician's professional competence or behavior do not have to be reported. For example, if a physician is denied appointment to the medical staff of a hospital because the hospital followed a properly prepared medical staff plan, that denial would not be reported. Withdrawal of an application for appointment or request for clinical privilege before the hospital board taking final action on the application or request does not have to be reported. Administrative suspensions of clinical privileges, for example, suspensions of failure to complete medical records, are not reportable. Voluntary relinquishment of privileges do not have to be reported unless that physician was under investigation for professional competence at the time of the relinquishment.

Access to the information in the databank is limited to hospitals, other healthcare entities, and state medical and dental licensing boards. Plaintiff attorneys, if they can prove that the hospital did not correctly access the databank, can also obtain this information. In addition, individual physicians and dentists can query the databank about themselves only. Failure to report a medical malpractice payment is punishable by a fine up to $10,000 for each violation. Failure of a medical board to do as it is stated could result in the loss of that board's powers. Failure of a hospital or other healthcare entity to comply with the reporting comments may result in the loss of immunity protection or pardon of the act for 3 years.

Change in the Delineation of Privileges

As has been clearly stated, a physician may voluntarily relinquish certain privileges at a hospital at any time without any fear of sanction. In general, medical staff membership and delineation of privileges are reviewed on a periodic basis, often every 2 years. This period may vary from state to state and hospital to hospital. It is perfectly reasonable at this time to change the privilege sheet, either to ask for new privileges or to relinquish old ones. In fact, if a physician no longer practices a certain procedure, it is probably advisable to relinquish that privilege. It is also possible for a hospital to sanction a physician by taking away certain privileges, which would be reportable to the databank. However, the physician may retain medical staff membership and other privileges.

The processes of privileging, delineation of privileging, and reappointment of privileges must be clearly stated and spelled out in the bylaws of the medical staff, along with the procedures for changing such delineation or procedures for taking away such privileges from a physician. In addition, the physician's rights with regard to hearings and appeal must also be clearly stated in the bylaws.

Recredentialing and Quality Assurance

Periodically all physicians are recredentialed. Not only is their medical staff membership looked at, but also, more acutely, each physician's privileges are scrutinized. This procedure is usually started at an anniversary date or at a periodic date set up by the hospital or state. At this time a physician is generally sent a reapplication form or, more precisely, a reappointment form. The reappointment form is similar to the original application form. Along with the demographic data, personal data, and information about licensure, the form asks for the narcotic registration number and any liability problems incurred in the preceding 2 years. In addition, the form may ask questions about the appointment requested, clinical privileges requested, health status, and continuing education. The reappointment application generally goes through the same committee process as the original application, with one significant change.

At the credentials committee level, the application is then mated with whatever quality assurance information there is about the physician and his or her practices in that hospital with recommendations from the department chair. The committee can provide several different answers to the request for reappointment. One is to have a favorable recommendation with no change. The other is to have a favorable recommendation with certain changes as delineated on the privilege list. There is also the possibility of unfavorable recommendation or a conditional reappointment. A recommendation can be made to reappoint a physician with certain conditions, for example, that the physician ceases to engage in certain types of disruptive behavior or agrees to take specific continuing medical education requirements. Time limits may be set on continuing medical education, and this limit is usually reappraised before the normal reapplication limit.

The quality assurance data reviewed are fairly comprehensive. In addition to normal adverse occurrence, there are requests for performance data. It is now possible to track such clinically significant parameters as frequency of procedures, length of stay, diagnostic-related group (DRG) data, severity trends, morbidity and mortality data, nosocomial infection rates, medical record timeliness, clinical pertinence, patient survey data, unplanned readmission rates, ancillary diagnostic testing, and laboratory service utilization data.

All of this information becomes part of the decision-making process of the credentials committee. These processes are no longer in the "rubber stamp" mode, but rather detailed, careful delineation on every member coming before the committee.

SUMMARY

This chapter delineated the application process and the credentialing and privilege granting processes and described several special issues with regard to credentialing. As has been stated repeatedly, all the policies concerning these elements of staff membership and privileges must be carefully delineated in the bylaws of the medical staff or in the regulations attached to such bylaws. These instruments are readily available to all physicians, and all applicants should read and understand thoroughly all bylaws and regulations of the hospital or health entity to which they are applying.

In the last 25 years the credentialing process has become more arduous, more systematic, and certainly more complete. An unsettling as this transition to greater accountability has been to date, it appears likely that a hospital medical staff that is able to adopt and maintain a proper type of credentialing process will be well positioned both against substandard medical practice from within and medical and legal scrutiny from without. It is arduous, time consuming, and necessary.

APPENDIX

A Delineation of Privileges Form

Department of Emergency Medicine

Physician's Name ______________________________

Check	Privileges	Education	Experience	References
		APPOINTMENT:	**REAPPOINTMENT:**	
_____	Diagnosis, management, and consultation for clinical conditions ordinarily classified as presumed or actual disease involving the specialty of emergency medicine (Emergency Medicine Core Content—American College of Emergency Physicians). In the case of a critical emergency, any physician shall be permitted to take action to save a life or prevent serious harm, regardless of delineated privileges.	__ Type I: Equivalency of an ACGME-approved residency in emergency medicine and emergency medicine board certification. OR __ Type II: Completion of an ACGME-approved residency in emergency medicine. It is expected that emergency medicine physicians on the BUMC staff will become board certified and will maintain that certification, OR	Sufficient number of cases to demonstrate current clinical competence	Emergency medicine board certification Letter from residency program training director documenting satisfactory completion of residency.
		__ Type III: a. Completion of approved ACGME residency in internal medicine, family practice, general surgery, pediatrics or obstetrics and gynecology. b. It is expected that emergency medicine physicians on the BUMC staff will become board certified and will maintain that certification. OR __ Type IV (double coverage): Emergency medicine, general surgery, or internal medicine residency of at least 1 year.		Letter from residency program training director documenting satisfactory completion of residency AND documentation of previous experience and satisfactory performance. Letter from director of department documenting duration of time in program and satisfactory performance and documentation of previous experience and satisfactory performance.

Check	Privileges	APPOINTMENT: Type I	Type II	Type III	Type IV	REAPPOINTMENT:	References
	Cardiac Pacing					Sufficient number of cases to demonstrate current clinical competence.	Letter from director of training program documenting satisfactory completion of residency or letter from director or previous experience documenting satisfactory performance.
_____	External	X	X	X			
_____	Internal	X	X	X			
_____	Transcutaneous	X	X	X			
_____	Cardioversion/defibrillation	X	X	X			
_____	Cardiopulmonary resuscitation	X	X	X			
_____	Intracardiac injection	X	X	X			

ACGME, Accreditation Committee on Graduate Medical Education; *BUMC*, Baylor University Medical Center; *IVP*, intravenous pyelography.

Physician's Name ____________________

Check	Privileges	Education				Experience	References
	Diagnostic Procedures						
____	Anoscopy	X	X	X			
____	Arthrocentesis	X	X	X			
____	Cystogram	X	X	X			
____	IVP Contrast	X	X	X			
____	Lumbar puncture	X	X	X	X		
		APPOINTMENT:				**REAPPOINTMENT:**	
	Airway Techniques	Type I	Type II	Type III	Type IV	Sufficient number of cases to demonstrate current clinical competence.	Letter from the director of training program documenting satisfactory completion of residency or letter from director or previous experience documenting satisfactory performance.
____	Cricothyrotomy	X	X	X			
____	Intubation	X	X	X			
____	Oral	X	X	X			
____	Nasal	X	X	X			
____	Mechanical ventilation	X	X	X			
____	Neuromuscular blockade	X	X	X			
	Anesthesia						
____	Local anesthesia	X	X	X	X		
	Regional Nerve Blocks						
____	Peripheral	X	X	X			
____	Orofacial	X	X	X			
	Cardiac Procedures						
	Cardiac Massage						
____	Closed	X	X	X	X		
____	Open	X	X	X			
		APPOINTMENT:				**REAPPOINTMENT:**	
	Thoracic Procedures	Type I	Type II	Type III	Type IV	Sufficient number of cases to demonstrate current clinical competence.	Letter from director of training program documenting satisfactory completion of residency or letter from director or previous experience documenting satisfactory performance.
____	Needle thoracostomy	X	X	X			
____	Tube thoracostomy	X	X	X			
____	Emergency thoracotomy	X	X	X			
____	Cardiorrhaphy	X	X	X			
	Other Techniques						
____	Foreign body removal	X	X	X	X		
____	Gastric lavage	X	X	X	X		
____	Incision drainage	X	X	X	X		
____	Perimortem skull trephination (burrhole)	X	X	X			
____	Wound repair	X	X	X	X		
		APPOINTMENT:				**REAPPOINTMENT:**	
	Arterial	Type I	Type II	Type III	Type IV	Sufficient number of cases to demonstrate current clinical competence.	Letter from director of training program documenting satisfactory completion of residency or letter from director or previous experience documenting satisfactory performance.
____	Arterial cannulation	X	X	X			
____	Arterial blood gases	X	X	X			
	Orthopedic Procedures						
	Fracture or Dislocation						
____	Immobilization	X	X	X	X		
____	Closed reduction	X	X	X			
____	Spine	X	X	X			
____	Cervical immobilization	X	X	X			
____	Cervical traction technique	X	X	X			
____	Trephination nail	X	X	X	X		
____	Injection of bursa or joint	X	X	X			
		APPOINTMENT:				**REAPPOINTMENT:**	
		Type I	Type II	Type III	Type IV	Sufficient number of cases to demonstrate current clinical competence.	Letter from director of training program documenting satisfactory completion of residency or letter from director or previous experience documenting satisfactory performance.
____	Suprapubic catheterization	X	X	X			
	Delivery of Newborn						
____	Precipitous delivery	X	X	X			
____	Culdocentesis	X	X	X			
	Head or Neck						
____	Epistaxis control	X	X	X	X		

Physician's Name ____________________

Check	Privileges	Education				Experience	References
____	Laryngoscopy	X	X	X			
	Hemodynamic Monitoring						
	Central Venous Access						
____	Subclavian	X	X	X			
____	Jugular	X	X	X			
____	Peripheral venisection	X	X	X			
____	Interosseous	X	X	X			
		APPOINTMENT:				REAPPOINTMENT:	
		Type I	Type II	Type III	Type IV	Sufficient number of cases to demonstrate current clinical competence.	Letter from director of training program documenting satisfactory completion of residency or letter from director or previous experience documenting satisfactory performance.
____	Paracentesis	X	X	X			
____	Nasogastric tube intubation	X	X	X	X		
____	Pericardiocentesis	X	X	X			
____	Peritoneal lavage	X	X	X			
____	Proctosigmoidoscopy	X	X	X			
____	Slit lamp examination	X	X	X	X		
____	Thoracentesis	X	X	X			
____	Tonometry	X	X	X	X		
	Genitourinary Techniques						
	Bladder Catheterization						
____	Filiform catheters	X	X	X			
____	Foley catheters	X	X	X	X		

____________________ ____________________

Physician's Signature Date Credentials Committee Signature Date

____________________ ____________________

Chief of Service Signature Date Board of Trustees Signature Date

77 Credentialing

John D. Dunn

OUTLINE

A major management focus for the 1980s and beyond is the question of competence of emergency department staff. Credentialing responsibilities lie ultimately with the board of trustees or the board of directors of the hospital, but the medical staff and the hospital management staff are delegated the responsibility of ensuring the competence and the qualifications of medical staff members and hospital staff professionals and nonprofessionals. This chapter outlines the issues and recommended methods for complying with management responsibilities to guarantee competence and the qualifications of professional and nonprofessional staff. The focus is the emergency department, but the principles are general.

LEGAL AND REGULATORY FACTORS

Parties responsible for the management of a hospital and its various departments ensure the competence and the qualifications of the personnel providing services in that institution. If a hospital has a responsibility to the public it serves, it is logical to assume that those managers of the institution are responsible for the acts of the employees of that institution.

The legal concept of *respondeat superior* is a tradition in the common law that loosely translated means that the master should respond to and be responsible for the acts of the servant. *Servant* generically in modern society means employees or agents. *Agents* in the legal meaning of the term are people who are engaged by the principal to act on behalf of that principal or for the benefit of that principal.

When servants are negligent, the master (in modern terms, the employer) will be legally liable for those acts of negligence. The legal rules are fairly clear in the case of employers and their employees. Problems develop in the area of agency. In many circumstances, professionals, contractors, vendors, and other providers of service act independently, and an institution or individual has no control over how they perform their duties. The courts look at the control exercised by the employer or the principal, whether the activities the engagement is designed for are routinely the responsibility of the institution, and what a reasonable customer should anticipate and expect.

In the hospital setting and in the emergency department, the law clearly creates responsibilities for an institution and its management.[1] Those responsibilities are measured in terms of what the usual business of the institution is, the charter of its corporation, and the expectations of the public. In the case of a hospital, the law has evolved to some degree. There is no debate about the responsibility of the institution for the competence and the acts of its employees. That creates two forms of potential liability for the institution. One would be a failure to properly credential and qualify, as well as train and orient the employees. The other liability transfers to the institution if those employees are negligent either by acts or omissions.

In the case of professional staff who are employees, even if they are physicians and nurses, the employee relationship imputes automatic liability for the institution. The liability questions develop in the area of professionals with unlimited licenses, such as physicians acting as contractors or even just as members of the medical staff.

HOSPITAL AND INSTITUTIONAL RESPONSIBILITY FOR MEDICAL STAFF MEMBERS

The seminal case in this area is *Darling v Charleston Community Hospital*,[2] which declared the hospital liable for failure to properly credential a physician in the area of orthopedic care. Allowing that physician to perform orthopedic care within the institutional setting created the expectation on the part of the public that the individual was qualified, generating responsibilities for the institution to guarantee that qualification.

A line of cases since *Darling v Charleston Community Hospital* has created liability for the institution in a failure to recredential or properly monitor medical staff members such as the notorious Dr. Nork in California.[3] The courts have commented in favor of creating liability for medical staff for failure to carry out their responsibilities as the delegated quality assurance and peer review agents of the hospital.[4] Therefore hospitals and their delegated agents in peer review, the medical staff, can be held liable for improper credentialing and improper peer review as they relate not only to members of the medical staff who are employees, but also to members of the medical staff who are considered independent.

APPARENT AGENCY

A more difficult area is the question of apparent agency as it relates to emergency physicians who are independent contractors. One interpretation emphasizes the fact that, as licensed professionals, physicians control the manner of provision of their professional services. This view emphasizes that hospitals do not tell physicians how to practice medicine, argues against any legal agency relationship, and creates separate and independent liability for a physician who is negligent. The only way a hospital could participate in the liability of an independent contractor physician would be voluntarily if it indemnified that physician or because of separate and independent liability for failure to properly credential that physician or monitor that physician's work. The hospital would still have responsibility for its employees involved in the care of the patient if those employees acted below the accepted standard of care.

An opposing interpretation is the plaintiff's bar, which argues that the patient who comes to the emergency department and is offered the emergency physician without any reasonable choice is in fact dealing with an institution that has an apparent agent, that is, the emergency physician. The innocent patient has reasonable expectations that the institution not only is ensuring the competence of the emergency physician but also is taking care of those responsibilities by providing an emergency physician who, therefore, becomes the agent of that institution. Many states have adopted this principle.[5] In some cases they have adopted it despite a state law that prohibits nonlicensed persons from controlling the acts of professionals.[6]

It would appear that the courts are weighing more heavily the responsibilities to the public than any technical interpretation of liability related to independent practicing professionals such as emergency physicians. The same tension exists with regard to hospital-based physicians in other specialties such as pathology, anesthesiology, or radiology, as well as emergency physicians. Credentialing responsibilities flow from all these legal principles—corporate liability for credentialing, agency, and apparent agency.

Separate from common law legal precedent, the hospital licensure law in all of the states, Conditions of Participation with Medicare,[7] which is a contract between the federal government and all hospitals that have a Medicare contract, as well as standards of accreditation from voluntary organizations such as the American Osteopathic Hospital Association and the Joint Commission on Accreditation of Healthcare Organizations (JCAHO) create formalized requirements in the area of credentialing, peer review, and recredentialing. Although one could view recredentialing as a separate area of responsibility, the same principles guide credentialing and recredentialing of medical staff and nonphysician staff of the hospital. Peer review in the hospital setting for nonphysician and physician staff involves an ongoing assessment of competence and will, necessarily, be a component of the recredentialing process. Recredentialing requires reassessment and evaluation of an individual's continuing competence, and peer review provides a basis for that evaluation if adequate measures of performance are in place.

CREDENTIALING OF NONPHYSICIAN PERSONNEL

Hospital management has a clear responsibility to ensure the qualifications and continued competence of employees; however, the responsibilities of physician medical directors are not so clear. JCAHO standards of accreditation require that physician directors be responsible for oversight in the area of personnel competence.[8] This requirement is in direct conflict with the fact that one cannot be responsible for that which one cannot control. Advisory positions for emergency department physician directors are classic examples of "neither fish nor fowl." The hospital relies on medical directors to provide physician supervision of hospital personnel; however, because physician directors usually do not have hiring, firing, or supervisory authority, they sometimes may have bark but no bite.

As a part of the "Agènda for Change," JCAHO standards of accreditation and JCAHO literature emphasize the importance of medical directors within the hospital environment.[8] This view is a mixed blessing for physicians who are offered the opportunity and challenge to reinsert physician influence into the hospital management structure. There is no doubt that meeting JCAHO standards of quality and accreditation requires an increased effort by physician medical directors of the various departments of the hospital. The product of the JCAHO emphasis is higher expectations, which frequently conflict with long-standing custom not to interfere with hospital operations and resistance from hospital staff to medical staff involvement in hospital operations and hospital personnel questions.

JCAHO standards on medical staff credentialing, hospital staff credentialing, continuing education for hospital staff, and proof of continued competence for medical staff are described briefly in this chapter.

PHYSICIAN CREDENTIALING

The Initial Application

Hospitals have the right, supported by the courts of this country, to set minimum criteria for membership on the medical staff.[9] Those minimum criteria are defined in terms of the following:

- Health
- Professional education and training
- Performance
- Professional liability insurance

Mental and physical capabilities of a member of the physician staff must be examined to ensure that a physician can perform up to the hospital's required standards. The hospital has the responsibility to reasonably define those parameters for the applicant. The Americans with Disabilities Act (ADA)[10] potentially can create some problems because it expands the requirement of employers to not restrict opportunities for employment based on medical conditions. The prudent manager must consider the application of a disabled physician in light of developing law. Only when a disability impairs necessary performance in a way that justifies rejection of the application should the health of the applicant be a factor in the application and recredentialing process. In other words the mental or physical health of applicants for medical staff privileges can become a reasonable issue if performance is or has been affected in such a way as to limit the competence or ability of the applicant.

In the case of the emergency department performance, minimal physical and mental health expectations cannot be ignored. An interesting question, given the hospital nature of emergency physician activity, would be whether the hospital has been required to modify its facilities or equipment to allow a disabled physician to perform as an emergency physician. Another consideration is whether a too burdensome change in facilities or equipment would prevent successful legal action by a disabled applicant. The balance of reasonable accommodation with reasonable public expectations of the capabilities of practitioners leaves the medical staff and the managers with a responsibility to define requirements and to act on those reasonable definitions. If the medical staff acts reasonably to protect the public expectation, its action to deny privileges would be defensible. The priorities are patient safety first, fairness and accommodation second.

EDUCATION AND TRAINING

A hospital can require minimum criteria such as board certification, residency training, or minimal levels of experience for emergency physicians. Short of that, because of the limited supply of emergency physicians, the hospital can reasonably require training and experience arbitrarily set out to balance expectations of expertise against the available supply of physicians for emergency department work.

The American College of Emergency Physicians (ACEP) has taken a position antagonistic to the idea of what is called *merit badge medicine*. Whenever a board certified emergency physician is also required to obtain short course certifications in areas such as pediatric advanced life support, advanced cardiac life support, or advanced trauma life support, the college position is that this training duplicates that expertise already earned through board certification in emergency medicine and would be similar to asking a general surgeon to take advanced trauma life support when the basic training covers the subject matter and curriculum of advanced trauma life support. Therefore ACEP and the American Board of Emergency Medicine are opposed to the use of short courses of training in emergency care as a requirement when someone already establishes expertise through board certification in emergency medicinc.[11] This issue will continue to be argued because many hospital contract groups require merit badges of expertise suggested in negotiations with their hospital clients.

PERFORMANCE

Measures of performance are certainly important in the recredentialing of an individual who is already a member of the medical staff, but they are also a reasonable portion of the initial application and initial credentialing evaluation of a new member of the medical staff. This two-step process involves a review and inquiry into past performance and an ongoing performance evaluation of the new member of the medical staff, who is usually placed on provisional or probationary status for a year or more before advancement to permanent privileges.

The emergency department physician director who ignores past performance does so at his or her own peril. It is not always easy, however, to obtain information about the real performance of a physician at previous locations. Standard reference letters and inquiries into status with the various state medical boards, certification, good standing with medical societies, and successful completion of formal training programs such as residencies are a part of the reasonable effort to evaluate the new applicant for medical staff privileges. The National Practitioner Data Bank and the state medical boards supervising practice in the states in which an individual has practiced and has been licensed before are also required resources in the background search for a new applicant. Extensive questionnaires on experience and exposure to clinical problems and procedures are used successfully by hospitals in the initial application.

Given the litigious nature of this society and the importance of professional reputation, many times previous medical staff and hospital performance is not easily discerned on the formal reference letter inquiry made by the medical staff reviewing an initial application. The best approach is to make some telephone calls and obtain some informal and more revealing information that might guide the credentialing process toward a more accurate assessment of the applicant. The usual response on the other end of the phone is "You're not going to quote me on this are you?" which leaves the medical staff in a quandary if they reject an individual's application. It is important to remember, however, that it is better to know than to not know. To reject an application, a careful investigation of the background of the individual is required. Also acceptance of an application, particularly for a hospital-based emergency physician, is much more discretionary for the medical staff and allows a stricter standard. To reject an independent practitioner in a nonhospital-based specialty, the medical staff must take a more elaborate and difficult approach, whereas because of the exclusive nature of an emergency department contract, an applicant for emergency department work can be almost arbitrarily rejected because emergency department contracts allow the hospital extraordinary control over acceptance of an application.

During the provisional or probationary status of a new member of the medical staff, the credentialing process continues. The emergency physician director must be conscious of the ongoing responsibility to evaluate incidents, untoward events, patient complaints, outcomes, and other parameters of performance.

INSURANCE

The hospital has the right to demand adequate liability insurance, by contract from the emergency physician and otherwise for any member of its medical staff.[12] Institutional financial integrity is the fiduciary duty of the board of directors or board of trustees, and the authority to require insurance comes from that fiduciary duty to ensure that the hospital is financially secure. Therefore the usual process of application requires that the emergency physician show adequate insurance coverage. Many hospitals have defined the amount of required insurance coverage, particularly for emergency physicians. Rarely, does a hospital not have a specific amount of malpractice included in the contract with the emergency group or with an individual emergency physician if the contract is between the hospital and the individual because, in most states, vicarious liability theories hold the hospital responsible for emergency physician malpractice.[13]

An interesting question arises in the area of insurance. If the contract is silent on the question of purchase of tail insurance, is the contract fatally flawed? It would be reasonable to require proof of insurance and a contractual requirement that emergency physicians buy tail insurance or some other insurance product that will provide for complete coverage for the period of the contract. See Chapter 57 for a more detailed explanation of tail coverage and some of the other emergency department malpractice insurance coverage issues.

NATIONAL PRACTITIONER DATA BANK

The National Practitioner Data Bank was created by Congress in the Health Care Quality Improvement Act of 1986.[14] This data bank was intended to be a repository for information on disciplinary and malpractice actions adverse to any practicing physician or dentist. Three enforcement tools are used to encourage hospitals and insurance companies to use the National Practitioner Data Bank and report disciplinary and malpractice events:

- Fines are assessed against any insurance company that fails to report a malpractice settlement or judgment.
- If a healthcare entity fails to make an inquiry with the National Data Bank at the time of credentialing or recredentialing, a plaintiff's attorney is given the legal right to include all data bank information as information that should have been known by the healthcare entity in its credentialing of the individual.
- Failure to report a disciplinary action voids the civil protections of this law. The Federation of State Medical Boards keeps information on malpractice suits and disciplinary actions in a separate data bank, which duplicates the information in the National Practitioner Data Bank, so that there are two potential sources of comprehensive information on an applicant for medical staff privileges.

The National Practitioner Data Bank includes information on malpractice judgments and settlements and a summary of the case. In addition, the data bank includes disciplinary actions that reduced clinical privileges for more than 30 days on the basis of competence or performance. Insurance companies are obligated to report any settlement or judgment along with a summary. The narrative of the summary is generated by the insurance company, but the physician defendant can affect the language of that summary before its submission to the National Practitioner Data Bank.

In addition, a physician can request the entry of an opposing point of view narrative if it is submitted in a timely manner (30 days) after a discretionary action is reported by a healthcare entity or society. After that the entry will include the physician's response to the original narrative as a part of the data bank record.

Hospitals are required to inquire with the National Practitioner Data Bank at the time of recredentialing. Fees have been increased to $10 per inquiry, and the National Practitioner Data Bank supplies a computer program for computer inquiries to facilitate inquiries from the hospital. Currently the American Medical Association wants to terminate the National Practitioner Data Bank, whereas Congress is interested in an expanded access to information that allows public inquiry. The National Practitioner Data Bank can respond only to inquiries by healthcare entities with legitimate credentialing responsibilities. It is difficult to determine how the National Practitioner Data Bank ensures itself of the legitimacy of an inquiry, given the tens of thousands of inquiries that they deal with from all sorts of healthcare entities. However, an inquiry by fraud is also subject to a fine.

EMERGENCY DEPARTMENT GROUP CREDENTIALING

Although it may seem a duplication of effort, emergency department groups actually do qualify as healthcare entities if they function as a formalized group with internal peer review. Therefore evaluation of the initial applicant, ongoing peer review, National Practitioner Data Bank inquiries, and recredentialing would be a part of reasonable medical group management practice. The qualifications of a contract physician for a group physician are the responsibility of those who use those physicians as agents or employees. Therefore most medical groups have developed internal credentialing programs that parallel the activities of hospitals, and contract groups would qualify as healthcare entities for the purpose of the National Practitioner Data Bank and this discussion.

PERFORMANCE EVALUATION

A necessary component of any peer review and credentialing process is a mechanism for disciplinary action, modification of behavior, and termination. As mentioned previously, emergency services contracts are unique, and the relationship of an emergency physician is affected by the exclusive nature of the contract. This creates two potential differences that are important to recognize. First the contract may provide for unilateral decisions by the hospital to remove a physician without disciplinary action. Second, the hospital may retain the authority to terminate privileges in emergency medicine for members of a contract group if the contract is terminated.

Terminations or removals may be without cause and are a mixed blessing. If the hospital can unilaterally request that a physician not be assigned shifts, formal disciplinary action can be avoided and the event not reported to the Board of Medical Examiners of that state or the National Practitioner Data Bank. If a termination of privileges occurs as the result of the termination of a contract and the result of that termination on the individual members of the group, that also is not a reportable event.

RECREDENTIALING PHYSICIANS

The recredentialing of physicians on a regular basis should verify continued health, competence, and insurance. Just as the initial credentialing process allows for a tremendous amount of flexibility within the hospital environment, so the recredentialing process must be realistic, oriented toward quality of care, and evenhanded. Hospitals, medical staffs, and supervising physicians are allowed a tremendous amount of flexibility in their judgment as to proof of continued competence and ability, but they are required to demonstrate attention to these parameters, consistency, and prudence. The legal standard applies to all liability situations: What would the reasonable person with the same responsibilities do? For example, the physician supervisor of emergency services should guarantee at the time of recredentialing that the subject physician delineate the following:

- Continued health adequate to the responsibilities of the position and the credentials requested
- Professional liability insurance coverage
- Continuing medical education or performance proof of continued competence in the privileges requested

Chapter 51 discuss internal quality assurance and peer review programs, which should be designed to evaluate performance of physicians during any credentialing period. Credentialing is usually performed annually or biannually, with most JCAHO-accredited hospitals going to biannual review of credentials. Specific procedures and areas of care for privileges should be specified in some detail. In the emergency care area all patients in all conditions must be addressed to ensure initial evaluation, identification of emergency conditions, and proper stabilization. In some hospitals, however, some procedures that would be the responsibility of emergency physicians, would be performed more properly at other hospitals by specialists and members of the medical staff with credentials for those procedures and those areas of care. Documentation of activity and evaluation of outcomes are the main competence components that should be reviewed.

An excellent example of evolving credentials changes for emergency physicians is the management of acute myocardial infarction, which requires timely thrombolytic intervention. The practice in the United States for timely thrombolytic treatment for acute myocardial infarction once the diagnosis is made argues against delays based on inappropriate requirements for credentials in thrombolytic therapy. These turf disputes are to a great extent proportionate to the expertise required, and consistency is essential. For example, if a delay in thrombolytic therapy occurred because of inappropriate reservation of credentials on the basis of turf battles, the hospital and those involved in the credentialing process might be subject to criticism and proportionate liability.

Turf disputes about trauma care, the care of critically ill patients of different age groups, or other situations in which emergency physician action necessarily invades the province of other specialties must be resolved in the credentialing process. This approach avoids exposing emergency physicians to criticism about doing too much, and at the same time ensures timely patient care.

The recredentialing process is an excellent vehicle for defining areas of responsibility and redefining those areas where practice and custom change. It is important for the director of emergency services to keep abreast of trends in emergency care so that the credentialing process reflects current practice and complies with recommended standards of emergency care. For example, most invasive procedures involve some inherent risk and, if specialists on the medical staff are available to perform invasive procedures in a timely basis, the emergency department may sometimes limit invasive procedures to those that are strictly defined as emergency and immediately necessary. A balance must be established on standards of care in procedures such as insertion of a temporary pacemaker, performance of emergency thoracotomy, and even the insertion of central lines. If medical staff response time is good and the definitive care is to be provided by another member of the medical staff, emergency physicians would be wise to coordinate triage, stabilization, and appropriate specialist care. Ill-defined procedural or medical care privileges could easily result in finger pointing in the case of an untoward outcome. Privileges should be well defined so that the medical staff cannot subsequently criticize emergency physicians for performing a procedure or managing cases beyond their delineated privileges.

DISCIPLINARY ACTIVITIES

The Health Care Quality Improvement Act[15] sets out an example of appropriate criteria for due process whenever a physician is subjected to disciplinary action. If a physician's permanent privileges or credentials are to be curtailed or terminated, he or she should be provided due process.

Due process in the United States is well defined as it relates to terminating or removing a person's rights or privileges. The right to practice medicine is considered to be a property right, and therefore termination of privileges must comply with these general principles of due process, which include substantive due process and procedural due process.

Substantive due process means that the substance of the activities are in compliance with fairness and impartiality. The standard is that the decisions must be made after thorough and complete investigation of the facts and disputes, and there must be no appearance of arbitrariness, capriciousness, or bias in the activities or decisions that are a product of those activities. Judicial review is available for these disciplinary actions, but only to a review of the record and whether the record shows no partiality, bias, or arbitrariness.

Procedural due process is a more technical part of the due process and involves the following components:

- Adequate notice and opportunity to respond to the notice of disciplinary action proposed
- A reasonable opportunity for review of all of the facts that are the basis for the proposed discipline
- Opportunity for a hearing with examination of facts and witnesses before an impartial officer or panel
- An opportunity to review a decision and the basis for that decision
- A procedure for interval appeal before a final disciplinary action is taken

The Health Care Quality Improvement Act also requires that a physician subjected to disciplinary action have the choice with regard to whether he or she wants to engage a lawyer or counsel such as physician counsel. It is difficult to defend oneself objectively and thoroughly when one is subjected to disciplinary action. If the hospital or medical staff is serious about a disciplinary action, it is wise to have a lawyer present for both sides to ensure proper conduct of the hearing.

Adequate notice under the Health Care Quality Improvement Act includes at least 30 days notice before the time of the hearing and enough information about the basis for a proposed disciplinary action to provide the subject physician an adequate opportunity to prepare a defense. Specification of the incidence, patient records, and the types of competence questions that will be raised in the disciplinary hearing are examples of information that should be made available.

CONDUCT OF THE DISCIPLINARY HEARING

A disciplinary hearing can be informal and still comply with due process requirements. The decision maker can be a panel of physicians or an arbitrator who is either a physician or a nonphysician. Or decisions can be made with a nonphysician or physician arbitrator making rulings on procedure and the decision-making power held by a panel or an individual. Many options are available. As long as the hospital avoids the appearance of unfairness, bias, or arbitrariness and as long as the decision is well founded and the rationale well articulated, the courts will defer to the decision.

Competitors of the subject physician create special problems. Competitors appearing as witnesses against the physician should be identified as such and should be weighed as potentially biased against the subject physician by those responsible for the decision making. Competitors should definitely not be a part of the decision-making panel or should not act as single decision makers on the question of disciplinary action. A gray zone is created by physicians who are not in a direct competition relationship with the subject physician but who might be consultants with, partners of, or close associates of any kind with potential competitors. The end result is that it is difficult, even on large medical staffs, to avoid the appearances of bias. Outside experts and hearing panels or officers may be a better choice.

The expertise of the panel or individual may or may not be appropriate to the medical issues involved, provided that the decision-making panel is offered adequate medical expertise and documentation on standards of care. A suggestion to the hospital or medical staff attempting this approach, to avoid having an outside panel hired, is an opportunity to review the outside expert witnesses' opinions at the hearing. One of the principles to be remembered in current legal thought is that surprises must be avoided and fairness of the hearing must be evident. Judicial review of these decisions is available to the subject physician and will be a review of the record on the due process issues recited here.

Reportable disciplinary actions are those that reduce the clinical privileges of a physician for more than 30 days on the basis of competence or performance.

Key concepts included in the language of the Health Care Quality Improvement Act that will help to protect the disciplinary body include a reasonable review of the facts,[16] an action taken "in the furtherance of quality patient care,"[17] and due process.

SUMMARY

Consumer and patient rights advocate groups argue that a significant percentage of physicians are incompetent or impaired in one way or another. They frequently use statistics in a casual way, based on studies of impairment in a general population. For example, it is not surprising to hear Dr. Sydney Wolfe of Public Citizen say that 10% of physicians are impaired. Whether there is a statistical basis for such projections is arguable. A suggestion that 10% of physicians are impaired presumes that a high-performance, high-achievement group is subject to the same level of impairment as the general population, which is a questionable thesis at best. Nonetheless, a certain level of competence and performance is expected of professionals, and professionals committed to providing quality healthcare services must continually monitor their abilities and competencies. The credentialing and recredentialing processes are the obvious foundation for maintaining professionalism, standards of excellence, and acceptable quality of care for patients. Responsibility for adequate credentialing and recredentialing lies in the hands of management physicians of all sorts across the spectrum of healthcare. Emergency department directors, regional directors for multicontract groups, and officers for medical groups and quality assurance and risk management directors for medical groups and hospitals are some examples of individuals responsible for adequate credentialing and recredentialing. Quality assurance is a toothless activity if it is not founded on good credentialing and recredentialing criteria, with its enforcement arm being the potential for termination or reduction of privileges.

REFERENCES

1. *Brownsville Medical Center v Gracia,* 704 S.W. 2d 68 (Tex App.—Corpus Christi 1985, ref. n.r.e.); *Nicholson v Memorial Hospital System,* 722 S.W. 2d 746 (Tex. App.—Houston 14 Dist. 1986, no writ).
2. *Darling v Charleston Community Memorial Hospital,* 33 Ill. 2d 326, 311 N.E. 2d 253 (1965).
3. *Gonzales v Nork* 60 Cal. App. 3d 728, 131 Cal. Rptr. 717 (Cal. App. 1971)
4. *Johnson v Misericordia Community Hospital* 294 N.W. 2d 501 (Wis. App. 1980) affd. 301 N.W. 2d 156 (Wis. 1981).
5. *Seneris v Haas,* 45 Cal. 2d 811, 291 P. 2d 915 (1955); *Jackson v Power,* 743 P. 2d 1376 (Alaska 1987); *Howard v Park* 37 Mich App. 496, 195 N.W. 2d 39 (1972).
6. Supra note 1. *Brownsville v Gracia;* Tex. Rev. Civ. Stat. Article 4505 (12), (15) and Art 4495 (b) Sec. 1.03(8), (Vernon Supp. 1990).
7. 42 CFR Parts 405, 412, 416, 417, 440, 441, 456, 482 and 489.
8. Accreditation Manual for Hospitals, MS 4.6, Joint Commission on Accreditation of Healthcare Organizations. Oakbrook Terrace, IL 1992.
9. *Christhilf v Annapolis Emergency Hospital Association, Inc,* 496v F. 2d 174 (4th Civ 1974). *Ascherman v San Francisco Medical Society* 114 Cal Reporter 681 (Cal. Ct. App. 1974). *Woodard v Porter Hospital,* Inc. 217 A2d 589 (N.H. Sup. Ct 1971) Cert. Denied 404 U.S. 995 (1971).
10. Americans with Disabilities Act of 1990, 42 U.S.C. Sec 12101 et. seq.
11. Certification in Emergency Medicine, Policy Summaries, p. 11, American College of Emergency Physicians, Dallas, 1993; Report to Diplomats Spring. 1993, p.3, American Board of Emergency Medicine, East Lansing, Mich.
12. *Courtney v Shore Memorial Hospital* 584 A.2d 817 (1990). *Stein v Tri-City Hospital Authority* 384 S.E. 2d 430 (1989).
13. Supra note 5.
14. 42 U.S.C. 11131-11137.
15. 42 U.S.C. 11101 et seq.
16. 42 U.S.C. 11112 (a) (2).
17. 42 U.S.C. 11112 (a) (1).

78 Nurse Credentialing

Catherine T. Kelly

OUTLINE

Credentialing terms
Certification organization/programs pertaining to emergency nursing
  Advantage of certification in emergency nursing
  Opposition to credentialing programs
Incorporating recognition of certified emergency nurses into the emergency department
  Special issues
Recredentialing
  Should continuing education be required?
Other verifications pertinent to emergency nursing
The future

To practice as a Registered Nurse (RN) in the United States, each individual must be licensed and registered. In addition, several voluntary certifications and verifications can be obtained after completing a required basic nursing education program, such as Pediatric Advanced Life Support (PALS) and the Trauma Nursing Core Course Provider (TNCC-P). Information about the most common credentials and their pertinence to emergency nursing practice are described in this chapter.

Benner[1] describes the growth of an individual nurse as he or she progresses from the novice stage to becoming an expert practitioner. Along this journey the nurse gains new knowledge and becomes more proficient in related skills. The basic credentials held by all registered nurses in the United States are a license and registration. Expert practitioners commonly attain specialty certifications.

In 1977, the Department of Health, Education, and Welfare (now the Department of Health and Human Services) issued a report on credentialing healthcare manpower.[2] Credentialing in this report referred to licensure and registration that was delegated to each state. General findings supported that a profession was served best by providing its own voluntary certification,[2] hence the inception and growth of nursing specialty certification programs.

CREDENTIALING TERMS

The American Nurses Association (ANA) recommends the following definition for licensure:

> Licensure is a process by which an agency or state government grants permission to individuals accountable for the practice of a profession to engage in the practice of that profession and prohibits all others from legally doing so. It permits use of a particular title. Its purpose is to protect the public by ensuring a minimum level of professional competence. Established standards and methods of evaluation are used to determine eligibility for initial licensure and for periodic renewal. Effective means are employed for taking action against licensees for acts of professional misconduct, incompetence, and/or negligence.[3]

Licensure is regulated by each state through a specific regulatory mechanism. As described previously, issuing a license to a registered nurse means the nurse has met the knowledge and practice requirements at the minimum level as evidenced by the successful completion of a national examination. Voluntary certifications (discussed later) focus on the attainment of additional knowledge and skills.

The ANA recommends the following definition for registration:

> Registration is a process by which qualified individuals are listed on an official roster maintained by a governmental or nongovernmental agency. It enables such persons to use a particular title and attests to employing agencies and individuals that minimum qualifications have been met and maintained.[3]

Registration addresses the concept of meeting minimum qualifications and maintaining the standards necessary to continue to practice. Some states require that a minimum number of continuing education hours be completed by the RN before registration can be renewed.

Neither licensure nor registration has any specific relationship to the practice of emergency nursing. The third type of credential, certification, is nursing specialty specific. The ANA delineates the differences between each of these credentials and describes certification as:

> a process by which a non-governmental agency or association certifies that an individual licensed to practice a profession has met certain predetermined standards specified by that profession for specialty practice. Its purpose is to assure various publics that an individual has mastered a body of knowledge and acquired skills in a particular specialty.[3]

In the early 1970s, discussion began among several professional nursing organizations about the need to set higher standards for nurses in specialty areas. The initial goal of establishing certification programs was the nursing profession's interest in providing safe and effective care and protecting the public's health.[4] The ANA led the way for American nurses and offered the first specialty certification examinations in 1974 for nurses practicing in geriatric and pediatric ambulatory care settings. The European nursing community also recognized the need to establish minimum standards for nursing education and agreed that specialist training be completed after demonstrating general proficiency in 1973.[5]

Credentialing agencies and specialty certifications have proliferated in the last 20 years. As of 1993, the American Hospital Association reported that there were 44 certifying agencies in healthcare, 13 of which were dedicated to nursing.[6] The American Nurses Credentialing Center (ANCC) offers 25 different certification programs. With more than 4.5 million nurses worldwide, there is great potential for certification programs to grow.[7]

Certification, along with licensure and current registration, provides a method of ensuring the public that a nurse has gained the necessary knowledge to provide a certain type or level of care. The public can recognize that an individual has attained a certain expertise or knowledge level by ascertaining whether an individual is certified. Certification is similar to recognizing the "Good Housekeeping" seal of approval.

In addition to protecting the public, it is generally accepted that an approved credentialing program gradually raises the standard of practice and increases the knowledge base of the nurse. Standards and recommendations for credentialing and certifying agencies have been established by voluntary organizations such as the National Organization for Competency Assurance (NOCA). The federal government also provides guidelines through the National Commission for Health Certifying Agencies (NCHCA). Box 78-1 lists the ANA recommendations for credentialing.

It is important to understand the criteria agencies use to certify their candidates so that the staffs' specific credentials can be evaluated. The manager needs to know: (1) the organization that offers the credential, (2) criteria used in awarding the credential, (3) method of obtaining the credential (i.e., examination or educational program), and (4) how it pertains to emergency nursing.

Four widely accepted steps are used in establishing a credentialing program. The specific competencies, required experience, knowledge, and skills are first identified. Next qualification requisites are established. The third step is individual assessment, which leads to the final step of achieving certification for the successful candidate.

CERTIFICATION ORGANIZATION/PROGRAMS PERTAINING TO EMERGENCY NURSING

The Certified Emergency Nurse (CEN) credential is offered by the Board of Certification for Emergency Nursing (BCEN). This certification program was established in 1980 and is internationally recognized as the credential that validates that the nurse has attained the specific knowledge required to practice emergency nursing.[8] The CEN examination is constructed by practicing emergency nurses from diverse practice environments (rural, urban, private hospital, university settings) and geographic locations. Each examination consists of 250 questions that are selected based on a role delineation study (RDS) of emergency nursing, which is conducted every 5 years to ensure that the examination tests current practice.[9] Table 78-1 lists the content areas that are tested for the CEN and Certified Flight Nurse (CFRN) credential.

The CEN credential is awarded for 4 years. Candidates may renew by examination or by a renewal option program (CEN-RO). The optional program requires the CEN to complete a self-assessment examination and 100 hours of continuing education within the 4-year cycle when recertification is due.

The BCEN also administers the Certified Flight Registered Nurse (CFRN) program. An extensive study, including RDS, was conducted by the BCEN and the National Flight Nurses Association (NFNA) in 1992 to compare emergency and flight nursing practice. Although these two areas shared a great deal of common knowledge, flight nursing emerged as a distinct specialty and the CFRN program was established.[10] Modification of the CEN examination content areas to reflect areas specific to flight nursing resulted (Table 78-1).

The American Association of Critical Care Nurses

BOX 78-1

RECOMMENDATIONS ON PRINCIPLES OF CREDENTIALING

The Committee for the Study of Credentialing in Nursing recommends that these principles be applied to credentialing in nursing:

The following principles derive from the basic premise that credentialing exists primarily to benefit and protect the public.

1. In addition to benefiting and protecting the public, credentialing also benefits those who are credentialed.
2. The legitimate interests of the involved occupation or institution and of the general public should be reflected in each credentialing mechanism.
3. Accountability should be an essential component of any credentialing process.
4. A system of checks and balances within the credentialing system should assure equitable treatment for all parties involved.
5. Periodic assessments with the potential for sanction are essential components of an effective credentialing mechanism.
6. Objective standards and criteria and persons competent in their use, are essential to the credentialing process.
7. Representation in credentialing systems of the community of interests directly affected by credentialing mechanisms should assure consideration of the legitimate concerns of each group.
8. Professional identity and responsibility should evolve from the credentialing process.
9. An effective system of role delineation is fundamental to any credentialing mechanism for individuals.
10. An effective system of program identification is fundamental to any credentialing mechanism for institutions.
11. Coordination of credentialing mechanisms should lead to efficiency and cost-effectiveness and avoid duplication.
12. Geographic, including interstate, mobility should be improved by the credentialing of the individual.
13. Widely accepted definitions and terminology are basic to an effective credentialing system.
14. Communication and understanding between health care providers and society should be facilitated through the credentialing process.

American Nurses Association: *Americans in nursing: contemporary developments and trends,* Kansas City, 1986, American Nurses Association.

Table 78-1 Examination Content Areas

	CEN	CFRN
Abdominal emergencies	5%	5%
Cardiovascular emergencies	9%	10%
Disaster management	2%	2%
Environmental emergencies	4%	4%
Maxillofacial emergencies	3%	2%
General medical emergencies/communicable diseases	8%	4%
Genitourinary and gynecologic emergencies	4%	1%
Neurologic emergencies	7%	8%
Obstetric emergencies	2.5%	5%
Ocular emergencies	2.5%	2%
Orthopedic emergencies	6%	4%
Mental health emergencies	4.5%	2%
Patient care management	9%	10%
Respiratory emergencies	9%	10%
Shock/multisystem trauma emergencies	7%	9%
Substance abuse/toxicologic emergencies	6%	3%
Wound management/surface trauma emergencies	4%	3%
Stabilization and transfer	2%	11%
Patient/community education	1.5%	1%
Legal issues	2%	2%
Organizational issues/quality improvement	2%	2%

From Board of Certification for Emergency Nursing: *CEN and CFRN handbook for candidates,* Park Ridge, Ill, 1996, BCEN.

(AACN) offers the Critical Care Registered Nurse (CCRN) credential for nurses who meet certain clinical eligibility requirements and initially pass an examination that focuses on critical care nursing knowledge. This certification is awarded for 3 years and candidates may recertify by examination or by meeting the requirements through the Continuing Education Recognition Point (CERP) program.[11] The emergency department is considered a critical care area by this program.

The American Nurses Association offers the largest number of certification programs through the ANCC. The overall goal of this certification program is "promoting and enhancing public health by certifying nurses . . . using ANA standards of nursing practice, nursing services and continuing education."[3] A specific credential is not offered for emergency nursing. However expertise in any of the identified practice areas would demonstrate the emergency nurse's ability to provide clinical care to specific patient populations or perform in a managerial role (Box 78-2). The ANCC offers certification in clinical areas, as well as administration, whereas the CEN and CCRN certifications are clinically based. Certification is awarded for 5 years; recertification can be achieved through reexamination or meeting continuing education requirements. Specific clinical eligibility requirements exist for each credential and a BSN degree (at a minimum) will be required in 1998 for eligibility.[3]

As the importance of specialty certification increases as a result of healthcare consumer awareness and economic incentives, new certification programs are emerging. The Canadian Nurses Association (CNA) has also developed a certification program for emergency nursing. This examination was first given in July, 1994.

Advantage of Certification in Emergency Nursing

Throughout the literature, one recurring theme evolves: protect the public. Donabedian writes:

> There is a social contract between society and the professions. Under its terms, society grants the professions authority over functions vital to itself and permits them considerable autonomy in the conduct of their own affairs. In return, the professions are expected to act responsibly, always mindful of the public trust. Self-regulation to assure quality in performance is at the heart of this relationship. It is the authentic hallmark of a mature profession.[12]

Attaining professional certification demonstrates the nurse has achieved a knowledge base that enhances his or her practice. It is imperative that the candidate and the employer know what the certification actually means in order to assess how that credential pertains to the nurse's practice.

The CEN has passed an examination that is reliable (the candidate will perform similarly on a comparable examination) and valid (measures emergency nursing knowledge). Currently the passing rate ranges between 69% and 72%; it is not an easy certification to achieve. In addition to demonstrating knowledge, the CEN/CFRN credential can increase a candidate's chance for being selected for a position or promotion.

Nurses who are certified may be held more accountable than uncertified peers. Several states require a certain percentage of staff to be certified to meet the requirements in order to be designated a trauma center.

The nurse who becomes certified has proven a commitment to professional development. Because certification is voluntary, an individual chooses to invest the time, energy, and money to achieve this goal.

Becoming certified increases the nurse's involvement in professional activities. The Groteleuschan Associates Technical report identified a consistent positive relationship between participation in continuing education and knowledge proficiency.[13] Reviewing previously learned material helps nurses remember information. This review process also assists with the learning of new material, as "old" information can be linked to new knowledge.

Professional recognition from peers and healthcare providers increases when certification is achieved. Congratulations are always offered in response to a new name plate and/or a certification pin. An individual's credibility increases, not only with co-workers but also with the public.

Mobility is enhanced by providing and attaining an internationally recognized certification. Nurses are highly mobile. Having to recertify for each state or country would be time consuming and a waste of economic resources. One internationally accepted credential removes multiple barriers from the recognition of emergency nurse specialty practice. As long as role delineation studies support that the practice of emergency nursing is comparable, there is no need to have a fragmented system. Lindquist[14] challenges us to "embrace the international concept as a framework." In this manner, we can influence healthcare globally. The 1985 International Congress of Nursing (ICN) study supports the development of multinational standards to increase uniformity of healthcare.[3]

The cost of individual certification varies. Box 78-3 lists

BOX 78-2

AMERICAN NURSES CREDENTIALING CENTER (ANCC)

PSYCHIATRIC AND MENTAL HEALTH NURSING

Clinical Specialist in Adult Psychiatric and Mental Health Nursing
Clinical Specialist in Child and Adolescent Psychiatric and Mental Health Nursing
Psychiatric and Mental Health Nursing

MEDICAL-SURGICAL NURSING

Medical-Surgical Nurse
Clinical Specialist in Medical-Surgical Nursing
Cardiac Rehabilitation Nurse

MATERNAL-CHILD NURSING

Pediatric Nurse Practitioner
Pediatric Nurse
Perinatal Nurse

COMMUNITY HEALTH NURSING

School Nurse Practitioner
Community Health Nurse
School Nurse
Clinical Specialist in Community Health Nursing
College Health Nurse
Home Health Nurse
Clinical Specialist in Home Health Nursing

GERONTOLOGICAL NURSING

Gerontological Nurse
Gerontological Nurse Practitioner
Clinical Specialist in Gerontological Nursing

NURSING ADMINISTRATION

Nursing Administration
Nursing Administration, Advanced

GENERAL NURSING PRACTICE

General Nursing Practice

PRIMARY CARE

Adult Nurse Practitioner
Family Nurse Practitioner

CONTINUING EDUCATION/STAFF DEVELOPMENT

Nursing Continuing Education/Staff Development

INFORMATICS NURSING

Informatics Nurse

ACUTE CARE NURSING

Acute Care Nurse Practitioner

American nurses credentialing center certification catalog; Washington, DC, 1996, American Nurses Credentialing Center.

BOX 78-3

CERTIFICATION COSTS

Examination fees and emergency nursing assoc. membership

	U.S.	Canada	Australia	NZ
Emergency nursing assoc. members currently CEN certified	$100	$145	NA	NA
Emergency nursing assoc. members **not** currently CEN certified	$110	$155	$155	$185
Emergency nursing non-assoc. members currently CEN certified	$200	$285	NA	NA
Emergency nursing non-assoc. members **not** currently CEN certified	$220	$315	$305	$375

CEN recertification by continuing education

Self assessment examination-all applicants: $60.00
Submission and evaluation of continuing education record:
ENA members: $60.00
non-ENA members: $160.00

American Association of Critical Care Nurses, CCRN certification exam

AACN member $120
non-AACN member $195

CCRN recertification

Exam
AACN member $120
non-AACN member $195
Continuing education recertification
AACN member $120
non-AACN member $195

pated that increased collaboration will occur as healthcare providers recognize the professional competency of the certified nurse.

RECREDENTIALING

Additional controversies surround the topic of recredentialing. Initial certification signifies the attainment of the knowledge base, whereas recertification provides documentation of ongoing knowledge acquisition. All nursing certifications require recertification. Debate continues as to whether recredentialing by examination, continuing education, or a combination of both is appropriate.

The CEN and CCRN programs have approached this area differently (Box 78-4). The BCENs' philosophy is that having a candidate take the examination every 8 years enhances the program by providing objective periodic reviews.

Change in practice is the primary justification for a continuing competency requirement. New information is constantly affecting the way we care for patients. Should recertification focus only on new information, or should it be comprehensive? At this time the major nursing certification programs have integrated new and old information.

Another controversy involves testing skills, as well as knowledge. The CCRN program requires documentation that candidates have performed a minimum of 17 interventions from a list of 30 within the certification period. These skills include activities such as cardioversion, caring for intubated patients, and the administration of thrombolytic agents. AACN selected these skills based on a role delineation study for critical care nursing performed in 1990.

Controversy continues with regard to clinical eligibility requirements. The majority of the certification programs require a minimum number of hours in clinical practice before one can take a certification examination. One must question how the minimum number of hours is chosen. The majority of nursing specialties identify experts within the specialty who discuss their opinions about the hour requirements and reach a consensus number agreed on by the group.

The BCEN conducted an extensive literature search about methods used to establish minimum clinical eligibility requirements. An objective mechanism for the establishment of clinical eligibility minimums was not identified. The BCEN elected to continue the recommendation, rather than initiating a requirement, that CEN candidates complete 2 years of emergency nursing practice before taking the examination. CEN examination statistics show that candidates with greater than 2 years experience pass at significantly higher rates than those with less experience.

BOX 78-4

CERTIFICATION AND RECERTIFICATION REQUIREMENTS CEN AND CCRN

CEN	Initial Certification: 2 years emergency nursing practice recommended.
CCRN	Initial certification: 1750 hours direct care of critically ill/injured patients required, 875 hours of care must have been provided within the previous year.
CEN	Recertification Every 4 years, every other certification must be attained by examination. In the interim years, completion of a self-assessment examination and 100 hours of continuing education (75% must be clinical) is required.
CCRN	Recertification 432 direct clinical care bedside nursing within the last 3 years (144 hours in the preceding year) and meet a list of clinical experiences.

Should Continuing Education be Required?

Wakeford et al.[15] believe that recertification should be closely linked to continuing education and professional development that is demonstrated by positive performance appraisals and self- and peer evaluations. In addition to written examinations, other recertification mechanisms include verbal examination, mandatory continuing education, peer/self-review, and a combination of any of these methods.

Continuing education that is guided (i.e., people taking a self-assessment examination) is most effective when concentrated in specific subject areas.[13] An interesting outcome in this study was that as participants increased their level of participation, their attitudes became more positive toward continuing education.[13]

The issues revolving around peer/self-review include bias and the individual's definition of competence. Evaluation should be well defined and as objective as possible. Current attention is focused on using a criterion-based evaluation. One example of such as tool, for the entry level emergency nurse, is noted in Figure 78-1. The CNA uses a combination of methods to certify nurses. The process involves peer/self-review, examination, and mandatory continuing education.

Costs of recertifying are also significant. In addition to the application fees, continuing education is expensive. Current changes in healthcare have resulted in a decrease of employer reimbursements for education, which increases the financial burden on each nurse planning recertification.

Nursing is not alone in recognizing the need to recertify its practitioners. Time-limited certification and recertification is required by nearly all 24 programs that participate with the American Board of Medical Specialists.[16] It is anticipated that physician certifications will be tied to financial returns. The American Board of Internal Medicine requires its members to recertify by examination every 10 years.[16]

OTHER VERIFICATIONS PERTINENT TO EMERGENCY NURSING

Other educational programs that verify knowledge and/or skill competency are appropriate for the practice of emergency nursing. Two of these programs are the following:

Trauma Nursing Care Course—Provider (TNCC-P) and Instructor level (TNCC-I). This course incorporates both lec-

SAINT FRANCIS HOSPITAL
POUGHKEEPSIE, NEW YORK 12601

RN II- EMERGENCY DEPARTMENT
JOB DESCRIPTION/PERFORMANCE APPRAISAL

	Rating
I. Position Description R.N. II: Emergency Department	
The RN II functions primarily in direct patient care, and demonstrates "competent" clinical practice. The RN II identifies and addresses typical patient/family care problems in terms of long range goals. The RN II appropriately assigns and plans work for designated emergency department staff.	______
II. Reporting Relationships:	
Position reports to Emergency Department Nursing Supervisor.	______
III. Supervision Exercised:	
A. Delegates work to Emergency Department technicians and reviews their compliance.	______
B. May provide input to the RN II, RN IV or supervisor regarding the evaluation of assigned support staff.	______
IV. Qualifications and Experience:	
A. ACLS certification or certification within one year of assignment to the Emergency Department staff.	______
B. Graduate from an accredited school of nursing and current licensure in New York State as a Registered Professional Nurse.	______
C. One year of continuous full time experience or 1750 hours of continuous part-time experience as professional registered nurse is necessary.	______
D. Demonstrated written and verbal communication skills:	
1. Passing grade on SFH Education Department medication test.	______
2. Completion of Blood transfusion therapy self-learning module.	______
V. Characteristic Duties and Responsibilities:	
A. Clinical Performance.	______
1. Assessment of the physical, psychological and social needs of patients and families:	
a. Uses effective interviewing skills to determine patients and families needs.	______
b. Uses physical assessment techniques (auscultation, percussion, palpation and observation) to identify patient's physical problems and patient-care needs. Recognizes self limitations and seeks out appropriate resources.	______
c. Identifies common variables affecting patient care; problems, symptoms, behavioral changes and deviations.	______
d. Demonstrates clinical competence in airway management, cardiac monitoring, IV therapy, blood gas analysis, venipuncture and physical assessment.	______
e. Reassesses patients health status and identifies significant changes in the patient's condition as appropriate.	______
f. Documents and communicates both baseline and ongoing patient assessments.	______
2. Plans Patient Care:	
a. Plans care that meets basic health needs of patient.	______
b. Interprets assessment data. Identifies problems and sets care priorities.	______
c. Individualizes plans of care.	______
d. Develops realistic, measurable expected outcomes (goals).	______
e. Develops intervention plans which will lead to achievement of the expected outcomes.	______
f. Includes independent and interdependent nursing interventions in care plan.	______
g. Coordinates the prescribed plan of care through collaboration with the health care team.	______
h. Documents plan of care.	______
i. Communicates pertinent aspects of plan to patient, family, or subsequent care givers.	______
j. Updates plan of care when there are changes in patient/family needs.	______
k. Initiates home health care referrals and interagency transfers.	______
l. Communicates rationale for nursing interventions utilizing sound nursing and scientific principles.	______

DNM - DOES NOT MEET* **ND** - NEEDS DEVELOPMENT* **MS** - MEETS STANDARDS (Quality Performance) **ES** - EXCEEDS STANDARDS*
***REQUIRES DOCUMENTATION**

FIGURE 78-1 Example of an evaluation form for the entry level emergency nurse.

the costs for the two most common certifications attained by emergency nurses, CEN and CCRN, in 1993.

Individuals may pay the entire amount or be partially to totally reimbursed by their employer. Many institutions ask the employee to pay the costs initially and then reimburse the employee if they are successful in passing the examination. This method creates a great deal of financial and testing pressure on the candidate. Successful candidates may be rewarded by an additional cash bonus at work and/or an increase in hourly wage. Financial rewards may also occur if attaining a certification is a component of a clinical ladder program in which the nurse attains a higher practice level. In some cases, certification may actually become a requirement of employment.

Third-party reimbursement may also be available to nurses who become certified in their specialties. Reimbursement requirements may take on added importance as the profession struggles to define advanced practice in nursing.

Employers who choose to financially support certification reimbursement receive several benefits. Staff members who perceive their employers are willing to make a personal investment in the personnel are more likely to invest their energies in supporting their employer. The increase in credibility, which is generated from other healthcare providers and the general public, can enhance the institution's image. The overall perception is the provision of programs to support the delivery of competent patient care.

Opposition to Credentialing Programs

Adherence to nationally recognized recommendations that establish minimal standards for certification programs ensures the consumer that the program is reliable and valid. Some programs may not follow these guidelines, leaving doubts as to whether a particular certification is worth obtaining.

Standards may be set below what would be considered the minimally competent level; on the other hand, the average practitioner may be penalized if standards are set too high. An RDS, which identifies the skills and knowledge needed by emergency nurses during their daily practice, ensures that the correct difficulty level is targeted and that current practice is tested.

Opposition is also encountered as people feel that opportunities are restricted for the noncertified. Innovation and individuality may be stifled as candidates may perceive that they are expected to fit a mold.

The financial cost of certification can be significant. Candidates and employers must consider the cost/benefit ratio. Eubanks[6] noted that certifications ranged in cost from $5 to $950.

A valid credential does not guarantee adequate performance by everyone who owns it; however, it does increase the likelihood of satisfactory services. Many people who oppose credentialing, along with those who support the process, object strenuously to grandpersoning. This mechanism allows individuals to gain a credential without meeting the new set of standards. This mechanism impairs the ability of the public to know that all practitioners meet the same standards.

INCORPORATING RECOGNITION OF CERTIFIED EMERGENCY NURSES INTO THE EMERGENCY DEPARTMENT

The first decision for managers is which certifications the department/administration will recognize. Factors influencing this choice include type of patient mix, acuity, and knowledge base expected of the RN staff.

For general emergency nurse practice, the CEN credential would be most appropriate. The content area tested covers newborns to geriatrics, along with the diverse health problems each of these groups encounters. Critical care transport teams and treatment areas that handle large numbers of critically ill patients may prefer the CCRN credential. The AACN corporation also offers an examination specifically geared for pediatric patients, which may be most appropriate within a pediatric center. The CFRN program specifically tests the nursing knowledge required to provide patient care in a rotor or fixed-wing aircraft. Clinical nurse specialists, educators, and others may find that certification through one of the ANA programs best meets their needs.

After choosing the certification program, the types of roles and responsibilities expected of the certified nurse must be distinguished. Certification may become one of the requirements to move up in a clinical ladder program, or certification may be required for a nurse assuming charge responsibilities. A CCRN may be required to care for any critical care patients who are being held or transferred. These decisions are based on patient population and availability of certified staff.

Special Issues

Certification may also be required for staff who provide education and participate in research. Management and education personnel are faced with several choices. Clinical certification would demonstrate they had achieved at a minimum the same knowledge base of the staff. This is possible with the CEN and CFRN program, but the CCRN program requires 432 hours in direct bedside care of the critically ill patient in the 3-year certification period[11] to renew. Other options for managers and educators include the ANA certifications, which focus on managerial and clinical specialist skills.

Incorporating recognition for certified personnel requires attention to the needs of noncertified peers and associated personnel. All RN staff must be given equal opportunity to attain certification. A certain amount of competition can be a strong motivator, leading to a cohesive unit. However, some nurses will not pass the examination. The manager must find a way to recognize these staff members in some other way if they are to remain in the unit. Associated personnel (e.g., aides, technicians) who are not eligible for professional certification programs can be encouraged to achieve skill verifications (such as Advanced Cardiac Life Support) and develop education programs for people with similar job descriptions. To date certification is not offered for emergency aides/technicians, although it is being discussed.

Collaborative practice can be encouraged by providing clear guidelines for staff and a role for everyone. Previously certified staff should help new members achieve this goal. As nurse credentialing becomes more common, it is antici-

SAINT FRANCIS HOSPITAL POUGHKEEPSIE, NEW YORK 12601	RN II- EMERGENCY DEPARTMENT JOB DESCRIPTION/PERFORMANCE APPRAISAL

	Rating
3. Implements the Plan of Care:	
a. Sets priorities and implements nursing measures which correlate with identified plan and standards of care.	______
b. Carries out nursing measures consistent with hospital's and nursing departments philosophies, policies, procedures.	______
c. Recognizes changes in patient's conditions and takes action to manage, reduce or eliminate symptoms and promote comfort.	______
d. Maintains open communication between caregiver and patient/family (responds promptly and courteously, introduces self, addresses patient by preferred title, keeps patient/family informed about patient's condition and progress towards goals).	______
e. Demonstrates respect for patients dignity and privacy (uses privacy drapes and closes doors appropriately, keeps patient covered, maintains confidentiality).	______
f. Documents nursing interventions and patient response consistent with the patient's condition, and legal and accreditation requirements.	______
g. Maintains a safe patient environment and takes actions to prevent risk situations (reports faulty equipment, uses side rails and restraints when appropriate, monitors for fire and electrical hazards, follows medication administration protocols).	______
4. Evaluates patients health status in relation to outcomes achieved as a result of nursing intervention and/or medical therapies.	______
a. Identifies, reports, and documents patient response to nursing interventions and/or medical therapies.	
b. Modifies nursing assessment measures and care plans as needed in response to changes in patients physical/emotional/mental status. Reports condition changes to M.D. and/or nursing supervisor as appropriate.	______
c. Determines the degree of achievement of outcomes.	______
d. Revises plan, seeks assistance as needed to establish alternative approaches when appropriate.	______
e. Transfer and discharge summaries include documentation of patient problem and care plan.	______
5. Provides patient/family education:	
a. Identifies patient/family learning needs, recognizes patients at risk and identifies discharge planning needs.	______
b. Plans and implements patient/family teaching for individuals.	______
c. Explains to patient and family, procedures, tests and treatments in understandable terms.	______
d. Utilizes available educational resource materials (i.e. pamphlets, a/v material, etc.)	______
e. Documents instructions given to patient's and their family.	______
B. Leadership Performance:	
1. Interpersonal skills:	
a. Communicates effectively with the following:	
1. Patients.	______
2. Visitors.	______
3. Peers.	______
4. Ancillary personnel	______
5. Physicians.	______
6. Management.	______
b. Assists other nurses in patient care activities.	______
c. Recognizes stress in self and co-workers and utilizes positive coping techniques.	______
d. Demonstrates respect for co-workers and contributes to a working atmosphere of trust and acceptance.	______
2. Organizational Skills:	
a. Accepts and completes delegated assignments.	______
b. Sets goals and prioritizes emergency nursing care to a group of patients according to individual patient acuity.	______
c. Delegates patient care and non-patient care to appropriate ancillary and nursing personnel.	______
d. Recognizes crisis situations and takes immediate action.	______
e. Demonstrates time management skills.	______

DNM - DOES NOT MEET* **ND** - NEEDS DEVELOPMENT* **MS** - MEETS STANDARDS (Quality Performance) **ES** - EXCEEDS STANDARDS*

***REQUIRES DOCUMENTATION**

FIGURE 78-1—cont'd. For legend see opposite page.

SAINT FRANCIS HOSPITAL POUGHKEEPSIE, NEW YORK 12601	RN II- EMERGENCY DEPARTMENT JOB DESCRIPTION/PERFORMANCE APPRAISAL

	Rating
3. Planning Skills:	
a. Plans care for assigned patients.	______
b. Participates in unit problem solving.	______
c. Supports and participates as needed within the Emergency Department.	______
4. Quality Assurance/Cost Control:	
a. Uses Emergency Department and nursing standards to guide practice.	______
b. Demonstrates knowledge of unit-based quality assurance activities.	______
c. Assists with quality assurance data collection as assigned.	______
d. Modifies own practice as recommended by QA Committee.	______
5. Accountability:	
a. Adheres to hospital policies and procedures regarding personal and professional conduct and image:	
1. Attendance.	______
2. Punctuality.	______
3. Scheduling.	______
4. Dress Code.	______
b. Attends 80% of departmental meetings and reviews minutes of those not attended.	______
c. Carries out physician orders accurately and promptly, when appropriate.	______
C. Professionalism: (The following criteria are mandatory)	
1. Professional Development:	
a. Continuing education:	
1. Participates in continuing education programs, documents participation on a monthly basis, and meets mandatory 15 hour annual minimum requirement.	______
2. Completes CPR recertification annually.	______
3. Completes ALS certification within 1 year of employment.	______
4. Attends mandatory hospital-sponsored inservices, including one infection control and one fire and electrical safety inservice annually.	______
5. Attends one patient care conference each year.	______
6. Prepares brief written description of a "critical incident" from the past year's practice (see definition).	______
b. Collaborates with performance evaluator to set goals for professional development based upon performance criteria.	______

DNM - DOES NOT MEET* **ND** - NEEDS DEVELOPMENT* **MS** - MEETS STANDARDS (Quality Performance) **ES** - EXCEEDS STANDARDS*
***REQUIRES DOCUMENTATION**

FIGURE 78-1—cont'd. For legend see page 688.

ture content and psychomotor skill training to prepare RNs to deliver trauma care. Verification is every 4 years.[17]

Emergency Nursing Pediatric Course—Provider (ENPC-P) and Instructor (ENPC-I). Incorporates lecture and psychomotor skills pertaining specifically to pediatric patients. Verification is every 4 years.[18]

Course in Advanced Trauma Nursing (CATN)—This program was initiated by the Emergency Nurses Association in 1996. The purpose of CATN is to strengthen critical decision making skills and optimally impact the outcomes of critically ill patients. Verification is contingent on successful completion of an oral examination. Renewal of verification is every four years through retesting.

If an emergency department unit employs prehospital care providers as staff members they must be appropriately credentialed. Each state establishes its own guidelines and requirements for prehospital care providers. The National Registry of Emergency Technicians provides national guidelines, although all states have not fully recognized this national credential. Three levels of certification are provided, each requiring demonstration of knowledge attainment and psychomotor skills. Emergency Medical Technicians (EMT) basic (B), EMT intermediate (I) and Paramedic (P).[19] Each level advances in complexity. The EMT-D credential is used to denote personnel who have received special training in order to provide automatic defibrillation.

THE FUTURE

The most pressing issue at this time is the delineation of advanced practice for nursing. Currently, advanced practitioners are considered to be nurse practitioners, clinical nurse specialists, nurse midwives, and nurse anesthetists. Programs exist that focus on the educational preparation for emergency nurse practitioners and clinical specialists, so this controversy affects the practice of emergency nursing.

Forty-two states currently have some type of regulation with regard to advanced nursing practice. The requirements are diverse, ranging from educational preparation (e.g., BS, MS, PhD) to physician collaboration, peer review, specialty certification, and proficiency examinations. The requirements for physician collaboration vary from formal approval and reporting mechanisms to joint practice agreements. Two systems have been proposed to designate advanced practice, a licensure mechanism and a system that requires specialty certification along with attainment of a master's degree. The proposed licensure system would require a separate and distinct second license for nurses practicing at the advanced level. Nursing would become the only profession with a secondary license requirement.

The strongest proponent of the two license system is the National Council of the State Boards of Nursing (NCSNB). They propose that advanced practice nurses have a minimum of a Master's degree and successfully complete a specific licensing examination. Specialty certification may be a qualification, but the state boards would establish the criteria for accepting the applicable certification.

There is currently great diversity with regard to how the State Boards of Nursing regulate the role of the advanced nurse practitioner. Proposals include the development of national standards; however, there is resistance to the perceived weakening of each state's independence. A comparative list of each states' current position on these legislative issues is available.[20]

The majority of the Nursing Specialties National Federation of Specialty Organizations (NFSNO), ANA, and Emergency Nurses Association (ENA) oppose a second license for advanced practice. All agree that standardization of titles needs to occur and that a candidate must have attained a master's degree along with specialty certification. The NFSNO and other specialty nursing organizations recommend that state boards defer to specialty organization credentialing mechanisms.

The recognition of advanced practice nurses will have a significant impact on reimbursement mechanisms. Direct reimbursement will increase the recognition and use of nurses as primary care providers.[21] The impact on emergency nursing may change the way that minor care areas are staffed, as well as the implementation of community outreach programs.

Many other issues related to credentialing are also being raised. As our healthcare system is streamlined and emphasis is placed on patient outcomes, appropriate credentialing will become increasingly important. Questions being asked of healthcare providers and consumers include the following:

- Should certification be required for nurses in specific roles such as teaching or supervision?
- Do nursing assistants need to be certified?
- Is a specific level of academic preparation needed?
- Is the purpose of certification to improve practice or for public protection?
- Should certification be viewed as a sign of clinical excellence or entry into practice?
- Is there a place for hospital or agency certification?
- How will the expanding scope of emergency nursing affect credentialing?

Because emergency nursing and the profession in general is changing rapidly, it is essential to critique each credential that a nurse attains for its validity and significance. The challenge is to foster the development of more uniform standards, which will facilitate the migratory freedom of nurses and promote a singular, international identification for nursing. As Margaretta Styles said, "Think of a world in which nursing speaks with one voice."[22]

REFERENCES

1. Benner P: *From novice to expert: excellence and power in nursing practice,* Menlo Park, CA, 1984, Addison-Wesley.
2. Grippando GM: *Nursing perspectives and issues,* New York 1986, Delmar Publishers.
3. American Nurses Association: *Credentialing in nursing: contemporary developments and trends,* Kansas City, MO, 1986, ANA.
4. Deloughery GL: *Issues and trends in nursing,* St Louis, 1991, Mosby.
5. Stallknecht K: Nursing in Europe, *Br Med J* 304:561-562, 1992.
6. Eubanks P: New guide clarifies health care wonder certifications, *Hospitals* 65:58-59, 1991.
7. Gosnell DJ: The international implication of nursing education and practice, *Int Nurs Rev* 32:105-108, 1985.
8. *Board of certification for emergency nursing. Candidates handbook,* Iowa City, 1993, ACT.
9. American College of Testing for the Board of Certification for Emergency Nursing: *Role delineation of emergency nursing,* Iowa City, 1990, ACT.
10. American College of Testing for the Board of Certification for Emergency Nursing: *Role delineation study of flight nursing,* Iowa City, 1992, ACT.
11. *Recertification handbook and application for critical care nurses,* 1992, AACN Certification Corporation,
12. Donabedian A: Foreword. In Phaneuf M: *The nursing audit and self recognition in nursing practice,* ed 2, New York, 1976, Appleton-Century-Crofts.
13. Groteleuschan Associates Inc. to the Mandatory Continuing Education Study Committee, State Board for Public Accountance, New York State Education Department. The effectiveness of mandatory continuing education for licensed accountants in public practice in the state of New York. New York 1990.
14. Lindquist GJ: Integration of international and transcultural content in nursing curricula: a process for change, *J Prof Nurs* 6:272-279, 1990.
15. Wakeford R, Jolly B, Newble D: Certification and recertification: college examiners and test experts meet, *Lancet* 338:1325-1326, 1991.
16. Frankel D: USA: compulsory recertification for internists, *Lancet* 340:1151-1152, 1992.
17. ENA, 1993 Trauma Nursing Core Course Application.
18. ENA, 1993 Emergency Nursing Pediatric Course Application.
19. The National Registry of Emergency Medical Technicians, National Registration Applications—EMT—Basic, EMT-Intermediate, EMT-Paramedic. National Registry of Emergency Medical Technicians, Columbus, OH 1993.
20. Pearson LJ: 1992-1993 update: how each state stands on legislative issues affecting advanced nursing practice, *Nurse Pract* 18:23-38, 1993.
21. Mittelstadt PC: Federal reimbursement of advanced practice nurses' services empowers the profession, *Nurse Pract* 18:43-49, 1993.
22. Styles MM: *On specialization in nursing: toward a new empowerment,* Kansas City, MO, 1989. American Nurse Association.

ADDITIONAL READING

American nurses credentialing center certification catalog; Washington, DC, 1993, American Nurses Credentialing Center.

Chaves DE, LaRochelle DR: The universality of nursing: a comprehensive framework for practice, *Int Nurs Rev* 32:10-13, 1985.

Cleland VS, McKibbin RC: *The economics of nursing,* Norwalk, Conn, 1990, Appleton & Lange.

Corcoran E: Two licenses for advanced practice nurses? ENA thinks not, *J Emerg Nurs* 19:78, 1993.

Fickelssen JL: 56 ways to get certified, *Am J Nurs* 90:50-56, 1990.

Staff. Specialty groups mobilize as boards weigh advanced practice licensure. *Am J Nurs* 92:90, 94, 1992.

Winter EJS, Pugh LC, Riley-Giomarlso O: Is certification for you? *Nursing '92,* 22:88-92, 1992.

79 Competency Based Nursing Orientation

Suzanne Rita

OUTLINE

An adequate orientation is the essential key to retention and recruitment of nurses in the emergency department. In the past, the practice has been to offer a standard orientation to all staff. Orientation was the same for the new graduate nurse or the experienced emergency department nurse. This practice causes job and patient dissatisfaction and problems with retention of nurses. It cannot be assumed that all nurses will be able to care competently for patients after a generic 4 week orientation. When the individual learning needs of the new staff nurse are not met in orientation, the nurse can become frustrated. Frustration can lead to an inability to retain nurses. Competency based nursing orientation allows the emergency department nurse to determine individual learning needs and allows management to set standard minimal behaviors that all nursing staff must exhibit. It is the ethical responsibility of nursing management to ensure that nurses who deliver patient care are competent to perform these tasks in a safe manner. This chapter discusses implementing a competency based orientation program, including the establishment of behaviors, teaching learning strategies to accomplish the demonstration of these behaviors, use of competencies as an evaluation tool, and strategies to maintain competency on a continuing basis.

COMPETENCY

In 1977, del Bueno and Altano[1] described an educational principle that established behaviors or competencies as the guide for learning needs assessment and evaluation. Competency is described as the ability to perform. The authors took this concept to another level when applying it to nursing and orientation. They developed a program by which managers established basic behaviors that are required for staff to be able to perform the job at a minimally competent level. Needs assessment tools were developed from these competencies to determine the education that a newly hired nurse would need to be able to function as a competent member of the healthcare team. Also involved in this concept is the use of various teaching strategies that support adult learning theory. Del Bueno and Altano[1] found this form of orientation decreased the time needed to adequately orient new employees, and provided an individualized orientation plan for each employee and an efficient orientation plan for experienced nurses.

Benner et al.[2] expanded on the del Bueno and Altano concept of competency. Using the Dreyfus model for skill acquisition and development, they described levels of competency in which nurses move from reliance on abstract principles to guide their decision making to using intuition and experience to make decisions. These levels are novice through expert and are detailed in Table 79-1. The understanding of this information is essential to the successful use of competency based orientation.

The Joint Commission on the Accreditation of Healthcare Organizations (JCAHO) supports the value of competency based education and orientation. As the standards for JCAHO have changed, an evolution to competency based education has occurred. In the *Accreditation Manual for Hospitals, 1995*,[3] orientation competency is addressed in the management of Human Resource Standard HR.4. This standard addresses the employee's competency to perform the job expectations. Competency assessment must include the age-specific tasks/knowledge required for the patient population served.

COMPETENCY BASED NURSING ORIENTATION

The purpose of orientation is to provide the orientee the appropriate learning experiences for the accomplishment of skills necessary to care for the emergency department patient and family. The nurse must possess knowledge about the science and art of nursing, including the nursing process and must be competent in skill performance to meet the needs of the emergency department patient. A competency based orientation program must begin with the development of a set of beliefs that can be accepted by the entire nursing staff. All team members must accept these beliefs to make the orientation program a success. The orientation program should include belief statements on the following:

1. Purpose and goals of competency based orientation
2. Roles and responsibilities of nursing team members
3. Communication among staff
4. Competency of the orientee
5. Enhancement of current skills/knowledge
6. Individualized orientation/self-evaluation
7. Preceptor/buddy-based program
8. Socialization into the emergency department culture
9. Adult learning as the educational theory
10. Flexibility related to meeting individual learning needs
11. Evaluation of the preceptor, preceptee, and the orientation program

The roles and responsibilities of the nursing team are defined in Box 79-1.

After the nursing team has agreed on a philosophy sup-

Table 79-1 Competency Model for Nursing of Benner et al.[2]

Competency level	Experience	Decision-making abilities
I. Novice	Limited	Task oriented. Lack of experience, limited decision-making capabilities. Uses pieces of information to make decisions. Lacks ability to synthesize.
II. Advanced beginner	6 months-2 years	Cannot plan ahead for complications, lacks flexibility. Does not anticipate life threat. Can begin to piece information together to make decisions but still relies on protocol to assist with decisions. Can accomplish tasks without difficulty. Follows actions of others.
III. Competent	At least 2 years	Able to plan as means of decision making. Can anticipate patient's needs.
IV. Proficient	At least 2 years	Synthesizes pieces of information into whole. Recognizes change in patient's condition and is flexible to change plan of care to meet needs.
V. Expert	Extensive experience	Focuses on important information only. Anticipates needs, implements care plan, and evaluates plan rapidly. Recognizes patterns from experience to assist with decision making. Possesses much self-confidence. More family oriented, not task oriented.

porting the orientation program, a competency assessment skills checklist should be developed. Behaviors that identify *minimal* competency should be defined. All members of the nursing team should be involved in the development of these behaviors. The checklist should be written according to outcome based criteria. This is an excellent tool to objectively evaluate the new orientee. It also ensures that expectations are consistent among the nursing staff.

The assessment skills checklist should be designed so that the new employee is able to adequately perform a self-assessment of the current knowledge and skill level, in order to develop an individualized orientation program. Mandatory skills for all caregivers (intravenous therapy, customer service, phlebotomy) should be included in the orientation program. Although the new employee may feel competent, some skills must be observed (intravenous therapy, medication administration, blood administration). Other skills that are low volume and high risk should be simulated (open heart defibrillation, autotransfusion, and emergency childbirth).

The format of the orientation must be flexible to meet the needs of each orientee. A nurse with experience at a level I trauma center and is at the expert stage will still need orientation to focus on hospital policy and procedure and socialization. A nurse that is a novice with pediatric patient care will need orientation to focus on the care of the pediatric patient.

The content of the orientation varies with every emergency department, but some components are the same because of JCAHO and Occupational Safety and Health Administration (OSHA) requirements.[4] The orientation should contain content necessary to deliver safe, quality patient care. The Emergency Nurses Association *Core Curriculum,* Standards *of Emergency Nursing Practice,*[5] and *Orientation To Emergency Nursing: Diversity In Practice* can be used as guides.

The new employee should be paired with an experienced nurse to facilitate the orientation process. The preceptor should be a proficient or expert nurse with excellent skills and knowledge. The preceptor must be a good role model, with a positive attitude about nursing and the emergency department. Knowledge and familiarity with emergency department and hospital policy, procedure, and culture are essential. An effective preceptor possesses good communication skills and enjoys teaching and guiding new employees through the orientation transition.[6]

The role of the preceptor is to assist the orientee in role mastery and acceptance as a peer by the team members. A preceptor is available to the new employee as a resource throughout the entire orientation. This relationship stimulates a camaraderie between both nurses. It is best that the nurses are paired according to personality types and needs of the orientee. Matching of preceptor/preceptee relationships should be guided by identifying personality styles and teaching/learning styles. Tools available to aid in this matching include the Myers Briggs Personality Inventory and Learning Style Inventory.

The preceptor is responsible for assisting the new employee in identifying personal needs and to develop a plan, along with other members of the nursing team, to meet these goals. Goals should be set each week and evaluated at the end of the week. The preceptor may change the orientation plan at any time to assist the new employee to meet their needs. The preceptor should alert the other nurses of the individual needs of the orientee so that if an experience the orientee needs is available, the preceptor is made aware.

A variety of teaching/learning strategies are available to assist the new employee to meet the goals of the orientation program. Self-learning packets are used to assist the new employee to attain new knowledge. Individuals can work at their own speed to meet the objectives of the self-learning packet. These may be used as mandatory information or as a tool that is available for a nurse that needs extra information on certain topics.

Case presentations are a good means to assess current knowledge and to teach new information. The orientee may present a patient situation to the preceptor who can then critique the nursing care. This strategy is to be used only for critique and not as a punitive measure. The preceptor may use case presentations to present new knowledge. The case presentation should include patient history (including presenting signs and symptoms) and past medical history. Assessment should be included and competing clinical hypotheses should be discussed. Appropriate interventions, includ-

BOX 79-1

ORIENTATION ROLES AND RESPONSIBILITIES

Emergency department manager/clinical nurse specialist

1. Assesses the orientation needs.
2. Identifies long- and short-term goals for orientation.
3. Develops and implements the orientation program.
4. Plans and monitors orientation.
5. Consults with the orientee and the preceptor at least on a weekly basis to evaluate individual orientee progress.
6. Evaluates the effectiveness of the orientation program.
7. Determines a plan to deal with disciplinary problems on an individual basis.

Preceptor

1. Assesses the orientation needs of the orientee.
2. Assists the orientee to identify short- and long-term goals.
3. Plans and monitors the evaluation.
4. Provides feedback to the orientee as needed.
5. Provides learning experiences for the orientee to accomplish role mastery.
6. Provides dialogue and experiences necessary to orient the orientee with the unit culture.
7. Communicates with leadership weekly.
   a. Reports on progress as determined by accomplishment of weekly goals.
   b. Documents progress through checklist and anecdotal notes.
   c. Provides input into evaluation of orientee by continuous assessments of strengths and weaknesses.
8. Demonstrates professional behavior.
   a. Provides support for the orientee.
   b. Acts as a role model and mentor to aid in the transition of the orientee.

Orientee

1. Identifies individualized learning needs.
   a. Completes self-assessment checklist.
   b. Seeks out appropriate resources.
   c. Participates in weekly goal setting and evaluation.
2. Completes orientation.
3. Evaluates orientation.
   a. Evaluates program.
   b. Evaluates preceptor.

ing rationale, should follow. Evaluation methods are then presented.

Another effective method is to have the orientee "talk aloud" about their decision making as they deliver nursing care. Orientees should be encouraged to cluster data as they are presented through subjective and objective assessment of the patient. This approach enables the orientee to test the competing clinical hypothesis (e.g., is the pain of cardiac or abdominal origin?)

Other educational forms can include video- and computer-assisted instruction. According to the needs of the new employee and the emergency department, these can be used as mandatory information or to augment the knowledge of the orientee. Each of these strategies should include participant objectives, a pretest to focus learning needs, and a posttest for evaluation.

Skill simulation and return demonstration is another teaching/learning strategy that is used in the orientation process. Some skills can be evaluated in the patient care setting during the daily care of the emergency department patient. Other high-risk, low-volume skills must be simulated in the laboratory setting or the orientee may be able to go to a nursing unit where the skill is performed frequently to gain competence.

DEVELOPING COMPETENCIES

A nurse is competent if she or he has the appropriate knowledge and skills to provide safe, quality nursing care. Competencies are developed to assess, achieve, and maintain skills and knowledge appropriate to the nursing performance standards of the unit. In the development of a competency based orientation program, personal performance standards are identified and are consistent with the unit standards. Standards may vary depending on the patient population and patient acuity levels. Some areas of basic competency will remain the same because of regulating agencies and the general role of the emergency department nurse. These basic competencies should include the following:[5]

1. Implementation of patient care depending on patient acuities
2. Safe drug and blood administration
3. Safe use of equipment
4. Safety practices (e.g., fire, bomb threat)
5. Safe performance of common emergency department procedures
6. Decision making and priority setting

A group representative of management and staff should work together to identify the basic skills that a staff nurse must possess to be deemed competent. Resources available to identify these skills include the Emergency Nurses Association *Core Curriculum* and *Standards of Emergency Nursing Practice*. Skills that are low volume but high risk should also be identified. The nurse should have knowledge of these procedures and the skills to perform them (Appendix A).

Competency outcomes are based on skill performance. Evaluation is simple to observe and is an objective measurement of performance. Outcome statements begin with verbs and address behaviors that can be observed. Examples include the following:

- Identify the location of
  - fire extinguishers
  - fire alarm
  - fire hose
  - evacuation plan.
- Describe the emergency department's disaster plan and your role if the plan is activated.
- Identify specific infection control measures used in the trauma room.

After the basic competencies are agreed on and described, the appropriate evaluation method must be considered. Observation will be used most often, but other methods include successful completion of self-learning packets, delivering case presentations, completing skill simulation and return demonstration, and viewing videotapes and completing computer-assisted instruction.

Competency based nursing orientation is an objective means by which to assess the nurse's ability to provide safe, quality patient care. Advantages of this orientation program include the following:

1. Goals and objectives of the program set clear expectations.
2. Self-assessed needs of the orientee will decrease the amount of time necessary to orient nurses through the development of a personalized orientation.
3. Cost effectiveness resulting from employee satisfaction and ultimately, retention.
4. Identification of learning needs can be accomplished early to determine length of orientation.
5. Several teaching/learning strategies can be implemented to meet the orientee's individual learning needs.

Competency based orientation does have disadvantages associated with its utilization. These include the following:

1. Time commitment to develop appropriate competencies. Developing personalized orientation plans requires time committed to develop a unique orientation for each new nurse.
2. Inability to adequately assess orientee's ability to complete self-assessment.
3. Scheduling problems resulting from flexibility of orientation for assessment of skills.
4. Support from management and staff to ensure success of the program.

MAINTAINING COMPETENCY

Once competency of skills has been established, it is important to maintain competency. Also, required competencies must be evaluated annually to accommodate competency changes to meet the needs of a changing healthcare environment. Competencies that should be examined on an annual basis include the following:[7]

1. Skills to coincide with emergency department goals and objectives
2. Quality assurance issues as identified through the quality improvement program
3. New skills or use of new equipment
4. High-volume, high-risk skills
5. Low-volume, high-risk skills

These skills can be completed at an annual "Skills Event" or on an individual basis throughout the year. Most often, skill simulation and return demonstration are used to observe competency. Self-learning packets and videotapes or computer-assisted programs with objectives and an evaluation tool may also be used.

Competency based nursing orientation is the most effective means to orient all nurses to the emergency department setting, novice to expert. Through the use of standardized competencies and an individualized self-assessment, each nurse will be able to create an orientation program that will meet his or her specific learning needs. Mastery of the role of staff nurse through a competency based nursing orientation will ensure nursing management that the nurse has the skills and knowledge to deliver safe, quality nursing care.

REFERENCES

1. Del Bueno DJ, Altano R: Competency-based education: no magic feather, *Nurs Manage* 15:48-53, 1984.
2. Benner P, Tanner C, Chesea C: From beginner to expert: gaining a differential clinical world in critical care nursing, *Adv Nurs Sci* 14:13-28, 1992.
3. Joint Commission of Accreditation of Health Care Organizations: Management of human resources. In *Accreditation manuel for hospitals,* Chicago, 1995, JCAHO.
4. Sedlak SK: Creative approaches to competency-based orientation and continuing education in the emergency department, *Leadersh Manage Emerg Nurs* 1:3-17, 1992.
5. Dunn SV: Orientation: the transition from novice to competent critical care nurse, *Crit Care Nurs Q* 15:69-77, 1992.
6. Asselin ME, Barber ED: Unit orientation for experienced nurses: process and evaluation, *J Nurs Staff Develop* 7:126-129, 1991.
7. Snyder-Halpern R, Buczkowski E: Performance based staff development: a baseline for clinical competence, *J Nursing Staff Develop* 6(1)7-12, 1990.

APPENDIX

A Sentara Hospital's Emergency Department's Registered Nurse Verification of Orientation Competencies

I. COMPETENCY: Complies with emergency procedures.

SELF ASSESSMENT N = NO EXP. E = EXP.	INSTRUCTION METHOD S = SLP C = CLASS CL = CLINICAL V = VIDEO	PERFORMANCE CRITERIA	COMPETENCY VERIFICATION Self Study (S) Written Test (WT) Observation (O) Verbalization (V) DATE/INITIALS
		• Demonstrates Code Cart readiness check.	
		• Demonstrates role in cardiac arrest through successful completion of Defib/Cardioversion or Megacode according to hospital standards.	
		• Discusses RACE procedure, locates fire equipment and O_2 shut valves according to hospital standards.	
		• State procedure to report a fire.	
		• Identified role in evacuation plans for the unit according to hospital standards.	
		• Identifies role in bomb threat according to hospital standards.	
		• Locate and discuss utilization of decontamination room.	
		• Verbalizes role in disaster (Radiation, Haz Mat, Internal & External).	
		• Verbalizes role in dealing with internal crisis - hostage situation, violent patients	
		• Verbalizes the role of security in the ED.	
		• Identifies security measures in place in the ED.	

Comments:

II. COMPETENCY: Complies with safety procedures.

SELF ASSESSMENT N = NO EXP. E = EXP.	INSTRUCTION METHOD S = SLP C = CLASS CL = CLINICAL V = VIDEO	PERFORMANCE CRITERIA	COMPETENCY VERIFICATION Self Study (S) Written Test (T) Observation (O) Verbalization (V) DATE/INITIALS
		• Demonstrate the use of :	
		- Universal Precautions, PPE	
		- HazMat Spill Kit including access, utilization and replacement.	
		- Panic Alarms	
		• Locate MSDS	
		• Demonstrates isolation techniques per guidelines.	
		• Demonstrates reporting of unsafe electrical equipment.	
		• Identifies the location and use of emergency electrical outlets	

Developed by C Abbott-Spears, RN; K Perry, RN; M Snyder, RN; E Rideout, RN; and S Rita, RN.

		• Demonstrates correct use of pediatric restraint.	
		• Demonstrates correct use of adult restraints.	
		• Utilize principles of safe patient care (siderails, positioning to prevent aspiration, call lights).	
Comments:			

III. COMPETENCY: Delivers patient care according to Administrative and Nursing policies and procedures and Emergency Guidelines of Care.

SELF ASSESSMENT N = NO EXP. E = EXP.	INSTRUCTION METHOD S = SLP C = CLASS CL = CLINICAL V = VIDEO	PERFORMANCE CRITERIA	COMPETENCY VERIFICATION Self Study (S) Written Test (T) Observation (O) Verbalization (V) DATE/INITIALS
		• Plans care for pediatric patients utilizing growth and development as a guideline of care.	
		• Demonstrates use of Guidelines of Care, Protocols, and Discharge Instruction sheets in planning patient care.	
		• Read appropriate policies and discuss with Preceptor, Team Coordinator/Manager or Educator. (separate list)	
		• Documents according to governmental laws and facility guidelines in dealing with: - Lifenet - Medical Examiner Case (including gunshots/stab wounds) - Policy Procedures * Collection of evidence, chain of custody. * Consent for care of a minor * Abuse, domestic violence, sexual assault * Animal bites * Legal blood alcohol	
Comments:			

IV. COMPETENCY: Complies with performance standards as a team member in the licensed Clinical Associate role..

SELF ASSESSMENT N = NO EXP. E = EXP.	INSTRUCTION METHOD S = SLP C = CLASS CL = CLINICAL V = VIDEO	PERFORMANCE CRITERIA	COMPETENCY VERIFICATION Self Study (S) Written Test (T) Observation (O) Verbalization (V) DATE/INITIALS
		• Effectively communicates with other members of the healthcare team using key principles of interaction management.	
		• Demonstrates leadership principles in the delivery of care.	
		• Meets with unit QI representative to discuss role and responsibilities with current and ongoing monitors and unit QI plan.	
		• Verbalizes the function of the Shared Governance Council.	

		• Demonstrates ability to prioritize care.	
		• Demonstrates ability to work independently by completing assignments as directed.	
		• Uses Core/Hear radios to communicate with prehospital providers.	
Comments:			

V. COMPETENCY: Complies with medication administration policies and procedures.			
SELF ASSESSMENT N = NO EXP. E = EXP.	**INSTRUCTION METHOD S = SLP C = CLASS CL = CLINICAL V = VIDEO**	**PERFORMANCE CRITERIA**	**COMPETENCY VERIFICATION Self Study (S) Written Test (T) Observation (O) Verbalization (V) DATE/INITIALS**
		• Administers medications per policy according to the five rights of medication administration.	
		• Assesses allergies to medications.	
		• Administers medications via the following routes:	
		- PO	
		- IM	
		- Subcutaneous	
		- Topical	
		- Ophthalmic	
		- Rectal	
		- Otic	
		- Sublingual	
		- IV Push Meds.	
		- IVPB	
		• Describe the process of the use of intra-osseous infusions in pediatric patients.	
		• Obtains medications from the Pyxis machines (if applicable).	
		• Administer medication to pediatric patients via the following routes:	
		- IM	
		- IV	
		- Otic	
		- PO	
		• Documents medication administration on E.D. chart.	
		• Assesses and documents effectiveness of medications/reassesses as needed.	
		• Administers IV conscious sedation per hospital policy and guideline of care.	
		• Documents discharge instructions according to hospital policy.	

Comments:

VI. COMPETENCY: Complies with IV Therapy policies and procedures.			
SELF ASSESSMENT **N = NO EXP.** **E = EXP**	**INSTRUCTION METHOD** **S = SLP** **C = CLASS** **CL = CLINICAL** **V = VIDEO**	**PERFORMANCE CRITERIA**	**COMPETENCY VERIFICATION** **Self Study (S)** **Written Test (T)** **Observation (O)** **Verbalization (V)** **DATE/INITIALS**
		• Completes IV therapy competency	
		• Completes Phlebotomy competency.	
		• Demonstrates use of correct IV administration set for Blood Administration, Pumps, Buretrols, Saline Lock.	
		• Demonstrates use and management of IV infusion pump according to hospital standards.	
		• Administers blood products according to hospital policies and procedures.	
		• Accesses VADS according to Guidelines of Care.	
		• Initiate and maintains IV access and maintenance for pediatric patients.	

Comments:

VII. COMPETENCY: Documents nursing care on the patient record according to hospital standards.			
SELF ASSESSMENT **N = NO EXP.** **E = EXP.**	**INSTRUCTION METHOD** **S = SLP** **C = CLASS** **CL = CLINICAL** **V = VIDEO**	**PERFORMANCE CRITERIA**	**COMPETENCY VERIFICATION** **Self Study (S)** **Written Test (T)** **Observation (O)** **Verbalization (V)** **DATE/INITIALS**
		• Completes initial triage assessment upon arrival and documents on triage form.	
		• Documentation reflects the category of the triaged acuity level.	
		• Performs primary and secondary assessment according to chief complaint and documents.	
		• Completes documentation of AMA.	
		• Completes documentation of patient transfer to outside institution.	
		• Complies with valuables policy.	
		• Discusses discharge instructions and followup with patient/SO.	
		• Completes documentation for patient discharge (nursing note, charges, acuity level).	
		• Discharges patient through Technicon.	

		• Communicates with other members of the health care team to provide continuity of care (nursing report).	

Comments:

VIII. COMPETENCY: Demonstrates primary and secondary assessment according to the chief complaint.

SELF ASSESSMENT N = NO EXP. E = EXP	INSTRUCTION METHOD S = SLP C = CLASS CL = CLINICAL V = VIDEO	PERFORMANCE CRITERIA	COMPETENCY VERIFICATION Self Study (S) Written Test (T) Observation (O) Verbalization DATE/INITIALS
		INITIAL ASSESSMENT (Appropriate Performance of the following)	
		• Demonstrate understanding of primary and secondary assessment .	
		• Interview and assess patient as appropriate to obtain and document a pertinent history.	
		• Uses records from transferring hospitals to assist with obtaining patient history.	
		• Demonstrate understanding of ED assessment document and guideline for its use. (Reviews document with preceptor).	

Comments:

IX. COMPETENCY: Demonstrates the nursing process in integumentary system care.

Self Assessment N = No Exp. E = Exp	Instruction Method S = SLP C = Class CL = Clinical V = VIDEO	PERFORMANCE CRITERIA	COMPETENCY VERIFICATION Self Study (S) Written Test (T) Observation (O) Verbalization (V) DATE/INITIALS
		• Implements wound care:	
		- Sets up suture tray and prepares patient for procedure.	
		- Wound irrigation/cleansing, pre and post examination and repair.	
		- Application of Steri Strips	
		- Suture/Staple Removal	
		- Dressing Applications/changes	
		- Burns: Debridement, application of dressing, dressing changes	
		• Performs and documents local infiltration per protocol. (SHGH)	
		• Performs and documents digital blocks per protocol. (SHGH)	

		• Evaluates patient's understanding of plan of care and expected outcomes as shown by verbalization of discharge instructions.	
		• Completes vaccination forms per protocol for all tetanus boosters.	
		• Assesses comfort and plans to alleviate discomfort.	
		• Implement and evaluate plan to alleviate discomfort.	
Comments:			

X. COMPETENCY: Demonstrates the nursing process in neurological patient care.

SELF ASSESSMENT N = NO EXP. E = EXP.	INSTRUCTION METHOD S = SLP C = CLASS CL = CLINICAL V = VIDEO	PERFORMANCE CRITERIA	COMPETENCY VERIFICATION Self Study (S) Written Test (T) Observation (O) Verbalization (V) DATE/INITIALS
		• Begins neuro assessment based on Triage/Admission forms.	
		• Performs secondary assessment and develops plan of care.	
		• Prepares patient for examination/surgery as indicated.	
		• Assists physician with lumbar puncture.	
		• Assesses pain and plans care to alleviate pain.	
		• Maintains cervical stabilization.	
		• Evaluate fetal heart tones.	
		• Obtains and interprets diagnostic lab values.	
		• Identifies and implements plan of care for patients experiencing neurological dysfunction.	
		• Administers neuromuscular blocking agents and sedatives safely and effectively.	
		• Monitors patient for physical and psychological needs.	
		• Provides nursing care per protocol/guidelines of care for patients with:	
		- Headaches	
		- Seizures	
		- CVA/TIA	
		- Concussion/Contusion	
		- Low Back Pain	
		- ICH or Bleeds	
		- Spinal Cord Injuries	
		- Skull Fractures	
		• Implement protocol for identification of potential organ donors.	
		• Provides patient/family education as indicated.	
		• Evaluates patient response to, and understanding of, plan of care and expected outcomes.	

Comments:

XI. COMPETENCY: Demonstrates the nursing process in cardiovascular care.			
SELF ASSESSMENT N = NO EXP. E = EXP.	INSTRUCTION METHOD S = SLP C = CLASS CL = CLINICAL V = VIDEO	PERFORMANCE CRITERIA	COMPETENCY VERIFICATION Self Study (S) Written Test (T) Observation (O) Verbalization (V) DATE/INITIALS
		• Begin assessment for the cardiovascular system according to triage criteria.	
		• Perform secondary assessment as indicated.	
		• Establishes level of chest pain according to 1 - 10 scale.	
		• Obtain and interpret diagnostic tests and Lab values: Cardiac Monitoring, Pulse Oximeter, ABGs, and 12-Lead EKG	
		• Identifies nursing diagnoses and plan of care for the patient with cardiovascular problems.	
		• Identifies:	
		- Sinus rhythm	
		- Supra-ventricular tachycardia	
		- Ventricular arrhythmias	
		- Heart block (1st, 2nd, and 3rd Degree)	
		- Aystole/PEA	
		- Atrial fibrillation/flutter	
		• Anticipate appropriate emergency response to life threatening dysrhythmia according to ACLS protocol.	
		• Implements cardiac clinical paths	
		• Implements care based on plan:	
		- Operation of external pacemaker (see competency).	
		- Administration of thrombolytic therapy.	
		Provides nursing care for the patient with the following:	
		- Sickle Cell	
		- Thrombophlebitis	
		- Congestive Heart Failure/Pulmonary Edema	
		- MI	
		- Angina	
		- Hypertension	
		• Evaluates patient response and understanding of plan of care and expected patient outcome.	

Comments:

XII. COMPETENCY: Demonstrates the nursing process in pulmonary care.

SELF ASSESSMENT N = NO EXP. E = EXP.	INSTRUCTION METHOD S = SLP C = CLASS V = VIDEO CL = CLINICAL	PERFORMANCE CRITERIA	COMPETENCY VERIFICATION Self Study (S) Written Test (T) Observation (O) Verbalization(V) DATE/INITIALS
		● Begins assessment for the respiratory system according to triage criteria.	
		● Performs primary and secondary assessment of the respiratory system.	
		● Obtains and interprets diagnostic tests and lab values (ABGs, and pulse oximeter).	
		● Identifies plan of care for respiratory patients according to standard of care.	
		● Implements care based on plan:	
		- Maintains a patent airway and adequate ventilation.	
		- Sets up and administers 0_2 (completes competency).	
		- Inserts and maintains oropharyngeal /nasopharyngeal airway.	
		- Sets up suction equipment (completes competency).	
		- Performs suction of patient: Oral, NT, ET, Tracheal, bulb syringe (infant).	
		● Demonstrates patient education on use of peak flow meter.	
		● Administers hand-held nebulizer (completes competency).	
		● Administers Meter Dose Inhaler (completes competency).	
		• Performs collection of sputum specimens.	
		• Performs collection of ABGs (completes competency). (SHGH)	
		• Demonstrates care of the mechanically ventilated patient.	
		• Obtains supplies and prepares patient, and assists with chest tube insertion.	
		● Complete TB SLP.	
		● Identify potential communicable diseases and implement isolation.	
		● Evaluates patient's response and understanding to plan of care and expected outcomes.	

Comments:

XIII. COMPETENCY: Demonstrates the nursing process in the care of GI emergencies.

SELF ASSESSMENT N = NO EXP. E = EXP.	INSTRUCTION METHOD S = SLP C = CLASS CL = CLINICAL V = VIDEO	PERFORMANCE CRITERIA	COMPETENCY VERIFICATION Self Study (S) Written Test (T) Observation (O) Verbalization (V) DATE/INITIALS
		• Begins assessment of gastrointestinal system and documents on Triage/ Admission form.	
		• Performs secondary assessment and develops plan of care.	
		• Prepares patient for examination.	
		• Obtains lab specimens requested.	
		• Collects specimens as indicated and documents appropriately: - Gastrocult/Hemocult (SHGH)	
		- Stool Specimen	
		• Performs the following correctly and documents appropriately results, patient tolerance, supplies used: - NG Tube	
		- Ewald Tube - Gastric Lavage	
		• Evaluates patient's response to medications, treatment.	

Comments:

XIV. COMPETENCY: Demonstrates the nursing process in general medical emergencies.

SELF ASSESSMENT N = NO EXP. E = EXP.	INSTRUCTION METHOD S = SLP C = CLASS CL = CLINICAL V = VIDEO	PERFORMANCE CRITERIA	COMPETENCY VERIFICATION Self Study (S) Written Test (T) Observation (O) Verbalization (V) DATE/INITIALS
		• Performs assessment of patient with communicable or infectious diseases, fluid and electrolyte disturbances, endocrine and hematologic disorders	
		• Obtains blood sugars with Glucometer according to hospital standards (see competency).	
		• Identifies nursing diagnoses and plan of care for patients with medical disorders.	

Comments:

XIV. COMPETENCY: Demonstrates the nursing process in orthopedic emergency care: Specific soft tissue - Contusions, Sprains, and Strains, Bony Skeleton - Dislocations, Fractures, Traumatic Amputation, Life Threatening: Hemorrhage from Fractures, Fat Embolism Syndrome, Compartment Syndrome.

SELF ASSESSMENT N = NO EXP. E = EXP.	INSTRUCTION METHOD S = SLP C = CLASS V = VIDEO CL = CLINICAL	PERFORMANCE CRITERIA	COMPETENCY VERIFICATION Self Study (S) Written Test (T) Observation (O) Verbalization (V) DATE/INITIALS
		• Performs primary and secondary assessment for musculoskeletal system (including neurovascular assessment).	
		• Obtains and interprets diagnostic lab values and tests.	
		• Identifies plan of care for patients with musculoskeletal conditions.	
		• Demonstrates need for and use of ring cutter.	
		• Applies and/or assesses immobilizers:	
		- Stiff Neck Collar	
		- Soft Cervical Collar	
		- Limb Immobilizers (slings, braces, etc.)	
		- Splints	
		• Provides care of partial and complete amputations.	
		• Recognizes and reports signs and symptoms of compartment syndrome.	
		• Assists with cast saw.	
		• Provides instruction and assists in the use of assistive devices:	
		- Canes	
		- Walkers	
		- Crutches	
		• Evaluates and prepares patient for surgery.	
		• Evaluates patient's response to and understanding of plan of care and expected outcomes.	

Comments:

XVI. COMPETENCY: Demonstrates the nursing process in genitourinary emergencies.

SELF ASSESSMENT N = NO EXP. E = EXP.	INSTRUCTION METHOD S = SLP C = CLASS CL = CLINICAL V = VIDEO	PERFORMANCE CRITERIA	COMPETENCY VERIFICATION Self Study (S) Written Test (T) Observation (O) Verbalization (V) DATE/INITIALS
		• Performs primary and secondary assessment for genitourinary system complaints.	
		• Identifies plan of care for renal care.	
		• Performs and maintains urinary catheters: Straight, Foley	

		• Provides care for patients with:	
		- Testicular Torsion	
		- Epididymitis	
		- UTI	
		- Renal Calculi	
		• Obtains urine specimen:	
		- Clean Catch	
		- Straight Catheterization	
		- Foley Catheterization	
		- Dipstick	
		• Evaluates patient's response to and understanding of plan of care and expected outcomes.	

Comments:

XVII.	**COMPETENCY:**	**Demonstrates the nursing process in obstetrical/gynecological emergencies.**	
SELF ASSESSMENT **N = NO EXP.** **E = EXP.**	**INSTRUCTION METHOD** **S = SLP** **C = CLASS** **CL = CLINICAL** **V = VIDEO**	**PERFORMANCE CRITERIA**	**COMPETENCY VERIFICATION** **Self Study (S)** **Written Test (T)** **Observation (O)** **Verbalization(V)** **DATE/INITIALS**
		• Performs primary and secondary (as indicated) assessment of reproductive system.	
		• Completes assessment of GYN history, maternal history for pregnant patient.	
		• Evaluate fetal heart tones	
		• Obtains and interprets diagnostic lab values and tests.	
		• Demonstrates ability to assist with pelvic exams and collect specimens.	
		• Demonstrates ability to conduct Perk exams.	
		• Demonstrates proper procedure for dealing with victims of sexual abuse.	
		- Provide emotional support	
		- Maintains chain of custody.	
		- Document accurately.	
		• Assesses fetal heart tone measurement.	
		• Implements care for the following based on plan including:	
		- STD/PID	
		- Post-abortion/miscarriage	
		- Ectopic Pregnancy	
		- Sexual Assault - Calls CONTACT or RESPONSE	

		- Obstetrical Emergencies	
		- Precipitant Deliveries (completes competency).	
		• Prepares patient for surgery as indicated.	
		• Evaluates pt. response to & understanding of plan of care & expected outcome.	

XVIII. COMPETENCY: Demonstrates the nursing process in psychiatric emergencies.

SELF ASSESSMENT N = NO EXP. E = EXP.	INSTRUCTION METHOD S = SLP C = CLASS CL = CLINICAL V = VIDEO	PERFORMANCE CRITERIA	COMPETENCY VERIFICATION Self Study (S) Written Test (T) Observation (O) Verbalization (V) DATE/INITIALS
		• Performs assessment for psychiatric complaints.	
		• Identifies nursing diagnoses and plan of care for psychosocial care.	
		• Provides nursing care for patient with Suicidal Behavior, Homicidal/Violent Behavior, Situational Crisis/Anxiety.	
		• Maintains confidentiality: performs patient care based on patient bill of rights.	
		• Demonstrates knowledge of local support agencies (Community Resource Book).	

Comments:

XIX. Demonstrates the nursing procession EENT Emergencies

		• Assess visual activity on all eye problems.	
		• Implement proper procedures for removal of contact lens	
		• Review policy re: ABA criteria for transfer	
		• Demonstrate proper use of Morgan lens for eye irrigation	
		• Initiate independent nursing actions to treat epistaxis	
		• Assist with nasal packing	

Comments:

XX. COMPETENCY: Demonstrates the nursing process in patient education.

SELF ASSESSMENT N = NO EXP. E = EXP.	INSTRUCTION METHOD S = SLP C = CLASS CL = CLINICAL V = VIDEO	PERFORMANCE CRITERIA	COMPETENCY VERIFICATION Self Study (S) Written Test (T) Observation (O) Verbalization (V) DATE/INITIALS
		• Determines patient's knowledge and needs re: discharge instructions/home care.	
		• Identifies teaching tools specific to patient diagnosis.	

		• Provides appropriate information to patient according to cognitive or educational need (discharge instruction sheets).	
		• Evaluates and documents patient/s.o. response to discharge instructions.	
Comments:			
XXI. Competency: Triage Nursing Care			
SELF ASSESSMENT N = NO EXP. E = EXP.	INSTRUCTION METHOD S = SLP C = CLASS CL = CLINICAL V = VIDEO	PERFORMANCE CRITERIA	COMPETENCY VERIFICATION **Self Study (S)** **Written Test (T)** **Observation (O)** **Verbalization (V)** DATE/INITIALS
		• Interview and assess as appropriate to obtain and document a pertinent history.	
		• Identify potential communicable diseases and implement isolation.	
		• Prioritize patients according to triage protocols.	
		• Triage patients to an appropriate area in the ED as swiftly as possible.	
		• Direct appropriate patients and families to crisis intervention.	
		• Demonstrate the proper use of the TTY Phone.	
		• Verbalizes use of the security panic button and identifies location.	
		• Identifies common characteristics of non-accidental trauma and states mechanism to report.	
Comments:			
XXII. Burn Nursing Care			
		• Appropriately calculate TBSA	
		• State Parkland formula for fluid resuscitation. Calculate 1 fluid resuscitation requirement (use scenario if necessary).	
		• Review policy re: ABA criteria for transfer.	
XXIII. Pediatric Trauma Nursing Care			
		• Complete pediatric trauma SLP	
		• Demonstrate usage of:	
		- Pediatric pulse oximeter	
		- Pediatric B/P cuff	
		- IO	
		- Braslow tape/bag	
		- Pedi u-bags	
		• State calculation for fluid resuscitation. Appropriately compute 2 scenarios	

		• Discuss the Pediatric CQI - Assess fluid volume status through 5 parameters of assessment (SNGH)	
		- Weight	
		- HR	
		- RR	
		- Lung sounds	
		- Capillary Refill	

XXIV. Competency: Trauma Nursing Care

SELF ASSESSMENT N = NO EXP. E = EXP.	INSTRUCTION METHOD S = SLP C = CLASS CL = CLINICAL V = VIDEO	PERFORMANCE CRITERIA	COMPETENCY VERIFICATION Self Study (S) Written Test (T) Observation (O) Verbalization (V) DATE/INITIALS
		• Describe infection control procedures used in the Trauma Bays including Room #2 (Burns)	
		• Locate in the Trauma Bay:	
		- masks, hats, gowns	
		- long sleeved gowns	
		- high top boots	
		- gloves (sterile & nonsterile)	
		• Locate trauma packs and name contents.	
		• Locate trauma log - complete x 2 - Tr pt # ________________ - Tr pt # ________________	
		• Relate difference between alpha and bravo traumas	
		• Complete trauma checklist x 3 - Date ________ - Date ________ - Date ________	
		• Demonstrates ability to complete all documentation on trauma flow sheet and trauma registry sheet x 3 - ____________ - ____________ - ____________	
		• Describe contents of anesthesia cabinet, state purpose for equipment, restock x 2 - Date ___________ - Date ___________	
		• Describe complete process to restock cabinet	
		• Locate the following items and describe purpose:	
		- thoracotomy trays	
		- combo tray	
		- ambu bags	
		- Life Pak 8	
		- Life Pak 10	

		- Atrium/chest tubes	
		- pressure infusers	
		- plastics and suture tray	
		• Identifies indications for peritoneal lavage.	
		- Locates equipment necessary for peritoneal lavage	
		• Identify situations that massive transfusion is indicated	
		• Describe the process to activate the massive transfusion protocol	
		• Complete SLPs	
		- Arterial pressure monitoring	
		- Ventriculostomy	
		- MAST	
		- Autotransfusion	
		- Internal defibrillation	

80 Nurse Retention and Development

Janet Gren Parker

OUTLINE

Retention and development are words used practically every day by someone in the nursing profession. In fact, they are used so frequently they are often no longer heard even when spoken. Initiating and maintaining the enthusiasm necessary to create an environment that fosters retention and development require dynamic, transforming leadership, not merely lip service.

What does retention really mean? If the emergency department's turnover rate is less than the current national norm is retention in the department satisfactory? Or does a certain percentage of nurses have to have been in the department for 10 years? There is no national standard by which retention is measured. The same is true for professional development. Each nurse in the department would probably define development differently. Some employees feel that the yearly mandatory inservices are development enough (they remind everyone every time they are "forced" to attend), whereas others think the hospital should have multiple degree programs readily available to them.

Leaders must have the ability to create a culture of excellence among the emergency department team. Attributes of excellence are encompassed in leaders who have power; are visionary; communicate ideas, values, and goals; and function as a team. Components of transformational leadership revolve around the attributes needed to create a culture of excellence. This culture is created by a leader with core values that are lived and clearly articulated. Most nurses see themselves as knowledgeable, respected professionals; but the nurses' self-image differs from what is perceived as the hospital's image of a nurse. Nurses believe that hospitals see them as workers or bureaucratic employees[1] (Table 80-1).

Today's challenge is to take the self-image of nurses and extrapolate that image to the culture of the department and/or hospital. Creating such a culture of excellence will have a significant impact on the retention and development of the nurse in the emergency department.

IDEALS TO ACHIEVE SUCCESS

New ways to achieve retention and promote development involve some revolutionary thinking and behavior by risk-taking leaders and empowered staff.

Organizational Structure

To create a culture that supports and encourages empowered employees, the actual organizational structure needs to be as "flat" as possible, promoting decision-making authority and accountability by staff. Three to five layers of leadership (Figure 80-1) between the staff and chief executive officer are preferable in an empowered environment. If there are more layers, empowerment is difficult, if not impossible.

The reporting relationship of leaders in the department has traditionally been along functional lines of responsibility. The feeling of teamwork and team building by empowered staff is difficult to create and maintain in such a structure. An organizational triad with multidisciplinary responsibilities is more conducive to a culture of excellence (Figure 80-1, *C*). Each discipline involved in the leadership of the emergency department is represented and works with each other to provide the necessary leadership for the department. This team or triad approach must occur with the leaders of the department or the team approach will not be successful at the bedside.

Leadership

Retention and development are enhanced with a high quality leadership team. Leaders should be creating vision, clarifying issues and generating enthusiasm in all staff. Visibility is extremely important. It is difficult, if not impossible, to create enthusiasm and clarify issues if no one ever sees the leadership team on an off shift or on the weekend. Leaders should follow through on daily events and be accessible, as needed, for any staff members. Staff need formal and informal interaction opportunities with their leaders. Risk taking needs to be allowed and encouraged. The promotion of staff leadership in the department has a positive impact on nursing job satisfaction and retention.

Management Styles

Professional staff do not need managers but require leaders. It does not matter whether the management style used is participatory, democratic, or autocratic; all of these styles will eventually fail. Facilitators, coordinators, or team leaders are more appropriate in the place of managers because staff should resolve issues rather than implement decisions from above.

Shared governance is a popular term that is used to describe management styles of the 1990s. Frequently, however, this term is verbalized and written about and held up as the style being used when final decisions are still made by some authority/management figure. Shared governance is certainly a concept that helps create a culture of excellence. The most devastating outcome is to espouse shared governance, but still have the management group approve each decision made by staff. If problem-solving issues are delegated to a group, that group must also have the accountability and authority that accompanies the outcome.

Self-governance is frequently used simultaneously with shared governance, but it is a different concept. In a self-governance model, the professional staff are totally autonomous, with no designated management position in place; They literally govern themselves. This approach requires a highly developed, motivated group of professionals. It may be the model of the future resulting from an outgrowth of departments that currently utilize shared governance.

Table 80-1 Image of Nursing

Attribute	Nurses' perception of own image	Hospitals' image
Knowledgeable professional	68%	20%
Humanitarian worker	14%	28%
Bureaucratic employee	4%	21%
Physician's handmaiden	2%	11%
Clerk/white-collar worker	2%	10%

From Kramer M, Schmalenberg C: *Nurs 91* 21:51-55, 1991.

Climate and Self-Image

The staff nurse role must be seen as one of competence, power, pride, and worth. With this view of themselves, nurses tend to have a high level of job satisfaction (defined as going home at the end of a shift and "feeling good"). Highly satisfied nurses tend to remain in their respective positions. In the emergency department, to create a positive climate and a strong self-image, nurses must be seen as respected colleagues and professional members of the healthcare team.

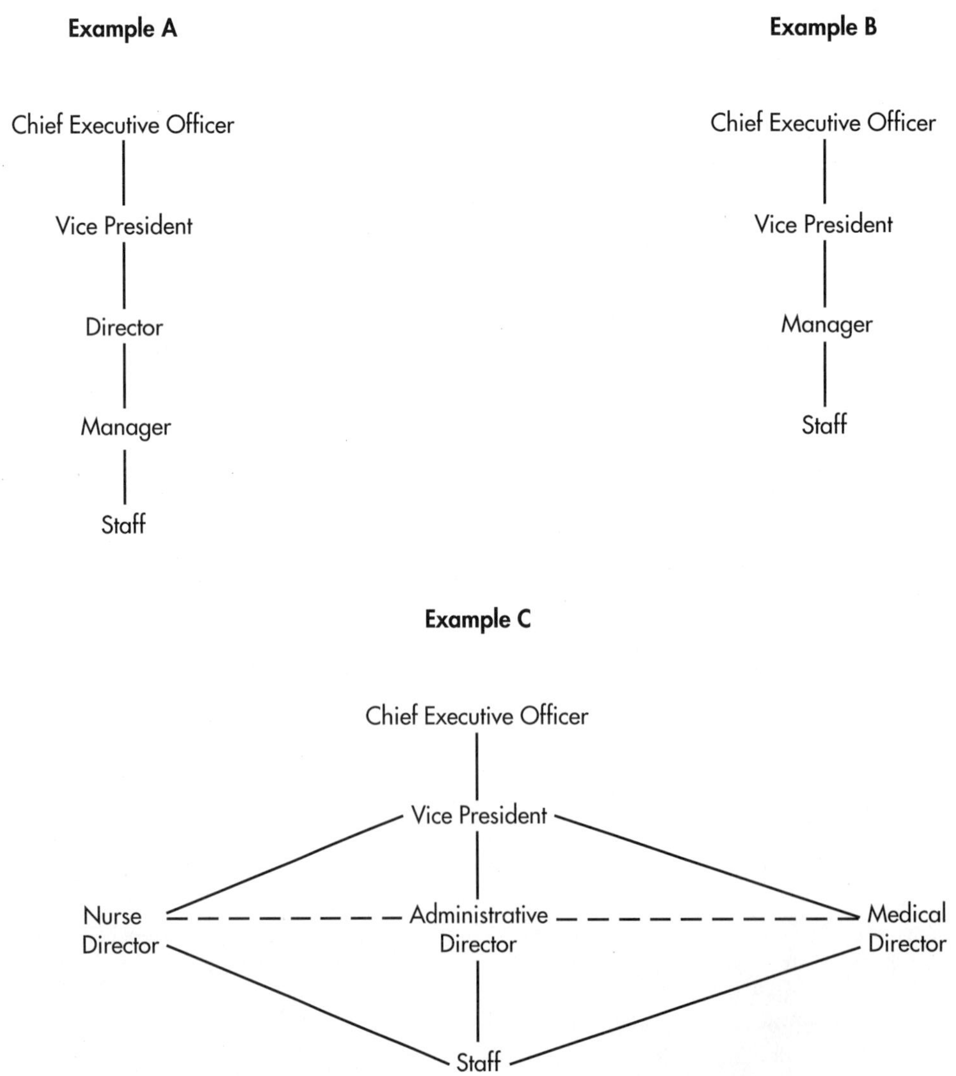

FIGURE 80-1 Leadership layers in empowered environments.

THE ECONOMIC PERSPECTIVE

Economic issues will be on the agenda of almost every meeting. Particularly as costs escalate and reimbursement declines, financial issues will remain a top priority. Direct costs related to retention and development are relatively easy to quantify. Indirect costs are more difficult to determine and quantify, but are just as important. Dollars spent on retention and development are easier to justify if one considers the dollars necessary to replace a nurse, particularly the dollars necessary to replace an experienced emergency nurse. Box 80-1 illustrates the direct and indirect cost factors that must be considered.

Turnover Costs

Turnover costs vary among institutions, depending on hourly wage rates, difficulty in replacing the staff nurse, institutional benefit costs, and whether the turnover or replacement involves an experienced nurse or a new graduate. Some institutions view turnover as "natural" or an expected cost of operation. These institutions do not include generic advertising and recruiting costs because these costs occur regardless of the turnover rate. Accumulated benefit payoffs for the departing nurse may not be included in some settings because these may be costed out on financial statements on a monthly basis as earned by each staff member. If this is the case, they should not be double counted when calculating turnover costs.

Orientation Costs

Table 80-2 illustrates one method of costing out orientation.[2] The dollar and hour amounts are arbitrary numbers used for this example. Institutional specific data would need to be inserted into the categories. This method illustrates the striking difference in costs between the new graduate and the experienced nurse. The learning curve difference between the two is not part of the model. Factoring in the time necessary to achieve total productivity during hours worked (learning curve) would highlight the differences even more between the new graduate and the experienced nurse.

Public Relations/Referral Impact

Frequently overlooked when examining the economic impact of retention is lost revenue related to dissatisfied patients, families, physicians, and Emergency Medical Services (EMS). This factor is extremely difficult to quantify and may be impossible to assess until enough time has elapsed to note changes in referral patterns and decreasing numbers of emergency department visits—unless, of course, a major referrer (such as a specialty physician or a particular EMS company) becomes dissatisfied and communicates changes directly to someone in the emergency department or hospital system. Monthly tracking of patient complaints and/or patients leaving without being seen might provide a more timely pattern, indicating a problem. If the department remains understaffed for a relatively long period, length of stay for patients may increase dramatically, influencing their satisfaction and willingness to return for other situations. This potential lost revenue should not be ignored as insignificant when justifying short-term staffing and higher staffing costs during periods of turnover.

MECHANISMS TO PROMOTE RETENTION AND DEVELOPMENT

Once the culture of excellence is established with the appropriate creative leaders in place, it is time to implement specific strategies to promote retention and development. These

BOX 80-1

ECONOMIC CONSIDERATIONS IN RECRUITMENT AND RETENTION

Direct cost factors

- Advertisements
- Use of recruitment firms
- Manager interview time
- Preceptor hours
- Educator hours
- Temporary replacement cost

Indirect cost factors

- Accumulated benefit payoff
- Nurse recruiter hours
- Processing cost of new employee (i.e., creating personnel file, physicial examination, processing benefit paperwork, etc.)
- Loss of efficiency and productivity of team as a result of temporary replacement staff in department
- Benefit cost of all hours including preceptor hours, educator hours, etc.
- Loss of patient revenue if patients, referring physicians, emergency medical services are dissatisfied

Table 80-2 Orientation Costs: New Graduate Versus Experienced Nurse

	New graduate	Experienced
Hourly salaries		
New hire	$14.00	$17.00
Preceptor	$18.00	$18.00
Instructor	$19.00	$19.00
Orientation hours		
Hospital	8	8
Nursing	80	40
Emergency department	160	120
Unit	240	130
TOTAL	488	298
Preceptor hours	220	100
Instructor hours	40	20
Total dollars		
Orientation	$6,832	$5,066
Preceptor	$3,960	$1,800
Instructor	$760	$380
Subtotal	$11,552	$7,246
Benefits (30%)	$3,466	$2,174
TOTAL	$15,018	$9,420

From Blaufuss J, Maynard J, Schollars G: *Nurs Manage* 5:56; 1992.

strategies should be examined for their fiscal implications. Several strategies may help the leaders and staff in the emergency department promote retention and development.

Professional Practice Milieu

The ultimate goal in creating a professional practice milieu is to provide nurses the control they desire over their own practice. Of 808 nurses surveyed by Kramer and Schmalenberg,[1] 82% rated professional practice as a very important aspect. Professional practice is supporting the nurse as an independent, competent decision maker, giving the nurse the freedom to act on what he or she knows. This empowerment, defined as involvement and commitment, ultimately leads to job satisfaction and increased productivity.

Standards of nursing practice and patient care guidelines should be developed and implemented by staff nurses themselves. They need to have the professional autonomy and leadership support to shape their own practice in the emergency department. By encouraging staff to become involved in these projects, personal growth and development are strengthened. The talents of each staff member should be highlighted (e.g., community outreach, research, injury prevention).

The delivery of care method used in the department must be determined by staff nurses in concert with ancillary staff and physicians (see Chapter 23). The delivery model should match staff mix with skill levels. Cross-training of staff is an idea that adds value and worth to the staff role and addresses their development at the same time.

At a minimum, there must be a committee, council, or group that is empowered to establish the delivery of care method in the department. This group may be multidisciplinary encompassing nurses, physicians, and other staff. It must have the freedom to establish the standards of practice and standards of care for the patient populations seen in the department.

Educational Resources

For professional development, some type of educational resources must be available to the department members. The department members are adult learners. This form of learning has been called *andragogy,* the art and science of helping adults learn.

From the theoretical base of andragogy, characteristics of adult learners may affect the resources needed in the department to support staff development. Adult learners have individualistic learning styles. Some like to learn through action and participation, whereas others accomplish more through quiet meditation and reading. There is a constant sensitivity about making mistakes in front of their younger colleagues or peers. This fear may lead to arrogance or quiet, withdrawn behavior. Another characteristic of adult learners is that of resistance to change. Development implies change, which can be threatening to the less flexible, less creative adult learner. Box 80-2 contains examples of resource possibilities for use in the development of emergency department staff.

Creativity is the key to help stimulate excitement in the area of development. Traditional methods such as lectures, seminars, discussion groups, and demonstrations are not as readily received as the more creative development methods that are available today. Examples of creative methods that may be used are listed in Box 80-3.

Evaluation Systems

If the nursing profession wishes to chart its own direction and maintain autonomous practice, it must develop effective methods to evaluate the performance of its members. There is a direct relationship between effective evaluation systems and increased motivation and satisfaction of staff nurses. The older systems, which are subjective, performed by a manager who rarely observes performance, and based on longevity instead of merit, rarely motivate, retain, or develop anyone.

Clinical ladders, developed in the early 1970s, helped recognize the expert bedside care provider. Unfortunately, they were frequently tied to degree attainment, subjective manager evaluations, and activities "above and beyond" the call of duty. Some institutions that implemented clinical ladders had a limited number of spots for level II, III, and IV. If these spots were full and a nurse achieved a new level, she or he may have had to wait for the promotion until a spot was available. Inherent in the use of clinical ladders is the necessity to build in a mechanism that ensures ongoing performance at the level awarded by the clinical ladder.

Peer review is an alternative to the more traditional evaluation methods. The American Nurses Association defines peer review as a process by which registered nurses, actively engaged in practice, assess and judge the performance of professional peers against predetermined standards.[3] Different methods and discussions of this concept can be readily found

BOX 80-2

EDUCATIONAL RESOURCES FOR DEVELOPMENT

Resource	Example
Institutional education specialist	Session on improving delegation skills
Emergency clinical nurse specialist	Design updated triage station
Trauma clinical nurse specialist	Injury prevention brochure development
Joint appointment faculty	Involvement in emergency nursing research
Physicians/staff nurses	Presentations about particular areas of clinical expertise
EMS Liaison Staff	Session on violence in the streets
Public Health Leaders	Update tuberculosis screening protocols
Area Emergency Department Leaders	Collaboration on discharge teaching material
Leadership Staff	Empowerment and shared governance sessions

throughout the nursing literature. There is widespread agreement that the use of peer review increases accountability and fosters a professional practice environment, thereby having a positive impact on retention and development.

Components of any peer review process include a staff nurse's self-evaluation related to accomplishments for the year, at least one peer's evaluation of the staff nurse, and a salary adjustment at the end of the process that is tied to performance or merit instead of longevity.

Financial Incentives

There is nothing more insulting in a culture of excellence and professional autonomy than punching a time clock or hourly reimbursement. The wave of the future is a salary model of compensation that reflects the fact that the professional nurse is reimbursed to do a job—no matter how much time it takes. This is certainly revolutionary thinking in some areas of nursing, but it has been in place for many years in settings such as ambulatory care and public health arenas. When designing a salaried model of compensation, the major issue is the lack of overtime payment and adequate compensation (comp) time.

One method of addressing compensation is bonus payments. Bonus payments also can be incorporated into the performance appraisal system and can replace the old clinical ladder system. One time bonus payments for additional hours over a set amount and/or for project completion and development above normal expectations allows professional nurses to feel justly rewarded for their professional practice.

Nursing group practice is a concept currently thriving, particularly on the East Coast. In this model, nurses form a group practice and contract with the institution to provide a certain number of nursing care hours at a certain price. The nurses hire others into their practice group and usually receive a bonus from the institution if they use fewer supplies and equipment than budgeted in providing care for patients in the department.

One of the biggest dissatisfiers is salary compression. The National Association of Health Care Recruiters states the difference between the average minimum and maximum staff nurse salary is $11,000. The American Hospital Association reports the figure as closer to $8300. [4] Salary compression certainly does not support retention. Salary decompression for nursing will continue to be one of the challenges in the next decade.

BOX 80-3

CREATIVE METHODS FOR DEVELOPMENT

Trivia quiz games
Computer simulation sessions
Interactive videotapes
Situational programed instruction
Journal clubs
Hospital education television channel

Staff Empowerment

Much has been said about staff empowerment in the 1990s. How does it actually work? What are some specific activities that can be used to actually empower staff? No magic formula works in all settings. One must remember that the human variable in empowerment leads to differential problem solving with different groups.

Several basic components of empowerment may be implemented in different ways at different institutions:

Committees or Councils. The backbone of empowerment is that problem solving and decision making are delegated to the affected groups. Some models call such groups committees, councils, task forces, quality circles, or quality improvement work groups. The group must be delegated the authority and accountability to problem solve and make decisions. Figures 80-2 and 80-3 illustrate empowered decision-making

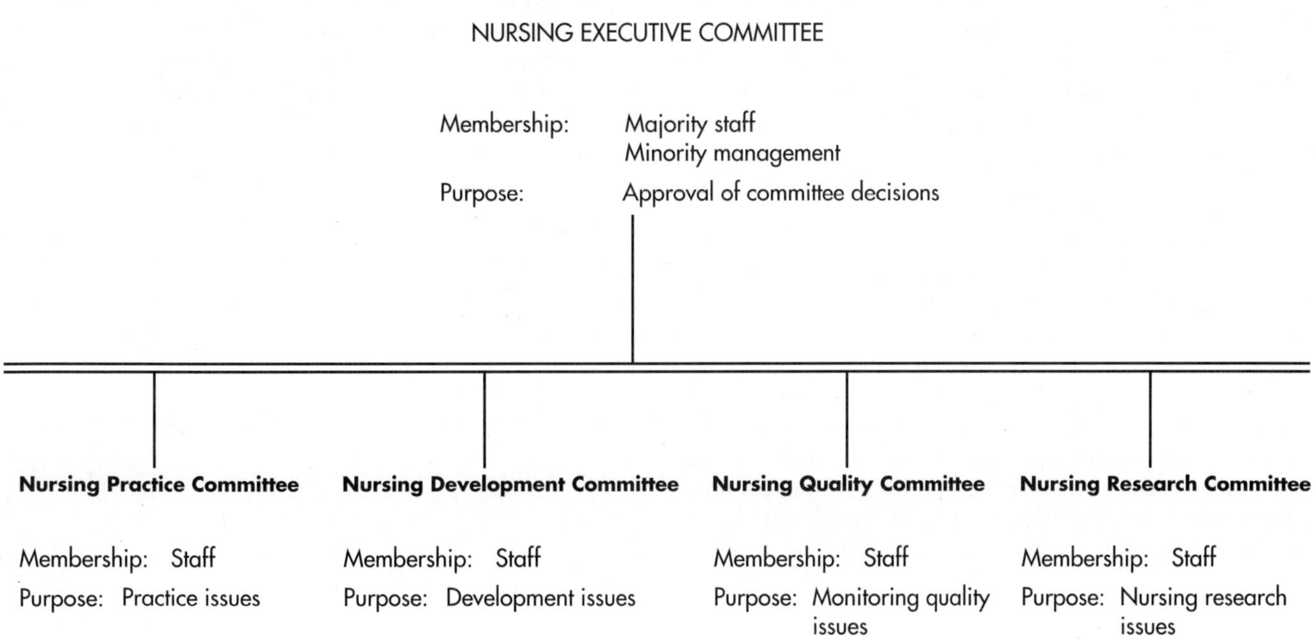
NURSING EXECUTIVE COMMITTEE
Membership: Majority staff
Minority management
Purpose: Approval of committee decisions
Nursing Practice Committee
Membership: Staff
Purpose: Practice issues
Nursing Development Committee
Membership: Staff
Purpose: Development issues
Nursing Quality Committee
Membership: Staff
Purpose: Monitoring quality issues
Nursing Research Committee
Membership: Staff
Purpose: Nursing research issues

FIGURE 80-2 Empowered decision-making model I.

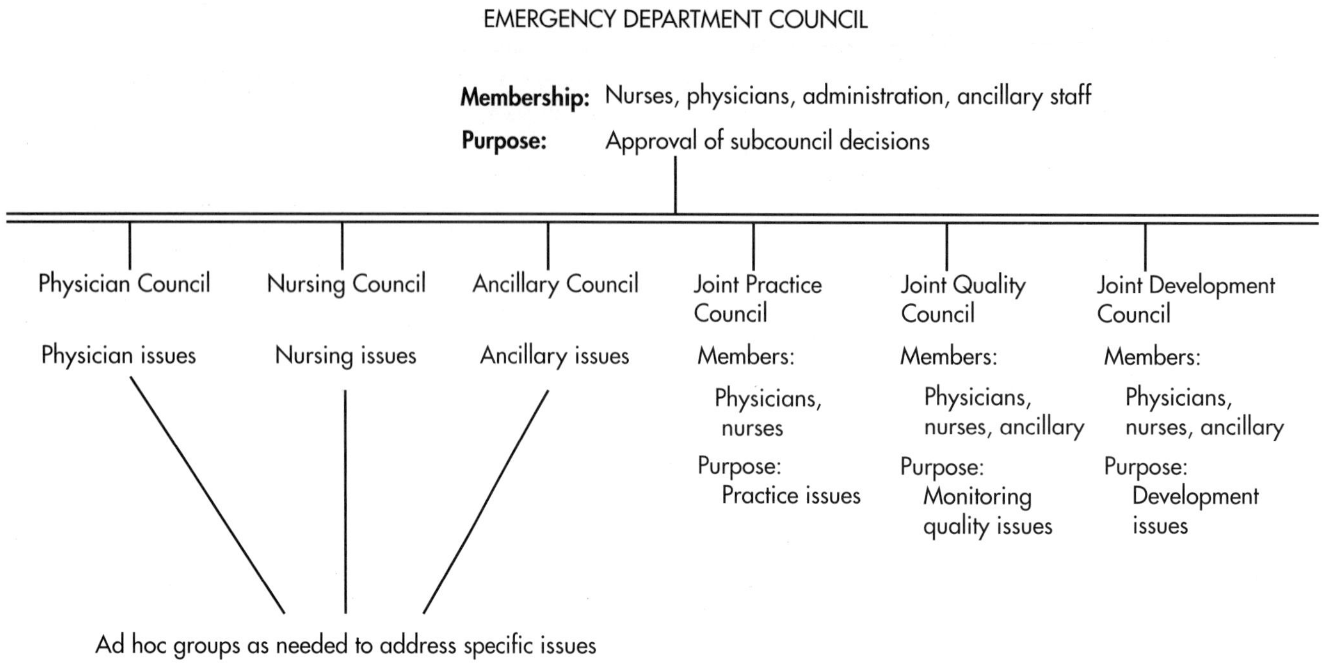

FIGURE 80-3 Empowered decision-making model II.

models. These models could be revised and individualized for specific emergency departments.

Self-Scheduling. Self-scheduling is defined as a process by which the staff of a unit collectively determine and implement their own monthly work schedule.[5] Established criteria are in place to ensure that staffing is adequate to deliver safe, quality patient care. Staff members usually rotate monthly as the schedule coordinator, each taking a turn in coordinating the final schedule. This process certainly provides a mechanism for staff to be responsible and accountable for scheduling. It creates an environment that decreases absenteeism, improves staff relationships, and increases job satisfaction.

Job-Sharing. Because the vast majority of nurses are female, part-time employment is attractive. Job-sharing is one method to make part-time employment as attractive to the institution as it is to certain staff. Job-sharing may offer a solution to the loss of valued staff who require less than full-time employment. It is not the same as two people working two part-time positions. Job-sharing means that two people split the position equally. Benefits are prorated and hours worked are split as are weekends worked, vacations worked, etc. Job-sharing nurses report the highest ratings for job satisfaction and physical health status.[6]

Self-Contained Department. Floating (working in other departments because of an administrative decision) is a source of great dissatisfaction among nurses. Increased job satisfaction is associated with working with other clinically competent nurses.[1] Some would argue that floating staff to critical care helps maintain particular skills and perhaps encourages development and decreases stress. Others would support maintenance of clinical competency from continual assignment to the same department working with the same team members. More creative ways are needed to maintain competence and decrease stress than floating to another unit. Varying assignments within the department, having staff participate in community educational events on paid time, or encouraging committee projects are better ways to promote competence and decrease stress than assigning staff to other units or departments.

SUMMARY

None of the presented principles will, by themselves, create a culture of excellence that encourages retention and development. It is the operation as a whole, the sum of all the principles, that creates and maintains the culture of excellence. It is the ability to synergize the staff to create a department that can synthesize and integrate these principles into a culture of excellence that leads to nurse retention and development. The nursing leader in the emergency department, in concert with the medical and administrative leaders of the department, must together build a culture of excellence for the next decade and beyond.

REFERENCES

1. Kramer M, Schmalenberg C: Job satisfaction and retention—insights for the '90s, Part 1 *Nurs 91* 21:51-55, 1991.
2. Blaufuss J, Maynard J, Schollars G: Methods of evaluating turnover costs, *Nurs Manage* 23:52-59, 1992.
3. *Peer review on nursing practice,* Kansas City, Mo, 1983, ANA.
4. Health care recruitment, *AHA News* 29:3, 1993.
5. Miller N: Job satisfaction through self-scheduling, *Nurs Manage* 23:96B-96D, 1992.
6. Kane D, Kartha A: Job sharing: impact on the general well-being of female nurses, *Can J Nurs Adm* 5:6-10, 1992.

81 Making Sense of Shift Work in Emergency Medicine

Dennis C. Whitehead and Rebecca Smith-Coggins

How can I then return in happy plight,
That am debarr'd the benefit of rest?
When day's oppression is not eas'd by night,
But day by night and night by day oppress'd?
And each, though enemies to either's reign,
Do in consent shake hands to torture me . . .

Shakespeare, *Sonnet* XXVIII

OUTLINE

- Circadian principles and physiology
- Sleep
  - Non-REM (NREM) sleep: brain idle, body mobile
  - REM sleep: brain on, body off
- Alertness and performance
- Changing shifts
- Clockwise versus counterclockwise
- Scheduling strategies
- Preventive countermeasures
  - Sleep hygiene
  - Diet
  - Exercise
- Napping
- Bright light exposure
- Pharmacologic considerations
- Social life
- Operational countermeasures
  - Physical activity
  - Environmental stimulation
- Summary

Shakespeare did not have shift work in mind when he wrote the above; indeed, shift work really was not feasible until the invention of the light bulb at the end of the nineteenth century. The mental torture he described was that of a lover's insomnia, the same anguish those of us who love emergency medicine experience as we work around the clock in service to our patients. The excitement and drama of our chosen specialty has a high price: there is no "down time."

Unless you are in an administrative position with bankers' hours, shift work is simply a fact of life for emergency physicians. Even the seldom practicing department chair with a straight daytime schedule must consider the effects of shift work when making duty rosters and arranging meetings. A large body of research deals with the problems of industrial shift work, a subject that is finally being addressed in the emergency medicine literature.

Shift work is *the* major stressor in emergency medicine. In an early unpublished study by the Behavioral Emergencies Committee of the American College of Emergency Physicians (ACEP), college members were asked to identify the most stressful aspect of emergency medicine. The most common response was "erratic schedule." Shift changes and scheduling difficulties are often cited as dominant causes of stress and career dissatisfaction in emergency medicine.[1,2]

Shift work is a principal reason for the high rate of attrition seen in emergency medicine and thus significantly contributes to the personnel shortage in our specialty. Data from ACEP show a 12% yearly rate of attrition among its members, with fewer than 10% expecting to be practicing emergency medicine in 10 years. This suggests the average full-time clinical practice career in emergency medicine lasts less than a decade, a much lower average than in other specialties.

ACEP leaders realized that this unacceptably high rate of attrition was only partly due to shift work, and that other factors were involved. From these concerns the Well-Being Committee was born. Over the last several years, the committee has identified other relevant factors, but the problem of shift work remains the most important.

To understand fully the best approaches to scheduling in emergency medicine, a brief overview of circadian science is necessary. One note on terminology: *biological rhythms,* such as circadian rhythms, are technically different from *biorhythms,* a term associated with the pseudoscience of forecasting events by means of intellectual, physical, and emotional "cycles." In actual practice, however, *biorhythms* is being used more and more as a substitute term for *biological rhythms,* and for convenience will be so used in this chapter.

CIRCADIAN PRINCIPLES AND PHYSIOLOGY

Observations about the rhythmic nature of animal functions date back at least to the time of Aristotle, who noted swelling of sea urchin ovaries during the full moon. "Sleep movements" of plants were also noted by the ancient Greeks, who ascribed the phenomenon to the presence of sunlight.

de Mairan, in 1729, conducted the first experiment designed to test circadian rhythms in plants. He demonstrated that plant leaves opened in the daytime, even when kept in total darkness. This was the first demonstration of an endogenous biologic clock functioning in the absence of *zeitgebers* ("time givers"). These findings in plants were confirmed by Duhamel in 1758.

The important concept of *free-running* in biologic clocks was discovered in 1832 by de Candolle, who placed *Mimosa* plants in constant bright light. After a few days, the leaves opened and closed on a 22-hour cycle. This showed the plant had its own independent day length. Free-running rhythms, many of them varying significantly from the 24-hour solar day, can be similarly demonstrated for any plant or animal species. In the 1950s Pittendrigh's experiments with fruit flies showed that these biologic clocks were innate and genetically transmitted.[3]

Experiments by many investigators have shown that humans have a *free-running 25-hour clock*.[4,5] Well-controlled studies by Weitzman and Czeisler over 6-month periods showed the 25-hour day to be constant and predictable in all subjects. All mammalian species seem to have their own independent day length. Higher animals also have *infradian* (>daily, as the menstrual cycle) and *ultradian* (<daily, as pulse and respirations) rhythms.

Hunter in 1778 reported a drop to temperature during sleep, which critics attributed to lack of physical activity. Kleitman[6] found that the temperature cycle is controlled by the biologic clock. If a subject is kept at rest in bed and awake for 24 hours, the temperature falls during the night and rises again the next day. Further studies by him showed if the subject is kept awake nights and sleeps during the day, the temperature cycle will eventually transpose to accommodate the new cycle.

Other physiologic functions follow the temperature cycle. Alertness and potassium excretion have a positive correlation, whereas accretion of growth hormone has a negative association with temperature. Cortisol has its own pattern, but follows a regular circadian cycle.

SLEEP

Sleep that knits up the ravell'd sleave of care,
The death of each day's life, sore labour's
bath, Balm of hurt minds, great nature's
second course, Chief nourisher in life's feast.

Shakespeare, *Macbeth,* Act II, Scene I

Definitions of sleep abound. The old maxim "the more the theories, the less the certainty" still applies. A generally accepted definition comes from Coleman:[7] "A state of inertia and loss of consciousness of a temporary nature from which one can easily be aroused."

Sleep occurs in discrete stages:[8]

Non-REM (NREM) Sleep: Brain Idle, Body Mobile

Stage 1. Stage 1 is a transition period that is usually completed within 10 minutes unless sleep disorder present. Brain activity slows and eyes roll slowly from side to side. Most sleep subjects awakened in stage 1 will claim they are not asleep. Automatic behavior, the rote performance of routine tasks performed without the subject's awareness or recollection, may be a prolonged form of this stage.

Stage 2. Stage 2 is somewhat deeper sleep; eye movements halt and the brain responds to a certain level of noise as seen in electroencephalographic (EEG) changes. About half of adult sleep is spent in stage 2, but there is less research on this stage than on any other. It usually lasts about 20 minutes before progressing to the next stage. Stage 2 separates blocks of other sleep stages and acts as the "glue" that maintains sleep architecture.

Stages 3 and 4. Stages 3 and 4 are characterized by deep sleep, commonly called *delta sleep* or *slow wave sleep* (SWS). It is characterized by cortical brain cells firing synchronously in slow large spikes. These stages are considered together because they are a continuum, stage 4 being the deepest stage of sleep. The bulk of SWS happens early in the sleep period, so it is often difficult to arouse someone an hour after onset of sleep. About 25% of adolescent sleep is SWS, and this percentage declines throughout adulthood until it may be absent in the elderly (Figure 81-1). Following sleep deprivation, this is the first stage to be made up. SWS is the most vital sleep component for physical recuperation, and those deprived of it will complain of fatigue and muscle aches. Growth hormone, vital for cellular repair, is secreted during stage 4.

REM Sleep: Brain On, Body Off

The usual onset of first rapid eye movement (REM) episode occurs after 90 to 120 minutes of NREM sleep. Hallmarks of REM sleep include a change in EEG to a pattern similar to wakefulness, dreams, rapid conjugate eye movements, irregular pulse and respiration, increase in O_2 consumption, increased cerebral blood flow (more than when awake), increased blood pressure, isolated muscle twitches, loss of facial muscle tone, and absent spinal reflexes. REM periods become longer as the night goes on, so the sleeper is likely to be in the midst of a dream when the alarm goes off. Most sleep periods will have 4 to 6 REM episodes. Infants spend more than 50% of sleep in REM; the percentage declines to about 25% around age 5 years and then stays fairly constant throughout life. REM sleep is vital for psychologic well-being, and those deprived of it complain of irritability and moodiness.[9] Because REM sleep has its own circadian variation (maximum at noon and nadir at midnight), it tends to cluster toward the end of the normal 7- to 8-hour sleep period. Those whose sleep tends to be shorter or more fragmented (such as shift workers) will likely be REM deprived.

Horne[10] refers to the first three SWS cycles (which occur during the first 3 to 4 hours and contain the bulk of each sleep period's SWS) as core sleep, with the rest of the sleep period considered "optional" sleep. Most subjects can function only on core sleep a maximum of 4 days without obtaining a full sleep period (restorative sleep).

Only about one third of lost sleep is made up. Lost sleep consists mostly of missing stage 4 SWS and about half of missing REM sleep. The sensation of sleepiness may have two components: that of missing core sleep (physiologic) and that of missing optional sleep (psychologic).

Researchers who measure sleepiness have found that alertness is lowest around 0300, with a diurnal trough also noted around 1400 (siesta time). Because of the circadian nature of REM sleep, a siesta produces better quality sleep than naps at other times.

ALERTNESS AND PERFORMANCE

Alertness is perhaps the greatest concern for industrial shift workers. Single vehicle commercial truck accidents increase by a factor of 8 between midnight and 0800, with the peak between 0300 and 0600. This is at the low point of alertness in the biologic day, and accident rates are highest even though this is the time when the fewest trucks are on the road.

Expressway driving is a good example of low-level per-

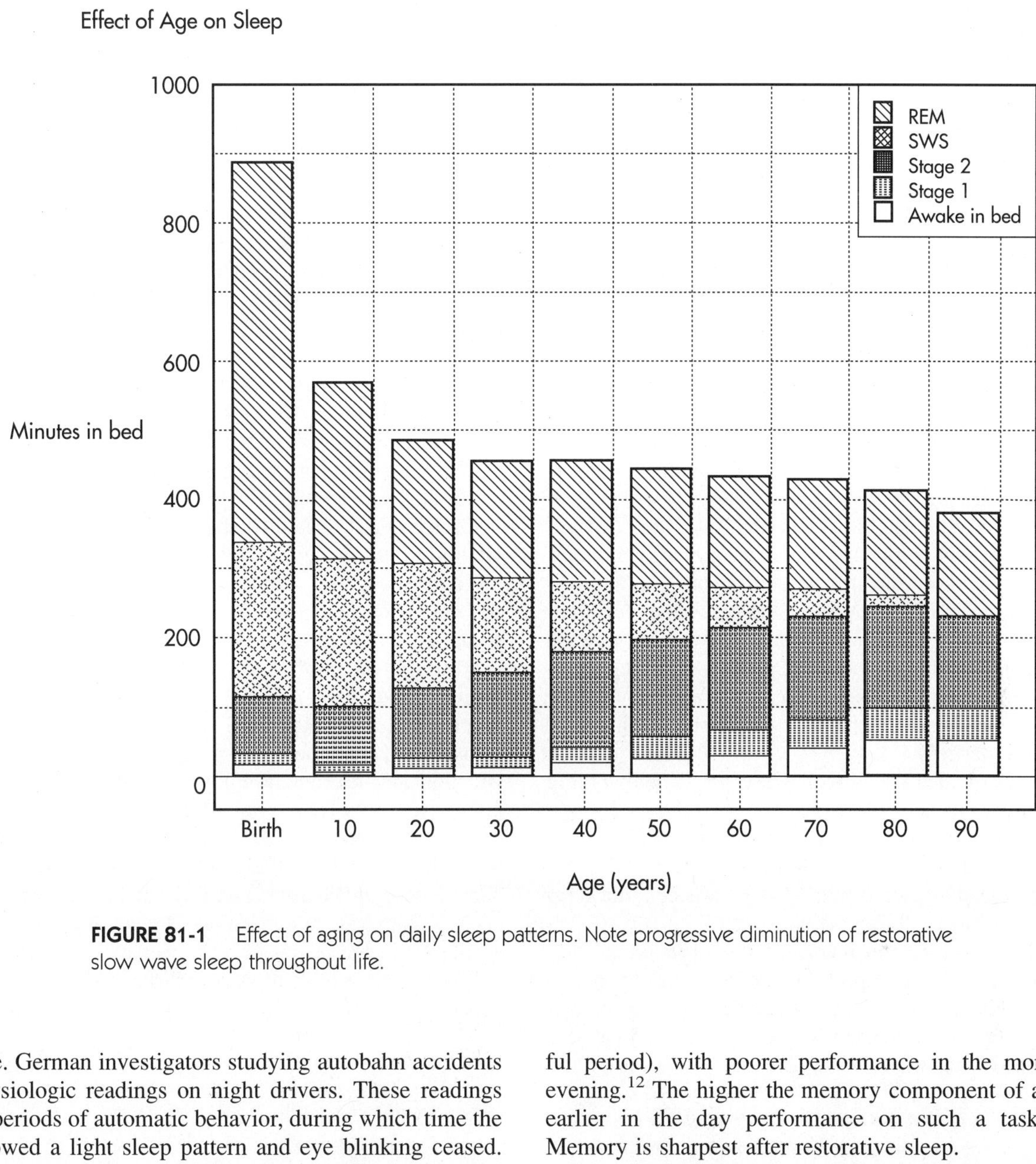

FIGURE 81-1 Effect of aging on daily sleep patterns. Note progressive diminution of restorative slow wave sleep throughout life.

formance. German investigators studying autobahn accidents took physiologic readings on night drivers. These readings showed periods of automatic behavior, during which time the EEG showed a light sleep pattern and eye blinking ceased. These periods lasted up to 20 minutes and subject recall for events was poor. Similar studies of night workers in the railroad, computer, and nursing industries have shown a corresponding tendency. When a sufficient stimulus occurs, the subject becomes awake on the EEG, but there is no anticipation of events while one is on autopilot.

The major determinants of daytime alertness include circadian phase, total sleep time the night before testing, the amount of SWS before testing, and the regularity and duration of the sleep and work schedule.

Performance for many tasks varies with the time of day.[11] Most performance curves can be brought into line with 24-hour temperature curves. Morning people (larks), who like to go to bed and get up early to accomplish things, usually have their temperature peak before noon. Evening people (owls), who like to get things done at night and then sleep in, have their temperature peak later in the day.[12]

There is a definite relationship between speed, accuracy, and reaction time to body temperature. People do best when their temperature is highest (usually the middle of the wakeful period), with poorer performance in the morning and evening.[12] The higher the memory component of a task, the earlier in the day performance on such a task peaks.[13] Memory is sharpest after restorative sleep.

"Post lunch dip" is an exception to the rules about performance. The precipitous fall in performance that occurs after lunch is not accompanied by a drop in body temperature.[14] This does coincide with the MSLT siesta trough.

Much has been written in the last 5 years about the issue of sleep deprivation in hours officers. A review of 27 articles showed significant decrements in moods and attitudes of house officers as a result of sleep deprivation in **all** articles. Performance tests requiring prolonged vigilance tended to deteriorate with sleep loss. There were minimal effects on most of the brief psychomotor tests measuring manual dexterity, reaction times, and short-term recall.[15]

CHANGING SHIFTS

Although shift work has been performed throughout history, the invention of the light bulb in 1883 made the practice of shift work feasible and economically desirable. Iron foundries and steel mills were among the first to implement the concept of shift rotation. The murderously difficult work schedules and frequent accidents gave much impetus to the rise of unions.

Henry Ford was one of the first industrialists to change from 12- to 8-hour shifts, increasing productivity in the process. Pressures from religious and social leaders in the 1920s helped reduce the average work week from 72.3 to 59.8 hours. The Walsh-Healey Act a few years later established the standard work week at 40 to 42 hours.

In the 1980s, about 26% of the male work force and 16% of the female work force had jobs that required some form of shift change. Of all shift workers, about 20% report no trouble changing shifts, 60% have moderate hardship, and 20% have such extreme difficulty that they abandon shift work altogether within 1 year.

Aging also disinclines a worker to rotate shifts, with most workers noting a marked increase in difficulty changing shifts after age 40. This seems to reflect the diminution of restorative SWS as life progresses. Approximately 100 minutes of nightly SWS is the threshold below which shift work (including permanent night work) becomes extraordinarily arduous. Because shift work is an intrinsic part of emergency medicine, and because most emergency physicians complete their residency training at about age 30, it is easy to see why the average full-time clinical practice career in emergency medicine lasts just 10 years. As the average age of emergency medicine's practitioners increases, shorter shift length may become more desirable.[16]

Monk[17] has divided the ill feeling one gets when working different shifts into two categories:

- *Circadian disharmony:* the "jet lag" malaise one experiences until adaption to a new shift occurs
- *Inappropriate phasing:* trying to stay awake or to sleep when the circadian clock says otherwise.

Research on insects and mammals forced to rotate their sleep/wake cycle showed up to 20% decrease in life span.[18] Shift workers have a higher rate of accidents on the job and greater risks of a fatal accident not only on the job but also driving to and from work. Work accident rates peak on the night shift.

Coleman's review of 200 studies on shift workers showed that 62% complained of a sleep disturbance, compared to 20% of day workers.[7] Shift workers average 5 hours sleep a day when on rotations, lasting less than 3 weeks, compared to 8 hours in day workers and in those whose shift rotations last longer than 3 weeks (which gives the body a chance to adjust).

Many studies show adverse effects of shift work on physical and mental health.[19-22] Shift workers have eight times the risk of developing stomach ulcers than those on day shifts. Depression and mood swings are up to 15 times more likely than in nonshift workers. Higher rates of drug and alcohol abuse, altered immune response, increased risk of chronic hypertension, increased cardiovascular mortality (risk worse than smoking a pack of cigarettes per day), increased infertility, increased rate of work-related accidents and errors, and higher divorce rates than for general population are also found in shift workers.

CLOCKWISE VERSUS COUNTERCLOCKWISE

For most of this century, the traditional shift rotation in industry has been a weekly counterclockwise rotation. This type of shift rotation is known variously as the Southern Swing, the Dow Schedule, the Hoover Schedule, and the Hanford Schedule. During the last 15 years it has fallen out of favor because research has shown that it leaves the biologic clock in shambles.

Why are weekly counterclockwise rotations undesirable?

1. Human free-running cycle is 25 hours, making it easier to delay sleeping than advancing it. The internal clock adjusts easily to a 2-hour sleep delay or advance, but little sleep will be had if sleep time is advanced 4 to 80 hours to accommodate the South Swing. (In like fashion, it is easier to adjust flying west than east across time zones.)
2. Shift workers on counterclockwise rotations take 1 to 2 weeks to reset their biologic clocks, so the weekly change of the Southern Swing means the worker never gets a chance to adjust to the new shift.
3. Weekly shift changes are enormously disruptive of family and social life.

Czeisler et al.[23] studied shift workers at a potash plant in Utah in the early 1980s. This plant used the weekly counterclockwise schedule, and the study was commissioned when the plant personnel director found that the most common complaint of workers was shift work. The researchers studied differing directions and lengths of rotations. Based on preliminary findings, Czeisler et al. tried a 3-week clockwise rotation for 2 years. With the new schedule, productivity increased 20%, and there was marked improvement in job satisfaction and sick time. Employee acceptance of this schedule after 1 year was 60%, growing to 90% after 2 years.

Czeisler's study of the Philadelphia Police Department, which had been using the Southern Swing, showed over half had sleeping difficulties, and 25% had an accident the preceding year. After a year of the 3-week clockwise rotation, accidents decreased by 40%, use of alcohol and hypnotics dropped 50%, and there was a marked drop in sleep disturbances.[24]

Many chronobiologists now recommend clockwise shift rotation, with at least a 1-month period between rotations to allow for circadian stabilization.[25,26]

SCHEDULING STRATEGIES

Many shift workers favor 12-hour shifts, and this type of shift is quite common in many emergency physician groups. Most industries on 12-hour shifts rotate weekly, but even when the rotations are longer, it takes longer to reset the biologic clock across a 12-hour change than it does for an 8-hour adjustment. In a demanding job such as emergency medicine, there is a tendency to fatigue in the last few hours of a 12-hour shift, especially if the hours occur on a new night rotation when alertness would be down anyway.

There is almost no mention in the literature about 24-hour shifts, a peculiar form of torture that all except emergency physicians have the sense to avoid. Common sense (sic) would suggest its use be reserved for low-volume emergency departments (<11,000 annual census), where the physician can reasonably expect to get at least 4 hours of uninterrupted core sleep.

Many European shift workers use the French System, which features a clockwise rotation through all three shifts over 3 successive days, on the theory that it is too difficult to reset the biologic clock. Therefore the sooner you get it over with the better. Circadian fatigue during night shifts is not addressed in this method.

The circadian "gold standard" for any industry requiring continuous coverage has been not to change shifts at all. Those working a night shift exclusively in this model must maintain the same sleep period, even during days off, to avoid disrupting their biologic clock. Most emergency physicians resist this idea, as it makes it difficult to participate in daytime family and social functions, or to be involved in medical staff activities. Some groups have tried to attract full-time night workers by paying them a premium to work these shifts exclusively. Conversely, in an attempt to retain valuable employees, some national emergency physician contract groups offer permanent day shifts (or at least no night shifts) to those with 10 to 15 years of continuous service. Relatively few physicians opt for the former category, and few qualify for the latter.

Objection to losing out on daytime activities is the primary reason some physicians also disparage the notion of monthly rotations, but in both cases there is a compromise of *anchor sleep,* which minimizes circadian desynchronization. Anchor sleep is a period of at least 4 hours during which one spends sleeping every day while on a particular shift rotation. For example, if you sleep from 0800 to 1600 after working nights, and from 0400 to 1200 on days off, the overlapping interval from 0800 to 1200 is anchor sleep (Figure 81-2). Sleeping until noon is preferable to sleeping all day for most people with families or other daytime commitments. By sleeping through at least half the time normally reserved for sleep, circadian rhythms are "anchored" to a particular schedule and minimally disrupted.

Some emergency physicians[27,28] have advocated a *single night shift system,* wherein each member of a group works a solitary night shift attached to "normal schedule." This system might work better for large groups, but a group of five people would still work at least every fifth night. Again, there is the issue of circadian fatigue during those single night shifts can be problematic.

In general, those who espouse the solitary night shift solution agree that the hazards of circadian disharmony outweigh the problem of inappropriate phasing, whereas the opposite is true for those who champion long rotations on a particular shift. It is important to note that the practice of weekly shift rotation, whether or not clockwise, is universally condemned in the recent literature.

Whitehead et al.[29] have proposed a system that combines longer night shift rotations with isolated night shifts. One member of the group works 1 month (or longer) on nights, and the other group members work isolated night shifts on their nights off. Small groups could work this system with little difficulty, and it would be attractive in a group where even only one member preferred working nights. Younger physicians, physiologically better able to withstand night shifts, may respond favorably to a pay bonus in return for permanent or prolonged night work.

For those working short stretches of nights, there is the compromise of *split sleep periods.* Because the short rotation will not allow for effective shift of the sleep/wake cycle, the goal is to prevent body rhythms from shifting and still stay awake and alert during the night. It is advisable to sleep in two 4-hour periods adjacent to the normal sleep time. If one normally sleeps from 2300 to 0700 and the night shift falls during that time, the best approach is to sleep for 4 hours immediately before and after work. Sleeping close to the beginning and the end of the normal sleep period maintains consistency in zeitgebers.

After working an isolated night shift, one should go to sleep as soon as possible after work and get up after 4 hours. This approach will result in sleepiness at the normal bedtime. Sleeping longer than 4 hours after working will significantly retard the next night's sleep, likely causing REM deprivation if one needs to be up early for day shift the next morning.

PREVENTIVE COUNTERMEASURES

Sleep Hygiene

There are individual differences to noise during sleep. Some need quiet to fall asleep, whereas others fall asleep best while listening to music or watching TV.[30] Sensitivity to noise becomes greater with age[31,32] and for women.[33] Occasional loud noise disturbs sleep even in people who do not remember the event in the morning. It increases the number of awakenings and thus increases the amount of stage 1 sleep. Wear-

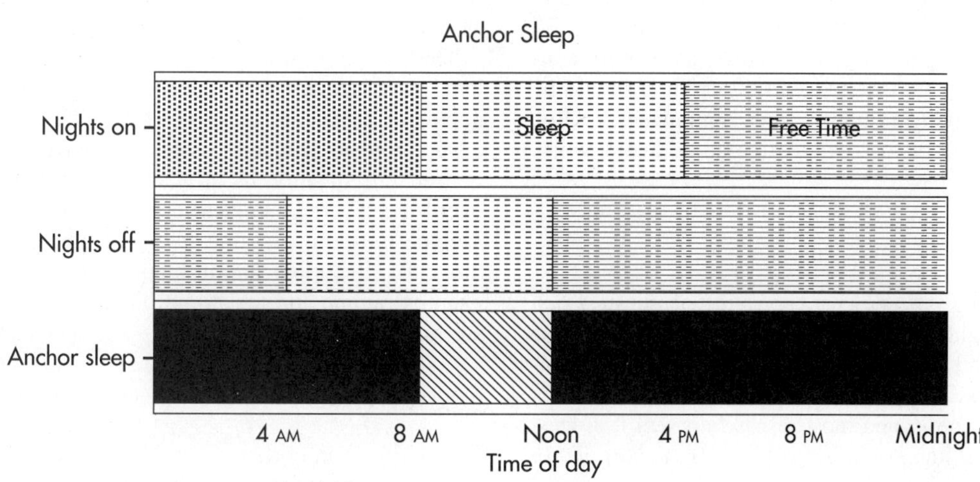

FIGURE 81-2 Daily 4-hour overlap in sleep period constitutes anchor sleep (crosshatch). Use of anchor sleep permits continuation of nocturnal entrainment on nights off.

ing earplugs, soundproofing the bedroom, and using a constant white noise may facilitate sleep in noisy environments.[34]

The ideal room temperature has not been determined; however, temperatures >24° C (75° F) seem to disturb sleep in humans,[35] and temperatures <20° C (68°F) were found to cause more emotional and unpleasant dreams.[36]

Anecdotally, most night shift workers favor sleeping on rainy or snowy days, and very high and low barometric pressures are associated with increased sleepiness during routine EEGs.[37]

There is little scientific evidence that the type of mattress (or lack thereof) plays much role in promoting sound sleep. The exception would be the individual requiring a certain specific surface for orthopedic reasons.[38-40]

Diet

Although there is no direct correlation between caloric intake and sleep, those who awaken too early in the morning might try a bedtime snack. Milk products seem to improve sleep.[41] Diet should be balanced and in harmony with circadian rhythms. Start "day" with a high protein meal, switching to complex carbohydrates toward bedtime. Maintaining regular meals during the waking period aids not only in sleep, but also in maintaining general alertness during the night shift. Caffeine and alcohol should be avoided within 3 to 4 hours of bedtime.

Exercise

Athletes enjoy more SWS than nonathletes, which has led some researchers to conclude that a steady exercise program deepens sleep.[42] However, a 1-day exercise binge may not deepen sleep that night. The time of day is important; exercise in the afternoon or early evening has more effect than exercise in the morning or late evening.[34,43] Therefore moderate exercise in the afternoon or early evening is recommended, especially if carried out over months. Exercise improves health and reduces stress. Additionally, vigorous aerobic exercise after awakening decreased the time needed to shift the circadian sleep/wake cycle from 8 to 1.5 days in one animal study,[44] a finding of great importance to those who are beginning a prolonged stretch of nights.

It is important to develop and practice a regular sleep ritual. Also, one should sleep only as much as is needed to be alert during wakefulness. If sleep does not occur in 30 minutes, it is best to get out of bed and do an activity conducive to sleep (e.g., read, watch TV). Sleep time should be kept sacred, care-giving responsibilities minimized. Finally, the bedroom should be used only for sleep: avoid work, worry, and exercise.

NAPPING

The role of napping is somewhat controversial. Siestas, rich in REM, are thought by most investigators to be psychologically refreshing and useful in promoting alertness during following night work. Napping before work seems to provide some subjective benefit, and most researchers feel it at least does no harm. It is suggested that at least 20 minutes elapse between awakening and starting work, so that *sleep inertia* has dissipated. (This phenomenon is readily noticed by those who nap during long shifts.)

Placement and length of naps are important. Power naps—for some reason a more palatable concept when referred to by that sobriquet—of 30 minutes or more can be helpful in maintaining alertness. Napping for longer than 1 hour can be detrimental, as it affects the next night's sleep. If you are to nap before a night shift, then a longer nap is useful. Napping should occur in an environment conducive to sleep.

The Japanese have for many years used preplanned naps during the night shift as a means of ameliorating the negative effects of night work. Those emergency physicians who share double coverage on night shift may be able to nap in this way when feasible.

BRIGHT LIGHT EXPOSURE

Exposure to bright light shifts the temperature nadir, changes the pattern of plasma cortisol concentration, effects subjective assessment of alertness, and improves cognitive performance in humans.[45-49] Shift workers exposed to 1000 lux ambient light had significantly higher levels of alertness and better cognitive performance across an 8-hour shift than shift workers in 1 to 20 lux or 100 lux ambient light.[37] Before daytime sleep, bright light should be avoided. After daytime sleep, 1 to 2 hours should be spent outside in bright sunlight. Full-spectrum lights are desirable at work stations where charting or other time-intensive activity is performed.

PHARMACOLOGIC CONSIDERATIONS

Although a single alcoholic drink can help tense people fall asleep,[50] alcohol actually causes poor sleep rather than ameliorating insomnia. Alcohol is the most potent inhibitor of REM sleep. Chronic alcoholics may approach 100% REM sleep during withdrawal, suggesting that delirium tremens may be a form of breakthrough REM. Alcohol causes greater sleep fragmentation, increasing the number of sleep stage changes per night from 40 to 50 to more than 100. Also, alcohol consumption makes nocturia more likely.

Caffeine and nicotine are both central nervous system stimulants and should be avoided for at least 4 hours before bedtime. They increase sleep fragmentation. Caffeine should be used at the 0200 to 0400 circadian trough and should be avoided close to the morning bedtime or after 0500. Caffeine should be used strategically. It should not be used immediately after starting a night shift or after a nap.

There are no miracle drugs to solve the shift work problem. As triazolam was being developed, there were great hopes for it because of its short half-life (1.5 to 2 hours). It is supposed to produce less of a hangover and as long as it is used infrequently, its efficacy does not seem to decrease over time. There is no clear objective evidence this benzodiazepine is free of the drawbacks common to other drugs in this class, including the problem of drug dependency.[51] Diphenhydramine and melatonin, now available commercially, are much safer alternatives.

SOCIAL LIFE

Social life is important for the shift worker, helping to relieve stress by maintaining close ties with family and friends. Planning for quality social time is a vital as planning for work. Close friends and relatives should be given a copy of the work schedule. Not being contacted by friends is sometimes worse than being awakened during sleep, and may add to the sense of temporal isolation that shift workers experience.

OPERATIONAL COUNTERMEASURES

Physical Activity

The best method for maintaining wakefulness is physical activity. When you feel tired, physically do something (e.g., walk around, talk to someone)

Environmental Stimulation

Use lighting and other stimuli to make the emergency department an activating environment during night shifts. Engage in interactions with others. Avoid monotonous, boring work. Vary activities.

SUMMARY

1. Classically, the best strategy has been to work the same shift all the time and to keep the same sleep pattern. This strategy is difficult to follow for most physicians who have families.
2. For those unable to maintain consistent sleep patterns, use of compromise strategies, such as anchor sleep and intelligent napping, may mitigate circadian disruptions.
3. Clockwise shift rotations are preferable to counterclockwise rotations, with 1 month minimum time per rotation recommended.
4. The concept of isolated night shifts has gained widespread acceptance. It may be difficult logistically for most small groups to use it exclusively, but it is recommended for large groups or in groups in which at least one member works nights full time. The main appeal is that the brevity of shift rotation does not disrupt circadian rhythms.
5. Sleep in a darkened room with minimal disruptions.
6. Start "day" with high-protein meal, switching to carbohydrate toward bedtime. Avoid caffeine and high calorie/high fat junk food before sleep. Eat meals regularly.
7. A bright light (10,000 lux for 2 hours after rising) is a useful adjunct for adjusting to new shifts.
8. Get regular exercise. Vigorous aerobic exercise after rising diminishes the time needed to adjust to new shifts. Regular exercise in the afternoon or early evening can improve sleep. Avoid heavy exertion just before sleep.
9. Work with family and friends to plan regular quality time together.
10. Do not try to live a day-shift lifestyle while working night shifts. Hold administrative meetings early in the morning or late in the afternoon when working night shifts.
11. Work shorter shifts.
12. You and you alone are responsible for your health and well-being. Stand up for your circadian rights and live longer and happier!

REFERENCES

1. Zun L, Kobernick M, Howes D: Emergency physician stress and morbidity, *Am J Emerg Med* 6:370-374, 1988.
2. Keller K, Koenig W: Sources of stress and satisfaction in emergency medicine, *J Emerg Med* 7:293-299, 1989.
3. Pittendrigh CS, Minis DH: Circadian systems: longevity as a function of circadian resonance in *Drosiphila melanogaster, Proc Natl Acad Sci (USA)* 69:1537-1539, 1972.
4. Aschoff J, Wever R: Spontanperiodik des Meschen bei Ausschluss alter Zeitgeber. *Naturwissenschaften* 49:337-342, 1962.
5. Czeisler CA: Human circadian physiology: internal organization of temperature, sleep-ware and neuroendocrine rhythms monitored in an environment free of time cues, doctoral dissertation, Palo Alto 1978, Stanford University.
6. Kleitman N: *Sleep and wakefulness,* ed 2, Chicago, 1963, University of Chicago Press.
7. Coleman RM: *Wide awake at 3:00 A.M.,* New York, 1986, Freeman and Co.
8. Baker TL: Introduction to sleep and sleep disorders, *Med Clin North Am*69:1123-1153, 1985.
9. McGrath MJ, Cohen DB: REM sleep facilitation of adaptive waking behavior: a review of the literature, *Psychol Bull* 85:24-57, 1978.
10. Horne J: *Why we sleep,* Oxford, England, 1988, Oxford University Press.
11. Blake MJF: Time of day effects on performance in a range of tasks, *Psycho Sci* 9:349-350,
12. Kleitman N: *Sleep and wakefulness,* Chicago, 1963, University of Chicago Press.
13. Folkard S: Diurnal variation in logical reasoning, *Br J Psychol* 66:1-8, 1975.
14. Lanuza DM: Circadian rhythms of mental efficiency and performance. *Nurs Clin North Am* 11:583-594, 1976.
15. Samkoff JS, Jacques CHM: A review of studies concerning effects of sleep deprivation and fatigue on residents' performance. *Acad Med* 1:687-693, 1991.
16. Thomas H Jr, Schwartz E, Whitehead DC: Eight- versus twelve-hour shifts: implications for emergency physicians, *Ann Emerg Med* 23:1096-1100, 1994.
17. Monk TH: Advantages and disadvantages of rapidly rotating shift schedules: a circadian viewpoint, *Hum Factors* 28:553-557, 1986.
18. Halberg F, Nelson W, Cadotte G: Living routine shifts sinulated on mice: biweekly manipulation of light/dark cycle. In *Twelfth International Conference Proceedings of the International Society of Chronobiology,* Milan, 1977, Il Ponte.
19. Frese M, Okonek K: Reasons to leave shiftwork and psychological and psychosomatic complaints of former shiftworkers, *J Appl Psychol* 69:509-514, 1984.
20. Milne D, Watkins F: An evaluation of the effects of shift rotation on nurses' stress, coping and strain, *Int J Nurs Stud* 23:139-146, 1986.
21. Davis P: Night nursing—an aspect of occupational stress, *Aust Nurs J* 13:46-47, 1984.
22. LaDou J: Health effects of shift work, *West J Med* 137:525-530, 1982.
23. Czeisler CA, Moore-Edy MC, Coleman RM: Rotating shift work schedules that disrupt sleep are improved by applying circadian principles, *Science* 217:460-463, 1982.
24. Raymond CA: Shifting work, sleep cycles are on the way to becoming another public health issue, *JAMA* 259:2958-2959, 1988.
25. Mitler MM, et al: Catastrophes, sleep, and public policy: consensus report, *Sleep* 11:100-109, 1988.
26. Winget CM, Hughes L, LaDon J: Physiological effects of rotational work shifting: a review, *J Occup Med* 20:204-210, 1978.
27. Michaels HE: Night shift work, *Ann Emerg Med* 13:201-202, 1984.
28. Thomas H: Coping with shift work, *North Carolina EPIC* 8, 1990.
29. Whitehead DC, Thomas H, Slapper DR: A rational approach to shift work in emergency medicine. *Ann Emerg Med* 21:1250-1258, 1992.
30. Robinson TM: Presleep activity and sleep quality of good and poor sleepers, Unpublished doctoral dissertation, June 1969, University of Chicago.
31. Lukas JS, Kryter KD: Awakening effects of simulated sonic booms and subsonic aircraft noise on six subjects, 7 to 72 years of age. NASA CR-1599, Palo Alto, 1970, Stanford Research Institute.
32. Roth T, Kramer M, Trinder J: The effect of noise during sleep on the sleep patterns of different age groups, *Can Psychiatr Assoc J* 197-201, 1972.

33. Dobbs ME: Behavioral responses during sleep of men and women to aircraft noises. 12th Annual Meeting of the Association for the Psychological Study of Sleep, Lake Minnewaska, New York, 1972.
34. Hauri P, Orr WC: *Current concepts: the sleep disorders,* Kalamazoo, Mich., 1982, The Upjohn Company.
35. Otto E: Physiological analysis of sleep disturbances induced by noise and increased room temperature. In Doella WP, Levin P, editors: *Sleep,* First European Congress on Sleep Research, Basel 1973,
36. Ziegler AJ: Dream emotings in relation to room temperature. In Doella WP, Levin P, editors: *Physiology, biochemistry, psychology, pharamacology, Clinical Applications,* First European Congress on Sleep Reserarch, Basel 1972,
37. Webb WB, Ades H: Sleep tendencies: effects of barometric pressure, *Science* 143:263-264, 1964.
38. Dement WC et al: Effects of the fluidized bed on sleep patterns of normal subjects. Paper presented at the First International Congress of the Association of the Psychophysiological Study of Sleep, Belgium, 1971.
39. Shurley JT: Effect of the air-fluidized bed on sleep patterns in healthy human subjects. In Artz CP, Haigert TS, editors: *Air-fluidized bed, clinical and research symposium,* Charleston, 1971, Medical Univ of South Carolina.
40. Rosekind M et al: Effects of waterbed surface on sleep: a pilot study. In Chase MH, Mitler MM, Walter PL, editors: *Sleep research.* Los Angeles, 1976, Brain Information Service/Brain Research Institute, UCLA.
41. Southwell PR, Evans CR, Hunt JN: Effect of a hot milk drink on movements during sleep, *Br Med J* 2:429-431, 1972.
42. Mrosovsky N, Salmon PA: A behavioural method for accelerating reentrainment of rhythms to new light-dark cycles, *Nature* 330:372-373, 1987.
43. Horne JA, Proter JM: Time of day effects with standardized exercise upon subsequent sleep, *Electroencephalogr Clin Neurophysiol* 40:178-184, 1976.
44. Griffen SJ, Trinder J: Physical fitness, exercise, and human sleep. *Soc Psychophysiol Res* 15:447-450, 1978.
45. Czeisler CA et al: Exposure to bright light and darkness to treat physiologic maladaptation to night work, *N Engl J Med* 322:1253-1259, 1990.
46. Campbell SS, Dawson D: Enhancement of nighttime alertness and performance with bright ambient light, *Physiol Behav* 48:317-320, 1990.
47. Badia P et al: Bright light effects on body temperature, alertness, EEG and behavior, *Physiol Behav* 50:583-588, 1991.
48. Dijk DJ, Cajochen C, Borbely AA: Effect of a single 3-hour exposure to bright light on core body temperature and sleep in humans, *Neurosci Lett* 121:59-62, 1991.
49. Dawson D, Campbell SS: Timed exposure to bright light improves sleep and alertness during simulated night shifts. *Sleep* 14:551-516, 1991.
50. Rundell OH et al: Alcohol and sleep in young adults. *Psychopharmacologia* 26:201-218, 1972.
51. Schneider-Helmert D: Why low-dose benzodiazepine-dependent insomniacs can't escape their sleeping pills, *Acta Psychiatr Scand* 78:706-711, 1988.

82 The Impaired Professional

Dennis C. Whitehead

OUTLINE

Few problems in emergency medicine are as vexing as dealing with an impaired professional. Following the old saw "Judge not lest ye too be judged" is often harmful not only to the patient, but also to the professional in question. Depending on the nature of the impairment, treatment is usually available that can resolve the problem, or at least make it manageable. A conspiracy of silence, although often the easier and more attractive course, is not an acceptable option when lives are at stake.

Impairment, defined here as a lessening of ability to perform professional duties, may be a result of several factors. In emergency medicine, most impairment in patients is due to substance abuse. Other diseases, both psychiatric and organic, are also in the differential diagnosis. Age itself may be a cause. All these factors need to be considered when evaluating the impaired professional.

This chapter addresses various causes of professional impairment, explores ways to determine the cause, and offers practical information about handling this thorny, life-threatening problem.

SCOPE OF THE PROBLEM

About 10% of all persons who use mood-altering substances become dependent on them. Studies of physicians indicate the incidence of addiction is higher, about 15%.[1] Physicians at greatest risk for addiction appear to be anesthesiologists, who have the easiest access to addictive substances. It is now thought that emergency physicians have the next highest risk, with some authorities believing they have moved into first place (Richard Bates, personal communication, 1988). Emergency services personnel, including physicians, nurses, and paramedics, have ready access to addicting drugs and the opportunity to use them and thus are at greater risk than the general population for developing the disease of chemical dependence. The demand for qualified emergency medicine personnel makes professional mobility easy and thus detection of the disease difficult. Because nearly all emergency physicians will at some point in their careers need to deal with the difficult problem of a chemically dependent colleague or employee, it is imperative to have as thorough an understanding of chemical dependence as with other common life-threatening diseases such as diabetes mellitus.

DISEASE MODEL OF CHEMICAL DEPENDENCE[2]

Chemical dependence which includes alcoholism, has been recognized as a disease by the medical profession since 1953.[3] Like other disease processes, chemical dependence possesses a characteristic symptom complex, clinical course, and treatment. Some aspects of the disorder that frustrate both those who have it and those who treat it are progression, denial, and a tendency to relapse. Victims of chemical dependence who are in the medical field are sometimes treated differently from the general population by their peers, as if their training should somehow make acquiring chemical dependence more a source of culpability than it would be for the nonprofessional.

Chemical dependence has been defined as "a cluster of cognitive, behavioral, and physiologic symptoms that indicate that the person has impaired control of psychoactive substance use and continues use of the substance despite adverse consequences. The symptoms of the dependence syndrome include, but are not limited to, the physiologic symptoms of tolerance and withdrawal.[4] Alcoholism, a specific form of chemical dependence, is defined by the National Council on Alcoholism as "a chronic, progressive, and potentially fatal disease characterized by tolerance and physical dependency or pathologic organ changes, or both—all the direct or indirect consequences of the alcohol ingested."

Chemical dependence is a complex psychosocial disease with a genetic component. All races, professions, and socioeconomic classes are affected. Susceptible individuals become addicted through a combination of chemical/alcohol use and biogenetic tendency. The disease does not appear without exposure to mood altering chemicals; thus it will not be seen in patients who never use such substances. The disease cannot be predicted otherwise on an individual basis.

Core Symptoms

Denial. Denial is the cardinal symptom of untreated chemical dependence. Denial manifests itself as displaced blame, wherein problems related to the disease are perceived by the victim as stemming from anything except chemical use. Continued denials mystify those around the addict, to whom the disease process is obvious. Recovering addicts say, "The disease tells you you don't have a disease."

Compulsion. Compulsion is the obsession to use despite real or potential adverse consequences. It is recognized by the addict when he or she admits complete inability to stop chemical use. The spirit may be willing, but the disease is too strong. Thoughts of use dominate waking hours and frequently intrude into dreams. There is the obvious insanity of "doing the same thing and expecting different results."

Progression. There is the inevitable deterioration of all aspects of life, spreading out from the addict like ripples in a pond. Social and family life disintegrate first, with the job usually the last thing to go. This is particularly true for professionals, whose only shred of self-respect as the world is collapsing around them is their work, which of course is also deteriorating.

Relapse. Chemical dependence is a powerful illness and has an relentless tendency to resurface no matter how long the period of recovery. Psychosocial deterioration, often difficult to detect behaviorally, usually precedes actual use. Relapse is generally due to a resurfacing of denial, the cardinal symptom. Addicts who have survived relapse speak of a failure to respect the disease and treat it appropriately. If detected early, relapse may be a positive experience for the addict.

Progression

By looking at advanced cases retrospectively, one can see that chemical dependence has a clear pattern of progression. It is difficult, however, to predict which drug users will progress to abuse and addiction. Early identification is important because of potential fatality. Chemical dependence generally exhibits the following pattern of progression:

1. Social use:
   - "Take it or leave it"
   - Does not preclude *infrequent* intoxication
   - Rare with intravenous drugs and smoked cocaine or heroin
2. Abuse:
   - Using interferes with life
   - Developing obsession with using
   - Frequent references to "getting loaded" noted
   - Increased solitary consumption
   - Absenteeism common
3. Addiction:
   - Life interferes with using
   - Obsessive/compulsive pattern well established
   - Waking state devoted to avoiding withdrawal
   - All other aspects of life (food, job) secondary
   - Institutionalization/insanity
4. Death: Either directly from toxicity or indirectly (accident, suicide)

The majority of abusers progress to addiction without intervention or treatment. Recovery may begin at any point in the process before death.

IDENTIFICATION OF IMPAIRED PROFESSIONALS

The most difficult aspect of helping the impaired professional is making the diagnosis. Denial is the cardinal symptom of the disease and may also be present in those close to the addict (e.g., spouse, business partner) who have an interest in protecting him or her from scrutiny. Chemical dependence is notoriously difficult for professional colleagues to detect in the early stages, as troubles at home or in the community may not be generally known.

Suspicions may be raised prospectively when a professional presents for credentialling in a new area. Ambiguous letters of reference, history of frequent job changes (geographic cure), prolonged periods between jobs, and overqualification for the position may be clues to chronic chemical dependency. The prospect may refuse to take a preemployment drug screen or may attempt to delay it by several days in hopes of producing a clean urine specimen. Most job prospects do not mind preemployment testing, and those successfully recovering from chemical dependency welcome it. A period of probation with random drug testing may be appropriate for a new employee with a known history of chemical dependency, especially if the period of recovery is less than 5 years.

It is the *pattern* of events, rather than a single precipitating incident, that aids in making the diagnosis of primary impairment. Although colleagues should be given the benefit of the doubt, there comes a time when action becomes necessary to protect the patient. There should be no compromise in this regard. Emergency medicine administrators must be familiar with *work-related* warning signs of chemical dependency, including those in Box 82-1.[5]

The situation is less difficult to identify when there is obvious alcohol or cannabis odor, slurred speech, ataxia, pinpoint pupils, etc. Chemical dependence is progressive, and work is almost always the last thing to deteriorate. Ample warning signs are usually evident to those who know the subject well before these signs occur on the job.

The medical profession has sometimes been accused of having a "code of silence" when it comes to dealing with its own members who have chemical dependence. Although this

BOX 82-1

WORK-RELATED WARNING SIGNS OF CHEMICAL DEPENDENCE

- Chronic tardiness
- Missing shifts or frequent last-minute rearrangements
- Sloppy charts
- Incomplete or altered medical records
- Variable handwriting quality
- Inappropriate orders
- Increasing complaints from patients and colleagues
- Won't answer phone when off duty
- Chronically broken beeper
- Excessive irritability when contacted at home
- Frequent use of strong cologne or breath mints
- Often prescribes controlled drugs for self or family
- Spends excessive time in bathroom
- Orders partial Tubex doses
- Carries saline vial and syringes on person at work
- Frequent visits to car during shift
- Erratic behavior with sudden wide mood swings
- Involvement in politics to detriment of medical practice
- Exaggerated exhilaration or negativism

Adapted from Whitaker GR: Keeping the emergency physician healthy and effective, *N Carolina EPIC* Spring: 1-2, 1990.

view may be extreme, physicians are commonly reluctant to pass judgment on a colleague's behavior. Nonetheless, our role as patient advocates supersedes these concerns. It is useful in such cases to remember that chemical dependence is a treatable disease and that the impaired professional is also a patient in need of care and compassion. According to the Ethics Manual of the American College of Emergency Physicians:

> The emergency physician may encounter colleagues or consulting physicians who are incompetent or impaired by drugs, alcohol, or psychiatric or medical conditions. The primary responsibility of the physician is to ensure patient safety. . . . . Having ensured patient safety, the emergency physician should attempt to help the impaired [professional].[6]

INTERVENTION

It is desirable to have medical staff or emergency medical system protocols in place proactively to deal with an acute patient safety problem in which immediate action is imperative. In most cases, however, intervention can and should be planned beforehand. Because most properly performed interventions are successful in getting the subject to admit to the problem, a treatment bed should be *immediately available.* If there is any delay, denial will quickly resurface and the window of opportunity may be lost.

A properly performed intervention can be life-saving. The person suffering from chemical dependence must be confronted by persons involved in all aspects of his or her life in such a way as to demolish the encircling wall of denial. This is the first step in recovery.

Procedure

1. Preintervention planning with a professional facilitator. Intervention is an emotionally taxing experience for all the participants, as the subject may initially claim that those present are betraying him or her. Thus preparation and rehearsal are imperative. Desired outcome will almost always be inpatient treatment, but participants also should be prepared for possible failure.
2. Include family, friends, professional colleagues, and successfully recovering persons the subject knows. It is especially important to include people the subject respects. Intervention should *never* be undertaken alone, as the subject is skilled at manipulating individuals to get out of jams.
3. The session is nonjudgmental, focusing on indisputable facts (absenteeism, poor work performance, bizarre behavior) rather than on the cause of the problems. The inevitable negative consequences of the subject's behavior should be stressed (job loss, licensing problems, marital discord) after concern and friendship are expressed and facts as known to the intervenor are reviewed. Intervenors must be emotionally prepared to follow through on the consequences specified if the subject does not agree to be helped. An intervention is not a time for bluffing.
4. Intervenors speak first, each to completion of statement. Interruptions from the subject should not be permitted.
5. Subject speaks last.
6. Treatment, or negative consequences should occur immediately as specified.

TREATMENT OF CHEMICAL DEPENDENCE

Most healthcare professionals require inpatient treatment, usually lasting 30 to 40 days. An initial assessment period of a few days may be necessary if the diagnosis is in doubt or if there are complicating psychiatric problems. Detoxification proceeds as indicated.

Treatment may be followed by some time in a recovery or halfway house, as professionals find it difficult to adopt a matter-of-fact attitude toward their disease the way that many lay persons can.

During treatment the patient is introduced to 12-step programs (e.g., AA, NA, OA) and group therapy. Frequent 12-step attendance is required. Counselors and physicians at the treatment facility will want to involve family and employers/colleagues throughout the process. Professional colleagues often need to be educated further about chemical dependence.

Relapse is a common feature of chemical dependence, and relapse prevention and planning should be thought out before discharge home. Treatment of relapse must be individualized and may have positive features, as the subject may then become convinced of the pervasive power of the disease.

Respect the confidentiality of the professional as with any patient, even though the problem will likely be well known. If asked, say the professional is on medical leave and is expected to recover.

RETURNING TO WORK

Attitude toward the returning professional is important, but recovery must come from within. Agreements with employer or medical staff should be formalized and specific, again focusing on patient welfare and the individual's recovery. There may be superseding licensing or legal requirements, which should be researched in advance of the need for action on a state-by-state basis.

Extremely important for the recovering professional is a structured aftercare program (Box 82-2). Not only is this of proven effectiveness for chemical dependency, but also ensures protection of patients treated by the recovering professional. The goal of aftercare is not punishment; rather its aim is to detect problems early when they are most amenable to correction. A brief relapse within the first year of recovery is

BOX 82-2

ELEMENTS OF AN AFTERCARE PROGRAM

1. Individualized
2. Written agreement, including plan if relapse occurs
3. 12-step meetings
4. Drug screening, randomized
5. Practice/prescribing monitoring
6. Continued contact with treating or other designated facility
7. Designated medical staff sponsor to ensure compliance
8. Advocacy for the professional when recovery is successful

not unusual for professionals and need not be greatly damaging if detected immediately.

In one recovery program, monitored physicians achieved a 96% recovery rate, compared to 64% when physicians were not monitored.[7] Because recovery rates for all healthcare professionals are higher than for the general population (perhaps as a result of closer monitoring), a similar high success rate can be expected for all properly monitored personnel recovering from chemical dependence.

SUMMARY

1. Chemical dependence is a treatable disease with a high rate of recovery in monitored healthcare professionals.
2. A prospective approach is important.
3. Early recognition and intervention are important for patient safety.
4. Successfully recovering professionals in monitored programs should be allowed to return to work when they are able.

REFERENCES

1. Talbott GD, Gallegos KV, Wilson PO, Porter TL: The Medical Association of Georgia's impaired physicians program, *JAMA* 257:2927-2930, 1987.
2. Jellinek EM: *The disease model of alcoholism,* Highland Park, Ill, 1960, Hellhouse Press.
3. American Medical Association Council on Mental Health: The sick physician: impairment by psychiatric disorders, including alcoholism and drug dependence, *JAMA* 233:684-687, 1973.
4. American Psychiatric Association: *Diagnostic and statistical manual of mental disorders,* ed 3, rev, Washington DC, 1987, American Psychiatric Association.
5. Whitaker GR: Keeping the emergency physician healthy and effective, *N C EPIC* 1-2, 1990.
6. Sanders AB et al: *Ethics manual,* Dallas, 1991, American College of Emergency Physicians.
7. Shore JH: The Oregon experience with impaired physicians on probation, *JAMA* 257:2931-2934, 1987.

83 Gender Influences and Issues in the Workplace

Roxane Spitzer-Lehmann

OUTLINE

Nursing is predominantly a female discipline. Most nurses, irrespective of their role in the organization, work in an environment where they continually interact with men who often are in positions of greater power and authority. Many women have accepted this relationship as the status quo in part because of gender stereotyping that permeated their nursing education and initial work experiences in the hospital environment. During their education, the role of student nurses, the majority of whom are female, was to follow the rules promulgated by administrators and physicians who were predominately men. It is no surprise that these gender stereotypes have remained the norm in many healthcare environments. Effective leadership behaviors are required for successful role implementation in the majority of nursing roles, whether at the bedside or in the boardroom. Gender influence is clearly evidenced by differences in communication, leadership styles, values, and acculturation in the workplace. The question remains, "How can we capitalize on these gender differences in the workplace as we effectively move nursing into the twenty-first century?"

Gender denotes a society's beliefs and perceptions about what is masculine and feminine. In our society "females have traditionally been socialized towards compassion, passivity, compliance, dependence, and supportiveness of others. . . . males have been socialized towards aggressiveness, independence, self reliance, activity and analytic skills."[1]

Because these perceptions about gender behaviors have been accepted as the cultural norm, there are numerous implications for enhanced interactions between the sexes in the workplace. These perceptions have their roots in our socialization, and for most of us they were learned and constantly reinforced during childhood. By the time we reached puberty, these values were operational in our daily behavior. Rules related to gender orientation and behaviors in the workplace have been evolving, but traditional values have been slow to change in most healthcare organizations. Peters[2] asserts that "gone are the days of women succeeding by learning to play men's games. Instead the time has come for men to move to learn to play women's games."

HOW IT ALL STARTED

Men and women grow up in the same environment, eating the same foods, watching the same movies, and going to school together; however, men and women live in disparate cultures and often do not share the same values. Gender-specific behaviors begin to develop at birth when parents often dress infants in color-coded clothes. Research studies validate the fact that infant girls are responded to more consistently than boys.[3] During childhood, mothers play with dolls with their daughters by holding the toy while the child comes to play with it. They roll a ball to their sons with the expectation that the child will return it to his mother before the game continues.

When parents think of boys, they think of rough, strong, firm, tough sports, competition, responsibility, etc. When parents think of girls the terms are significantly different—gentle, sweet, pretty, caring, sensitive, comforting, and nurturing. These images remain with the child while he or she develops and are consistently reinforced by society. Children learn to fulfill their prescribed roles in play, in learning and in relating to all those around them.[4] Children at an early age begin to play together, but by a very different set of rules. Boys learn to be competitive; girls learn to be warm and nurturing.

Business behaviors are often played out by the sexes in much the same way childhood games were played. Men view business as a team sport; women view it as a series of one-to-one encounters. Both sexes have characteristics of the other gender's behavior, but often don't know how to use them effectively without compromising their own values. Understanding these differences may allow us to generate additional and perhaps different approaches to some of the dilemmas we face daily in the workplace. Heim[5] has succinctly articulated the lessons we learned as children (Box 83-1).

The gender differences are clearly evident in childhood play. Boys play outside in groups that are hierarchically structured. Status is negotiated by giving orders and making them stick. Rules govern play and players are highly competitive. On the other hand, girls play in small groups or pairs and intimacy is the key. Everyone gets a turn to play and there

BOX 83-1

LESSONS CHILDREN LEARN

Girls learn
- Playing one-to-one usually with a best friend
- Getting along without direct conflict so everyone wins
- Fairness through compromise
- Play as a process often without an outcome
- Negotiation by group concensus
- Cooperation in a network

Boys learn
- Playing in large groups is vital and stimulating
- Coaches are necessary and must be followed
- Aggressiveness, or posturing it, contributes to power plays
- Feedback is connected with improving performance
- Focusing on goals and winning is important
- Strategy is vital to success.

From Heim P, Golant S: *Hardball for women,* Los Angeles, 1992, Lowell House.

are rarely winners or losers. Most of the time they sit and talk. Girls are more concerned about being liked than having status.

As girls continue to mature, traditionally feminine skills are frequently manifested in manipulative behavior, behind the scenes manuveuring, gossip, and discreet jockeying for favorable positions. Popularity and acceptance lead many women to value their ability to please, to look good, to be liked, and to act pleasantly. Capabilities critical to leadership—negotiation, persistence, expert power, negotiation, and conflict resolution—are often not part of women's developmentally learned skills.[6] Both sexes, irrespective of their acculturated gender differences, bring diverse strengths to business; women often bring their competent interpersonal skills and interactive relationship skills, whereas men bring their learned ability to downplay relationships in favor of bringing their aggressive, competitive, winning behaviors.

Tannen[7] views male and female differences from the perspective of gender differences in one's communication style. She cites that when one watches women move into positions of authority, keeping old behaviors or changing styles and talking like men are equally ineffective. Women, who speak and hear a language of connection and intimacy, and men, who speak and hear a language of status and independence, notice interactions between them seem difficult to understand, because the participants, speak different genderlects. By understanding each other's styles and our own options, we can find opportunities for a shared language in interactions to negotiate positive individual and organizational outcomes.

Gender as a concept will remain. As Goffman[8] states, it is "one of the most deeply seated traits of man. We create masculinity and femininity in our ways of behaving, all the while believing we are simply acting normally." In our society men are often seen to women as adults are to children. The male protector is often viewed as competent and capable of commanding respect, whereas the female is often viewed as incompetent, incapable, and desiring of indulgence. Being protected is often associated with the loss of independence, respect, and being treated as not equal.[5]

CROSS-GENDER COMMUNICATION STRATEGIES

Opening of communication, whether in one's personal or work life, focuses on accepting the differences in style without placing blame. Interpreting the other gender's messages and explaining one's own in a way that can be understood may be much more realistic and effective than changing one's own style. Understanding differences can open communication lines and makes it possible to change one's own style when desired.

Successful communication is predicated on assessing the goals and process of the communication. These include the perceived success of the communication and maintaining participant relationships as well as the process of communication which involves a message, a sender, a receiver and the interpretation of the message. Men are often more effective at addressing the task goal of communication, whereas women more easily attend to relationships of the interaction. Emphasis must often be placed on a goal that is not culturally impoverished as a result of gender affiliation so that the desired change and outcomes are attained during the interaction. Communication can be enhanced by paying attention to assertive communication patterns, nonverbal communication and incongruent messages often sent by body language, control of the environment, and image projection. The literature is replete with information about these strategies and techniques to enhance communication. Practice, evaluation, and continued pursuit of aiming for control or shared control of the conversation often enhance an individual's effectiveness. Some men and women find it helpful to run a movie in their minds or role play an interaction with a peer in preparation for a significant meeting. This preparation enhances self-confidence and allows the opportunity to practice new responses, using gender-based responses when they are effective and replacing gender-related patterns and responses when they hinder effective interactions.

GENDER INFLUENCES/ISSUES IN THE EMERGENCY DEPARTMENT

Gender influences and issues are often apparent in the emergency department because of the intensity of the experience for caregivers, patients, and their significant others. The environment is crisis oriented and the pace rapid; the work is intermittent and episodic. Gender behaviors may not be seen as an issue at the time of crisis or service delivery. During an in-depth analysis of situations, one often finds that in stressful interactions both genders revert to previously learned gender dominant behavioral patterns. Female nurses often become more passive, which weakens their opportunity to be effective as collaborative partners with physicians and administration.

THE FEMALE ADVANTAGE

Businesses of the 1990s will be flatter, more flexible, less structured, team oriented, and able to redesign or change on a moment's notice. One group, women, has the advantage of being effective in these new environments because of their inherent strengths, which are the antithesis of those often portrayed by successful men.

- Hierarchy is out. Redesigned organizations are based on networks and relationships.
- The firm is no longer the center of the universe. Organizations are conceived of only in relationships to outsiders and the interrelationships that are critical to success.
- The team always comes before the star. High performing, self-managed, cross-functional teams that cut across all boundaries will be the work unit of the future.
- The new job is never done. Continual improvements in quality and customer service coupled with change will be the focus of organizational cultures.
- Process is at least as important as result. Organizations will be driven by long-term relationships and partnerships.
- Values dominate rules. Focusing on key values and creating an environment that supports and rewards lifelong learning will be benchmarks of success.
- Voluntarism underpins the company's pact with every employee. Leadership focuses on enhancing the commitment of knowledge workers to daily improvement: Value added comes from the head.
- Employee empowerment determines managerial success. In nonhierarchical fluid organizations, those at the point of service must have information, skills, and resources to do the job unsupervised.
- Teamwork leads to success. Those who can work successfully on cross-functional teams across traditional organizational boundaries will be successful.
- Lovers of ambiguity shine. Success will be a measure of thriving with ambiguity.[2]

These traits hardly reflect the environment in most organizations today, but organizations are beginning to move in this direction. Men and women take different approaches. Each can learn from the other. Success in the future will not be dictated by maleness or femaleness, but by the blending of styles and a seamlessness between the values in one's life and one's work. Perhaps the most frequently discussed aspect of cultural diversity is gender differences, which is not surprising considering that women constitute more than half the work force. Male talent has remained untapped as well because of gender stereotyping. Hegelson[9] points out that men are having to learn to become more multifaceted in their identity, less identified solely with their position on the job, also taking identity from their personal and community life.

SHATTERING THE GLASS CEILING

Successful personnel must gain access to career opportunities and have the necessary skills. Key to success in shattering the glass ceiling in healthcare organizations is gaining experience, ongoing self-assessment of strengths and weaknesses, developing unquestionable talent, and becoming visible.[10] To follow this path strengths and weaknesses must be assessed. Feedback from a superior, mentor, peers, and subordinates should be solicited. Participate in a career development workshop with the outcome of identifying skill gaps, capabilities, and the strategies needed to achieve your goals. Make your talent unquestionable through both formal training and skills building; gain experience in both line and staff roles; modify your job; take risks; volunteer for projects and task forces; participate in government or community group activities. Network through *women's networks* when campaigning for a leadership position. Don't overlook the "old boy's network" as an entrée to advancement. Visibility outside of one's institution enhances one's ability to join the ranks of the profession's key players. Committee and task force participation in professional and healthcare organizations at the local and state levels is a positive action step to attain enhanced visibility.

Success in today's healthcare environment is not only about gender issues. It is a question of who has the best tools and who knows how best to use them. Just as important in today's downsized organizations is positioning oneself to be employable. Any role you are in today will change markedly in the future. Focusing on lifelong learning and building many well-developed skills that can be used in a variety of settings contributes to success and ongoing employability. One must set goals and chart the course to obtain them.

FEMALE SEX ROLE STEREOTYPING

Power is a critical issue that surfaces when discussing sex role stereotypes. Most women aren't used to having people working with or for them, whether that person is a member of a patient care team or the administrative assistant to a female nurse and physician executive. Often a dichotomy in female behaviors results in a woman either being seen as too busy to provide adequate leadership or too bossy as a result of her perceived or actual position of power within the organization. Generally accepted women's sex role stereotypes include the mother role, Queen Bee, and Aunt Tom phenomena. Mother roles in the work environment are played out by women who

- Give advice
- Foster dependence
- Interfere in conflicts
- Are passive
- Don't set limits
- Take care of everyone without promoting herself.

Queen Bees are characterized by their:

- Identification with those above themselves
- Alignment with the establishment and resistance to change
- Antifeminist behavior
- Desire to "run the show"
- Independent working habits
- Positive view of systems positively
- Siding with physicians

The Aunt Tom phenomenon as played out by women focuses on:

- The belief that authority comes from longevity and an eagerness to help others
- Blind compliance to male bosses coupled with interference with other women's work
- The assumption of an emissary role
- Destructiveness to females

Women often assume these roles unconsciously, as a result of observing other women's behavior in these sex-stereotyped roles. These roles can be counterproductive to women when they block the effective use of power and their leadership potential in an organization.

MENTORING

Few of us, whether male or female, succeed without a coach. Most men seek out and find an experienced coach or mentor to facilitate their development and advancement in an organization. Women report some of the positive benefits of a mentoring relationship as protection and support, role modeling of leadership/management behaviors, career planning, and sponsorship within the organization.[11] Women, on the other hand, who have not been acculturated to use a coach, may not seek out a mentoring relationship. In a research study of those in top roles in organizations, all the women in executive roles had a mentor.[11] Men may be reluctant to mentor a woman. Men tend to mentor another man because of a shared identity and common background and the likelihood of promoting another man. On the other hand, women who have a male mentor may run the risk of coping with cultural mores related to cross gender relationships, which may not support the intense interpersonal relationships that evolve during the usual 8- to 10-year span of a mentoring relationship.

POWER AND POLITICS

Gender differences about power are apparent in today's organizations. Adjectives commonly used to describe power in traditional organizations include *control, self-reliant, secure, capable,* and *risk taker.* In an empowered setting, power is viewed as *delegating, sharing information, providing assistance, reinforcing others strengths, trusting others,* and *providing challenging assignments and support for their completion.* Most men relate to each other in terms of rank and status. In today's work world when a male leader does not show his power often, his subordinates feel uncomfortable. Men use power to support and confirm their leadership position; in the female culture, use of power to confirm a leadership position may cause one to lose power, especially with female staff. Nevertheless, making requests and demands of those around her as a means to demonstrate power may be critical to a female's success in a top leadership position. The old adage use it or lose it is true about power for both men and women in leadership positions in today's hierarchical organizations. Power is merely the ability to get things done, a critical success factor in most positions in today's healthcare organizations.

In empowered organizations, where effective use of power is viewed as sharing power, the female style of being people oriented, expressing a desire to share resources, and build interdependent relationships reflects the traditional way women have been socialized to use power in this country. Women have learned in their roles as wives and mothers to serve as a resource and a source of support to those around them, a skill transferred by many women to the workplace. Women have also learned that by facilitating success for others they are respected and consulted. Often the mere act of empowerment increases one's personal power, a critical concept in today's transformed healthcare organizations.

Political behavior is clearly associated with power and can be used positively or have deleterious manifestations in an organization. Political behavior is most apparent in competitive situations, where there is limited resources, uncertainty, or lack of concensus about resource allocation. In these situations, power is used to influence behaviors that promote one's self or group interests. Men are often more astute than women in political situations as a result of the gender differences previously discussed related to competition and conflict resolution.

Because politics really centers on competition and resources, political behavior may be manifested by an array of behaviors. These behaviors may include building dominance and superiority, building alliances to enhance a power base, scapegoating behaviors, gaining support from higher levels and aligning with powerful others, using information as a political tool by withholding information, distorting information, overwhelming another with information or whistle blowing, amassing real or symbolic resources, exchanging favors to create obligations, outside professional activity; negotiating compromises in regard to issues or policies, and possessing knowledge of gatekeepers and power centers within the organization.

Irrespective of gender, key questions to consider related to political behavior in an organization include the following:

- Who has legitimate power?
- Who has the real power?
- Who makes and implements decisions?
- Who talks to whom?
- Where can I get important information?
- Who supports whom in the organization?
- How is cultural diversity handled in the organization?

Increased awareness of the politics in an organization will enable you to play political games more successfully to attain positive outcomes and increase your ability to avoid their negative impact on you.

SUBTLE SEXISM AND SEXUAL HARASSMENT

Subtle sexism may be less blatant but just as damaging to one's career. As more women are joining the ranks of upper management in flattened, less hierarchical organizations, fewer positions are available to men. Men are not prepared for these changes and often respond by telling sophomoric jokes, talking about sports, forgetting to introduce women at meetings, and stealing women's ideas. None of these behaviors are illegal, but they can adversely affect a career. Strategies to combat this subtle sexism might include ignoring the joke or leaving the room, introducing yourself before the meeting begins, reading the sports page and participating in the conversation, and publicly taking credit for your stolen ideas.[12]

Sexual harassment is a form of discrimination, but not all discrimination is sexual harassment. Every organization should define which behaviors move from sexual nonharassment to sexual harassment.

Today's courts have identified two types of sexual harassment:

- *Quid pro quo* of "Tangible benefit loss" type of harassment, which involves loss of job benefits by an individual because of rejection of unwanted sexual overtures

- The "hostile work environment" in which an employer creates or allows an intimidating, hostile, or defensive environment including such things as sexist jokes, sexually orienting photography displayed in the workplace, or bantering that creates a work environment that is hostile or abusive and interferes with a person's work performance.[13]

According to a recent study of Fortune 500 human resources executives and readers of *Working Woman,* 84% of women respondents knew what sexual harassment involved. More than 60% said they had been harassed, and more than 33% knew someone who had been harassed. More than 90% of respondents thought their companies should do more to prevent and stop harassment. Only one of five female respondents thought complaints were treated fairly. Of those who reported harassment, 83% claimed to have suffered ill effects.[14]

Six Steps for Preventing Sexual Harassment

Historically, sexual harassment has been manifested in gender inequality through misuse of power. Today, sexual harassment is everyone's problem in an organization. Employees must be able to report harassment without fear of recrimination; investigation must be objective, data-based, and conducted in a timely fashion.

Benchmarks of successful programs incorporate support of top management, including executive support. Involvement in shaping policy influences the way the organization approaches the problem. Written posted policies are visible and communicated and include the organization's position, legal definitions of harassment, and behavior descriptions of harassment, as well as the procedure for reporting and handling complaints and disciplinary action. Procedures should include time frames that address the issues quickly and provide responses to the alleged victim, alleged harasser, and work group. Training programs should focus on behavioral changes and be customized so that all executives, managers, and staff know how to prevent and report harassment. Ongoing employee follow-up education and introductory training for all new employees are key elements to a program's success.[14]

Costs: Individual and Organizations

Sexual harassment affects the work group, as well as individuals involved. The price paid in decreased efficiency, poor morale, absenteeism, and turnover far outweigh legal costs in the workplace. Sexual harassment costs the average large corporation $6.7 million annually in decreased productivity, increased absenteeism, and employee turnover.[15] Harassment has been manifested in gender inequality through the misuse of power. Although predominately a female issue, men are now filing sexual harassment complaints against women. Individual and organizational costs can be affected by (1) changes in behavior of potential harassers who think twice before acting, (2) those with alleged complaints who speak up quickly, and (3) executives who seek advice from human resource specialists and legal counsel about this problem in the workplace.

FUTURE SUCCESS

No one can attain success alone. We must shape our styles to promote success irrespective of our role in an organization or society. We often do not provide support to each other to cope with gender issues in the workplace. Flexible, adaptable organizations will be key to organizational success in the future. Organizations that can redesign on a moment's notice, address consumer demands, remain competitive, and adapt to a changing environment will be successful. Understanding gender differences and issues in the workplace and our personal lives and learning how to use gender differences synergistically will enhance chances for success in these organizations and in our personal lives.

REFERENCES

1. Edwards JB, Lentz CL: The influence of gender on communication for nurse leaders, *Nurs Adm Q* 15:49-55, 1990.
2. Peters T: The best managers will listen, motivate, support. Isn't that just like a woman?, *Working Woman* 142-143, 216-217, 1990.
3. Stewart R, Morain R: Sibling relations: the role of conceptual perspective—taking on the ontogeny of sibling congruency, *Child Dev* 55:1322-1332, 1984.
4. Pogrebin L: *Growing up free: raising your child in the 80's,* New York, 1980, McGraw Hill.
5. Heim P, Galant S: *Hardball for women,* Los Angeles, 1992, Lowell House.
6. Porter-O'Grady T: *Creative nursing administration,* Rockville, MD, 1986, Aspen Publications.
7. Tannen D: *You just don't understand,* New York, 1990, Ballantine Books.
8. Goffman E: *Gender advertisements,* New York, 1979, Harper & Row.
9. Hegelson S: *The female advantage,* New York, 1990, Doubleday.
10. Eubanks P: The experts career advice to women: aspire, plan, act, *Hospitals* 65:19, 1991.
11. Morrison A et al: *Breaking the glass ceiling,* New York, 1992, Addison-Wesley.
12. Scheele A: Career strategies—subtle sexism, *Working Woman* 16-17, 1992.
13. Bravo E, Cassidy E: *The 9-5 guide to combatting sexual harassment,* New York, 1992, Wiley & Sons.
14. Sandroff R: Sexual harassment: the inside story, *Working Woman* 47-51, 1992.
15. Fisher A: Sexual harassment: what to do, *Fortune* 128:84-88, 1993.

PART EIGHT
Practice Diversification

84 Chest Pain Emergency Departments

Vince P. Verdile and Richard F. Salluzzo

OUTLINE

Few clinical conditions define the practice of emergency medicine as well as acute cardiovascular diseases and especially acute myocardial infarction (AMI). Beginning with the prehospital care directed by emergency physicians, through the emergency department interventions, the emergency healthcare system is focused on the recognition and treatment of AMI and its complications. Recently, however, the emergency department care rendered to these patients has been the subject of some criticism, particularly with regard to the timely administration of thrombolytic therapy.[1-4]

Many factors come into play when a patient presumed to be suffering from an AMI enters the emergency department. Not only do the nurses and physicians need to be anticipating the patient's medical needs, but also many individuals and processes outside of the department's control must be prepared to act quickly on the patient's behalf. For instance, the electrocardiogram (ECG) must be performed and interpreted, the laboratory must be able to provide the results of the cardiac isoenzyme tests, thrombolytic therapy must be available and administered in a timely fashion, and the cardiologist and coronary care unit (CCU) must be ready to take over the care of the patient once emergency department treatment and stabilization are completed.

In an effort to streamline the process of caring for patients with AMI some emergency departments have developed chest pain emergency departments (CPED) within or adjacent to the primary emergency department. Although the formation of a CPED is frequently associated with a marketing blitz in the surrounding community, the impetus for its creation was initially not marketing but an effort to enhance care for patients with AMI. Besides the issues surrounding the immediate care of the patient in the emergency department with AMI, CPED programs are also committed to public information and education.

This chapter discusses the CPED concept as a practice diversification for emergency physicians. The basis for the implementation of the services and the anticipated impact for the emergency department are described.

THE EVOLUTION OF CHEST PAIN EMERGENCY DEPARTMENTS

Although death from coronary heart disease has declined significantly over the last few decades, still about 1.25 million people experience AMI annually, resulting in approximately 500,000 deaths. Nearly half these cardiac events occur outside of the hospital.[5] A significant number of patients therefore will access the emergency department as the portal of entry into the healthcare system for their AMI or related problems.

Many time delays are identified in the early care of patients with AMI. Some delays are attributed to the patients, some to the emergency medical services (EMS) system, and some to the emergency department. Attempts to enhance patient awareness of the symptoms of AMI in order to decrease the time for seeking medical care has had limited but not sustained success.[6-9] EMS systems have facilitated public access through 9-1-1 services, expanded the scope of practice of basic life support providers in allowing the development of automatic external defibrillator programs, and successfully performed prehospital ECGs to facilitate early recognition of AMI in an effort to enhance patient care.[10-13] Unfortunately, the time from EMS access to hospital arrival still offers some irreducible delays related to dispatch, assessment, intervention, and transport that inevitably add to the overall delay in obtaining definitive treatment (i.e., thrombolysis) for some patients.[1]

Consequently, and under the direct purview of the physician manager, addressing the obstacles to the timely treatment of AMI patients in the emergency department is paramount. It is well recognized that earlier administration of thrombolytic therapy improves efficacy.[14-18] Therefore the impetus for change should be in reducing delays in the emergency department for the administration of thrombolytic therapy for patients with AMI. This statement, however, has many different and separate individual facets that must be aligned to achieve success. It was with this goal in mind that CPED originated.

Obviously, not all patients with chest pain who present to an emergency department are having AMI.[19-22] The central role of the emergency physician, however, is determining as expeditiously as possible, which patients are at risk or are actually having AMI and which are not. Focusing the emergency department and the ancillary staff on the needs of the patient with chest pain, analogous to what has occurred with the evaluation and care of the trauma patient, is the challenge being met by CPED programs.

COMPONENTS OF A CHEST PAIN EMERGENCY DEPARTMENT

Fundamental building blocks are necessary for a successful CPED. Although a variety of permutations is possible, the minimum structure and function are outlined below and listed in Box 84-1.

Physical Space

Although a distinct area in or near the emergency department is desirable for a CPED, it is not entirely necessary. Some programs have not only a distinct area, but also a separate entrance and staff, which is the model of the original CPED at St. Agnes Hospital in Baltimore, Maryland.[23] The proponents of a separate physical space argue that it streamlines the entire process from triage and registration to the administration of thrombolytic therapy by having a dedicated and specially trained staff. One might counter that it is unrealistic to expend money on such a luxury when in reality the CPED program is much more a concept than a new physical structure.

Some CPED programs have both an initial evaluation area for patients with chest pain and an observation area for patients not meeting criteria for thrombolytic therapy, yet without a clear etiology of their chest pain.[24-26] These observation units can also be in, adjacent to, or remote from the main emergency department, which will of course dictate staffing and equipment needs. Because more than 50% of patients in the multicenter chest pain study group required an extended evaluation to determine the presence or absence of AMI, it is not surprising that observational units have become integral to successful CPED programs.[27]

Staffing

Much like other aspects of emergency department patient care, the CPED requires a collaborative, medical-nursing model to be successful. Assigning the appropriate number of nurses and physicians is patient-volume dependent. Staffing patterns are discussed elsewhere in this textbook (see Chapters 21 and 24). In light of the potential seriousness of the condition of patients triaged to a CPED, at least initially nurse staffing should be commensurate with this level of potential patient acuity.

Ancillary Support

Integral to the development of a CPED is the commitment to an expeditious response from the ancillary service necessary to facilitate the diagnosis and treatment of AMI. These are primarily clinical laboratory services, ECG services, and pharmacy services.

Clinical laboratory services must be able to provide the results of the cardiac isoenzymes, specifically creatinine phosphokinase-MB (CK-MB) in 30 to 60 minutes, 24 hours a day. For patients with atypical histories or ECGs, the cardiac isoenzymes can be a critical piece of information required for appropriate patient disposition. Some of the newer monoclonal antibody-based CK-MB assays have proved to be extremely effective and economical.[27,28] Using this assay, Gibler et al.[28] were able to detect which patients with chest pain were experiencing myocardial ischemia in less than 3 hours from emergency department presentation 96% of the time.[28]

Furthermore, serial CK-MB testing has become the cornerstone to a successful short stay or CPED observation units.[29] Subforms of CK-MB may prove to be a more sensitive and rapid methodology for detecting AMI and thus should be an integral part of CPED programs.[30]

The ECG remains the single most important diagnostic tool in the initial evaluation of patients with chest pain. A successful CPED will have the ability to perform and interpret the ECG almost instantaneously after the patient's arrival. The ECG not only is an important indicator of AMI, but also can portend AMI complications.[31] Some CPEDs have cross-trained nurses or nursing assistants in the performance of ECGs or put in place a dedicated ECG machine in the CPED to facilitate acquisition. Regardless of how it is accomplished, an ECG performed at the time of presentation to the emergency department is paramount if the remainder of the care delivered to patients with chest pain is to be optimized.

Together, the initial ECG and CK-MB can identify at best three fourths of AMI cases.[32] This is precisely why CPEDs have incorporated observation units to help identify AMI patients. Gibler et al.[29] and others[33,34] have demonstrated that protocol-driven patient care and compressed serial ECG and CK-MB testing are an effective and feasible means to arrive at a rule-out-AMI end point within 9 to 12 hours after presentation to the emergency department.

The last ancillary service that must come into play for a successful CPED is the pharmacy. There can no longer be a question of the increasing efficacy of thrombolytic agents with decreasing time to administration. Therefore no obstacle should stand in the way of the prompt administration of thrombolytic agent to CPED patients meeting the criteria. Several strategies can be used to accomplish this time-dependent task.

First, and optimally, all nursing staff can be trained to prepare and administer the thrombolytic agents, which would be stored in the emergency department medication room. Alternatively, a pneumatic tube system could be installed between the emergency department and the pharmacy to expedite the delivery of the thrombolytic agent to the department once it is ordered. Finally, and perhaps least efficient, a courier system could be established between the emergency department and the pharmacy to minimize the time it takes to hand-carry the thrombolytic agents from one point to the other. Although seemingly trivial, the availability of thrombolytic agents can represent a serious barrier to timely administration if a specific system is not thoughtfully developed in advance.[35]

Some CPEDs have gone beyond the routine evaluation of

BOX 84-1

COMPONENTS OF CPED

- Physical space
- Dedicated staff
- Ancillary support
- Observation capabilities
- Marketing and outreach

chest pain patients and incorporated more advanced, noninvasive diagnostic testing to further aid in the detection of AMI. Continuous ECG S-T segment monitoring, echocardiograms, exercise stress testing, stress thallium testing, and technetium sestamibi imaging are examples of some of the other diagnostic tools currently being used by some CPED programs to enhance the risk stratification of chest pain patients.[36-39]

Marketing and Outreach

One of the criticisms often voiced about CPED programs is that they are more about marketing and increasing a hospital's market share of chest pain patients than about patient care and reducing mortality from AMI. Not surprising, a significant part of a CPED program must extend beyond the emergency department. Heightening the public's awareness of the symptoms of AMI, the importance of early evaluation for such symptoms and the benefits of these prudent actions are a logical extension of a CPED program. All of these efforts, combined with reducing the time to thrombolytic therapy, are aimed at the same end point: reducing the morbidity and mortality from AMI.

Of course, this aspect of the CPED will cost up to $50,000 initially on marketing efforts by one estimate.[40] In light of the limited but not sustained success of some programs to change the public's behavior with regard to seeking medical care for early symptoms of AMI,[6-9] additional and ongoing public information and education programs will reinforce the importance of seeking medical assistance promptly. The Early Heart Attack Care (EHAC) program of St. Agnes Hospital is an excellent prototype of a multifaceted approach to public education, which includes videotapes, deputization programs, and school programs as mediums.[41]

CHEST PAIN EMERGENCY DEPARTMENT IMPACT

With nearly 500 CPED programs in operation,[39] it is unfortunate that a precise financial or patient outcome analysis has yet to be performed. There is a suggestion, however, that CPEDs will benefit the hospital and the emergency department in its ability to recruit new patients and subsequently influence the referral patterns of the patient's physicians.[40,42] A small 65-bed community hospital increased the number of cardiac patients per month by 56% since opening a CPED.[40] St. Agnes Hospital, the first to have the CPED program in the country, noted an approximately 65% increase in both CCU admissions and total number of chest pain patients seen in the emergency department from 1980 to 1986.[43]

If the CPED includes an observation unit, thereby limiting the actual number of patients admitted to the hospital, recent reports reveal up to a $1500 per patient savings.[33,44,45] These CPED programs are protocol driven, with compressed laboratory analysis, resulting in an emergency department stay of 8 to 12 hours rather than a several day hospitalization to rule out AMI. Assuming that the per patient savings is only $500, for a 300- to 400-bed hospital, the annual variable cost savings will be nearly $200,000 (30% less chest pain admissions combined with the $500 variable cost savings per patient).[46] The increased number of patients, combined with the cost savings, argues favorably for CPED programs in any healthcare delivery venue.

Shesser and Smith,[47] on the other hand, present a compelling argument that CPEDs are too costly per life saved. Although conceding that the care rendered to patients with chest pain in traditional emergency departments requires modification, these authors estimate that the cost associated with setting up a CPED in every hospital-based emergency department in the country (approximately 4500), is $378,000 to $3.78 million per life saved. They concluded that the cost-benefit analysis based on the data garnered from a variety of sources does not support widespread implementation of CPEDs.

The most flawed aspect about the Shesser and Smith analysis, however, is the assumption that all 4500 emergency departments in this country will have a CPED. The true number of CPED programs needed in any given community, much like the true number of trauma centers, has not been accurately ascertained. CPEDs, currently numbering nearly 500 nationwide, have probably not yet succumbed to true market forces of supply and demand. Managed care organizations may ultimately have some influence in this regard.

CPEDs have been successfully implemented in community hospitals,[40,43] university-affiliated hospitals[48] and academic health science centers.[49] Fundamental to the success of the CPED in any hospital is the multidisciplinary medical/surgical oversight and continuous quality improvement.[48-50] It appears that no hospital-based emergency department is incapable of establishing a CPED program. The first CPED in a given community, however, would have some advantage from a marketing standpoint, as it would be the first to be recognized as a facility with special interest in treating patients with chest pain.[40]

The final potential impact of CPED is the risk management gains. Emergency physicians fail to diagnosis a significant number (4% to 7%) of patients having chest pain with AMI.[51-53] In addition, missed AMI constitutes 20% of the malpractice awards against emergency physicians.[54] These facts make a compelling case for establishing a CPED, especially one that provides an observation unit component, to enhance the emergency physician's ability to accurately diagnosis patients with chest pain.

SUMMARY

CPEDs are growing in number throughout the country. The ability to streamline the care provided to patients having chest pain, provide a period of observation with serial ECGs and CK-MBs testing, and reduce the chances of misdiagnosis are all valid reasons for hospitals to create CPEDs. Emergency department physician managers must be an integral part of the medical and administrative oversight of such CPED programs. Although some costs are involved with the start up of the CPED, the cost savings and lives saved as a result of an optimal delivery of diagnostic and therapeutic process will create a rewarding practice venue for emergency physicians.

REFERENCES

1. Kereiakes DJ, Weaver WD, Anderson JL et al: Time delays in the diagnosis and treatment of acute myocardial infarction: a tail of eight cities. Report from the Pre-hospital Study Group and the Cincinnati Heart Project, *Am Heart J* 120:773-780, 1990.

2. Sharkey SW, Brunette DD, Ruiz E et al: An analysis of time delays preceding thrombolysis for acute myocardial infarction, *JAMA* 262:3171-3174, 1989.
3. Turi ZG, Stone PH, Muller JE et al: Implications for acute intervention related to time of hospital arrival in acute myocardial infarction, *Am J Cardiol* 57:203-209, 1986.
4. Moses HW, Bartolozzi JJ, Koester DL et al: Reducing delays in the emergency room in administration of thrombolytic therapy for myocardial infarction associated with ST elevation, *Am J Cardiol* 68:251-253, 1991.
5. The National Heart, Lung, and Blood Institute. Morbidity and Mortality: *Chart book on cardiovascular, lung and blood diseases,* Bethesda, MD, 1994, U.S. Department of Health and Human Services, Public Health Service, National Institutes of Health.
6. Eppler E, Eisenberg MS, Schaeffer S et al: 911 and Emergency Department use for chest pain: results of a media campaign, *Ann Emerg Med* 24:202-208, 1994.
7. Moses HW, Engelking N, Taylor GJ et al: Effect of a two-year public education campaign on reducing response time of patients with symptoms of acute myocardial infarction, *Am J Cardiol* 68:249-251, 1991.
8. Ho MT, Eisenberg MS, Litwin PE et al: Delay between onset of chest pain and seeking medical care: the effect of public education, *Ann Emerg Med* 18:727-731, 1989.
9. Mitic WR, Perkins RRT: The effect at a media campaign on heart attack delay and decision times, *Can J Public Health* 75:414-418, 1984.
10. Auble TE, Menegazzi JJ, Paris PM: Effect of out of hospital defibrilation by basic life support providers on cardiac arrest mortality: a Meta-analysis, *Ann Emerg Med* 25:642-648, 1995.
11. Aufderheidi TP, Keelan MH, Hendley GE et al: Milwaukee prehospital chest pain project-phase I: Feasibility and accuracy of prehospital thrombolytic candidate selection, *Am J Cardiol* 69:991-996, 1992.
12. Weaver WD, Eisenberg MS, Martin JS et al: Myocardial infarction, triage and intervention project-phase I: patient characteristics and feasibility of prehospital initiation of thrombolytic therapy, *J Am Coll Cardiol* 15:925-931, 1990.
13. National Heart Attack Alert Program Coordinating Committee: Staffing and equipping emergency medical services systems: rapid identification and treatment of acute myocardial infarction, *Am J Emerg Med* 13:58-66, 1995.
14. Weaver WD, Cerqueira M, Hallstrom AP et al: Prehospital-initiated vs. hospital initiated thrombolytic therapy: the Myocardial Infarction Triage Intervention Trial, *JAMA* 270:1211-1216, 1993.
15. White HD, Norris RM, Brown NA et al: Effect of intravenous streptokinase on left ventricular function and early survival after acute myocardial infarction, *N Engl J Med* 317:850-855, 1987.
16. ISIS-2 (Second International Study of Infarct Survival) collaborative group: Randomize trial of intravenous streptokinase, oral aspirin, both, or neither among 17,187 cases of suspected acute myocardial infarction: ISIS-2, *Lancet* 2:349-360, 1988.
17. Midgett AS, O'Connor GT, Baron JA et al: Effect of intravenous streptokinase on early mortality in patients with suspected acute myocardial infarction, *Ann Intern Med* 113:961-968, 1990.
18. Gruppo Italiano per Lo Studio Della Sopravvivenza Nel'Infarto Miocardico. GISSI-2: A factorial randomized trial of alteplase versus streptokinase and heparin versus no heparin among 12,490 patients with acute myocardial infarction, *Lancet* 336:65-75, 1990.
19. Lee TH, Cook EF, Weisberg M et al: Acute chest pain in the emergency room, identification and examination of low risk patients, *Arch Intern Med* 145:65-69, 1985.
20. Carney RM, Freedland KE, Ludbrook PA et al: Major depression, panic disorder, and mitral valve prolapse in patients who complain of chest pain, *Am J Med* 89:757-760, 1990.
21. Nevens F, Janssens J, Piessens J et al: Prospective study on prevalence of esophageal chest pain in patients referred on an elective basis to a cardiac unit for suspected myocardial ischemia, *Dig Dis Sci* 36:229-235, 1991.
22. Beitman BD, Basha I, Flaker G et al: Atypical or non anginal chest pain, panic disorder or coronary artery disease? *Arch Intern Med* 147:1548-1552, 1987.
23. Bahr RD: The chest pain emergency room, *Md Med J* 28:79-82, 1979.
24. Gibler WB: Chest pain evaluation in the emergency department: beyond triage, *Am J Emerg Med* 12:121-122, 1994.
25. Gaspoz JM, Lee TH, Cook EF et al: Outcome of patients who are admitted to a new short stay unit to "rule out" myocardial infarction, *Am J Cardiol* 68:145-149, 1991.
26. Fineburg HV, Scadden D, Goldman L: Care of patients with low probability of acute myocardial infarction: cost effectiveness of alternatives to coronary care unit admission, *N Engl J Med* 310:1301-1307, 1984.
27. Apple FS, Preesse LM, Riley L et al: Financial impact of a rapid CK-MB specific immunoassay on the diagnosis of myocardial infarction, *Arch Pathol Lab Med* 114:1017-1020, 1990.
28. Gibler WB, Lewis LM, Erb RE et al: Early detection of acute myocardial infarction in patients presenting with chest pain and nondiagnostic ECGs: serial CK-MB sampling in the emergency department, *Ann Emerg Med* 19:1359-1366, 1990.
29. Gibler WB, Young GP, Hedges JR et al: Acute myocardial infarction in chest pain patients with nondiagnostic ECG's: serial CK-MB sampling in the emergency department, *Ann Emerg Med* 21:504-512, 1992.
30. Puley RR, Meyer D, Wathen C et al: Use of a rapid assay of subforms of creatine kinase MB to diagnosis or rule out acute myocardial infarction, *N Engl J Med* 331:561-566, 1994.
31. Brush JE, Brand DA, Acampora D et al: Use of the initial electrocardiogram to predict in-hospital complications of acute myocardial infarction, *N Engl J Med* 312:1137-1141, 1985.
32. Young GY, Green TR: The role of single ECG, creatine kinase and CK-MB in diagnosing patients with acute chest pain, *Am J Emerg Med* 11:444-449, 1993.
33. Hoekastra JW, Gibler WB, Levy RC et al: Emergency department diagnosis of acute myocardial infarction and ischemi: a cost analysis, *Acad Emerg Med* 1:103-110, 1994.
34. DeLeon AC, Farmer CA, King G et al: Chest pain evaluation unit: a cost effective approach for ruling out acute myocardial infarction, *South Med J* 82:1083-1089, 1989.
35. The National Heart Attack Alert Program Coordinating Committee 60 Minutes to Treatment Working Group. Emergency department: Rapid identification and treatment of patients with acute myocardial infarction, *Ann Emerg Med* 23:311-329, 1994.
36. Tsakonis JS, Shesser R, Rosenthal R et al: Safety of immediate treadmill testing and selected emergency department patients with chest pain: a preliminary report, *Am J Emerg Med* 9:557-559, 1991.
37. Kirk JD, Turnipseed S, Lewis WR et al: A new approach to management of low risk patients presenting to the emergency room with chest pain: the immediate exercise treadmill test, (abstract), *J Am Coll Cardiol* 25:171A, 1995.
38. Varetto T, Cantalupi D, Altieri A et al: Emergency room technetium sestamibi imaging to rule out acute myocardial ischemic events in patients with nondiagnostic electrocardiograms, *J Am Coll Cardiol* 22:1804-1808, 1993.
39. Bahr RD: Wiping out heart disease before the year 2000: an obtainable goal, a prediction for the future, *J Cardiovasc Manag* 3:40-43, 1993.
40. Berg E: Treating chest pains brings big financial gains, *Mod Healthc* 21:32-33, 1991.
41. Bahr RD: Access to early cardiac care: chest pain as a risk factor for heart attacks, and the emergents of early cardiac care centers, *Md Med J* 41:133-137, 1992.
42. Gombeski WR, Carroll PA, Lester JA: Influencing decision-making of referring physicians, *J Health Care Marketing* 10:56-60, 1990.
43. Bahr RD: Chest pain emergency rooms: an idea whose time has come, *J Cardiovasc Manag* 9:1-6, 1991.
44. Sayre MR, Bender AL, Chayan C et al: Evaluating chest pain patients in an emergency department rapid diagnostic and treatment center is cost effective, (abstract), *Acad Emerg Med* 1:A45, 1994.
45. Gaspoz JM, Lee TH, Weinstein MC et al: Cost effectiveness of a new short stay unit to "rule out" acute myocardial infarction in low risk patients, *J Am Cardiol* 24:1249-1259, 1994.
46. Field JL: Emergency evaluation of chest pain: an economic case for definitive MI rule out in the ED, *Clinician* 13:48-51, 1995.
47. Shesser R, Smith M: The chest pain emergency department and the outpatient chest pain evaluation center: revolution or evolution? *Ann Emerg Med* 23:334-341, 1994.

48. Ellestad MH, Stavinsky Y, Easley B et al: Five year experience with a chest pain center in a university-affiliated community hospital, *Clinician* 13:17-20, 1995.
49. Barish RA, Doherty RJ: Establishing a chest pain center in an academic medical center: the University of Maryland experience. *Clinician* 13:39-43, 1995.
50. Espinosa JA: Quality management of the chest pain unit: practical chest pain center QM tragedy, tools, and pitfalls, *Clinician* 13:68-71, 1995.
51. Lee TH, Rouan GW, Weisberg MC et al: Clinical characteristics and natural history of patients with acute myocardial infarction sent home from the emergency room, *Am J Cardiol* 60:219-224, 187.
52. Schor S, Behar S, Modan B et al: Disposition of presumed coronary patients from an emergency room, *JAMA* 236:941-943, 1976.
53. Zarling EJ, Sexton H, Milnor P: Failure to diagnosis acute myocardial infarction, *JAMA* 250:1177-1181, 1982.
54. Rusnak RA, Stair TO, Hansen K et al: Litigation against the emergency physician: Common features in cases of missed myocardial infarction, *Ann Emerg Med* 18:1029-1034, 1989.

85 Trauma Center Care

Thom A. Mayer

Among the opportunities available for practice diversification in emergency medicine, trauma center care is at once full of potential and problematic. Virtually all emergency departments across the country handle some level of trauma care, ranging from minor injuries to the most severe major trauma patients. Regardless of whether formal verification or designation as a trauma center is pursued, most emergency departments will continue to see substantial volumes of trauma care because data indicate that, even in the face of trauma system development, only 10% to 15% of the most severely injured patients need to be cared for in a referral trauma institution.[1] Commitment to the process of verification and/or designation as a trauma center involves a substantial investment of resources, energy, capital, and ongoing management. Such a task should not be undertaken without a clear understanding of the magnitude of change involved, the necessity for careful integration both within and outside of the hospital, and the potential dilemmas that lie therein.

This chapter defines trauma center verification and designation, describes differences between trauma centers and trauma systems, describes the general requirements for trauma center diversification, and identifies specific emergency department issues that relate to practicing in a trauma center environment.

TRAUMA CENTER VERIFICATION AND DESIGNATION

In 1976 a task force of the American College of Surgeons' (ACS) Committee on Trauma published a report that delineated the commitment required of hospitals and healthcare institutions wanting to address the problems of seriously injured patients.[2] After the publication of this report, many hospitals sought to hold themselves out as *trauma centers,* the meaning of which varied from simply applying a label to the institution to a detailed commitment to the care of the seriously ill and injured patient. From the late 1970s through the 1980s, various state and local entities passed legislation governing the circumstances under which hospitals could legitimately call themselves trauma centers. This legislation varied from nonbinding site review by review teams from governmental agencies and/or professional societies to detailed processes of verification and designation.[3-6]

Trauma center verification refers to a voluntary process of review by appropriately conducted teams from either legislative agencies or professional groups (usually the ACS of Verification/Consultation Program) indicating that the institution has met the minimum requirements for level 1, 2, or 3 trauma center status. In most cases, this process has not meant that multiple institutions within a given service area could be prevented from simultaneously pursuing such verification. Thus verification simply refers to the verifying agency indicating that the hospital has met the requirements in certain clearly specified areas. This process often produced trauma centers heavily concentrated within large urban areas, often with as many as six or seven level 1 trauma centers in a given geographic area.[6,7]

Trauma center designation refers to a quasipolitical process through which legislative bodies or foundations determined which of several competing institutions would be granted trauma center status, often in a competitive fashion. Thus if two hospitals desired to be a level 1 trauma center in a specific location, site survey teams reviewed these two hospitals and issued reports indicating which they felt qualified as the most appropriate institution for trauma center designation. Understandably, this system often led to contentious and sometimes vituperative situations.[8,9]

The Committee on Trauma later revised their original document to a much more detailed and comprehensive document originally published in 1990, and revised in 1993.[10,11] The current document identifies 108 essential criteria for level 1 trauma centers and somewhat fewer for level 2 and level 3 verification. Mitchell et al.[12] reported incisively on the experience of the ACS verification/consultation program in a recent report. This report detailed the ACS experience with 120 trauma center reviews, focusing on reasons for criteria deficiencies for each hospital. The most common reasons for unsuccessful verification reviews are summarized in Table 85-1. Of the 120 trauma center reviews, 54 hospitals failed verification. The most important reasons, in order of frequency, were (1) lack of a quality improvement program, (2) no identified trauma service, (3) failure to document trauma surgeon presence in the emergency department, (4) trauma surgeon continuing medical education, (5) neurosurgeon availability, and (6) other specific failures to document a functioning trauma service.

In 1987 the American College of Emergency Physicians (ACEP) published its Guidelines for Trauma Systems,[13] which have since been revised in 1993[14] and expanded with appropriate appendices.[15-17] The ACEP document appropriately focused on the role of trauma centers within the overall trauma system, and indicated specific areas of commit-

Table 85-1 Criterion Deficiencies of 54 Unsuccessful Verification Reviews

Criterion deficiency	Number (%) of Hospitals	Additional deficiencies	Number (%) verified at second visit	No re-review
Quality improvement	40 (74)	5.1	15 (38)	19 (48)
Trauma service	25 (46)	6.8	8 (32)	11 (44)
Trauma surgeon in emergency department	22 (41)	4.7	7 (32)	12 (55)
Trauma surgeon continuing medical education	22 (41)	6.5	6 (27)	15 (68)
Neurosurgeon available	19 (35)	6.5	8 (42)	6 (32)
Trauma coordinator	17 (31)	8.2	5 (29)	8 (47)
Trauma registry	15 (28)	7	6 (40)	7 (47)
Surgical commitment	14 (26)	6.9	2 (15)	10 (71)
24-hour operating room	13 (24)	4.4	2 (15)	7 (54)
Research*	10 (19)	4.8	4 (40)	5 (50)
Anesthesiology in-house 24 hours	9 (17)	7.6	1 (12)	5 (56)
Trauma surg ICU response	9 (17)	6.4	4 (45)	5 (56)
Trauma director	8 (15)	7.5	4 (50)	4 (50)
Outreach program	8 (15)	8.9	1 (13)	7 (88)
CT technician in-house 24 hours*	7 (13)	4.9	4 (57)	3 (43)
Trauma surgeon credentials	7 (13)	5.7	1 (15)	4 (57)
Public education	7 (13)	8.4	1 (15)	3 (43)
Continuing education	7 (13)	8.9	0 (0)	3 (43)
In-house surgeon	6 (11)	6.8	0 (0)	4 (67)
Quality of care	5 (9)	5.4	1 (20)	3 (60)
Admits to nonsurgical service	5 (9)	6.8	1 (20)	3 (60)
Hospital commitment	3 (5)	8	0 (0)	2 (67)
Attending surgeon in OR*	2 (4)	6.5	1 (50)	1 (50)
Surgical director of ICU	2 (4)	6	0 (0)	2 (100)
Emergency department equipment	2 (4)	9.5	0 (0)	1 (50)
Laboratory delays	2 (4)	10.5	0 (0)	2 (100)
Rehabilitation	1 (2)	14	0 (0)	1 (100)
ICU equipment	1 (2)	14	0 (0)	1 (100)

From Mitchell FL, Thal ER, Wolferth CC: *J Trauma* 37:557-564, 1994.
*Level I facilities only.

ment and expertise required for a functioning trauma system (Figure 85-1). Both the ACS and ACEP guidelines have been included in federal legislation governing trauma services,[18] and the expertise of each of these specialty groups has been widely accepted as a template for development of trauma centers and trauma systems.

An essential initial step for any emergency department considering diversification into trauma center services should be a careful review of the ACS and ACEP documents, as well as the article by Mitchell et al. In-depth understanding of these criteria is essential for emergency department team members to understand the high level of specificity required for commitment as a trauma center/system.

REQUIREMENTS FOR TRAUMA CENTER DIVERSIFICATION

Diversification to trauma center status requires a multidisciplinary obligation to provide the facilities, training, and commitment necessary to care for ill and injured patients (Figure 85-2). The order of magnitude of complexity in marshalling these resources, even for level 2 or level 3 verification, is truly massive. The process should always begin with a clear understanding of how such a verification/designation process fits within the institution's overall goals and objectives. The verification teams routinely assess the institution's level of commitment to the trauma program as an essential component of site review. This institutional commitment must exist all the way from the board level, to administration, to the medical staff, to the day-to-day providers of clinical trauma care. Too often, trauma center verification is sought as a "window dressing" in which administration or medical staff leadership desires such verification, but the providers of care have not been willing to integrate it within the institution's overall mission. The strategy for affecting trauma center status should be discussed carefully with hospital governance, administration, and appropriate levels of the medical staff. Because of the substantial amount of resources of a capital-intensive nature necessary to operate a trauma center, it is important to ensure that this level of commitment is discussed objectively throughout the organization.

To ensure that a functioning trauma service exists, it is necessary to provide the appropriate infrastructure necessary for the care of large numbers of trauma patients. An identified trauma service must exist within the institution, and as is indicated by the study of Mitchell et al.,[12] the need for a clearly identified leader of such a service is an essential component. The trauma service provides multiple functions, including the critical aspect of guidance in oversight of the continuous quality improvement program. In initiating and monitoring trauma operations, close cooperation and integration with the emergency department are essential. Indeed, the ACS guide-

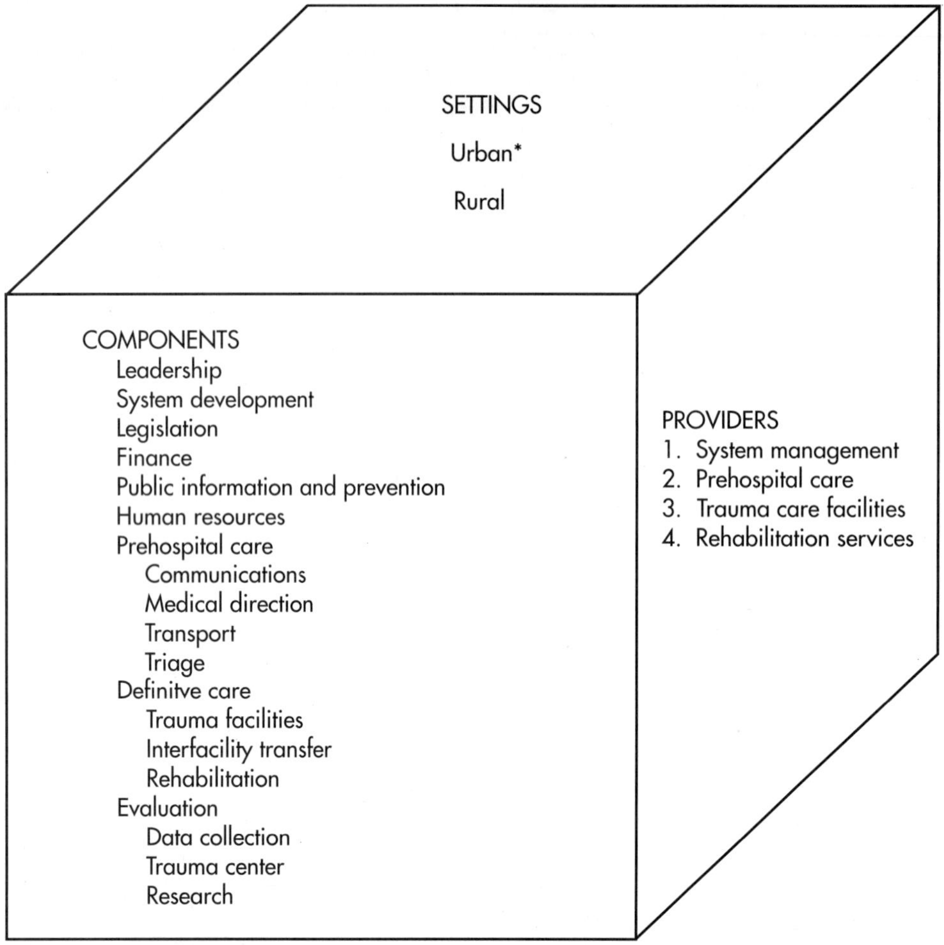

FIGURE 85-1 The three dimensions of trauma care systems.

(Adapted from American College of Emergency Physicians: Guidelines for trauma care systems, *Ann Emerg Med,* June 1993; 22:1079-1100.)

lines require integration of the emergency department physician as team members in the response to the trauma patient.[10,11] Even more important, the emergency department nursing staff will provide an indispensable role in the evaluation and management of such trauma patients. Trauma patients are substantially disintegrative to emergency department operations and will involve pulling the resources of the emergency department physicians, nurses, and laboratory and radiographic services away from other patients within the department.

In organizing the trauma service, there must be a substantial level of commitment from surgical subspecialists, including neurosurgery, orthopedic surgery, plastic surgery, and other surgical subspecialists. A detailed quality improvement structure that assesses the impact of the trauma program on the care of injured patients is a critical part of the planning for trauma center verification/designation and was the most commonly noted deficiency in the ACS study. The ACEP Trauma Systems Guidelines have also emphasized the need for a detailed quality improvement initiative to ensure that appropriate patients for the system receive the best possible level of care.[15]

Even when the issues within the hospital itself have been addressed in detail, the trauma center must address substantial extramural issues, including integration with emergency medical services (EMS) providers, education for EMS, outreach education programs to the community, trauma research programs, and the trauma center's role in disaster planning and other trauma system issues.

IDENTIFYING THE COST OF TRAUMA CENTER DIVERSIFICATION

An institution's decision to approach trauma center designation involves a substantial investment of resources, including facilities, training, and the requisite commitment necessary for verification. The 108 ACS criteria do not each have an incremental cost associated with them; however, there substantial costs are involved.

From an administrative standpoint, it is quite clear that a formal trauma service, including a detailed quality improvement program, must be in place for verification as a trauma center. This almost always involves protected administrative time for at least the surgeon in charge of the trauma service, as well as appropriate support staff, trauma coordinator, and secretarial support. In level 1 centers, a research program

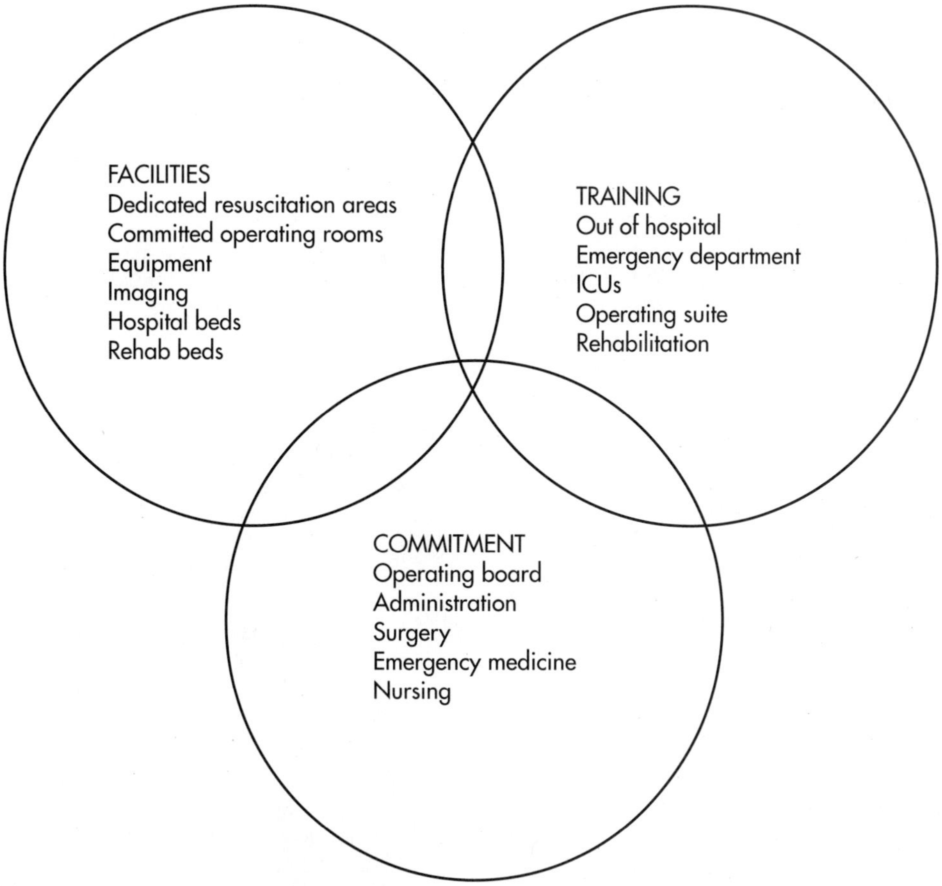

FIGURE 85-2 The facilities, training, and commitment (FTC) approach to ensuring that adequate resources are available for trauma system diversification.
(Courtesy John Shea, MD.)

must also be supported, as well as substantial resources for implementation and maintenance of the trauma registry, outreach education, public relations, and other programs. In most cases the appropriate equipment will be available, although there may be some increased incremental staffing costs in areas such as maintaining a computed tomography (CT) technician in-house 24 hours a day for level 1 centers. Appropriate continuing medical education for trauma surgeons and emergency physicians must also be budgeted.

Verification as a trauma center can substantially alter staffing relationships in the emergency department and must be taken into consideration when diversification into trauma center operations is considered. It is critical to understand that trauma patients are substantially disintegrative patients for the emergency department. Because of the nature and acuity involved in trauma patients, they require substantial resources from the trauma surgeon, emergency physician, emergency department nursing staff, and all ancillary services. In effect, in many emergency departments, the laboratory, radiology, and much of the physician and nursing resources for the emergency department virtually shut down when even a single major trauma patient presents to the emergency department. The effect of such trauma patients can be dramatic on nontrauma patients in the emergency department and is an important aspect of consideration of trauma center diversification. Because of the dramatic nature of the response to the trauma patient, patients, families, and even medical staff members present in the emergency department are often well aware of the disintegrative effect that such patients have. Careful planning for the need for increased resources and ensuring that trauma patients are handled in the fastest, most efficient manner can help allay some of this effect; nevertheless, the resources required for the care of the major trauma patient is substantial.

The cost of the care of the trauma patient can be diminished somewhat by using a tiered trauma response, combining physiologic data, anatomic data, and mechanism of injury criteria. Boxes 85-1 and 85-2 illustrate the response used at Fairfax Hospital, delineating both the criteria for tiered response and the staff involved. Such a system decreased costs for care of the trauma patient by more than $1000 per patient, and the quality of care of the patients was maintained at an appropriate level.[19] A tiered response requires a careful quality improvement ongoing study to ensure that the needs of the injured patient are met in the most cost-effective fashion available. It is likely that such tiered responses will be necessary to maintain the resources for trauma center verification and to ensure that emergency department flow patterns for nontrauma patients are maintained.

The emergency department physician group must create a staffing pattern that considers the trauma patient. Even with the presence of surgical residents (which are usually needed

BOX 85-1

HEALTHCARE PERSONNEL IN ATTENDANCE FOR CODE BLUE AND CODE YELLOW

Code Yellow	Code Blue
Emergency physician	Emergency physician
Emergency resident	Emergency resident
Senior surgical resident	Trauma surgeon
Trauma critical care fellow	Senior surgical resident
Emergency trauma nurse (Two)	Trauma critical care fellow
Respiratory therapist	Anesthesiologist
Radiography technician	Emergency trauma nurse
Total: 8	ICU trauma nurse responder
Trauma surgeon-notified	Recorder nurse
Anesthesiologist-notified	Emergency technician
Social service-notified	Respiratory therapist (two)
	Radiography technician (two)
	Laboratory technician
	Social service
	Total: 16

From DeKeyser FG, Paratore A, Seneca RP, Trask A: *Ann Emerg Med* 23:841-844, 1994.

in level 2 and level 3 centers), the trauma patient will require more of the emergency department physician's time in virtually all cases. Thus a change or increase in the staffing may be needed to ensure adequate emergency physician coverage, both for the trauma patient and for maintaining flow in nontrauma emergency department visits. In some cases, emergency departments have seen decreases in nontrauma revenues because of the perception in the community that turnaround times lengthen in the presence of substantial numbers of trauma patients in the emergency department. Nonetheless, this perception is often balanced by a nonquantifiable yet perceptible halo effect that many communities feel about their trauma centers. It has never been conclusively shown that verification of a trauma center has any substantial marketing effect, but there may be some perception on the part of the public that trauma centers offer a higher level of care.

BOX 85-2

CRITERIA FOR ASSIGNING A TWO-TIERED (CODE BLUE, MOST SEVERE; CODE YELLOW, LESS SEVERE) TRAUMA SYSTEM, BASED ON PHYSIOLOGIC, ANATOMIC, MECHANISM OF INJURY CRITERIA.

Code blue criteria

- Airway and breathing emergencies
- Systolic BP ≤ 85
- GCS ≤ 8
- Paralysis
- Penetrating injuries
  - Head
  - Neck
  - Torso
- Crush to torso/upper thighs
- Major amputations

Code yellow criteria

Physiologic alterations

- Loss of consciousness
- Pregnancy = 3 months or more

Anatomic alterations

- Maxillo-facial trauma
- Significant subcutaneous air
- Evidence of pelvic instability
- Two or more long-bone deformities
- Major lacerations involving fascia

Mechanism of injury

- Ejection from vehicle
- Pedestrian/MVA/motorcyclist
- Burns > 20%
- Suspected respiratory burns
- High-energy dissipation
- Significant vehicle damage
- Prolonged extrication > 20 minutes
- Documented falls > 20 feet or 2 stories

BP, blood pressure; GCS, Glascow Coma Scale; MVA, motor vehicle accident.

TRAUMA CENTER DIVERSIFICATION: YES OR NO?

Perhaps the most important issue to address in deciding whether to pursue trauma center designation is how such a commitment fits with the institution's overall mission. Is the hospital operating board, administration, and medical staff committed to the development and deployment of resources necessary for trauma center status? The ACS verification study clearly identified a discrete subset of hospitals in which administration and/or the board desired trauma center verification, but there was a lack of commitment by the medical staff to the program.[12] Such programs uniformly failed their verification visits and were similarly unsuccessful on reverification efforts. It is critical to determine whether the level of commitment is present and if the trauma center status meets the overall mission of the institution at all levels before requesting verification. It is important to balance such issues as the quality of patient care, institutional mission, and community commitment to the trauma patient with the time, energy, effort, and diversion of resources from other areas that will be involved in a practical fashion in implementing trauma center status.

Integrating trauma surgery with the emergency department is extremely important in developing trauma center status. Although the interaction of emergency physicians and surgeons occurs routinely even in nontrauma centers, development of a formal trauma program means that there will be an even higher level of integration required of the trauma surgeons and emergency physicians, because the initial resuscitation of the trauma patient nearly always occurs in the emergency department setting. This involves a complex interaction of the emergency physicians, emergency department nurses, and trauma surgeons. In addition, those programs that include surgical residents have an even higher level of potential disintegrative effect. Such surgical residents are often not well oriented to the dictates of the trauma program and rotate through the service every few months. This presents an essential paradox: The surgical resident is a critical part of the trauma resuscitation team, but is often seen by the "permanent" staff in the emergency department (emergency physicians, nurses, laboratory, radiology) as having less than a clear understanding of the overall operations of the trauma service. The leadership of the emergency department and trauma surgery program must work closely together to ensure that the element of integrating the residents into the program is addressed in a careful and ongoing fashion. Careful orientation, quality improvement monitoring, and mentoring are all necessary to ensure this problem is addressed.

Integration of the trauma service with the emergency department nursing staff is also an extraordinarily important issue. Addressing the potential effect on emergency department flow is an important beginning in this regard, because at least one and many times two emergency department nurses must be pulled out of the staffing pattern to care for the major trauma patient. Appropriate protocol and inservice education must occur to ensure that the nursing staff is aware of the specific ways in which trauma patients differ from general emergency department patients. Key personnel should have access to advanced trauma life support courses, and a specific trauma nurse specialist program should be developed. Many emergency departments have developed a core group of trauma responders from the emergency department nursing personnel. Although this arrangement results in a high degree of education among relatively few members of the staff and can give predictability to the trauma nursing response, it can also have an additional substantially disintegrative effect on the nursing staff. If the trauma nurses are viewed as elite nurses, this can create understandable resentments to those who are not among the chosen group of trauma responders. Instead, many trauma centers have ensured that all nurses within the emergency department are required to be trained to work as trauma responders. In addition to having an integrative effect, this strategy also helps ensure that appropriate resources are available at any given time to care for multiple trauma patients. It also has a salutary effect on the ability of the nursing management to schedule appropriately because all nurses are trauma responders in such a program.

Development of a multidisciplinary trauma conference, which includes emergency department nurses, can be an important step in ensuring the acceptance of the trauma program among emergency department personnel. Emergency department budgets should be planned in such a way that multidisciplinary meetings are either strongly encouraged or required of the nursing staff.

When trauma services are initiated, it is not uncommon for such a service to be viewed as an outsider, separate and distinct in some respects from the general operations of the emergency department. At times the magnitude of this reaction approaches the transplantation analogy, in which a true graft-versus-host reaction occurs. Appropriate administrative time and effort need to be prospectively budgeted to ensure that these issues are aired, addressed, and worked through so that the staff can cooperate fully in the care of the major trauma patient.

Designation as a trauma center can have a substantially positive effect on the emergency department physician group for several reasons. First, most emergency physicians view trauma as an essential emergency department disease, and there is a substantial amount of pride among many emergency physicians in being a part of the care of the major trauma victim. The drama and magnitude often associated with the major trauma victim can have a positive effect on the emergency department physician group. Conversely, because of the substantial violence associated with many trauma victims, there is also an important psychologic effect that must be considered. Particularly in environments in which substantial penetrating trauma occurs, the emotional toll on the emergency physician and nurse can be an important consideration.

Second, although it is not well documented, most physicians practicing in major trauma centers believe that caring for the major trauma victim helps improve the emergency physician's ability to care for both minor trauma and other patients with nontraumatic critical care diseases. The more frequently emergency physicians care for victims with major physiologic alterations, the more likely they are to be able to care for other patients with a high level of skill, including both cognitive and technical aspects of care.

Third, combining these factors may result in the ability to recruit high quality emergency department physicians and nurses to the trauma center, which helps improve both staffing and morale in the department. Finally, for many emergency physicians practicing in trauma centers, there is a deep sense of contribution to the community's mission because the emergency department functions at all possible levels in the care of the most severely injured victims. In this sense, it is often gratifying for the emergency physician and other personnel to feel that they are functioning in a real emergency department.

SUMMARY

There is a rich experience in the development and implementation of trauma center diversification in emergency medicine. Although well-known and quantifiable costs are involved for the hospital in the emergency department in entering into such a product line, there are also well-described, definable benefits for the institution. This substantial disintegrative effect of the trauma patient on overall flow in the emergency department should be kept in mind, and should be communicated appropriately to the administration, medical staff, and emergency department patient. Most patients and families can appreciate that the major trauma patient is labor intensive; few people want to see such patients substantially delay their progress in moving through the emergency department.

Most important, diversification as a trauma center requires a major *team* effort among the trauma surgeons, emergency physicians, emergency department nurses, and ancillary services, as well as the highest levels of governance, administration, and medical staff. If the institution is not willing to ensure that there are appropriate facilities, training, and commitment to trauma center diversification, the project should be seriously reconsidered. Nonetheless, when such commitment is available, operating as a designated trauma center can be a highly successful strategy for emergency department diversification.

REFERENCES

1. Knopp R, Yanagi A, Kallsen G et al: Mechanism of injury criteria for prehospital trauma triage, *Ann Emerg Med* 17:895-902, 1988.
2. American College of Surgeons: *Optimal hospital resources for care of the seriously injured,* Chicago, 1976, American College of Surgeons.
3. Pennsylvania Trauma Systems Foundation: Standards for trauma center accreditation, Mechanicsburg, Pa, 1996.
4. West JG, William MJ, Trunkie DD et al: Trauma systems current status—future challenges, *JAMA* 259:3597-3600, 1988.
5. Kales RH, Trunkie DD: Preventable trauma deaths: a review of trauma care systems development, *JAMA* 254:1059-1063, 1985.
6. Espisoto TJ, Lazear SE, Maier RV: Trauma care systems development: evolution in current transperiod. In Maull KI, editor: *Advances in trauma and critical care,* vol 6, Chicago, 1991, Yearbook Medical Publishers.
7. Shackford SR, Hollingsworth-Fridlund P, Cooper GF et al: The effect of regionalization upon the quality of trauma care as assessed by concurrent audit before and after institution of trauma system: a preliminary report, *J Trauma* 26:812-8230, 1986.
8. Shapiro MJ, Keegan M, Copeland J: The misconception of trauma reimbursement, *Arch Surg* 124:1237-1240, 1989.
9. Jacobs LM, Schwartz RJ: The impact and prospectrum reimbursement on trauma centers: an alternative payment plan, *Arch Surg* 121:479-483, 1986.
10. Committee on Trauma, American College of Surgeons: *Resources for optimal care of the injured patient,* Chicago, 1990, American College of Surgeons.
11. Committee on Trauma, American College of Surgeons: *Resources for optimal care of the injured patient—1993,* Chicago, 1993, American College of Surgeons.
12. Mitchell FL, Thal ER, Wolferth CC: American College of Surgeons verification/consultation program: analysis of unsuccessful verification reviews, *J Trauma* 37:557-564, 1994.
13. American College of Emergency Physicians: Guidelines for trauma systems, *Ann Emerg Med* 16:459-463, 1987.
14. American College of Emergency Physicians: Guidelines for trauma care systems, *Ann Emerg Med* 22:1070-1085, 1993.
15. American College of Emergency Physicians: Guidelines for trauma care systems: Appendix C: quality improvement, *Ann Emerg Med* 22:1096-1100, 1993.
16. American College of Emergency Physicians: Guidelines for trauma care systems: Appendix A: trauma triage algorithms, *Ann Emerg Med* 22:1085-1090, 1993.
17. American College of Emergency Physicians: *Guidelines for trauma care systems:* Appendix B: injury control, *Ann Emerg Med* 22:1091-1096, 1993.
18. The Third National Injury Control Conference: *Setting the national agenda for injury control in the 1990s.* Atlanta, Georgia, 1992, Centers for Disease Control.
19. DeKeyser FG, Paratore A, Seneca RP, Trask A: Decreasing the cost of trauma care: a system of secondary in inhospital triage, *Ann Emerg Med* 23:841-844, 1994.

86 Poison Control Centers

Paul M. Wax and Robert S. Hoffman

OUTLINE

Background
Poison control center operations
 Staffing
 Information and management guidance
 Data collection
 Education
Poison control center funding: mechanisms and justification
Development of medical toxicology
 Scope of practice
 Training programs
Emergency physicians and poison control centers
Future trends

Over the last few years, an increasing number of emergency medicine physicians have developed an area of special expertise in medical toxicology. Accordingly, emergency medicine has had an impact on the growing subspecialty of medical toxicology. Emergency medicine physicians now account for 50% of medical toxicologists.[1] Emergency medicine/medical toxicologists divide their time between their practice of emergency medicine and medical toxicology. Medical toxicology activities may include medical direction of a poison control center, teaching of medical toxicology to medical students, emergency medicine, pediatric, internal medicine housestaff, and paramedics, toxicologic research, and the participation in a consultative and/or inpatient medical toxicology service. Practice diversification into toxicology provides an opportunity for the emergency medicine practitioner to develop a subspecialty niche while continuing to confront the challenges of a diverse emergency medicine practice. This chapter discusses opportunities for emergency medicine physicians in poison control centers and medical toxicology practices.

BACKGROUND

Poison control centers developed in the early 1950s as a means of centralizing information about toxic drugs and chemicals. As the number of available drugs and chemicals multiplied after World War II, individual physicians found it increasingly difficult to keep fully informed on product information and treatment recommendations for the growing number of potentially toxic agents available around the home and workplace. Simultaneously, household poisoning became increasingly recognized as a problem area, especially among young children. A 1952 study showed that potentially poisonous ingestions accounted for more than 50% of childhood accidents.[2] Responding to these developments, the first poison center opened in Chicago in 1953 as a collaborative effort among several local pediatric departments to meet the informational needs of local pediatricians.

Over the next few years, the poison control center concept rapidly spread across the country. These first centers provided toxicity information on drugs and household products and made management recommendations to healthcare professionals. The National Clearinghouse for Poison Control Centers, established in 1957, helped standardize poison center informational resources by disseminating 5″ × 8″ index cards containing poison information to the various centers. In turn, the poison centers collected demographic information on toxic exposures that was tabulated by the Clearinghouse. As more centers opened, it became apparent that poison center services would also prove useful to the general public. Accordingly, the public became the most frequent user at many centers.

By 1978 there were 661 poison control centers in the United States. Many of these centers consisted of a part-time telephone service located in the back of the emergency department for pharmacy, often staffed by anyone who could be freed from other responsibilities.[3] In 1978, the American Association of Poison Control Centers (AAPCC) introduced standards of regional poison center designation in an attempt to upgrade poison control center operations and offer a national standard of service. Obtaining this designation required poison centers to be staffed by full-time poison specialists dedicated exclusively to poison center activities 24 hours a day. Such centers were required to have a medical toxicologist as its medical director and to serve a catchment area of between 1 and 10 million people.[4]

In response to these rigorous guidelines for poison control centers, a rapid consolidation among centers resulted. Currently 87 poison centers are operating, 38 of which have obtained regional certification.[5] Supporting the premise that regional centers provide better care, several studies have now demonstrated that advice provided by regional poison control centers is more competent than advice provided from nonregional poison centers.[6,7] When compared to nonregional poison control centers, regional poison control centers are more likely to serve a large population base, receive a greater number of calls, have more certified specialists in poison information, and have more qualified medical and administrative leadership.[8]

POISON CONTROL CENTER OPERATIONS

A survey of poison control centers in 1993 demonstrated that regional poison control centers (RPCCs) handle on average 38,000 human exposure cases a year, with a range of 12,000 to 78,000.[5] Thirty-four percent of RPCCs are affiliated with a university medical center, 42% are affiliated with a university-affiliated hospital, 8% are affiliated with a hospital that is without university affiliation, and 16% have other institutional affiliations.

Staffing

During the early years of the poison control centers, staffing was often provided by personnel with little special training in toxicology. Some of the staff may have consisted of nurses or pharmacists who were designated to answer the "poison phone" when time permitted them to be away from their primary responsibilities. Other staff may have had no formal health-related education and answered poison calls as part of a telephone crisis hotline.

As part of the growth and development of poison control centers, professionalization of the staff occurred. The personnel who currently answer the telephone at regionally designated poison control centers are referred to as specialists in poison information (SPI). Eligible candidates for such a position are required to have an RN, RPh, or MD degree. A recent survey of SPIs revealed that 56% were nurses, 36% were pharmacists, and 8% were classified as other.[9] Newly hired specialists in poison information undergo extensive didactics and closely supervised on-the-job training. Since 1983 the AAPCC has offered a credentialing examination for specialists in poison information to enhance the rigor and standards of poison control centers.[10] Candidates for the examination must have handled at least 2000 poison exposure calls. The average full-time specialist in poison information handles more than 3400 human exposure calls a year. An average of 10 full-time specialists in poison information (range 4 to 22) are employed at regional poison control centers. About 60% of the specialists in poison information have received AAPCC certification.[5]

Poison control centers are operated under the direction of a physician medical toxicologist who serves as medical director. The first medical directors were predominantly pediatricians whose emphasis was on accidental childhood ingestions.[11] Over the years, more and more emergency medicine physicians have taken leadership roles in poison control centers. In 1989 only 30% of medical directors had emergency medicine board certification.[12] This percentage had increased to 47% by 1994.[5] Medical directors of regional poison control centers spent on average 45% of their professional time allotted to poison center activities.

Poison centers may also employ an administrative managing director and public health educator. Managing directors usually have an advanced degree in pharmacy, pharmacology, or nursing. A rigorous credentialing examination offered by the American Board of Applied Toxicology is now available for nonphysician managing directors. Public health educators who work for poison control centers often have an advanced degree in education.

Information and Management Guidance

Daily operations of the poison control center include (1) the 24-hour delivery of sophisticated information and current treatment advice to health professionals (physicians, nurses, paramedics, pharmacists, hazardous material response teams) and the lay public, (2) data collection, and (3) professional and public education.[13] Telephone calls are initially received by the SPI who collects basic demographic and toxic exposure data. For the vast majority of information inquiries, the specialist in poison information can adeptly answer the callers' questions. Major advances in the storage and retrieval of poison information permit the poison specialist to have immediate access to data on the vast majority of toxic or potentially toxic products used by physicians or consumers. One of the most valuable references is the POISINDEX, which is accessible by computer on CD-ROM. This reference, which is updated quarterly, is particularly useful for product information and its extensive list of references. TOMES is another computerized database that has extensive information about chemicals and industrial hazards. Other standard poison center references include toxicology textbooks, current toxicology journal literature, books on toxicokinetics, and plant and animal toxins. Emergency physicians are well represented as authors and editors of many of these textbooks and journals.

Poison centers also use a variety of consultants in selective situations such as in cases of life-threatening toxicities or when the caller specifically requests a consultant. The primary consultant is the physician medical toxicologist, who may be the medical director, assistant medical director, or other faculty members associated with the poison control center. At poison centers with medical toxicology fellowships, the medical toxicology fellows actively participate in both telephone and bedside consultations. Seasoned backup for the fellows is always available from board-certified medical toxicologists. Because many of these fellows are recent graduates of emergency medicine residencies, consultation is usually offered with an emergency medicine perspective. Other consultants include botanists, mycologists, zoologists, herpetologists, entomologists, and marine biologists who may assist in the identification of poisonous plants and animals. Close cooperation with local hyperbaric experts may expedite the provision of hyperbaric therapy. Poison centers may also, on occasion, call on other medical specialists such as nephrologists and anesthesiologists to assist with particularly problematic cases.

One of the most important recommendations from the poison center involves the decision to treat the patient at home or refer them to the hospital. In 1993, approximately 80% of the calls to the poison control center originated in a nonhealthcare facility (usually the home). After poison control center consultation, only 12% of these cases were referred to a healthcare facility for management.[14] Recommendations for already hospitalized patients includes assisting with differential diagnosis, determining appropriate utilization of tests, analyzing test results, and advising on different treatment modalities. Follow-up telephone calls to the home or hospital on all potentially significant exposures is another important facet of poison center operations. During follow-up calls, the poison specialist or medical toxicologist seeks to establish whether treatment recommendations have been properly followed, appraises their impact, and/or counsels on appropriate poison prevention strategy.

Data Collection

In addition to providing information to the caller, an important function of the poison control center is to collect epidemiologic data on toxic exposures. The AAPCC has set up the Toxic Exposure Surveillance System (TESS), which collates calls from poison centers around the country. In 1993 1.75 million calls were reported to the TESS database from

64 participating poison centers.[14] The collected data provide toxin-specific demographic and morbidity and mortality information. They also provide for surveillance of adverse effects from marketed products, drugs, and other chemicals. Regulatory agencies and industry use this information to monitor product safety. Analysis of the database may uncover important new toxicologic problems, as well as focus preventive and treatment strategies on the more frequently encountered highly toxic problems.

The integrity of the database requires routine reporting of cases encountered in the emergency department. A close relationship between the emergency department and regional poison control center is essential in maintaining the optimal flow of information from the poison control center to the emergency department and from the emergency department to the poison control center. Collaborative efforts among emergency medicine colleagues situated in both sites exemplifies a team approach among emergency physicians to provide optimal patient care.

Education

Poison control centers also serve as important educational resources for health professionals and the general public. Poison control centers offer a unique training environment for the teaching of medical toxicology to physicians, pharmacists, and nurses.[15] The large array of clinical cases, vast informational resources, presence of board-certified medical toxicology consultants, and ongoing research endeavors provided by a regional poison control center offer a rich environment for focused study of medical toxicology. Most of the fellowship programs in medical toxicology are closely affiliated with their local regional poison control center. Poison centers also provide a productive training exposure for housestaff and medical students rotating on a medical toxicology elective. In particular, many emergency medicine residency programs use a regional poison control center as a site for a core rotation in toxicology. During such rotations, residents and students usually take part in poison center call backs, supervised handling of poison center calls, didactic conferences, bedside toxicology teaching, and research projects. Poison control centers also may offer continuing education programs for local physicians, pharmacists, nurses, and other health professionals.

Public education is another important poison center responsibility. Many poison centers employ full-time educators who work extensively with schools and a variety of outreach organizations to address poison prevention issues and orient people to the functions of the poison control center. Areas of emphasis include education on handling and storage of drugs and household chemicals, understanding safety packaging, instructions on first aid interventions, and accessing poison prevention services. Close cooperation with the local media and participation at community health fairs are also important components of public education operations.

POISON CONTROL CENTER FUNDING: MECHANISMS AND JUSTIFICATION

Recently, an increasing number of poison control centers have encountered funding difficulties.[5] Maintaining stable funding resources has been problematic. Funding sources for poison control centers varies considerably among centers. Because poison control center services to the public are nonreimbursable, operations tend to rely on a variety of benefactors from both the public and private sectors. According to a 1993 survey of poison control centers, 11% of regional poison centers received non-Medicaid federal funding, 11% received Medicaid support, 76% received state government funding, 21% received county or city funding, and 39% received private hospital funding.[5] Some of these poison control centers received several different sources of funding. Other types of support included donations from corporations (21%), donations from community service organizations (16%), industry contracts (34%), grants (21%), and support from other healthcare facilities (29%). The total direct funding of regional poison centers averaged $845,000, with a range of $262,000 to $1,870,000. The total cost per human exposure averaged $29.27.

State funding mechanisms include state legislative appropriations, state department of health block grants, excise tax on residential and business telephone use,[16] and surcharges on emergency department and/or inpatient admissions at the parent hospital of the poison control center. Private funding sources include philanthropic organizations (e.g., United Way), direct mail solicitation of contributions from poison center users,[17] contractual arrangements with private industry, partnerships with a chain drug store corporation,[18] and underwriting by hospitals and universities. To generate needed revenue, some poison centers have organized affiliate member hospital programs that charge annual fees to member hospitals and fee-for-service to nonmember hospitals for poison control center services.[19]

The rationale to fund poison control centers stems, in part, from the poison center's ability to decrease healthcare costs by discouraging unnecessary emergency department visits for accidental exposures to nontoxic and/or minimally toxic substances. Although somewhat counterintuitive to the usual emergency department practice of not making treatment decisions over the telephone and encouraging all telephone callers to seek medical attention in a timely fashion, poison control centers will advise parents to keep their children at home if the exposure is not thought to be significantly toxic. Approximately 85% of telephone inquiries to the poison control center involve nontoxic or minimally toxic exposures.[20] The specialist in poison information is quite adept at supervising the administration of syrup of ipecac or other basic decontamination strategies, or deciding that no treatment is required when the exposure is judged to be minimally toxic over the telephone. It has been estimated that for patients with exposures that only require dilution or reassurance, medical costs can be decreased by 75% to 80% when the patient uses the poison control center.[21] Further costs may be saved by decreasing unnecessary hospital admissions and unnecessary use of the emergency medical services (EMS) system.

Regional poison control centers have been shown to reduce excess emergency department visits for childhood poisonings. In a retrospective review, Chafee-Bahamon and Lovejoy[22] demonstrated that noncallers to the poison control center were much more likely to be seen at the emergency department than callers to the poison control center. In this study, noncallers to the poison center represented the vast majority of emergency department visits for pediatric poisoning episodes.

One of the best studies on the cost impact of the poison

control center was performed as the result of the unfortunate closing of the poison control center in Baton Rouge, Louisiana, which serviced the entire state.[23] The costs for unnecessary outpatient services resulting from "self-referral" to healthcare facilities increased significantly after the poison center closed. Self-referral of poison exposure cases to healthcare facilities increased by four times during this period. A cost analysis showed that the expenditures from unnecessary outpatient usage was estimated to be $1.4 million, an amount three times greater than the previous state appropriation for the poison control center.

Emergency medicine physicians who are involved in managing a poison center and/or serve as a poison center consultant are able to have a significant impact on improving appropriate patient use of emergency departments. Such physicians bring to the poison center an important perspective on the needs of the emergency department and emergency department patients. Decreasing inappropriate visits to the emergency department may decrease waiting times in the emergency department, increase availability of EMS for the transport of truly sick and injured patients, and increase the quality of emergency department care to patients in real need of emergency services. The involvement of emergency physicians in a healthcare approach that results in decreased costs is important in these days of a rapidly changing medical delivery system.

DEVELOPMENT OF MEDICAL TOXICOLOGY

Analogous to emergency medicine, medical toxicology is one of medicine's newest subspecialties. The first physicians to develop a strong interest in toxicology were pediatricians who became active in attacking the problems of childhood poisonings during the 1950s and 1960s, a period that predates the origins of emergency medicine. With the development of the specialty of emergency medicine, emergency physicians have played an increasingly visible and important role in the development of medical toxicology. A recent survey of medical toxicologists revealed that 50% were board certified in emergency medicine, 24% were board certified in pediatrics, 21% were board certified in internal medicine, 4% were board certified in preventive medicine, and 10% were board certified in other specialties or were non-board certified.[1] Obviously, emergency medicine board-certified physicians are greatly overrepresented in medical toxicology given that board certified emergency medicine physicians constitute only 2.6% of all board-certified physicians.

In 1968 the American Academy of Clinical Toxicology (ACCT) was founded by a group of toxicologists to improve the national standards of care of the poisoned patient.[24] Medical toxicology first established itself as a medical subspecialty in 1974, when the ACCT established the American Board of Medical Toxicology (ABMT). This board was founded to recognize the physician practitioner of medical toxicology.[25] A certifying examination was implemented, and by 1992, 212 physicians were board certified by the American Board of Medical Toxicology.

Because the American Board of Medical Toxicology developed outside the jurisdiction of the American Board of Medical Specialties (ABMS), an attempt was made in the early 1990s to obtain formal ABMS recognition for the field of medical toxicology. Despite the relatively small number of medical toxicologists, in 1992 the ABMS granted formal subspecialty recognition to medical toxicology. Medical toxicology is now recognized as a formal subspecialty of emergency medicine, pediatrics, and occupational medicine. Hence, medical toxicology joins pediatric emergency medicine as the two ABMS-approved subspecialties of emergency medicine. Beginning in late 1994, an ABMS-sponsored certifying examination in medical toxicology was offered to eligible candidates. Those eligible to sit for the board examination in medical toxicology include those previously certified by the now defunct ABMT, those who complete a fellowship in medical toxicology, and, for a limited time, those who fulfill the requirements of a practice track option.

Scope of Practice

A recent survey of medical toxicologists attempted to better define the scope of medical toxicology practice.[1] According to this survey, more than half the respondents were involved in telephone consultation, didactic teaching, direct patient care, bedside teaching, and toxicologic research (Table 86-1). Fifty-three percent of medical toxicologists spent less than 25% of their professional time on toxicologic activities, and 14% spent greater than 75% of their professional time on toxicologic activities. Furthermore, 79% of respondents were affiliated with a poison control center. Toxicologists affiliated with a poison control center spent on average 12 hours a week on this activity.[2]

Table 86-1 Toxicologic Activities Performed by Medical Toxicologists

Activity	% practicing	Average hours per week	Range of hours per week
Phone consultation	82	4.3	0.1-40
Didactic teaching	81	3.8	0.1-80
Direct patient care	79	6.9	0.25-30
Bedside teaching	63	5.0	0.5-36
Research	58	6.5	0.5-40
Administration	50	7.3	0.25-45
Legal consults	44	3.9	0.1-30
Public health policy	17	4.8	0.5-40
Clinical laboratory	7	11.4	1-54

Adapted from Donovan JW, Goldfrank LR. Medical toxicologist practice characteristics, specialty certifications and manpower needs. Presented at 1992 AAPCC/AACT/ABMT/CAPCC Annual Scientific Meeting, Tampa, FL.[1]

Training Programs

As the emerging field of medical toxicology has matured over the last two decades, training programs in medical toxicology have developed at several institutions across the country. As of 1993, there were 22 fellowship programs in medical toxicology in the United States.[26] The majority of these programs were operated under the auspices of departments or divisions of emergency medicine. Board eligibility in a medical specialty is the primary prerequisite, and fellowship programs usually run for a minimum of 2 years. Although many candidates have trained in emergency medicine, given the broad scope of medical toxicology, graduates of pediatrics, occupational medicine, internal medicine, and other residency programs are also eligible for medical toxicology fellowships.

EMERGENCY PHYSICIANS AND POISON CONTROL CENTERS

Several recent studies have analyzed interactions between emergency medicine physicians and poison control centers. In a study of Utah emergency physicians, Caravati and McElwee[27] showed that 53% of emergency physicians frequently called the poison control center for cases of acute symptomatic drug overdoses, whereas only 15% frequently called for cases of occupational exposure, 13% frequently called for chronic poisoning, and 5% frequently called for adverse drug reactions. The most common reasons for calling the poison control center included the desire for toxicity information and management recommendations. Thirty-two percent of physicians called the poison center for consultation with a physician toxicologist. Less than 10% of physicians called the poison center to report a case to the AAPCC database.

A recent phenomenon among emergency departments has been the purchase of the POISINDEX for the emergency department. Several different studies have shown that 23% of emergency departments have their own Poisindex.[27-29] From 75% to 83% of respondents have suggested that access to an emergency department Poisindex decreases their use of the poison control center. The concern generated from these studies suggests that physician-generated calls to poison control centers may decline as more emergency departments purchase Poisindex. Fewer calls to the poison control center, particularly with regard to significantly toxic exposures, may decrease the validity of the AAPCC database. Healthcare providers who choose to rely on their own Poisindex may not be privy to important local epidemiologic trends in drug use and poisoning that the poison center can provide. Several recent studies have suggested that a notable number of in-hospital poisoning deaths were not reported to the poison control center.[30,31] In a review of 121 in-hospital poisoning deaths in Rhode Island, only 27% were reported to the poison control center.[31] This underuse of the poison control center has generated significant concern.[32] Increased emphasis on the other resources of the poison control center including prompt consultation with a medical toxicologist is required to optimize emergency physician use of the poison control center.

In a survey study about emergency physician's perceptions of poison centers, Misra et al.[33] showed that 78% of emergency physicians surveyed thought their calls to the poison control center contributed to better patient management. Forty percent of physicians surveyed, however, did not even know the technical training of the person responding on the telephone. Respondents to this survey most desired that poison control centers upgrade the sophistication of their response on occupational and environmental toxicology issues.

FUTURE TRENDS

Although the field of medical toxicology has grown significantly in the last few years, the financial crisis affecting poison control centers has become more acute with each passing year. It is hoped that healthcare reform will provide the much needed long-term financial commitment to poison control centers in recognition of their ability to curb unnecessary healthcare expenditures. Perhaps managed care providers will recognize that poison control centers play a useful "gatekeeper" role by determining when an appropriate need exists for hospital-based medical evaluation of patients with a possible poisoning exposure.[34]

Nevertheless, further consolidation of poison control centers is most likely inevitable. Although the presence of 60 regional poison control centers has been suggested as an optimal number of centers nationwide,[20] the final number of adequately funded centers may be considerably lower. Although these trends suggest that the number of positions for medical toxicologists in poison control centers may not be on the rise, other opportunities for medical toxicologists, such as direct care of toxicologic patients on a fee-for-service basis, are evolving.

Recently growing enthusiasm has developed in the United States among medical toxicologists (including many medical toxicologists/emergency physicians) to establish regional toxicology treatment centers. Such centers have existed in several European cities including Edinburgh, Birmingham, Paris, Brussels, and Marseilles for many years, but have not as of yet established a firm footing in this country.[35] As distinguished from regional poison control centers, which offer telephone consultative services, toxicology treatment centers will serve as referral centers for patients requiring advanced toxicology evaluation and treatment. The goals of the toxicology treatment center is to enhance care of the poisoned patient, strengthen toxicology training, and facilitate research.[36] These centers will be staffed by board-certified physician medical toxicologists and nurse specialists. Direct inpatient, outpatient, and consultative services will be provided. Somewhat akin to trauma centers, the toxicology treatment center will require financial commitments, a critical mass of appropriate patients, and EMS cooperation to optimize its operations.

A career combining medical toxicology and emergency medicine is an exciting vocational alternative for the emergency medicine physician, particularly for the emergency medicine physician seeking a subspecialty niche to complement the broad-based approach of emergency medicine. Medical toxicology offers the opportunity to develop an expertise in a well-defined discipline firmly rooted in basic science that has fallen outside the confines of traditional medical specialties. Because so many toxicologic problems are first recognized by the emergency medicine physician, practice diversification into medical toxicology is but a small step. Medical toxicology as a medical subspecialty is still in its infancy. Nurturing by its many different practitioners (including the considerable number of emergency medicine physicians involved in this field) will undoubtedly influence its growth and development in the years ahead.

REFERENCES

1. Donovan JW, Goldfrank LR: Medical toxicologist practice characteristics, specialty certifications and manpower needs, (abstract), *Vet Hum Toxicol* 34:336, 1992.
2. Crotty JJ, Verhulst HL: Organization and delivery of poison information in the United States, *Pediatr Clin North Am* 17:741-747, 1970.
3. Scherz RG, Robertson WO: The history of poison control centers in the United States, *Clin Toxicol* 12:291-296, 1978.
4. Manoguerra AS, Temple AR: Observations on the current status of poison control centers in the United States, *Emerg Med Clin North Am* 2:185-197, 1983.
5. Litovitz T, Kearney TE, Holm K et al: Poison control centers: is there an antidote for budget cuts? *Am J Emerg Med* 12:585-599, 1994.
6. Thompson DF, Trammel HL, Robertson NJ, Reigart JR: Evaluation of regional and nonregional poison centers, *N Engl J Med* 308:191-194, 1983.
7. Geller RJ, Fisher JG, Leeper JD et al: Poison centers in America: how well do they perform? *Vet Hum Toxicol* 32:240-245, 1990.
8. Geller RJ, Fisher JG, Leeper JD, Ranganathan S: American poison control centers: still not all the same? *Ann Emerg Med* 17:599-603, 1988.
9. Mrvos R, Dean BS, Krenzelok EP: A demographic profile of the specialist in poison information, *Vet Hum Toxicol* 36:330-331, 1994.
10. Certification examination for poison information specialists, *Vet Hum Toxicol* 25:54-55, 1983.
11. Robertson WO: National organizations and agencies in poison control programs: a commentary, *Clin Toxicol* 12:297-302, 1978.
12. Manoguerra AS: The status of poison control centers in the United States, 1989: a report from the American Association of Poison Control Centers, *Vet Hum Toxicol* 33:131-150, 1991.
13. Lovejoy FH, Caplan DL, Rowland T, Fazen L: A statewide plan for care of the poisoned patient: the Massachusetts poison control system, *N Engl J Med* 300:363-365, 1979.
14. Litovitz TL, Clark LR, Soloway RA: 1993 Annual report of the American Association of Poison Control Centers Toxic Exposure Surveillance System, *Am J Emerg Med* 12:546-584, 1994.
15. Lovejoy FH, Edlin AL, Goldman P: Utilization of the poison center for the teaching of clinical toxicology to medical and pharmacy students, housestaff, and health care professionals, *Clin Toxicol* 15:393-400, 1979.
16. Bobbink S: Consolidating a poison network via total state funding, (abstract), *Vet Hum Toxicol* 35:324, 1993.
17. Trestrail JH, McCoy DJ: Direct mail solicitation of contributions from poison center users-success or failure? *Vet Hum Toxicol* 27:506, 1985.
18. Wanke LA, Burton B, Putnam TS: Financial support for poison control centers: a unique partnership with a chain drug store corporation, *Vet Hum Toxicol* 30:475-479, 1988.
19. Dean BS, Tibbs IS, Krenzelok EP: Toxicology consultation fees to health care facilities: a successful revenue generating program for poison centers, *Vet Hum Toxicol* 34:166-167, 1992.
20. McIntire MS, Angle CR: Regional poison-control centers improve patient care, (editorial), *N Engl J Med* 308:219-220, 1983.
21. Geller RJ, Looser RW: Cost saving from poison center use by medial consumers, *Vet Hum Toxicol* 27:521, 1985.
22. Chaffee-Bahamon C, Lovejoy FH: Effectiveness of a regional poison center in reducing excess emergency room visits from children's poisonings, *Pediatrics* 72:164-169, 1983.
23. King WD, Palmisano PA: Poison control centers: can their value be measured? *South Med J* 84:722-726, 1991.
24. Rumack B, Ford P, Sbarbaro J et al: Regionalization of poison centers: a rational role model, *Clin Toxicol* 12:367-375, 1978.
25. The American Board of Medical Toxicology. *Vet Hum Toxicol* 29:510, 1987.
26. Fellowship programs in medical toxicology. *Ann Emerg Med* 22:1428-1430, 1993.
27. Caravati EM, McElwee NE: Use of clinical toxicology resources by emergency physicians and its impact on poison control centers, *Ann Emerg Med* 20:147-150, 1991.
28. Wax PM, Rodewald L, Lawrence R: The arrival of the emergency department based POISINDEX: perceived impact on poison control center utilization, *Am J Emerg Med* 12:537-540, 1994.
29. Byars T, Patton J, King W, Nichols M: Utilization of the poison control center by emergency departments with POISINDEX, (abstract), *Vet Hum Toxicol* 36:353, 1994.
30. Soslow AR, Woolf AD: Reliability of data sources for poisoning deaths in Massachusetts. *Am J Emerg Med* 10:124-127, 1992.
31. Linakis JG, Frederick KA: Poisoning deaths not reported to the regional poison control center, *Ann Emerg Med* 22:1822-1828, 1993.
32. Goldfrank LR: Data, epidemiology, and the future strength of emergency medicine, (editorial), *Ann Emerg Med* 22:1859-1860, 1993.
33. Misra S, Haulman J, Robertson WO: Washington ER physicians' perceptions of poison centers, *Vet Hum Toxicol* 35:164-165, 1993.
34. Bonfiglio F, Rainey S, Seger D: Health care reform—managed care or managed chaos: what's in store for poison centers? *Vet Hum Toxicol* 36:354, 1994.
35. Donovan JW, Martin TG: Regional poison systems—roles and titles, (editorial), *J Toxicol Clin Toxicol* 31:221-222, 1993.
36. American Academy of Clinical Toxicology facility assessment guidelines for regional toxicology treatment centers, *J Toxicol Clin Toxicol* 31:209-210, 1993.

87 Sports Medicine

James M. Ellis, Jr.

OUTLINE

Emergency physicians are widely recognized as having a broad base of training comprising virtually all elements of acute care medicine, as well as blending elements of primary care medicine. This diversity in training and expertise can be extremely helpful in developing practice diversification opportunities. Such diversification may be helpful in addressing the attrition of physicians in emergency medicine, which has been attributed to a wide variety of causes including shift work and psychologic stress.[1-5] As emergency department physician groups look to avenues of diversification to allow for additional income sources and, more important, further areas of expressing their personal interests and expertise, sports medicine offers an important opportunity because emergency physicians are well trained and comfortable with the acute care aspects of evaluation and treatment of such injuries.

Sports medicine has traditionally been the domain of the orthopedic surgeon, but has become more accessible to physicians from other specialties. Sports medicine fellowships have become available to physicians other than orthopedists, including family practitioners and emergency physicians.[6] Sports medicine in the context of this chapter is a broader topic than just team physicians. Most physicians think of sports medicine being limited to acute injury care, physical rehabilitation, and some aspects of preventive medicine, with most of the expertise in this area traditionally lying within the practice of orthopedic surgery. The role of a team physician may include, but is certainly not limited to, these areas. Venue medicine is another realm within the sports medicine arena; however, it has received little attention either in the medical literature or within the physician community, at least until recently.

Emergency physicians are uniquely trained to handle all emergencies whether minor or major. No other specialty has that distinction. In sporting events, care for both the spectator and the athlete often includes primary orthopedic injuries, as well as general medical problems including life-threatening emergency conditions and injuries. Airway problems, head injuries, cervical spine injuries, cardiac arrest, cardiac arrhythmias, respiratory distress, intraabdominal trauma, dehydration, heat illness, allergic reactions, and even the diagnosis and treatment of dermatologic diseases may all be diagnosed by the physician practicing sports medicine. In most events, care of the athlete has typically been the orthopedist's responsibility, and emergency medical services (EMS) and/or nurses have delivered spectator care. Spectator care in most cases, has received minimal physician involvement. All too often, the choice of physicians to provide spectator care has not been based on knowledge and ability, but simply familiarity with the event organizers. With an increased emphasis on risk management and professional liability, consideration and selection of physicians to provide spectator care have become more important.

Opportunities in sports medicine for the emergency physician are vast. The biggest obstacle has been the issue of reimbursement. In many cases, both as team physicians and in providing spectator care, the medical community is called on to simply donate its time. For example, in surveying team physicians, it is not uncommon to learn that they spend 75% of their time with the athletic team, but only receive 25% of their income for this time. Addressing the question of reimbursement is a difficult task, but must be considered carefully before diversification into sports medicine becomes a viable strategy for an emergency physician group. In negotiating reimbursement, stressing the need for quality medical care in the diverse clinical entities that may present, as well as the role of risk management in our litigious society, may be of benefit.

THE EMERGENCY PHYSICIAN AS A TEAM PHYSICIAN

Historical Perspective

The origin of sports medicine arose from orthopedic surgery. This historical perspective is understandable, as the definitive management of severe orthopedic injuries, whether operative or nonoperative, is clearly the province of the orthopedic surgeon. Although the unquestioned expert in the field of musculoskeletal injuries, orthopedic surgeons are often faced with athletes who have nonorthopedic injuries. Team physicians also have other responsibilities, which may include but are not limited to preseason physicals, medical illnesses, acute neurosurgical problems, lacerations, and heat illnesses.

Several teams have recently realized this increased need for a broader scope of medical care and have begun to use internists, family practitioners, or emergency physicians to fill this void. Of these, the emergency physician clearly has better training for the diversity of clinical problems that may occur. Physicians trained in internal medicine may not be as comfortable with traumatic injury and rarely treat heat illnesses or life-threatening illnesses. Although physicians trained in family practice have a broad range of training, they may not have the depth of training and experience to manage severely injured patients in a multiple or major trauma situation. Airway management and cardiac arrhythmia recognition and treatment are invaluable skills of the emergency physician that may be needed even at a junior high school or high school level of care. This combination makes the emergency physician an obvious choice as the most qualified candidate for serving as a team physician.

Training and Experience

Developing a strategy for practice diversification in sports medicine for emergency physicians can be approached in a number of ways and includes virtually all levels of play—high school, college, and professional sports. Most teams want one person who is responsible for the medical care so that they may have one path to approach with concerns, problems, or feedback. Although this may be a requirement or request for the team, to allow maximum flexibility, multiple physicians within an emergency department group may be used for coverage, which offers substantial advantages. The team will probably request that one physician still be the main contact person for the entire group. The most important factor other than training and experience in emergency medicine is an interest in the particular sport that the physician is covering. Being a team physician can be most gratifying, particularly when the team enjoys success and the team physician feels part of it.

As mentioned, three fellowships are currently available for emergency physicians to train in sports medicine. (Box 87-1). Although this is ideal training, it certainly is not a requirement to act as a team physician. The background and training of emergency physician allow them to possess the appropriate knowledge in this field. Selected readings from the orthopedic literature are a substantial benefit in the role as a team physician on the high school level.[7,8] Higher levels of expertise may be expected and required in the college and professional ranks.

The flexibility of an emergency physician would allow coverage at most events in which the team participates, but this must be considered when one has other job commitments. As stated, an interest in the sport that one covers is one of the most critical aspects of being a team physician. Each sport has its individual rules and regulations, as well as particular injuries that are most common. For example, some sports require the referee to clear the athlete for medical intervention. If assistance is offered on the field of play without following the proper guidelines, the athlete may be disqualified. A number of sports have recently developed policies on the bleeding athlete in an effort to address concerns over HIV exposure. It is imperative that the team physician understand all of these policies and be prepared for them. There will be a need for an agreement with an orthopedic surgeon for referral in the case of complicated injuries. The orthopedic surgeon must be an integral part of the medical team for continuity of care and should be someone with whom the emergency physician is familiar and comfortable.

BOX 87-1

SPORTS MEDICINE FELLOWSHIPS

California

Steven M. Green, M.D.
Loma Linda University
Department of Emergency Medicine
A-108
Loma Linda, CA 92354
Phone: 909-824-4085
Fax: 909-478-4121
Length: 1 year

North Carolina

Robert W. Schafermeyer, M.D.
Division of Sports Medicine
Department of Emergency Medicine
P.O. Box 32861
Charlotte, NC 28232-2861
Phone: 704-355-3181
Fax: 704-355-5609
Length: 1 year

Earl Schwartz, M.D.
Department of Emergency Medicine
Bowman Gray School of Medicine
Medical Center Boulevard
Winston-Salem, NC 27157-1089
Phone: 919-716-3947
Fax: 919-716-5438
Length: 1 year

How to Organize

The best approach to finding a position in sports medicine is to obtain direct contact with someone within the team's organization who makes the medical decisions. This person could be a trainer, principal, head coach, athletic director, chancellor, owner, or the current team physician who may or may not be an orthopedic surgeon. The contact person obviously depends on the level of a team with which one is working. The best way to prepare for all medical problems of the team is to have a referral base for specific illnesses or injuries similar to what happens in the day-to-day practice of emergency medicine. The process would need to begin with a written medical plan that includes policies and procedures for all situations. These protocols should include preseason physicals, referrals, on-call availability during practices, and attendance at the games. The team may want to select its own panel of physicians somewhat like a managed care organization for referrals, or it may want the team physician to undertake this task.

One way to extend a broader scope of care would be to include a hospital in the package. With hospitals looking for ways to increase their market share, this arrangement could be treated like a managed care situation, and the hospital could help in providing services and equipment. Although the prevalence of this type agreement is rare, it could prove advantageous for a hospital to "sponsor" a team. The level of sponsorship and commitment would obviously vary according to the hospital's desire to help and the possibility of a benefits package that the team could offer.

Medical Plan

The most important aspect in preparing to be a team physician is the development of a written medical plan, which would be all inclusive of one's role as a team physician and should document why the physician would be an asset to the team as the team physician.

Of paramount importance to the program is the availability of the physician,[7] not only during the games but also during the team's practice. As with emergency medicine, this may include a 24-hour commitment. The advantage of emergency medicine is that team members may be identified as such and present to the emergency department if an understanding with one's group has been reached.

The medical plan itself must address the broad base of knowledge seen in athletic competition including medical injuries and illnesses, psychologic problems, pharmacologic intervention, and exercise physiology, as well as rehabilitation and biomechanics.[7] The athlete should be treated the same medically as anyone else presenting to an emergency physician. The only exception would be any banned substance from the sport's governing body. There are also particular protective devices that may not be used by the athlete.

The medical plan should include policies, procedures, and protocols not only for specific injuries, but also for particular settings such as games, practices, and if extended to the highest level, nonathletic-related injury and illness. Continuity and consistency are critical in this regard. For example, if one athlete on the team has a second-degree ankle sprain, the way in which that athlete is cared for should be consistent with the treatment of other athletes who have had similar injuries.

The plan should also include ways for the team physician to be contacted 24 hours a day or should delineate the understanding with the emergency department to cover during night-time hours. There should also be a referral list for injury and illness outside the scope of the team emergency physician. The orthopedic surgeon is the most integral part of this picture, but other subspecialists must also be available.

A number of people may be needed in addition to the emergency physician. Residents may be helpful in covering games if this arrangement is acceptable to the team. Although their expertise is limited, they may be adequate under appropriate supervision. The role of the qualified athletic trainer should not be underestimated. They typically have an outstanding knowledge base and can be an invaluable asset in dealing with the team. For the emergency physician, the trainer must be considered another integral part of the overall management team in the medical plan.

A team physician must understand the athletes themselves, the potential for injury, and any preexisting conditions that may be important in a treatment plan.[9] A list of appropriate equipment and supplies that will be used in various situations including games and practices must also be included in the medical plan.[10] Finally, there must be a plan of action to be followed if the athlete needs transportation to the hospital, either via the local 911 emergency system, county EMS system, or private transport service that may be onsite during the games. The medical plan should allow for the proper assessment, treatment, and stabilization of the athlete so that they may have the best outcome in the event of injury or illness.[9] Joseph F. Waeckerle, MD, FACEP gave an outstanding lecture, "The Team Physician—How to Manage Common Sports Injuries," at the 1994 ACEP Scientific Assembly, which summarizes the benchmark treatment of the injured athlete.

Acquisition

The emergency physician group has an advantage over other physicians. The group may have a larger physician base to offer a sports team. A larger number of emergency physicians has the ability to pursue more acquisitions. One must thoroughly understand and consider the amount of commitment required to be a team physician when acquiring teams for which they will be responsible. The most approachable teams are obviously the lower level ones such as high schools that may not have any significant medical coverage already in place. As one moves up the scale to college and professional teams, more comprehensive coverage is typically requested and medically needed. Certainly the stepping stone to the college or professional level may be one's performance on the high school level. Therefore an effort should be made not to compromise any one team in favor of another.

The appropriate person to approach depends on the level of the team. The most important aspect of presenting one's self for consideration as a team physician should be the written medical plan explaining all of the comprehensive details of the medical service. Important points to stress are the broad scope of expertise offered by the emergency physician and 24-hour availability of the individual or the group at the hospital emergency department. Specific examples of conditions that may require this extensive coverage include head injuries with or without seizures, cardiac contusions with cardiac arrhythmias, heat-related illness and injury including heat stroke, cardiac arrest, intraabdominal trauma, expertise in airway management, and the overall background of the emergency physician to treat all types of medical illness and injury, as well as critical care knowledge. Finally, the team must consider the liability factor. The training of the emergency physician lessens the team's liability in comparison to someone who has no training in trauma or the nonemergency physician attempting to care for injuries and illnesses with which they are not familiar.

Management/Maintenance

Management and maintenance of the agreement are paramount. Teams want a single person with whom they can identify and go to when a problem surfaces. The availability of quality medical care is imperative and should be stressed so that the team feels confident that someone is willing to help them even for their most minor problems. A sound quality assurance program should be developed into the medical plan. Rehabilitation is a part of the program because the goal of both the athlete and coaches is to get the athlete back on the field of play as soon as possible. This component is also important for referral physicians in areas where the emergency physician may not have expertise. When approaching a team about providing medical coverage and being the team physician, the physician should stress interest in the sport; possible background or participation in the sport; the wide variety of expertise, knowledge, and understanding of the injuries unique to that sport; and the ability to handle all conditions including urgent, minor, or true emergencies. A thorough quality assurance program should be developed in the medical plan, and its results should be shared with the team. This provides the team with ongoing evaluation of the services and expertise they are receiving.

Although the emergency physician is well trained and will deliver outstanding medical care to teams, remember that lay people typically do not know good medicine, but they do know good people. Therefore although providing quality medical care should be one's ultimate goal, providing a customer service attitude and meeting the needs and expectations of customers will keep the relationship with the team positive.

VENUE MEDICINE

Historical Perspective

In contrast to the paucity of articles that exist in the emergency medicine literature about team physicians, a recent increase in literature that outlines venue medicine and medical care at mass gatherings has occurred.[11-18] In addition, the American College of Emergency Physicians has published an excellent paper on medical care at mass gatherings.[19] In the past, most venues have been covered in agreements or private contracts with the owner of the venue or the government agency that manages the venue. This has become somewhat of a "political contract" and may be founded not on the level of expertise, but based on local factors such as political connections, contact with stadium owners or managers, or relationships with important decision makers on the prevalent team at the venue. Because of the aforementioned level of training and experience, the emergency physician is the obvious choice for organizing and supervising medical care at venues for mass gatherings including athletic events and rock concerts.

When evaluating a venue to determine the level of care needed and the staffing numbers, several factors must be considered. Peter T. Pons, MD, FACEP delivered a comprehensive lecture on mass gatherings at the 1994 ACEP Scientific Assembly. He gave a complete overview of mass gatherings, which included an excellent example of practical application with the visit of Pope John Paul II.[20] He summarized the factors influencing medical coverage at a venue including indoor versus outdoor, seated versus nonseated, environmental conditions, event site, attendance, attendees, particular type of event and the availability of food, water, alcohol and drugs[20] (Table 87-1). These factors will mandate flexibility in the staffing guidelines that are cited in the literature and should be adaptable to the specific venue or stadium to be covered.[19]

Unfortunately stadiums are not designed for medical care.

Table 87-1 Factors Affecting Usage of Medical Service

	More use	Less use
Environment	Heat	Cold
Seating arrangement	Unseated event	Seated event
Age (no alcohol)	Older	Younger
Event	Football, concert	Baseball, basketball
Alcohol	Available	Unavailable

The ideal situation would be to assist the architect in designing the stadium with an emphasis on safety issues, adequate space for medical response, and location and design of medical stations. More often than not, however, medical stations are an afterthought and providers must use available space and design a response with the predetermined architectural constraints of the venue.

Training and Experience

There are no specific training programs for venue medicine, although the principles of emergency medicine and disaster medicine are applicable for venue medical care. Venue medicine has typically been the domain of the EMS community or a nonemergency physician who has a desire to attend the event and watch the activity, but not necessarily participate in spectator medical care. Venues may be indoor stadiums, outdoor stadiums, or an outdoor concert seating arrangement that is not within an enclosed stadium, but rather within an enclosed perimeter. Venues may contain sporting events, rock concerts, conventions, and a wide variety of events that may attract crowds ranging from a few hundred to greater than 100,000 people. Although there is some information about the incidence of injuries and summaries of medical care at mass gatherings, there is little specific literature about the level of training of personnel.[11-15] Fortunately, the emergency physician does not need any specific training, except a knowledge of the area and a desire to participate in the care of the injured or ill spectator. The training for the emergency physician consists of evaluating all areas of the venue in an effort to become familiar with the multitude of variables unique to the venue that will affect the medical response. After this training is completed, a comprehensive plan specific to that particular venue can be developed. The full spectrum of illness and injury seen in the emergency department may be encountered in the venue; therefore, appropriate preparations must be made after determination of the level of care to be rendered for each situation.

How to Organize

Each venue that has a coordinated medical team should have a medical plan that is developed specifically for the venue. This plan will again depend on the type of venue (indoor versus outdoor) and size of the venue. It should provide flexibility to accommodate for the many variables that will affect the medical response in the venue. During the organizational phase, it is certainly appropriate to use some approximation and general guidelines, but the specific plan must be tailored to fit the venue in question with an accurate working knowledge of its individual nuances. The plan should delineate the specific flexibility to downsize or upgrade staff based on the different crowd expectations or conditions at the venue. Although the literature is replete with guidelines and approximations with regard to the number of physicians, nurses, and paramedics and/or EMTs that may be used at sporting events, the individual venue must be evaluated to determine any road blocks that may come up when applying these numbers. For example, there is an unwritten rule of verticality that may increase staffing needs because of multiple levels of the stadium. Also, although two areas of a stadium may appear to be in close approximation with one another, an artificial barrier may create an access problem, thereby increasing staffing needs more than normally projected for the crowd size. The organization of a venue plan must include appropriate personnel with specific training, and the implementation must be with personnel that can be trusted. If the emergency physician group has an EMS service for which they serve as medical director, it may want to consider a partnership to deliver venue medical care in addition to the emergency physician.

Since the setting is similar to a field setting, the paramedic and EMT appear to be the best personnel to use in a venue. Considering there may be a need for more that one physician on occasion, certainly other members of an emergency medicine group may be used at various times. Also with large venues that frequently have events, it may not be possible for one physician to cover all of them. In addition to personnel flexibility, equipment flexibility must be evaluated. The configuration of a given venue (e.g., stadium, road race, etc.) may dictate the various types of transportation and response vehicles needed. Numerous substitutes for ambulances have been used including medically configured golf carts, all-terrain vehicles, and bicycles.

Finally, the level of care to be delivered must be determined. Obviously, basic first aid and advanced life support are the two areas that must be supplied. Everything in between is optional depending on the setting, level of expertise, and expectations of the venue management. This level of care will determine the personnel, supplies, and equipment needed. Decisions must be made with regard to treatments such as suturing, respiratory rebulizers, narcotic pain medication, and possibly thrombolytic therapy. Although one of the goals of venue medicine is to lesson the impact on hospitals and the local EMS entities, there are limitations as to what can be managed adequately within the venue.

Medical Plan

Dr Ricardo Martinez, MD, FACEP, of Medical Sports Group has been the Medical Consultant to the NFL for the Super Bowl. He has found that few venues have a written or well-structured plan. Although no one format will work well in all venues, specific areas must be addressed to minimize risks and maximize quality medical care. This led Dr. Martinez to develop a template so that each venue may be adapted specifically to fit within a basic plan. This template consists of administration, providers, first responders, training, triage, transportation, communication, medical direction, medical aid stations, hospitals, equipment and supplies, access, and quality assurance[21,22] (Box 87-2). These areas are specifically addressed here.

One person must be responsible for determining the appropriate level of care at the venue. This person must be adept at working with others at the venue including the venue administration, security, ushers, and vendors. Choices for this position can be either the physician in charge (medical director) or someone in a high ranking position with the EMS service (EMS director) who is working with the emergency physician. Ideally, the choice should be the medical director; however the director must be prepared not only for administrative meetings but also for frequent questions and concerns of the administration at the venue. If the medical director chooses to delegate this responsibility to the EMS director, the emergency physician should be aware of and have a hand in every critical decision made by the EMS personnel.

> **BOX 87-2**
>
> **TEMPLATE TO DEVELOP MEDICAL PLANS FOR VENUES**
>
> **Spectator care**
>
> Injury control
> Medical response
> Disaster planning
>
> **Medical response**
>
> Administration
> Providers
> First responders
> Training
> Triage
> Transportation
> Communications
> Medical direction
> Medical aid stations
> Hospitals
> Access
> Equipment
> Quality assurance

Paramedics and EMTs are the best providers in this arena because it is similar to a field setting. Nurses work well in a fixed medical aid station. The emergency physician is without question the best trained physician to provide medical care at these events because of the aforementioned spectrum of medical issues. Finally, one must consider other personnel such as administrative people or clerical staff who may help not only in the aid station but as runners if more supplies or equipment is needed. In addition, someone familiar with the stadium and the concept of dispatch should be in charge of dispatching mobile teams to the scene of needed medical care in the stadium.

First responders at the venues may be anyone from ushers or security people to vendors. When interacting with the other personnel at the venue, it is important to realize that these people can be trained in CPR through a hospital or the American Red Cross. Some stadiums use American Red Cross trained people as first responders in venues. If this group is used they must have excellent back up from paramedics, EMTs, or nurses for delivering a higher level of care. There has also been some success in training first responders to use automated external defibrillators.[15]

Most of the education should focus on familiarization of

personnel with the venue itself and the medical plan. Paramedics and EMTs used as response teams within the venue should know the areas they will be responsible for and understand the interaction with security and ushers. They must know all of the appropriate markings for determining section, row, and location for any response within the stadium, but must especially be familiar with their assigned area for that particular day. Response times to the area for which they are responsible should be approximately 4 to 5 minutes or less.

Triage at the venue should be developed under the direction of the physician in charge. Whether someone is treated at the seat and not seen at the medical station, transported to the medical station, or transported directly to the ambulance and to the hospital is the decision of the physician who is providing medical control at the venue. There should be adequate protocols and guidelines developed in which paramedics and nurses may treat minor injury and illness without a physician actually seeing a patient, but the physician should be aware of each encounter as much as possible to limit liability and improve quality of care. Some medical plans include a self-treatment option for patients requesting aspirin, Tylenol, or Band-aids; but spectators must sign a liability release form.

Transportation consists of two areas: transportation from a seat to a medical station and transportation by ambulance to the hospital. Ambulance stretchers may be placed at various locations within the venue, or they may be dispatched from the medical aid station to the site if transportation is deemed necessary. Use of wheel chairs and specifically designed stair chairs for stadiums also may be necessary. The number of ambulances required has been reported as low as one vehicle for every 10,000 spectators. Some states have laws that determine this level. A more reasonable number appears to be at least one ambulance for every 20,000 spectators. With small venues that may only have 20,000 or less, there certainly should be a protocol in place for replacement of this vehicle if the only ambulance leaves with a transport. The location of the ambulance is determined somewhat by security. Optimally it should be located in close proximity to the first aid station on the ground level. Most venues have an employee entrance or a loading dock that is typically a good site to park the ambulance. If there is not a good site, staging of an ambulance may occur in a different area, with communication available to bring the ambulance into a designated location close to the venue when needed for transport.

All routine communications should occur on a single channel. Preferably, the dispatcher should be located in a central command post along with administration of the venue including head of operations, head of security, the supervisor of the ushers, and any other appropriate agencies. This dispatcher should be able to communicate with all medical personnel in the venue on a single frequency. The medical director should have two frequencies, one for communicating with medical personnel and a separate frequency for communicating with the command staff in case of a disaster situation. The supervisor of the EMS personnel may require a separate frequency. The response teams should have at least one hand-held radio per team. Each of the mobile stations also should have a radio. These stations may also benefit from having a telephone line. Some stadiums use ring down phones that connect only to the command staff and vice versa. If a more traditional phone line is used, it should be a two-line system that will allow the aid station to receive a second in-coming call while on the phone so that there will be no interruption in communication. Talk on the radio system should be kept to a minimum and should be used only for pertinent exchange of information.

Typically, physicians responsible for medical direction have been unqualified, unavailable, underused, or uninformed. Therefore medical direction for the venue should come under the control of the emergency physician on-site. There may be some need for base station medical control for different cases with smaller crowds in attendance if a physician is not needed on site. If that is not possible, then off-line medical control can be used with standing order protocols that have been set up by the physician medical director. As stated, optimally the physician should be on site and should be an emergency physician. This will decrease liability, as well as provide a higher level of medical care for the spectators. The medical director should be intimately involved in all decision making at the venue and during the event should be either in the main aid station treating patients or in the central command post if multiple physicians are used.

Medical aid stations should be set up as a microcosm of the emergency department. Required equipment and supplies depend on the scope of care. The scope of care should be determined by the emergency physician medical director. Adequate space should be secured, with at least the ability to treat two simultaneous cardiac arrests in the same area. There are no specific square footage requirements, but a minimum of 800 square feet is needed to treat patients adequately. There should be one station on each level of the stadium. If one level of a stadium has more than 30,000 to 40,000 people, a second station should be considered. An outdoor venue that may be spread out and may not have levels should place stations in locations based on concentrations of crowds and distance between stations. Patients should not have to walk more than 5 minutes or approximately ⅛ of a mile to get to an aid station.[19] In the case of a marathon, for example, stations should be set up along certain mile increments, with increasing number of stations and shrinking increments toward the end of the race. The concentration of medical personnel should be greatest at the end of the race. This arrangement is best not only for the spectators, but also for the athletes.[23] An often overlooked but important topic is signage. Spectators must know where to go to seek medical care or how to activate the system if in an enclosed suite. Adequate signage should be a venue-wide priority. The ability for the spectator to self-present will decrease the use of mobile team responses for nonurgent medical problems.

An agreement should be undertaken with an appropriate hospital for transportation of the spectators to that hospital and supplies and equipment. Preferably, this hospital should be the one nearest to the venue, although that is not necessarily a requirement. Certainly a hospital that is farther away may be used for the majority of transports, but the nearest hospital will always be a consideration and is essential in the case of life-threatening emergencies. If the area has a trauma system, the predetermined trauma hospital must be on alert on days of specific events. The stable patient who is to be transported may designate a specific hospital of choice.

Unlimited access to all areas of the venue is imperative. Security must be familiar with medical personnel and understand that a cardiac arrest can happen anywhere in the venue, leaving no area off limits to the medical providers. When credentials are being issued, unlimited access must be requested for all medical personnel throughout the venue, although there may be some limitations on the field of play. If the same medical team is responsible for the field of play, it must be given credentials specific to the field of play. Usually athletic teams have their own medical support staff to respond to the athletes. In this case, there should be an agreement with them and an understanding that backup is available in the form of an emergency physician and/or EMS personnel.

The supply and equipment list can be developed in accordance with the services offered at the venue. As stated earlier, there may be a desire or need to suture at the venue and this would obviously change the supply list. Venues in the future may be able to administer thrombolytic therapy before transport. The specific supplies and equipment to be stocked include equipment and drugs for advance cardiac life support (ACLS). Every medical aid station should have intubation equipment, a defibrillator, and the full supply of ACLS drugs. Intravenous fluids, specifically normal saline, should be available for trauma victims in traumatic resuscitation. The American College of Emergency Physicians has an excellent supply and equipment list in their publication on medical care at mass gatherings.[19]

Quality assurance, an important part of venue medical care, should be the responsibility of the medical director. The quality assurance program should provide ongoing review of the medical care delivered, identifying problem areas and making an effort to correct them. Documentation of each encounter must be logged. A documentation form should be available for both paramedics and EMTs and physicians. There should be a follow-up instruction form in addition to an AMA form for anyone wishing to refuse medical care. Review of these forms may be undertaken by both the emergency physician medical director and the EMS director. The form may be used in working with the administration at the venue if any patient-related problems arise. It is also important from a medicolegal standpoint. The cornerstone of quality assurance is proper record keeping and strong medical direction.

Each venue should have a disaster plan that delineates appropriate response within the venue. There should also be a plan for using outside sources to help with a larger scale disaster. This plan should be discussed with the local officials in charge of disaster planning for that particular area.

Staffing the venue is an inexact science. The many factors discussed earlier make it difficult to predict the number of encounters to be expected. Different studies acknowledge the wide variation in medical encounters, which are determined variables such as the site, environment, crowd size, crowd demographics, and alcohol availability.[11-14,16,17,19,20] The previously published numbers range from 1.6% to less than .01% of attendees seeking medical care. With the aforementioned wide range of variability, .01% to .05% (1/1000 to 5/1000) is a safe starting point. Approximately 2% to 4% of the patients encountered may eventually be transported.

A paramedic/EMT team can easily cover between 10,000 to 20,000 spectators if they are not spread over too large of an area. There should be at least one medical aid station on each level of the stadium, and there may be consideration for two if it is a large venue or if there are more than 30,000 people on one level. The best guideline for physician staffing is 1 to 2 physicians for every 50,000 spectators.[12] With a high profile event like the Super Bowl in Atlanta, we used one physician in every aid station (four levels), as well as a supervisory physician.

Rather than concentrating on the number of spectators, another approach is to look at time response. Originally, 4 minutes for basic life support and 8 minutes for advanced life support (ALS) were considered acceptable guidelines.[12] More recent literature recommends ALS within 5 minutes.[14] Obviously the faster the response, the better the chance for survival in cases of cardiac arrest.

Acquisition

A contract for a venue may be acquired in several ways. It can be approached through the emergency physician group. Often one needs a number of personnel to cover the venue depending on the frequency of the events. There also may be a need to have more than one physician at the venue depending on the size of the event. Other personnel involved may include paramedics, EMTs, and nurses. Before approaching a venue, an agreement must be reached between the involved parties who will be participating in the proposed medical plan at the venue. All involved should have a thorough understanding of their role. The contract should be initiated with the head of operations of the venue or their designated person. This may be through city, county, or state government agencies or through a private company. The approach may be with a physician group, an EMS service, or with a hospital. Compensation will depend on the normal rates for that particular person's full-time employment. Approximately 50% of the normal rate works well for physician payment. Nurses and paramedics may require the usual hourly rate they receive on their full-time job. The financial agreement is difficult to execute, but to ensure quality medical care it must be well planned and negotiated from a strong position. Some facilities recommend passing the cost on to the primary tenant or the promoter of each individual event.

When pursuing an agreement with a venue, quality must be stressed. The physician component should be clearly delineated so that the high level of care the venue will receive is understood. Some contracts are put out to bid. An estimate must include personnel and supplies. Once a venue contract is acquired, an excellent track record can be developed leading to other contracts.

Management/Maintenance

Maintenance of the contract is best accomplished through communications with the head of operations based on the recommendation of the administration of the venue. Some will desire a more hands-on approach and need frequent feedback including a report after every event. Others prefer quarterly or yearly reports. Included in the report should be a summary of the number of patients treated, their respective diagnoses, number of people transported, and any complications that may occur during these events. A close working relationship with security and the ushers is imperative. One must have full and total access in the stadium to render quality care. The authority should feel that they have one person that is a contact person for each concern and should not have to deal with different people for various problems. Communication is key.

The quality assurance plan should be used for ongoing feedback to the administration. The administration must feel that their venue is perceived as important and that they receive quality medical care for their expense. If problems arise, communication should be undertaken as soon as possible to resolve any outstanding issues important to the authority.

REIMBURSEMENT

In the words of Dr. Martinez, "form follows finance." Reimbursement as a team physician or with venue medical care is usually the exception rather than the rule. The importance of quality medical care for athletes and spectators is expected, but everyone seems to believe that physicians should donate their time. In the past, physicians have obliged, and because of the lack of a reimbursement agreement, care of the athlete and the spectator has sometimes been suboptimal. As the old saying goes, "you get what you pay for." If premium medical care with a true customer service approach is the goal, then reimbursement is essential. Without reimbursement, the relationship will probably be short lived. With athletic teams, interest is eventually lost and enthusiasm turns to apathy. With venues, there are the minor events such as dog shows and tractor pulls, which may not receive as much attention and support within a physician group unless there is monetary reimbursement.

There is no specific way in which to negotiate the monetary necessity of these efforts, but the primary objective is to sell quality. Certainly the issue of risk management should be discussed, especially in the venue setting where there is a significant potential for liability. The actual reimbursement amount is difficult to ascertain. Nurses, paramedics, and EMTs must be paid approximately 75% to 100% of their hourly wage at their full-time job. Physicians receiving 50% of their typical wage seem to be attracted enough to cover the event. Higher profile events such as major sporting events or concerts, in which individuals may have a greater interest, are easier to staff; if these were the only events covered, reimbursement may not be necessary. Unfortunately, even these events after a certain period of time become more of a chore than a pleasure, and reimbursement will eventually become an issue.

Team physicians can either negotiate a flat yearly rate or bill hourly for the time invested in caring for the team. Team orthopedists are able to generate income with surgical and office procedures. Unfortunately even that does not adequately reimburse them for the amount of time they spend with the team. An emergency physician who has limited invasive credentialing must find an alternative. If the flat rate or hourly bill is unacceptable, then each encounter with an athlete must be billed. This approach should be closely studied, however, because hospital and/or group contracts may prohibit this type of arrangement.

Until the practice of reimbursing physicians becomes widespread within venue medicine and athletic team physicians, it is up to the individual to sell his or her services. The three areas that must be promoted are quality medical care, risk management, and liability protection, with a customer service approach.

SUMMARY

The emergency physician as a team physician or as a venue physician is an enjoyable alternative to the daily grind of seeing patients nonstop in the emergency department. There also may be the significant perks of good vantage points for events at the venue and close personal contact with athletes if the physician has an interest in that particular sport. With reimbursement still difficult to achieve, it requires significant motivation and success to reach a comfortable financial situation that would allow a full-time sports medicine practice. The area of venue medicine should certainly be the exclusive domain of the emergency physician. In addition, the emergency physician can act as a team physician in a close relationship with an orthopedic surgeon.

REFERENCES

1. Whitley TW, Allison EJ Jr, Gallery ME et al: Work-related stress and depression among practicing emergency physicians: an international study, *Ann Emerg Med* 23:1068-1071, 1994.
2. Whitley TW, Gallery ME, Allison EJ Jr et al: Factors associated with stress among emergency medicine residents, *Ann Emerg Med* 20:1157-1161, 1991.
3. Keller KL, Koenig WJ: Management of stress and prevention of burnout in emergency physicians, *Ann Emerg Med* 18:42-47, 1989.
4. Gallery ME, Whitley TW, Klonis LK et al: A study of occupational stress and depression among emergency physicians, *Ann Emerg Med* 21:58-64, 1992.
5. Hall KN, Wakeman MA, Levy RC et al: Factors associated with career longevity in residency-trained emergency physicians, *Ann Emerg Med* 21:291-297, 1992.
6. Sports medicine fellowships for primary care physicians. *Phys Sportsmed* 1992; 20:(3):217-221.
7. Mellion MB, Walsh WM, Shelton GL: *The team physician's handbook*, St Louis, 1990, Mosby.
8. Samples P: The team physician: no official job description, *Phys Sportsmed* 16:169-175, 1988.
9. Waeckerle JF: The team physician: how to manage common sports injuries: 1994 Scientific Assembly, Orlando, Fla.
10. Howe WB: What I take to the game. *Phys Sportsmed* 18:61-66, 1990.
11. Baker WM, Simone DM, Niemann JT et al: Special events medical care: the 1984 Los Angeles Summer Olympics Experience, *Ann Emerg Med* 15:185-190, 1986.
12. Sanders AB, Criss E, Steckl P et al: An analysis of medical care at mass gatherings, *Ann Emerg Med* 15:515-519, 1986.
13. Ounanian LL, Salinas C, Shear CL et al: Medical care at the 1982 U.S. Festival, *Ann Emerg Med* 15:520-527, 1986.
14. Spaite DW, Criss EA, Valenzuela TD et al: A new model for providing prehospital medical care in large stadiums, *Ann Emerg Med* 17:825-828, 1988.
15. Weaver WD, Sutherland K, Wirkus MJ, Bachman R: Emergency medial care requirements for large public assemblies and a new strategy for managing cardiac arrest in this setting, *Ann Emerg Med* 18:155-160, 1989.
16. Thompson JM, Savoia G, Powell G et al: Level of medical care required for mass gatherings: the XV Winter Olympic Games in Calgary, Canada, *Ann Emerg Med* 20:385-390, 1991.
17. Bowdish GE, Cordell WH, Bock HC, Vukov LF: Using regression analysis to predict emergency patient volume at the Indianapolis 500 mile race, *Ann Emerg Med* 21:1200-1203, 1992.
18. Bock HC, Cordell WH, Hawk AC, Bowdish GE: Demographics of emergency medical care at the Indianapolis 500 mile race (1983-1990), *Ann Emerg Med* 21:1204-1207, 1992.

19. Leonard RB, Petrilli R, Noji EK, Calabro JJ: *Provision of emergency medical care for crowds,* Dallas 1990, American College of Emergency Physicians.
20. Pons PT: Mass gatherings world youth day and the visit of Pope John Paul II. 1994 Scientific Assembly, Orlando, Fla.
21. Martinez R: Medically alert, *Athletic Business* 9:53-56, 1992.
22. Martinez R: Super Bowl safety, *Emerg Med Serv* 21:1-4, 1992.
23. Ellis DG, Verdile VP, Paris PM et al: Medical coverage of a marathon: establishing guidelines for deployment of health care resources, *Prehospital Disaster Med* 6:435-441, 1991.

88 The Role of Air Medical Services

Luis F. Eljaiek, Jr. and Thom A. Mayer

OUTLINE

Qualifications and experience
Emergency department diversification in air medical services
Emergency physician as medical director
Administrative and hospital integration
Outside relations
Emergency physician as a flight crew member
Integration within the emergency department physician group
Summary

The field of emergency medicine and the roles of the emergency physician have changed rapidly over the last 25 years. One of the areas of growth has been in subspecialties within emergency medicine. Transport medicine and air medical services are areas of practice diversification that have a rich history for emergency physicians and provide substantial opportunities for emergency department groups and the physicians comprising them. The mid to late 1980s saw a tremendous growth in the number of air transport programs, primarily in rotor wing aircraft. This growth was due to an increase in the number of trauma centers and related tertiary care programs in this country, as well as the funding mechanisms to offset their operating costs. There was a major emphasis in healthcare on the care of the traumatized patient and other critically ill patient populations, including cardiac, neonatal, pediatric, and other intensive care unit patients. As more hospitals incorporated trauma and acute care and the infrastructure of trauma systems grew, so did the need for a rapid and reliable method of transport coupled with delivery of critical care capabilities in the aircraft. Thus the medivac model from the Korean and Vietnam wars was adopted into civilian practice. However, hospital-based medivac programs also included highly trained critical care crews capable of substantial interventions far beyond that available in the military model.

The goals for most medivac programs are to provide a rapid method of transportation and to initiate the resuscitation and stabilization of the patient until the patient receives definitive care. These mission goals are strikingly similar to those seen in emergency medicine. Therefore the emergency physician is by training and experience ideally suited to be involved in air medical services. In addition, the emergency physician group is readily available at all times to provide on-line medical direction and support for air medical crews. To varying degrees, patients transported by air medical services are resuscitated and stabilized in emergency department settings before admission to the trauma service or critical care units. For these reasons, the majority of physicians involved in medical direction for air medical services are emergency physicians.[1]

Emergency physicians pursuing the subspecialty of air medical services have several options: participation as a full- or part-time medical director, involvement as a member of the flight crew itself, or participation as a member of the emergency department group providing medical direction to the hospital's helicopter service. In many cases, these roles overlap substantially and some programs have elements of all three combined into their service. The role of the medical director in particular provides the emergency physician with substantial opportunities for career expansion as a physician manager.

QUALIFICATIONS AND EXPERIENCE

Involvement in air medical service requires a high degree of clinical expertise in all aspects of emergency medicine because most flight programs transport a broad diversity of patients. Residency training or board certification in emergency medicine provides the basic background required for such clinical expertise. Emergency physicians participating in flight services also should be well aware of the overall strategic mission and operating goals of the hospital because the air medical services is a logical extension of such goals and objectives. Further, a working knowledge of hospital operations beyond the emergency department, including the contribution of critical care services to the hospital's overall bottom line, is also important for physicians involved in air medical services. In addition, working knowledge of the operations of the critical care units who will be receiving the patients is also of benefit, although not necessarily a prerequisite for involvement in the service.

Beyond these baseline qualifications, the emergency physician needs to establish a scientific foundation in the field of aeronautics and air medicine. There is a rich literature dealing with both of these areas.[2,3] In addition, emergency medicine residency programs established at institutions that provide air medical services can offer the resident an insight into this subspecialty. Fellowships in air medical services are, at present, uncommon. Professional organizations also help provide the foundation necessary to be involved in air medical services and include the Air Medical Physician Association,* the Association of Air Medical Services,†and the National Association of Emergency Medical Services Physicians.‡

*Critical Care Medicine, LDS Hospital, Eighth Avenue & C Streets, Salt Lake City, UT 84143.
†35 South Raymond, Suite 205, Pasadena, CA 91105.
‡230 McKee Place, Suite 500, Pittsburgh, PA 15213.

EMERGENCY DEPARTMENT DIVERSIFICATION IN AIR MEDICAL SERVICES

Why should an individual physician or an emergency department group consider diversification into air medical services (Box 88-1)? First, most hospitals do not enter into air medical services without a clear understanding of their strategic importance toward extending the market of the hospital far beyond its existing boundaries. In this sense, it allows the emergency physician group, and the medical director specifically, to participate in meeting the hospital's strategic needs in a critical area of service. Second, because critical care air medical services extend the hospital's service area, they help integrate the emergency department group within the overall mission and long-term plan of the hospital. Third, air medical services are an extremely visible symbol of the hospital's presence within the community and are often featured in media accounts of the hospital's service. Emergency physician involvement in such a visible service is an important aspect of care. In addition, air medical services are substantially cost intensive, allowing the emergency physician and or emergency physician group to gain additional expertise in financial management and analysis. Similarly, this experience also ensures that the medical director of the service and, to a lesser extent, the other emergency physicians in the group have a broader entree into the field of physician management (see Chapters 1 and 9).

Finally, because the emergency physicians usually provide on-line medical direction for the critical care patients flown in by the helicopter, the skills and abilities of the entire physician group are broadened with regard to these critically ill and injured patients. In most settings, all trauma patients and some of the critical care patients are evaluated, resuscitated, and stabilized in the emergency department anyway, so an early familiarity with these patients can be helpful from a clinical standpoint.

Although there are substantial advantages to diversifying in air medical services, there are also some potential disadvantages (Box 88-2). First, the time, energy, and effort necessary for providing medical direction for the service must be factored into the group structure. If administrative time is created for the medical director who is a member of the emergency physician group, this time must be compensated, usually in some form of administrative stipend from the hospital. The clinical time that the medical director would have spent needs to be accounted for in the overall structure of the group's clinical services. Second, the mere fact that a critical care flight service exists can lead to some disintegration in the emergency department only because the trauma and critical care patients that are flown require the use of emergency department resources (to the extent that they are evaluated and resuscitated in that area). As all emergency physicians recognize, trauma patients are disintegrative to emergency medicine services and can result in pulling clinical and ancillary resources away from existing emergency department patients. Third, medical direction of the helicopter on an on-line basis requires some time and effort by the emergency physician on duty at the time that the helicopter flies. Although this is not a substantial amount of time or effort, it is one more demand on the emergency physician's already precious time. Despite these potential difficulties, one final fact needs to be kept in mind. If the hospital is already providing air medical services the emergency department physician group and the emergency department staff will be required to work with this service anyway. In most cases, it is far preferable to ensure that prospective controlling guidance is provided by the emergency physician group as opposed to physicians and/or staff from other areas of the hospital. For this and for other reasons, there are few circumstances in which the emergency department group will not find it beneficial to provide medical direction for helicopter services.

EMERGENCY PHYSICIAN AS MEDICAL DIRECTOR

The medical director of the flight service must assume many new roles and responsibilities including transition from clinician to physician manager (Chapters 1 and 7). These skills include leadership development, motivation theory, development and implementation of mission statements, conflict resolution, financial analysis, and negotiation skills. In addition, the following skills are specific for the clinical and administrative aspects of air medical services:

1. Clinical and administrative supervision of the air medical crew
2. Integration with the hospital's administrative structure
3. Establishing relationships with tertiary care specialists within the hospital

BOX 88-1

DIVERSIFICATION ADVANTAGES

1. Allows the medical director to participate in the hospital's strategic planning.
2. Allows the emergency department to integrate within the hospital's long-term planning and mission goals.
3. Emergency medicine and the hospital's visibility is enhanced within the community via the media coverage of air medical services.
4. Allows the medical director and other emergency physicians in the group to have an entry path into the field of physician management.

BOX 88-2

DIVERSIFICATION DISADVANTAGES

1. Roles and responsibilities of the medical director need to be included in the group's structure.
2. Administrative time needs to be compensated, usually from the hospital.
3. Critically ill and injured patients flown to the emergency department can demand resources (clinical and ancillary) away from the existing patients.
4. Medical direction for on-line control and service coordination can place greater demands on the emergency physician on duty.

4. Establishing relationships with ground emergency medical services within the hospital's service area
5. Establishing relationships with outlying physicians and hospitals
6. Involvement in community relations
7. Marketing
8. Knowledge in air physiology
9. Knowledge of aircraft capabilities, aeronautical principles and regulations
10. Managing relations between the emergency and flight departments

As with all areas of supervision and management, time is probably the most important consideration. The medical director needs to assess the level of involvement within the flight program and the many tasks that will be demanded by outside forces. For these reasons, there should be a negotiated protected time to meet these various obligations.

Along with protected time, reimbursement of this valuable position needs to be negotiated. The time spent on nonclinical or administrative time can be met by either the emergency medicine group or the hospital. This is a 24-hour, on-call job for any administrative or medical issues that may need immediate attention. Also, funds should be set aside for the director to attend relevant meetings, continuing medical education, and other special circumstances that may be relevant to the program operation. Professional liability insurance issues also must be addressed in the form of an added rider to the physicians' existing policy or indemnification by the hospital for medical direction and supervision of the air crew.

Medical direction for the air crew is usually done off-line. The medical guidelines should ideally be written by the flight crew and medical director to achieve a comfort level and balance of medical and clinical skills. Development of such protocols is a labor-intensive but critical aspect of the start up of the program. The guidelines will require periodic revisions, as the nature of the specialty and medicine in general changes.

Operational protocols also should be developed in a cooperative fashion with the air medical crew, communications specialists, and pilots. This approach results in an optimum level of operations and delivery of medical care.

ADMINISTRATIVE AND HOSPITAL INTEGRATION

The didactic and skills training of the air medical crew rests with the medical director. Some of these areas may be delegated to others, and any specialty training that is beyond the usual scope of the medical director needs to be delegated.

The way in which the medical director interacts with the rest of the emergency department group is also important. The on-duty emergency physician at times may be called on to offer on-line medical control, depending on circumstances. Therefore the medical director must be able to offer assistance and guidance to other emergency department physicians. There are many ways to communicate the activities and operations of the flight program back to the emergency department, including regularly scheduled department meetings, newsletters, or memos.

Integration into the hospital's administrative structure is particularly important. The administrative suite needs to understand how vital the air medical program is to the overall goals and success of the institution. This integration places the medical director in the role of a physician manager. The medical director must always maintain the best interest of the patient, but at the same time must skillfully balance the goals and interests of the institution.

The medical director wears two hats. On one hand, the clinical model addresses the care of the patient and the relationship between the patient and physician. On the other hand, the managerial model deals with the overall goals of the department or institution and is not established on a personal level. The successful medical director is able to merge these two differing schools of thoughts and evolve them into a new one. Some of the new duties of the medical director include resource allocation, departmental budgets, hospital administrative policies, and management of personnel.

The relationship to other members of the medical staff is also important. The medical director must be able to address the concerns of the primary care physicians and the specialty or tertiary care physicians who use the flight program. The key is to establish a service that delivers high quality medical care and is flexible to meet the expectations of others who depend on the flight service.

One way to establish a forum for communication is to establish a medical advisory committee for the flight program. The members should include key representatives for the users of the flight program and others who may be vital to the success of the program. In this fashion, there is a collaborative exchange of ideas and knowledge. This forum is particularly valuable for the review and revision of the medical guidelines. It is also particularly important to ensure that at every phase of interaction with services in the hospital it is made clear that the medical director should be informed of *any* problems or concerns with regard to clinical or administrative issues of the flight service. This approach helps ensure that all medical staff members and their administrative counterparts are aware that the management of the flight program is interested in hearing any concerns or feedback that can improve service.

OUTSIDE RELATIONS

The focus areas outside the institution are primarily the referring ground emergency medical services, physicians, and hospitals. Each of these areas is unique and consequently must be dealt with differently.

The ground emergency medical system provides a doorway to that community's particular tertiary medical needs. The medical director must understand and work within the existing structure. It is always best to work in a collaborative fashion rather than dictate policy. The contact established also provides the referring community with a glimpse into the flight program's institution.

The medical director should offer the institution and flight program's resources to the referring system, including ongoing medical education, case reviews, and training.

The medical director's relations with referring physicians and hospitals is also important. Ideally, there should be clear communication between all involved parties. Specific topics that should be part of the relationship include medically necessary transfers, medical guidelines for transferring of patients, and costs involved with air medical transports.

EMERGENCY PHYSICIAN AS A FLIGHT CREW MEMBER

The vast majority of flight programs in this country do not routinely fly with physicians as crew members.[1] The majority fly in a flight nurse-paramedic configuration, with a smaller number flying either flight nurse-flight nurse, paramedic-paramedic, or single paramedic configurations. In some circumstances, however, emergency physicians may be involved as flight crew members, usually on an "as needed" basis for only the most critically ill or injured patients. Emergency physicians who are directly involved with patient care during the flight process are technically part of the air medical crew. Supervision of the program still rests with the medical director, but there is greater autonomy than is typically seen in a team without a flight physician. Under such circumstances when a physician is flying, there is the implied sense that the medical protocols can be exceeded, at the judgment of the physician on the flight itself.

When physicians are used on flight, it is critical that they be part of the group that staffs the flight program's emergency department or are otherwise highly familiar with the aircraft and its operations. The stresses of flight, the physiology involved in flight medicine, and other changes make it radically different to participate as a flight crew member than to simply assume that it is an extension of the emergency department.

Most flight crews have had the experience of having physicians unfamiliar with the aircraft become a hindrance to delivery of quality patient care, as opposed to complementing quality patient care. This problem can be avoided by ensuring that physicians know the limitations of patient care within the aircraft and have in-depth familiarity with the aircraft's operation. Safety features are paramount when *anyone* is on the aircraft on an infrequent basis, and it should include all of the standard precautions used routinely by the flight crew, including wearing flame-retardant material and helmets.

When services are contracted through the flight department, several key areas may need to be addressed. The most time-consuming and problematic issue is conflicting schedules. Most flight programs require 8 hours of rest before starting flight duty. If an emergency physician is going to be involved as a flight crew member, this schedule must be followed. Otherwise, it is extremely difficult to maintain appropriate discipline and adherence to standard operating procedures if "all rules are off" when an emergency physician is flying. Malpractice, disability, and life insurance also need to be negotiated and rated for this line of work.

INTEGRATION WITHIN THE EMERGENCY DEPARTMENT PHYSICIAN GROUP

Participation in flight medicine is usually advantageous not only to the medical director but the entire physician group. Nonetheless, other members of the physician group must be made aware of its importance. Because the medical director usually has protected administrative time and therefore provides less clinical service than other emergency physicians, the advantages of the program to the entire group must be discussed openly and clearly. This will prevent resentments or concerns developing as a result of the decreased clinical hours of the medical director. Routine follow-up needs to be provided to the members of the emergency physician group with regard to the progress of the flight program, changes in medical protocols, and role of the flight program in advancing the strategic goals and objectives of the emergency physician group.

SUMMARY

The diversification of the emergency physician and emergency department into air medical services is relatively new, but is rich in opportunity both for the individual and for the emergency department physician group. It provides a high profile and exciting subspecialty to emergency physicians. For the medical director, there is ample opportunity to branch out into management and administration. This merging of skills and disciplines provides the physician manager the opportunity to work with many diverse customers in differing roles and functions in a collaborative fashion.

REFERENCES

1. Cady G: 1993 Air medical program survey, *Air Med J* 12:306-312, 1993.
2. Benson NH, Low RB, Chisholm CD et al: Air medical transport: an annotated bibliography of the recent literature, *Am J Emerg Med* 9:510-519, 1991.
3. Norton EG: Model curriculum in air medical transport for emergency medicine residencies, *Ann Emerg Med* 20:431-432, 1991.

89 Pediatric Emergency Medicine

Michael F. Altieri and Thom A. Mayer

OUTLINE

Evolution of pediatric emergency medicine
Pediatric emergency medicine in other countries
Advantages and disadvantages of practice diversification in pediatric emergency medicine
Components of a pediatric emergency medicine section
- Emergency physicians
- Nursing
- Administrative support
- Ancillary personnel
- Physical plant
- Equipment
- Laboratory support

Treatment guidelines
Quality improvement
Education
Summary

Of the 92 million emergency department visits in the United States, pediatric patients (less than 16 years old) comprise nearly one third.[1] Of these, only 10% to 15% are seen in children's hospitals, which means that up to 25 million pediatric patients a year are seen in general emergency departments throughout the country.[2] Although many of these patients have minor illnesses or injuries, large numbers of pediatric patients with life-threatening diseases experience an initial resuscitation and stabilization in the general emergency department setting. To have the greatest impact on pediatric emergency care, effort should focus on improving pediatric care delivered in the general emergency department.

Although the development of emergency medicine as a speciality has helped ensure that sufficient numbers of board-certified emergency physicians are available to staff emergency departments across the county, evidence indicates that the supply is insufficient to meet the demand.[3,4] Furthermore, two other factors have made it difficult to ensure that the pediatric emergency care needs of communities are met. First, emergency medicine residencies are 3 years long, of which as little as 3 months may be spent specifically in pediatric emergency medicine.[5] Second, as the subspecialty of pediatric emergency medicine grows, the knowledge base has expanded rapidly, making it difficult even for board-certified or residency-trained emergency physicians to stay abreast of the clinical and management developments in the specialty. For example, principles of conscious sedation and rapid sequence intubation have changed fairly dramatically during the last several years as they relate to the care of pediatric emergency patients.[5,6]

Because of these factors, diversification in pediatric emergency medicine is a logical strategy to help improve emergency department care for children. With the development of fellowship training programs specifically for physicians already trained in emergency medicine, the potential to have general emergency departments with at least one physician subspecialty trained in pediatric emergency medicine, but whose original training was in general emergency medicine, is becoming a reality (see below). Further, because virtually all emergency departments have substantial numbers of pediatric patients, diversification into pediatric emergency medicine is an obtainable goal for those emergency departments willing to commit the necessary time, energy, and money.

EVOLUTION OF PEDIATRIC EMERGENCY MEDICINE

Pediatric emergency medicine came into being as a true subspecialty in the early 1980s, when Sections of Pediatric Emergency Medicine were developed in the American Academy of Pediatrics and the American College of Emergency Physicians. Formal training programs developed as postgraduate training fellowships in the early 1980s. These fellowships were 1 to 2 years long, primarily based at children's hospitals, almost exclusively offered to graduates of pediatric training programs, and began turning out fellows as early as 1982. Subspecialty board certification first became available through the American Board of Pediatrics and the American Board of Emergency Medicine in 1992. Since then, subspecialty board certification examinations have been offered in pediatric emergency medicine every 2 years. Qualifications to sit for the examination include either a fellowship track (requiring a formal 2-year fellowship in pediatric emergency medicine) or a practice track (in which the appropriate number of hours of pediatric emergency care must have been completed before July 1, 1996). After that date, graduates of emergency medicine residencies must complete a formal 2-year fellowship program in pediatric emergency medicine for board eligibility, and pediatric graduates seeking certification in this subspecialty, as granted by the American Board of Pediatrics, will be required to complete 3 years of fellowship training, beginning in 1995. Applications and information about subspecialty certification in emergency medicine should be obtained from the board in which the physician is primarily certified.* Core content documents have been prepared for both graduates of pediatric and emergency medicine residency training programs.[8]

*American Board of Emergency Medicine, 3000 Coolidge Road, East Lansing, MI 48823, 517/332-4800; American Board of Pediatrics, 111 Silver Cedar Court, Chapel Hill, NC 27514, 919/929-0461.

The Section of Pediatric Emergency Medicine of the American Academy of Pediatrics is the fastest growing section in the Academy. There is also a large and active Section of Pediatric Emergency Medicine in the American College of Emergency Physicians. Over the years, both these bodies have developed guidelines and treatment protocols for the emergency treatment of children, as well as equipment lists addressing the needs of a pediatric emergency department and the needs of prehospital care providers.[9-12]

A large emphasis to propagate training guidelines for pediatric emergency care came with the publication of the report of the Institute of Medicine in 1993,[9] which defined the dismal state of pediatric emergency care in the United States. This report detailed the inadequacies of pediatric emergency care in this country, commenting on the lack of training of some emergency physicians as far as their ability to care for sick and injured children, a lack of proper equipment in emergency departments, the lack of training of many prehospital providers, and the failure of many emergency medical services (EMS) systems to provide a specific pediatric component. Added effort has been put toward refinement of pediatric emergency care since then, and many emergency departments have developed sections of pediatric emergency medicine that help integrate into the general emergency department setting.

PEDIATRIC EMERGENCY MEDICINE IN OTHER COUNTRIES

The need for pediatric emergency care is not only recognized in the United States. The medical literature is replete with articles dating back more than 20 years that define the need for pediatric emergency care in both developed and developing countries. In 1975 Ogundipe[13] published an article that defined the need for pediatric emergency centers in Nigeria. He stated that the emergency unit care would serve a need "to cater to a large number of children who could be very ill and promptly dealt with," and in many cases formal hospitalization would not be necessary. Diseases such as gastroenteritis with dehydration, pneumonia, malaria, respiratory illnesses, and kwashiorkor were some of the medical problems that he thought could be dealt with initially in the emergency department. Ogundipe thought that the emergency department should have its own site or building, that there "should be special emergency personnel," and that the department should be equipped with the "drugs and tools" to deal with acutely ill children. He also noted the importance of keeping good medical records in the emergency unit and that a simple and easily applied system of doing so should be adopted for both doctors and nurses. The point was also made that the operation of an emergency department is not inexpensive, and that the expenditure of money is justifiable on two grounds. First, humanity demands that we alleviate suffering, especially in the young; second "should the public feel that we are calloused to their children in those anxious moments, we will never reach out to them to carry out the most important aspect of delivery of healthcare which is prevention."

Several advances in pediatric emergency care have occurred in the United Kingdom. In England it is estimated that between 20% and 25% of the pediatric population is treated in accident or emergency departments, which translates to between 2 and 2.5 million children a year.[14,15] In most general emergency departments annually, such as those in the United States, 20% to 30% of their patient population are children. The largest group of children treated are those with major and minor trauma. Approximately 15% of the pediatric patients in the emergency departments are there for medical conditions, ranging from the seriously ill to trivial illnesses. A joint statement produced in 1988 by the British Pediatric Association and the British Association of Pediatric Surgeons and the Causality Surgeons Association recommended that pediatric accident and emergency medicine should develop a specialty with the aim of establishing consultant posts in pediatric emergency medicine in children's hospitals. The statement also recommended that there should be at least one pediatric accident and emergency unit in each region or large urban area based in either a children's hospital or a large accident and emergency unit within a general hospital. Presently there are five pediatric emergency units in England and Wales, two in Scotland, one in Northern Ireland, and two in the Republic of Ireland. The rationale for the existence of pediatric emergency units in the United Kingdom is as follows:[14]

1. As a teaching and training resource for medical, nursing, and other staff.
2. For research into epidemiology and pathology of acute illness and injury.
3. For the development of management strategies for acutely ill and injured children.

ADVANTAGES AND DISADVANTAGES OF PRACTICE DIVERSIFICATION IN PEDIATRIC EMERGENCY MEDICINE

Before entering into any sort of practice diversification, it is essential to consider both the advantages and disadvantages from a strategic and practical standpoint. There are several advantages to practice diversification in pediatric emergency medicine. First, and most important, if properly designed and implemented, diversification should result in a general increase in the level of care for children in the emergency department, because it involves a direct commitment to the facilities and training, to care for such children. Ideally, all emergency physicians and nurses should be assigned to the department, although there are almost always "standard bearers" among both the physician and nursing staffs with regard to their interest and expertise in pediatric emergency medicine. Practical experience indicates that a detailed quality improvement approach can readily document improvements in care of pediatric patients when pediatric emergency medicine diversification is implemented. These improvements are palpable, discrete, and important to the improvements in the clinical care of children.

Second, the majority of emergency physicians and nursing staff will see such diversification as an advantage; those who where responsible for administering this service are usually charged with ensuring that all members of the department are kept abreast of the rapid developments in the speciality of pediatric emergency medicine. For example, if one of the emergency physicians is performing duties as the EMS medical director, he or she should be able to rely on the expertise of the pediatric emergency physician to help develop the EMS component of care. Similarly, the educational component of the program should be a welcome addition to the inservices for the nursing and technical staffs of the department.

Third, because the educational component is such an important part of diversification in pediatric emergency medicine, it helps establish the groundwork and develop a format for other such educational forms, which can be extraordinarily helpful in pursuing other areas of emergency medicine practice diversification. Fourth, when properly implemented, the development of the section of pediatric emergency medicine can have substantial benefit in improving the relationship with pediatricians in the community. A central goal of the person responsible for the pediatric emergency section should be a close liaison relationship with the pediatricians in the community, including regular feedback to them (see the following discussion). Fifth, diversification can have an important effect on market share for the emergency department. If a section is developed that has recognized expertise in pediatric emergency medicine care that is shared by members of that department, pediatricians, emergency medical services, referring hospitals, and the community in general can be made to understand that the emergency department, with an active diversification in pediatric emergency medicine offers substantial advantages. Finally, diversification almost invariably improves the relationship with the EMS services in the community. Prehospital care providers are well known to be concerned about their ability to provide the best possible care for severely ill or injured children. When the diversification program is actively educating them with regard to both clinical care and equipment care needs, it is a natural consequence that relationships with EMS providers improve substantially.

It is also important to recognize the potential disadvantages to diversification. The first and most common disadvantage is the natural resistance to change inherent in any program, including developing new levels of expertise and new policies and procedures. The science of change management has become increasingly recognized (see Chapters 1 and 13), and strategies to help reduce resistance to change should be implemented.[16,17] Second, it is extremely important to recognize that there is often specific resentment from existing emergency physicians, emergency department nurses, and, in some cases, even the pediatricians in the community. For example, for a residency-trained, board-certified emergency physician, there may be some inherent resistance to the concept that a "subspecialist" in pediatric emergency medicine has skills, abilities, and expertise that exceed those of someone who has not completed such a fellowship. There can also be resistance among nurses and emergency department support staff, such as, "We take excellent care of children and have for years! Who are you to tell us to do things differently?" Managing this relationship requires firm commitment at all levels of the emergency department and the hospital, including hospital administration. Ensuring that the pediatric emergency medicine program is being implemented to help augment and facilitate improvements in care is critical. When resistance occurs, it should be recognized and addressed in a straightforward and aggressive fashion.

An additional disadvantage to diversification in pediatric emergency medicine is that it can often be seen as a potential threat to other area emergency departments who have not made the commitment to such diversification. Finally, involvement in a pediatric emergency medicine program requires an substantial investment of time, money, energy, and effort. Any emergency department considering such a diversification process should look at this decision in a careful and strategic fashion, which includes an analysis of the specific advantages and disadvantages for the individual emergency department.

COMPONENTS OF A PEDIATRIC EMERGENCY MEDICINE SECTION

Emergency Physicians

Not every pediatric patient who comes into an emergency department must be seen by a specially trained pediatric emergency physician. However, every section of pediatric emergency medicine must have a minimum of one physician who has formal training or experience in pediatric emergency care. It is the responsibility of this physician to set the standard of care for children in the department. This person should develop the guidelines and treatment protocols for the department, ensure that the proper equipment is available to deliver pediatric emergency care, and assist in the further training of all emergency physicians and nurses in the department to deliver a high level of pediatric emergency care. This physician should also monitor the care rendered to children in his or her department. This can be accomplished through quality insurance mechanisms, chart reviews, and dealing with physician and patient complaints concerning the pediatric care given in the department.

A staffing pattern for the pediatric emergency physicians is easily developed by studying the flow of children into the department over time. A study such as this was carried out in our institution over the last 8 years. A consistent finding was that children present to the emergency department mainly in the evening hours (Figure 89-1), with peak hours being between 7:00 PM and midnight. These are the hours that a pediatric emergency physician should be on duty. During the other hours when there is a lesser flow of pediatric patients, children can be adequately cared for by physicians trained in emergency medicine and further trained and assisted by the pediatric emergency physicians in their group. A pediatric emergency physician should always be available for consultation, at least over the telephone, so that all emergency physicians have access to information to help deliver the best possible care to the pediatric patient. In addition, as part of the routine emergency department meetings, pediatric inservices on evolving topics in pediatric emergency care can be helpful in ensuring that there is a true team approach to the care of the pediatric patient among the emergency physicians in the group. Where appropriate, protocols can be helpful in ensuring as much uniformity of care as possible (see Appendix A).

Nursing

The nursing care rendered to the pediatric patient in the emergency department is critical. The nurse must be comfortable with the care of children, adept at procedures such as blood drawing, starting intravenous lines, placing Foley catheters,

1994	0-1 Yrs	Admits	1-4 Yrs	Admits	5-10 Yrs	Admits	11-17 Yrs	Admits	Total Month	Total Admits	Percent
12MN-3AM	21	3	47	3	16	2	28	4	112	12	10.7%
3AM-6AM	9	4	24	7	8	3	6	0	47	14	29.8%
6AM-9AM	12	3	13	3	10	2	18	1	53	9	17.0%
9AM-12N	25	7	43	4	23	4	40	10	131	25	19.1%
12N-3PM	27	4	54	5	45	2	71	4	197	15	7.6%
3PM-6PM	30	6	71	10	39	5	72	4	212	25	11.8%
6PM-9PM	28	5	80	8	82	6	108	12	298	31	10.4%
9PM-12MN	49	14	83	8	35	3	63	8	230	33	14.3%
TOTAL	201	46	415	48	258	27	406	43	1280	164	12.8%

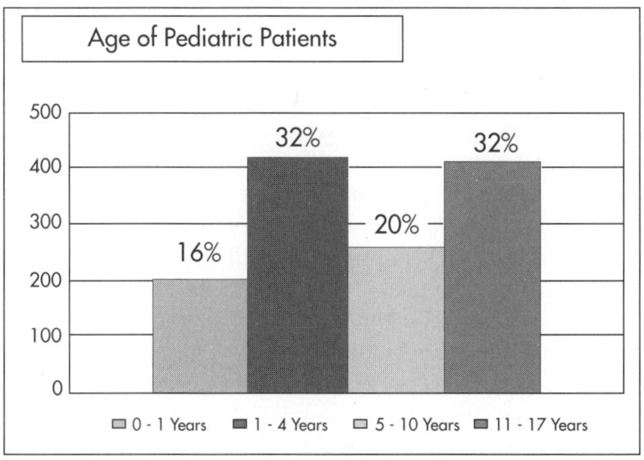

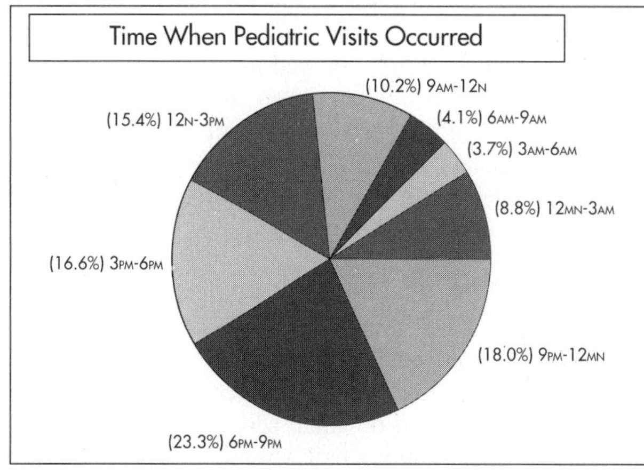

FIGURE 89-1 Fairfax Hospital Pediatric Totals October 1994.
(Courtesy, Fairfax Hospital Emergency Department, Falls Church, Va.)

and restraining small children for emergency department procedures. Nurses in triage need to be aware of serious problems particular to small children and to be able to sort out the very sick from the not so sick children who present to the emergency department. For example, all triage nurses should be aware of the sometimes subtle symptom pattern of intussusception and the need for prompt therapy. Similarly, the presence of bilious vomiting in a newborn should alert the nurse to the possibility of midgut volvulus and the need for urgent evaluation.

It is widely recognized that a greater degree of nursing time and involvement is needed to care for pediatric patients than for the typical adult patients. It takes longer to obtain vital signs in an uncooperative child, procedures are by and large more difficult to perform on smaller children, and nearly every child needs to be restrained for nearly every procedure; the nurse must assist the physician in these undertakings. A study in 1984 in the emergency department at the Childrens Hospital of Philadelphia showed that patients with complex problems required extensive nursing time, and the staffing patterns were inadequate to meet the needs of the complex patients.[3] The study determined the nursing time necessary to care for individual patients who presented to the emergency department with several different problems. These problems were categorized based on the nursing time required. This type of nursing assessment should be performed in every department with a pediatric section, and ongoing surveillance of the nursing requirements should be evaluated so that the proper staffing is made available to meet the needs of the various types of pediatric emergency patients presenting for care.

A nursing leadership role should be defined within the pediatric section. This nurse along with the pediatric emergency physician chief should develop patient care guidelines for the pediatric patients. Nonpediatric nurses should have inservice instruction on how to triage children, perform certain procedures such as intravenous line placement and interosseous needle insertion, restrain patients properly, and perform various other procedures pertinent to pediatric emergency care. This nurse should have paid administrative time and be able to function in a quality insurance or overseer capacity to ensure that the proper pediatric care is being rendered by the entire nursing staff. Nursing inservices are a critical part of the evolution of diversification into pediatric emergency medicine. For example, even the process of triage must be looked at somewhat differently in an emergency department committing to raising the standards of care for pediatric emergency patients. Specific inservices on intussusception, radial head subluxation, fever in the neonate, and other areas can be helpful to ensure that all nursing staff working in triage are aware of the necessity for dealing with these entities in an appropriate fashion.

The nursing staff should be encouraged to become pediatric advanced life support (PALS) certified, and be offered various other pediatric nursing courses such as the Emergency Pediatric Nursing Course sponsored by the Emergency Nurses Association. The pediatric emergency nurse coordinator should also act as a liaison to the nursing components in the pediatric intensive care unit, the pediatric ward, and the trauma service if pediatric trauma patients are cared for in that particular institution.

Administrative Support

Although it is not necessary to have a specific administrator for the section of pediatric emergency medicine, it is extremely important to ensure that the administrators responsible for the emergency department and pediatric aspects of the hospital are jointly committed to, informed of, and cooperate with the rules and objectives of the diversification into the pediatric emergency medicine. These administrators are critical with regard to keeping the overall administrative team informed about the purpose and progress within the section, as well as ensuring that appropriate budgetary measures are taken to meet the needs of the development of the section. A cooperative, team approach (see Chapters 1, 3, and 14) is necessary because the section can be successful only if the efforts of many people are closely and cooperatively aligned.

Ancillary Personnel

All ancillary personnel who interact with emergency department patients should be adept and comfortable in dealing with the pediatric patient. Laboratory personnel should have the ability to draw blood on small patients and perform microtechniques so that only small amounts of blood are necessary. Radiology technicians should be able to perform radiographic examinations on children so that quality films are available to physicians. Radiologists should be able to perform the various techniques particular to children for shooting the films and shielding patients. Respiratory technicians should have the appropriate equipment to deliver respiratory care to children, should be familiar with pediatric dosing of the various medications used for respiratory care, and should have the ability to teach the pediatric patient and parent various therapies such as the use of an inhaler with an aerochamber, chest physiotherapy, and peak flow meter. Emergency department technicians should be able to apply adequate dressings to children's wounds, be able to splint the limbs of small children, and be able to generally interact well with a child and the parent. People who fail to recognize the various developmental stages of children and their capabilities with regard to interaction should not be caring for the pediatric patient. The pediatric emergency physician and pediatric emergency nurses must ensure that all ancillary personnel interact appropriately with the child-parent unit and to provide instruction when necessary.

Physical Plant

When designing the "bricks and mortar" of an emergency department, which will contain a specialized pediatric section, several considerations must be kept in mind. First the facility should be designed so that high levels of care can be delivered in the most effective, least taxing, and most cost effective way. It is not necessary to have a separate facility to care for pediatric emergency patients, but separating the children from the adult patients who may potentially become violent or abusive is of the utmost importance. This goal can be achieved by clustering the pediatric rooms in one area, or by using a dedicated hallway of rooms for the pediatric section.

It is also important to separate treatment areas by walls, not curtains, and to close off each room from outside noise and visual stimuli. Fear, apprehension, and crying in the child being treated or examined is very contagious and can easily spread from one patient to another if these patients are in a large treatment area separated only by curtains or screens. It is also disconcerting for parents waiting outside the treatment area to hear the crying and the screams of their child and feel helpless to comfort them.

Each of the rooms used in treating children should be adequately equipped with the tools necessary to perform routine pediatric examinations. Rooms used to care for sicker children should be equipped with airway management supplies and monitoring equipment, such as a cardiorespiratory monitor and pulse oximeter, and should have adequate supplies for starting intravenous lines, drawing blood, and any other supplies deemed necessary for responding to an acute cardiorespiratory emergency. These rooms should also contain the supplies used to meet the practical needs of the patient (e.g., diapers, child-sized gowns, wipes). It is also a good idea to have such things as children's books, coloring books, and safe, washable toys within the room so that parents can entertain the children while they are waiting to be seen or waiting for laboratory results. The room should also be "child friendly." Using bright colors, designs, pictures, and various other decorations camouflage the sterile, medical look of an examination room.

A major resuscitation room or trauma room should be available for pediatric use. This room also could be capable of supporting adult trauma and cardiopulmonary resuscitation. Pediatric equipment needed for a trauma or medical resuscitation should be readily available and, if at all possible, stocked in the room separate from the adult supplies. Monitoring, radiography, and other support equipment can serve both the adult and pediatric patient. One important consideration in the pediatric trauma or resuscitation room is control of the thermal environment of the small child, which usually requires an overhead warmer or a bank of heating lamps that can be used when an infant needs to be resuscitated.

For many of the same reasons that it is important to have a treatment area for children separate from that of the adults, it is also important that the waiting area for children be segregated from the area used by adult patients. These pediatric waiting areas are deficient in many hospitals. In a 1985 survey in England, only 25% of hospitals provided separate waiting areas for children; anecdotally this seems similar to the experience in the United States.[15] The pediatric waiting area should be capable of isolating pediatric patients from any adult patients who are exhibiting violent or abusive behavior, while at the same time allow for parental observation and supervision of these children. The waiting area should also contain things such as children's books, coloring books, and various toys so that the children may entertain themselves in what sometimes is a long wait to be seen in the emergency department.[18] It is also advisable for the pediatric waiting area to have its own television/VCR combination so that children's movies and television shows may be viewed. This setup also allows for the nursing staff to show child care videos for parents in the waiting area to help educate them in the care of common pediatric problems.

The triage function is an integral part of pediatric emergency services. It is at this point that most patients first enter the system and where the severity of the child's illness is determined. There is no need to have a separate triage area for the pediatric patients as long as the general triage area is appropriately equipped to deal with pediatric patients. The capability of obtaining blood pressures, pulse oximetry, and a complete set of vital signs should be present in the triage area. There also should be an area in triage where a patient may be isolated if he or she has a highly contagious illness, such as chickenpox or measles. The triage area should also be equipped with emergency airway equipment and have the ability to rapidly alert the pediatric emergency physician when a patient presents in extremis. When an appropriately equipped triage area is staffed by nursing personnel who are trained in pediatric triage assessment and who have at their disposal adequate ancillary help to deal with sick and uncooperative children, this important function can be carried out effectively and rapidly.

Equipment

The appropriate tools to care for ill and injured children must be readily available. Much has been written about the appropriate equipment necessary in pediatric emergency departments to adequately care for children.[10] Both individuals and the pediatric section of the American Academy of Pediatrics have recommended equipment lists (Box 89-1).

Emergency and resuscitation equipment must be both present and easily accessible. Its location must be known to all the nursing staff, and its working order continually monitored. In addition to emergency or resuscitation equipment, a large amount of other equipment is needed for the pediatric patient including small ear speculums, appropriately sized gowns for the pediatric patients, diapers, formula and oral fluids, small-gauge catheters, and infusion pumps.

A pediatric "crash cart" must be available in the pediatric section. It should have the ability to move to any of the rooms in which a pediatric patient may be seen. The contents of this cart may vary among institutions but the basic contents are similar to the listing in Boxes 89-2 and 89-3.[19]

Laboratory Support

The laboratory plays a vital role in the emergency care of the pediatric patient. The laboratory that supports the emergency department should be able to use micromethods and whole blood determinations to minimize the amount of blood necessary to perform tests and to reduce the response time. Laboratory tests that should be available on a "stat" basis, with results available in a few minutes, are a complete blood count, blood gases, blood chemistries (including calcium), and urinalysis. Other tests that should be available on a stat basis that may take slightly longer to perform should include total protein, erythrocyte sedimentation rate, liver function tests, serum osmolarity, spinal fluid analysis (including protein, glucose, cell count, and differential), serum anticonvulsant levels, and urine and toxicology screens.[20] In departments that see pediatric trauma, blood bank support with rapid cross-match of blood is also necessary, as well as the clotting studies of prothrombin time and partial prothrombin time. It is also necessary to be supported by the bacteriology laboratory because several cultures of blood, urine, spinal fluid, and other body fluids are often necessary in the evaluation of many pediatric problems. Blood cultures to rule out occult bacteremia are common in the pediatric emergency department and the department relies on the laboratory not only to process the cultures but to provide immediate feedback to the emergency physician about results of a positive blood culture so that immediate follow-up can take place. Various other specialty laboratory functions may be necessary in some departments, including the collection of various cultures and specimens with a documented chain of evidence for examinations in the forensic evaluation of children for possible sexual molestation. These special needs, as well as the special documentation needs for this type of laboratory support, must be in place before doing such evaluations.

TREATMENT GUIDELINES

One of the first tasks for the pediatric section chief and the head pediatric emergency nurse is to develop treatment and/or practice guidelines for both physician and nursing staff. It is important to develop "guidelines" and not protocols, thereby allowing individual physicians the freedom and leeway to practice medicine as they are comfortable, while remaining well within the standards of care set forth by the medical community.

These guidelines can be framed in may different manners. They may take the form of algorithms with suggestions for various therapeutic entities (Figures 89-2 and 89-3), of a hospital policy (Appendices A and B), or of a didactic such as that illustrated in Tables 89-1 and Boxes 89-2, 89-3, and 89-4. All treatment guidelines should be consistent with existing hospital policy, standard of care practiced in the community, and previously published treatment guidelines from organizations such as the American Academy of Pediatrics, the American College of Emergency Physicians, and the American Medical Association.

QUALITY IMPROVEMENT

Quality improvement has become an integral part in all medical practices and in all medical specialties.[10] Pediatric emergency medicine is no exception. The most effective way to achieve ongoing quality improvement in the pediatric section of a general emergency department is to integrate the pediatric quality improvement into the quality improvement functions for the whole department. This may include periodic chart review by the chief of the pediatric section; treatment audits of various pediatric disease entities such as asthma, otitis media, and occult bacteremia; and the review of various procedures, such as blood drawings, spinal taps, and suturing.

Quality improvement is also an area in which communication with referring physicians, private pediatricians, and referring hospitals can be monitored so that gaps or shortcomings in this vital link to institutions providing referrals and individuals providing follow-up can be identified. The key is not to expend time, effort, and money in reinventing the wheel to provide pediatric quality improvement. Incorporating these functions into already existing systems will allow for a better product with a minimal increased expenditure in resources.

BOX 89-1

PEDIATRIC EQUIPMENT GUIDELINES FOR THE GENERAL HOSPITAL EMERGENCY DEPARTMENT

The following supplies and equipment are recommended for pediatric patients in a general emergency department. Recommended guidelines are shown in parentheses.

An emergency cart or other system to house all supplies, equipment, and drugs for a designated pediatric resuscitation area should be available.

Monitoring devices
- ECG monitor-defibrillator/cardioverter with pediatric and adult-sized paddles and hard copy recording capability
- Otoscope/ophthalmoscope/stethoscope
- Pulse oximeter with pediatric adaptor
- Sphygmomanometer and Doppler ultrasound blood pressure devices
- Arterial and venous pressure monitoring equipment immediately available to emergency department
- Rectal temperature probe
- Hypothermia thermometer
- Blood pressure cuffs (neonatal; infant; child; adult-arm, thigh)
- End-tidal PCO_2 monitor
- Blood gas kit
- Peak flow meter

Vascular access supplies and equipment
- CVP kits, 18-22 gauge (4)
- Catheter-over-needle devices, 16, 18, 20, 22, 24 (2 each)
- Butterflies, 18, 21, 23, 25 (4 each)
- Intraosseous needles, 16 gauge (4)
- Tourniquets (3), rubber bands
- 4×4 sponges
- Povidone-iodine swabs (10)
- Alcohol swabs (10)
- Tape, waterproof—½, 1.2 in. (1 roll each)
- Stopcocks (2)
- T-connectors (3)
- IV tubing, 30 inches (2)
- Armboards (2 each size)
- Tincture of benzoin
- Povidone prep solution
- Betadine ointment (2)
- IV fluid/blood warmer
- Infusion pumps, drip or volumetric, with microinfusion capability
- IV administration sets and extension tubing
- IV solutions
  - Normal saline
  - 10% dextrose in normal saline
  - 5% dextrose in 0.25 normal saline
  - 5% dextrose in 0.5 normal saline
  - Ringer's lactate
  - Mannitol, 20%
  - Albumin, 5%, 25%

Respiratory equipment and supplies
- Bag-valve-mask resuscitator, self-inflating (infant, child, and adult)
- Suction devices
- Laryngoscope handle
- Laryngoscope blades
  - Curved: 2,3
  - Straight or Miller: 0, 1, 2, 3
- Stylets for endotracheal tubes (infant and adult) (1 each)
- Magill forceps
- Endotracheal tubes
  - Uncuffed sizes: 2.5, 3.0, 3.5, 4.0, 4.5, 5.0 (2 each)
  - Cuffed sizes: 5.5, 6.0, 6.5, 7.0, 7.5, 8.0 (2 each)
- Tracheostomy tubes
  - Shiley tube sizes: 00, 0, 1, 2, 3, 4, 6
- Oral airways
  - Sizes: 0, 1, 2, 3, 4, 5
- Nasopharyngeal airways
  - Sizes: 12, 16, 20, 24, 28, 30 Fr
- Clear oxygen masks
  - Standard and nonrebreathing (neonatal, infant, child, adult)
- Nasal cannulae (child and adult) (2 each)
- Oxygen cylinder, flow meter, tubing
- Suction catheters
  - Sizes: 6, 8, 10, 14 Fr (2 each)
- Yankauer suction tips (4)
- NG tubes
  - Sizes: 6, 8, 10, 12, 14, 16 Fr (2 each)
- Tongue blades (5)
- Lubricant (K-Y jelly) (4)
- Nebulizer

Medications (unit dose prepackaged—2 of each)
- Atropine, 0.1 mg/ml—10 ml
- Calcium chloride, 10%—10 ml
- Dextrose, 25%—10 ml
- Diazepam, 5 mg/ml
- Lorazepam, 2 or 4 mg/ml
- Epinephrine, 1:10,000—10 ml and 1:1000—30 ml
- Lidocaine, 1%—10 ml
- Naloxone, 0.4 mg/mL or 1 mg/ml
- Phenobarbital, 65 mg/ml
- Phenytoin, 50 mg/ml
- Sodium bicarbonate, 8.4%—50 ml
- Sodium bicarbonate, 4.2%—10 ml
- Related supplies/equipment
  - Medication chart, tape, or other system to assure ready access to information on proper per kilogram dose for resuscitation drugs and equipment sizes

Adapted from tables in American Academy of Pediatrics, Committee on Pediatric Emergency Medicine: *Emergency Medical Services for Children: The Role of the Primary Care Provider* Elk Grove, Ill, 1995, American Academy of Pediatrics; and American College of Emergency Physicians: Policy Statement; *Pediatric Equipment Guidelines for a General Emergency Department,* Dallas, 1994, ACEP.

BOX 89-1

PEDIATRIC EQUIPMENT GUIDELINES FOR THE GENERAL HOSPITAL EMERGENCY DEPARTMENT—cont'd

Syringes: TB, 3, 5, 10, 20, 30, 60 mL (5 each)
Needles: 21, 23, 25 gauge (5 each)
Feeding tubes (for endotracheal drugs)
  Sizes: 3.5, 5, 8 FR (2 each)
Activated charcoal
Albuterol for nebulization 5 mg/ml

Specialized pediatric trays for the following procedures:
  Tube thoracostomy and water seal drainage
  Thoracotomy tray with chest tubes
    Sizes 8-40 Fr
  Cricothyrotomy including needle cricothyrotomy
  Peritoneal lavage
  Venous cutdown
  Lumbar puncture
  Umbilical vessel cannulation
  Catheterization: Foley catheters
    Sizes: 5-12 Fr (2 each)
  Obstetric pack
  Newborn kit

Fracture management devices
  Spine board (child and adult)
  Femur splint (Hare traction) (child and adult)
  Spine board
  Semirigid neck collars (child and adult)
  Cervical spine immobilization device
  Extremity splints, various sizes

Miscellaneous equipment
  Infant scale
  Heating source, overhead warmer preferred
  Cardiac backboard
  MAST trousers (toddler, child, adult)

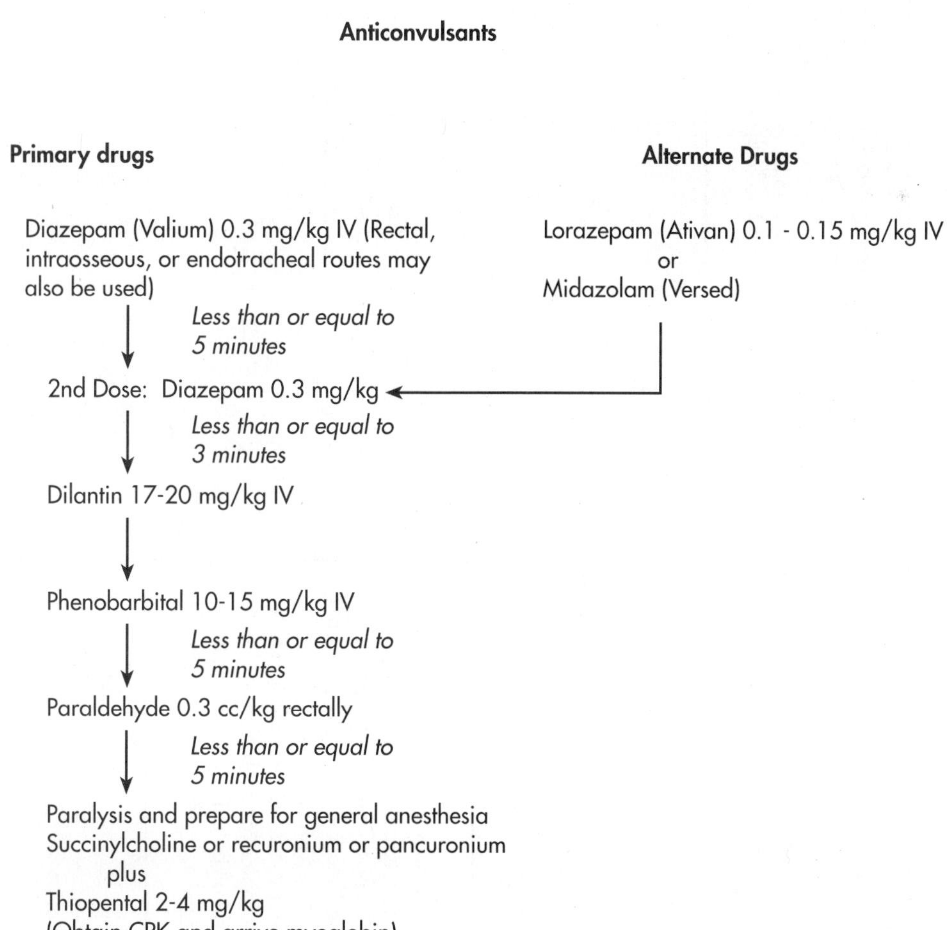

FIGURE 89-2 Anticonvulsant use in status epilepticus. Algorithms can be helpful in ensuring that pediatric patients are treated more uniformly, guided by such clinical pathways.

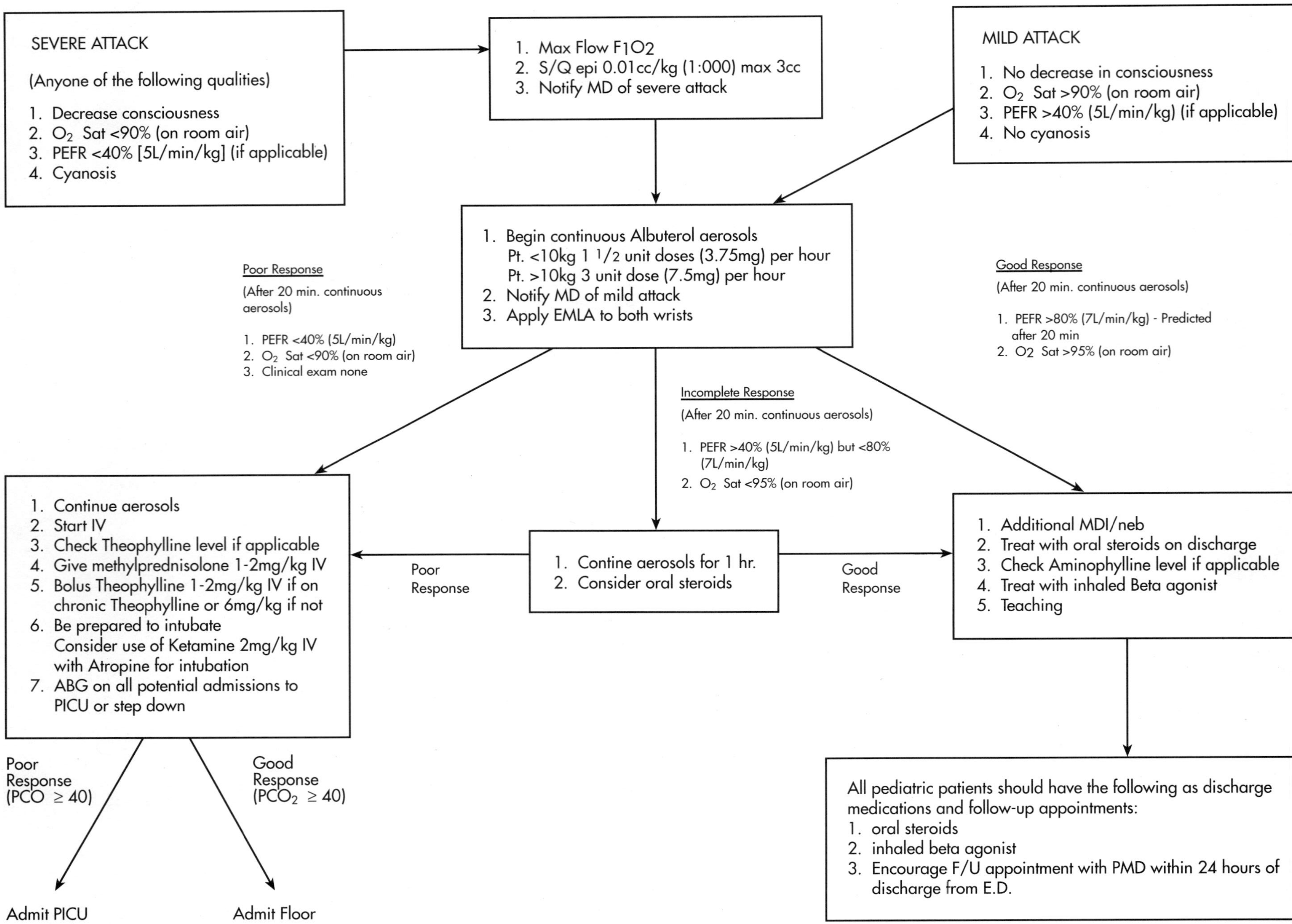

FIGURE 89-3 Fairfax Hospital Emergency Department Pediatric Asthma Treatment Guidelines.
(Courtesy, Fairfax Hospital Emergency Department, Falls Church, Va.)

Table 89-1 Medication List for Pediatric Immediate Care Cart

	Name	How supplied	Remarks
Pediatric resuscitation drugs	Atropine sulfate	0.1 mg/ml solution 1 mg/ml solution	Prefilled syringes
	Epinephrine HCL	1:10,000 1:1,000	Prefilled syringes
	Lidocaine	20 mg/ml (2%)	Prefilled syringes
	Sodium bicarbonate	1 mEq/ml (8.4%)	Prefilled syringes
Pediatric supplemental drugs	Aminophylline	250 mg/ml	
	Dextrose, 50%	500 mg/ml	
	Dextrose, 25%	Not supplied	Must dilute 50% dextrose 1:1 with sterile water or normal saline solution
	Diazepam	5 mg/ml	
	Diphenhydramine	50 mg/ml	
	Mannitol, 25%	250 mg/ml	
	Morphine sulfate	5, 8, 10, 15 mg/ml	
	Naloxone	0.4 mg/ml 0.1 mg/ml neonatal	
	Syrup of ipecac		

BOX 89-2

PEDIATRIC IMMEDIATE CARE CART EQUIPMENT

Monitor-defibrillator	With infant and child paddles (4.5 cm and 8.0 cm)
Bag-valve-mask resuscitator (masks for above)	750 ml. Delivers 100% oxygen: infant, child, small adult
Blood pressure cuffs	Infant, child, small adult
Back board (spinal immobilization)*	
Stiff neck collars*	Small, medium, large
Sand bags*	
Femur splint, pediatric*	
Antishock trousers	Pediatric
Laryngoscope	Curved and straight blades, sizes: 0, 1, 2
Endotracheal tube stylets	6 Fr and 14 Fr
MacGill forceps	Pediatric
Stethoscope	2-sided, pediatric
Pediatric emergency drug dosage book or chart	Dosage by weight
Chest tube tray with pediatric-sized chest tubes	8 Fr through 16 Fr
Cricothyrotomy and tracheostomy tray with pediatric tubes	
Cutdown tray	

*Although it is recommended that all equipment possible be actually in or on the cart, the items with stars are very bulky and could be stored within the emergency department if space on the cart was not available. However, there should be a notation on the cart itself to indicate exactly where these items are to be found, and these items should be accounted for each shift when the cart is checked.

EDUCATION

The personnel of the pediatric section must provide educational resources not only for the components of the system that delivers pediatric emergency care but also to the individuals who consume their services.

The first level of education is for the attending level physicians involved in delivering pediatric emergency care, both the nonpediatric emergency physicians and the pediatricians who practice in the community. Educational interactions with these physicians could include presentation in a grand rounds setting of various commonly encountered problems in the pediatric emergency department and the latest method of treatment. The emergency physician also should function as a resource for distributing the latest pediatric emergency literature among the other emergency physicians in the group. The emergency physician also should be available to consult with pediatricians in their offices and to provide inservice training in such areas as cardiopulmonary resuscitation, respiratory emergencies, and assistance in office preparedness for emergency care.

Probably the most effective way of imparting information to an individual physician is on a one-to-one basis, often precipitated by a patient problem encountered in the department and picked up on chart review. In such sessions the pediatric emergency physician must take great care to respect his or her colleagues' medical abilities and deliver suggestions con-

BOX 89-3

PEDIATRIC IMMEDIATE CARE CART SUPPLIES

IV Supplies	
Normal saline solution	(This is the currently recommended pediatric emergency IV solution. Hospitals may elect to stock other fluids as well)
Minidrip burette	All pediatric IV lines should be on an infusion controller as well
Over-the-needle catheters	24, 22, 20, 18 Gauge
Butterfly needles	25, 23, 21 Gauge
Jamshidi needles (for interosseous infusion)	15, 18 Gauge
Armboards	Infant, short, long
Oral airways	Sizes 0-5
Pediatric O_2 masks, nasal cannulas	
Endotracheal tubes	
Uncuffed	2.3, 3.0, 3.5, 4.0, 4.5, 5.0, 5.5, 6.0
Cuffed	6.5, 7.0, 7.5, 8.0 (For use in children more than 8 years of age)
Suction catheters	6Fr, 8Fr, 10Fr, 14Fr, Yankauer
Pediatric lumbar puncture tray	1½ inch, 22 Gauge spinal needle
Peritoneal lavage kit	
Foley catheter tray	
Foley catheters	8-14 Fr
Central venous pressure catheters	Pediatric sizes
Nasogastric tubes and infant feeding tubes	Assorted sizes 5 Fr through 14 Fr
Pleurevac, pediatric	

BOX 89-4

PEDIATRIC IMMEDIATE CARE CART SUGGESTED OUTLINE FOR DRAWER SET-UP

Top of cart

Monitor/defibrillator (unless already at each bedside or on separate cart)
Infant/pediatric paddles in storage case

Drawer no. 1

Pediatric emergency drugs
Dosage by weight chart or booklet

Drawer No. 2

Intubation equipment
- Laryngoscope handle and blades
- Endotracheal tubes and stylets
- Lubricant, Xylocaine jelly

MacGill forceps
Trach tubes and tray
Cricothyroidotomy needles
Oral and nasopharyngeal airways
Suction catheters

Drawer No. 3

NG Tubes/infant feeding tubes
Foley tray and catheters
U-bags
Chest tray and chest tubes
Cutdown tray

Drawer No. 4

IV Supplies (needles, catheters, tubing, tape, armboards, skin swabs, tournequets, etc.)
Burette
Assorted syringes and needles
Jamshidi needles (for interosseous infusion)
Extra LP needles
Central lines

Drawer No. 5

IV Solutions
Pediatric lumbar puncture tray
0_2 Tubing, masks, cannulas
Peritoneal lavage kit
Blood pressure cuffs
Pediatric stethoscope

Large bottom bin

Antishock trousers
Infant and pediatric resuscitation devices in cases with assorted masks (these may also be hung from hooks on the sides of the cart, which will leave room for sandbags and stiff neck collars)
Pleurevac

structively so as not to alienate the physician or make him or her less open to constructive criticism.

Another area for which the pediatric emergency physician must take responsibility is the training of prehospital or EMS personnel. As demonstrated in the 1993 Institute of Medicine report, the pediatric training of prehospital personnel in many cases is extremely deficient.[9] The pediatric emergency physician is charged with the development of treatment protocols, the development of training modules, and participation in emergency medical technician and paramedic training courses to help fill the gap in pediatric prehospital care training and experience.

As mentioned earlier, the pediatric emergency physician in conjunction with the pediatric emergency nurse must provide for the entire nursing staff inservice training to cover the many aspects of pediatric emergency care as well as inservice instruction on the implementation of the newly developed pediatric care guidelines. The initial investment of time in these inservice sessions is usually considerable, but decreases over time as the nursing staff becomes more familiar with and more adept with pediatric emergency care. After a few years only periodic refresher courses are usually needed.

In many settings residents and medical students are trained in the emergency department. These individuals must be provided the basics in pediatric emergency care, and usually in most community hospital settings they need to receive a supervised clinical experience in pediatric emergency care. This experience is best gained by seeing several pediatric patients from the severely ill to the not so ill and being directly supervised by a pediatric emergency physician.

Finally, especially in the community setting, the community turns to the pediatric emergency physician to provide instruction to parents and participate in school and safety activities and also take the lead in such organizations as Safe Kids Coalitions and community wellness programs.

The pediatric emergency physician is also called on to participate in organized educational activities such as Pediatric Advanced Life Support (PALS) and Advanced Pediatric Life Support (APLS) if they are available in the area in which they practice. If they are not available, it is often up to the pediatric emergency physician to organize such courses.

SUMMARY

Because pediatric patients comprise up to one third of the volume of general emergency departments, diversification in the pediatric emergency medicine will be a logical choice for many institutions. As the availability of well-trained specialists in pediatric emergency medicine with concomitant training in general emergency medicine increases, the development of practice diversification in pediatric emergency medicine will become more widespread. The advantages and disadvantages of such a program should be carefully weighed; commitment from the medical staff, administration, and nursing components are essential for its success. Integrating the pediatric emergency physician into the overall emergency physician group structure is also an important aspect of this diversification.

Despite the considerable time, energy, and cost necessary to develop pediatric emergency medicine diversification, this approach offers rich opportunities for combining progress and patient care with progress and career and group development.

REFERENCES

1. Mayer TA: Pediatric care in the general emergency department. In Swartz GR et al, Editors: *Principles in practice of emergency medicine*, ed 3, Philadelphia, 1992, Lea and Febiger.
2. National Association of Children's Hospitals and Related Institutions: Annual Report—1993, Alexandria, Virginia.
3. Kromash EJ: Patient classification and required nursing time in a pediatric emergency department, *J Emerg Nurs,* 10:69-73, 1984.
4. Luten RC: *Recognition of the sick child: problems in pediatric emergency medicine,* New York, 1988, Churchill Livingston.
5. Ludwig S et al: Pediatric training in emergency medicine programs, *Ann Emerg Med* 114:170-174, 1982.
6. Yamamoto LG, Yim GK, Britten AG: Rapid sequence anesthesia induction for emergency intubation, *Pediatr Emerg Care* 6:200-208, 1990.
7. Curriculum Sub-Committee Section of Emergency Medicine, American Academy of Pediatrics: Pediatric emergency medicine (PEM) fellowship curriculum statement, *Pediatr Emerg Care* 7:48-53, 1991.
8. King CK, Nilsen GJ, Henretig FM, Wagner DK: Proposed core content for pediatric emergency medicine fellowship training of emergency medicine graduates, *Ann Emerg Med* 24:825-835, 1994.
9. Durch P, Lohr J, editors: *Institute of Medicine report on emergency medical services for children. Committee on Pediatric Emergency Medical Services,* Washington, DC 1993, National Academy Press,
10. Mellick LB, Dierking BH: One size doesn't fit all, *J Emerg Med Serv JEMS,* 21:28-36, 1991.
11. Baraff LJ, Bass JW, Fleisher GR et al: Practice guideline for the management of infants and children 0 to 36 months of age with fever without source, *Ann Emerg Med* 22:1198-1210, 1993.
12. Dieckmann RA: Rectal diazepam for pre-hospital pediatric status epilepticus, *Ann Emerg Med* 23:216-224, 1994.
13. Ogundipe O: Organization of emergency pediatric units, *Environ Child Health* 10:32-37, 1975.
14. Phillips BM, Robson WJ: Pediatrics in the accident and emergency department, *Arch Dis Child* 67:560-564, 1992.
15. Richmond PW, Evans RC, Silbert JR: Improving facilities for childrens in an accident department, *Arch Dis Child* 62:299-301, 1987.
16. Schein EH: How can organizations learn faster? The challenge of entering the green room, *Sloan Manage Rev* 34:85-92, 1993.
17. Senge PM: The leaders new work: building learning organizations, *Sloan Manage Rev* 31:7-23, 1990.
18. Liptak GS, Super DM, Baker N, Roghamann KJ: An analysis of waiting times in a pediatric emergency department, *Clin Pediatr* 24:1985.
19. Wayland BW, Rowland MC: Pediatric immediate care cart, *J Emerg Nurs* 14:91-95, 1988.
20. Braggion F, Ceriotti, F, Churmello G: Pediatric emergency laboratory, *Z Med Lab Diagn* 32:32-36, 1990.

APPENDIX

A

Adult/*Pediatric* Emergency Department Asthma Treatment Guidelines

Regular, Adult & Pediatric
Italic, Unique to Pediatric

Initial Assessment

↓

Triage - If a room is unavailable, page the respiratory therapist to evaluate and begin treatment at Triage.

History
Physical Exam
Pulse Oximetry
PEFR (Mandatory)
Theophylline Level (If Indicated)

↓

Hydration as Appropriate
Supplemental O_2

Triage → 60-90 Minutes Maximum

Moderate to Severe
PEFR < 200

PEFR < 50% Predicted *(5L/Kg/Mg)* or Personal Best
Cyanosis, Decreased LOC
O_2 Sat < 90% on Room Air

1. One Hour of Continuous Nebulized Treatment with:
   - Beta-adrenergic (Albuterol)
   - Anticholinergics (Atrovent * 250-500 mcgrms)
2. IV Corticosteroids *(Methylprednisolone 1-2 mg/kg)*
3. Optimize Theophylline if Clinically Indicated
4. *Apply EMLA to Both Wrists*
5. *Reassess within 20 Minutes*

Mild to Moderate
PEFR > 200

PEFR > 50% Predicted or Personal Best
No Cyanosis or Decreased LOC
O_2 Sat > 90%

1. One Hour of Continuous Nebulized Treatment with:
   - Beta-adrenergic (Albuterol)
   - Anticholinergics (Atrovent * 250-500 mcgrms)
2. IV *or PO* Corticosteroids if Patient on Maintenance or Clinically Indicated *(1-2 mg/kg Prednisone)*
3. Consider Theophylline

Pediatric Albuterol Dosage
< 10 kg 1 1/2 Unit Doses (3.75 mg/Hr)
> 10 kg 3 Unit Doses (7.5 mg/Hr)

Pediatric Theophylline Dosage
(Bolus Theophylline 1-2/mg/kg IV
If on Chronic Therapy or 6 mg/kg if not)

Reassess (Consider MDI in Place of HHN Where Appropriate)

Hour

Respiratory Failure

Extreme Distress
PEFR ≤ 100 ≤ 25% Predicted or Personal Best
Hypoxia (or Sat < 90%)
Be Prepared to Intubate (Ketamine 2mg/kg IV with Atropine for Intubation)
ABG

Poor Response

Marked Diffuse Wheezes
Continued SOB
PEFR ≤ 200 ≤ 50% Predicted or Personal Best
O_2 Sat 90-95%

Incomplete Response

Mild Persistent Wheezing
PEFR ≤ 300 ≤ 75% Predicted or Personal Best
O_2 Sat 90-95%

Good Response

Symptom Free
Near Baseline
PEFR ≥ 300 ≥ 75% Predicted or Personal Best
O_2 Sat > 95% on Room Air

Consult Admitting Physician Re: Impending Admission

Total Time 2-2.5 Hours

Respiratory Failure:
- *$pCO_2 \geq 40$* → ADMIT TO ICU or *PICU*
- *$pCO_2 < 40$* → *ADMIT FLOOR*

Continuous Nebulized Beta-adrenergic with Anticholinergic
Assess pCO_2 as Clinically indicated
Consider Alternate Therapies

Continued Wheezing
PEFR ≤ 200
or
≤ 50% Predicted or Personal Best

↓

ADMIT

Improved
PEFR 200-300
(50-75% Predicted or Personal Best)

Consider:

1. Continued Therapy
2. Consult PCP
3. Admission/Discharge Based on Clinical Indications

↓

Reassess

Good Response → Education

↓

DISCHARGE ON:
- Oral Steroids if Indicated
- Inhaled Beta Agonist
- Encourage Appointment within 24 Hours

* In patients with or at risk for glaucoma, medication/mist should not contact the eyes or conjunctival

draft 1/96
adasthma.prs

APPENDIX

B Fairfax Hospital Care of Patients Under Intravenous Conscious Sedation

Purpose

To promote consistent care for the patient undergoing a procedure or diagnostic exam under IV conscious sedation at Fairfax Hospital.

Definitions

General anesthesia is a medically controlled state of unconsciousness accompanied by a loss of protective reflexes, including the inability to maintain a patent airway independently and respond purposefully to physical stimulation or verbal command.

Deep sedation is a medically controlled state of depressed consciousness or unconsciousness from which the patient is not easily aroused. It may be accompanied by a partial or complete loss of protective reflexes, and includes the inability to maintain a patent airway independently and respond purposefully to physical stimulation or verbal command.

Conscious sedation is a medically controlled, minimally depressed level of consciousness that retains the patient's ability to maintain a patent airway independently and continuously respond appropriately to physical stimulation and/or verbal command. The stipulation that loss of consciousness should be unlikely is a particularly important part of the definition of conscious sedation, and the drugs and techniques used should carry a margin of safety wide enough to render unintended loss of consciousness unlikely.

This guideline is designed to assist the practitioner in those situations in which the intent is conscious sedation in patients undergoing a diagnostic or therapeutic procedure. It is not prescriptive for patients who are not undergoing a diagnostic or therapeutic procedure (e.g., post-operative analgesia, sedation for treatment of insomnia, anxiolysis, drug/alcohol withdrawal prophylaxis, treatment of seizure disorders or other medically necessary circumstances) or for situations where it is anticipated that the required sedation will eradicate the purposeful response to verbal commands or tactile stimulation (as distinct from reflex withdrawal from a painful stimulus).

Goals of IV Conscious Sedation

The goals of IV conscious sedation include, but are not limited to:

1. Patient Safety
2. Control of the Patient's Behavior
3. Production of Positive Psychological Response to Treatment
4. Return to Pretreatment Level of Consciousness (If Discharged)

Responsible Persons For Administration of IV Conscious Sedation

- MD performing procedure
- RN under the direction of the physician performing the procedure

Responsible Persons for the Care of the Patient Under IV Conscious Sedation

A physician, registered nurse, or other healthcare provider(s) trained in the recognition of and intervention in potential complications associated with IV conscious sedation.

Equipment

The following equipment must be readily available:

- Approved hospital resuscitation cart
- Defibrillator
- Oxygen source, cannulas and masks
- Suction, with catheters and Yankauer tips
- Ambu bag with fitting masks
- Monitors:
  1. ECG monitor
  2. Blood pressure monitor
- Pulse oximeter
- Equipment to institute intravenous access

Agents Used for IV Conscious Sedation

See Addendum A.

1. Midazolam (Versed)
2. Diazepam (Valium)
3. Lorazepam (Ativan)
4. Morphine
5. Meperidine (Demerol)
6. Fentanyl
7. Phenergan

Agents Used for Reversal of IV Conscious Sedation

See Addendum A.

1. Flumazenil
2. Naloxone

Standard I Personnel

The physician responsible for the procedure shall be immediately available throughout the duration of the procedure requiring IV conscious sedation. There shall be a professional or other trained healthcare provider in attendance to monitor the patient during and after the procedure. The RN or healthcare provider trained in the care of a patient receiving IV conscious sedation shall demonstrate competency of the following:

- Knowledge of age specific parameters of cardiac and respiratory rates
- Knowledge of role in the procedure(s) performed
- Knowledge of the pharmacology of the medication(s) used and their reversal agent(s) by identifying actions, dose, route, side effects, and reversal agents(s)
- Skills necessary to recognize and treat complications of IV conscious sedation
- Cardiac dysrhythmia recognition
- Basic cardiac life support (BCLS)

Standard II Monitoring

All patients receiving IV conscious sedation will have intravenous access established before the administration of the sedative of choice.

Baseline physiologic status should be documented before the procedure. During IV conscious sedation, the patient's oxygenation, ventilation, circulation, and level of consciousness (verbal or tactile stimuli response) should be continually evaluated, at least every 5 minutes. Post-procedure vital signs should be recorded every 15 minutes until stable or return to baseline. Assessment methods include the following:

Oxygenation: Continuous pulse oximetry should be used to evaluate the patient's oxygen saturation.

Ventilation: Continual clinical observation of chest excursions and respiratory rate.

Circulation: Continually assess cardiac monitor with continuous display. Measurement of blood pressure, heart rate, and pulse.

At the direction of the attending physician, or in cases in which pulse oximetry falls below presedation baseline, the nurse or designee will immediately provide oxygen therapy. The physician will immediately be notified.

Similarly, if the patient demonstrates cardiovascular instability (hypotension, tachycardia, dysrhythmia, or bradycardia) the nurse or designee will immediately notify the physician performing the procedure.

Standard III Documentation

The patient's record should contain the following documentation:

- History and physical
- Informed consent for procedure
- Procedure performed
- Monitors employed and physiologic data obtained, (e.g., oxygen saturation, vital signs, cardiac rhythm)
- Medications administered, dose, time, route, effect
- IV fluids administered
- Estimated blood loss (when applicable)
- Complications and management
- Status of patient at conclusion of procedure

If patient is being discharged to home, documentation should include the following:

- Status of patient at discharge, including level of consciousness
- Name of physician who discharged patient
- Criteria used for discharge

Standard IV Discharge

The patient may be discharged or the healthcare provider may leave the patient's room when the following criteria are met:

- The patient is fully awake and aware
- Stable cardiopulmonary system to preprocedure status:
  - Stable blood pressure within 20% of preprocedure value
  - Heart/respiratory rate and rhythm within normal range for age and history
  - Breath sounds audible and clear or as preprocedure status
  - Oxygen saturation $\geq$ 95 on RA or $\geq$ preprocedure level
- Satisfactory modified Aldrete score*—10 or same as pre-op. See Addendum B.
- No adverse reactions to medications
- Minimal nausea, vomiting, dizziness
- Dressing checked (no excessive bleeding or drainage present)

If the patient is being discharged to home, the following criteria must also be met:

- Able to ambulate without assistance and without dizziness
- Able to tolerate oral fluids (unless contraindicated by procedure)
- Patient and/or responsible adult given and understands written discharge instructions
- Prescriptions sent home with patient, if ordered
- Responsible adult present to escort patient home
- Physician's and emergency phone numbers given to patient

Standard versus Quality Measurement

Ongoing review will be maintained in each area administering IV conscious sedation to ensure consistent medication administration and patient monitoring.

President, Medical Staff of the Fairfax Hospital　　Date:

Approved:　　Effective Date:　　Replaces:

ADDENDUM A

IV Conscious Sedation Agents and Dosages Guidelines

The dosages indicated here are intended to serve as guidelines for the administration of IV conscious sedation without the loss of protective reflexes. Each patient is unique and individual clinical history and status should be taken into consideration when determining dosages. When these agents are used in combination, dosages may need to be decreased.

Drug	Pediatric dose	Adults <60 years old	Adults >60 years old, chronically ill and/or debilitated, and patients with reduced pulmonary reserve	Notes
Midazolam	Initial Dose: 0.05-0.2 mg/kg Maximum dose of 4 mg generally adequate	Initial Dose: 1 to 2 mg Titrate in 1 to 2 mg increments q 2-3 minutes Total dose of 5 mg generally adequate, however, rarely may go up to 10 mg.	1 to 1.5 mg Titrate in 0.5 to 1 mg increments q 2-3 minutes. Total dose of 3.5 mg usually adequate	Decrease dose by 30 to 50% when used concurrently with an opiate agonist.
Diazepam	Initial Dose: 0.07-0.09 mg/kg Max Dose of 10 mg generally adequate	Initial dose: 2 to 10 mg Total dose of 10 mg generally adequate but may go up to 20 mg.	Not recommended in >60 years due to long half life	Decrease dose when used concurrently with an opiate agonist.
Lorazepam	Initial Dose: 0.02-0.05 mg/kg Max Dose of 2 mg generally adequate.	Initial Dose: 0.044 mg/kg (up to 2 mg) Up to 4 mg in some patients	Generally do not exceed 2 mg in patients >50 years old.	
Meperidine	Initial Dose: 1-2 mg/kg Maximum dose of 100 mg	Initial dose 50 to 150 mg	Initial dose 25-75 mg	Not recommended in >60 due to active metabolite nonmeperidine
Morphine	Initial Dose: 0.1-0.2 mg/kg Maximum of 10 mg.	Initial Dose: 2.5 to 10 mg Maximum dose of 20 mg may be used	Initial Dose: 1.25 to 5.0 mg. Maximum dose of 10 mg may be used	
Reversal agents				
Flumazenil	<20 kg: 0.01 mg/kg up to 0.2 Mg. repeat doses of 0.005 mg/kg. 20-40 Kg: 0.2 mg. repeat doses of 0.005 mg/kg >40 kg: Use adult dosages	Dose: 0.2 mg; repeat 0.2 mg at ~ 60 second intervals up to maximum total dose of 1 mg in 20 minutes. If resedation occurs, doses may be repeated at 20 minute intervals. No more than 3 mg should be administered in 1 hour.	Same as Adult dosages.	
Naloxone	0.005 to 0.01 mg at 2 to 3 minute intervals to desired degree of reversal.	0.1 to 0.2 mg IV at 2 to 3 minute intervals. Titrate to desired degree of reversal.	Same as Adult dosages.	

ADDENDUM B
Modified Aldrete Scoring System

Airway	
Maintains Airway	2
Oral/Nasal Airway	1
Endotracheal Tube	0

Movement	
Moves Purposefully	2
Moves Involuntarily	1
Not Moving	0

Respiration	
Deep Breathes and Coughs	2
Shallow Breathing	1
Apnea	0

Color	
Satisfactory Color	2
Dusky, Blotchy	1
Cyanotic	0

Awareness	
Awake and Aware	2
Arousable	1
Not Responding	0

90 Hyperbaric Medicine as a Career Alternative for the Emergency Physician

Larry D. Weiss, Jean G. Brannon, and Keith W. Van Meter

OUTLINE

Clinical Overview
- Background
- Physics and physiology
- Risks and complications
- Contraindications
- Emergency medicine indications
- Nonurgent indications
- Future applications

Management
- Establishing a clinical hyperbaric service
- Feasibility study
- Equipment and installation
- Personnel
- Physician training
- Marketing
- Billing and reimbursement
- Other administrative responsibilities

Summary

Hyperbaric medicine offers an opportunity for career diversification for the emergency physician. Many of the clinical indications for hyperbaric oxygen therapy (HBOT) involve clinical conditions often encountered in emergency medicine. In addition, the training of an emergency physician allows for a relatively easy transition into the clinical practice of hyperbaric medicine, much like it does for toxicology, emergency medical services, and sports medicine. Unlike physicians from other disciplines, the emergency physician finds it easier to divide his or her time among multiple activities. A designated number of days per month can be devoted toward the emergency department and a hyperbaric practice.

There are many advantages to developing a hyperbaric medicine service. Perhaps the greatest advantage is the opportunity for career diversification. "Burnout" caused by chronic stress is a major concern for emergency physicians.[1-3] In addition to having an interesting caseload, the hyperbaric physician is usually working in a low-stress environment. Even when the service is very busy, most patients are stable and not difficult to manage.

Developing expertise in a small, relatively esoteric area of medicine can add to job satisfaction. Generally, the emergency physician has knowledge that is spread over a vast area and is usually not consulted by other physicians. The hyperbaric physician, on the other hand, provides a service in an area in which few physicians have much knowledge. If the service is properly marketed, it can become an important source of new patients for the hospital, thereby enhancing the importance of an emergency physician group within the hospital.

Emergency physicians have become well represented in hyperbaric medicine. Currently, emergency physicians comprise approximately 15% of the membership of the Undersea and Hyperbaric Medical Society (UHMS). Along with internal medicine and anesthesiology/critical care medicine, emergency medicine is among the most heavily represented specialties in the UHMS (UHMS personal communication, February 1991). The UHMS recognized the important association between emergency medicine and hyperbaric medicine when they convened a symposium, *Hyperbaric Oxygen in Emergency Medical Care,* in 1983.[4]

This chapter is not a comprehensive review of hyperbaric medicine. Many reviews of diving medicine[5-8] and clinical hyperbaric medicine[9-13] have already been written. Rather, it examines the relevance of HBOT to emergency medicine and provides guidelines for establishing a hyperbaric medicine service within an emergency medicine department or group. It is necessary, however, to begin with a brief discussion of the background, basic physics, and physiology of HBOT.

CLINICAL OVERVIEW

Background

Clinical hyperbaric chambers were probably first used in the mid-1840s in France. They were used initially to treat cases of decompression sickness that were contracted by coal miners who were working in a compressed air environment.[14] These chambers used compressed air; oxygen was not commonly used until the latter half of the twentieth century. The first widespread use of recompression chambers occurred in 1889 during the construction of the Hudson River Tunnel in New York City. Within the next several years, chambers were commonly used across the United States to treat compressed air workers.

The first U.S. Navy (USN) treatment tables were developed in 1924.[15] They were further refined in 1946 when the Navy formally developed "Treatment Tables I-IV."[16] A detailed description of these tables can be found in the original USN sources.[16-19] These tables all used compressed air and down through the years had a considerable failure rate. They were widely used until the mid-1960s.

Yarborough and Behnke began to study the use of compressed oxygen in the late 1930s.[17-19] The use of oxygen was resisted for many years because of the fear of oxygen toxicity and the presumed fire hazard. In 1964 Goodman and Workman[20,21] developed USN Treatment Tables 5 and 6 using compressed oxygen. These were adopted by the Navy in the late 1960s. Tables 6A (for gas embolism) and 7 (for extraordinary exposures) were added later. The Navy has just added a Table 8 for divers who deteriorate while receiving a Table 6 or 6A treatment.

The modern era of clinical hyperbaric medicine began approximately 30 years ago with the appearance of two landmark papers. In 1960, Boerema et al.[22] published a study in which severely phlebotomized dogs survived when exposed to hyperbaric oxygen. In 1961, Brummelkamp et al.[23] first reported the successful use of HBOT in patients with life-threatening clostridial infections.

This overview demonstrates that HBOT is not a new technology but rather new applications for an old technology. Hyperbaric therapy fell into relative obscurity after the early 1900s and again in the late 1960s because some proponents of hyperbaric medicine made exaggerated and unsubstantiated claims about its efficacy. Only in recent years has a concerted effort been made to scientifically delineate the clinical efficacy of HBOT.

Physics and Physiology

Box 91-1 is a list of pressure equivalents. The SCUBA diver is exposed to one atmosphere absolute (ATA) at sea level. Every 33 feet of sea water (FSW) adds another atmosphere of pressure. By using the diver as an example, we can better understand the principles of HBOT in other clinical settings.

For the purposes of this discussion, it is necessary to review two basic laws of physics: Boyle's law and Henry's law. Boyle's law ($PV = K$) states that an inverse relationship exists between the pressure (P) and volume (V) of an ideal gas. As a diver ascends, the gas in the lungs expands because the pressure is decreasing.

As an example, suppose a diver runs out of air at 66 FSW (3 ATA). If the diver takes one last deep breath and rapidly ascends, the gas in the lungs will expand rapidly and potentially rupture the lungs. Air may be directly insufflated into a pulmonary vein, return to the left side of the heart, and probably travel to the brain, resulting in a cerebral air embolism.

Boyle's law explains not only the pathophysiology of a gas embolism but also the rationale for treatment. Recompression in a hyperbaric chamber will decrease the size of the bubble through a direct pressure effect, and the use of oxygen will accelerate nitrogen washout, further decreasing the size of the bubble.

Henry's Law ($C = n\ [Pg]$) states that the amount of an ideal gas that is physically dissolved in solution is directly proportional to the partial pressure of the gas. For example, large amounts of carbon dioxide are dissolved under pressure in softdrink bottles. When the cap is suddenly removed, the ambient pressure in the bottle is dramatically reduced. As a result, millions of microscopic bubbles come out of solution.

Although oversimplified, this situation is essentially analogous to decompression sickness. A diver may go underwater too deep, stay too long, or ascend too quickly. As a result, nitrogen (in divers breathing compressed air) comes out of solution and bubbles form in the circulation and tissues. Henry's law also explains the rationale for treating decompression sickness in a hyperbaric chamber. Recompression in a hyperbaric chamber can redissolve microscopic gas bubbles, allowing for a more controlled decompression. A description of the various recompression treatment tables is beyond the scope of this discussion.

BOX 90-1

PRESSURE EQUIVALENTS

1 atmosphere (ATM)
0.1013 megapascals (MPa)*
1.013247 bar (10 meters of sea water)
33 feet of sea water (FSW)
34 feet of fresh water (FFW)
14.7 pounds per square inch (psi)
760 mm Hg

*Preferred SI (International System of Units) measurement.

Physiologically, hyperoxia produces several other effects. Hunt and others have demonstrated in a number of experimental models and clinical studies that elevated tissue wound oxygen tensions result in accelerated healing and more rapid resolution of infection.[24-27] Hyperoxia increases angiogenesis, fibroblast proliferation, collagen formation, epithelialization, and the ability of white blood cells to kill bacteria.[28-32] Intermittent hyperoxia is probably optimal because intervening periods of relative hypoxia are needed for maximal angiogenesis and stimulation of fibroblasts and macrophages.[33,34]

Hyperoxia causes vasoconstriction, which may be beneficial in a patient with a crush injury and/or compartment syndrome. The vasoconstriction decreases edema and compartment pressures while hyperoxygenating endangered muscle tissue.[35,36]

At very high oxygen tensions, oxygen has an antitoxin effect with regard to carbon monoxide,[37-41] clostridial exotoxin,[42-45] and possibly cyanide,[46-50] hydrogen sulfide,[51] and carbon tetrachloride.[52,53] In addition to a general antibacterial effect,[26,27,54] hyperoxia is especially effective with regard to anaerobic infections[43,55-58] and enhances the effect of antibiotics in experimental models.[59-63]

Risks and Complications

Treatment in a hyperbaric chamber is extremely safe. Fire is theoretically more of a risk in a monoplace chamber (Figure 90-1), although no fires have occurred in a clinical monoplace chamber in the United States. Such a fire would certainly be fatal. In its usual configuration, the monoplace chamber is pressurized with compressed 100% oxygen.

Claustrophobia is a more significant problem in monoplace chambers than in multiplace chambers (Figure 90-2) where the incidence is approximately one in every 2000 patients.[64] Theoretically, multiplace chambers are less of a fire hazard, although some fires have been associated with these chambers.[65] Multiplace chambers are pressurized with compressed air. Patients breathe oxygen intermittently through tight-fitting aviator masks or hoods. Some monoplace chambers can be reconfigured in this manner (i.e., they can be pressurized with air, and patients can breath oxygen through a hood or mask).

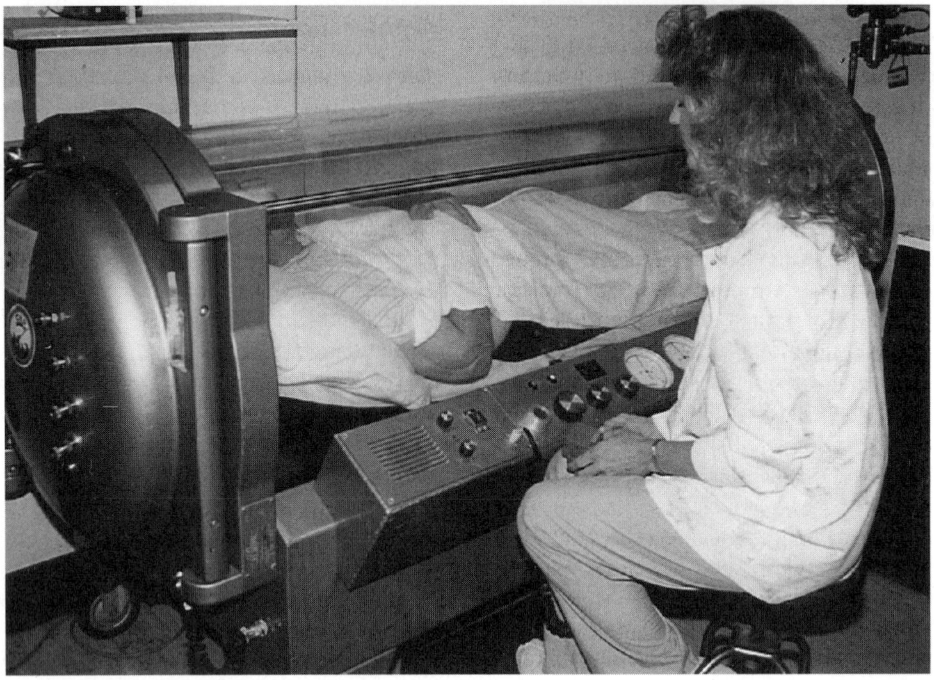

FIGURE 90-1 Monoplace hyperbaric chamber.
(From Weiss LD, Van Meter KW: *Am J Emerg Med* 10:558-568, 1992.)

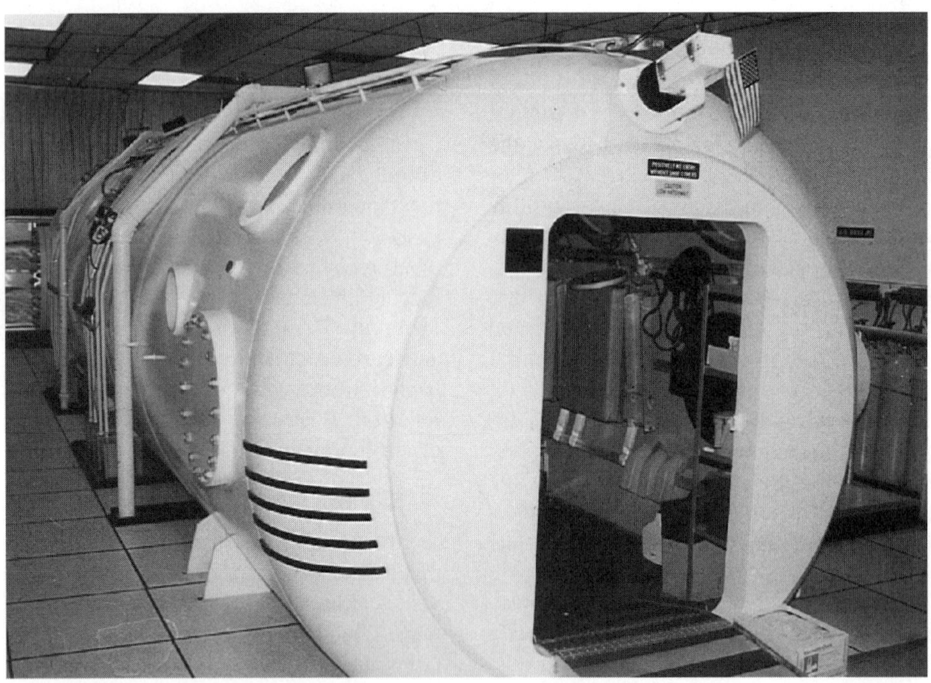

FIGURE 90-2 Multiplace hyperbaric chamber.
(From Weiss LD, Van Meter KW: *Am J Emerg Med* 10:558-568, 1992.)

Barotrauma, especially to the middle ear, is probably the most common complication but is usually mild. In Davis' experience, 0.37% (1 in 270) had barotrauma significant enough to interrupt their treatments, but even in most of these cases the injury was mild.[64] Some cases may result in the development of a middle ear effusion, which may be hemorrhagic. Infrequently, a ruptured tympanic membrane may result. If a patient requires repetitive treatments and cannot perform pressure equalization (modified Valsalva or Frenzyl maneuver), PE (pressure-equalization) tubes can be inserted in the tympanic membranes. Barotrauma to other areas in the respiratory tree is unusual in the clinical setting.

Decompression sickness can occur in a patient or inside tender in the hyperbaric chamber but is exceedingly rare. Decompression sickness is a complication of breathing inert gas (e.g., nitrogen in compressed air) and therefore is not possible in a patient being treated in a monoplace chamber that is compressed with oxygen.

In a multiplace chamber, patients are breathing 100% oxygen except for 5- to 10-minute air breaks (depending on the treatment table). Nitrogen that accumulates during the brief air breaks is quickly off-gassed during the oxygen-breathing periods. However, inside tenders in a multiplace chamber breathe compressed air. They are more susceptible to decompression sickness. This is obviated by exposing the tenders to 100% oxygen toward the end of the treatment and staying within the USN safe diving guidelines.[66]

Although rare, acute central nervous system (CNS) oxygen toxicity is the most feared complication of HBOT. Davis et al.[64] estimated the incidence of oxygen seizures at 1 in 11,000 treatments. When a patient is exposed to 3 ATA of oxygen for a prolonged time, a seizure is almost certain. At 2 ATA, seizures are extremely rare. Seizures are unpredictable, as patients have a variable susceptibility to oxygen toxicity. Most current treatment tables for nondiving indications limit the pressure to 2.0 to 2.8 ATA for 90 to 120 minutes.

Subacute pulmonary oxygen toxicity is extremely rare with current treatment tables. For several years we closely followed patients with serial spirometry but did not find a single case of even mild toxicity (unpublished observation). This is entirely consistent with experience in the literature.[67,68] We would currently recommend serial spirometry only in patients with active pulmonary disease.

Hyperoxia has mild ocular side effects. There are several anecdotal reports of accelerated cataract growth,[69] but HBOT has never been shown to cause cataracts. A reversible myopia develops in 20% to 40% of patients who are treated repetitively.[70] Vision returns to pretreatment levels within several weeks after the cessation of HBOT.[71]

We routinely use vitamins C and E for their antioxidant effects.[72-75] There is no proof that they can prevent oxygen toxicity, but because of their low potential for toxicity, they are commonly used in this setting (also, both may accelerate wound healing). An important technique to prevent acute CNS oxygen toxicity is to administer oxygen intermittently. This technique is most easily accomplished in a multiplace chamber. If a seizure does occur, it is most easily managed in the multiplace chamber. The inside tender can simply remove the mask or hood from the patient. The seizure usually terminates abruptly when the patient is no longer exposed to 100% oxygen.

Contraindications

The only absolute contraindication to HBOT is an untreated pneumothorax. Relative contraindications include obstructive lung disease (especially CO_2 retainers), previous ear surgery or injury (patients may need PE tubes), significant upper respiratory infections (patients may have difficulty with pressure equalization), fever (may lower seizure threshold), and claustrophobia. Preexisting cataracts and optic neuritis are often listed as relative contraindications based on anecdotal reports of decreased visual acuity in patients after HBOT.[69-71,76]

Pregnancy was previously considered a strong relative contraindication to HBOT because of the presumed adverse effects of hyperoxia on fetal development. However, Soviet researchers have published more than 700 cases of pregnant women who were treated with HBOT without complications.[77-79] Indeed, because animal studies have shown that fetal hemoglobin has a higher affinity for carbon monoxide, it has recently been recommended that the threshold for treating pregnant women in this setting be lower than for the general population.[80]

Patients with idiopathic seizure disorders, a history of chest surgery or pneumothorax, and altered sensorium should be treated with caution. Glucose levels should be closely monitored in persons with diabetes because of the tendency of HBOT to cause hypoglycemia in some patients.[81,82] Steroids, amphetamines, catecholamines, insulin, and thyroid hormone may enhance CNS oxygen toxicity. Patients receiving these medications should be closely monitored for any untoward effects.

Emergency Medicine Indications

Box 90-2 lists the indications for HBOT that are currently approved by the UHMS. The UHMS has a Hyperbaric Oxygen Committee, which updates its official recommendations approximately every 3 years.[83] The members of the Committee are all actively involved in hyperbaric medicine (either experimentally or clinically). A detailed explanation of their approval process is contained in the preface of their report.[83]

The four traditional indications for HBOT (decompression sickness, acute gas embolism, carbon monoxide poisoning, and gas gangrene), as well as many of the more recent indications, are conditions encountered in emergency medicine practice. Each of the indications, the rationale for HBOT, and the evidence for its efficacy are presented.

Decompression Sickness and Acute Gas Embolism. Decompression sickness and acute gas embolism (AGE) have already been discussed in sufficient detail for the scope of this chapter. The efficacy of HBOT in this setting was extensively studied by the USN.[17-21,84] High-flow oxygen and rehydration at the scene are helpful, but HBOT is the only treatment modality that is efficacious in treating these conditions.

BOX 90-2

CURRENT UHMS-APPROVED INDICATIONS FOR HYPERBARIC OXYGEN THERAPY (CATEGORY 1)

1. Gas embolism
2. Decompression sickness
3. Carbon monoxide poisoning
4. Clostridial gas gangrene
5. Cyanide poisoning (with coexisting CO poisoning)
6. Crush injuries, compartment syndromes, acute traumatic ischemia
7. Selected refractory problem wounds
8. Necrotizing soft-tissue infections
9. Chronic refractory osteomyelitis
10. Osteoradionecrosis
11. Compromised skin grafts and flaps
12. Thermal burns
13. Brown recluse spider bites

There are many nondiving etiologies of AGE, many of them iatrogenic. Approximately 20,000 cases of AGE occur each year in the United States.[85] It is difficult to determine the relative incidence of the various etiologies of AGE, but diving contributes only a small percentage of cases.

Nondiving etiologies of AGE include mechanical ventilation, invasive medical procedures, surgery (especially craniotomies, carotid endarterectomies, and cardiovascular procedures), trauma (especially penetrating chest trauma), central venous catheterization, dialysis, angiography, status asthmaticus, and forceful cunnilingus during pregnancy.[86] Cardiac arrest after penetrating chest trauma should alert the physician to the possibility of coronary artery air emboli.[87-89] The appearance of a new neurologic finding after cardiovascular or neurologic surgery, dialysis, or instrumentation should alert one to the possibility of AGE. Regardless of the etiology, HBOT can rapidly decrease the size of gas bubbles in the circulatory system and in many cases eliminate them altogether.

Carbon Monoxide Poisoning. Carbon monoxide (CO) poisoning is widely believed to be the most common cause of death in the United States (and worldwide) from poisoning. Few people would question the efficacy of 100% oxygen in this setting because of the ability of oxygen to compete with CO at the hemoglobin and cytochrome binding sites.

The efficacy of oxygen in this setting, however, has never been proven. A randomized prospective controlled clinical trial has never been performed to compare 100% oxygen to room air in CO-poisoned patients. On the other hand, the theoretic rationale (as well as the accumulated clinical experience) for the use of high-flow oxygen is overwhelming. The half-life of carboxyhemoglobin (COHb) is largely dependent on minute ventilation. There is much individual variability, but the half-life of COHb is 6 to 8 hours while breathing room air and only 80 minutes on 100% oxygen. On 3 ATA of oxygen in a hyperbaric chamber, the half-life may be as low as 23 minutes.[38,90,91]

For the last several decades, physiologists have argued whether the primary site of CO toxicity was at the hemoglobin or cytochrome binding site. Recent evidence has shown that much of the neurotoxicity of CO may be due to its ability to cause lipid peroxidation in the CNS.[92] Hyperbaric oxygen was demonstrated in an experimental model to prevent this process, whereas 100% oxygen at surface pressure (i.e., 1 ATA of oxygen) failed to do so.[40,41]

Most deaths from CO poisoning occur at the scene. The exception is the patient who has profound neurologic injury and never regains consciousness. The other major clinical problem after CO exposure is the presence of persistent neuropsychiatric sequelae.[93-96] These sequelae are often described as "subtle" or "minor" but can cause significant long-term morbidity. In most cases, the rationale for vigorously treating CO-poisoned patients is to prevent these so-called mild sequelae.

Gross neurologic impairment occurs in 2% to 10% of patients.[96-98] However, more subtle psychiatric sequelae occur in up to 40% of patients.[96,99] The most common complications are memory loss, personality deterioration (usually depression), and prolonged mild organic brain dysfunction (i.e., delirium).

Therefore, perhaps the most important aspect of emergency department evaluation in stable patients is the mental status examination. Several brief examinations, such as the Folstein Mini-Mental Status Examination, are amenable to emergency department use.[100,101] Several abbreviated batteries of psychometric tests have been developed for use in this setting.[95]

When evaluating efficacy of a treatment modality for CO poisoning, the main questions are the overall mortality and the incidence of complications. Because most deaths occur in the prehospital setting, the presence of neuropsychiatric sequelae is probably the most significant (and sensitive) parameter by which to evaluate various treatment modalities.

Much experimental data[38,91,102-104] and clinical experience[98,99,105-112] suggest that HBOT is superior to 100% oxygen. The most significant evidence demonstrating the efficacy of HBOT was published by Myers et al.[99] This study was prospective and controlled but not randomized. In addition to not being randomized, another problem with this study was the use of COHb levels to assess severity of exposure (although the primary determinent of severity in this study was the presence or absence of neuropsychologic impairment). COHb levels have never been shown to closely correlate with severity.

In this study, patients with signs or symptoms of neuropsychologic impairment were treated with HBOT regardless of COHb level. Those without neuropsychologic impairment and a COHb level of <30% were treated with 100% oxygen. Even though the design of the study was strongly biased against HBOT (i.e., the more severely poisoned patients were treated with HBOT), patients who were treated with HBOT had a better outcome. These patients had no neuropsychologic impairment. The mildly poisoned patients who were treated with 100% oxygen had a 12% incidence of sequelae. The most common complications were chronic headaches, irritability, personality changes, confusion, and memory loss.

In a recent widely quoted study, Raphael et al.[113] published the first prospective, controlled, randomized study comparing HBOT to 100% oxygen. They classified patients as mildly or severely intoxicated simply on the absence or presence of unconsciousness. Mildly poisoned patients were randomized to receive 100% oxygen or HBOT. Severely poisoned patients were randomized to receive one or two HBOT treatments.

The authors concluded that HBOT offered no additional benefit in mildly poisoned patients. They also concluded that an additional HBO treatment offered no advantage in severely poisoned patients, but that these patients should receive one HBO treatment.

There are many flaws with regard to the design and methods of this study. Only mildly poisoned patients were randomized into 100% oxygen versus HBOT groups. HBOT is not recommended in mildly poisoned patients. It is not surprising that no differences were found between the two groups. The study was not truly randomized because patients who refused such randomization were still included in the study. Only minimal patient follow-up was performed. Follow-up examinations consisted of a self-questionnaire and a general physical examination by the patients' personal physician (not by one of the authors) 1 month postexposure. Mental status examinations were not performed.

Thom et al.[114] are currently involved in a randomized prospective controlled study comparing HBOT to 100% oxygen in symptomatic patients with CO poisoning. When they first presented their preliminary data in 1992, they had entered 27 patients into the study. The HBOT treated group had a significantly lower incidence of neuropsychologic sequelae. As of July 1993, they had entered 65 patients into the study (personal communication) and they are still collecting data.

What recommendations can be made based on the currently available data? The UHMS recommends HBOT if the patient has any signs of acute end-organ damage (e.g., altered mental status, neurologic signs, or cardiovascular dysfunction) regardless of the COHb level. The COHb level is a poor prognostic indicator. Nevertheless, if the level is greater than 25% in the locality of a hyperbaric chamber (or >40% elsewhere), the UHMS recommends that the patient be transferred for evaluation and possible HBO therapy. Until more definitive data are available, these recommendations appear to be both prudent and conservative.

Cyanide Poisoning. The UHMS currently recommends HBO in cases of combined CO and cyanide poisoning. This combination is not uncommon in cases of smoke inhalation.[115,116] Some evidence suggests that cyanide and CO have synergistic toxic effects.[117]

Most prehospital cases of cyanide poisoning involve exposures that are rapidly fatal. Cases in which survival is long enough for the patient to reach the hospital are rare. It is possible that HBOT is efficacious for isolated cyanide exposures, but this would be extremely difficult to prove in a randomized prospective study.

On the other hand, iatrogenic cases in hospitalized patients (e.g., from nitroprusside infusions) usually involve relatively low levels of cyanide exposure that can be readily treated with standard antidotes. Therefore HBOT is recommended only in cases of cyanide poisoning complicated by significant CO exposure. It would be prudent to lower the threshold for treating CO poisoning when concomitant exposure to cyanide is known or presumed.

Clostridial Gas Gangrene. There are no known randomized, prospective, controlled clinical trials dealing with any aspect of the treatment of gas gangrene. Because of its rarity in civilian populations (and its severity), such a study would only be possible in military populations during wartime. Randomization in such a setting would be quite difficult.

In addition to a strong theoretic rationale and extensive clinical experience, animal studies have demonstrated the efficacy of HBOT in the treatment of gas gangrene. Perhaps the most elaborate and best controlled study was that performed by DeMello et al.[118] A total of 187 dogs were injected with spores of *Clostridium perfringens.* They were divided into eight groups according to treatment. Surgery, antibiotics, HBOT, and every possible combination of these modalities were compared (as well as a control group that received no treatment).

By far, the highest survival rate (95%) occurred in dogs that received all three modes of therapy. The difference was statistically significant ($P<0.01$). Surgery and antibiotics were demonstrated to be absolutely essential, but dogs that received only these two modalities had a survival rate of 70%. None of the control dogs survived. HBOT was shown to be valuable adjunctive therapy that enhanced survival.

The theoretic rationale for the use of HBOT is based on the ability of hyperoxia to interfere with clostridial spore formation and α-exotoxin production. Clostridia are *facultative* anaerobes. They can multiply freely in tissues with an oxygen tension up to 30 mm and can grow in a restricted manner in oxygen tensions up to 70 mm.[119] At an oxygen tension of 250 mm, spore formation and α-exotoxin production cease.[39] Tissue oxygen tensions of more than 300 mm can be produced when the patient is exposed to 3 ATA of oxygen in the hyperbaric chamber.[120]

Several papers in the surgical literature have attested to the efficacy of perioperative HBOT and the ability of HBOT to delineate healthy from necrotic tissue.[23,121-128] The result is often a less drastic amputation. Without HBOT, the delineation between viable and necrotic muscle tissue is indistinct. This would necessitate a more drastic amputation to ensure complete excision of contaminated tissue.

Considering the high morbidity and mortality from this disease, aggressive therapy with surgery, antibiotics, and HBOT is certainly indicated. In addition to a strong rationale for the use of HBOT, animal studies and an extensive amount of clinical experience in the literature support its use.[23,117,120-127]

Other Surgical Infections. A variety of other extremely aggressive gas-forming infections have had traditionally high mortality rates. These clinical entities are difficult to classify, and many of their manifestations overlap. Necrotizing fasciitis, synergistic bacterial gangrene, Meleney's ulcer, crepitant anaerobic cellulitis, nonclostridial myonecrosis, and Fournier's gangrene may have some subtle differences but have much in common. Nonclostridial myonecrosis is an invasive, highly destructive infection that has much in common with clostridial gas gangrene. The other entities are also serious, but are usually more superficial.

They are all mixed infections, extremely aggressive, tissue-destructive, and most are gas-producing. Aggressive surgical debridement and wide-spectrum antibiotics are standard therapy. In some centers where it is available, HBOT is a valuable adjunct in the treatment of these conditions.

As with gas gangrene, no aspect of the treatment of these conditions has been subjected to randomized, prospective, controlled clinical trials. These entities are all rare and difficult to classify, and most patients have a variety of underlying diseases that make it difficult to randomize them into equivalent populations. Because of the explosive nature of these conditions, it is generally accepted that heroic measures are indicated if the patient is to survive.

A common denominator in all of these infections is tissue hypoxia in a compromised host. HBOT can reverse tissue hypoxia, enhance polymorphonuclear leukocyte killing ability, promote angiogenesis and fibroblast proliferation, and have a direct inhibitory effect on anaerobic organisms. Published clinical series have shown a lower than expected mortality rate when HBOT was used for these conditions (12.5% to 25%) compared with cases where HBOT was not used (33% to 67%).[129-134]

The UHMS recommends that HBOT be used as an adjunct to surgery and antibiotics in compromised patients or in any life-threatening situation. If antibiotics and surgery are effective in a localized non-life-threatening crepitant infection, HBOT is not needed.

Crush Injuries, Compartment Syndromes, and Posttraumatic Ischemia. Nylander et al.[35] demonstrated that HBOT significantly reduced postischemic edema in a controlled rat model ($P < 0.001$). Strauss et al.[36] used a dog model to produce a compartment syndrome. Dogs treated with HBOT had significantly less necrosis compared to untreated controls ($P < 0.01$).

Because there has not yet been a controlled, randomized, clinical study evaluating HBOT in this setting, it should probably be reserved for limb-threatening cases, or cases in which a massive amount of muscle debridement is contemplated. HBOT has the ability to oxygenate muscle tissue while constricting blood vessels. The vasoconstriction results in a decrease in posttraumatic edema and compartment pressures. Even though blood flow is initially decreased by 20%, tissue oxygen tensions increase up to tenfold.[135]

Anemia From Exceptional Blood Loss. This term refers to cases of blood loss sufficient to cause cardiovascular or respiratory insufficiency in a patient who cannot or will not receive a blood transfusion. The patient may have antibodies resulting in incompatibilities with banked blood or may belong to a religious sect that bans transfusions. Also, there is increasing concern among the lay public about the safety of transfusions.

The body requires six volumes-percent of oxygen to satisfy basic metabolic needs. A patient with a dramatically lowered hematocrit may not have this oxygen-carrying capacity even when exposed to 100% oxygen. At 3 ATA of oxygen, almost seven volumes-percent of oxygen is physically dissolved in plasma. Basic oxygen requirements are fulfilled without the need for hemoglobin to carry any oxygen.

Because of the rare and extraordinary nature of this problem, randomized prospective trials have not been performed. Several experimental studies[22,136-140] and clinical series[141-144] have been published that demonstrate rapid improvement in hemodynamic parameters and surprisingly low mortality rates.

We have been involved in several cases of Jehovah's Witnesses who refused postoperative transfusions. One case was a 31-year-old otherwise healthy woman who presented with a lower gastrointestinal bleed. She continued to bleed postoperatively until her hematocrit decreased to 5.0. Despite the administration of 100% oxygen, she had continued episodes of chest pain, shortness of breath, and ventricular dysrhythmias.

Folate, vitamin B_{12}, and iron injections were administered daily; and the patient was treated in the hyperbaric chamber at 2.8 ATA for 2 hours three times a day. The HBOT allowed us to provide sufficient oxygen to sustain this patient until her hematocrit could be increased by the other treatment modalities. Her symptoms rapidly resolved, and 3 days later HBOT was discontinued. It is only for such extraordinary cases that HBOT has been recommended.

Burns. It was not until 1989 that the UHMS gave full approval for the use of HBOT in burn patients. Much of the experimental and clinical data supporting the use of HBOT is more than 10 years old. The delay in granting approval was due to the controversy involved.

The rationale for using HBOT in this setting is to decrease edema, preserve marginally viable tissue, promote wound closure, and to enhance host defenses.[83] Well-controlled animal studies have demonstrated these effects.[30,145-148] Many published uncontrolled clinical series appear to demonstrate beneficial effects of HBOT in burn patients. The number of such reports is so large that a discussion of their results is beyond the scope of this chapter.

Two randomized, prospective, controlled clinical trials demonstrate the efficacy of HBOT in burn patients. Hart et al.[149] studied the effects of HBOT in burn patients in a prospective, randomized, controlled, double-blinded setting. They were able to simulate the effects of pressure in the control group by slightly pressurizing the chamber to 10 FSW and then allowing the pressure to slowly drift back to 1 ATA. Therefore the control population essentially received 100% oxygen. Hart et al demonstrated decreased fluid requirements and more rapid wound healing in the HBOT treated group. Only 16 patients were entered into this study, but results were statistically significant ($P < 0.005$). In another randomized study, Merola and Piscatilli[150] demonstrated improved healing in 37 patients with partial-thickness burns compared to 37 controls.

There is at present a great polarization of opinion about the efficacy of HBOT in burn management. Those who have a great deal of experience with HBOT in this setting feel that it would be unethical to expose their patients to further randomization. On the other hand, most burn units in the United States do not use HBOT. Perhaps in this setting a much larger randomized study can be performed to definitively resolve this controversy. Until such a study is performed, the controversy will remain, regardless of UHMS approval.

Nonurgent Indications

Even though many of the indications for HBOT involve emergent conditions, most patients in the United States who receive HBOT have chronic refractory wounds, including patients with refractory venous stasis ulcers, marginal diabetic ulcers, and arterial insufficiency ulcers that persist after vascular reconstruction. Other nonacute wounds that may benefit from HBOT include compromised skin grafts and flaps, osteoradionecrosis, and chronic refractory osteomyelitis.

Some of the strongest clinical evidence supporting the efficacy of HBOT was reported in patients with refractory wounds. In a randomized, prospective, controlled clinical trial, Perrins[151] demonstrated an improved outcome in HBOT-treated patients compared with controls. Marx[152] reported a similar outcome in a randomized, prospective, controlled clinical trial of HBOT in patients with osteoradionecrosis of the mandible. Baroni et al.,[153] in a prospective and controlled (but not randomized) study, showed an improved outcome in HBOT-treated patients with diabetic foot ulcers.

This chapter cannot describe in detail the management of patients with chronic wounds. However, most hyperbaric physicians spend much of their day managing chronic wounds. This is an area where the emergency physician may need additional training before being able to function as a hyperbaric physician.

Future Applications

Currently, there is much interest in providing more definitive data for the indications designated as "currently indicated" by the UHMS. The need for such studies is greatest with regard to carbon monoxide poisoning and some of the nonemergent indications for HBO therapy (selected problem wounds, chronic refractory osteomyelitis, and compromised grafts and flaps). Data with regard to osteoradionecrosis are quite definitive.[151]

Until 1989, the UHMS designated a Category 2 for experimental indications (Box 90-3). This category was created

BOX 90-3

EXPERIMENTAL INDICATIONS (CATEGORY 2)

This category was eliminated by the UHMS in 1989. It was originally developed to stimulate interest in research.

1. Anaerobic brain abscesses
2. Carbon tetrachloride poisoning
3. Cerebrovascular accidents
4. Closed-head injuries/cerebral edema
5. Nonunion of fractures and bone grafts
6. Hydrogen sulfide poisoning
7. Hansen disease (leprosy)
8. Meningitis
9. Multiple sclerosis
10. Pyoderma gangrenosum
11. Pseudomembranous colitis
12. Radiation enteritis and proctitis
13. Radiation myelitis
14. Central retinal artery occlusion
15. Selected refractory mycoses
16. Intraabdominal abscesses
17. Sepsis
18. Sickle cell anemia crises
19. Brown recluse spider bites
20. Spinal cord injuries

to help stimulate interest in research. At present there is little interest in some of the entities on this list, and a great deal of interest in some entities not included on the list. In 1989 Category 2 was eliminated, and the UHMS merely updated its list of approved indications.

There is presently a great deal of interest in the use of HBOT after a documented myocardial infarction. Earlier work has shown a beneficial effect of high-flow surface oxygen in reducing infarct size.[153] Thomas et al.[154] recently studied mongrel dogs that were given HBOT, recombinant tissue plasminogen activator (r-tPA), or both after experimental occlusion of the left anterior descending coronary artery. Controls were untreated. The best results were obtained in the group that received HBOT and r-tPA. In this group there was a 96.9% restoration of oxidative enzyme activity (reflecting a reduction in injury) compared to the control group ($P < 0.001$).

Hart et al.[155] and Messina et al.[156] are currently engaged in a prospective, randomized, controlled trial using HBOT in patients receiving tPA. After initiating tPA therapy, patients are randomized into groups receiving HBOT (experimental group) and high-flow surface pressure oxygen (control group). Other researchers are currently studying the effects of HBOT during cardiac arrest[157] and in patients with unstable angina.[158]

There was a great deal of interest in the use of HBOT in patients with multiple sclerosis after a study by Fischer et al.[159] demonstrated short-term benefits. This study was prospective, randomized, controlled, and double-blinded. Subsequent prospective, randomized, controlled trials[160,161] and many nonrandomized studies have shown no efficacy of HBOT. Fischer's results have not yet been reproduced, and the UHMS does not currently recommend HBOT for patients with multiple sclerosis.

Other current areas of interest include cerebral vascular accidents,[162-167] subarachnoid hemorrhage,[168,169] central retinal artery occlusion, anaerobic sepsis,[170] migraine and cluster headaches[171,172] blunt head and spinal cord injury,[173,174] peripheral nerve injuries[175] and carbon tetrachloride[52,53] and hydrogen sulfide poisoning.[51,176-179] In a randomized, prospective, controlled, double-blinded study in patients with severe brain injury, the HBOT-treated group had a 17% mortality rate compared to 32% for the control group ($P=0.037$).[180] However, among survivors, HBOT did not improve neurologic outcome. The authors used an abbreviated HBOT schedule and postulated that perhaps with a different treatment schedule, neurologic outcome would have been different. Nevertheless, they were able to demonstrate a positive effect of HBOT in this setting. Further studies are necessary to better delineate any possible role for HBOT in the management of acute or chronic brain injury.

MANAGEMENT

Establishing a Clinical Hyperbaric Service

There are many logical reasons for emergency physicians to get involved in hyperbaric medicine. Development of a hyperbaric service may provide many benefits for an emergency physician group. It can augment income, provide diversity within the practice, enhance the value of the emergency physician group within the hospital, provide a change of pace for the emergency physician, increase job satisfaction, and perhaps help avoid "burnout."

The decision to establish a clinical hyperbaric service should begin with a feasibility study. Other important issues are cost of equipment and installation, physician training, management of personnel, marketing, reimbursement, and quality assurance.

Feasibility Study

Several different mathematical models have been developed for estimating the need for hyperbaric services within a community. One model, developed by Perry Baromedical Services (Riviera Beach, Florida), estimates a need of one HBOT/day per 100,000 people in a referral area (i.e., in an urban metropolitan area). Another model, developed by Hyperbaric Oxygen Treatment Systems ("H.O.T.S.," San Diego, California) estimates a need of 4.25 treatments/year per 1000 people.

For example, in a metropolitan area containing 1 million people, the Perry model would yield an estimated need of 10 HBOTs a day. The HOTS model would yield an estimate of 4250 treatments a year, or 12 treatments a day. In our experience, both models yield a very conservative estimate of the potential need for HBOT in a community. They are useful in providing a "worst-case scenario" in terms of patient flow and financial viability of a hyperbaric service. Patient flow can be favorably influenced by an effective marketing system, positive clinical interactions, and favorable patient results (the best possible marketing technique).

The U.S. Air Force has also developed a model for carrying out feasibility studies.[181] It is somewhat cumbersome to use and is based on ICD-9 numbers derived from inpatient discharge diagnoses. It may not accurately predict the number of outpatients that may require HBOT.

Equipment and Installation

The most important decision with regard to equipment is whether to install a multiplace or monoplace chamber. The difference between these two types of chambers has been discussed previously. A new monoplace chamber costs approximately $80,000. Installation costs depend largely on the distance between the proposed facility and the hospital's air and oxygen storage tanks. Based on our experience, the installation of one or two monoplace chambers will cost $50,000 to 75,000 in current dollars.

The cost of a multiplace chamber can vary widely depending on the manufacturer and size and specifications of an individual chamber. A typical chamber suitable for clinical use and large enough to treat eight patients (perhaps 30 to 35 feet long and 8 to 10 feet wide) may cost $400,000 to 500,000. The cost of compressors, plumbing, and installation can bring the total cost to approximately $1.5 million.

A multiplace chamber becomes cost-effective when treating a large number of patients. It may also be preferable to a monoplace chamber for diving-related injuries, unstable critical-care patients, and patients with claustrophobia. Otherwise, most patients can be treated in a monoplace chamber.

In many cases, it may be more logical to start with monoplace chambers. We recommend starting with at least two monoplace chambers. It is extremely difficult to generate much revenue with only one monoplace chamber, and the same number of personnel can manage at least two chambers. It is not difficult to add additional monoplace chambers as the patient census increases. A monoplace chamber can easily be placed in an average-sized emergency department room.

Another approach is to begin with monoplace chambers and to add a multiplace chamber when the patient census increases. Having both types of chambers allows for maximal flexibility. Most patients prefer being treated in a multiplace chamber, but some patients prefer the privacy of a monoplace chamber. We have found the monoplace chamber valuable in treating many emergencies, allowing the routine treatments in a multiplace chamber to proceed without interruption. A single patient who requires emergent treatment after normal working hours (e.g., a stable patient with carbon monoxide poisoning) can be treated just as effectively in a monoplace chamber with less personnel (only one chamber technician will be needed).

Both types of chambers can be located conveniently within or near an emergency department. As most hyperbaric patients are outpatients, this is an ideal setting that allows for cross-coverage by the emergency physician if necessary and cross-training of emergency and hyperbaric personnel.

Most equipment manufacturers will assist with design of the hyperbaric facility (i.e., engineering specifications, floor space, and installation). The facility must conform to federal engineering, fire, and safety standards.[182,183] Most manufacturers will make a site visit and provide architectural drawings.[184,185] In addition to providing adequate space for the chamber(s), additional space should be provided for a small waiting area, dressing/locker rooms, restrooms, and a wound management room.[181, 185]

Many hyperbaric treatment schedules involve daily treatments for several weeks. In many cases, patient compliance may become a problem. We have found it to be cost-effective to purchase and operate a transportation van. We also have an annual contract with a taxicab company to transport ambulatory patients. The cost of providing transportation is more than justified by the resulting increase in compliance.

Personnel

The most vital ingredient of a successful hyperbaric service is a highly motivated and well-trained physician-director (or team of physicians). Successful marketing strategies must involve direct contact with other physicians to generate referrals. The largest group of patients will be those with chronic refractory wounds. Daily vigorous wound management by the hyperbaric physician is often necessary for a successful outcome.

A monoplace facility may require only one chamber technician and a nurse for wound care. A nurse can be trained easily to function as a monoplace hyperbaric technician. National standards now exist for the training of hyperbaric technicians, and the National Board of Diving and Hyperbaric Medical Technology has been granting certification since 1991.[186] Therefore a physician may manage a monoplace facility with one or two nurses (or a nurse and a hyperbaric technician). A secretary will be needed, perhaps on a part-time basis, for a small facility. If additional monoplace chambers are added, the need for additional personnel will increase incrementally.

A multiplace facility, or a service with many monoplace chambers, will need a head nurse/clinical manager, a wound care nurse, and several technicians. Most multiplace chambers require two technicians for optimal chamber operation. Most technicians trained by the military or the offshore oil industry can easily provide maintenance services for the chamber and compressors.

Multiplace treatments also require an inside observer. The observer may be a paramedic or a nurse. Our policies require a registered nurse if the patient requires ventilator support, an intravenous infusion, or cardiac monitoring during the HBOT. Therefore the operation of a multiplace chamber requires significantly more personnel.

The duties of the nurse-manager can include overall supervision of other personnel, scheduling patient treatments and transportation, and coordinating all other aspects of patient care. A capable manager can be a valuable asset to the hyperbaric physician by interfacing with other hospital departments in a positive manner, assisting with marketing, documentation, and quality assurance activities.

Physician Training

At the present time, there are no training programs in hyperbaric medicine that are recognized by the ACGME (Accreditation Council on Graduate Medical Education). The UHMS is currently working with the American Board of Preventive Medicine to sponsor a certification examination.[187] The American College of Hyperbaric Medicine is also developing a process for board certification.

Currently, there is a section of Hyperbaric Medicine in the American College of Emergency Physicians (ACEP). The American Board of Emergency Medicine has explored the possibility of developing a subspecialty examination in hyperbaric medicine, but this is not being pursued at the present time. If hyperbaric medicine were adopted by a primary board, formal training programs with standardized curricula and a certification examination could then be developed.

Several 1- or 2-year research fellowships in hyperbaric medicine are available in the United States. Most of these programs have a clinical component. The Navy and Air Force have comprehensive training programs in hyperbaric medicine. Also, the National Oceanic and Atmospheric Administration (NOAA) has an annual training program in diving medicine, perhaps the most comprehensive program in diving medicine available to civilian physicians in the United States.

The UHMS sponsors several 1-week introductory courses at various locations around the United States. A schedule of upcoming courses can be obtained from the Society. These courses are designed as a basic introduction, not as a means of "licensing" or "certifying" physicians to practice hyperbaric medicine. It may be necessary to recruit a full-time medical director if no one in the emergency physician group has training or experience in hyperbaric medicine.

Marketing

An effective and comprehensive marketing program can often be the determining factor in establishing a successful hyperbaric service. Marketing should be a continuous process. It is logical to begin marketing within the institution, and then on a local and regional level.

The primary marketing audience to target are potential referring physicians. Referrals are most likely to come from general, vascular, and plastic surgeons. Other likely referral sources include maxillofacial surgeons, otolaryngologists, orthopedic surgeons, and radiation oncologists. Providing lectures to the medical staff is a time-honored technique to generate referrals. The most successful marketing tool is to provide a high quality of service to the hospital and to return successfully treated patients to their referring physicians.

Local and regional marketing can also involve direct contact with targeted specialists. A newsletter and direct mailings can also be productive. Regional marketing can involve direct contact with other emergency departments, poison control centers, firefighters, burn units, and wound care centers. Contact with dive shops, dive clubs, or diving contractors can be productive if the hospital is located near an area of significant diving activity.

Billing and Reimbursement

Reimbursement varies widely among regions. Even national programs such as Medicare and Medicaid have regional variations in their payment schedules. It is difficult therefore to provide estimates of third-party reimbursement. It would be prudent to contact local third-party payors to determine potential remuneration for HBOT.

Future calculation of payments by federal programs is a topic of much speculation. In January 1993, the Health Care Financing Administration (HCFA) eliminated physician reimbursement for HBOT. This decision was reversed several months later.[188,189] A change in billing and reimbursement is expected to occur in 1994 for hyperbaric services. Current Procedural Terminology (CPT) code 99183 has been designated as the billing code for HBOT beginning in 1994 (replacing codes 99180 and 99182). CPT defines this code as "physician attendance and supervision of hyperbaric oxygen therapy, per session." Medical services and/or procedures (e.g., wound debridement) provided in conjunction with HBOT should be reported separately.

Even though a limited number of CPT codes are used for hyperbaric services, billing personnel must be carefully selected and trained. Third-party payors often refuse to reimburse for HBOT on initial request, as they are often unfamiliar with hyperbaric medicine. Follow-up letters must often be sent to insurance companies, occasionally by the physician. In most cases, this type of interaction with the insurance companies will have positive results.

The physician must be physically present to bill for services. The hospital usually bills for the technical component (use of the equipment). If the equipment is owned by the physicians, they may bill third-party payors for the technical component, except Medicare and Medicaid. Some physician-owned units have arranged to have the hospital bill Medicare and Medicaid for the technical component, pay a fee to the hospital for billing services, and have the hospital reimburse the rest to the physicians. Another possibility is to rent the chamber to the hospital and allow the hospital to keep whatever collections they receive from the technical component.

In general, collections are much better for outpatients. Third-party payors that use a Diagnostic-Related Group (DRG) method of payment will not provide any additional reimbursement (for the technical component) for inpatients that receive HBOT. Many referring physicians are not aware that HBOT can be arranged on an outpatient basis. It is wise to routinely inform the referring physician of this option and to encourage him or her to discharge the patient when possible. In some cases, patients can be transferred to a skilled nursing facility. Reimbursement by Medicare (for the technical component) is then based on cost and in most regions is usually reimbursed for both inpatients and outpatients.

If a physician group plans to purchase the equipment and lease it to the hospital, a healthcare attorney should review the contract between the group and the hospital to ensure that federal fraud and abuse legislation is not being violated. Representative Pete Stark (D-CA) has sponsored a series of bills designed to discourage "self-referral" of patients. His 1987 bill provided for civil penalties in cases where physicians self-referred Medicare patients (e.g., to their own laboratories, outpatient radiology centers). In 1993, Congress passed the Comprehensive Physician Ownership and Referral Act ("Stark II"). This statute expands the self-referral prohibition to all patients (not just Medicare patients). Any arrangement between hyperbaric physicians and their hospitals must conform to these statutes.

Other Administrative Responsibilities

The Joint Commission on Accreditation of Healthcare Organizations (JCAHO) does not have specific requirements for hyperbaric facilities. However, it would be prudent to maintain a policy and procedure manual, institute a quality assurance/continuous quality improvement (CQI) program, and to conform to general safety guidelines in the hospital. JCAHO generally requires that clinical departments maintain these standards. The policy and procedure manual should include all HBOT treatment schedules, job descriptions, and procedures routinely performed in the hyperbaric department, as well as all equipment that should be routinely available.

CQI is the the mechanism of quality assessment that is currently preferred by the JCAHO. It is a prospective, system-oriented method (as opposed to department-oriented). When a problem is identified, it should be taken through an administrative "loop" that results in resolution. Indicators that may be used include appropriateness of diagnoses and patient selection, appropriateness of diagnostic evaluation, conformity with departmental guidelines, and monitoring of sentinal events (e.g., barotrauma, oxygen toxicity, hypoglycemia, mortality, overuse of HBOT).

SUMMARY

The development of a hyperbaric medicine service can add an exciting dimension to an emergency medicine practice. Emergency physicians are particularly well suited to serve as hyperbaric physicians because of their broad background and immediate availability within the hospital and because most of the current indications for HBOT involve emergent conditions. A hyperbaric service can improve job satisfaction, diversify an emergency medicine practice, augment income, and perhaps help to avoid "burnout" by decreasing stress.

An emergency medicine group that is contemplating establishment of a hyperbaric medicine practice should begin with a feasibility study. Purchasing a monoplace or multiplace chamber is perhaps the most important and fundamental decision to make during the planning phase. Personnel will then have to be recruited and/or trained, including the physicians. An intensive wound management program is necessary for establishing a successful service, as well as an ongoing marketing program. It is also essential to have well-trained and well-motivated billing personnel who are familiar with the unique aspects of reimbursement for hyperbaric services. Such comprehensive preparation will ensure the successful development of a hyperbaric medicine service.

REFERENCES

1. Freudenberger HJ: The ups and downs of emergency medicine, *ACEP News* 9:3-14, 1990.
2. Patten TH: Stress management. In *Comprehensive guide to effective practice management,* Dallas, 1986, American College of Emergency Physicians.
3. Slapper D: Emergency medicine is here to stay. What about emergency physicians? *ACEP News* 10:16-17, 1991.
4. Hamilton RW, Peirce EC, editors: *Hyperbaric oxygen in emergency medical care,* Bethesda, 1983, Undersea Medical Society.
5. Arthur DC, Margulies RA: A short course in diving medicine, *Ann Emerg Med* 16:689-701, 1987.
6. Bove AA, Davis JC, Editors: *Diving medicine,* ed 2, Philadelphia, 1990, WB Saunders.
7. Kizer KW: Diving medicine, *Emerg Med Clin North Am* 2:513-530, 1984.
8. Strauss RH: Diving medicine, *Am Rev Respir Dis* 119:1001-1023, 1979.
9. Fischer B, Jain KK, Braun E et al: *Handbook of hyperbaric medicine,* ed 1, Berlin, 1988, Springer-Verlag.
10. Myers RAM, Baker T, Cowley RA: Hyperbaric medicine: state of the art, *Am Surg* 48:487-494, 1982.
11. Thom SR: Hyperbaric oxygen therapy, *Emerg Med Care* 6:1-8, 1986.
12. Thom SR: Hyperbaric oxygen therapy, *J Intensive Care Med* 4:58-74, 1989.
13. Weiss LD, Van Meter KW: The applications of hyperbaric oxygen therapy in emergency medicine, *Am J Emerg Med* 10:558-568, 1992.
14. Pol B, Wattel JJ: Memoire sur les effets de la compression de l'air, *Ann d'Hyg Pub et de Med Leg* 1:241-249, 1854.
15. US Navy Department, Bureau of Construction and Repair: *Diving manual,* Washington DC, 1924, US Government Printing Office.
16. Van Der Aue OE, White WA, Hayter R et al: Physiological factors underlying the prevention and treatment of decompression sickness, Bethesda, rep no. 1, Project X-443, 1945, Naval Medical Research Institute.
17. Behnke AR et al: The effect of oxygen on man at pressures from one to four atmospheres, *Am J Physiol* 110:565-572, 1935.
18. Behnke AR: Effects of high pressure, prevention and treatment of compressed air sickness, *Med Clin North Am* 26:1213-1226, 1942.
19. Yarbrough OD, Behnke AR: The treatment of compressed air illness utilizing oxygen, *J Indust Hyg Toxicol* 21:213-218, 1939.
20. Goodman MW, Workman RD: *Minimal recompression, oxygen-breathing approach to treatment of decompression sickness in divers and aviators,* Washington DC, Research Report 5-65, 1965, US Navy Experimental Diving Unit.
21. Workman RD: Treatment of bends with oxygen at high pressure, *Aerosp Med* 39:1076-1083, 1968.
22. Boerema I, Meyne NG, Brummelkamp WD et al: Life without blood. *Arch Chir Neerl* 11:70-83, 1959.
23. Brummelkamp WD, Hogendijk J, Boerema I: Treatment of anaerobic infections (clostridial myositis) by drenching the tissues with oxygen under high pressure, *Surgery* 49:299-302, 1961.
24. Hohn DC, Mackay RD, Halliday B et al: The effect of O_2 tension on the microbicidal function of leukocytes in wounds and in vitro, *Surg Forum* 27:18-20, 1976.
25. Hunt TK, Linsey M, Grislis G et al: The effect of differing ambient oxygen tensions on wound infection, *Ann Surg* 181:35-39, 1975.
26. Knighton DR, Halliday B, Hunt TK: Oxygen as an antibiotic: a comparison of inspired oxygen concentration and antibiotic administration on in vivo bacterial clearance, *Arch Surg* 121:191-195, 1986.
27. Knighton DR, Halliday, Hunt TK: Oxygen as an antibiotic: the effect of inspired oxygen on infection, *Arch Surg* 119:199-204, 1984.
28. Hunt TK, Pai MP: The effect of varying ambient oxygen tensions on wound metabolism and collagen synthesis, *Surg Gynecol Obstet* 135:561-567, 1972.
29. Hunt TK, Zederfeldt BH, Goldstick TK: Oxygen and healing, *Am J Surg* 118:521-525, 1969.
30. Ketchum SA, Thomas AN, Hall AD: Angiographic studies of the effects of hyperbaric oxygen on burn wound revascularization. In *Proceedings of the Fourth International Congress on Hyperbaric Medicine,* Tokyo, 1970, Igaku Shoin.
31. Klebanoff S: Oxygen metabolism and the toxic properties of phagocytes, *Ann Intern Med* 93:480-489, 1980.
32. Mandell G: Bactericidal activity of aerobic and anaerobic polymorphonuclear neutrophils, *Infect Immun* 9:337-341, 1974.
33. Chvapil M, Hurych J, Mirejovska E: Effect of long-term hypoxia on protein synthesis in granuloma and some organs in rats, *Proc Soc Exp Biol Med* 135:613-616, 1966.
34. Juva K, Prockop DJ, Cooper GW et al: Hydroxylation of proline and the intracellular accumulation of a polypeptide precursor of collagen, *Science* 152:92-96, 1966.
35. Nylander G et al: Reduction of post-ischemic edema with hyperbaric oxygen, *Plast Reconstr Surg* 76:596-603, 1985.
36. Strauss MB, Hargens AR, Gershuni DH et al: Reduction of skeletal muscle necrosis using intermittent hyperbaric oxygen in a model compartment syndrome. *J Bone Joint Surg* 65A:656-662, 1983.
37. Ball EG, Strittmatter CF, Cooper O: The reaction of cytochrome oxidase with carbon monoxide, *J Biol Chem* 193:635-647, 1951.
38. Britten JS, Myers RAM: Effects of hyperbaric oxygen on carbon monoxide elimination in humans, *Undersea Biomed Res* 12:431-437, 1985.
39. Young LJ, Caughey WS: Oxygenation of carbon monoxide by bovine heart cytochrome c oxidase, *Biochemistry* 25:152-161, 1986.

40. Thom SR: Antagonism of carbon monoxide-mediated brain lipid peroxidation by hyperbaric oxygen, *Toxicol Appl Pharmacol* 105:340-344, 1990.
41. Thom SR, Elbuken ME: Oxygen-dependent antagonism of lipid peroxidation, *Free Radic Biol Med* 10:413-426, 1991.
42. DeMello FJ, Hasimoto T, Hitchcock CR et al: The effect of hyperbaric oxygen on the germination and toxin production of *Clostridium perfringens* spores. In *Proceedings of the Fourth International Congress on Hyperbaric Medicine,* Tokyo, 1970, Igaku Shoin.
43. Hill GB, Osterhaut S: Experimental effects of hyperbaric oxygen on selected clostridial species. I. In-vitro studies, *J Infect Dis* 125:17-25, 1972.
44. MacLennan JD: The histotoxic clostridial infections of man, *Bacteriol Rev* 26:177-276, 1962.
45. Van Unnik AJM: Inhibition of toxin production in *Clostridium perfringens* in-vitro by hyperbaric oxygen, *Antonie Van Leeuwenhoek* 31:181-186, 1965.
46. Cope C: The importance of oxygen in the treatment of cyanide poisoning, *JAMA* 175:1061-1064, 1961.
47. Isom GE, Way JL: Effect of oxygen on cyanide intoxication: reactivation of cyanide inhibited glucose metabolism, *J Pharmacol Exp Ther* 189:235-243, 1974.
48. Ivanov KP: The effect of elevated oxygen pressure on animals poisoned with potassium cyanide, *Pharmacol Toxicol* 22:476-479, 1959.
49. Skene WG, Norman JN, Smith G: Effect of hyperbaric oxygen in cyanide poisoning. In Brown IW, Cox B, editors: *Proceedings of the Third International Congress on Hyperbaric Medicine,* Washington DC, 1966, National Academy of Sciences, National Research Council.
50. Takano T, Miyazaki Y, Nashimoto I et al: Effect of hyperbaric oxygen on cyanide intoxication: in situ changes in intracellular oxidation reduction, *Undersea Biomed Res* 7:191-197, 1980.
51. Ravizza AG, Caruga D, Cerchiari EL et al: The treatment of hydrogen sulfide intoxication: oxygen vs nitrites, *Vet Hum Toxicol* 24:241-242, 1982.
52. Bernacchi A, Myers R, Trump BF et al: Protection of hepatocytes with hyperoxia against carbon tetrachloride-induced injury, *Toxicol Pathol* 12:315-323, 1984.
53. Merolla L, Bimonte D, Cacciator L et al: Observations of the influence of hyperbaric oxygenation in acute poisoning of the rat by carbon tetrachloride, *Boll Soc Ital Biol Sper* 43:1760-1762, 1967.
54. Mader JT, Brown GL, Guckian JC et al: A mechanism for the amelioration by hyperbaric oxygen of experimental staphylococcal osteomyelitis in rabbits, *J Infect Dis* 142:915-922, 1980.
55. Hill GB: Hyperbaric oxygen exposure for intrahepatic abscesses produced in mice by non-spore-forming anaerobic bacteria, *Antimicrob Agents Chemother* 9:312-317, 1976.
56. Nowicki S, Parks M, Mader JT: Bactericidal activity of aerobic and anaerobic leukocytes against *Bacteroides fragilis* (abstr), *Undersea Biomed Res* 18(suppl):82, 1991.
57. Schreiner A, Tonjum S, Digranes A: Hyperbaric oxygen therapy in *Bacteriodes* infections, *Acta Chir Scand* 140:73-76, 1974.
58. Wallyn RJ, Gumbiner SH, Goldfein S et al: Treatment of anaerobic infections with hyperbaric oxygen, *Surg Clin North Am* 44:107-112, 1964.
59. Adams KR, Sutton TE, Mader JT: Aminoglycoside potentiation with adjunctive hyperbaric oxygen therapy in experimental *Ps. aeruginosa* osteomyelitis (abstr), *Undersea Biomed Res* 14(supp):37-38, 1987.
60. Haft JR, Cleary TJ: The potentiation of the aminoglycoside tobramycin by hyperbaric oxygen therapy in an animal model of chronic *Pseudomonas aeruginosa* pneumonia (abstr), *Undersea Biomed Res* 18(suppl):40, 1991.
61. Norden CW, Kleti E: Experimental osteomyelitis caused by *Pseudomonas aeruginosa, J Infect Dis* 141:71-75, 1980.
62. Keck PE, Gottleib SF, Conley J: Interaction of increased pressures of oxygen and sulfonamides on the in vitro and in vivo growth of pathogenic bacteria, *Undersea Biomed Res* 7:95-106, 1980.
63. Park MK, Muhvich KH, Myers RAM et al: Hyperoxic enhancement of the aminoglycoside-induced postantibiotic effect in *Pseudomonas aeruginosa, Undersea Biomed Res* 18(suppl):42, 1991.
64. Davis JC: Hyperbaric oxygen therapy, *J Intensive Care Med* 4:55-57, 1989.
65. Youn BA, Gordon D, Moran C et al: Fire in the multiplace hyperbaric chamber, *J Hyperbaric Med* 4:63-67, 1989.
66. *U.S. Navy diver's handbook,* San Pedro CA, 1993, Best Publishing Co.
67. Rusca F, Ambrosio F, Garetto G et al: Lack of modifications in pulmonary function tests after HBO therapeutic expositions (abstr), *Undersea Biomed Res* 16(supp):33-34, 1989.
68. Rusca F, Garetto G, Ambrosio F et al: HBO therapy and pulmonary function tests, *Undersea Biomed Res* 18(supp):112, 1991.
69. Palmquist BM, Phillipson B, Barr PO: Nuclear cataract and myopia during hyperbaric therapy, *Br J Ophthalmol* 68:113-117, 1984.
70. Anderson B, Farmer JC: Hyperoxic myopia, *Trans Am Ophthalmol Soc* 76:116-124, 1978.
71. Lynn AJ: Ocular effects of hyperbaric oxygen therapy, *Trans Ophthalmol Soc UK* 98:66-68, 1978.
72. Bieri JG, Corash L, Hubbard VS: Medical uses of vitamin E, *N Engl J Med* 308:1063-1069, 1983.
73. Levine M: New concepts in the biology and biochemistry of ascorbic acid, *N Engl J Med* 314:892-901, 1986.
74. North LN, Mathias MM, Schatte CL: Effect of dietary vitamin E or selenium on prostaglandin dehydrogenase in hyperoxic rat lung, *Aviat Space Environ Med* 55:617-619, 1984.
75. Roberts JH: Perspective on vitamin E as therapy, *JAMA* 246:129-131, 1981.
76. Nichols CW, Lambertsen CJ, Clark JM: Transient unilateral loss of vision associated with oxygen at high pressure, *Arch Ophthalmol* 81:548-552, 1969.
77. Molzhaninov YV, Chayka VK, Domanova AI et al: Experience and prospects of using hyperbaric oxygenation in obstetrical practice. In *Proceedings of the Seventh International Congress on Hyperbaric Medicine,* vol I, Moscow, 1983, Nauka Public.
78. Pobedinskiy NM, Proshina IV, Fanchenko NO et al: Application of hyperbaric oxygenation in certain disruptions of the reproductive functions in women. In *Proceedings of the Seventh International Congress on Hyperbaric Medicine,* vol I, Moscow, 1983, Nauka Public.
79. Vanina LV, Yefuni SN, Beylin AL et al: Obstetric aid under conditions of hyperbaric oxygenation. In *Proceedings of the Seventh International Congress on Hyperbaric Medicine,* vol I, 1983, Nauka Public.
80. Van Hoesen KB, Camporesi EM, Moon RE et al: Should hyperbaric oxygen be used to treat the pregnant patient for acute carbon monoxide poisoning? *JAMA* 261:1039-1043, 1989.
81. Beckman DL, Crittenden DJ, Overton DH, et al: Influence of blood glucose on convulsive seizures from hyperbaric oxygen, *Life Sci* 31:45-49, 1982.
82. Springer R: The importance of glucometer testing of diabetic patients pre and post dive (abstr), *Undersea Biomed Res* 18(suppl):20, 1991.
83. Thom SR, editor: *Hyperbaric oxygen therapy: a committee report,* Bethesda, 1992, Undersea and Hyperbaric Medical Society.
84. Waite CL, Mazzone WF: *Cerebral air embolism. 1. Basic studies,* Washington DC, Research Report 493, 1967, US Navy.
85. Fischer B, Jain KK, Braun E, editors: *Handbook of hyperbaric medicine,* ed 1, Berlin, 1988, Springer-Verlag.
86. Bray P, Myers RAM, Cowley RA: Orogenital sex as a case of nonfatal air embolism during pregnancy, *Obstet Gynecol* 61:653-657, 1983.
87. Halpern P, Greenstein A, Melamed Y et al: Arterial air embolism after penetrating lung injury, *Crit Care Med* 11:392-393, 1983.
88. Ponn RB, Zatarain G, Gerzberg L et al: Systemic air embolism in experimental penetrating lung injuries, *J Thorac Cardiovasc Surg* 74:766-773, 1977.
89. Thomas AN, Stephens BG: Air embolism: a cause of morbidity and death after penetrating chest trauma, *J Trauma* 14:633-638, 1974.
90. Pace N, Strajman E, Walker EL: Acceleration of carbon monoxide elimination in man by high pressure oxygen, *Science* 111:652-654, 1950.
91. Sasaki T: On half-clearance time of CO-hemoglobin in blood during hyperbaric oxygen therapy, *Bull Tokyo Med Dent Univ* 22:63-77, 1975.
92. Thom SR: Carbon monoxide-mediated brain lipid peroxidation in the rat, *J Appl Physiol* 63:997-1003, 1990.

93. Beard RR, Grandstaff N: Carbon monoxide exposure and cerebral function, *Ann NY Acad Sci* 174:385-395, 1970.
94. Myers RAM, Messier LD: The development of a neuropsychological screening battery for use in the clinical assessment of carbon monoxide-intoxicated patients. In *Proceedings of the Eighth International Congress on Hyperbaric Medicine,* Bethesda, 1984, Undersea Medical Society.
95. Myers RAM, Messier LD, Jones DW et al: New directions in the research and treatment of carbon monoxide exposure, *Am J Emerg Med* 2:226-230, 1983.
96. Smith JS, Brandon S: Morbidity from acute carbon monoxide poisoning at three-year follow-up, *Br Med J* 1:318-321, 1973.
97. Choi IS: Delayed neurologic sequelae in carbon monoxide poisoning, *Arch Neurol* 40:433-435, 1983.
98. Norkool DM, Kirkpatrick JN: Treatment of acute carbon monoxide poisoning with hyperbaric oxygen therapy: a review of 115 cases, *Ann Emerg Med* 14:1168-1171, 1985.
99. Myers RAM, Snyder SK, Emhoff TA: Subacute sequelae of carbon monoxide poisoning, *Ann Emerg Med* 14:1163-1167, 1985.
100. Folstein MF, Folstein SE, McHugh PR: Mini-mental state: a practical method for grading the cognitive state of patients for the clinician, *J Psychiatr Res* 12:189-198, 1975.
101. Zun L, Howes DS: The mental status evaluation: application in the emergency department, *Am J Emerg Med* 6:165-172, 1988.
102. Koyama K: Acute experimental carbon monoxide poisoning and hyperbaric oxygenation, *Tokyo Jikeikai Med J* 91:195-215, 1976.
103. Ogawa M, Shimazaki S, Tanaka N et al: Blood volume changes in experimental carbon monoxide poisoning. *Ind Health* 12:121-125, 1974.
104. Sukoff MH, Hollin SA, Jacobson JH: The protective effect of hyperbaric oxygenation in experimentally produced cerebral edema and compression, *Surgery* 62:40-46, 1967.
105. Goulon M, Barios A, Rapin M et al: Carbon monoxide poisoning and acute anoxia due to breathing coal gas and hydrocarbons (english translation), *J Hyperbaric Med* 1:23-41, 1986.
106. Gozal D, Ziser A, Shupak A et al: Accidental carbon monoxide poisoning: emphasis on hyperbaric oxygen treatment, *Clin Pediatr* 24:132-135, 1985.
107. Mathieu D, Nolf M, Durocher A et al: Acute carbon monoxide poisoning: risk of late sequelae and treatment by hyperbaric oxygen, *Clin Toxicol* 23:315-324, 1985.
108. Myers RAM et al: Value of hyperbaric oxygen in suspected carbon monoxide poisoning, *JAMA* 246:2478-2480, 1981.
109. Onji Y, Sugimoto T, Ogawa M et al: Clinical study on carbon monoxide poisoning with special reference to hyperbaric oxygen. In *Proceedings of the Fifth International Hyperbaric Congress,* Burnaby, Canada, 1976, Simon Fraser University.
110. Smith GI, Sharp GR: Treatment of carbon monoxide poisoning with oxygen under pressure, *Lancet* 2:905-906, 1960.
111. Yee LM, Brandon GK: Successful reversal of presumed carbon monoxide-induced semicoma, *Aviat Space Environ Med* 54:641-643, 1983.
112. Ziser A, Shupak A, Halpern P et al: Delayed hyperbaric oxygen treatment for acute carbon monoxide poisoning, *Br Med J* 1:289, 1984.
113. Raphael JC, Elkharrat D, Jars-Guincestre MC et al: Trial of normobaric and hyperbaric oxygen for acute carbon monoxide intoxication, *Lancet* 1:414-419, 1989.
114. Thom SR, Taber RL, Mendguren I, et al: Delayed neuropsychiatric sequelae following CO poisoning and the role of treatment with 100% O_2 or hyperbaric oxygen: a prospective, randomized, clinical study (abstr), *Undersea Biomed Res* 19:47(Suppl), 1992.
115. Clark CJ, Campbell D, Reid WH: Blood carboxyhaemoglobin and cyanide levels in fire survivors, *Lancet* 1:1332-1335, 1981.
116. Wetherell HR: The occurrence of cyanide in the blood of fire victims, *J Forensic Sci* 11:167-173, 1966.
117. Norris JC, Moore SJ, Hume AS: Synergistic lethality induced by the combination of carbon monoxide and cyanide, *Toxicology* 40:121-129, 1986.
118. DeMello FJ, Haglin JJ, Hitchcock CR: Comparative study of experimental *Clostridium perfringens* infection in dogs treated with antibiotics, surgery, and hyperbaric oxygen, *Surgery* 73:936-941, 1973.
119. McLeod JW: Variations in the periods of exposure to air and oxygen necessary to kill anaerobic bacteria, *Acta Pathol Microbiol Scand* 3(suppl):255, 1930.
120. Kivisaari J, Niinikoski J: Use of Silastic tube and capillary sampling technique in the measurement of tissue pO_2 and pCO_2, *Am J Surg* 125:623-627, 1973.
121. Brummelkamp WH: Considerations on hyperbaric oxygen therapy at three atmospheres absolute for clostridial infections type *welchii, Ann NY Acad Sci* 117:688-699, 1965.
122. Du Toit DF, Pretorius CF, Esterhuizen N et al: Gasgangreen, *S Afr Med J* 68:760-762, 1985.
123. Guidi ML, Proletti R, Carducci P, et al: The combined use of hyperbaric oxygen, antibiotics and surgery in the treatment of gas gangrene, *Resuscitation* 9:267-273, 1981.
124. Hart GB, Lamb RC, Strauss MB: Gas gangrene. II. A 15-year experience with hyperbaric oxygen, *J Trauma* 23:995-1000, 1983.
125. Hitchcock CR, Demello FJ, Haglin JJ: Gangrene infection: new approaches to an old disease, *Surg Clin North Am* 55:1403-1410, 1975.
126. Schweigel JF, Shim SS: A comparison of the treatment of gas gangrene with and without hyperbaric oxygen, *Surg Gynecol Obstet* 136:969-970, 1973.
127. Shupak A, Halpern P, Ziser A et al: Hyperbaric oxygen therapy for gas gangrene casualties in the Lebanon war, *Israel J Med Sci* 20:323-326, 1984.
128. Unsworth IP, Sharp PA: Gas gangrene. An 11-year review of 73 cases managed with hyperbaric oxygen, *Med J Aust* 140:256-259, 1984.
129. Bakker DJ: Pure and mixed aerobic and anaerobic soft tissue infections, *Hyperbaric Oxygen Rev* 6:65-95, 1985.
130. Gozal D, Ziser A, Shupak A et al: Necrotizing fasciitis, *Arch Surg* 121:233-235, 1986.
131. Radaelli F, DellaVolpe A, Colombi M et al: Acute gangrene of the scrotum and penis in four hematologic patients, *Cancer* 60:1462-1464, 1987.
132. Riegels-Nielsen P, Hesselfeldt-Nielsen J, Bang-Jensen E et al: Fournier's gangrene: five patients treated with hyperbaric oxygen, *J Urol* 132:918-920, 1984.
133. Zanetti CL: Necrotizing soft tissue infection and adjunctive hyperbaric oxygen, *Chest* 92:670-671, 1988.
134. Ziser A, Girsh Z, Gozal D et al: Hyperbaric oxygen therapy for Fournier's gangrene, *Crit Care Med* 13:773-774, 1985.
135. Bird AD, Telfer ABM: Effect of hyperbaric oxygen on limb circulation, *Lancet* 1:355-356, 1965.
136. Attar S, Esmond WG, Cowley RA: Hyperbaric oxygen in vascular collapse, *J Thorac Cardiovasc Surg* 44:759-770, 1962.
137. Blair E, Henning G, Esmond WG et al: The effect of hyperbaric oxygenation on three forms of shock: traumatic, hemorrhagic and septic, *J Trauma* 4:652-663, 1964.
138. Elliot DP, Paton BC: Effect of 100% oxygen at one and three atmospheres on dogs subjected to hemorrhagic hypotension, *Surgery* 57:401-408, 1965.
139. Ledingham IM: Hyperbaric oxygen in shock, *Int Anesthesiol Clin* 7:819-839, 1969.
140. Navarro RU, Ferguson CC: Treatment of experimental shock by the combined use of hyperbaric oxygen and low molecular weight dextran, *Surgery* 63:775-781, 1968.
141. Amonic RS, Cockett ATK, Thompson JC et al: Hyperbaric oxygen therapy in chronic hemorrhagic shock, *JAMA* 208:2051-2054, 1969.
142. Hart GB: Exceptional blood loss anemia: treatment with hyperbaric oxygen, *JAMA* 228:1028-1029, 1974.
143. Hart GB, Lennon PA, Strauss MB: Hyperbaric oxygen in exceptional acute blood-loss anemia, *J Hyperbaric Med* 2:205-210, 1987.
144. Myking O, Schreiner A: Hyperbaric oxygen in hemolytic crisis, *JAMA* 227:1161-1162, 1974.
145. Kethchum SA, Zubrin JR, Thomas AN et al: Effect of hyperbaric oxygen on small first, second and third degree burns, *Surg Forum* 18:65-67, 1967.
146. Korn HN, Wheeler ES, Miller TA: Effect of hyperbaric oxygen on second-degree burn wound healing, *Arch Surg* 112:732-737, 1977.

147. Nylander G, Nordstrom H, Eriksson E: Effects of hyperbaric oxygen on oedema formation after a scald burn, *Burns Incl Therm Inj* 10:193-196, 1984.
148. Wells CH, Hilton JG: Effects of hyperbaric oxygen on post-burn plasma extravasation. In Davis JC, Hunt TK, editors: *Hyperbaric oxygen therapy,* Bethesda, 1977, Undersea Medical Society.
149. Hart GB, O'Reilly RR, Broussard ND et al: Treatment of burns with hyperbaric oxygen, *Surg Obstet Gynecol* 139:693-696, 1974.
150. Merola L, Piscatelli F: Considerazioni e prospettive sull'impiego dell'ossigeno ad aumentata pressione nel trattamento della malattia da ustione, *Ann Med Nav (Roma)* 83:515-526, 1978.
151. Perrins DJD: Influence of hyperbaric oxygen on the survival of split skin grafts, *Lancet* 1:868-871, 1967.
152. Marx RE, Johnson RP, Kline SN: Prevention of osteoradionecrosis: a randomized prospective clinical trial of hyperbaric oxygen versus penicillin, *J Am Dent Assoc* 111:49-54, 1985.
153. Baroni G, Porro T, Faglia E, et al: Hyperbaric oxygen in diabetic gangrene treatment, *Diabetes Care* 10:81-86, 1987.
154. Maroko PR, Radvany P, Braunwald E et al: Reduction of infarct size by oxygen inhalation following acute coronary occlusion, *Circulation* 52:360-368, 1975.
155. Thomas MP, Brown LA, Sponseller DR et al: Myocardial infarct size reduction by the synergistic effect of hyperbaric oxygen and recombinant tissue plasminogen activator, *Am Heart J* 120:791-800, 1990.
156. Hart GB, Shandling AH, Ellestad MH: Hyperbaric oxygen (HBO) and thrombolysis in myocardial infarction: a preliminary report (abstr), *Undersea Biomed Res* 17(suppl):65, 1990.
157. Messina V, Hart GB: Clinical experience in an HBO/t-PA myocardial infarction study (abstr), *Undersea Biomed Res* 17(suppl):103-104, 1990.
158. Van Meter K, Gottleib SF, Whidden SJ: Hyperbaric oxygen as an adjunct in ACLS on guinea pigs after 15 minutes of cardiopulmonary arrest (abstr), *Undersea Biomed Res* 15(suppl):55, 1988.
159. Kugel HL, Neubauer RA, Gottlieb SF: Hyperbaric oxygen therapy in unstable angina (abstr), *Undersea Biomed Res* 18(suppl):104, 1991.
160. Fischer BH, Marks M, Reich T: Hyperbaric oxygen treatment of multiple sclerosis: a randomized, placebo-controlled, double-blind study, *N Engl J Med* 308:181-186, 1983.
161. Barnes MP, Bates D, Cartlidge NEF et al: Hyperbaric oxygen and multiple sclerosis: short-term results of a placebo-controlled, double-blind trial, *Lancet* 1:297-300, 1985.
162. Harpur GD, Suke R, Bass BH et al: Hyperbaric oxygen therapy in chronic stable multiple sclerosis: double-blind study, *Neurology* 36:988-991, 1986.
163. Jain KK: Effect of hyperbaric oxygenation on spasticity in stroke patients, *J Hyperbaric Med* 4:55-61, 1989.
164. Marano P, Pallotta R, Longobardi P et al: Use of TRH-T during HBO and physiotherapy treatments of stroke (abstr), *Undersea Biomed Res* 18(suppl):34-35, 1991.
165. Marroni A: Hyperbaric oxygen and in-water rehabilitation in complete stroke, *J Hyperbaric Med* 3:15-23, 1988.
166. Nagayoshi I, Kawashima M, Tamura H et al: The effect of hyperbaric oxygen therapy for cerebral embolism (abstr), *Undersea Biomed Res* 18(suppl):35, 1991.
167. Neubauer RA, End E: Hyperbaric oxygenation as an adjunct therapy in strokes due to thrombosis, *Stroke* 11:297-300, 1980.
168. Reitan JA, Kien NG, Thorup S et al: Hyperbaric oxygen increases survival following carotid ligation in gerbils, *Stroke* 21:119-123, 1990.
169. Ohta H, Hadeisha H, Nemoto M et al: Transient effect of hyperbaric oxygen on cerebral blood flow and intracranial pressure, *J Hyperbaric Med* 5:3-13, 1990.
170. Kawamura S, Ohta H, Yasui N, et al: Effects of hyperbaric oxygenation in patients with subarachnoid hemorrhage, *J Hyperbaric Med* 3:243-256, 1988.
171. Thom SR: Hyperbaric oxygen therapy in septicemia, *J Hyperbaric Med* 2:141-146, 1987.
172. Fife WP, Fife CE: Treatment of migraine with hyperbaric oxygen, *J Hyperbaric Med* 4:7-15, 1989.
173. Weiss LD, Ramasastry SS, Eidelman BH: Treatment of a cluster headache patient in a hyperbaric chamber, *Headache* 29:109-110, 1989.
174. Gamache FW, Myers RAM, Ducker TB et al: The clinical application of hyperbaric oxygen therapy in spinal cord injury; a preliminary report, *Surg Neurol* 15:85-87, 1981.
175. Sukoff MH, Ragatz RE: Hyperbaric oxygenation for the treatment of acute cerebral edema, *Neurosurgery* 10:29-38, 1982.
176. Zamboni WA, Brown R, Roth AC et al: Effect of hyperbaric oxygen on peripheral nerve regeneration (abstr), *Undersea Biomed Res* 18(suppl):43, 1991.
177. Hoidal CR, Hall AH, Robinson MD et al: Hydrogen sulfide poisoning from toxic inhalations of roofing asphalt fumes, *Ann Emerg Med* 15:826-830, 1986.
178. Hsu P, Li HW, Lin YT: Acute hydrogen sulfide poisoning treated with hyperbaric oxygen, *J Hyperbaric Med* 2:215-221, 1987.
179. Smilkstein MJ, Bronstein AC, Manning Picket H et al: Hyperbaric oxygen therapy for severe hydrogen sulfide poisoning, *J Emerg Med* 3:27-30, 1985.
180. Whitcraft DD, Bailey TD, Hart GB: Hydrogen sulfide poisoning treated with hyperbaric oxygen, *J Emerg Med* 3:23-25, 1985.
181. Rockswold GL, Ford SE, Anderson DC et al: Results of a prospective randomized trial for treatment of severely brain-injured patients with hyperbaric oxygen, *J Neurosurg* 76:929-934, 1992.
182. Workman WT, Robinette MD, Laird TD et al. Medical planning criteria for implementation of clinical hyperbaric facilities, Brooks AFB, Texas, 1984, USAF School of Aerospace Medicine.
183. Monoplace chamber safety guidelines published, *Pressure* (UHMS newsletter) 20(6):1-3, 1991.
184. National fire codes, vol 5, Section 99, pp 123-132, Quincy MA, 1990, National Fire Protection Association.
185. *Introduction to hyperbaric oxygen therapy,* Chula Vista, CA, 1983, Hyperbaric Oxygen Therapy Systems.
186. *Technical instructions and installation requirements,* Anaheim, CA, 1985, Sechrist Industries.
187. *Board certification in hyperbaric technology,* New Orleans, 1991, National Board of Diving and Hyperbaric Medical Technology.
188. Certification examination may become reality by '92, *Pressure* 20(1):1, 1991.
189. College wins major victory on medicare fees. *Hyperbaric Horizons* (Amer Coll of Hyperbaric Med newsletter) 1(1):1-4, 1993.
190. Cianci P: HCFA rescinds action on HBO, *Pressure* 21(3):1, 1992.

91 Practice Diversification in Emergency Nursing

Mark B. Parshall

OUTLINE

Scope of emergency nursing practice
Verification programs
Advanced cardiac life support and pediatric advanced life support
Trauma nursing core course and emergency nursing pediatric course
Course in advanced trauma nursing
Certification programs
Department issues
Diversified roles
Competency based roles
Other competency based roles
Poison information specialist
Forensic Nursing
Advanced practice roles
Emergency nurse practitioner
Clinical nurse specialist
Future Directions

To the uninitiated, the variety of titles related to nursing education and licensure, specialty credentials, and skills verification is often perplexing. Unlike medicine, basic nursing education consists of multiple pathways. Nurses have no requirement for residency or board-certification before employment in virtually any setting. Basic nursing education and licensure are intended to produce and validate nurses who are competent for basic, safe, entry-level nursing practice. Most basic nursing curricula do not provide more than superficial exposure to specialty practice. Nevertheless, the American Nurses Association (ANA) acknowledges "that most nursing practice is general nursing in a specialized area, having a specialized population or focus."[1] Orientation to a particular clinical area and subsequent on-the-job training remain the norm, within nursing, for entry into more specialized practice. Consequently, when one hears a nurse say, "I'm an emergency nurse," the statement lacks context. How experienced is this nurse? How does one judge whether this nurse possesses sufficient breadth and depth of knowledge to back up such a claim?

To understand the diversification of emergency nursing practice, considerable attention must first be devoted to defining the generalist emergency nurse—the most significant role, in terms of the number of nurses and of patients served in emergency nursing practice. Adequate evidence of a sound foundation in generalist emergency nursing practice must be established before branching out into diversified emergency nursing roles. A combination of experience, course-completion verifications, and specialty certification constitutes the ideal base for identifying the generalist emergency nurse.[2]

Role diversification arises from this generalist base in response to identified special needs of discrete populations or settings, to changes in knowledge or technology, or by virtue of focused interest—or the recognition of new opportunities—by nurses in the specialty. Diversification is spontaneous and relatively unregulated. Diversified roles tend to be locally or regionally defined, and practice boundaries are mutable. It is not possible to create an exhaustive catalog of diversified emergency nursing roles. Rather, we shall examine various stages of diversification and specialization in the hope that innovative practice ideas will be recognized, supported, and nurtured.

"Specialization means a narrowed focus on a part of the whole field of nursing."[1] Typically, specialization occurs over time as sufficient numbers of nurses whose practice has diversified in congruent directions identify a core domain with discrete boundaries and practice standards. Hallmarks of a mature specialty include a national specialty organization, nationally based practice standards, a certification program, focused research, specialty publications, and graduate nursing programs in the specialty.[3] As with medicine, nursing has become so complex and diverse, the boards of nursing cannot have sufficient expertise to judge qualifications in all specialty areas. Nor do the ANA, specialty nursing organizations, or graduate faculties create specialties. Rather, these groups codify, standardize, certify, and teach nursing content that has developed a sufficient base in clinical practice.[1]

Styles[3] described a decades-long process of restructuring nursing along vertical and horizontal axes. The vertical axis corresponds to the multiple tiers of licensure and of educational preparation. The horizontal axis corresponds to the formation of specialties and subspecialties in nursing. The largest specialty groups originally developed along lines suggested by the structure of hospitals, nursing homes, and the public health sector. Increasingly, nurses identify areas of need and create the structures and roles to address them.

All specialties also have dimensions of setting, population, and experience by which they are defined. Setting includes elements of the place, intent, and scope of the services rendered. Populations may be based in a specific body system or disease process, developmental stage, gender, or other defining characteristic(s).[4] Experience refers to the qualifications of a given nurse with respect to a particular type of setting or population. By way of example, Benner observes that an experienced, masters-prepared clinical specialist in adult critical care might well initially function at a novice level in a neonatal intensive care unit.[5]

One third of nursing's "social contract" is devoted to specialization. According to the ANA Social Policy Statement,[1] specialization arises in five main ways:

- The amount and complexity of knowledge and technology create a demand for a few professionals to give special attention to applications in delimited practice areas.
- A few . . . pioneers seek to obtain greater depth of understanding of phenomena related to a segment of nursing and to test new practices. . . .
- Public attention and available funds become focused on an area of practice in which heretofore there has been a lack of interest, knowledge, and skilled practitioners.
- The complexity of services exceeds . . . prevailing knowledge and skills of general practitioners, and . . . is approached by intense personal studies or post-basic study by a few interested professionals.
- Part of a professional field expands, and . . . some of its members seek ways for expanded use of their intellectual and other capacities.[1]

Diversification of clinical practice from a generalist base is the first step in developing a critical mass of practitioners and practice-based knowledge.

SCOPE OF EMERGENCY NURSING PRACTICE

Emergency nursing is practiced in multiple settings: prehospital systems, emergency departments, free-standing urgent care facilities, ambulatory clinics, military, occupational, educational, and correctional settings. The intent of services is provision of nursing care to persons with "perceived actual or potential sudden or urgent physical or psychosocial problems that are primarily episodic or acute. . . ."[4] The scope of these services ranges from preventive to immediate, life- and limb-saving measures. Rather than being based in a specific population defined by age, body system, disease, etc., the population in which emergency nursing is based is defined by the perception by a patient or others of a situation that requires immediate care. Emergency nurses must have sufficient experience and education to enable them to triage, prioritize, stabilize, resuscitate, and perform all phases of the nursing process with patients of all ages and underlying conditions, often with a limited, or unreliable database. They must be able to prepare for and intervene in disasters and other unpredictable situations, where resources may be severely limited relative to demand for services.[4]

Obviously, such experience must be acquired over a considerable period of time. Various means have been contrived to validate skills and performance in regard to populations that are significant in terms of patient volume (e.g., pediatrics) or degree of inherent risk (e.g., cardiac arrest). Typically, such validation occurs by means of local or regional credentialling (e.g., mobile intensive care nurse) or nationally developed and marketed verification programs such as Advanced Cardiac Life Support (ACLS), Pediatric Advanced Life Support (PALS), Trauma Nursing Core Course (TNCC), and Emergency Nursing Pediatric Course (ENPC). Validation of a sufficient knowledge base for competence across the breadth of emergency nursing, or related specialties, is obtained through national certification programs.

VERIFICATION PROGRAMS

Advanced Cardiac Life Support and Pediatric Advanced Life Support

The most established skills verification program relevant to emergency nursing is the ACLS course of the American Heart Association (AHA). In some jurisdictions, this course is mandated by statute or regulation for prehospital and hospital-based emergency care providers. In other locales, it is mandated by institutional policy.

Over the years, the content has undergone considerable refinement and modification. What originally were termed *Standards* have, since 1980, been termed *Guidelines*.[6] The AHA explicitly disclaims any intent to "certify" the competence of individuals. Rather, it conducts the meetings from which the recommendations are generated, publishes and promulgates the guidelines, and, through its affiliates, trains faculty, administers and markets the course, and verifies course completion. The AHA takes the position that certification of clinical competency is the responsibility of "licensing agencies, . . . specialty boards, hospitals, health departments, and EMS authorities."[6]

Despite explicit disclaimers that treatment algorithms have been developed for instructional purposes only, the *Guidelines for Cardiopulmonary Resuscitation and Emergency Cardiac Care* is the yardstick by which, from both a medical and legal standpoint, adherence to standards of practice is likely to be judged. In terms of any type of emergency nursing practice, this content is so essential with regard to the frequency of and degree of risk inherent in resuscitations that "course completion" (provider) status is indispensable. Course completion is considered desirable, as well, for those involved in the management, administration, regulation, or evaluation of emergency services.[6] Experienced emergency nurses often become ACLS instructors as one means of demonstrating clinical leadership.

Early versions of the guidelines did not adequately address guidelines for the resuscitation of neonates, infants, and children. Since 1983, guidelines for and courses in neonatal resuscitation, and pediatric basic life support (BLS) and advanced life support (ALS) have been developed under the joint auspices of the AHA and the American Academy of Pediatrics. As with ACLS, these courses verify "course completion," not certification. Increasingly, emergency departments and prehospital systems expect that nurses and other providers obtain PALS verification in addition to ACLS. Current national recommendations for trauma nursing are that PALS is essential for nurses involved in trauma resuscitation in levels I and II trauma centers and desirable for those in level III centers.[7] For other emergency nurses (those working in hospitals not designated as trauma centers), it is recommended that at least 50% of the nurses in a given department be verified as PALS providers.[7] It is especially important that in smaller departments, in which pediatric and neonatal intensive care services may not be available and frequency of pediatric or neonatal resuscitation situations is low, every effort is made to ensure that adequate that numbers of emergency nurses have completed these courses.

TNCC and ENPC Trauma Nursing Core Course and Emergency Nursing Pediatric Course

TNCC and ENPC have been developed by the Emergency Nurses Association (ENA) in response to the distinct, physiologic, and psychosocial needs of these two emergency populations. These courses are designed to teach a standardized knowledge base and clinical approach. Each course is 16 hours long and includes didactic components and skills practica. Each recommends a minimum of 6 months, emergency nursing experience before taking the course. "Provider" verification is by means of written and psychomotor skills testing. The reverification interval for both courses is 4 years.

TNCC provider verification is considered essential for all trauma resuscitation nurses regardless of trauma center level. For emergency nurses working in hospitals not designated as trauma centers, it is recommended that in a given department at least 50% of the nurses be verified as TNCC providers.[7] As suggested earlier, maintaining an adequate cadre of verified TNCC providers is especially important in rural hospitals, regardless of whether they are designated trauma centers. In the rural setting, facility capabilities for definitive care of major trauma victims may be limited, and ancillary services may not be immediately available 24 hours a day. The ability of emergency nurses to assess, stabilize, prioritize care, and facilitate transfer rapidly can mean the difference between life and death for a trauma victim whose "golden hour" may well have elapsed before the arrival of Emergency Medical Services (EMS) at the scene. At times, grant money is available through the ENA or through State EMS Bureaus to help subsidize costs of mounting TNCC courses for rural nurses. TNCC is also highly recommended for nurses involved in any phase of trauma care, not just emergency nurses.

The ENPC program was constructed along parallel lines to TNCC to train adequate numbers of emergency nurses in the emergency care of children by means of standardized didactic and skills-verification components. The course is recommended by the ENA for all emergency nurses whose work entails pediatric emergency care.

Course verifications do not certify proficiency or expertise. Their value consists in creating and maintaining a reliable level of skill, knowledge, and organizational readiness with respect to high-frequency/high-risk populations. They reflect a national, acceptable medicolegal standard of care to which emergency nurses and departments will likely be held. Every effort, including budgeting for adequate time off and reimbursement, should be made to effect the recommended departmental dissemination thresholds for these courses.

Course in Advanced Trauma Nursing

After several years of development, the ENA has created a Course in Advanced Trauma Nursing (CATN). The course represents a significant change from past emphasis on algorithmic didactic instruction and skills verification. A minimum of 2 years of experience in trauma nursing and current verification as a TNCC provider are strongly recommended as prerequisites. CATN uses a case-based learning approach structured around concepts such as oxygenation/ventilation, transport/perfusion, mobility/sensation, tissue integrity, pain, consciousness, collaboration, and ethics. The thrust of the course is toward fostering critical thinking and critical decision making within a biopsychosocial conceptual framework. The primary emphasis is on satisfactory course completion as evidenced by the ability to integrate and apply the conceptual, critical thinking, and decision-making components in case studies through all phases of the trauma cycle. Initial response of those who have taken the course has been highly positive. An optional verification component is available, but is not the principal intent of the course. The verification process involves a rigorous oral examination that requires substantial grounding in physiologic and psychosocial sciences (S. Talbert, personal communication).

CERTIFICATION PROGRAMS

Certification in emergency nursing and flight nursing are treated more extensively elsewhere in this text (see Chapter 88). These certifications are the *sine qua non* for objective validation that a nurse possesses the essential knowledge base of either field. The Board of Certification for Emergency Nursing (BCEN), which administers both certification programs, subscribes to the National Specialty Nursing Certifying Organization definition of certification as "the process by which a nongovernmental agency or association validates, based on predetermined standards, an individual Registered Nurse's qualifications and knowledge for practice in a defined or clinical area of nursing."[8] The content of both examinations has been validated by appropriate role delineation studies. The reliability of the Certification Examination in Emergency Nursing (CEEN) is well demonstrated. The first sitting for the Certified Flight Registered Nurse (CFEN) exam was in July 1993. Reliability data for the CFRN examination is accruing as increasing numbers of flight nurses take the examination. Previously, many flight nursing services would require either the Certified Emergency Nurse (CEN) or Critical Care Registered Nurse (CCRN) credential within a specified interval from time of hire. Now that a national credential particular to the specialty of flight nursing exists it will undoubtedly become the essential certification for flight nurses; CEN or CCRN credentials will continue to be viewed as desirable.

The ENA endorses attainment of the CEN credential by all emergency nurses.[9] *The Resource Document for Nursing Care of the Trauma Patient* states that the CEN or CCRN credential be considered desirable for all trauma resuscitation nurses regardless of trauma center level, and that for non-trauma center emergency nurses, the desired threshold be at least 50% of a given department's emergency nurses.[7]

The BCEN, ENA, and National Flight Nurses Association (NFNA) recommend that nurses sitting for either the CEN or CFRN examination have a minimum of 2 years experience in the respective field. This comports well with the "competent" level of skills acquisition described by Benner.[5] This is not to say that nurses lacking these credentials are not competent, merely that their acquisition of the core knowledge of their specialty has not been independently and objectively tested and validated. The "competent" nurse in Benner's model is one who is able to use steps of the nursing process to prioritize and perform "based on considerable conscious, abstract, analytic contemplation" of a given situation.[5] Essentially what is being validated is that the nurse has a sufficient knowledge base to be considered a generalist within the specialty. The ENA takes the position that the CEN credential should "be incorporated into professional advancement models, be recognized, supported, and valued by institutions as the certification credential for all nurses practicing in emergency care settings."[9]

Department Issues

Department-based orientation and competency verification are less objective than course verifications or certification and are subject to institutional pressures to upgrade marginal performers. The recommended dissemination thresholds described previously need to be interpreted in light of usual staffing patterns. A 50% threshold for TNCC dissemination in a department that staffs six to ten nurses a shift will likely ensure an adequate number of TNCC provider nurses on any given shift. However, the same threshold in a rural department that staffs only one or two registered nurses per shift would mean that for some proportion of shifts, no TNCC-verified nurse would be on duty. Therefore a 50% threshold may be too few in a smaller department.

There are logistical and economic difficulties for individual nurses and their departments in obtaining and maintaining multiple credentials. Managers and administrators need to resist any temptation to think of credentials as window dressing (i.e., nice, but not necessary). These credentials are widely recognized as the national standard by which competency in the specialty is judged. Any suggestion that these standards apply only to larger, better-funded, or academically affiliated emergency departments amounts to an argument that one's own service population either needs or deserves some lesser standard.

In addition, it should be recalled that orientation costs per nurse typically run to several thousand dollars, an investment that no hospital can afford to squander. There is widespread agreement in nursing that retention of qualified nurses is cost-effective compared to recruitment and replacement costs. For example, a study of retention of registered nurses in rural community hospitals (defined as having no metropolitan statistical area in the hospital's county or in any adjacent county) showed that among short- and long-term rural registered nurses (respectively, those who anticipated leaving their current position within 1 year or remaining for greater than 5 years) the extent to which the hospital did not "reward . . . advanced training and education" was a source of job-dissatisfaction (72.8% and 65.8% dissatisfied, respectively) second only to pay scale (86.9% and 83.2% dissatisfied, respectively).[10] Creating a departmental culture that values professionalism and "rewards advanced training and education," may well be a cost-effective means of decreasing turnover and orientation costs.

DIVERSIFIED ROLES

A series of essays published in 1980 described the following emergency nursing roles: flight nurse, EMS consultant, observation/holding unit nurse, writer, clinical specialist, independent educator/consultant, EMS administrator, psychiatric clinical specialist, rural nurse, contracted emergency nursing service, victim counselor, and emergency nursing educator.[11] A subsequent article elaborated the role of emergency nurse practitioner.[12] No systematic attempt was made at the time to organize these roles under distinct rubrics. These roles can be subsumed in the categories: flight nursing, prehospital nursing, emergency nursing entrepreneurs, diversified or advanced practice emergency nursing, and nursing education. All of these roles have, to some degree, persisted and evolved. The reader is invited to consult these articles and compare the observations therein with the reader's own as regards specialization and diversification since 1980.

For the purposes of this discussion, it is helpful to divide roles into two broad categories. Competency based roles are defined through some combination of local, regional, state, or national criteria, but do not require a masters degree for entry into the role. Advanced practice roles (e.g., clinical nurse specialist, nurse practitioner) require a minimum of a master's degree or legally recognized advanced practice certification. This division corresponds to the "vertical" axis (level of education and licensure) previously described.[3] Within each category, the degree to which a given role represents either a subspecialty of emergency nursing or has become—or is moving toward—a distinct specialty (i.e., the "horizontal" axis described earlier) is identified. In addition, the dimensions of setting, population, and requisite experience are discussed.

Competency Based Roles

Prehospital Nursing. Emergency nurses have always been involved in all levels of prehospital care: providers, EMS dispatch, mobile intensive care nurses (MICN), EMS education and administration. In each of these areas, specific competencies—with closer ties to emergency nursing than to any other nursing specialty—are needed. Historically, the MICN and other prehospital nursing roles have been defined at the state, regional, or local level. Apart from the MICN, a regionally defined nursing role that coordinates care in the field and links communication between the field and receiving facilities, there has been considerable controversy about whether emergency nurses in prehospital settings need to be certified/registered as EMTs or paramedics. Before the existence of defined education and practice standards for prehospital nurses, EMS systems, and nurses themselves necessarily used existing EMT and paramedic standards to demonstrate competency.[13] Often prehospital nurses in regions without MICN titling were, and in some jurisdictions still are, required to practice under EMT or paramedic regulations that create numerous problems in terms of job description and authority to regulate practice. The Emergency Nurses Association and National Flight Nurses Association take the position that:

> Registered Nurses practicing in the prehospital environment should not be required to certify as emergency medical technicians, at any level, before assuming a nursing role in the prehospital environment, provided they have obtained the appropriate knowledge and demonstrated skill proficiency unique to the delivery of prehospital care.
>
> . . . . Focused education and subsequent maintenance of specifically identified and recognized prehospital knowledge and skills must be a prerequisite for Registered Nurses who practice in this environment.[14]

Further, as with all nursing practice, ultimate regulatory authority resides with state boards of nursing.[14] Flight nursing practice standards,[15] and nationally sanctioned curricula for air medical crew[16] and prehospital nursing[17] adequately address the needs of prehospital nurses for education and skills training beyond postbasic nursing education. The *National Standard Guidelines for Prehospital Nursing Curriculum* was developed by the ENA and published in 1991. These guidelines are neither a course nor a certification program. Rather, they are intended for use at the state or regional level in the development of educational and credentialing programs. While acknowledging that various jurisdictions have different patterns of both EMS and nursing regulation, the guidelines affirm that authority for regulation of all nursing practice derives from state Nurse Practice Acts.[18] According to a 1993 report, the ENA guidelines were used in Maryland to develop a prehospital nursing curriculum under the auspices of the state board of nursing. Of interest, a survey of emergency nurses undertaken before curriculum development found that the greatest interest was among nurses already affiliated with volunteer EMS systems. It was neither the intent of the program nor of the interested nurses to encroach on the practice of paid emergency medical technicians (EMTs) and paramedics.[19]

In an era of increasing financial constraint, there is no clinical or economic justification for redundancies in educational requirements and levels of regulation. It is entirely reasonable to insist that nurses or physicians possess the same knowledge and skills as their EMT or paramedic counterparts, but it is neither necessary nor desirable to require that they retake courses whose content is routine to their basic professional education.

Flight Nursing. The role of the flight nurse is included under "competency based roles" because, although a distinct specialty with its own specialty organization, practice standards, certification, and graduate-level study, entry into flight nursing does not require a masters degree. Expected qualifications include RN licensure, graduation from an accredited program (BSN preferred, but the NFNA acknowledges 'grandmothering' of non-BSN RNs), at least 2 years of experience in emergency or critical care nursing, verification in BLS and ACLS, and trauma course verification (by means of TNCC, Basic Trauma Life Support (BTLS), or prehospital trauma life support).[7] Course completion in the Flight Nurse Advanced Trauma Course (FNATC) is desirable.[7] Specific competencies expected of flight nurses, for which flight programs develop didactic and skills modules and verification/reverification processes include scene response and stabilization, endotracheal intubation, cricothyrotomy, thoracic decompression, and central line insertion.[7]

Inclusion of the role of flight nurse in this discussion should in no way be construed as implying any kind of subordination to, or subspecialty status within, emergency nursing. It is included because it shares many commonalities in its scope of practice with emergency nursing and because emergency nursing is one of the two largest pools from which flight programs draw their nurses. That the NFNA chose to contract with the BCEN for administrative services for the certification examination in flight nursing further suggests a close relationship of the two specialties.

Trauma Nursing Roles. Trauma resuscitation nurses and their recommended qualifications have been alluded to previously. The structure of and qualifications for members of trauma resuscitation teams vary considerably, but the common denominator is that nurses who are identified as trauma resuscitation nurses must, at a minimum, possess the knowledge, skills, and communication ability to assume primary nursing responsibility for the seriously injured through all phases of resuscitative care.[20] An excellent example of the functional roles of all members of the trauma team in initial resuscitation can be found in the *Resource Document: Nursing Care of the Trauma Patient.*[7]

In many areas of the country, before the advent of TNCC in 1986, trauma nursing curricula were developed under the auspices of level I trauma centers, regional, or state agencies, which paralleled or incorporated the content of the Basic and Advanced Trauma Life Support courses of the American College of Surgeons Committee on Trauma (ACSCOT). Participants who completed the training—a combination of didactic instruction, clinical practica, and skills modules, typically lasting a month—were accorded a title of Trauma Nurse Specialist (TNS). TNS courses go well beyond the scope of TNCC. Some centers or regulatory authorities require these courses for trauma resuscitation nurses or flight nurses. In other regions, it has been considered desirable, although not required. Accordingly, there is a potential lack of 'portability' of such a credential from the region where it was earned to another region. The title trauma nurse specialist is also problematic. By way of example, there is no index citation for trauma nurse specialist in either of two major textbooks on trauma nursing.[21,22] Further, use of the term *specialist* to refer to a non–masters-prepared nurse conflicts with the ANA definition of a clinical nurse specialist.[1] Nevertheless, many nurses who have completed such courses have found them valuable, particularly trauma coordinators in centers that do not require a masters degree for the role.

The role of trauma coordinator, or trauma nurse coordinator, as it was originally called in some areas,[7] arose as a practical necessity out of the trauma center designation process.[23] Designation created urgent needs: for trauma team policies and procedures; for staff development; for trauma registry, research, and quality assurance activities; and for maintenance of liaison between departments and between facilities in the system.[23] As early as 1971, it was recognized that professional nurses were uniquely qualified in terms of education, skills, and communication ability to create and perform a role that addressed all these needs.[24] The evolution of the title to *trauma coordinator* merely reflects that what is being coordinated is a multidisciplinary team, not just nurses. Nevertheless, the trauma coordinator should always be a registered nurse.[7]

> The Trauma Coordinator promotes optimal trauma care in the context of a regionalized trauma care system through: clinical activities; professional and public education; research activities; quality assurance activities; [and] administrative functions.[25]

Recommended qualifications include RN licensure, a minimum of a BSN (Masters preferred), a minimum of 5 years experience in trauma nursing, documented recent trauma continuing education, and experience in quality assurance. Certification as a CEN, CCRN, or CFRN is desirable.[7] The combination of role expectations—clinical expertise, staff-development, quality assurance, and research—bears a striking similarity to the role of the clinical nurse specialist and shares with that role a type of expertise explicitly intended to cut across departmental and bureaucratic boundaries in the interests of better trauma care. The relative emphasis given by the trauma coordinator to the various component subroles tends to vary with the maturity of the position within a given system. In systems where the role is less established, greater emphasis is given to staff and policy development. In more established systems, the role tends to broaden and emphasize more of the consultative, quality assurance, research and administrative aspects of the role.[4] A case management approach to structuring trauma services under the direction of the trauma coordinator has also been described.[26]

OTHER COMPETENCY BASED ROLES

Poison Information Specialist

Poison and drug information centers use registered nurses, pharmacists, and physicians as poison information specialists. For nurses, a strong background in emergency or critical care nursing is desirable. As virtually all consultations are by telephone, and inquiries come from the general public as well as health professionals, excellent communication and history-taking skills and the ability to handle stress and function in an autonomous role are musts.[27] Certification as a specialist in poison information is by means of an examination administered by the American Association of Poison Control Centers. Requirements for taking the examination include current employment by a poison center, a minimum of 2000 hours experience handling phone consultations, and a minimum of having handled 2000 calls under supervision. A recommendation from a medical director of a poison center is also required. Finally, the candidate must pass a written examination.[28] The recertification interval is 5 years. Recertification is by examination. Potential strengths that emergency nurses bring to the role include their assessment skills with an incomplete or unreliable database and practical experience in management of particular toxicologic situations.

Forensic Nursing

In many areas of the country, registered nurses from a variety of specialty backgrounds, including emergency nursing, women's health, and psychiatric nursing,[29] have taken a leadership role in the development of Sexual Assault Response Teams (SARTs). The role of Sexual Assault Nurse Examiner/Clinician (SANE/SANC) arose in response to the needs of victims for timely, expert, compassionate care. In the absence of a SART program, sexual assault victims, despite the best intentions of emergency department personnel, often endure unconscionable delays in receiving an evidentiary examination. Delays arise from the "time-consuming, cumbersome succession of examiners from different disciplines in the emergency department,"[30] and the logistical difficulty of arranging an uninterrupted block of examination time to maintain the chain of evidence.

A SART program assures the victim of prompt assessment and examination by a qualified sexual assault nurse clinician whose exclusive focus is the victim. Programs typically involve close collaboration between community-based sexual assault victim-advocacy programs, law enforcement agencies, professional counselors, registered nurses, and physicians. Some programs use free-standing centers for all services except those required by victims who have sustained injuries that necessitate emergency medical treatment. Other programs have on-call teams that respond to various emergency departments in their jurisdiction. A resource list of programs and contact persons is maintained by the ENA to facilitate networking.[31]

Core services include medical/forensic examination and treatment, crisis-intervention, pregnancy screening, sexually transmitted disease screening and prophylaxis, victim-advocacy and counseling, social services, expert testimony, follow-up treatment, and referrals. Several programs in California have nurse examiners trained in colposcopic examination and photography by means of which subtle, but characteristic patterns of injury not visible in routine pelvic examination have been identified and documented, resulting in much higher rates of objective physical findings of vulvovaginal injury than had ever been reported previously.[32] The credibility of nurse examiners in court has generally been found to be at least as high as that of physician examiners.[29]

Training of SANE's is a vital aspect of every program and typically includes didactic and clinical practicum components. For nurses interested in starting SART programs in regions where they have not yet been developed, some training programs accept qualified applicants from out-of-state, and a resource manual on how to start a program has been published.[33]

The International Association of Forensic Nurses has become instrumental in defining the role and setting standards for providers and programs. They define forensic nursing as, "the application of the forensic aspects of health care, combined with the bio-psychosocial education of the Registered Nurse in the scientific investigation and treatment of trauma- . . . or death-related medicolegal issues."[34]

ADVANCED PRACTICE ROLES

Emergency Nurse Practitioner

Over the last 20 years, several roles and settings have been proposed for Emergency Nurse Practitioners (ENPs), including primary care providers in rural settings,[35] advanced triage and primary care in urban hospitals,[36,37] free-standing emergency and urgent care centers,[12] hospital-based "fast-tracks,"[38-42] and as substitutes for or augmentation of house staff.[43,44] The majority of these reports emphasize the ENP as serving the primary care population of their respective places of employment, although a case management role within a trauma service—inpatient and outpatient—has been described,[44] and there is increasing interest in acute care roles for the nurse practitioner.[45]

A historical peculiarity of the ENP literature is its bimodal time distribution. In 1982, funding was withdrawn from non-primary care nurse practitioner programs; the ENP programs did not survive.[46] No further reports of the ENP were published between 1984 and 1992, although nurse practitioners continued to be involved in emergency care in some settings.[47] Some data suggest that as of 1990, most ENP practice focused on primary care populations.[48,49]

Since the early 1990s, there has been a tremendous increase in interest in using nurse practitioners in emergency care. Several trends are contributing to this renewed interest including case management, managed care, emergency department overcrowding, and limitations on house staff hours. In addition, several reports of collaborative or group practice arrangements have been published.[47,50] As of 1994, an estimated 320 nurse practitioners were working in emergency settings.[46] Many of them had trained as primary care nurse practitioners but had emergency nursing experience, or had received special training within a given emergency or urgent care setting.[38] At present, there is one graduate program with a specific Emergency Nurse Practitioner curriculum, the University of Texas Health Sciences Center, Houston.[51] The ENP role is treated extensively elsewhere in this text (see Chapter 23).

Clinical Nurse Specialist

The clinical nurse specialist (CNS) is a registered nurse "who through study and supervised clinical practice at the graduate level (masters or doctorate), has become an expert in a defined area of knowledge and practice in a selected clinical area of nursing."[1] The clinical specialist "is an expert in clinical practice, an educator, a consultant, a researcher, and may be an administrator."[52]

Traditionally, the distinction between the nurse practitioner and the CNS is said to be that the former is concerned primarily with the provision of care in a primary care setting, and the latter specializes in a client-centered practice (typically based in age, disease process or organ system) in a secondary- or tertiary-care setting.[53] Obviously this distinction is problematic with respect to emergency nursing because emergency care settings take care of multiple populations spanning all ages and ranging from primary care to resuscitative care.

Acknowledging that the role of the emergency CNS was "poorly developed . . . and underutilized,"[54] the ENA undertook to clarify the role by means of guidelines, sample job descriptions and evaluation tools, an annotated bibliography and a networking resource list, which were published in 1991.[54] New advanced emergency nursing practice guidelines that cover both clinical specialist and nurse practitioner roles are due to be published by the ENA in late 1996. The 1991 guidelines[54] provided examples of Emergency CNS behaviors in each of five traditional domains of CNS practice:

1. **Expert clinician:** Uses advanced concepts in all phases of the nursing process across the full scope of emergency nursing practice, assumes a leadership role in the development and implementation of practice standards and role-models excellence in emergency nursing practice to foster clinical growth among emergency nurses.
2. **Educator:** Mentors emergency nurses, participates in the development of emergency nursing curricula at the institutional level or through academic affiliation, contributes to professional literature in the specialty, develops client-teaching and discharge planning materials, and is a resource to patients and the community in the dissemination of information relating emergency care, health, and prevention.
3. **Consultant:** Deals with clients, other healthcare professionals and organizations, and with legislative and regulatory bodies with respect to complex clinical situations and systems issues.
4. **Researcher:** Conducts, collaborates in, and disseminates current research.
5. **Administrator/Leader:** Takes a leadership role in the development and periodic review of emergency nursing policies and procedures at the departmental, institutional, and systems levels; develops and implements quality assurance programs; participates in employee performance evaluations; and is involved in budgetary decision making with respect to emergency care.[54]

A secondary analysis of 1990 emergency nursing role delineation data obtained from the BCEN indicated that masters-prepared CENs (who possessed credentials sufficient for an advanced practice role irrespective of job title) had different patterns of clinical practice than non–masters-prepared emergency staff nurses controlling for experience, certification, and hours per week in clinical practice. Among the masters-prepared CENs was a substantial evidence of a greater clinical focus on high-acuity and high-risk patients (e.g., shock, toxicologic emergencies, mental health emergencies, and care of sexual assault victims). Masters-prepared CENs also had significantly more involvement in research and staff development activities than staff nurses.[48,49]

Specific CNS functions may include patient-advocacy, crisis intervention, and case management; oversight of planned change; improving documentation; and development, implementation, and evaluation of orientation, staff-development, and cost-containment programs.[55] Given widespread concerns about the adequacy of emergency services available to pediatric and psychiatric populations, persuasive arguments have been put forward for the use of pediatric and psychiatric CNSs in general emergency departments.[56-58] Common sense suggests that departments publicly identified as providers of specialized emergency services (e.g., pediatrics, chest pain emergency departments, trauma centers) should use CNSs as one means of supporting their claims of expertise.

More has been published about implementation of the CNS role than about clinical outcomes.[53] Published outcome studies focus on inpatient or specialty clinic populations for which clinical and cost indicators such as complication and infection rates, readmission rates, and length of stay appropriately lend themselves to measurement. Ease of measurement, however, does not guarantee that the quality of care is being measured. Given the broad scope of emergency nursing practice and its episodic nature, determining valid, reliable outcome measures that lend themselves to objective measurement is extremely difficult. There are no published outcome studies to validate either the clinical or cost effectiveness of the emergency CNS. There is clearly a need for research in this area. Nevertheless, it is hard to imagine a service industry outside of nursing with 'round-the-clock organizational demands of similar complexity that does not require in-house expertise.

FUTURE DIRECTIONS

In the future, the role of generalist emergency staff nurse will continue to be the most common and essential role in emergency nursing. Flight nursing and forensic nursing will evolve as distinct specialties, but prehospital nursing roles will continue to depend on and vary according to local and regional political factors. With greater emphasis on managed care and justification of clinical outcomes, the freedom to identify and create new emergency nursing practice roles laterally[3] (i.e., on the basis of certification or skills verification) may be constrained. Certification and skills verification programs will remain vitally important as a means of documenting standard knowledge and skills in the specialty, but are not a substitute for advanced (i.e., graduate level) education.

On the other hand, increased emphasis on integrated healthcare delivery systems should lead to increased opportunities for graduate-prepared advanced practice nurses in emergency settings, especially in primary care and case management roles.[59] Advanced practice emergency nurses will likely blend CNS and nurse practitioner roles to focus on the needs of particular high volume, high risk, or problematic patient populations in their particular work settings. Increased entrepreneurialism in advanced practice nursing may lead to greater numbers of independent advanced practice nurse-contractors, or collaborative practice arrangements with emergency medicine group practices for providing specialized or primary care services.[41] Rural and other underserved areas may begin to have greater access to the expertise of advanced practice emergency nurses via participation in integrated healthcare networks. Legal, clinical, and ethical imperatives will stimulate further role diversification among advanced practice emergency and psychiatric nurses specializing in emergency mental health assessment and crisis intervention.

Finally, as pressures mount within the healthcare system to demonstrate good clinical outcomes while cutting costs, it is imperative to generate more research-based knowledge by emergency nurses in regard to clinical outcomes, primary prevention, and the structure and operations of emergency care services. In the past, except in teaching hospitals with a major commitment to research, the role of researcher in emergency nursing has been discussed, if at all, as a subset of CNS or trauma coordinator practice, or in terms of quality assurance activities. In recent years, however, there has been a marked increase in the amount of emergency nursing research being performed and published. Because the clinical focus of emergency care settings is on relatively brief, episodic care, under conditions of high stress for patients and providers alike, emergency nursing research poses enormous challenges to investigators and policy makers. The role of nurse researcher, with doctoral preparation in research methods and data analysis, will take on greater importance as all providers of emergency care are called on increasingly to demonstrate sound, cost-effective clinical outcomes.

REFERENCES

1. American Nurses Association: *Nursing: a social policy statement,* Kansas City, 1980, ANA.
2. Emergency Nurses Association: *Standards of emergency nursing practice,* ed 2, St Louis, 1991, Mosby.
3. Styles M: Clinical nurse specialists and the future of nursing. In Sparacino PSA, Cooper DM, Minarik PA, Editors: *The clinical nurse specialist: implementation and impact,* Norwalk CT, 1990, Appleton & Lange.
4. Emergency Nurses Association: Scope of emergency nursing practice, Chicago, 1993, ENA.
5. Benner P: *From novice to expert: excellence and power in clinical nursing practice,* Menlo Park, CA, 1984, Addison-Wesley.
6. Emergency Cardiac Care Committee and Subcommittees, American Heart Association: Guidelines for cardiopulmonary resuscitation and emergency cardiac care, *JAMA* 268:2171-2302, 1992.
7. Trauma Nursing Coalition: Resource document: nursing care of the trauma patient, 1992, TNC.
8. CEN: *Certification examination for flight nurses, 1994 handbook for candidates,* Chicago, 1993, BCEN.
9. Emergency Nurses Association: Position statement: CEN credentialing and review courses, 1991.
10. Muus KJ et al: Retaining registered nurses in rural community hospitals, *J Nurs Admin* 23:38-43, 1993.
11. Hart MA et al: The various roles of EDNA nurses, *J Emerg Nurs* 6:40-61, 1980.
12. Widhalm SA, Anderson LA: Emergency nurse practitioners: motivators, barriers, and autonomy in role performance, *J Emerg Nurs* 8:67-74, 1982.
13. Lyle N: Prehospital nurse clinician: job description and evaluation tool, *J Emerg Med* 12:365, 1986.
14. Emergency Nurses Association, National Flight Nurses Association: *Joint position statement: role of the registered nurse in the prehospital environment,* Chicago, 1993, ENA/NFNA.
15. National Flight Nurses Association: *Practice standards for flight nursing,* Rapid City, 1986, NFNA.
16. U.S. Department of Transportation: *Air medical crew national standard curriculum,* Pasadena CA, 1988, ASHBEAMS.
17. Emergency Nurses Association: *National standard guidelines for prehospital nursing curriculum,* Chicago, 1991, ENA.
18. Robinson K: Development of the ENA national standard guidelines for prehospital nursing curriculum, *J Emerg Nurs* 18:48-53, 1992.
19. Miller PM, Epifanio PC: Development of a prehospital nursing curriculum in Maryland, *J Emerg Nurs* 19:206-208, 1993.
20. Snyder JA: Evolution of trauma care. In Neff JA, Kidd PS, editors: *Trauma nursing: the art and science,* St Louis, 1993, Mosby.
21. Cardona VD et al: Trauma nursing: from resuscitation through rehabilitation, Philadelphia, 1988, WB Saunders.
22. Neff JA, Kidd PS: *Trauma nursing: the art and science,* St Louis, 1993, Mosby.
23. McArdle M, Murrin P: Role of the trauma nurse coordinator, *Nurs Clin North Am* 21:673-675, 1986.
24. Beachley M et al: Developing trauma care systems: the trauma nurse coordinator, *J Nurs Admin* 18:34-42, 1988.
25. Flint CB: The role of the trauma coordinator: a position paper, *J Trauma* 28:1673, 1988.
26. Songne EA, Holmquist P: Comprehensive care by trauma nurse providers: Mission Hospital's ten-year experience, *J Emerg Nurs* 17:73-79, 1991.
27. Litovitz T et al: Poison information providers, *Am J Emerg Med* 2:129-135, 1983.
28. American Association of Poison Control Centers: AAPCC 1993 Certification exam for specialists in poison information, *Vet Hum Toxicol* 35:81-86, 1993.
29. Ledray LE: The sexual assault nurse clinician: a fifteen year experience in Minneapolis, *J Emerg Nurs* 18:217-222, 1992.
30. Pisarcik-Lenehan G: Sexual assault nurse examiners: a SANE way to care for rape victims, *J Emerg Nurs* 17:1-2, 1991.
31. Emergency Nurses Association: ENA sexual assault nurse examiners resource list, J Emerg Nurs 17:31A-35A, 1991.
32. Slaughter L, Brown CRV: Colposcopy to establish physical findings in rape victims, *Am J Obstet Gynecol* 166(1 Part 1):83-86, 1992.
33. Forensic Nursing Services: *The SART/SANE orientation guide and The SART/Sane institute implementation guide,* Santa Cruz, CA, Forensic Nursing Services.
34. Lynch V: Forensic nursing: a clinical approach to law and medicine, 1992. In *On the edge* (Newsletter) North Pacific Region, IAFN, 1(2):1, 1993.
35. Geolot D et al: Emergency nurse practitioner: an answer to an emergency care crisis in rural hospitals, *Ann Emerg Med* 6:355-357, 1977.
36. Roglieri JL: Multiple expanded roles for nurses in urban emergency rooms, *Arch Intern Med* 135:1401-1404, 1975.
37. Fincke MK: A new dimension in emergency nursing, *J Emerg Nurs* 1:45-52, 1975.

38. Covington C et al: Implementation of a nurse practitioner-staffed fast track, *J Emerg Nurs* 18:124-131, 1992.
39. Hazen M: The emergency room walk-in clinic (WIC): the multidimensional nursing role within an ambulatory care setting. In Goetzen IE, editor: *Differentiating nursing practice into the twenty-first century,* New York, 1991, ANA-Publ-Am-Acad-Nurs.
40. Meislin HW et al: Fast track: urgent care within a teaching hospital emergency department: can it work? *Ann Emerg Med* 17:453-456, 1988.
41. Pisarcik-Lenehan G: Timing is everything: the growing need for emergency nurse practitioners, *J Emerg Nurs* 19:269-270, 1993.
42. Wright et al: Fast track in the emergency department: a one-year experience with nurse practitioners, *J Emerg Med* 10:367-373, 1992.
43. Silver HK, McAtee P: Should nurses substitute for house staff? *Am J Nurs* 88:1671-1673, 1988.
44. Spisso J et al: Improved quality of care and reduction of housestaff workload using trauma nurse practitioners, *J Trauma* 30:660-665, 1990.
45. Keane A, Richmond T: Tertiary nurse practitioners, *Image* 25:281-284, 1993.
46. Curry J: Nurse practitioners in the emergency department: current issues, *J Emerg Nurs* 20:207-212, 1994.
47. Lumb E, McCabe P, Rice A et al: Successful ED nurse practitioner group advocates more general nurse practitioner program [letter], *J Emerg Nurs* 20:7-8, 1994.
48. Parshall MB: Advanced emergency nursing practice: A pilot role delineation study, unpublished master's thesis, Lexington, 1994, University of Kentucky.
49. Parshall MB: Advanced emergency nursing practice: a preliminary role delineation (abstract), *J Emerg Nurs* 21:378-379, 1995.
50. Wilson C, Farrell M, Bove S: Emergency department nurse practitioners: the AtlantiCare Medical Center program in review, *J Emerg Nurs* 20:195-198, 1994.
51. Cole F, Abel C: New emergency nurse practitioner course announced (letter), *J Emerg Nurs* 20:256-257, 1994.
52. American Nurses Association: *The role of the clinical nurse specialist,* Washington DC, 1986, ANA.
53. Sparacino PSA: A historical perspective on the development of the clinical nurse specialist role. In Sparacino PSA, Cooper DM, Minarik PA, editors: *The clinical nurse specialist: implementation and impact,* Norwalk, CT, 1990, Appleton & Lange.
54. Emergency Nurses Association: Emergency clinical nurse specialist guidelines, Chicago, 1991, ENA.
55. Schrader et al: Role of the clinical nurse specialist in emergency care, *Top Emerg Med* 13:47-61, 1991.
56. Gross RP: The role of a pediatric clinical nurse specialist in a general emergency department, *Clin Nurse Spec* 5:144-148, 1991.
57. Jacoby LE, Jones SL: The psychiatric clinical nurse specialist in the emergency room, *J Psychosoc Nurs Ment Health Serv* 22:8-13, 1984.
58. Pisarcik G: The psychiatric nurse in the ED, *J Emerg Nurs* 6:51-54, 1980. (cf. *J Emerg Nurs* 18:535, 1992 and *J Emerg Nurs* 19:377, 392; 1993.
59. Daleiden AL: The CNS as trauma case manager, *Clin Nurse Spec* 7:295-298, 1993.

PART NINE
Professional Relations

92 Public Relations

David J. Pillow

This chapter explores the interactions between the emergency department and the public it serves. The public, for the purposes of this discussion, is any individual who has dealings with the emergency department, but is not a member of the staff. This would include but not be limited to patients, their families, the medical staff, hospital administration, personnel from other departments in the hospital, prehospital care providers, and vendors.

This chapter provides the means to thoughtfully create a relationship with the public. It first examines how relationships can just happen in a way that requires no creativity. Then how to thoughtfully design a public relations campaign for the emergency department and how to provide the leadership to implement it are described. The chapter provides practical examples of how to use the concepts presented in the everyday functioning of the emergency departments.

ORDINARY RELATIONSHIPS

A relationship already exists between the public and the emergency department. For one patient it is the place where her life was saved, and a place she honors, respects, and deeply appreciates. For another, it is the place where the patient or family was treated rudely, a place that appears not to care about people. For a member of the medical staff, the emergency department is a hectic and unfriendly place, where everyone seems too busy to help. For other members of the medical staff, it is a place where dependable care occurs for their patients and a place that can be trusted. Each individual who interacts with the emergency department develops a perception. The perception is based on past experience and interpretation of these experiences and is sustained in memory. Psychoanalytical thinking strongly emphasizes the idea that humans remain most importantly influenced, in their present patterns of living, by their past experiences.[1]

In any visit to the emergency department, a multitude of experiences occur, any one of which may become the basis for the relationship with the whole department. The relationship between the emergency department and the public is not a tangible object with substance and form that can be physically touched. It exists in language and is therefore fragile, malleable, constantly changing, and subject to interpretation. The challenge is to mold and shape the relationship with the public so that it is advantageous to the emergency department.

CREATING A DEPARTMENTAL IDENTITY

The first step in designing the relationship is to decide how it should be perceived. What would you want the public to say about you and the service you provide?

This step is relatively easy to accomplish. A mandatory staff meeting should be scheduled in which the following question is posed to the staff: If your mother, father, or best friend came to our emergency department for treatment, what would you want them to say to you about their experience in our department? The people who work in the department always come up with an inspiring vision of how they want to be perceived. They want the patient to be happy with their care and to leave with an experience of being treated with dignity, compassion, and respect. In addition, they want the patient to experience technically excellent care and to say that the people who staffed the department seemed to be a group of high-quality people who cared about each other, respected each other, and worked well together. They want the patient to say the business side of the encounter also was handled with integrity and excellence. In this exercise, the emergency department staff literally create who and what they are committed to being as a department. They are expressing what they value and stand for as a group of professionals.

In the Continuous Quality Improvement/Total Quality Management (CQI/TQM) paradigm, workers are trained to work in teams to improve quality using a variety of new tools. Their new tool box contains Pareto diagrams, histograms, cause and effect diagrams, control charts, flow charts, nominal group techniques, brainstorming, and many others too numerous to mention.[2] What is evolving is the importance of basing these "hard technologies" on a foundation comprised of the values of the people who do the work. A vision can be such a foundation, and having one can be key to both the quality of work life, and the quality of the goods or services being produced by those working.[3]

This principle was beautifully expressed by C. Philip Alexander, a specialist in quality and human systems development: "Quality will begin internally as a vision, as an awareness of a creative impulse to express values and ideals. . . . Quality will become the manifestation of human intellect and ability in its myriad forms. And we will know the quality product or service for what it truly is—the visible and tangible expression of human excellence."[4]

The next challenge for the physician-manager is to give these values a physical existence outside of memory. This step can also be relatively easy to accomplish. It should be written down and labeled the vision statement for the emergency department. It should be written concisely so that it can be easily remembered. An example is shown in Box 92-1.

Step 1 of designing the relationship is now complete. The emergency department staff have thoughtfully and intentionally created how it wants to be perceived by the public. It has declared what it stands for, designed who it is going to be, and given it an existence outside of memory. The department is saying to the public, "This is who we are for you, this is what you can count on us for in our relationship."

BECOMING KNOWN

The challenge now facing the emergency department is to be perceived by the public in the fashion it has designed for itself. To achieve this goal, the department must find ways to give people experiences consistent with that vision. If the department says it is a place where people are treated with compassion, dignity, and respect, but people say it is a place where they are treated coldly and rudely, the staff have failed to follow the vision for the department.

The department becomes known to the public simply by telling them who it is and what they can expect. The challenge is to find many different ways to share the vision with the public. Little in the existing literature specifically addresses this issue. The following section describes a variety of ways that I have tried over the years and found effective.

The vision should be prominently displayed in the waiting room of the emergency department. This begins the process of creating a relationship with each person who reads it. At the same time, the physical details of the display and the physical environment of the waiting room should be addressed. A shoddy display in a cluttered, dirty waiting room will not be perceived in the same way as a quality display in a neat and clean waiting room. An enhancement is to post pictures of the staff around the vision statement. Doing so sends many unspoken but powerful messages that create a relationship with the public. These messages might include the following: We care enough about you to show you who will be taking care of you, we want you to know us and feel comfortable with us, and we are professionals and caring human beings. People may feel they already know the staff because they have seen their pictures in the waiting room. Their anxiety may be lessened because they know the department and to what it is committed.

Patient rooms should have plaques that further communicates who the emergency department is and what can expected from it. I have used such a promise (Box 92-2) modified from one I found years ago advertised in a catalog of items for dentists' offices.

OPERATING WITH INTEGRITY

The next challenge is on a personal level. The staff must discipline themselves and encourage themselves to operate consistent with the vision. To meet this challenge, the vision statement should become the steering wheel for action as the staff function in the emergency department.[6] This metaphor of a steering wheel invites creativity. Daily practices should be developed that express the vision of the department and set an example for the staff. Each shift can be an opportunity to practice expressing this vision.

PERSONAL PRACTICES

During my career as an emergency physician, I have been constantly on the lookout for practices that leave patients with an experience of being treated with compassion, dignity, and respect. It is challenging to build a relationship with a patient that imparts vision in the hectic environment of the emergency department.

The patient's experience with the physician begins the moment he or she walks into the room. I use my appearance to begin to instill a sense that patients are being treated by a professional in whom they can have confidence. I intentionally wear a crisp clean white coat, a dress shirt, tie, and shoes recently shined. I might be more comfortable in blue jeans, tennis shoes, and a polo shirt; but that attire would not communicate the message I am committed to delivering. I take a moment to introduce myself to the patient and family members and then sit down at the patient's side. The nature of language is that what is not spoken communicates powerfully and richly. In this simple act I communicate to the patient

BOX 92-1

ELSEWHERE MEMORIAL HOSPITAL EMERGENCY DEPARTMENT VISION STATEMENT

Our staff stands committed:

- To providing **quality emergency care** to each of our patients
- To treating our patients and each other with **compassion, dignity, and respect**
- To functioning in partnership with other providers and our staff as a **championship team**
- To bringing the same **excellence and integrity** to our business practices as we bring to our patient care[5]

BOX 92-2

OUR PROMISE

We have the desire and interest to listen, really listen, to what you are saying. Please don't ever hesitate to ask about anything you don't understand.

You will be dealing with members of a professional team whose primary job is to care for you.

We promise to treat you with dignity and respect.

and family that they are important, that I care, that I have time for their problem, and that they now have my undivided attention. I let the patient tell me about the problem without interruption before I begin directing the interview. I let people know what will happen next, and how long it usually takes. I use the patient's name multiple times in my communications. I express my concern at any opportunity with statements such as, "I'm worried that your pain might be due to a kidney stone," or "I'm concerned that you may have pneumonia." I end each encounter with the question, "Is there anything else you have a question about, or is there anything else I can do for you today?" The important point is to develop practices that give people the opportunity to experience you as you are committed to being perceived.

DEPARTMENTAL PRACTICES

The next challenge is perhaps even larger. How can the staff be stimulated to develop practices that reflect the vision of the emergency department? The answer begins with leadership finding ways to keep the mission and vision alive and present in the minds of the department personnel.[7] Here is an opportunity to be creative. The physician group can create a "Nurse Excellence Award" to recognize a nurse who is a fine example of operating consistent with the departmental vision. We give a $1000 educational grant, award it with great fanfare at our yearly Christmas party, and place the nurse's name on a plaque. The physicians write a personal letter to that nurse, and a copy is framed and placed on a wall in the break room, next to the departmental vision statement and the plaque. Every 2 to 3 months, the physicians give a small gift to the nurses, expressing appreciation for their high-quality care. At the monthly staff meeting, positive comments from patient surveys are read and appreciation is expressed to the individuals involved for functioning consistent with our vision. Performance evaluations are structured to evaluate whether the employee is practicing in a fashion consistent with each area of the vision statement. Another means to encourage expression of the vision is to set up contests. We have held contests to judge who could perform the most transfers with perfect documentation, who could have the fewest patient complaints, and who could have the most patients cared for in less than 2 hours from triage to discharge. All employee counseling should take place with the vision statement in mind. In addition, inservices on guest relations should be held regularly. Leadership must be constantly looking for and designing new ways to keep the vision alive and present. The vision lives only in language and must be constantly respoken and acted out, or it disappears.

RELATING TO THE MEDICAL STAFF

Another important segment of the public is the medical staff of the hospital. The challenge is to establish a relationship in which the vision is communicated. We have used the minutes of our quality assurance meetings as a vehicle to communicate with key members of the medical staff. They are included in the packet sent to each member of the executive committee of the hospital before their monthly meeting. We start each quality assurance meeting with a declaration that this meeting is our opportunity to come together as a team and work on improving the quality of care in the emergency department. We report the actions we have completed to improve care and the actions we will be taking the next month. We use the minutes as an opportunity to share both our vision for quality emergency care and the work we are doing to make that vision real.

When we send out cards asking the private staff if and how they prefer to be called when their patients use the emergency department, we include a cover letter that creates a relationship by letting them know we are committed to functioning as their partners in the care of their patients.

Once a year we prepare an annual report that we send to the officers of the executive committee and the chair of each department. In that annual report we communicate our vision statement and the results of all the work we have done consistent with it. We also make it a practice to greet the private physicians when they are in the department and ask if they need anything.

Every emergency physician is on a hospital committee to do the work of the committee and be an ambassador for the emergency department. Furthermore, we never miss a chance to be written up in the hospital newsletter. We resolve every staff physician complaint with a personal telephone call and letter, and in resolving the complaint share our vision for the department.

Once the commitment is made to being known as the vision, a million opportunities to share the vision of the department with the public will become apparent.

RELATING TO HOSPITAL ADMINISTRATION

Another segment of the public is the hospital administration. Ingenuity in making the emergency department known in this arena is key to success in improving the department. If the hospital perceives the department as a necessary evil, it is difficult to get funding and support for needed staffing, equipment, and space. In today's economic environment, it is important that the administration perceives the department as a financial plus as well as an environment in which quality care is compassionately rendered. The challenge is to design a dialogue that leads to that perception.

At our hospital the chief financial officer prepares a quarterly report in which we look at the incremental revenue generated for the hospital by each admission from the emergency department. When it was discovered that each admission was worth approximately $2000 in incremental revenue, there was new interest in ideas for building volume and admissions. We send the hospital administration a statistical report each month so that they know the percentage of volume that is admitted, the percentage of hospital admissions that come through the emergency department, and any increases that are occurring. We meet with our chief financial officer and set yearly goals for increases in volume and admissions and talk about the increase in revenue that will occur for the hospital if we meet these goals. We send the annual report discussed in the previous section to administration, so they are reminded of our vision and made aware of the results of our work. We are then able to talk about investments in the emergency department and the potential returns on that investment, rather than our need for administration to increase their expenses.

MORE ON INTEGRITY

Throughout this chapter, public relations has been presented as a means of letting the public know who the emergency department is and to act accordingly. It does no good and probably damages the relationship with the public to say the department is one thing and then act in another way. Operating with integrity is the basis for success. However, most of us are not saints. We can become angry with patients who are not behaving as we think they should. Some staff members occasionally make fun of certain types of patients behind their backs and say derogatory things about their coworkers and others. We forget that our reason for being is our patients and instead the triage bell ringing becomes an occasion to mutter "oh no, not another one." At times we react with anger when people return for follow-up in the emergency department when we told them to go to a particular physician's office if they continued to have problems. We all have many reactions like these, yet when we are thoughtful and think about how we want to be, an inspiring vision emerges. Leadership's job is to encourage action consistent with that vision by constantly finding ways to recognize and express it.[8]

THE CONVERSATION THAT BUILDS RELATIONSHIP

Public relations is the development of relationships with the public. We have noted that relationships are created by word and deed and are not a thing with a tangible existence. Relationships can be created by saying, "This is who I am for you, and this is who you are for me." The nature of this declaration is that it is a speech act, which not only announces but creates. I declare that I am committed to treating you with dignity and respect. My commitment is not an object with a tangible existence, which I am now describing to you. The commitment to treat you with dignity and respect is created in the declaration. The declaration will be valid if I strive to treat you with dignity and respect, and invalid if I do not.

PREVENTING EROSION

Another vital part of public relations is the ability to resolve complaints and dissatisfaction. In all relationships over time there are conflicts to resolve, and failure to resolve them erodes the relationship. We must strive to develop practices that at least provide a chance to resolve dissatisfaction and restore the relationship with the public. All patient and staff complaints must be investigated. In our practice, we make personal contact with the person expressing the complaint and let them know we take their complaint seriously. We have an intention to resolve it in a manner that is satisfactory to them, even though that is not possible in every case. We investigate the complaint thoroughly and communicate in person our findings and conclusions and follow up with a letter. Leadership should be trained in a variety of methodologies for conflict resolution.

SUMMARY

To build a relationship thoughtfully, the first step is to decide how one is going to be in the relationship and then commit to being that way. Next one must let the other person or persons know what can be expected in the relationship. Finally, it is important to operate with integrity in the relationship. The medium for building the relationship is language, and the action is declaration. There is the freedom to declare how one is committed to being as an individual or as a department. There is the freedom to creatively find ways to share oneself, to let the public know in word and deed who one is. There is the challenge of operating with integrity, being in action as who one says one is.

REFERENCES

1. Ellis A, Harper R: *A new guide to rational living,* New York, 1975, Wilshire.
2. Scholtes P: *The team handbook,* New York, 1988, Joiner Associates.
3. Jones A: Team Psychology. In American College of Emergency Physicians: *Managing the emergency department: a team approach,* Dallas, 1992, ACEP.
4. Dixon G, Swiler J: *Total quality handbook: the executive guide to the new American way of doing business,* Philadelphia, 1990, Lakewood Books.
5. From the company vision statement of Metroplex Emergency Physician Associates (MEPA), Dallas, Texas, 1989.
6. Covey S: *The 7 habits of highly effective people,* New York, 1990, Fireside (Simon & Schuster).
7. Scott C, Jaffe D, Tobe G: *Organizational vision, values, and mission,* Chicago, 1993, Crisp Publications.
8. Clemmer J: *Firing on all cylinders,* Dallas, 1992, Business One Irwin.

ADDITIONAL READINGS

Winograd T, Flores F: *Understanding computers and cognition,* Norwood, NJ 1986, Ablex.

Henry G: *Emergency medicine risk management,* Dallas, 1991, ACEP.

American College of Emergency Physicians: *Managing the emergency department: a team approach,* Dallas, 1992, ACEP.

Bennis W, Nanus B: *Leaders: the strategies for taking charge,* New York, 1985, Harper & Row.

Blanchard K, Peale N: *The power of ethical management,* New York, 1988, Fawcett Crest.

Searle J: *Speech acts: an essay in the philosophy of language,* New York, 1969, Cambridge University Press.

93 Medical Staff Relations

Michael J. Peikert, Robert Strauss, and David T. Overton

OUTLINE

Becoming clinically indispensable
Becoming administratively indispensable
Medical staff organization
  Bylaws
  Hospital committee structure
Emergency department organization
  Departmental status
  Medical director/department chair
  Emergency department nursing director
  Emergency department quality committee
  Emergency department policies and procedures
Special skills for emergency physicians
  Communication
Summary

Developing and maintaining an effective working relationship between emergency physicians and the rest of the hospital medical staff can be a challenging experience. Nonetheless, substantial rewards can be gained from the effort. An aging population, a continuing move to outpatient medicine, an increasing number of uninsured patients, and a trend toward group practices have all contributed to an increased volume and an increased severity of illness of patients seen in emergency departments. Although these trends have placed an increased burden on emergency physicians, they have also provided them significant opportunities.

This chapter discusses some of the administrative and organizational skills needed to take full advantage of these opportunities (i.e., how emergency physicians can become more indispensable members of the medical staff). Such "indispensability" is in the eye of the beholder. Emergency physicians should strive to be viewed as indispensable by others, but avoid falling into the trap of viewing themselves that way.

BECOMING CLINICALLY INDISPENSABLE

Emergency medicine is in many ways a unique specialty. The rapid growth and assimilation of the specialty into the mainstream of organized medicine came about because emergency medicine filled a unique void in the healthcare system. The discipline's major strong point remains its ability to provide high quality care to large numbers of patients, regardless of medical condition, ability to pay, or time of presentation. Despite the sometimes extraordinary administrative efforts expended by emergency physicians, the foundation of the specialty, and thus, our relationships with the medical staff, still lie with our critical role as members of the healthcare team.

Practicing emergency medicine has often been likened to practicing medicine in a fishbowl. The emergency physician's methods, manners, and medical care are easily viewed by patients, families, hospital staff, hospital administration, and fellow medical staff members.

With this burden however, comes an opportunity. The emergency department fishbowl not only allows others to see in, but allows the emergency physician to see out. From this vantage point, emergency physicians often know the strengths and weaknesses of the entire medical community. Continuous interaction with prehospital care providers, private physicians, hospital-based medical specialists, and hospital departments such as radiology, surgery, laboratory, and admitting allows the emergency physician to identify opportunities for improvement. Knowledge is power. Because healthcare is moving from traditional methods of quality assurance to a strategy of total quality management, the positive use of this knowledge can substantially improve patient care, allowing the emergency physician to gain respect in the eyes of the hospital medical staff and administration.

BECOMING ADMINISTRATIVELY INDISPENSABLE

Hospitals and hospital medical staffs are complex organizations that require tremendous energy to keep them running efficiently and effectively. Once emergency physicians are viewed as clinically indispensable to the institution, they can then focus on becoming perceived as administratively indispensable as well.

Hospitals frequently add new departments or services to provide improved care to their communities. These new services often require medical input and direction. This need creates a void that can often be effectively filled by skilled emergency physicians. Examples of such services include medical educational programs, prehospital care systems, poison control centers, air medical systems, ambulatory care centers, ACLS/BCLS/ATLS/APLS/PALS education, disaster management, research programs, medical coverage of sporting or fitness events, and community educational programs.

Providing medical direction to such programs serves a number of useful purposes. Emergency physicians are often the most knowledgeable members of the medical staff with regard to the subject matter involved in these programs and thus provide the most authoritative input about program organization and operation. These high profile positions allow the emergency physician to become more visible to the hospital administration, medical staff, and community. This visibility allows the physician's talents, perhaps previously unrecognized, to be acknowledged and appreciated. Finally, medical directors must work closely with members of the medical staff from various specialties, allowing cooperative interaction between the emergency physician and other influential staff members. An effective way to foster stronger medical staff relationships is by being a contributing team player (and especially by being the team captain).

Keep in mind, of course, that until a positive reputation as an administrative leader has been developed, the emergency physician may have to actively pursue such positions. Once the reputation has been established, however, the physician may not need be so proactive, and indeed, may have to pick and choose from numerous opportunities.

MEDICAL STAFF ORGANIZATION

Bylaws

Hospital medical staffs are complex social organizations. The emergency physician should understand both the formal and informal makeup of the medical staff and become an integral part of it.

Today's medical staff structure and the relationship between the medical staff and the hospital were developed early in the twentieth century. Leaders of the American College of Surgeons were vocal in seeking improvements in patient care[1] and in 1919 published a one page *Minimum Standard for Hospitals*.[2]

From these recommendations emerged the organized hospital medical staff. The organized medical staff was envisioned as a patient-protective mechanism to ensure the community of dependable medical care and was governed by rules and regulations adopted "with approval of the governing board of the hospital."[2] The hospital's governing board became legally and ethically compelled to safeguard patients, and its relationship with the organized medical staff became the primary mechanism for fulfilling this social contract.

The now traditional two bylaw model for hospitals (corporate bylaws and medical staff bylaws) evolved from this relationship between the governing board and the organized medical staff. The hospital's ownership and governance are defined by corporate bylaws. Through provisions of that document, the organized medical staff is named and created. As frequently occurs, tradition has become law, so that today a hospital cannot be licensed by the state[3] or accredited by the Joint Commission on Accreditation of Healthcare Organizations (JCAHO)[4] without an organized medical staff.

The medical staff is a legal entity that is formally defined and governed by a set of medical staff bylaws that supplement the hospital's corporate bylaws. The medical staff bylaws define not only the structure of the medical staff, but the rights and responsibilities of its members. Bylaws usually cover topics such as departmental structure, medical staff committee structure, election of officers, dues, meeting attendance requirements, credentialling and privileging, physician quality/performance assessment, and fair hearing mechanisms. Moreover, bylaws are not static documents; they can and should be changed as the organization grows and matures.

Tedious as it may seem, every physician should become familiar with the medical staff bylaws. These bylaws are analogous to the rules of a game. Just as it is difficult to participate in a game without knowing the rules, it is difficult to fully participate in a medical staff organization without understanding its bylaws. Unfortunately, ignorance does not grant immunity from being governed. In practice, a lack of thorough knowledge of the medical staff bylaws is really an abdication of power.

Hospital Committee Structure

The structure of the organized medical staff is usually defined by several standing committees. These committees carry out the day to day responsibilities of the medical staff in overseeing the quality of patient care. Although organizational structures and committee names/roles may vary somewhat among institutions, these committees usually include a medical executive committee, a credentials committee, a quality committee, a pharmacy and therapeutics committee, and a medical records committee. In addition ad hoc task forces may be appointed, as needed.

The medical executive committee's membership is defined by the medical staff bylaws and usually includes the chief-of-staff, the chief-of-staff elect, departmental chair, and assorted members at large. Its functions are to oversee the work of other medical staff committees and to report to the hospital board.

The credentials committee's membership usually includes the chief-of-staff, the chief-of-staff elect, and other established leaders of the medical staff, as defined in the medical staff bylaws. Its function is to recommend the appointments and privileges of medical staff members to the hospital board and in some institutions to set the minimum criteria for credentialling in a given area.

The quality committee usually includes departmental and/or divisional quality assurance officers, as well as nonphysician representation from nursing, respiratory care, radiology, medical records, and other clinical departments. Representation from centralized quality-related hospital departments, if any, may also be included. Its function is to develop quality indicators, review clinical data and outcomes, and report its findings to the medical executive committee or the hospital governing board.

The pharmacy and therapeutics committee usually consists of physicians appointed by the chief-of-staff, as well as representatives from pharmacy, nursing, and other applicable hospital departments. Its functions include maintaining and updating the hospital formulary and reviewing drug utilization patterns and adverse drug reactions.

The medical records committee usually includes physicians appointed by the chief-of-staff, as well as representatives from the medical records department, nursing, and other clinical departments. Its function is to establish and monitor compliance with rules and regulations pertaining to hospital records.

Various ad hoc task forces may be appointed as needed. Their membership and function are usually determined by the chief-of-staff.

Although participation in these committees is time consuming and can be tedious, the long-term value of emergency physician participation is considerable. Emergency department interests are more likely to be represented in hospital policy when emergency physicians are active in these committees. Emergency physicians' status will increase when they actively participate in medical staff affairs. Finally, committee participation is an opportunity for emergency physicians to "pay their dues," allowing them to rise through the ranks of the medical staff hierarchy. Committee participation is usually necessary before an individual is appointed committee chair or gains sufficient support to be elected to a medical staff leadership position, such as chief-of-staff. Even if such positions are not an ultimate goal, the collegiality of working with other physicians toward a common goal can build beneficial bridges for the individual emergency physician and the department as a whole.

EMERGENCY DEPARTMENT ORGANIZATION

The nature of the contractual relationship between emergency physicians and the hospital, although often not under the direct control of the individual emergency physician, can directly affect relations with the rest of the medical staff. Human nature dictates that people are most comfortable with the familiar, and acceptance by the medical staff generally occurs most readily when emergency physicians have contractual relationships most similar to their own. Thus physicians employed by remote contracting groups may be viewed as outsiders, and hospital-employed physicians may not be accepted as peers by medical staff in private practice. A medical staff predominantly made up of private practitioners are most likely to accept emergency physicians who belong to a local group of incorporated emergency physicians who bill independently for their services.

Regardless of the service arrangement between the emergency physicians and the hospital, the most important factor leading to good working relationships between emergency physicians and the rest of the medical staff remains an organized, efficient emergency department with established policies that deal with common problems. The rest of this section describes the important components of these policies.

Departmental Status

Independent departmental status within the institution is extremely important. Departmental status symbolically puts emergency medicine on equal ground with other clinical disciplines and allows the emergency department medical director to sit on the medical executive committee and have a direct voice and vote on this high ranking medical staff committee. Independent departmental status within medical schools is an equally laudable but separate goal. University hospitals and their associated medical schools usually have separate organizational structures, and it is not uncommon for emergency medicine to have full departmental status within the hospital, but sectional or divisional status within the university.

Medical Director/Department Chair

Regardless of specific title, this individual needs to be an excellent and respected clinician with good leadership, organizational, administrative, and communication skills. The medical director not only works closely with the emergency department administrative staff, nursing staff, and ancillary personnel, but represents the department to the rest of the medical staff and hospital administration.

Emergency Department Nursing Director

The nursing director also needs excellent clinical and administrative skills. This individual represents the emergency department when dealing with other clinical departments and should feel comfortable communicating with medical staff physicians about issues concerning emergency department operations. The nursing director must set the tone for the professional performance of the emergency department nursing staff.

Emergency Department Quality Committee

Whether labeled quality assurance or continuous quality improvement, this committee should be composed of full-time emergency physicians and nurses and is primarily concerned with monitoring and improving patient care. This committee is often chaired by the medical director, although some departments designate a separate physician to fill this role.

Emergency Department Policies and Procedures

To improve long-term relations between emergency physicians and the rest of the medical staff, it is important to establish a comprehensive and widely understood set of policies that cover frequently occurring or high-risk situations.

Admittedly, short-term friction between disciplines may increase by directly and openly discussing points of disagreement and conflict. However, the long-term benefits of avoiding frequent night-time telephone squabbles and resultant simmering resentment are substantial and more than worth the initial effort.

Appropriate issues for such policies may be identified by any physician, nurse, or administrator who deals with the emergency department. These policies frequently address the following:

- Notification of medical staff physicians of their patients' presence in the emergency department
- Handling of managed care patients
- Telephone narcotic orders
- Notification of medical staff physicians of abnormal test reports on discharged patients
- On-call lists, including admitting responsibilities for patients without physicians
- Responsibilities for writing admitting orders
- Restricted procedures
- Expected response times for consultants
- Referral of patients to specialists

Many of these potential conflicts stem from the presentation, evaluation, treatment, and referral of "private" patients in the emergency department. Understandably, physicians responsible for follow-up care or who have gatekeeping responsibilities under managed care plans have a special interest in the emergency department care of their patient. However, this interest must be carefully balanced with the care that is determined appropriate by the treating emergency physician.

Thus departmental policies dealing with these issues should be proactively developed by representatives of all interested parties and ultimately approved by the appropriate hospital authority. The existence and dissemination of these written policies should give all concerned individuals a clear understanding of what is expected when a controversial situation arises. The American College of Emergency Physicians (ACEP) has adopted and published policy statements that relate to many of these issues. Reference to these positions papers can be quite useful and influential when dealing with (and educating) the medical staff regarding these issues.

Medical staff responsibility for emergency department patients[5] outlines medical staff responsibilities about the availability and timeliness of consultant and follow-up services, as well as the circumstances under which private physicians care for patients in the emergency department. Other ACEP Policy Statements address the responsibilities for writing admission orders,[6] telephone orders,[7] procedures with regard to the care of managed care patients,[8] and emergency physicians' patient care responsibilities outside the emergency department.[9]

SPECIAL SKILLS FOR EMERGENCY PHYSICIANS

Communication

Emergency physicians should be skilled in keeping the lines of communication open to the rest of the medical staff. This goal can be accomplished through both verbal and written methods.

Emergency physicians should regularly interact face-to-face with as many medical staff members as possible. Whether termed "schmoozing" or the more fashionable "networking," such interactions with other physicians in the emergency department, cafeteria, staff lounge, or at committee meetings or social events can build valuable and beneficial relationships for the emergency physician.

Telephone communication with physicians about the care of their patients in the emergency department is another important form of verbal communication. A thoughtful telephone call about a patient who needs office follow-up or referral to a specialist, or has had an abnormal test result return after discharge is good medical care and simple common courtesy, and it reflects a caring, conscientious attitude.

A further use of telephone communication is "rumor control." An informal telephone call to a physician rumored to be unhappy with the emergency department can often prevent a minor problem from blossoming into a major one.

Written communication also provides an effective bridge between the emergency department and the rest of the medical staff. Memos or newsletters to the medical staff can efficiently keep them informed of new emergency physicians or new policies that may affect them. It is also wise to send follow-up letters to medical staff members documenting verbal agreements. This practice will ensure that both individuals have the same understanding of the outcome and will provide a written reference if the problem should recur.

Dictated, transcribed emergency department records, along with a reliable and timely method of delivering them to the medical staff, is (in our anecdotal experience) one of the most effective ways that emergency physicians can improve their medical staff relationships. Typed, legible emergency department records make life much easier for the medical staff and, by their very appearance, portray the emergency care delivered as being professional and of high quality.

Other valuable communication skills for emergency physicians are the abilities to make effective group presentations and to conduct efficient committee meetings. Both skills enable the emergency physician to more effectively represent the emergency department's interests to the medical staff.

SUMMARY

Strong medical staff relationships are based on both clinical and administrative factors. Emergency medicine's rapid growth in size and stature has occurred primarily because of the provision of high quality care to an underserved population in the healthcare system. Clinical excellence has always been our strongest bond with our medical staff colleagues.

Close behind this clinical strength is the ability to be an administratively contributing member of the medical staff. A hospital and its medical staff require an enormous amount of energy to function effectively. By understanding the structure and needs of the medical staff, emergency physicians can position themselves as key organizational players. The contribution of time and knowledge to committees, the provision of medical director services, and the development of emergency department policies are all ways that emergency physicians can simultaneously improve patient care and medical staff relations.

REFERENCES

1. Codman EA: The product of a hospital, *Surg Gynecol Obstet* 118:491-496, 1914.
2. The *minimum standard for hospitals,* Chicago, 1919, American College of Surgeons.
3. Thompson RE, Haddad L: *The medical staff organization: 1990's answers to twenty tough questions,* Dallas, 1990 TMA.
4. *The accreditation manual for hospitals (AMH),* 1993 Edition, Governing Body Standard GB. 1.2.6., Oakbrook, Ill, 1993, JCAHO.
5. *Medical staff responsibility for emergency department patients,* Dallas, June, 1993, American College of Emergency Physicians.
6. Writing admission orders, *Ann Emerg Med* 19:599, 1990.
7. *Telephone orders in the emergency department,* Dallas, 1992, American College of Emergency Physicians.
8. *Managed health care plans and emergency care,* Dallas, 1993, American College of Emergency Physicians.
9. *Emergency physicians' patient care responsibilities outside of the emergency department,* Dallas, 1992, American College of Emergency Physicians.

94 Marketing and Outreach

Richard V. Aghababian and Gregory A. Volturo

OUTLINE

Marketing technique
Outreach services

Increasing competition for patients, budgetary constraints, and a greater expectation for optimal patient outcome have inspired hospitals to market services and to seek out new ways to reach their customers. The marketing of emergency services has become a viable means to increase a hospital's market share of its service area. Patients who have a positive experience in the emergency department frequently will continue to use the hospital for other services. The emergency department is the "hospital's window to the public," and a high quality emergency department will enhance the image of the hospital in the community. Furthermore, higher emergency department volumes will generally increase the hospital's inpatient census, as a percentage of emergency department patients will require admission to the hospital.

The key to developing an effective marketing strategy is to define a product line (service) or several product lines that can be offered in your emergency department. Service development or department expansion should be guided by customer demand. Specific community needs can be addressed with specific programs (e.g., sports medicine, occupational medicine). In designing a product line, one needs to view the service from a patient's perspective. Patients prefer services that are close to home, with convenient hours of operation, little or no waiting time, and low out of pocket cost. In addition, patients tend to have confidence in physicians based on past positive experiences or their perceived reputation. Basic marketing principles in emergency medicine are essentially the same as in any other business. The four "Ps" of marketing are product development, price structure, place service is offered, and promotion.[1]

MARKETING TECHNIQUE

In developing an emergency department marketing plan, consideration should be given to the overall marketing plan of the hospital. The emergency department marketing plan should follow and enhance the marketing plan of the hospital and should be flexible so that revisions can be made after it is implemented or as the hospital plan changes.

In writing a marketing plan, several key elements must be included (Box 94-1). The plan should begin with an introduction. This section should include the reasons for starting the marketing process. A complete description of the new service to be provided or the old service to be promoted also should be included in this area of the plan. At this point, it is also important to identify the members of the marketing committee, as well as the structure and terms of the committee. The marketing committee should consist of members from the emergency department, medical and nursing staff, the emergency department medical director and nurse manager, hospital administration, and public relations/marketing department.

The second element of a marketing plan is the situation analysis. All other phases of marketing depend on a thorough and accurate analysis of data. The first task is to identify the customers or target audience of the program being marketed (e.g., patients, physicians, industry, etc.) and to consider all actual and potential markets. One must then view the patient as a potential customer of the service to be offered. Customers needs and preferences are identified and the demand for the service determined. The strengths and weaknesses of the emergency department should be identified, including the physical plant as viewed from a patient's perspective. The type of professional services being offered (e.g., full-service emergency department, obstetrics, pediatrics, trauma, etc.) and the product lines within the scope of your professional services also should be identified.

A thorough look at the competition within the service area is also necessary at this time. Their strengths and weaknesses, costs, and the resources they use should be learned. Included in the assessment of competitors are ambulatory services offered at your hospital, local physicians' offices, and home maintenance organizations, as well as similar services offered by other hospitals. The medical staff should be surveyed about their needs and perception of the service that is to be marketed. In addition, patients, community members, industry, emergency medical services (EMS), and all other sources of referrals or potential customers should be surveyed.

Next, it is important to assess the business environment. The cost, resources needed, legal constraints, and all anticipated sources of revenue should be estimated. Review patient demographics, payor mix, patient records, and emergency department log books should be assessed potential volume. The population of the service area, their geographic distribution, and the overall emergency department trends for the previous 3 to 5 years, should be determined as well as the emergency department volume at the hospital and at competing hospitals. From this information, the percentage of market share can be calculated and the goals by which the progress of the marketing initiative will be judged can be determined. In addition, the percentage of emergency department patients who are actually seen by the emergency physicians and the patient acuity level should be determined. To further determine revenue, the emergency physician pay structure, average patient charge, and overall emergency department collection rate are reviewed.

BOX 94-1

KEY ELEMENTS OF THE EMERGENCY DEPARTMENT MARKETING PLAN

I. Introduction
   1. Identify need
   2. Identify members of the marketing committee
   3. Define structure of the committee
   4. Identify service which is to be marketed
II. Situation Analysis
   1. Identify customer needs and preferences
   2. Review data regarding your hospital and program
   3. Review data regarding external forces and competition
   4. Assess business environment
III. Design
   1. Develop marketing objectives
   2. Develop marketing strategies
   3. Develop a time table and assign responsibilities
   4. Develop budget
IV. Promotion
   1. Public relations
   2. Advertisement
   3. Educational programs
V. Evaluation
   1. An evaluation plan for each strategy should be established
VI. Summary

In the design phase of a marketing plan, marketing objectives are outlined and strategies are developed. Marketing goals and a timetable should be established to meet goals. All objectives should first be presented to and discussed with the marketing team. Objectives should be stated in quantifiable terms (e.g., target volume and time frame) and should be capable of being supported by a specific marketing strategy. Strategies should be established to enable the attainment of marketing objectives and the identification of the individual who is responsible for execution of each strategy. Finally, a marketing budget must also be developed that allows sufficient funds to complete each strategy. The emergency director must take a central role in the strategic planning process as it relates to marketing objectives. It is also the director's responsibility to enlist the support of the emergency department physician staff and convince them that their participation is worthwhile. The emergency department director should also serve as a liaison to the hospital's medical staff, enlisting their support for the marketing program.

The next phase of marketing is the promotion of the service or services being offered. Promotional activities inform the customer of the available services. These activities can be as broad as the imagination and budget will allow and includes activities such as advertising, public relations, direct mail campaigns, special events, brochures, and education of emergency department user groups. The most important advertising, however, is person-to-person contact in the emergency department. The interaction of the patient and all hospital and physician staff must be positive. The patient's first impression of the department must be designed to be a good impression. It is the responsibility of the emergency department director and nurse manager to counsel their respective staff to have a positive attitude to all patients. In addition, standards should be established to ensure that the appearance of both the physician and nursing staff is always neat and professional.

The development of educational programs for the general public may introduce the hospital, as well as the services offered, to potential patients (see Appendix A). Patients tend to use hospitals where they feel comfortable or have familiarity. Orienting potential customers to an emergency department program when they are not in need of service will keep the hospital in their minds when an actual need arises. Programs such as cardiopulmonary resuscitation training, emergency medical technician (EMT) training, skiing safety, and baby sitting may meet some of the marketing needs of the emergency department, as well as provide a worthwhile community service. Other activities that may introduce the service to new patients include free blood pressure checks and cholesterol screening, radio call-in shows, or other public education and information venues.

Patient follow-up calls solidify existing patient relationships and potentially prevent spreading bad reviews from dissatisfied patients. Although it is difficult to provide follow-up calls to all patients who present to a busy emergency department, if funding and staff permit, follow-up calls can be made to patients with select diagnoses and those who may have had a problem in the department and were dissatisfied with their service. This is not only a good public relations tool, but also may be rewarding to emergency department staff by providing some follow-up information and benefit to the patient by reinforcing follow-up instructions.[2,3]

The use of the media to promote the service should also be considered. Direct advertising in local newspapers, television, or radio may be beneficial. Advertising the service in conjunction with the provision of a public service announcement on radio or television may be more acceptable. The emergency department director could provide weekly or monthly articles to a local newspaper discussing topics such as sprains, back injury, and pediatric fever, which may also promote services at the hospital. Directly addressing the business community by offering special services for business customers, such as drug screening and workers compensation evaluation, may also promote the services to a new patient population.

Establishing communication with local physicians, healthcare groups, and other healthcare providers is another important facet of emergency department marketing, which may lead to increased referrals for services that the department provides. An emergency department newsletter to hospital staff may educate the medical staff about services available in the emergency department, as well as promote overall better relations with other departments. A routine call-back system to alert physicians of the status of their patients after they have been evaluated in the emergency department not only promotes continuity of care, but prevents misunderstandings between the emergency department physicians and the hospital medical staff. The rapid delivery of a copy of the emergency department medical record either by fax or mail is well received by all healthcare providers and may promote increased referrals.

The last phase of a marketing plan is the evaluation phase. An evaluation system for each strategy should be established to measure the attainment of goals. The evaluation should include follow-up with the customer to determine that their needs are being met. In addition, monitoring patient complaints, turnaround times, left-without-being-seen patients, and the payor mix can be useful. A patient satisfaction survey also may be helpful to evaluate success. In addition the competition's response to the marketing plan should be monitored. During this phase the marketing plan should be reassessed and modified as needed.

OUTREACH SERVICES

Identification of local market niches enables the hospital to focus efforts on product lines that are in most demand and most profitable. Outreach services not only potentially increase patient volume in the emergency department, but also may result in an increase in inpatient admissions for the hospital.

Marketing of fast track services, for example, can be rewarding to the hospital and the emergency department. An emergency department fast track offers an alternative for patients to obtain convenient medical care for minor injuries and illnesses. It may supplement care, which is usually rendered in the regular physician's office, during hours when the office is closed or when the office is too busy, and should be marketed to patients, physicians, and insurers for this purpose. Fast track services should also offer reduced cost to patients and insurers, making them an attractive alternative to the traditional emergency department. If the hospital serves a large pediatric population, it may be advantageous to separate pediatric and adult fast track services. Offering pediatric specific fast track services staffed with pediatric nurses and physicians experienced in pediatric care is attractive to parents and referring pediatricians, which may allow this area to flourish on its own (see Chapter 90).

If the community already has free-standing urgent care centers, networking with these centers may be a better alternative than competing with them. An agreement with an urgent care center to treat patients who need a higher level of service can be positive for both the urgent care center and the hospital.

The establishment of specialty emergency departments may offer a unique niche for the hospital, establishing it as a referral center for other hospitals and as a center of excellence to the public. If the hospital is equipped and prepared to care rapidly for patients with specific problems such as stroke, chest pain, burn care, pediatric emergencies, psychiatric emergencies, or geriatric medicine, the designation of specific space and staff to establish a speciality emergency department may be an excellent marketing tool. However, if a speciality service is marketed, it must truly be provided. For example, in establishing a chest pain emergency department, a cardiologist must be immediately available to the emergency physician, and technologies such as bedside echocardiogram, hemodynamic monitoring, and thrombolytics must be available in the emergency department.

Establishment of a trauma center at the hospital may elevate the stature of the hospital in the community and surrounding referral areas. Patients who are referred there for trauma services may continue to use the service after their initial exposure to the hospital. The establishment of a trauma center, however, is costly and requires the total commitment of the hospital administration, medical staff, and the regional EMS system.

Emergency department-based toxicology services can be a bonus for both the hospital and the emergency department. Ideally, at least one-board certified medical toxicologist should be on staff, and comprehensive toxicology laboratory services should be available. Promoting the service to other hospitals and also directly to patients will increase direct emergency department volume, as well as inpatient admissions, particularly to critical care areas.

Emergency transportation services offer another option to promote the emergency service at the hospital. Patients may associate the use of an ambulance with the institution. In addition, emergency transportation services may allow the hospital to provide a community service if the community does not have a dedicated professional emergency transportation service. These services not only include ground ambulance transportation, but also emergency helicopter transportation and low acuity "medi-van" transportation services. Generally, most of these transportation services can be staffed with paramedics and EMTs; however, with helicopter transport, where there may be a significant amount of interhospital transportation business, having a physician as part of the flight team may be better received by customers.

Other programs that may also promote emergency services include services such as school support services, occupational medicine and worker compensation services, adolescent services, travelers services, sports injuries, and the provision of routine urgent care, which may be enhanced by adding specific space, equipment, and staff. Physician referral services and courtesy service for staff physicians may also promote the emergency department, as well as improve relationships between the emergency department and the hospital medical staff. Preferred patient registration programs, in which patients complete a form with critical information to allow immediate treatment, which is kept on file in the emergency department, may help introduce patients to the emergency service before it is actually needed. Finally, hospitality programs for the emergency department staff to aid in improving their skills in dealing with the public may be one of the most important facets of your marketing plan.

Marketing, once unknown in medicine, has become a necessary survival strategy in the rapidly changing healthcare environment. If approached in an organized and stepwise fashion, marketing can be rewarding for all involved.

REFERENCES

1. Mayer TA, Tilson W, Hemingway J: Marketing and public relations in the emergency department, *Emerg Med Clin North Am* 5(1):83-102, 1987.
2. Chande VT, Exum V: Follow-up phone calls after an emergency department visit, *Pediatrics* 93(3):513-514, 1994.
3. Shesser R, Smith M, Adam S, Walls R, Paxton M: The effectiveness of an organized emergency department follow-up system, *Ann Emerg Med* 15(8):911-915, 1986.

ADDITIONAL READINGS

Berl RL, Hooper R, Sweeney RE: Product lines in a hospital emergency room, *J Ambul Care Mark* 2(2):9-34, 1988.

Buschiazzo L: Marketing the emergency department, *Nurs Manage* 16(9):30B-30D, 1985.

Cardello DM: Implementation of a one-hour fast-track service: one hospital's experience, *J Emerg Nurs* 18(3):239-243, 1992.

Cole G, Brown C: Product-line management: concept to reality, *Top Health Care Financ* 14(3):62-75, 1988.

Frank IC: Marketing the emergency department, *Nurs Manage* 16(4):10-11, 1985.

Nelson LJ, Staebell SL, Cooper JW: Marketing and public relations for the emergency department. In van de Leuv JH, editor: *Management of emergency services* Rockville, Md, 1987, Aspen.

Ramsey FE: *Marketing emergency services,* Dallas, 1986, American College of Emergency Physicians.

van de Leuv JH: Public relations in the emergency department. In van de Leuv, editor: *Management of emergency services,* Rockville, Md, 1987, Aspen.

Vestal KW: Marketing concepts for the emergency department, *J Emerg Nurs* 10(5):174-276, 1984.

Widra LS, Fottler MD: Survival of the hospital emergency department: strategic alternatives for the future, *Health Care Manage Rev* 13(3):73-893, 1988.

APPENDIX

A Public Relations/Patient Information Available from the American College of Emergency Physicians

I. Patient Brochures/Handouts
   1. Medicine's Frontline Folder
      Emergency Physicians as Medicine's Frontline
   2. Home Organizer for Medical Emergencies
   3. Frontlines Newsletter
      Current Topics in Emergency Medicine
   4. What You Should Know about Emergency Care
      Recognizing, Preparing For and Handling of Emergencies
   5. Public Education Handouts
      When to Call an Ambulance
      Home Safety Checklist
      Travel First Aid Kit, etc.

II. Public Service Announcements
   1. TV: Chest Pain, Drunk Driving, and Emergency Medicine
   2. Radio: Preventing Child Abuse, Warning Signs of a Medical Emergency, How to Call For Help, Low Back Pain

III. Feature Columns
   Warning Signs of a Medical Emergency, Safety Tips for Travel, Sore Throat, Why Work Out? Prevention Keeps Kids Safe

Call ACEP Public Relations at 202-728-0610 for full catalog.

PART TEN

Prehospital Care

95 Emergency Medical Services Systems:

AN EMERGENCY PHYSICIAN'S GUIDE TO ACQUISITION AND ENHANCEMENT

John C. Johnson

OUTLINE

EMERGENCY MEDICAL SERVICES SYSTEM DEFINED

Historical Perspectives

In 1965, accidents became the leading cause of death among persons under 37 years of age and the fourth leading cause of death in all age groups in the United States. Motor vehicles (cars, trucks, and motorcycles) were the leading cause of death among those under 75 years old. A total of 107,000 persons died from accidents that year[1] (Box 95-1).

One in four Americans, more than 52 millions persons, were injured in accidents; 4% of them required hospitalization. They averaged 11 days per admission and occupied 65,000 beds, 1 in every 8 beds occupied that year. These 22 million bed days exceeded those required by cardiac patients and were more than four times the bed days required by cancer patients that year.[1]

This information was published by the National Academy of Science/National Research Council in the 1966 report, *Accidental Death and Dying: the Neglected Disease of Modern Society.* As a result the Eighty-Sixth Congress adopted the Highway Safety Act of 1966 (Title 23, U.S.C.). The intent of this law and its application are perhaps best expressed in the report of the House Committee on Public Works:

> When accidents occur, it is essential that every available resource be mobilized to save lives, lessen the severity of injuries, protect property, and restore movement of traffic. An essential part of the State safety program should be the development (an) of emergency facilities system. This will require the advice and services of experts and personnel in medicine,* [1]law, engineering, communications and law enforcement, as a minimum.[2]

The law authorized the Secretary of Transportation to develop a comprehensive Highway Traffic Safety Program, which would serve as a guide to states developing their own programs. Although the word "guide" was used, participation and compliance with the Highway Safety Program guidelines ensured that states would *not* have their federal highway funds reduced in future years. The *Highway Safety Program Manual* consisted of 19 volumes of guidelines. Only one, Volume 11, *Emergency Medical Services,* dealt with medical care.[3]

Although the thrust of the program was obviously directed at the reduction of lives lost on the nation's highways, the program was not totally myopic. Within the pages of Volume 11, *Emergency Medical Services,* it was recognized that support for the victims of highway accidents is only one of several demands placed on an Emergency Medical Services (EMS) system and, as such, the program outline attempted to provide States with enough flexibility to design their EMS system to meet their particular state, regional, and local needs.[3] The Federal initiative was not designed to simply provide an ambulance, but rather to provide a *system* of medical care.

The system guidelines designed by the Department of Transportation/National Highway Traffic Safety Administration (DOT/NHTSA) defined three objectives for States:

1. To provide prompt identification and response to crashes under a range of emergency conditions.
2. To sustain and prolong life through proper first aid and emergency care measures, both at the scene and in transit.
3. To provide the coordination, transportation, and communications necessary to bring the injured person and definitive medical care together in the shortest practicable time, without simultaneously creating additional hazards."[3]

DOT/NHTSA provided not only the threat of a loss of general federal highway funding, but, under Section 402 of Title 23, the opportunity for states to obtain funds for EMS system development, resulting in both punitive and carrot-and-stick motivation.

States responded to the initiative at varying rates and to varying degrees, with California adopting the first act

*Please note the inclusion of "medicine".

BOX 95-1

ACCIDENTAL DEATH—1965: THE IMPETUS FOR EMERGENCY MEDICAL SERVICES IN THE UNITED STATES

Cause	*Deaths (%)*
Motor vehicle	49,000 (46%)
Home related	28,500 (27%)
Work related	14,100 (13%)
Miscellaneous	15,400 (14%)

From National Academy of Sciences, National Research Council: *Accidental death and disability: the neglected disease of modern society,* Washington, DC, 1966, NAS/NRC.

BOX 95-2

EMS SYSTEM COMPONENTS

Current	1973
1. Medical direction	nm
2. Protocols	nm
3. Financing	nm
4. Education	Training
5. Communication	Communication
6. Prehospital transport	Transportation
7. Interfacility transport	Patient Transfer
8. Receiving facilities	Emergency Facilities
9. Specialty care units	Critical Care Units
10. Dispatch	Access to Care
11. Public information, education	public information, education
12. Audit, quality assurance, continuous quality improvement	System review, evaluation
13. Disaster planning	Disaster planning
14. Mutual aid	Mutual aid
nm	Manpower
nm	Public safety agencies
nm	Consumer participation
nm	Standardized record keeping

From Roush WR, editor: *Principles of EMS systems: a comprehensive text for physicians,* American College of Emergency Physicians.
nm, Not mentioned.

(Wedworth-Townsend) promoting EMS and paramedics in 1970, which was signed by then Governor Ronald Reagan. In some parts of the country, grass roots efforts often predated state actions. Such early EMS development moved forward without the authorization or protection of law. William Grace, MD, Director of Medicine at St Vincent's Hospital (New York City), is credited with the first U.S. mobile intensive care unit (MICU). His program was modeled after J. Frank Pantridge's program in Belfast, Northern Ireland, which had begun in the early 1960s. Eugene Nagel, MD, brought telemetry on line from the streets of Miami, with a unit weighing a mere 54 pounds housed originally in a milk crate. J. Michael Criley, MD, (Los Angeles), John Suelzer, MD, (Indianapolis), and Leonard Cobb, MD, (Seattle) were all EMS pioneers in their respective urban centers. Ralph Feichter, MD, refused to believe that EMS was purely an urban phenomenon and began the first rural paramedic services in Haywood County, North Carolina.[4]

With this growing interest and demonstrated activity in prehospital care came a series of initiatives among medical professionals, which furthered the cause. The American College of Cardiology hosted the Sixth Bethesda Conference, Early Care of the Acute Coronary Patient, which focused in part on the prehospital needs of cardiac patients. The combined 1969 Arlie Conference of the American College of Surgeons and the American Academy of Orthopedic Surgeons (AAOS) heralded the successes of early EMS programs and promoted the continued expansion of EMS and EMS systems for the general welfare of U.S. citizens. As an offshoot of the American Medical Association's efforts in this regard, the National Registry of EMTs was formed in June 1970 in response to a President's Committee on Highway Safety recommendation to nationally standardize the certification and registration of prehospital personnel. The DOT developed a standardized training curriculum for EMS personnel in 1970, with the AAOS following quickly in 1971 with the first EMT text, *Emergency Care and Transportation of the Sick and Injured.* The first paramedic curriculum was later released in 1975. The 1972 National Conference on CPR and Emergency Cardiac Care highlighted the fact that 350,000 of 600,000 citizens dying of cardiac disease die *before* reaching the hospital. Momentum was building.

In November 1973, the Ninety-Third Congress passed the Emergency Medical Services Act (P.L. 93-154), which focused specifically on EMS systems development through the Department of Health, Education and Welfare (currently, Health and Human Services). Although not specifically designed to foster EMS activities, the Ninety-Third Congress later passed in 1974 the National Health Planning and Resources Development Act (P.L. 93-641), which helped promote a regional approach to EMS system development within state boundaries.

Although physicians (medicine) was referenced in the 1966 Public Works Committee Report and the efforts that heightened the awareness of the real and potential benefits of expanded EMS services were provided by physicians and physician organizations, the original 15 components of an EMS system as defined by the 1973 legislation failed to mention physician involvement (direction) in prehospital care. It was not until the 1981 National Research Council Report, *Medical Control in Emergency Medical Services Systems,* that the issue of medical control received its proper emphasis[5] (Box 95-2).[6]

Modern EMS System Components

A system of EMS can be as large or as small as it wishes to define itself. At one extreme is the isolated rural EMS service, with only one ambulance and several volunteer personnel who attempt to meet their local area's prehospital medical needs. Although remote, that singular service will usually need to rely on some other agency for dispatch (e.g., law enforcement or fire service), the local hospital for primary transport, a tertiary facility for transporting more complicated cases, coordination with civil defense or the Red Cross for disasters, or assistance from surrounding services. All of this requires that the isolated service either develop its own system for EMS or become part of a larger system. At the other extreme, a national EMS system provides for coordinated teams, such as the Disaster Medical Assistance Teams (DMAT), to respond to large-scale disasters as part of a National Disaster Medical Service (NDMS), which maintains linkages, structure, and levels of command in all 50 states.

On a state level, a State Emergency Medical Services or Emergency Management Agency is responsible for coordinating EMS activities within the state. Depending on the size and demographics of the state, it may be further subdivided into regions that generally will have natural catchment areas for EMS services related to receiving facilities (hospitals) and specialty care units (tertiary hospitals) or the transport modes used to access specialty care in the region. Indiana, for example, provides for a single statewide EMS system with state government, tertiary facilities, and transportation focused to the center of the state (Indianapolis). At the corners of the state, the closest major urban medical centers are in surrounding states. Thus, although the Indiana EMS System maintains coordination from Indianapolis, there is regional referral outside the state. In larger states, several regions may exist within the state, which provide for natural interaction, coordination, and transfer. Texas (Dallas, Houston, San Antonio) and California (Los Angeles, San Diego, San Francisco) are examples of this type of organization.

Regardless of their size and organization, *all* EMS systems need to address each of the 14 modern system components to be effective. In fact, every single EMS service within a larger EMS system should itself strive to address all 14 components.

Medical Direction. Prehospital care is medical care and, as such, should be under the control and licensure (certification) of a physician medical director. By law, all states require that advanced life support (ALS) level care is provided under the direction of a physician licensed in that state. Many states further require that care provided at the basic life support (BLS) level similarly have medical input and direction. At least one physician by law is then ultimately responsible for the patient care provided.

Generally, medical direction is divided into at least two categories: off-line medical control, and on-line medical direction.[7]

Off-line medical control is an administrative function wherein a physician is responsible for the development and ongoing monitoring and evaluation of the system, as well as the provision and continuous improvement of the care and service rendered to patients. In addition, off-line control has oversight responsibility for on-line direction. The role of off-line medical direction is embodied in several of the 14 components of a modern EMS system.

On-line direction is the interpersonal communication that occurs at the time of or immediately after a patient contact. Prehospital providers receive assistance and immediate feedback relative to the care that they are providing to a particular patient. On-line direction may be provided by a physician in direct communication or physical contact with the EMS personnel. If the communication function is delegated to another individual (e.g., nurse, paramedic), a physician retains responsibility for the quality and appropriateness of the communication and is ultimately responsible and liable for the actions of the delegated on-line personnel communicating with the prehospital providers.

Protocols. A protocol is a defined method or procedure for accomplishing a task. It can be as simple as a procedure for unlocking the ambulance door or as complicated as managing a traumatic cardiac arrest. Each service and in turn each EMS system has protocols that define, as a minimum, (1) dispatch procedures, (2) communications, (3) patient treatment, (4) transport or destination, and (5) quality assurance (QA) or continuous quality improvement (CQI) procedures. In addition, the service is likely to have protocols, or standard operating procedures, for the many administrative tasks required to keep the service running properly.

A subset of protocols related to patient treatment or medical care is often referred to as standing orders. The protocol defines the complete procedure for assessing or providing care and stabilization of a specific patient problem. The complete protocol is used for primary education, continuing education, and quality assurance. The portion of the protocol that the prehospital personnel are authorized to follow in the absence of on-line medical direction is referred to as *standing orders*. In a particular EMS system, a suspected cardiac patient, for example, may be sat upright, given oxygen, undergo electrocardiography and monitoring of vital signs, have a keep-open intravenous line of dextrose solution established, and may be transported to the nearest available hospital without prior communication with on-line medical direction. The use of nitroglycerin (sublingual or intravenous), opiates (meperidine or morphine), or inhalation analgesics (nitrous oxide), on the other hand, may be restricted to a direct physician order for each patient. In another system, the use of these medications maybe included in the standing orders. The protocol for suspected cardiac patients in either system is the same, but the standing orders vary based on the off-line medical director's treatment philosophy, confidence with the involved EMS personnel, and demographic considerations such as transport time and communication limitations.

Financing. Financing deals with the issue of paying for the service or system. Tax subsidy, user fees (fee-for-service), grants, and volunteerism in isolation or combination must be considered. The off-line medical director should be involved with financial planning decisions about the selection and purchase of patient care equipment and supplies, staffing patterns, and other factors that directly or indirectly affect patient care and also have a financial implication.

Education. Although EMS initially may have sought to train individuals to do a limited number of rote tasks, the current thrust of EMS is to educate healthcare professionals who can address the many service needs of the patients they encounter. Education can be divided into two levels: (1) primary education and (2) continuing education.

In the ideal EMS system, the off-line medical director is involved with the primary education of all personnel functioning under the physician's license. In reality, many systems frequently hire personnel trained elsewhere or do not have the resources to provide their own education and must rely on other systems or programs for the primary education of their personnel. In the case of hiring previously trained prehospital providers, the definition of education should include the evaluation of these potential incoming personnel as part of the hiring process. Knowledge and skills testing, a preceptorship, and a test to ensure understanding of local protocols should be a routine part of the hiring process. In the case of systems that contract for training technically outside of the system, an affiliation should be maintained to allow for the monitoring of the contracted primary education process by the medical leadership.

Continuing education should occur in all systems regardless of their source of primary education. Continuing education should be based on guidelines and desired outcomes within the system monitored through the system's continuous CQI program. ACLS may be repeated biannually to meet the standards adopted by the ACLS affiliate faculty or at some other frequency to meet local standards (hospital or EMS system). Rapid evaluation and transport of trauma patients could be emphasized quarterly to target achievement of an on-scene time standard established by local medical control to improve trauma patient outcomes. For example, barring the need for prolonged extrication, the goal may be to have all major trauma patients en route to the hospital in no more than 10 minutes from the time of arrival of EMS personnel at the scene. CQI monitoring may detect that children with respiratory distress become more compromised en route to the hospital. Assessment skills may need to be enhanced and treatment options discussed to improve the performance of the prehospital providers.

Communication. Communication is an important component of any EMS system, as it both facilitates patient care and interaction within the system at multiple levels. Communication begins with the ability of a victim or someone discovering a victim initially to contact a source for help. This is followed by dispatch (a separate component discussed later) where one or more units (ambulance or other primary response vehicle) or services (EMS, fire, law enforcement, rescue) are sent to meet the victim's immediate needs. Ongoing communication with the victim or the caller until help arrives takes on an increasingly important role today, providing BLS assistance until dispatched units arrive. Communication among the responding EMS units (one or more), law enforcement, fire service, and other public safety agencies is also crucial. Communication between the responding medical personnel and the hospital or on-line medical direction must be available. In a disaster situation, many additional public and private entities must be considered for inclusion in the EMS communication system.

Prehospital Transport. Once the patient has been discovered, response has occurred and care provided, a mechanism for transporting the patient (e.g., land vehicle, aeromedical) and defining a destination (e.g., nearest available facility, trauma center only, pediatric center) must be in place.

Interfacility Transport. In most systems throughout the United States, communities will not possess the hospital resources to meet the needs of every potential patient problem that can be encountered. Even if a community would normally have all resources at hand, at times, the resources may be used to capacity, and the patient must be moved to another facility. Given the mobility of individuals today, there may also be indications for transporting patients, once stable, to their or their healthcare payor's choice of facility. All of these examples require a mechanism to be in place, in advance, to facilitate the transfer of patients from one healthcare facility to another, whether proximate or remote. In addition, the system requires protocols or standards to dictate when and how the transfer shall be effected, communication between facilities, and the level of care and supervision present during the transfer.

Patient transfer should not be taken lightly. Federal law specifies the need for initial evaluation and stabilization, when possible, for all patients at the initial receiving facility before transport. Interfacility transport, when indicated, must then appropriately anticipate the patient's needs en route. Patient transfer is discussed in greater detail in Chapter 61.

Receiving Facilities. In general, the receiving facility will be a hospital emergency department that accepts ambulance patients. Although less common, nonhospital facilities in remote areas may serve a stabilizing role as part of an integrated healthcare system. In yet other areas, transport of specific types of patients may be directed away from hospital facilities to nonhospital healthcare entities. With current healthcare reform initiatives being discussed in Washington, D.C. and the board rooms of healthcare payors, business, and industry, alternative transport destinations can be anticipated more frequently. Transport, regardless of destination, should be defined by protocol. The capabilities of each type of facility that receives a patient should be defined by the system to ensure that a minimum level of care is present when the patient arrives. Without this standard, the care available in the back of the transport vehicle provided by prehospital personnel could exceed the capabilities of the facility agreeing to receive the patient.

Specialty Care Units. A facility that provides specialty care (e.g., cardiac, trauma, pediatric, obstetric, neonatal, burn, neurospinal, reimplantation) should also meet a minimum standard with regard to facilities, equipment, and personnel to qualify to receive patients transported by EMS services. Each system needs to define their specialty care needs and then arrange for the availability of that care, either within the system or through contractual arrangements with facilities outside of the region's normal geographic or catchment area.

Dispatch. Dispatch is more than mere verbal communications to send an ambulance. It must genuinely integrate the needs of all public safety agencies to provide for an ever present network to facilitate, in this case, the emergency medical needs of the community. Access to a dispatch center (e.g., Enhanced 911 or similar uniform number), protocols for a defined response to a given complaint or predicament (e.g., first responder, BLS, ALS, dual response, etc.), defined ancillary support services (e.g., extrication, fire suppression/prevention, traffic control, utility company assistance, etc.), assistance to the initial caller until arrival of rescue and emergency personnel, and CQI evaluation of the program concurrently and retrospectively all must become a part of a bona fide dispatch component of an EMS system.

Public Information and Education. At one time public information focused on educating citizens to access their local EMS services. In today's cost-conscious environment, the role of public information and education must share time with the appropriate access of emergency and other healthcare resources. Although prehospital services are often used as a taxi to a clinic or hospital, their appropriate, cost-effective use merit increasing devotion. Safety- and prevention-related education to minimize injuries and illness will take on a greater meaning to preserve resources and funding for those who unavoidably require a full EMS response.

Audit, QA, and CQI. The ultimate outcomes goal of an EMS system is to improve the life and livelihood of its citizens. Through proper application of the components of an EMS system and the ongoing assessment of the delivery of those components within the system, EMS can continually improve. CQI will in turn minimize the morbidity and mortality of the citizens who access the EMS system. Issues of patient care, dispatch time, on-scene times, adherence to protocols, use of resources, and location of resources are just a few of the areas worthy of monitoring and evaluation.

Disaster Planning. Even the community that will never have a hurricane, flood, train derailment, terrorist attack, or other national media event may experience a boiler explosion in the local school, a school bus accident, or a large passenger jet dropping in unannounced. In fact, a multiple vehicle accident may meet the definition of a disaster in many communities. A disaster occurs when an EMS system's resources are not sufficient to meet the patient care needs of an incident. As a result, alternative plans must be implemented to overcome the immediate problem. Disaster situations must be anticipated, contingency arrangements made and formalized, and the overall disaster plan practiced to maintain a state of readiness.

Mutual Aid. If every EMS system is viewed by its personnel and management as an island unto itself and the eventuality of a need for outside assistance is therefore never anticipated, the program can easily become overtaxed. A multiple victim accident or a fire with casualties may occur, which can be handled by existing system resources. The remaining citizens, however, who are normally served by those same EMS services may now be underserved. It is necessary to anticipate situations commonly thought to be less than disastrous in proportion. A mere shifting of resources from one system or service to a position closer to the boundaries of an overextended service may provide adequate coverage until the normal resources can be returned to service. A defined plan and contractual relationships, which can be easily activated in time of need, should be established as part of a system's planning.

ROLES AND RESPONSIBILITIES IN AN EMS SYSTEM

EMS Physician Medical Director

The physician should be cognizant of and involved in all phases of the development and ongoing administration of an EMS system. Given the obligations and demands placed on the schedules, business and personal, of most physicians involved with emergency medicine this omniscience is not always possible. The statement should stand, however, as the ideal. What the EMS system medical director must accomplish to be effective depends on the system, its resources, and the ability of the medical director to attract and retain personnel with whom he or she can work to accomplish the *medical* management of the system.

Medical management has been highlighted on purpose. Although some physicians may have the time, energy, and expertise to manage literally all aspects of an EMS system, in most cases this will not occur. The nonpatient care aspects should be managed by someone other than the medical director. The relationship between the physician and nonphysician-manager must be firm. An agreement should be reached in the beginning of the relationship, which should adhere to the following principles, in general:

> The physician Medical Director will be ultimately responsible and will have authority over all aspects of the system and the services provided within the system that deal with patient care.
>
> The administrative director will be ultimately responsible for have authority over all aspects of the system and services provided within the system which do not involve hands on patient care.
>
> The responsibility for any areas of the system or service which overlap will be jointly administered by the physician and non-physician manager. Components or services which are predominately patient oriented will be the ultimate responsibility of the physician director with strong input and consideration from the non-physician director. Components or services which are *not* predominately patient oriented will be the ultimate responsibility of the non-physician director with strong input and consideration from the physician director.
>
> The physician and the non-physician directors will establish their areas of responsibility and channels of communication and oversight at the beginning of their relationship. Neither party may unilaterally alter the agreement until both parties have an opportunity to meet and make appropriate, mutually acceptable modifications to the original principles governing their relationship.

Restated, the physician should be cognizant of and involved in all phases of the development and ongoing administration of an EMS system to include all 14 of the current components. The medical director should not take on this responsibility alone, however. To be effective as a medical director, to preserve time for business and family, and to retain one's sanity, the medical director must be willing and capable of effectively delegating (sharing) responsibilities with other individuals or groups of individuals. In addition to the personal benefits gained by such delegation, the EMS system will also benefit from the broader input and support that it receives. Risk or liability will also be shared, in the case of a committee, among a group of individuals whose collective wisdom will most likely be more compelling than a single individual's as it relates to the development of policy, standards, and performance expectations.

Table 95-1 lists the 14 modern components of an EMS system. Although the principles and components listed refer specifically to formal EMS systems, they may also be directly applied to individual services or subunits of a formal EMS system. The individual, either medical director or administrator, who should be ultimately responsible for that component or subcategory is listed. In several cases, the ultimate responsibility should be shared. In addition, suggestions for delegation to an individual or committee are referenced by superscript and defined below. As the reader becomes involved with an EMS system or service, the actual division of responsibilities between the medical director and the administrator and the involvement of other persons and committees will need to be defined based on the attributes of the system (service) and the persons involved. Table 96-1 is merely a point of reference. The medical director and the administrator of the EMS system should strongly consider developing and using these or similar resources.

Table 95-1 Division of Roles in an EMS System

Component	Subcategory	Ultimate responsibility
Medical direction	Off-line	Medical director*
	On-line	Medical director*
Protocols	Dispatch	Shared*
(Procedures)	Assessment	Medical director*
	Treatment	Medical director*
	Transport	Medical director*
	Operational	Administrator
Financing		Administrator
Education	Primary education	Medical director†
	Hiring assessment	Medical director†
	Continuing education	Medical director†
	Nonpatient care	Administrator
Communication	On-line	Medical director*
	Operational	Administrator
Prehospital transport	Patient related	Medical director*
	Vehicular	Administrator
Interfacility transport	Patient related	Medical director*
	Vehicular	Administrator
Receiving facilities	Qualifications	Medical director*,‡
	Designation	Medical director*,‡
	Destination	Medical director[a]
Specialty care units	Qualifications	Medical director*,‡
	Designation	Medical director*,‡
	Destination	Medical director*
Dispatch	Dispatch	Administrator
	Caller assistance	Medical director*
Public information, education	Content	Medical director*
	Delivery	Shared*
Audit, QA, CQI	Patient related	Medical director†
	Operational	Administrator
Disaster planning	Overall planning	Shared*§
	Patient related	Medical director*
	Facility involvement	Medical director*,‡
	Operational	Administrator
Mutual aid	Needs assessment	Shared*

*EMS medical advisory committee.
†EMS educational coordinator.
‡EMS facilities advisory committee.
§EMS hospital/community medical disaster committee.

EMS Medical Advisory Committee

The EMS Medical Advisory Committee (MAC) deals with patient care issues. It can be composed of physicians only or may include other healthcare professionals that interact with the prehospital personnel and their patients. In the case of systems with multiple hospitals, each emergency department should have the opportunity to send at least one physician representative (e.g., emergency department medical director) to serve as a voting member of the MAC. EMS educators, EMS administrators, emergency department nursing unit directors, emergency department nursing educators, specialty care unit physicians, or nursing managers who represent units that frequently interact with EMS (e.g., ICU/CCU for transfers, neonatal ICU, trauma service) are all considered for membership on the MAC.

It is extremely beneficial to include as members of the MAC several representatives of the EMS personnel (so called "street-wise medics") who are selected by vote of their nonmanagerial peers. The winners of this electoral process are generally experienced medics who are trusted by the other members of the service. This has been done successfully with the original intent of providing insight into the realities of "street medicine." It has also proven beneficial during the implementation phase of new protocols, policies, and procedures. These EMS representatives can accurately convey at a peer level the discussions that occurred in the MAC and the purpose of the new mandate, as well as their participation and input into the process. Although it is imperative that the EMS medical director has had firsthand experience with EMS personnel at the scene practicing "street medicine," it is unlikely that many of the other members of the MAC will have this perspective. Participation by these elected EMS personnel brings reality to the table during discussions.

The MAC may engage in discussions related to all of the components indicated with an asterisk in Table 96-1 or only those that the medical director determines to be appropriate.

The medical director, not the committee, retains ultimate responsibility for the defined component, but can share some of this responsibility and liability with the members. The goal is to delegate *some* of the authority to other appropriate involved individuals without abdicating responsibility. Certain members of the consolidated MAC may be inappropriate for all of the activities listed. It may be more efficient and effective to develop subcommittees or task forces within the MAC that focus on particular issues.

EMS Education Director

The EMS education director is an individual who is responsible for the development of curriculum, securing of resources and overall coordination of educational programs, both primary and continuing. The individual should have a strong background in prehospital care generally at the ALS level unless the system is only BLS and will always remain at the BLS level. Depending on the availability of physicians and other clinical instructors, the EMS education coordinator may be responsible for a portion of the teaching required within the system. The medical director, however, should participate to some degree as an instructor and an evaluator in the training programs.

The education director is also appropriate to evaluate, through written and skills testing, the applicants who seek a patient care position within the EMS system. The results of such evaluation will be coordinated with the medical director's interview and personal evaluation of the candidate. With education being directed by the system's protocols and continuing education being largely directed at issues discovered during QA/CQI activities, the education director is the appropriate person to manage the assessment activities as they relate to patient care and outcomes. In many systems, the administrator, medical director, and education director form the management team responsible for the system's structure, function, and overall performance.

EMS Facilities Committee

Depending on the size of the system, the number of medical facilities (e.g., hospitals, clinics) to which transport occurs and the medical/political arena in which the system must operate, it may be prudent to form an EMS facilities committee composed of appropriate representatives from the facilities within the region that interact with EMS. The facilities committee would adopt national criteria (e.g., American College of Surgeons Trauma System Guidelines [see Suggested Reading]), when they exist, or develop local criteria, which define the level of commitment necessary for a facility to participate within the EMS system. They must then design, when appropriate, or adopt a designation process to determine which facilities will be used and under what circumstances. In smaller EMS systems, the MAC may serve as an EMS facilities committee.

EMS Disaster Committee

The Joint Commission for the Accreditation of Healthcare Organizations requires the presence of a hospital disaster committee, which interacts with the community's disaster preparedness efforts. Although the EMS medical director retains ultimate authority for the EMS system's disaster program and response as it relates to patient care, much of the effort can be shared with the existing disaster preparedness program currently in place at the facility or within the community.

DEVELOPING A NEW SYSTEM VERSUS ENHANCING AN EXISTING SYSTEM

Developing a New EMS System

A new medical director for a system would need to develop a system from scratch in an area that (1) has no form of EMS currently available, or (2) has either just lost its EMS system entirely or has a system in such disrepair that it is best to start anew. Although either scenario is possible, it is unlikely that a new medical director will inherit such an area for development in the United States.

As mentioned earlier, the system components discussed are applicable to any size system. They are also applicable to a single service. A medical director may be asked to develop a new EMS service. Again, the principles and components outlined here should apply to both an individual EMS service and to an entire EMS system. In this case, it is quite likely that the new service will replace a prior service. For example, a for-profit service may cancel its contract or a municipal service can no longer fund its involvement through the tax base resulting in the impetus for a "new" EMS service.

This following outline assumes that the new system or service being developed will occur at a regional, county, or local level within an existing state EMS system.

Steps to Develop a New EMS System (Service)

1. Obtain and review copies of the following applicable documents, as a minimum:
   a. Current state code (law) applicable to EMS
   b. Current state administrative code (rules and regulations) applicable to EMS
   c. Current state EMS plan
   d. Current applicable credentialing (certification or licensure) criteria for EMS personnel (state-specific criteria or national registry of EMTs' standards, as appropriate)
   e. Guidelines for Emergency Medical Services Systems (see Appendix A)
   f. Standard Guide for Structures and Responsibilities of Emergency Medical Services Systems Organizations (ASTMF-1086-87).*
2. Understand fully the key components of each of the preceding documents as they apply to the system to be developed. Seek counsel from other physicians, either within the area or with appropriate expertise, if questions arise.
3. Meet with the state EMS or emergency management agency director and, if applicable, medical director to discuss state requirements, as well as any local history or perspective relative to the new system's development.
4. Determine the individuals who would be described as influential within the healthcare and lay community in which the system is to be developed.
5. Select the individual who is most influential, most inter-

*This document may be obtained directly from ASTM by writing or calling: ASTM, 1916 Race Street, Philadelphia, PA 19103; (215)299-5400.

ested, or who will stand to gain the most by the development of the EMS system and ask him or her to host a meeting of the key players delineated in paragraph four, above. The purpose of the meeting should be threefold:
a. Introductory (a chance to meet the key players),
b. Data gathering (learn what resources are available, their degree of availability, and the willingness of the key players to participate), and
c. Focus (Given the totality of system development contained in the 14 components, to which area or areas should the initial efforts be directed?)
6. Reaffirm the information gathered and the focus selected through the process described in paragraph five through one or more meetings with pivotal persons within the community (e.g., county commissioners, mayor, city council leaders, hospital emergency department director and administrator).
7. Obtain sponsorship from within the community for a meeting of all key individuals involved in the various components of an EMS system. The most influential players in paragraphs five and six along with the state EMS director and, if applicable, medical director, may serve on a panel seated at the front of the meeting room. Their presence will add credibility to your efforts, provide comments, and also serve as informational resources if questions arise about the authority or process.
   The purpose of this meeting is fivefold:
   a. Introductory (introduce yourself and the concept of system development)
   b. Focus (outline the initial focus established for the system development process)
   c. Support (gain support from the key players who must participate in the system's development and its ongoing administration and function)
   d. Commitment (establish committees that will oversee the development and implementation of the various components of the system)
   e. Time frame (establish a time frame for periodic reporting on achievements and completion of tasks)
8. Establish a steering committee consisting of the chairs of the various committees formed and several key players to share information, trouble shoot problems, and maintain momentum.
9. Schedule frequent meetings with the key players outlined in paragraphs five and six to keep them up to date on the progress of systems development, maintain their support, and seek guidance as problems occur.
10. Ultimately implement all 14 components of an EMS system as currently defined beginning with those priorities established during the initial meetings and subsequently expanded as the development process continues.

As obstacles are encountered, recognize that those same obstacles have probably been encountered by at least one other EMS system medical director, more likely many, over the years. Establish early on a networking environment among other medical directors within the region, state, and country. Although ego may try to dictate "I can do this myself," there is no need for self-sacrifice. Given the pioneer spirit in which EMS has developed in the United States, someone has probably already encountered the same or similar problem and will be quite free to discuss potential solutions and their merits. The state chapter of the American College of Emergency Physicians (ACEP), national ACEP and its section on Emergency Medical Services, the National Association of EMS Physicians (NAEMSP), National Association of State EMS Directors (NASEMSD), and the National Council of State EMS Training Coordinators (NCSEMSTC) are just a few of the available resources. See Appendix B for contact information regarding these and related organizations.

Enhancing an Existing EMS System

It is more likely that the new medical director will inherit an existing system. In the case of a good system, the medical director may be blessed with the need for little or no change. In the case of the poorly performing system, the medical director may wish that he or she could start over. It is also possible that the new service will be an enhancement of the current BLS service, which is upgrading to ALS—an opportunity that is much desired by both the personnel and the community.

In any case, initial data gathering for a new system or existing system is similar and is identical to that described for a new EMS system items 1 through 3. In addition, for an existing system, the new Medical Director will need to meet with the state officials to discuss any prior problems and to gain their perspective on the local system's history and its need for modification or future enhancement.

Documents to be collected and reviewed as part of the current system's analysis include the following:

- Local EMS system plan
- Local disaster plan
- EMS protocols (BLS and ALS) to include patient care protocols, standing orders, nonpatient care operational or administrative protocols (e.g., procedures, rules, regulations), transport and destination protocols
- Personnel policies and procedures, if applicable.
- Budget, financial projections, capital equipment list (to include age) and anticipated capital equipment purchases.
- Curriculum for courses offered in the system, and primary and continuing education.
- Documentation of current certification and participation in continuing education and QA/CQI activities by all personnel currently providing patient care within the system.
- Communication logs, dispatch protocols, and logs.
- Standard equipment and medication allotments for each vehicle and the type(s) and number of vehicles within the system.
- Criteria for qualification or designation as a receiving hospital and a specialty care unit within the system.
- List of designated receiving and specialty hospitals, date of designation, and date for reevaluation.
- Copies of public information programs and education materials undertaken and provided.
- Copies of favorable and unfavorable media coverage in the recent past (e.g., 6 months to 1 year).
- Copies of mutual aid agreements currently in effect.

Basic information of any existing system should be reviewed. The new medical director should review the following list of data. The system will need to ensure access to the necessary data and assistance in interpreting data for which the meaning is not readily apparent or the context in which it was collected is unknown.

- Run data (volume, types of runs, acuities, payor mix, point of origin, response time data, garaging location, or system status management data)
- Copies of all death, resuscitation, critical trauma, and critical pediatric patient charts (EMS and emergency department) for the past 6 months. (Note: Given the run volume for the system, the new medical director may not wish to review all such charts. They should be presented to the director, nonetheless, so that he or she can determine which charts will be reviewed. Discovery of a chart included in the time frame that was not available for review should provide cause for a more thorough chart review. The quality or the content of the charts may encourage the review of more or fewer charts to further substantiate trends noted during the initial review.)
- Copies of nontransport or AMA (refusal—against medical advice) charts for the last 6 months. (Note: The number of months depends on the volume of refusals. In a system in which EMS must transport all patients except refusals, 6 months is a suggested time frame. In a system in which noncritical or nonurgent patients can be denied transport, a representative sample should be reviewed.)
- Copies of all or a representative random sampling of run sheets for the prior 6 months based on, for example, every fifth chart or random numbers. (The number of charts is based on run volume and the resources available to review them.)
- Copies of the minutes of QA/CQI meetings documenting both pleasures and concerns noted and commendations provided and corrective action taken.
- Copies of all incident reports regarding patient care for the prior 6 months.
- Copies of all current patient care related personnel files.

The preceding data specifications assume that the new medical director is inheriting a small to moderately sized EMS system or a single EMS service. If the system or service is substantial in size, either the quantity of materials requested for review needs to be modified; or, more appropriately, trusted personnel will need to be available or put in place under the medical director's authority to assist with the review. All of the data in paragraph 5 may not need to be reviewed in detail. The purpose of the review is to determine recurrent problem areas and general trends. The review is also designed to generally familiarize the new medical director with the system (service) and its function.

Once the rules, regulations, and protocols have been understood and the current system's performance reviewed in light of the preceding documents or any others thought to be appropriate, the medical director should be prepared to draw some conclusions about the system's current function, strong points, and room for improvement.

Next, the new medical director must reaffirm the information gathered and conclusions drawn by the process described previously through one or more meetings with pivotal persons within the community (e.g., county commissioners, mayor, city council leaders, your own hospital emergency department director and administrator, other hospital emergency department directors and administrators, other physicians, the current or recent EMS administrators, nonmanagerial EMS personnel).

The goals for the future should now be established, prioritized, and a time frame set for their accomplishment. It must be decided whether the system requires a major overhaul or if less drastic changes are required over time. In the case of a major revision, steps 8 through 10 in the discussion Steps to Develop a New EMS System should be followed. If the required changes deal with only limited areas of the system or are less drastic, consider obtaining sponsorship from within the community for a meeting of all key individuals involved in the various components of the EMS system for which change is anticipated and desired. Influential members of the community along with the state EMS director and, if applicable, medical director may serve on a panel present at the front of the meeting room as discussed previously. An inappropriate "show of force" for a relatively minor system enhancement may be an overkill and may lead to either suspicion or criticism. Minor changes to a satisfactorily functioning current system may be accomplished best without fanfare. A small meeting with only the key players should suffice to define the areas for change, and gain support for assistance with change and to implement the new program. As always, a time frame should be established and communicated.

Finally, a steering committee consisting of the chair of any committees formed to share information, troubleshoot problems, and maintain momentum should be established. The medical director should not shoulder all of the responsibility and therefore liability. Others should be appropriately involved, but the medical director should maintain control of the process and the desired outcome.

FUTURE EMS SYSTEMS

Twenty-five years ago, EMS was merely a vision held by a limited number of individuals across the country who were privy to the data and who participated in the conferences described at the beginning of the chapter. Several others joined the cause as a result of conversations initiated by these individuals. If not for the images of Roy DeSoto and Johnny Gage entering our homes since the 1970s on the television show **Emergency** once a week, however, few would have understood the meaning and importance of EMS to each of our lives. Today, EMS is taken for granted, a right demanded of our municipal leaders throughout most of the United States.

In the beginning, those of us who served as medical directors almost literally gathered up everything used in the emergency department or had endured as part of a first-aid training program over the years and tossed it into the back of the ambulance. There was no research with regard to the equipment or prehospital use of the equipment or medications to validate or invalidate this early practice. As a result, everything in the emergency room became a part of the EMS armamentarium, and there was also a proliferation of new prehospital equipment.

Physician involvement in the early days was also limited. What involvement did occur was generally not recognized as attested to the failure to include "medical direction" in the 1973 federal legislation. There was also a lack of physician understanding of the concepts, strengths and, weaknesses of prehospital medical care. Many shunned its existence as a fleeting fancy, whereas others sought, but were unable to find, a true education. Most early prehospital medical and administrative education was obtained by learning through trial and error. The ability of EMS to grow from a gratuitous service provided by funeral directors in most communities to a multi-billion dollar industry is quite remarkable. This proliferation along with that of all of healthcare, however, will warrant the need for careful scrutiny and change in the near future.

EMS and EMS systems will change over the next 5 to 10 years, as will healthcare in general. Although EMS has not been earmarked for major change in the current Washington proposals, the current outcomes data in EMS supports only a limited number of interventions. In fact, there is limited data to make any decisions. Without supportive data, the system is vulnerable to major modification.

Although some EMS systems are extremely busy and understaffed, many systems have excess capacity. They are a resource located in the community that frequently spends much of its time waiting to be needed. The potential for using this resource during down time will undoubtedly be explored: Immunization programs, home visits, and home treatment with no transport are only a few of the possibilities.

While it is difficult to predict the future of EMS, change will most certainly occur. The current structure and function of EMS will need to be modified, and modification will likely be governed by the following principles:

- Does it work? Do the treatments provided or the equipment utilized in prehospital medicine make a difference?
- Is there any adverse effect to withholding care? Although the treatments or equipment may be effective when applied to the prehospital patient, will the patient actually benefit from the interaction, *or* can treatment be safely withheld until arrival at a hospital or clinic* or physician's* office where definitive evaluation and care are performed?
- Is it cost effective? Does the treatment or the transportation to whatever prescribed facility provide cost-effective care of the patient's problem? For example, should the treatment, if any, be provided at the scene and transportation refused requiring the patient to seek his or her own means of access to the healthcare system?
- Does it add to the patient's quality of life? If the outcome of the treatment and transport is unlikely to improve the patient's quality of life, should it not be withheld? For example, should cardiac arrest patients or trauma patients who do not respond at the scene after "XX" minutes be left for dead, the coroner called, and the patient not transported?

These and other questions will become more important in EMS system's thinking over the next few years and will dictate to a large degree the future of prehospital care and the individuals who have dedicated their life to this profession.

It is imperative that the physician and the personnel be introduced to the concept of change and that all involved personnel be given the opportunity to participate in the local deliberations that ultimately effect those changes. Through involvement, open communication, and understanding, the medical director will be able to demonstrate his or her leadership role within the system, minimizing the confusion and hostility that will otherwise occur as the inevitable changes occur in healthcare.

*EMS transport has been traditionally directed to hospital facilities with full-service emergency departments. It would be anticipated that EMS services will follow modified transport protocols requiring noncritical patient transport to facilities defined by healthcare payors as less expensive.

SUMMARY

At one time only a limited number of physicians across the country became truly involved in the evolving area of prehospital medicine. Based on public demand fanned by federal initiative and television, in many communities the availability of EMS services spread quickly. Often, they spread in the absence of medical direction because of a lack of time, understanding, funding, or commitment. As a result, several systems evolved without medical leadership other than a quick signature, a rubber stamp, to make it all appear correct.

Today, EMS for prehospital providers has become a profession no longer dominated by those looking for merely a quick ride with lights ablaze and sirens blaring. It is no longer perceived as a short career of several years. Today individuals enter the EMS field with the intention that this will be their life's work, their profession.

EMS for physicians has become an area of special expertise and anticipated subspecialty board certification. It is no longer the "reward" in some systems for being the newest member of the emergency department group or medical staff, the lowest member on the totem pole. It is a position requiring special needs, skills, and dedication.

Although the components of an EMS system may change for reasons largely out of prehospital medicine's current control, the requirement for continued involvement, analysis, introspection, and leadership cannot be overstated. This chapter has attempted to outline the existing components of an EMS system, large or small, which are also applicable to individual services. It has defined the role of the physician director in classic systems and encouraged the use of support personnel to refine the medical director's job to a manageable task—a leader, but also a mentor and coordinator of resources. It has provided guidance on the evaluation of existing structures and direction for effecting change. Finally, this chapter has anticipated change and the need for the medical direction process.

It is impossible to anticipate the needs of every community or EMS system within the confines of a single chapter in a text. The availability of resources within the EMS community, many of whom have grown into their present position by trial and error, should be remembered as questions arise.

REFERENCES

1. National Academy of Sciences, National Research Council: *Accidental death and disability: the neglected disease of modern society,* Washington, DC, 1966, NAS/NRC.
2. US House of Representatives Report 1700, 89th Congress, 2d Session, p. 19.
3. Highway Safety Program Standard 11: *Emergency Medical Services,* Washington, DC, April 15, 1974, US Department of Transportation, National Highway Traffic Safety Administration.
4. Page JO: *The paramedics,* Morristown, NJ, 1979, Backdraft Publications.
5. Subcommittee on Medical Control, Committee on Emergency Medical Services, Assembly of Life Sciences, National Research Council: *Medical control in emergency medical services systems,* Washington, DC, 1981, National Academy Press.
6. Roush WR, Editor: *Principles of EMS systems: a comprehensive text for physicians,* Dallas, 1989, American College of Emergency Physicians.
7. Polsky S, Krohmer J, Maningas P et al: Guidelines for medical direction of prehospital EMS, *Ann Emerg Med* 22:742-744, 1993.

APPENDIX

A American College of Emergency Physicians Information Paper

Guidelines for Emergency Medical Services Systems—1994

PREAMBLE

Emergency Medical Services (EMS) in the United States originated from the concept that appropriate treatment of the sick and injured "in the field" could reduce morbidity and mortality. This concept was further developed in the 1960s and, by the early 1970s, emergency medical service systems (EMSS) were born. The EMSS Act of 1973 (PL 93-154) initially defined a model EMS system and identified 15 essential component requirements of a basic system. The components were identified to assist government officials, system administrators, and the public in the development and implementation of local EMS programs.

The practice and scope of emergency medical services have grown dramatically since passage of the landmark EMSS Act. As the field of EMS continues to grow and evolve, basic principles and guidelines must be reviewed periodically to ensure currency and appropriateness. With this in mind, the American College of Emergency Physicians issues the "Guidelines for Emergency Medical Services Systems—1994."

These guidelines are the result of ACEP's continuing interest and support in the field of EMS. They are the result of extensive work by the ACEP EMS Committee, composed not only of ACEP members but also of representatives from a spectrum of organizations at the national level. Current guideline documents from other pertinent fields are referenced and incorporated.

"Guidelines for Emergency Medical Services Systems—1994" represents the current view of what constitutes the necessary components of a comprehensive EMS system. These guidelines are intended as a reference document for those who seek to develop new EMS systems or to review, evaluate, and revise existing systems.

SYSTEM ORGANIZATION

A. Authority and Responsibility
   1. EMS systems must strive to assure excellence in patient care by coordination of all components within the system.
   2. Each system must have authority commensurate with its responsibility to provide emergency services including, but not limited to, the ability to seek enabling legislation and appropriate rules and regulations (when required), appropriate rules/regulations, and the development and implementation of patient care standards, quality management activities, educational programs, contract negotiations, and funding sources.

B. System Administrative Lead Agency
   1. Each system should be headed by an administrative lead agency. This agency is responsible for system management.
   2. The lead agency should be receptive to comments from a broad-based group of providers and consumers.
   3. The lead agency should approve a master plan for the system, including operational standards for each approved component.
   4. The lead agency should develop a method to evaluate:
      a. Medical accountability
      b. System effectiveness
      c. Compliance with operational policy
   5. The system should appoint a medical control board with the ultimate responsibility of overseeing all aspects of patient care.
   6. The medical control board should approve the appointment of the medical director(s) who should be solely responsible to the medical control board.
   7. The lead agency should retain an adequate number of qualified administrative staff and personnel with special qualifications to assure implementation of operational policies as developed by the agency.
   8. The lead agency should develop a budget that identifies resources and expenses, by line item, for planning, implementation, operation, and evaluation.
   9. The lead agency should ensure the system is operated in compliance with all federal, state, and local requirements.

C. Medical Direction[1,2]
   1. Qualifications
      To optimize medical direction of all out-of-hospital emergency medical services, these services should be directed by physicians who have demonstrated the following:
      a. Essential:
         (1) License to practice medicine or osteopathy
         (2) Familiarity with the design and operation of EMS systems.
         (3) Experience or training in the out-of-hospital emergency care of the acutely ill or injured patient.
         (4) Experience or training in medical direction of out-of-hospital emergency units.
         (5) Active participation in the emergency management of the acutely ill or injured patient.
         (6) Experience or training in the education of out-of-hospital personnel

(7) Experience or training in the EMS quality improvement process.
(8) Knowledge of EMS laws and regulations.
(9) Knowledge of EMS dispatch and communications systems.
(10) Knowledge of local mass casualty/major incident and disaster plans.

b. Desirable:
(1) Board certification in emergency medicine.

2. Responsibilities:
a. Serve as patient advocate in the EMS system.
b. Set and ensure compliance with patient care standards including communications standards and dispatch and medical protocols.
c. Develop and implement protocols and standing orders under which the out-of-hospital care providers function.
d. Develop and implement the process for the provision of concurrent medical direction.
e. Ensure the appropriateness of initial qualifications of out-of-hospital personnel involved in patient care and dispatch.
f. Ensure the qualifications of out-of-hospital personnel involved in patient care and dispatch are maintained on an ongoing basis through education, testing, and credentialing.
g. Develop and implement an effective quality improvement program for continuous system and patient care improvement.
h. Promote EMS research.
i. Maintain liaison with the medical community including, but not limited to, hospitals, emergency departments, physicians, out-of-hospital providers, and nurses.
j. Interact with state, regional, and local EMS authorities to ensure that standards, needs, and requirements are met and resource utilization is optimized.
k. Be involved with coordination of activities such as mutual aid, disaster planning and management, and hazardous materials response.
l. Be involved with the promulgation of public education and information on the prevention of emergencies.
m. Maintain knowledge levels appropriate for an EMS medical director through continued education.

3. Authority
The medical director must have authority over all clinical and patient care aspects of the EMS system including, but not limited to, the following:
a. Recommend certification, recertification, and decertification of nonphysician out-of-hospital personnel to the appropriate certifying agency.
b. Establish, implement, revise, and authorize systemwide protocols, policies, and procedures for all patient care activities from dispatch through triage, treatment, and transport.
c. Establish criteria for level of initial emergency response (e.g., first responder, Basic EMT, EMT-Intermediate, Paramedic).
d. Establish criteria for determining patient destination.
e. Ensure the competency of personnel who provide concurrent medical direction to out-of-hospital personnel including, but not limited to, physicians, nurses and EMTs.
f. Establish procedures or protocols under which non-transport of patients may occur.
g. Require education and testing to the level of proficiency approved for the following personnel within the EMS system:
(1) First responders
(2) EMTs, all levels
(3) Nurses involved in out-of-hospital care
(4) Dispatchers
(5) Educational coordinators
(6) Physicians providing on-line (concurrent) medical direction
(7) Physicians providing off-line (prospective and retrospective) medical direction
h. Implement and supervise an effective quality improvement program. The medical director shall have access to all relevant records needed to accomplish this task, including out-of-hospital and hospital records.
i. Remove a provider from medical care duties for due cause using an appropriate review and appeals mechanism.
j. Set or approve hiring standards for personnel involved in patient care.
k. Set or approve standards for equipment used in patient care.

4. Obligations of the EMS system
a. Compensation for the time required.
b. Provision of material and personnel resources necessary to fulfill responsibilities.
c. Liability insurance for duties/actions performed by the medical director.
d. A written agreement that delineates the medical director's authority and responsibilities and the EMS system's obligations.

D. Communications:
There should be a comprehensive communication plan for the following:
1. EMS communications fully integrated with other public safety agencies.
2. Adequate spectrum and frequency allocation for EMS use.
3. Minimum radio dead space.
4. Minimum vehicle communication equipment defined to assure communication capability with all vehicles and aircraft operating in the system.
5. Minimum communication educational requirements for providers within the system.
6. Protocols for the appropriate utilization of communications equipment and frequencies.
7. Designated frequencies for communications:
a. Dispatch
b. Medical direction
c. Inter-vehicle
d. Inter-agency
e. Mass casualty/major incident

8. Ensured system access by some public convenience method such as 911 or a single well-posted number.
9. Centralized dispatch for all public service agencies (where possible).
10. Established training and certification standards for EMS dispatchers.
11. Provision of on-line (concurrent) medical direction by trained personnel.
12. Established communications quality improvement program that includes continuous evaluation of dispatch and on-line (concurrent) medical direction operations.

OPERATIONAL POLICIES

The system should develop operational policies for the following:

1. System administration
2. Medical direction
3. Out-of-hospital transport
4. Interfacility transport
5. Dispatch
6. Communications
7. Protocols
   a. Triage
   b. Treatment
   c. Transport and non-transport
   d. Transfer
   e. Diversion[3]
   f. Limitation of care (e.g., Do-Not-Attempt-Resuscitation)
8. Receiving facilities
9. Specialty care units
10. Education
11. Financing
12. Audit and quality improvement
13. Mass casualty/major incident
14. Public information and education
15. Mutual aid integration with other regional EMS
16. Infection Control
17. Hazardous materials response

HUMAN RESOURCES AND EDUCATION

A. The lead agency should assure that programs exist for volunteer and career recruitment in out-of-hospital and hospital disciplines.
B. The lead agency should assure the availability of educational programs. These should include:
   1. Primary programs for all levels of providers in the system that should:
      a. Be under the direction of a physician experienced and involved in EMS systems.
      b. Meet or exceed the national standard curriculum.
      c. Contain additional curriculum addressing specific needs identified by the system.
      d. Be assured of adequate funding.
      e. Have sufficient experienced staff.
      f. Be affiliated with an institution of higher learning (desirable).
   2. Continuing education programs for EMTs, physicians, nurses, medical dispatchers, and other specialty providers. The curricula of these programs should meet or exceed recertification requirements as mandated and address system needs identified through the quality improvement process.
   3. Recognized educational programs for physicians providing medical direction.
   4. Public education programs to provide information regarding system access and use.
C. The lead agency should provide for critical incident stress debriefing and other support services.

TRANSPORTATION

A. The lead agency has the authority to allow transport services to function within the system.
   1. Vehicles must be licensed according to approved standards.
   2. Equipment lists must be consistent with system standards.
   3. Personnel must be certified consistent with system standards.
   4. Number of responders must be consistent with system standards.
B. The lead agency will develop an ambulance placement plan that includes the following:
   1. Response time standards for appropriate triage acuity (measured on a percentile basis).
   2. Predetermined response boundaries.
C. All agencies providing emergency transports within the system, including public, private, air, and water, should be coordinated by the lead agency.
D. Transportation will be to appropriate receiving facilities according to destination and diversion policies established by the medical director(s) and the agency.
E. Provision for medically supervised transport, including interfacility transport, should exist.

FACILITIES*

A. The lead agency should identify appropriate facilities that are capable of providing diagnosis and stabilization of ill and injured patients.[4,5] Receiving facilities' capabilities include:
   1. Emergency department with emergency physician staffing
   2. Surgical facility availability
   3. Laboratory, blood bank, and x-ray availability
   4. Critical and intensive care unit availability
   5. Documented commitment to participation in the EMS system
   6. Willingness to accept all emergency patients regardless of their ability to pay for services
   7. Provision of medical audit to ensure quality improvement and medical accountability
   8. Integration in mass casualty/major incident preparedness plans

*In some rural areas it may be necessary to deliver patients to emergency facilities in accordance with the EMS system protocols that do not meet all of the criteria.

†Burn, trauma, pediatric, etc.

B. Specialty Care†
   1. Each system should identify facilities capable of providing specialty care for the subset of emergency patients requiring such treatment. Specialty care within the system should include:
      a. Trauma[6,7]
      b. Burns
      c. Cardiac
      d. Pediatric
      e. Perinatal and high-risk obstetrics
      f. Psychiatric/Behavioral
      g. Spinal[8]
      h. Poison control center[9] (need not be receiving facility)
      i. Environmental (hyperbaric, hypothermia, hazardous materials, etc.)
      j. Rehabilitation
   2. Utilization according to protocols and policies developed by the agency, coordinated by the medical director of the system.
   3. Helicopter landing capability as necessary.
   4. If specialty facilities do not exist within the system, formal transfer agreements should be developed by the EMS system.[10]
   5. Participation in medical audit to ensure quality improvement and medical accountability
   6. Integration in mass casualty/major incident preparedness plans

PUBLIC INFORMATION AND EDUCATION

A. Public education—A critical ingredient to an optimal EMS system is Public education. It is the responsibility of the EMS system to educate the public in matters regarding EMS and health matters in general. This should include:
   1. EMS service availability, level of service, and access
   2. CPR and first aid training
   3. General health care issues, including early problem recognition
   4. Injury and illness prevention
B. Recognition and response—The system must educate the public regarding recognition and response to illness or injury including:
   1. Immediate recognition of an illness or injury
   2. System access, such as 911 or a single, widely disseminated telephone number
   3. First aid and CPR, either via post-dispatch EMD instructions or previous lay person training.
   4. Appropriate utilization of resources
C. Other services—There are other services integral to the totality of emergency patient care, including, but not limited to:
   1. Suicide counseling
   2. Counseling for victims of domestic violence
   3. Child and elder abuse information
   4. Sexual assault
   5. Poison control
   6. Community mental health resources
   7. Critical Incident Stress Debriefing (CISD)
D. Media Interaction—Effective education and interaction with media resources is critical to an EMS system's ability to disseminate information to the public.

QUALITY IMPROVEMENT

The provision of high quality EMS care requires that a system be in place to assess patient care rendered, assure accountability, and facilitate continuous improvement. A quality improvement process must be a fundamental part of the EMS system, and have the unwavering support of system leaders and field personnel, the financial support of the organization, and a broad scope to evaluate all activities of the system. System evaluation and improvement must be driven by data.

A. Data Collection
   The process of data collection should include:
   1. Standardization of EMS data elements and definitions.
   2. Standardization of data collection forms including patient care records, dispatch records, and medical direction records.
   3. Agreements with receiving facilities to furnish outcome information as a necessary part of participation in the EMS system.
   4. Agreements with the local medical examiner to furnish autopsy data on EMS-related cases.
   5. Record handling to protect the confidentiality of patients and providers.
   6. Computerized data acquisition, reporting and manipulation (desirable).
   7. Statistical consultation for design of data collection and utilization (desirable).
B. Data Assessment
   The process of data assessment should include:
   1. EMS system assessment parameters which are both process and outcome directed.
   2. A comprehensive approach to the evaluation of care rendered on both a system-wide and individual provider basis.
   3. A broadly focused assessment that evaluates system performance from access to delivery to definitive care. Key elements include:
      a. Access
      b. Dispatch
      c. First response
      d. BLS care
      e. ALS care
      f. Medical direction
   4. Data assessment strategies that empower front-line personnel to participate and direct efforts to improve quality.
C. Modification of Existing Standards
   The process by which the results of data assessment are used to modify existing standards should include:
   1. A commitment on the part of management to support and implement improvements identified as necessary through assessment techniques.
   2. Ongoing assessment and improvement mechanisms and support personnel as a fundamental part of the EMS system
   3. A direct and ongoing relationship between system assessment and education components.

D. EMS Research
Maturation of the EMS system and the field of EMS as a whole demands that the system allow for scholarly inquiry into care rendered through quality out-of-hospital research. EMS systems should supply:
1. Pragmatic and philosophical support of EMS research as a means to allow for growth of the scientific basis for EMS.
2. Policies to allow for ethical and appropriate EMS studies.
3. Oversight of field EMS studies to protect the rights and welfare of patients.
4. Opportunities for investigators to cooperate with local system members for participation in multicenter studies as appropriate.

DISASTER MANAGEMENT AND MASS CASUALTY/MAJOR INCIDENT PLANNING

Each EMS system should develop a disaster management or mass casualty/major incident plan that addresses unusual or unexpected emergencies that exceed system resources. The plan will address:

A. Planning of EMS response:
1. Mass gathering events known to routinely occur in the community (eg, concerts, stadiums, schools).
2. Known potential mass casualty/major incident events (eg, transportation accidents, industrial settings).
3. Known potential hazards (eg, hazardous materials).

B. Integration of EMS with all public safety agencies involved in disaster response under the incident command system.

C. Organization of the EMS response within the overall response.

D. Coordination of all out-of-hospital and hospital components of the response.

E. Coordinated communications at all levels of the response.

F. Mutual aid resources at local, regional, state, and national levels.
1. Interface with National Disaster Medical System (NDMS)

G. Regular training of EMS personnel in disaster response activities:
1. Response structure based on incident command system.
2. Patient care activities, including triage, on-scene treatment, transportation.

H. Regular multi-agency drills to test disaster preparedness.

REFERENCES

1. American College of Emergency Physicians: *Medical Direction of Emergency Medical Services.* Dallas, Texas, ACEP, 1993.
2. American College of Emergency Physicians: Medical Direction of prehospital Emergency Medical Services Dallas, Texas ACEP, 1992.
3. American College of Emergency Physicians: Ambulance diversion/destination policies. *ACEP News* January 1992: insert.
4. American College of Emergency Physicians: Emergency care guidelines (revised). *Ann Emerg Med* 1991;20:1389-1395.
5. Emergency Nurses Association: *Standards of Emergency Nursing Practices Second Edition,* St. Louis, W Mosley Co, 1991.
6. American College of Emergency Physicians: Guidelines for trauma care systems. Dallas, Texas ACEP, 1992.
7. American College of Surgeons: *Resources for Optimal Care of the Injured Patient,* Chicago, ACS, 1990.
8. American Spinal Injury Association Foundation: *Guidelines for Facility Categorization and Standards of Care; Spinal Cord Injury,* Chicago, ASIAF, 1981.
9. American Association of Poison Control Centers: Criteria for designation as a regional poison control center. Adopted by American College of Emergency Physicians, April 1982.
10. American College of Emergency Physicians: Appropriate Interhospital Patient Transfer. Dallas, Texas ACEP, 1992.

APPENDIX

B EMS Resource Organizations

1. State EMS or Emergency Management Agency
   Contact your State office building for address and telephone number.
2. State chapter of the American College of Emergency Physicians
   Contact National ACEP (see below) for state address, telephone and contact person.
3. American College of Emergency Physicians (ACEP)
   P.O. 619911
   Dallas, Texas 75261-9911
   1- 800/798-1822
   1- 214/550-0911
4. ACEP Section on Emergency Medical Services
   Contact National ACEP (see above).
5. National Association of EMS Physicians (NAEMSP)
   230 McKee Place, Suite 500
   Pittsburgh, PA 15213
   1-800/228-3677
   1- 412/578-3222
6. National Association of State EMS Directors (NASEMSD)
   1947 Camino Vida Roble, Suite 202
   Carlsbad, CA 92008
   1-619/431-7054
7. National Council of State EMS Training Coordinators (NCSEMSTC)
   P.O. Box 11910
   Iron Works Pike
   Lexington, KY 40578-1910
   1-606/231-1923
8. National Highway Traffic Safety Division (Department of Transportation) (NHTSA)
   DOT/NHTSA - EMS Office
   NHTSA NTS 42
   400 7th Street, S.W.
   Washington, D.C. 20590
   1-202/366-5440

96 Medical Command Facility Responsibilities

Richard M. McDowell

OUTLINE

This chapter describes the responsibilities of a medical command facility, which translates directly to the roles and responsibilities of a medical command facility medical director. This follows because the medical director is responsible for all activities that relate to patient care, which is the facility's raison d'etre. The challenge of this chapter is that the multitude of different emergency medical services (EMS) system configurations in the United States offer many possible models for a successful medical command facility. No single model can be used because the facility must match the EMS system into which it is integrated.

With this problem in mind, certain fundamental principles of medical command facility structure and function should always be followed regardless of the specific local EMS configuration. These fundamental principles are discussed first in each section, and they should be used as guidelines in all systems. A menu of variations and different options follows the fundamental principles to allow choices that can be selected to fit a specific local EMS system configuration.

Because of the wide range of available configurations of EMS systems, a flexible approach is required in designing an effective medical command facility. For example, EMS systems can be rural, suburban, or urban, all of which can be anticipated to have very different transport times. One medical command facility can serve multiple receiving facilities, or all the receiving emergency departments may be designated medical command facilities. Direct (on-line) medical command may be available from many different emergency physicians in one or several emergency departments, or it may be provided by a finite number of emergency physicians with portable radios from home or work. In some systems, direct medical command may rarely be needed if paramedics function on standing orders within protocols. Paramedics may be volunteer, full-time employees of a hospital-based service, employees of small local or large multistate private ambulance company, unionized firefighters, or employees in a public utility model.

Although many factors can make one system different from another, fundamental principles must be applied to all systems. There are two good general reference textbooks on EMS systems and EMS medical direction, the former by the American College of Emergency Physicians (ACEP), and the latter by the National Association of EMS Physicians (NAEMSP).[1,2] The content of these textbooks far exceeds the scope of this chapter and therefore they should be a reference for any medical director of a medical command facility.

MEDICAL DIRECTION

Fundamentals

The medical command facility provides the critical interface between the medical director who is responsible for medical command and the EMS providers. ACEP's policy statement on medical direction of prehospital emergency medical services requires that all aspects of the organization and provision of EMS have the active involvement of physicians and defines the primary role of the medical director to be ensuring quality patient care.[3] Guidelines for physician direction of EMS have been published and include a detailed explanation of the fundamentally important concepts of indirect (off-line) and direct (on-line) medical direction using prospective, concurrent, and retrospective methods.[4] Although these guidelines were not specifically written for medical command facility medical directors, the principles of medical direction are the same.

Note also that medical direction is critical not only for advanced life support (ALS) services, but also for basic life support (BLS) services. This would be particularly true in EMS systems where BLS providers render a significant amount of trauma care or provide automated external defibrillation.[5] In addition, some state statutes and pursuant rules and regulations provide more specific guidelines for medical command facilities and their directors, which must be considered.[6]

Out-of-hospital medical care should be directed by protocols that are best developed jointly between physicians and providers using national standards and current medical literature as references. These protocols serve as templates against which direct physician orders and EMS provider treatment can be compared. Deviations from the protocols can be identified and then judged as appropriate or inappropriate through the quality management program.

It is important not to confuse protocols with standing orders, which are a subset of protocols. The protocol is a set of medical treatments that govern a certain condition (e.g., treating chest pain of presumed cardiac origin with oxygen, nitroglycerin). The standing orders component of protocols can be executed by the ALS provider without first contacting online medical command (e.g., defibrillation, intubation).

Variations

The medical director may delegate some responsibility for medical direction to surrogates (e.g., other command physicians, nurses, or paramedics). Most EMS systems have a paramedic coordinator or supervisor and other emergency physicians serving as command physicians. The NAEMSP has published a position paper on online medical control for EMS medical command facilities, which makes recommendations for the medical command facility medical director and command physicians' requirements, as well as the different options for on-line medical command.[7]

One of the most powerful medical director surrogate models is 24-hour coverage by specially chosen paramedic supervisors who respond to high risk or problem patient scenes. This allows for concurrent on-line medical direction and is the best way to monitor out-of-hospital patient care and individual provider skills. Some systems, such as the City of Pittsburgh, Bureau of EMS, actually use physicians or emergency medicine residents in this capacity.[8]

The medical director of the medical command facility may not be the medical director of the BLS or ALS services that receive command. Some services may have a service medical director and receive command from several different facilities, each with a separate medical director. Nevertheless, the medical command facility medical director must have direct input into the medical care rendered by the BLS/ALS services that receive direct command.

QUALITY ASSURANCE/QUALITY IMPROVEMENT

Fundamentals

This section on quality assurance/quality improvement (QA/QI) is continuation of the previous section on medical direction; both concepts are intimately connected. In a landmark article Holroyd et al.[9] equated medical control with QA: "Medical control is a system of physician-directed quality assurance that provides professional and public accountability for medical care provided in the prehospital setting." They continued to describe the components of medical control, breaking it down into prospective, immediate (on-line) or concurrent, and retrospective.

Prospective medical control or QA includes EMS legislation, medical/triage/operational protocols, training, and certification of providers. Immediate or concurrent medical control or QA includes voice contact on-line and presence on scene. Retrospective medical control or QA includes trip report review, case reviews, and statistical review of the EMS system.

There has been significant interest in incorporating the principles of continuous quality improvement (CQI) into EMS systems, and two books on EMS quality management have been published recently by both ACEP and NAEMSP.[10,11] One of the fundamental lessons of CQI when applied to EMS is to include significant input from the EMS providers. This is best accomplished by providing for direct contact with the medical director on a regular and structured basis. EMS provider input into the CQI program should not be filtered through medical director surrogates. Although there are many methods to solicit input, it can readily be accomplished with a regular schedule of field ride-alongs and medical command facility meetings, which include all EMS providers. The methodologies of CQI are covered more extensively elsewhere in this textbook.

Retrospective review should include audits of patient care reports (PCRs) and medical command logs. Ideally, these audits should involve an initial review by the field providers in a peer review atmosphere, with final review by the medical command facility medical director. The process by which retrospective reviews are performed should be outlined in a written QA/QI plan, which includes certain high risk patient encounters such as cardiac arrests, trauma, intubations, and refusal of care. Regularly scheduled medical command facility meetings can include tape reviews, case reviews, protocol discussions, and general problem solving to enhance the delivery of out-of-hospital medical care.

Variations

In EMS systems where multiple emergency physicians provide medical command, the medical command facility meeting is the perfect forum to achieve concordance in the quality of medical command and to enforce adherence to protocols that are mutually approved by providers and command physicians. In systems where there is little on-line activity, the presence of the medical command physicians is less significant, because protocol development and problem solving are mainly accomplished prospectively between the providers and the medical command facility medical director. Command facilities that interface with multiple BLS/ALS services, each having a different service medical director, should involve these physicians or their surrogates to achieve agreement with treatment and operational protocols.

EDUCATION

Fundamentals

Because the medical command facility is the hub of the wheel of activity between the EMS providers and the command physicians, it should also be the primary venue for educational programs. This educational role serves to advance the standard of care for EMS medical practice and ensures consistency with current medical literature and practice. It also facilitates the relationship between the EMS providers and physicians by emphasizing patient-centered care and the overall mission of the EMS system. An ideal situation is to offer the emergency department of the medical command facility as a venue for the EMS providers to work one on one with an emergency physician to enhance skills of patient assessment and medical decision making.

Variations

Educational programs at the medical command facility may be designed in several ways. If all the ALS/BLS services are volunteer, they can serve as the main source of low cost continuing medical education (CME) as a regular monthly or quarterly didactic presentation. Tape reviews of interesting patients may be included, with positive goals and peer review principles in mind. Even if the majority of local EMS services are at the other end of the spectrum as large, consolidated programs with full-time providers and an in-house complement of educational programs, the medical command facility needs to be integrated into the overall educational program. The monthly medical command facility meeting is an excellent venue for regular education, peer review, and protocol development.

CREDENTIALING MEDICS

Fundamentals

The certification (or licensing) of EMS providers is governed by state regulation and is rarely the responsibility of a medical command facility. In some cases, the facility will be involved in hiring providers, but in other cases the providers are either hired by an independent ALS/BLS service or are volunteer. Therefore issues of certification and employment may never be of concern to the medical command facility, but the agreement to provide medical command for a provider is always required. This agreement may be called *granting command privileges,* but whatever the legal term, it represents an agreement that the medical command facility medical director will provide direct medical command to the paramedic provider. This means that the medical command facility has reviewed the provider's credentials and will monitor performance, including the review of current certifications(s), skills and procedures, adequacy of assessments, and adherence to protocols (including medical and operational). The exact role and responsibility of the medical command facility medical director regarding the credentialing or recredentialing of EMS providers may be articulated more clearly in state statute. The medical director must be familiar with the state and local regulations and ordinances governing this process.

Variations

The review and monitoring of EMS providers can be accomplished in several ways. Traditionally, they involve retrospective review of PCRs and the tabulation of actual procedures in the field. There may be established CME requirements, and in some systems retesting is involved.

One of the best ways of credentialing and documenting field performance is concurrent QA (i.e., direct field observation). This process can be delegated to EMS physicians, but is more realistically and perhaps more effectively accomplished by specially chosen paramedic supervisors. An EMS system that provides 24-hour paramedic supervisors (or physicians) who are the delegated representatives of the system or command facility medical director represents the most sophisticated structure of oversight, medical command, and QA/QI. It provides a contemporaneous evaluation process with the opportunity for intervention when needed to provide safe and effective patient care.

CREDENTIALING PHYSICIANS

Fundamentals

If physicians at a medical command facility are to give direct medical command, they can do so automatically once they are hired as emergency department physicians. This would also be true for physicians trained in emergency medicine residency programs, as the EMS education has been found to be quite variable.[12] Physicians must be credentialed for the specific role of providing direct medical command and for other roles they might be expected to perform as a member of the medical command facility. Even in systems that operate largely on standing orders, there must be a method for immediate consultation between the EMS provider and a command physician on-line if a patient problem or medical care question arises.[13]

Because system protocols serve not only as guidelines for treatment and operations, but also as standards to guide retrospective QA/QI of patient care, they can be used to monitor the activities of command physicians, as well as EMS providers. Direct medical command activity must be monitored for compliance with the accepted protocols. Feedback to the physicians with regard to their compliance should be part of the quality management program.

Variations

Items for credentialing command physicians can be included in a mandatory orientation to the medical command facility. A review of protocols, communications, QA/QI activities, and a ride-along program can be mandated. Continuing requirements for reappointment may include continued ride-along time, attendance at medical command facility meetings, teaching of CME courses, and participation in other QA/QI activities. Individual state statutes and pursuant regulations may also guide credentialing, as does the NAEMSP position paper on EMS command facilities.[6,7]

COMMUNICATIONS

Fundamentals

The basic concept of a medical command facility was initially to provide a mechanism by which paramedics could communicate directly with emergency physicians with regard to patient care and receive direct orders contemporaneously. Although in some systems a great majority of ALS care may actually be provided by medics using standing orders within defined protocols, a direct pipeline from the field to a medical command physician must always be available.[13,14]

Variations

Communication is usually with an emergency department staff of medical command physicians known as a medical command facility. However, communication may be designed to be received by an individual EMS physician who may not actually be located in an emergency department or even in one single location. For example, the physician could be in a separate EMS building or even completely mobile, including taking direct medical command responsibility from home on a portable radio or cellular telephone.[14,15]

Communications hardware should be chosen based on several factors, including topography, costs, cellular telephone capabilities, and requirements for telemetry transmission including the use of 12-lead ECGs in the field. Cellular telephones with one or several dedicated lines into the medical command facility that have automatic audiotaping capabilities are an excellent communication system. Other EMS systems still use radio communications (UHF), which were the standard until cellular systems proliferated. No single communication system will fulfill the needs of every medical command facility. The most reliable, cost-effective means to ensure consistent communication between the EMS providers and the physician, however, remains paramount.

RECORDKEEPING

Fundamentals

A record of the medical care must be rendered to patients in the field; this is usually the paramedic PCR or run sheet. It should be completed on all dispatches, whether or not there is patient transport or even patient contact. When the dispatch center sends the provider out after a request for EMS service, the system has been invoked and the results of that dispatch must be documented. The details of where and how long to keep these records are usually governed by state regulation. Frequently, the PCR becomes part of the patient's medical record when the patient is transported to a receiving facility. When there is no patient transport or no patient contact, the PCR may be submitted to the ALS medical director and/or medical command facility medical director for evaluation of statistical data, protocol adherence, and QA/QI. Data on nontransports are particularly important because of risk management issues, which can possibly include exposure to violating federal antidumping regulations (Emergency Medical Treatment and Active Labor Act [EMTALA] [see Chapter 61]) for ALS services owned by hospitals.[16] Beyond this, the nontransport patient contact has been shown to frequently involve seriously ill or injured patients. These types of patient encounters warrant close scrutiny in the overall EMS systems QA/QI program.[17,18]

In addition to the paramedic trip sheet, systems can require documentation of the medical command activities for patients in the out-of-hospital phase of care. Although this documentation may be included on the PCR documented by the paramedics and cosigned by the physician, the physician may also have to complete a separate medical command report. In some systems, it is also included as part of the patient's hospital medical record. The medical command report can be a variety of forms or checklist worksheets depending on the requirements stipulated in the regulations of the EMS jurisdiction (Figure 96-1).

Medical command audiotapes are useful tools for education and quality improvement. They are also used in some systems for risk management and legal purposes, so their storage and maintenance is often governed by state regulations.[6]

Variations

The PCR will usually be part of a patient's medical record at the receiving hospital. In addition, it will be reviewed as part of the QA/QI process for nontransported patients. It may not be feasible, however, to require the medical command documentation forms to be part of the medical record if patients are transported to a facility different from the medical command facility. In some systems, direct medical command may be required so rarely that these forms will not be routinely collected and submitted for incorporation into the patient's medical record.

In the case of medical command audiotapes, the local or regional dispatch center may be the legal repository, and the command facility may access them only when necessary for QA/QI purposes. Individual state statutes and pursuant regulations may guide recordkeeping requirements.[6]

DISPATCH AND COMMUNICATIONS CENTERS

Fundamentals

The communication center(s) and dispatch policies in an EMS system are critically important for ensuring an efficient, appropriate, and timely response. Unfortunately, an EMS system may have to compete for operational authority in a 911 center with other services such as police and fire. Furthermore, some centers have inadequate or nonexistent medical direction. Ideally, the dispatch center should have a medical director or medical oversight committee that can work with the EMS system and the medical command facility medical director(s) to provide a seamless system of call taking and dispatching. Just like every other component of the EMS system, the communication centers must be subjected to rigorous quality control measures.

Variations

The medical command facility medical director along with the local or regional EMS system medical director should have input into the design and function of the communication center. The ideal situation is a dispatch center medical director who is EMS knowledgeable and who reports to or works closely with the other EMS physicians in the system. Each medical command facility, however, must have a clear role and responsibility in its relationship with the communication center for both routine EMS operations and disaster/mass casualty situations.

RECEIVING FACILITIES

Fundamentals

Emergency departments that receive EMS patients must be designated. That process is usually governed by statute or regulation specific to the EMS system. The emergency de-

Albany Medical Center - Department of Emergency Medicine

Advanced Life Support Medical Control Record

☐ TAPE REVIEW REQUESTED

MD Signature: ____________ MD#: ____________ Date: ____________ Time: ____________

Type of call: ____________ Going to: ____________

ALS Squad: ____________ Paramedic # : ____________ REMAC Run # ____________

Age: ________ Male ☐ Female ☐ Weight: ____________ PMD: ____________

Complaint and HPI: ____________

____

____

Meds: ____________ Allergies: ____________

Examination: BP: ____________ P: ____________ RR: ____________

A & O x 3 ☐ Other: ____________ Other Findings: ____________

Pupils: PERL ☐ Other: ____________ ____________

Skin: ____________ Treatment: ____________

Lungs: ____________ Oxygen: ____________ L/min by: ____________

Pedal Edema: ☐ JVD: ☐ IV: ____________ at rate: ____________ ☐:KVO

GCS: ________ TS: ________ EKG: ____________ MAST: ____________

ORDERS AND PATIENT STATUS

TIME	BP	P	RR	TREATMENT AND RESPONSE
				STANDING ORDER DRUGS GIVEN:

Draft 7/18/91
Rev. 4/93

Receiving MD/RN: ____________ ETA: ____________ min.

FIGURE 96-1 Example of a medical command log.
(Courtesy Albany Medical Center.)

partments should be integrated into the system with preestablished requirements to receive patients. The National Highway Traffic and Safety Administration has been instrumental in assisting the development of EMS systems on a statewide level, including the categorizing of receiving facilities.[19] The medical command facility must be cognizant of the capabilities of the receiving facilities to optimize patient distribution and care.

Variations

The manner in which local emergency departments are included or excluded from the EMS system varies dramatically. In some systems, all local emergency departments attached to a licensed hospital may receive patients. In some cases, every receiving facility is also a medical command facility. For example, in a large county there may be 30 or more emergency departments, each of which is also a medical command facility for a countywide EMS system. In contrast, in other areas, the emergency departments must be designated to receive patients or certain types of patients and must meet stringent requirements that may even include specific physician and nurse staffing levels. An example of this situation is New York City, which has extraordinarily detailed requirements for emergency departments that receive EMS patients written by a special group called the 911 Committee.[14,20]

SUMMARY

The medical director of a medical command facility must be fully conversant with the principles of EMS medical direction. The medical command facility must be fully integrated into the local EMS system configuration in every regard. Medical direction is a system of physician-directed QA/QI, which provides professional and public accountability for out-of-hospital medical care. The medical director of the medical command facility is responsible for creating an effective interface between medical command and EMS providers to ensure quality medical care for the people who call the EMS system for help, and in doing so, become our patients.

REFERENCES

1. Roush WR: *Principles of EMS systems,* ed 2, Dallas, 1994, American College of Emergency Physicians.
2. Kuehl AE: *Prehospital systems and medical oversight,* ed 2, St Louis, 1994, Mosby.
3. American College of Emergency Physicians: Medical direction of prehospital emergency medical services. *Ann Emerg Med* 22:767-768, 1993.
4. Polsky S, Krohmer J, Maningas P et al: Guidelines for medical direction of prehospital EMS, *Ann Emerg Med* 22:742-744, 1993.
5. McDowell R, Krohmer J, Spaite D et al: Guidelines for implementation of early defibrillation/automated external defibrillator programs, *Ann Emerg Med* 22:740-741, 1993.
6. PA Department of Health: Emergency medical services regulations. *Pa Bull* 19(Part II):2843-2884, 1989.
7. National Association of Emergency Medical Services Physicians: EMS base station function and design: on-line medical control, *Prehospital Disaster Med* 4:53-56, 1989.
8. Stewart RD, Paris PM, Heller MB: Design of a resident in-field experience for an emergency medicine residency curriculum, *Ann Emerg Med* 16:175-179, 1987.
9. Holroyd B, Knopp R, Kallsen G: Medical control: quality assurance in prehospital care, *JAMA* 256:1027-1031, 1986.
10. Polsky S, Culhane DE, McDowell et al: *Continuous quality improvement in EMS,* Dallas, 1992, American College of Emergency Physicians.
11. Swor RA, Rottman SJ, Pirrallo RG, Davis E: *Quality management in prehospital care,* St Louis, 1993, Mosby.
12. Paris PM, Benson NH: Education about prehospital care during emergency education residency training. *Prehospital Disaster Med* 5:209-205, 1990.
13. Wuerz R, Swope G, Holliman CJ, Miguel GV: On-line medical direction: a prospective study, *Prehospital Disaster Med* 10:51-54, 1995.
14. Braun O: Direct medical control. In Khuel AE, editor: *Prehospital systems and medical oversight,* 2nd ed, St Louis, 1994, Mosby.
15. Stewart C: Communication with emergency medical services providers, *Emerg Med Clin North Am* 8:103-117, 1990.
16. Emergency Medical Treatment and Active Labor Act, 42 USC; pursuant regulations effective July 22, 1994.
17. Sucov A, Verdile VP, Garettson D et al: The outcome of patients refusing prehospital transportation, *Prehospital Disaster Med* 7:365-371, 1992.
18. Zachariah BS, Bryan D, Pepe PE et al: Follow-up and outcome of patients who decline or are denied transport by EMS, *Prehospital Disaster Med* 7:359-364, 1992.
19. Snyder JA, Baren JM, Ryan SD et al: Emergency medical service system development: results of the statewide emergency medical service technical assessment program, *Ann Emerg Med* 25:768-775, 1995.
20. New York City Health and Hospitals Corporation: Emergency Medical Service Emergency Department Standards. ed 5, October, 1986, Prepared by the Standards Subcommittee of the 911 Receiving Hospital Advisory Committee and the New York City Emergency Medical Service Staff.

97 Prehospital Personnel and Technology

Edward T. Dickinson

OUTLINE

Emergency medical services (EMS) and the emergency department maintain a symbiotic relationship mandated by the very nature of both entities. As in any symbiotic system, both EMS and the emergency department benefit from their relationship.

For EMS units, the emergency department is the end point of their patient care encounter. In the eyes of prehospital providers, the emergency department is also the hub of the medical universe as their source of medical control, medical feedback on the patient care they deliver, and the resupply depot for certain supplies.

For the emergency department, EMS units provide a steady flow of patients. Approximately 16% of emergency department patients arrive by ambulance.[1] Because the emergency department has more routine contact with EMS than virtually any other healthcare entity, a fundamental understanding of EMS personnel, equipment, and operations is essential knowledge for the emergency department physician manager.

EMS AGENCIES

The types and organizational structures of EMS agencies vary widely among states. Municipal agencies, fire departments, hospital-based units, volunteer rescue squads, and private corporations are examples of organizations that provide prehospital emergency care.

The diversity of EMS agencies providing prehospital care has led to an equally diverse variety of EMS systems around the country.[2] In some parts of the nation, all prehospital patient care is provided by a single agency. The same agency dispatches the call, provides medical care, and subsequently transports the patient to the emergency department. In other jurisdictions, several agencies provide a combined, or *tiered,* response to patient care. A typical tiered response system would be composed of fire department response of the nearest fire engine staffed by basic EMTs, response of a nontransporting fire department paramedic unit, and the use of a private ambulance service for transportation of the patient and the fire department paramedic to the hospital.

Fire department-based EMS systems have become increasingly widespread over the last two decades. Several factors have contributed to the emergence of EMS within the fire service. The Emergency Medical Services ACT of 1973 provided broad-based federal funding for EMS system development. The increased availability of funding for EMS systems throughout the 1970s was paralleled by a steady decrease in the number of actual fire calls around the nation. Fire department managers and firefighter unions, sensitive to issues of job security in light of decreased fire suppression duties, took advantage of federal funding to aggressively integrate EMS into the United States fire service. Today, EMS has now become the mainstay of many fire departments. In some cases, EMS medical responses account for more than 70% of the fire departments' total call volume.[3]

Traditionally, fire department EMS response has used firefighters cross-trained as either EMTs or paramedics operating in a tiered system such as the one described earlier. Recent trends, however, are toward fire departments providing ambulance service in addition to first response nontransporting care. This trend is largely financially driven, as municipalities, which have traditionally relied on tax-based system financing, have begun to seek out fee-for-service transport revenues that have traditionally been lost to private ambulance services in a tiered system.[4]

EMS agencies that are not fire department based are often referred to as *third service* agencies. Municipal EMS departments, private corporations, hospital-based units, and volunteer rescue squads are examples of third service agencies. Municipal agencies and volunteer rescue squads are typically empowered to provide emergency medical services by local or state legislative mandates, whereas private corporations and hospital-based services frequently provide EMS as a result of competitive bids to local jurisdictions.

An inescapable dichotomy of EMS agencies is the separation of career versus volunteer-based services. Volunteer rescue squads and ambulance corps have a long-standing tradition in EMS, especially in rural and suburban areas. These agencies' members donate many hours of noncompensated time to both emergency responses and training and continuing education. Volunteer agencies are in a constant struggle to maintain funding, recruit and retain members, and remain in compliance with state and local standards that rarely delineate between them and their monetarily compensated counterparts in EMS.

Issues of patient care, quality assurance (QA), and EMS system management often mandate emergency department physician administrators to meet with the chief officers and/or administrators of local EMS agencies. Because of the wide variety of EMS agencies, the dynamics of the interface between emergency department administration (both medical and nonmedical) and the administrators of EMS agencies need to be carefully tailored to the local EMS environment. In large catchment areas, with multiple prehospital agencies, this may require a squad by squad approach. Furthermore, the logistics of dealing with a large unionized city fire department is vastly different from that required for a 25 member volunteer rescue squad. For example, the manner in which a physician emergency department manager would resolve the QA issues surrounding a prehospital esophageal intubation would differ greatly between a large municipal fire department with a full-time medical director in charge of the department's QA program and a small volunteer rural rescue squad that lacks a formal QA mechanism.

PREHOSPITAL PROVIDERS

The didactic and clinical training of prehospital providers varies depending on the level of care delivered (Table 97-1).[5] Similarly, the medical capabilities of EMS providers also vary widely, but are generally directly proportional to their length of training and thus, level of certification (Table 97-2).[6,7] Levels of prehospital patient care are generically separated into basic life support (BLS) and advanced life support (ALS). Traditionally BLS care has included basic assessment skills (taking vital signs), basic airway management, splinting, hemorrhage control, cardiopulmonary resuscitation (CPR), and oxygen administration. ALS care has denoted more invasive skills such as defibrillation, endotracheal intubation, advanced assessment skills (breath and heart sounds), and drug administration. Recently, the distinction between BLS and ALS care has become more hazy with the introduction of modalities such as rapid defibrillation, with automatic external defibrillators (AEDs) being introduced at the first responder and EMT-Basic levels. Indeed, orotracheal intubation is now contained as an optional skill in the national EMT-Basic curriculum.[7]

The most rudimentary nationally recognized level of EMS provider certification is the first responder. First responders undergo an approximately 45-hour course in which they are trained in the equivalent of advanced first aid with the addition of determination of vital signs including blood pressures and certain other skills designed to assist the EMT or paramedic who will subsequently assume the patient's care. Because first responders are almost by definition the first on the scene of medical emergencies, there is currently great emphasis on equipping these responders with AEDs.

Beyond the first responder level of training is the emergency medical technician or EMT certification. Three levels of EMTs are nationally recognized: the EMT-Basic, the EMT-Intermediate (EMT-I), and the EMT-Paramedic (EMT-P). The federal department of transportation sets the minimal training curriculum for each of these EMT classifications, and specific scopes of practice and protocols are determined by state and local EMS authorities. Certification of EMTs is provided by the states, although the National Registry of Emergency Medical Technicians does provide competency based testing, which allows EMTs at all levels to become nationally registered. Conditions of reciprocity are determined on a state by state basis.

The EMT-Basic has emerged as the backbone of prehos-

Table 97-1 Average Training of Prehospital Personnel

	First responder	EMT-Basic	EMT-Intermediate	EMT-Paramedic
Didactic training	40 hr	85 hr	89 hr*	283 hr*
Hospital training	0-10 hr	10 hr	36 hr*	125 hr*
Practical training	17 hr	39 hr	26 hr*	155 hr*

From *Training and certification of EMS personnel. 1989, The National Association of EMS Directors, Falls Church, Va.*
*In addition to EMT-Basic Training.

Table 97-2 Sample Capabilities of EMS Providers

Skills	First responder	EMT-Basic	EMT-Intermediate	EMT-Paramedic
Assessment				
Obtains vital signs	optional	yes	yes	yes
Determines breath sounds (presence/absence)	no	yes	yes	yes
Determines breath sounds (type/quality)	no	no	yes	yes
Care skills				
CPR	yes	yes	yes	yes
Oropharyngeal airway use	yes	yes	yes	yes
Orotracheal intubation	no	optional	yes	yes
ACLS Drugs	no	no	optional	yes
Defibrillation	optional	yes	yes	yes
Surgical airway	no	no	no	yes

From National EMS Education and Practice Blueprint Task Force: *National Emergency Medical Services Education and Practice Blueprint,* Washington, D.C., 1993, National Highway Traffic Safety Administration; and *EMT-basic curriculum,* Washington, D.C., 1994, Department of Transportation.
ACLS, Advanced cardiac life support.

pital care, being the nationally accepted minimal level of training that personnel staffing an ambulance should hold. Traditionally, EMTs have provided the basic life support skills including spinal immobilization, hemorrhage control, CPR, and oxygen administration. In recent years these traditional BLS skills have been augmented by those advanced life support skills deemed so crucial to good patient care that they have been introduced into the EMTs armamentarium. Specific examples include the use of Military Anti-Shock Trousers (MAST) in the 1980s and the use of AEDs in the 1990s.

The EMT-I is a person who has already obtained certification as a basic EMT and has received more advanced training in more invasive advanced life support modalities such as intravenous techniques and endotracheal intubation.

Although intravenous and advanced airway management are currently the national standards for EMT-Is, many states have advanced EMT certifications that exceed these minimal standards yet fall short of a full-fledged paramedic. Critical care technicians and cardiac technicians are examples of this class of provider, who, in addition to providing intravenous and airway management, also provide basic advanced cardiac life support (ACLS) type care including standard cardiac arrest medications as put forth by American Heart Association ACLS guidelines.

The EMT-P is the top level of certification for prehospital providers. Most paramedic training programs exceed 1000 hours of classroom, clinical, and internship training. Didactic teaching of paramedics includes vectored instruction in medical, pediatric, obstetrics/gynecology, and surgical emergencies; and their clinical exposure routinely involves rotations through anesthesia, intensive care units, labor and delivery, and the emergency department. In practice, the paramedic is the physician's eyes, ears, and hands in the field. The EMT-P's advanced assessment skills include determination of breath and heart sounds and recognition of salient physical findings such as jugular venous distention or subcutaneous emphysema. The scope of paramedic practice varies from region to region, but routinely includes all the skills of the EMT-Basic plus electrocardiogram recognition, administration of all standard emergency medications, and emergency surgical interventions, such as needle decompression of tension pneumothorax and needle of surgical cricothyroidotomy.

COMMUNICATION SYSTEMS

It is safe to say that modern emergency medical services could not exist without a well-organized communication systems. From the patient's initial telephone call to the dispatch center to request assistance, to the radio dispatch of EMS units, to the use of biotelemetry between physicians and paramedics, EMS and communication systems are inseparable.

The first human link in most EMS systems is the dispatcher/call-taker who receives the initial call for help. During the 1980s, both dispatch centers and dispatchers were raised to new levels of sophistication. The widespread adoption of centralized 911 communications and the evolution of the enhanced 911 phone system that automatically gives the dispatcher not only the caller's phone number, but also the street address was central to this process. Today, about 75% of the US population is served by the 911 system.[8] In addition, through the pioneering work of Dr. Jeff Clawson, the EMS dispatcher was transformed from a passive conduit of scant caller information, to an emergency medical dispatcher (EMD). The EMD is trained to elicit relevant medical information from the caller and to use prearrival instructions to provide medical guidance to the caller before the arrival of the dispatched EMS unit.[9]

A basic understanding of EMS communication systems is essential for emergency department management. The most relevant aspects of EMS communications that affect the emergency department are that they provide the department with notification of incoming patients and allow the emergency physician to provide medical direction to advanced EMTs in the field.

The Federal Communications Commission (FCC) allocates specific radio frequencies to EMS applications such as dispatch, unit to unit, unit to hospital, and biotelemetry. The FCC is also responsible for licensing EMS agencies and hospitals to use these specific frequencies. The emergency department's radio capabilities will likely be mandated by the EMS system(s) that surrounds the hospital. Routinely, the most frequently used radio frequencies for hospital communications are the very high frequency (VHF) band and the ultrahigh frequency (UHF) band.

Traditionally VHF radio has been used for routine EMS to hospital notification, and UHF has been reserved for biotelemetry and medical command functions, but local variations exist.

Finally, the recent widespread use of cellular phone technology has driven many EMS agencies to use cellular communications with greater frequency. The establishment of a dedicated phone line in the emergency department to be used solely for incoming EMS telephone communications has proven a valuable addition for many emergency departments, particularly in areas where UHF and VHF radios are inconsistent methods of communication.

EMS EQUIPMENT

The specific equipment carried by EMS vehicles is determined by both state and local regulations and by the levels of training of prehospital providers. Current technologies have greatly expanded the variety of both ALS and BLS equipment carried by ambulances and rescue vehicles.

From the emergency department perspective, use of both low- and high-tech equipment by prehospital providers in patients who subsequently arrive in the department creates certain specific logistical challenges of resupply and space considerations. In practical terms, prehospital equipment that is used on patients that arrive in the emergency department can be divided into "leave behind" items and disposable and exchangeable items.

Leave behind items include equipment such as backboards, head immobilizers, and traction splints. These items tend to remain on the patient long after the EMS unit has left the emergency department, and are thus left behind by prehospital providers on a regular basis. Such items are uniformly both bulky and relatively expensive, necessitating provisions within the department for a secure and adequately sized storage area. Some emergency departments use a formal tracking system for each piece of leave behind equipment, whereas others are much less compulsive in dealing with these items. Because these items are almost exclusively attached to trauma patients, the department also needs to have a system for at least grossly decontaminating these devices of substances such as blood and vomitus before placing them in storage. A decontamination shower area can be an ideal location for cleaning these items.

Disposable and exchangeable equipment used by EMS units creates another set of emergency department logistical challenges. The primary focus is the issue of which items the department is willing to restock for the EMS units, and, of those items, which ones the department will restock gratis and which ones it will charge to either the EMS agency or the patient. Nationally, approaches run the entire spectrum on this issue, from restocking none of the items to restocking all items from gauze pads costing a few cents to external pacer pads costing $45. Which of these items the department bills for is also quite variable, but as a general rule all advanced life support supplies such as drugs and intravenous equipment are restocked to the units and the cost passed on to the patient's emergency department charges. In these systems the EMS providers usually complete some type of formal requisition form, which includes the patient's name and a detailed list of the supplies used. These forms are subsequently either reviewed by the nursing staff and incorporated into the determination of emergency department visit "level" or passed along for separate itemized billing.

The actual system by which EMS providers restock their supplies within the emergency department must be clearly delineated by each emergency department. Open, unlocked cabinets filled with supplies such as medications, intravenous and airway supplies are a set-up for larceny. However, the other extreme—sending a paramedic through the bowels of the hospital to the central pharmacy to restock a single prefilled syringe of epinephrine—is also far from optimal, as it may put the EMS unit out of service for a prolonged time. In general, the assignment of an EMS contact person (usually a nurse) on each shift best facilitates accurate exchange of information and supplies. The EMS contact person can coordinate the return of "leave behinds" to their rightful owners, supervise the restocking of medications and other supplies, and ensure that the appropriate documentation for billing of supplies is placed on the patient's chart.

INFECTIOUS DISEASE ISSUES

All emergency departments must make provisions for various infectious disease issues relating to EMS. The emergency department needs to make policy and provisions for the biomedical waste and contaminated sharps generated by EMS services. Such guidelines must meet Occupational Safety and Health Administration (OSHA) standards where applicable and be clearly understood by emergency department staff and EMS providers. In some circumstances, the emergency department may develop specific exchange systems with EMS agencies to assist the agencies in meeting certain infection control mandates. An example would be exchanging a contaminated laryngoscope blade with an agency for a hospital autoclaved laryngoscope blade, thus alleviating that agency's need to decontaminate the blade to OSHA standards in the station setting.[10] In addition, recent federal legislation mandates that hospitals must evaluate and disclose relevant information concerning the exposure of EMS providers to specific airborne and blood-borne infectious diseases.[11] This responsibility will likely rest within the medical administration of the emergency department.

DOCUMENTATION

Documentation of the treatment EMS units deliver to their patients is critical medical and legal information. The emergency department is generally obligated to provide some space for EMTs to complete their mandated documentation of the patient encounter. Similarly, the department should have a system in place which ensures that the prehospital care reports are not only available to the emergency department's medical and clerical staff, but also guarantees that records are incorporated into the permanent hospital records.

Documentation of the medical direction provided by physicians over the base station radio is also important. In some regions of the country, this documentation may be used to generate additional revenues for the emergency department. In all cases, written documentation of base station activity should be stored and maintained because audio documentation of base station transmissions is either nonexistent or erased on a regular basis by communication centers.

Finally, analysis of patient care reports and base station records, combined with physician and staff observations, can be an integral part of the quality assurance feedback loop to EMS providers.

SUMMARY

Prehospital emergency medical services and the emergency department share a truly intimate relationship. A well-rounded understanding of the training, equipment, and motivations of prehospital providers is essential to both patient care and smooth emergency department operations and management.

REFERENCES

1. *U.S. emergency medicine statistical profile,* Dallas, 1993, American College of Emergency Physicians.
2. EMS in the United States: a survey of providers in the 200 most populous cities. *J Emerg Med Serv* 18:72-85, 1993.
3. City of Albany Fire Department: *1993 Run Tabulations,* Albany, NY, 1993, Albany Fire Department.
4. Stout JL: System financing. In Kuehl AE (editor): *Principles of EMS systems,* ed 2, Dallas, 1994, American College of Emergency Physicians.
5. *Training and certification of EMS personnel,* Falls Church, Va, 1989, The National Association of EMS Directors,
6. *National Emergency Medical Services Education and Practice Blueprint,* 1993, National EMS Education and Practice Blueprint Task Force.
7. EMT-Basic Curriculum, Department of Transportation, 1994.
8. Lumpe D: Calling 911: who will answer the call? *Emerg Med News* XV:10-14, 1993.
9. Clawson J, Dernocoeur K: *Principals of emergency medical dispatch,* Englewood Cliffs, 1988, Brady-Prentice Hall.
10. Stern A, Dickinson ET: Soak that scope. Cleaning laryngoscope blades. *J Emerg Med Serv* 8:64-66, 1993.
11. Title IV, Subtitle B of the Ryan White Comprehensive AIDS Resources Emergency Act of 1990 (Ryan White Act), *Fed Reg* 54:1994.

98 Prehospital Therapies

Peter T. Pons

OUTLINE

Philosophy of prehospital therapies
Prehospital therapies
- Overview
- Trauma
- Nontrauma
- Pediatric

Summary

From its pioneering roots in the mobile coronary care unit initiated by Pantridge[1,2] in Belfast, Ireland, in the late 1960s, prehospital emergency medical care has undergone a revolution in the last 20 to 25 years. Where once the only real purpose for calling an ambulance was to obtain rapid transportation to a hospital, we have now come to expect the arrival of trained professional technicians who bring to the patient many of the treatments that formerly were available only in the hospital and provided only by physicians. This chapter reviews the current status of prehospital interventions provided by Emergency Medical Services (EMS) agencies in the United States.

PHILOSOPHY OF PREHOSPITAL THERAPIES

It is appropriate to first discuss what may be considered the philosophy of prehospital, or what some are now referring to as out-of-hospital, emergency medical care. EMS should provide two crucial components of medical care. The first is access to a medical care system that rapidly evaluates the nature and urgency of the patient complaint and matches that complaint to the available and appropriate resources in the community. Second, the EMS system is still responsible for providing transportation of the patient to the healthcare delivery site.

In addition to accomplishing these two goals, EMS systems now provide a wide variety of advanced interventions including drug therapy, airway management, and invasive procedures. It is imperative to decide what is appropriate to be performed in the field setting and what should be delayed until arrival at the hospital. Even though many interventions can be accomplished in an ambulance, not all of them should be done in the field. As a general rule, field interventions should be limited to those that can be easily maintained, be performed with relative speed, have a low risk/benefit ratio, and positively affect patient outcome.

Difficulties have been encountered in the prehospital setting with regard to the last criterion—positively affecting patient outcome. In numerous instances, a particular procedure, piece of equipment, or therapy has been introduced into the field setting, gathered widespread acceptance, and in some cases even been mandated by law before any prospective, controlled studies have documented the efficacy of the intervention. Only recently has it been recognized that research and critical evaluation of the role of planned additions to the prehospital provider's armamentarium are needed and that these studies should be accomplished before, and not after, formal endorsement of the additional procedure or therapy.

Prehospital emergency medical care is the practice of emergency medicine out of the hospital by providers performing their function under the extended license of a physician as required by law in every state in the United States. Therefore physicians must be involved in the development, maintenance, and updating of the medical protocols these personnel operate under, as well as participate in the quality improvement activities of the service agency. The service agency must grant adequate authority to match this responsibility. Beyond the medical care issues, the role of the physician medical director can be, and often is, debated. How much the physician is involved in other administrative activities depends on the individual agency; however, it is essential that the medical supervisory role for patient care not be delegated or diluted.

PREHOSPITAL THERAPIES

Overview

Fundamental to the prehospital management of any patient is the recognition that patients fall into two general categories: those who have sustained injury (from whatever mechanism) and those who have called for assistance for nontrauma-related diseases. At one time, all patients were treated the same by the EMS system. This practice was shown to be detrimental to some groups of patients. Definitive care for the victim of trauma, for instance, is related to the control of hemorrhage, usually operatively, and replacement of circulating blood volume. This can be accomplished only in the hospital. Therefore the field management of the trauma patient must prioritize expeditious evacuation and transport to an appropriate destination. On the other hand, the nontrauma patient, in particular those with acute cardiac problems, can often be stabilized in the prehospital setting before transport. Thus it is acceptable for the medical care provider to intervene more comprehensively in these cases at the scene.

Although it is often not considered a component of prehospital therapy, the choice of destination has a profound effect on patient outcome. In EMS systems that have more than one destination to choose from, policies should be in place that define criteria, based on medical need, for choosing one institution over another. Ideally, political and financial considerations should be subordinated to the fact that all hospitals do not provide every therapy, and patient need is the ultimate determinant of destination. To that end, the following is a general protocol for choosing a destination:

- Patients who are critically ill or injured and have a special medical need should be taken to the closest facility that can provide for that need.
- Patients who are critically ill without a special need should be taken to the closest appropriate facility.
- Everybody else should receive their choice of destination or the closest facility if they have no expressed preference.

In this way, the EMS system and the medical community recognize that there are cases (usually no more than 2% to 10%) where the patient should be directed to a destination because of the need for specialized or immediate care, whereas the rest of the patients, who often have preexisting relationships with physicians or hospitals, can have their choice of destination or can go to the closest hospital if they do not have a choice.

Trauma

Airway. It has generally been accepted that airway management of the trauma patient is a priority and is one of the few procedures that should be performed at the scene.[3] Traditional dogma has taught that if the mechanism of injury is such that the potential for cervical spine injury exists, the spine should be kept immobile and the airway managed by any means available other than oral endotracheal intubation. These patients were thus treated with nasotracheal intubation, esophageal obturator airways, and assorted other airway devices. Review of the literature failed to substantiate the concern that oral intubation was unsafe if appropriate precautions were taken. Therefore the current recommendation is that oral endotracheal intubation is the procedure of choice, with in-line stabilization of the spine when the mechanism of injury suggests potential spinal injury.

Transport. As mentioned earlier in this chapter, definitive care of the trauma patient is based on control of hemorrhage from injured organs such as the torn or ruptured spleen, liver, blood vessel, or other site and restoration of the patient's blood volume by transfusion when necessary. These interventions can only occur at the hospital; therefore rapid transport of the patient to an appropriate destination must be considered an integral component of prehospital trauma care and every bit as important as any other direct therapy performed by the provider.[4]

Intravenous and Fluid Administration. Treatment of shock in the trauma patient has undergone significant scrutiny in the last several years, bringing into question whether traditional intervention is appropriate or perhaps even detrimental. Field management of traumatic shock has revolved around Pneumatic Anti-Shock Garment (PASG) application, venous access, and crystalloid fluid administration.

PNEUMATIC ANTISHOCK GARMENT. Nowhere has the issue of appropriate (or inappropriate) evaluation of a prehospital intervention before widespread implementation been better illustrated than in the case of the PASG. Twenty years ago, the PASG was introduced to EMS and immediately hailed as the answer to the need for a simple device that could be used in the field to raise the blood pressure of patients in shock.[5-9] In a short time, it was considered an essential piece of equipment on ambulances and was mandated in many states by inclusion in the EMS statutes.

Research demonstrated that the device did in fact raise blood pressure[6,7]; however the effect on patient outcome was not studied in a prospective fashion until recently. Mattox et al.[10,11] showed that contrary to popular belief the PASG did not improve outcome and in cases of thoracic trauma actually increased mortality. Other studies have documented similar findings.[12] It has been suggested that the garment may be beneficial in victims who have sustained abdominal or pelvic injury because the device can conceivably compress the bleeding site under the garment. However, additional work is needed to prove or disprove this theory, especially in the nonurban EMS environment where transport time is long and provider skill may be different from that found in the urban setting.

INTRAVENOUS ACCESS. Numerous studies in the early and mid 1980s questioned whether prehospital providers could rapidly initiate intravenous access in trauma victims where every minute spent in the field was costly for the patient.[3,13-18] These studies reported that paramedics were taking as long as 13 minutes to obtain venous access.[3] Others documented that paramedics in systems with strong medical control and quality assessment programs could start an intravenous (IV) line in 1 to 4 minutes.[19,20] In addition, O'Gorman et al.[21] demonstrated that paramedics could obtain venous access in a moving ambulance as successfully as in a stationary site. Thus it appears that if prehospital providers can expeditiously access a vein, it is acceptable to do so, and in most cases the procedure should be initiated after transport has been initiated.

FLUID RESUSCITATION. Once a vein has been cannulated, traditional teaching has been to administer crystalloid to the patient in shock in an effort to normalize blood pressure. As with the PASG, the effect on outcome was never evaluated or questioned. Recent animal studies have suggested that instead of improving outcome, rapid infusion of large volumes of crystalloid may accelerate the rate of on-going hemorrhage and increase morbidity and mortality.[22] A recent human study undertaken to evaluate this question demonstrated no statistical difference in outcome between those patients who received traditional field resuscitation and those who had delayed crystalloid administration.[23] Continued study is necessary to answer this question; at present, the usual practice is to initiate crystalloid resuscitation and restore the systolic blood pressure to 90 to 110 mm Hg.

Miscellaneous Trauma Techniques. Several invasive procedures are taught to prehospital providers and often performed on trauma victims, including needle thoracostomy for suspected tension pneumothorax and pericardiocentesis for suspected cardiac tamponade. As has been mentioned, no studies have been performed that demonstrate the effectiveness of these procedures in the field setting.

Nontrauma

Airway. Airway management in cases of non-trauma-related disease is generally accepted as appropriate for the prehospital setting. Oral or nasal endotracheal intubation is the procedures of choice when airway control is necessary.

IV and Fluid Administration. Obtaining venous access is not a controversial procedure for the medical patient. Many patients will require pharmacologic treatment as soon as possible to stabilize or treat the presenting symptoms or disease process. When indicated, crystalloid administration may be initiated in the field for the patient who is volume depleted.

Pharmacology and Procedures

CARDIAC. Advanced life support (ALS) efforts in prehospital care had their origins in cardiac care. The first reported ALS ambulance was developed and implemented by Pantridge in Belfast to decrease the mortality rate from out-of-hospital cardiac arrest.[2] Since then, treatment of the cardiac patient and the patient who has sustained cardiac arrest has been the subject of significant investigation. Current treatment of the cardiac patient is guided by the recommendations of the American Heart Association.

Once cardiac arrest has occurred, the time to electrical defibrillation of the fibrillating heart is the only intervention that has been shown to positively affect patient outcome.[24] Emergency medical services efforts to treat cardiac arrest in a given community must be directed toward providing defibrillation as soon as possible.[25,26] Patient survival is optimized if defibrillation is provided within 8 minutes or less from the time of arrest. Technologic advances in computer algorithms have now brought this intervention to the lay person. Automated defibrillators, which can analyze a cardiac rhythm, determine if a shock is needed, and either deliver that shock or advise the operator to deliver the shock, are now widely available and obviate the need for training in rhythm recognition and manual defibrillation.[27]

Transcutaneous cardiac pacing for the prehospital setting was initially met with great enthusiasm. It appeared that a method had been developed that would permit the application of pacing to a much wider population than was previously available. Unfortunately, this reaction has since been tempered by the reality that in the majority of cases for which it was anticipated to be of benefit, in fact, transcutaneous pacing has not provided a significant impact.[28]

The pharmacology of prehospital cardiac arrest care also has undergone a reevaluation.[29] Just as various techniques are being critically studies to determine their efficacy, so too are the drug interventions.[30,31] The American Heart Association has now classified the "standard" cardiac arrest drugs, which for so long have been used with minimal science to guide their administration, into several groups based on their documented action and efficacy. Drugs such as epinephrine, atropine, and adenosine have defined indications for use. Other drugs such as sodium bicarbonate and isoproterenol have limited use.

Of particular interest and importance is work in the area of prehospital treatment of myocardial infarction. Several studies have shown that, as with trauma, the time to definitive care of the heart attack victim is crucial to the final outcome. In the case of myocardial infarction, this is the time to diagnosis and initiation of thrombolysis. Administering thrombolytic medications in the field and obtaining prehospital 12-lead electrocardiograms have significantly shortened the time to treatment.[32,33]

Finally, several studies have begun the process of evaluating the role of prehospital pharmacologic intervention in other cardiac-related situations not involving cardiac arrest. Hoffman and Reynolds[34] compared several treatment regimens for out-of-hospital management of pulmonary edema and Meador and Wuerz[35] evaluated the prehospital care provided to patients diagnosed in the field with congestive heart failure. Each of these studies demonstrated that although significant benefit can be obtained from appropriate prehospital pharmacologic treatment, limitations remain. The optimal combination of drugs for management has yet to be determined. Correctly diagnosing the presenting condition to provide appropriate treatment is difficult. Each of these concerns is also valid for the host of other medical conditions prehospital providers are expected to evaluate and treat.

RESPIRATORY. One of the most common respiratory related complaints treated by prehospital providers is shortness of breath due to asthma or chronic obstructive pulmonary disease. The mainstays of therapy were once epinephrine and aminophylline. These drugs have largely been supplanted by the aerosolized preparations such as albuterol and metaproterenol. Both drugs are easily administered in an ambulance and can be obtained prepackaged in a unit dose for ease of preparation.

OTHER. Although prehospital providers are confronted with a wide variety of presenting complaints and diseases, three bear mentioning because of their frequency and the ability to treat them in the field with relative ease. Many diabetic patients have episodes of hypoglycemia resulting from their antidiabetes agent, whether oral or parenteral. Reversal of symptoms is easily accomplished in the field by the administration of 50% dextrose intravenously. The second group of patients are those who have seizures. Although the majority of patients will have an isolated seizure that is over by the time the ambulance arrives, some will go on to have status epilepticus. In most cases the seizure can be aborted in the field by the administration of a benzodiazepine parenterally. Finally, patients who have overdosed on opiates and present with central nervous system depression or respiratory arrest can be easily reversed with the administration of naloxone.

Pediatric

Overview. The physiology of the infant and child are different from that of the adult. Knowledge of normal variations in vital signs and compensatory mechanisms is essential in assessing these patients. The ability of the provider to adequately evaluate the patient and determine organ system dysfunction is more important than arriving at a differential or final diagnosis. Prehospital providers must be aware that pediatric patients more often sustain cardiac arrest secondarily as a complication of respiratory problems rather than primary cardiac disease. Pediatric patients require specially sized equipment, and drug doses and fluid volume must be modified based on size and weight. Finally, knowing when to transport rather than spend a great deal of time attempting to intervene is probably just as important as the variety of prehospital therapies that can be performed.

Airway. Perhaps the most important intervention that can be performed in the prehospital setting when treating a pediatric patient is ensuring a patent airway and maintaining adequate oxygenation. As mentioned earlier, primary respiratory failure is the most common cause of cardiac arrest in children. At the same time, the prehospital provider must know when airway management is not needed as an emergency. For example, most children with seizures do not need active airway intervention. Most children with croup and epiglottitis can be adequately managed by allowing them to assume a position of comfort and providing rapid transport. The ability of the provider to assess the physiologic status of the child is crucial in making airway intervention decisions.

IV and Fluid Administration. In contrast to adults, the need to start an IV line in children to restore volume in the prehospital setting is rare. Instead, IV access is usually necessary only when medications must be given; these situations are generally limited to cardiac arrest and anaphylaxis. Unfortunately, IV access in the pediatric patient is often technically difficult to obtain, and the patient in whom the line is desired the most is the most troublesome. Intraosseus placement is a viable alternative for IV access in the pediatric patient and in many cases may be faster than continued attempts at venous cannulation.

When the decision is made to administer crystalloid, the volume must be determined by a strict milliliter per kilogram of weight calculation. Failure to do so may cause life-threatening complications such as pulmonary edema.

Pharmacology. In the overwhelming majority of pediatric patients, pharmacologic therapy is not needed in the prehospital setting. Exceptions include the patient who has sustained cardiac arrest or is having an anaphylactic reaction. As is the case with fluid administration, drug doses must also be calculated on a per kilogram of weight basis to prevent underdosing one patient and overdosing another.

SUMMARY

The prehospital treatment of adults and children has undergone a revolution in the last 25 years. To paraphrase Abraham Lincoln, the dogmas of the quiet past are inadequate for the present. That which is considered acceptable today will no doubt be the discard of tomorrow. Yet as we participate in the evolution of this aspect of our specialty, a number of points must be made.

As new drugs, tools, and interventions are introduced to the practice of medicine, they must be carefully evaluated in the prehospital setting and their efficacy determined based on patient outcome before widespread acceptance and implementation occurs. Even when efficacy has been determined, each prehospital agency must evaluate the logistics and cost of implementation. The cost is not only financial. There is an associated cost in resource availability and prehospital time whenever a change in practice occurs. These must be balanced with the potential benefit of introducing the change.

REFERENCES

1. Pantridge JF, Geddes JS: Cardiac arrest after myocardial infarction, *Lancet* 1:807, 1966.
2. Pantridge JF, Geddes JS: A mobile intensive-care unit in the management of myocardial infarction, *Lancet* 2:271-273, 1967.
3. Smith JP, Bodai BI, Hill AS et al: Prehospital stabilization of critically injured patients: a failed concept, *J Trauma* 25:65, 1985.
4. West J, Trunkey D: Systems of trauma care: a study of two counties, *Arch Surg* 114:455, 1979.
5. Civetta JM, Nussenfeld SR, Rowe TR et al: Prehospital use of the military anti-shock trouser (MAST), *J Am Coll Emerg Phys* 5:581, 1976.
6. Kaback KR, Sanders AB, Meislin HW: MAST suit update, *JAMA* 252:2598, 1984.
7. McSwain NE: Pneumatic trousers and the management of shock, *J Trauma* 17:719, 1977.
8. McSwain NE: Pneumatic anti-shock garment: state of the art 1988, *Ann Emerg Med* 17:506, 1988.
9. Soler J, Muller HA, Kennedy TJ: Clinical use of the "G-Suit", *J Am Coll Emerg Phys* 5:609, 1976.
10. Mattox KL, Bickell WH, Pepe PE et al: Prospective randomized evaluation of antishock MAST in post-traumatic hypotension, *J Trauma* 26:779, 1986.
11. Mattox KL, Bickell W, Pepe PE et al: Prospective MAST study in 911 patients, *J Trauma* 29:1104, 1989.
12. Honigman B, Lowenstein SR, Moore EE et al: The role of the pneumatic antishock garment in penetrating cardiac wounds, *JAMA* 266:2398, 1991.
13. Aprahamian C, Thompson BM, Towne JB et al: The effect of a paramedic system on mortality of major open intra-abdominal vascular trauma, *J Trauma* 23:687, 1983.
14. Clevenger FW, Yarbrough DR, Reines HD: Resuscitative thoracotomy: the effect of field time on outcome, *J Trauma* 28:441, 1988.
15. Cwinn AA, Pons PT, Moore EE et al: Prehospital advanced trauma life support for critical blunt trauma victims, *Ann Emerg Med* 16:399, 1987.
16. Gervin AS, Fischer RP: The importance of prompt transport in salvage of patients with penetrating heart wounds, *J Trauma* 22:443, 1982.
17. Smith JP, Bodai BI: The urban paramedic's scope of practice, *JAMA* 253:544, 1985.
18. Spaite DW, Tse DJ, Valenzuela TD et al: The impact of injury severity and prehospital procedures on scene time in victims of major trauma, *Ann Emerg Med* 20:1299, 1991.
19. Jones SE, Nesper TP, Alcouloumre E: Prehospital intravenous line placement: a prospective study, *Ann Emerg Med* 18:244, 1989.
20. Pons PT, Moore EE, Cusick JM et al: Prehospital venous access in an urban paramedic system: a prospective on-scene analysis, *J Trauma* 28:1460, 1988.
21. O'Gorman M, Trabulsy P, Pilcher DB: Zero-time prehospital IV, *J Trauma* 29:84, 1989.
22. Kowalenko T, Stern S, Dronen S et al: Improved outcome with hypotensive resuscitation of uncontrolled hemorrhagic shock in a swine model, *J Trauma* 33:349, 1992.
23. Martin RR, Bickell WH, Pepe PE et al: Prospective evaluation of preoperative fluid resuscitation in hypotensive patients with penetrating truncal injury: a preliminary report, *J Trauma* 33:354, 1992.
24. Dean NC, Haug PJ, Hawker PJ: Effect of mobile paramedic units on outcome in patients with myocardial infarction, *Ann Emerg Med* 17:1034, 1988.
25. Eisenberg MS, Horwood BT, Cummins RO et al: Cardiac arrest and resuscitation: a tale of 29 cities, *Ann Emerg Med* 19:179, 1990.
26. Olson DW, LaRochelle J, Fark D et al: EMT-defibrillation: the Wisconsin experience, *Ann Emerg Med* 18:806, 1989.
27. Weaver WD, Hill D, Fahrenbruch CE et al: Use of the automatic external defibrillator in the management of out-of-hospital cardiac arrest, *N Engl J Med* 319:661, 1988.
28. Barthell E, Troiano P, Olson D et al: Prehospital external cardiac pacing: a prospective, controlled clinical trial, *Ann Emerg Med* 17:1221, 1988.
29. Shuster M, Chong J: Pharmacologic intervention in prehospital care: a critical appraisal, *Ann Emerg Med* 18:192, 1989.
30. Brown CG, Martin DR, Pepe PE et al: A comparison of standard-dose and high-dose epinephrine in cardiac arrest outside the hospital, *N Engl J Med* 327:1051, 1992.
31. Stiell IG, Hebert PC, Weitzman BN et al: High-dose epinephrine in adult cardiac arrest, *N Engl J Med* 327:1045, 1992.
32. Belgian Eminase Prehospital Study Collaborative Group: Prehospital thrombolysis in acute myocardial infarction: the Belgian Eminase prehospital study, *Eur Heart J* 12:965, 1991.
33. Weaver WD, Eisenberg MS, Martin JS et al: Myocardial infarction triage and intervention project—Phase I: Patient characteristics and feasibility of prehospital initiation of thrombolytic therapy, *J Am Coll Cardiol* 15:925, 1990.
34. Hoffman JR, Reynolds S: Comparison of nitroglycerin, morphine and furosemide in treatment of presumed pre-hospital pulmonary edema, *Chest* 92:586, 1987.
35. Wuerz RC, Meador SA: Effects of prehospital medications on mortality and length of stay in congestive heart failure, *Ann Emerg Med* 21:669, 1992.

99 Diversion and Bypass

Jon R. Krohmer

OUTLINE

In recent years increasing numbers of patients have been seeking care in emergency departments in the United States. Reasons for this increasing census include lack of primary care resources, larger numbers of patients sustaining traumatic injuries, and the desire of the population to receive medical care in a manner most convenient to them. Many of these reasons have prompted the current initiative for health-care reform. This increased census frequently causes emergency departments to face situations in which the department is "overcrowded," potentially stressing available resources to a critical level. Although this formerly affected primarily large, urban teaching hospitals, the overcrowding phenomenon has begun to affect suburban areas as well. When this occurs, the hospital must address the issue of "closing" the hospital or emergency department to Emergency Medical Services (EMS) traffic, forcing the institution to "divert" ambulances from that hospital. The overcrowding then becomes an issue for the affected hospital and EMS system and, ultimately, the other hospitals participating in that EMS system. The overall goal of the EMS system is to ensure that patient transport occurs to the closest facility with the most appropriate resources for the patient's needs.[1-3]

The EMS system, working with emergency department managers of the participating institutions, must develop mechanisms to identify situations in which needed hospital resources are not available and in which temporary diversion of EMS patients from that hospital is acceptable; notify system participants of those situations; and provide for the safe, appropriate, and time-efficient care of patients entering the EMS system. Mechanisms for accomplishing those goals are discussed in this chapter.

Often, confusion exists between destination protocols and diversion policies. Many times those terms are used interchangeably; destination protocols and diversion policies are often referred to collectively as "diversion" or "bypass." For purposes of this chapter, a distinction is made between an EMS destination protocol and a diversion policy (Box 99-1).

SYSTEM OVERCROWDING

A number of articles have outlined the overcrowding issue in emergency departments.[4-7] More patients are seeking care in emergency departments with increasing numbers of hospital admissions arising in the department. Those who are subsequently admitted are often more seriously ill.[8] A number of factors are contributing to this emergency department overcrowding problem (Box 99-2).

Overcrowding leads to significant congestion in emergency departments and severely limits both the timely access to emergency care and the quality of care that can be provided. Mechanisms that have been suggested for managing this overcrowding include restricting access to some types of patients, actively transferring patients to other facilities, refusing to accept transfers from other facilities, and diverting ambulances.[2-4] Obviously there are significant medical, legal, and financial implications of all of those choices.

DESTINATION POLICIES

It is generally well accepted that the patient has the right to select his or her physician and hospital; most EMS systems support this principle. EMS systems, however, also recognize that certain groups of patients are best served by being transported to institutions that have the appropriate resources to care for the patient's particular needs. This may be necessary even if a particular center is neither the patient's primary choice nor the closest institution. In most cases, when that occurs, it is in the patient's best interest that the transport occur directly to that specialty center without stopping at another institution (either by patient preference or proximity) initially. This is most evident in the use of trauma and burn centers when those resources are necessary and available. Other, similar situations may occur in the case of specialized pediatric care, psychiatric problems, high-risk obstetric care, and the need for hyperbaric oxygen therapy. Those types of decisions for direct transport to specialty care centers should be established by policy by the EMS system, in cooperation with the participating hospitals and emergency departments, with the patient's best interest in mind.[1]

To function effectively, these policies should be prospectively established before the destination decision must be made by out-of-hospital personnel for any particular patient. The designation of particular institutions as specialty care centers should be made based on prior review by the EMS system of the institutions' resources using preexisting criteria. These criteria may be established by the local EMS system or by state (e.g., state health department) or national organizations (e.g., American College of Surgeons or trauma center criteria). Certification or verification by a state or national organization may serve in place of the local review.

BOX 99-1

DISTINCTION BETWEEN DESTINATION PROTOCOL AND DIVERSION POLICY

Destination protocol: An EMS protocol that prospectively establishes, by policy and protocol, certain categories of patients who should be transported directly to specialty care centers (e.g., burn unit or trauma center)

Diversion policy: A policy that establishes a mechanism for an EMS system to transport patients, for preestablished reasons, to facilities other than those to which the patients would normally have been transported if the defined reasons did not exist (e.g., "no room at the inn")

BOX 99-2

REASONS FOR OVERCROWDING

- Insufficient number of beds
- Hospital and emergency department closures of other institutions in the geographic area
- Shortage of healthcare professionals (difficulty recruiting and retaining nurses and physicians in needed areas)
- Changes in patient populations using emergency departments: (e.g., victims of violence, drug abuse)
- Increased number of elderly and homeless persons
- Inadequate healthcare resources
- Large uninsured patient population

BOX 99-3

REASONS FOR REQUESTING DIVERSION STATUS

- Emergency department resources are overwhelmed.
- No critical care beds are available.
- Trauma team or operating suites are not available.
- No hospital beds are available (specific type or in general)
- Critical functional component of the hospital is incapacitated.
- Physical plant failure (fire, flood, power failure, or evacuation) has occurred.
- Internal disaster occurring.

Once the receiving hospital designations have been made, the EMS protocols must be established identifying for out-of-hospital personnel those patients who should be transported to the specialty care center. Those protocols should include medically relevant criteria identifying measurable or observable parameters (e.g., vital sign abnormalities, mechanisms of injury, and stage of pregnancy) that can be easily identified in the field based on patient presentation. Those criteria should explicitly describe the findings or signs that are required to trigger the decision by out-of-hospital personnel to transport directly to the specialty care center. Review of the criteria, destination protocols, and hospital designations must be routinely reviewed as part of the EMS system's Quality Improvement program.

DIVERSION POLICIES

As previously noted, a diversion policy provides a mechanism for a hospital to inform the EMS system, its providers and personnel, and the medical direction component that the hospital does not wish to receive patients. This may apply either to certain types of patients (e.g., head-injured patients only) or to all EMS-transported patients. Diversion status may be requested for a number of reasons (Box 99-3).

The American College of Emergency Physicians has identified a series of guidelines that can be used when developing a diversion policy.[1] The National Association of EMS Physicians is also finalizing such guidelines. In addition, many local EMS systems have policies in place that could be used as models.

Diversion status can be requested when the staff of the institution believe that they are not able to adequately care for an increased patient load. The process by which a hospital requests diversion status must be established prospectively. Generally the criteria used are established by the EMS lead agency (e.g., medical control authority) with input from and cooperation of all the out-of-hospital agencies and hospitals in the EMS system. The criteria should apply equally to all the participating institutions. It is important that all hospitals within the EMS system work together to ensure appropriate bed utilization (both inpatient and emergency department beds). In addition to establishing the criteria to qualify for diversion status, the EMS system lead agency must have a plan for reviewing resources and categorizing receiving facilities to allow for appropriate destination decisions when diversions are in effect.

The criteria established for requesting diversion should be based on exceeding the hospital's capabilities for providing needed services. They should not be based on such factors as protection of beds for elective cases or unforeseen needs (e.g., walk-ins or in-house patient deterioration) or a desire not to call in additional staff. Obviously no diversion should occur because of a patient's financial resources. Hospitals should exhaust all internal mechanisms to relieve the precipitating situation before requesting diversion status. To ensure that all attempts have been made to internally alleviate the situation, responsible hospital administrative and clinical personnel should carefully review the situation before requesting diversion status. That request should be made to the EMS system by hospital personnel who have been prospectively "approved" by the EMS system to submit such a request. Limiting the number of persons who can request a diversion ensures that in-house communication with appropriate administrative and clinical personnel occurs before the diversion request is declared.

Categories of acceptable diversion must also be defined by the EMS system. Categories most commonly used include critical care patients, selected patients (e.g., pediatrics, head injuries, burns, or cardiovascular diseases, etc), routine admissions, and all patients.

Once the criteria have been met, the hospital may request diversion status. Before granting the diversion request, the EMS system must ensure that the hospital's services are, in fact, limited or *not* available (by requesting sufficient information from the institution and documenting that the established criteria are met) and that patient transport to other hospitals can be safely accomplished in a timely manner with the available EMS resources.

After the diversion status has been granted, all components of the EMS system (e.g., personnel, agencies, and other hospitals) must be notified in a timely manner. This can occur via communication with all the hospitals and out-of-hospital agencies involved in the system. A Computerized Hospital On-line Resources Allocation Link (CHORAL) system has been developed that links all hospitals and communications centers together and provides immediate information about the status of all institutions operating in the system and the consequences of diversion.[9,10]

While the diversion exists, the system must ensure that patients are distributed to the other hospitals in such a manner that none of those hospitals become overloaded. Should all other hospitals in the system become overloaded, all hospitals will begin receiving patients. In that event the EMS system may have to function in a "disaster" mode with all hospitals receiving patients in an organized manner. The diversion policy should also allow provisions for the prehospital personnel to override a hospital's "diversion status" if it is in the interest of the patient to do so (e.g., critically ill patient). That patient can later be transferred from the original institution after initial stabilization.

Diversions should occur only on a temporary basis for limited periods of time. Some systems consider an automatic return to normal status after a defined period (e.g., 8 hours). During that time the hospital must make every attempt to overcome the factors necessitating the original diversion request. This may necessitate transferring patients, selectively screening admissions, calling in additional personnel, or ensuring timely equipment repair.

The EMS system must closely monitor the diversion status of participating hospitals. A regular review and updating of statuses must occur. The EMS lead agency should receive a written report of each diversion request that includes the type of diversion, the reason, anticipated or actual time of diversion activation and deactivation, and names of administrative personnel requesting and rescinding the diversion. Likewise, any variations from the diversion policy must be immediately reported to the EMS lead agency, and the variations investigated. Periodic review of the frequency of and reasons for diversions should occur as a routine part of the EMS system's Quality Improvement program.

The potential exists for ambulance diversions to significantly affect the EMS system and patient care issues. Neely and others[9] noted that transport times were longer for diverted patients and they traveled longer distances than non-diverted patients in the authors' system. In addition, the health maintenance organization–related hospitals had the highest number of hours of resource unavailability. They also had the largest number of diverted patients in the study. This was particularly true for patients participating in managed care programs. This study[9] did not report on the impact of those diversions on patient outcomes or on the overall impact on the EMS system resources.

COBRA IMPACT

The relationship between the requirements of the COBRA/OBRA regulations and hospital diversion policies is unclear. The federal "antidumping" regulations do not apply specifically to out-of-hospital agencies. There is, however, confusion regarding whether they apply when the hospital may have a "relationship" with the patient. Certainly, OBRA prevents hospitals from diverting patients simply for financial reasons (see Chapter 61).

Confusion exists regarding whether a patient has the "right" to demand to be transported to a hospital that is currently on diversion status. Certainly, not going to the "patient's hospital" has the potential to negatively affect the patient's care (e.g., no medical records available and not being able to be cared for by the personal physician). However, it is incumbent on the EMS personnel to appropriately inform the patient about the hospital's status, including possible negative consequences of being transported to that hospital, so that the patient can make an "informed" decision. The patient must understand that it may not be in his or her best interest to go to the hospital on diversion status. Obviously this information must be well documented in the out-of-hospital and emergency department records.

A second potential concern regarding diversion status centers around the issue of a hospital on diversion status providing on-line medical direction to out-of-hospital personnel. In the case of Johnson versus University of Chicago Hospital,[11] paramedics established on-line medical direction with the closest hospital before initiating transport of a child in cardiac arrest to that hospital. Because that hospital did not have any pediatric intensive care unit beds available, it diverted the patient to another nearby hospital. The patient was initially resuscitated and transferred to a third institution where he subsequently died. A charge of a COBRA violation was brought forward, using the argument that by establishing on-line medical direction, the out-of-hospital personnel had "presented" the patient to the emergency department of the closest hospital and therefore the hospital was responsible for that patient's care. The hospital was initially found to be at fault. Following several appeals, however, the courts have held that establishing on-line direction is not equivalent to physically presenting to the hospital. Nonetheless, this case does raise the issue as to whether it is in the hospital's best interest to not provide on-line direction for EMS patients while the hospital is on diversion status if the EMS system has a contingency mechanism to accomplish it.

SUMMARY

An EMS system must acknowledge that there are situations in which it is not in the best interest of patients to transport them to particular institutions. Such a situation may occur because of a lack of resources at those institutions, either on a routine or sporadic basis. The EMS system, working with participating hospitals and emergency departments, must establish a mechanism to address these situations, either through destination or diversion policies. When prospectively established criteria have been met, the information must be communicated to all participants in the EMS system. This would allow direct transport of patients to appropriate specialty care centers (e.g., destination protocols) or diversion of patients (diversion policy) when extenuating circumstances dictate the need for such. The EMS lead agency must be responsible for ensuring that all available resources are used to provide the most appropriate care needed to the citizens accessing the system.

REFERENCES

1. American College of Emergency Physicians: *Ambulance diversion/destination policies: policy statement and guidelines,* Dallas, 1991, ACEP.
2. American College of Emergency Physicians: Hospital and emergency department overcrowding: position statement, *Ann Emerg Med* 19(3):336, 1990.
3. American College of Emergency Physicians: Principles of appropriate patient transfer: position statement, *Ann Emerg Med* 19(3):337-338, 1990.
4. Andrulis DP, Kellermann A, Hintz EA et al: Emergency departments and crowding in United States teaching hospitals, *Ann Emerg Med* 20:980-986, 1991.
5. Baker DW, Stevens CD, Brook RH: Patients who leave a public hospital emergency department without being seen by a physician, *JAMA* 266:1085-1090, 1991.
6. Beck M, Glick JN, Katel J: State of emergency, *Newsweek,* pp 52-53, Oct 14, 1991.
7. Gibbs N: Do you want to die? *Time,* pp 58-65, May 28, 1990.
8. Bindman AB, Grumbach K, Keane D et al: Consequences of queuing for care at a public hospital emergency department, *JAMA* 266:1091-1096, 1991.
9. Neely, KW, Norton RL, Young GP: The effect of hospital resource unavailability and ambulance diversion on the EMS system, *Prehosp Disas Med* 9:172-177, 1994.
10. Neely KW, Bennison A, Acker J et al: Computerized Hospital On-line Resource Allocation Link (CHORAL): a mechanism to monitor and establish policy for hospital ambulance diversions, *Prehosp Disas Med* 6:459-462, 1991.
11. Reader's Forum: *Emerg Department Law* 4:1, 1993.

ADDITIONAL READINGS

Health care crisis coming to a head in the next decade. *Emerg Department Manage* 4:4-8, 1992.

Frew SA, Aranosian RD: Medical-legal concerns of EMS. In *Principles of EMS systems,* ed 2, Dallas, 1994, ACEP.

Frew SA, Roush WR, LaGreca K: COBRA: implications for emergency medicine, *Ann Emerg Med* 17:835-837, 1988.

Garza MA: Dangerous detours: ambulance diversions stall patient delivery, *J Emerg Med Serv* 14:42, 1989.

Shanaberger C: Understanding COBRA's twists and turns, *J Emerg Med Serv* 16:101-103, 1991.

Zydlo S: Diversions and bypass. In Kuehl AE, editor: *EMS medical directors' handbook,* St Louis, 1989, Mosby.

100 Improving Quality in EMS

Edgardo J. Rivera-Rivera and Robert A. Swor

OUTLINE

OVERVIEW OF QUALITY EFFORTS IN HEALTHCARE

Efforts to ensure and improve the quality of medical care are as old as the time of the ancient Egyptian pharaohs, who ordered their physicians buried with them at their deaths. No doubt, this approach to the ancient medical practitioner has influenced our view of quality efforts. Since that time a number of medical leaders have sought to improve patient care through a systematic review of care rendered. The modern era of "institutionalized" quality efforts began in the 1950s with the formation of the Joint Commission on Accreditation of Healthcare Organizations (JCAHO). This institution was formed on a voluntary basis by hospitals to develop standards generally agreed to be associated with high-quality institutions. With the inception of the Medicare program in the 1960s and its mandate that hospitals be JCAHO accredited to receive Medicare reimbursement, the issues of quality medical care and funding have become inextricably intertwined. This relationship must be remembered in any discussion of quality efforts in Emergency Medical Services (EMS).

Quality efforts in EMS, much like in general medical care, are intended to serve two vital functions. Accountability is demanded of all healthcare providers, and furthermore, the public expects that quality medical care be continuously reviewed and improved: hence the development of the disciplines of Quality Assurance (QA, to ensure quality) and Quality Improvement (QI, to improve quality), which are institutionalized in healthcare and are now being applied to EMS. There is scant research on QA in EMS and even less on QI in EMS.[1] The lack of a well-defined approach to quality methods (defined collectively in this chapter as Quality Management [QM]) coupled with the interest of the entire industry, will result in a myriad of approaches to this issue.

Quality Assurance versus Quality Improvement

Quality Assurance. Quality Assurance in healthcare has been well defined by Donabedian[2] and elsewhere in this textbook (see Chapters 52 to 55). It is responsible for key concepts in the evaluation of care, including peer review and systematic, analytic evaluation of care (prospective, concurrent, and retrospective evaluations). Quality Assurance ensures accountability, is oriented to individual providers and outcomes, and generates valuable data about care. Its limitations are that the QA focus on individuals can be perceived as punitive and that outcome evaluation is often difficult. Furthermore, QA is an "add-on" function for organizations and results are not easily integrated. Despite its benefits, it limitations have led to QA falling into disfavor in some parts of the medical community.

Quality Improvement. During the 1980s an emphasis on "QI" has pervaded American industry and is being widely implemented in healthcare as well.[3,4] Key features of QI include the following: (1) a philosophy that employees work diligently to perform their duties, (2) an emphasis that faulty processes must be improved if care is to improve, (3) a commitment to quality from senior management, and (4) empowerment of caregivers to improve the system of care. Quality in the QI approach is determined solely by the customer, with customers originating both internally and externally to an organization.

Quality Improvement philosophy as articulated by Deming[5] and others assumes that most problems (85%) are process or system in origin, rather than individual provider problems. Thus the key to quality is continuous improvement of efficient, user-friendly processes. This focus on processes is unique in that it crosses traditional boundaries in healthcare. For instance, trauma care involves EMS providers, nurses, physicians, ancillary laboratory and radiology personnel, operating rooms, and intensive care units. Quality Improvement methods focus on *data-driven* evaluations that examine the processes dealing with the complete care of the patient, not on the performance of individual disciplines. The effective implementation of QI requires an integrated organization and a management structure that is willing and able to coordinate the evaluation and provide the resources for this effort. The lack of commitment by management of adequate resources could potentially be a limitation in efforts to apply QI to EMS care.

The EMS environment holds unique challenges for physicians trying to improve quality. They must have an appreciation of the limitations and challenges of EMS systems. The purpose of this chapter is to review methods presently used in EMS and address new concepts as they may be applied to prehospital care.

The Emergency Medical Services Environment

EMS system structure plays a crucial role in the ability to adequately evaluate and improve care. Grants provided for by the EMS Act of 1973 (1200-series grants) called for development of 303 EMS regions (each of approximately 750,000 population) throughout the country. These 1200-series grants provided funding for the following: (1) feasibility studies (nos. 1201 and 1202), (2) initial operations (no. 1203), (3) expansion and improvement (no. 1204), and research (no. 1205). As these grants were used and ongoing funding dried up, improvement, expansion, and research suffered primarily.[6]

Another result of the 1973 EMS Act was the development of many different EMS system types. For medium-sized cities single-service EMS organizations evolved, facilitating coordination of resources and minimizing redundancies.[7] For other regions small municipalities were forced together, to form a single region and to compete for funding. The result was a patchwork of large and small providers for many regions of the country.

EMS care can be provided by many different agencies. The common agencies providing EMS service include firefighting services; municipal "third-service" agencies, which are neither police nor fire; public safety officers, who are police, firefighters, and EMS; private agencies; franchisees; volunteers services; and any combination of these. On a single patient encounter the system that cares for a patient may include a police dispatcher, a volunteer first responder, a firefighter to provide extrication, a private-agency paramedic to render hands-on care, and a physician from hospital A rendering medical direction for care that will be continued by a physician at hospital B. This complex approach to prehospital patient care demands an innovative approach to evaluation and QM strategies.

The administrative structure for EMS organizations is complex and similar to the hospital model of care. Operational issues of equipment, staffing, discipline, and supervisory hierarchy may be the responsibility of an owner, a fire or police chief, or a manager. Responsibility for medical care, however, including protocols, medications used, on-line supervisory responsibility, and QM, classically falls to a system medical director, who often by law is ultimately responsible for care rendered. The medical director's responsibility may be delegated in some instances to a medical board or an oversight committee, which represents the medical community of the EMS region. This structure requires a close working relationship between the medical and operational entities to resolve the many operational issues that are not directly "medical care issues" (e.g., location of emergency vehicles) but clearly impact patient care.

Scope of Authority

The initial problem an EMS system faces in developing a QM plan is defining the scope of its authority. As described earlier, patient care may often be rendered by multiple organizations over which the EMS system leadership may have limited authority. Many states provide EMS agencies authority only for care rendered by paramedics. Recently, first responders and basic providers have been acknowledged as needing EMS lead agency supervision, too. Similarly, 911 centers (also known as Public Safety Answering Points [PSAPs]), are often staffed by police agencies that have little knowledge of or experience or interest in EMS patient care. As dispatch is becoming recognized as serving a critical role in the provision of EMS care, an interest in providing medical direction for PSAPs is evolving. Statutory authority, however, may not always exist to allow implementation of training standards, dispatch protocols, and QA programs for PSAPs.

Authority for receiving facilities is similarly ill defined. For states with strong trauma legislation in place, the EMS lead agency can have responsibility for the trauma system as well. A contractual agreement with receiving hospitals is established to provide a certain level of care for trauma patients in the emergency department and throughout the hospital. In the absence of such a well-defined relationship the role of the EMS lead agency may be limited to developing standards for receiving emergency departments, or just to exerting peer pressure on hospitals to provide a uniform level of training and personnel.

Ambulance transfer of critical care patients by paramedics or Emergency Medical Technicians (EMTs) and interfacility transfers are often issues for EMS systems for a number of reasons. This service is usually provided by EMS providers that are licensed or credentialed by the EMS system. These transports, however, may require skills not normally taught to paramedics, and may take emergency vehicles out of service during times of peak demand. Patient complications are invariably handled by the EMS providers, which could have a medical governance different from that of the referring facility. In addition, interhospital transfers can be financially more attractive and therefore affect reimbursement strategies and competition for patients. For these reasons responsibility for these transports must be defined by the EMS system leadership.

DATA COLLECTION AND HANDLING

Coordination of the varied sources of data collection and evaluation is a major logistic burden for the EMS system. Sources of patient care data include standardized EMS "runsheets," agency dispatch logs, police and fire department reports, base station order sheets, emergency department records, inpatient charts, and pathology reports. Agreements must be obtained to allow data access or submission with all these varied organizations. Concrete assurances must be given that confidentiality will be maintained. Collation of various sources of data for a single patient may be a difficult, exceedingly complex task for an entire system. Centralization of record handling with proper controls for these records is critical for QM program development.

Sophisticated methods of data collection, such as optical scanning of EMS runsheets as developed by Joyce and others,[8] have led to efforts to develop large EMS databases in a number of states such as Arizona, Mississippi, Colorado, and

Pennsylvania. Some areas have used other computerized methods such as bar coding and handheld electronic recording devices. Common data elements for both EMS care and QM activities must be identified early in the development of a QM program.[9] No method of data handling is effective unless common data elements are well defined throughout the system and expectations are developed for data recording.

DEVELOPING STANDARDS FOR EMERGENCY MEDICAL SERVICES

The role of standards in EMS is variable; few standards are well defined throughout the country. National standards for individual patients for a given level of provider are equally applicable to urban, suburban, and rural systems. Performance standards for training are also similar. Structural standards for a system have been delineated by Stout[10,11] and others and may be used as references in local development. Local standards should include the number of personnel, types of equipment, medications used, and so forth. Of particular importance in each environment is the process of standard development, which must address local realities. Key considerations include resource availability, medical community support, geographic constraints, statutory mandates, and political issues. For example, a published national standard of an 8-minute response time for 90% of all calls is meaningless in a predominately rural community. Similarly, mutual aid agreements mandating response of a closest vehicle to an emergency may be precluded by a municipality's ordinance that forbids response of an ambulance outside its city limits.

Many agencies have unique needs and constraints in their ability to adhere to standards. Therefore a broad-based consensus approach to standard development with exhaustive discussion is absolutely vital if standards are to be enforceable throughout the EMS region. Unless this political process is adhered to, retrospective enforcement of standards is doomed to failure. Specific standards such as training, staffing levels, continuing education, and patient care protocols must all be addressed. A failure to have appropriate standards may serve as a basis for malpractice actions against an EMS system.[12]

Standards for documentation, radio communications, and data collection are often overlooked and should be developed. Key elements of information for radio reports and runsheets should be identified for all cases and for specific case types. These standards serve as a model for inculcating new EMTs into the system and for retrospective review of patient care. A manual addressing these topics is a valuable supporting document and is used in many large systems.

EVALUATION OF SYSTEM COMPONENTS

System-Based versus Service-Based Review

Evaluation of system components must take place both at the level of the individual service and regionwide. Confidentiality and logistic factors favor the use of in-house, service-based activities to evaluate compliance with standards, performance of invasive procedures, minor incidents, and appropriate documentation. In general, service-based activities assess care rendered to individual patients. System-based activity, on the other hand, evaluates care rendered by the entire system. Evaluations are conducted by an independent agency to provide impartial confirmation of standard compliance, review major incidents, review triage protocols and adherence to them, and assess system parameters that cross agency boundaries.[13]

Prospective Evaluation

Prospective evaluation is the major means by which quality of care has been ensured in EMS systems. The assurance that the components are in place to provide quality EMS care is critically important. It is also logistically less burdensome than other methods of review. Key parameters to review include system structure, key policies and procedures for patient care, standing orders for direct patient care, and credentialing of providers at the many different levels of care.

Credentialing of providers is an important task and to a large extent dictates the standard of care that will be provided in a system. Requirements for paramedics in most systems include initial training requirements and further local training demands. Advanced Cardiac Life Support (ACLS) and Basic Trauma Life Support (BTLS) certification are two of the most common additional training requirements. Many systems also require practical or didactic testing at the time of recertification. Documentation of procedural proficiency is required by some large systems. Alamada County, California, and King County, Washington, require that a minimum number of intubations be performed, to qualify for recertification. This practice makes particular sense in systems that have a relatively large number of paramedics and Advanced Life Support units (e.g., suburban systems), which dilute each individual's procedural expertise, or in systems with low run volumes. "Hands-on" refresher courses are a reasonable alternative for this purpose.

Requirements for basic EMTs and first responders are less well defined. The large number of first responders makes this task particularly difficult. With the development of automatic defibrillator programs, attention will be placed on credentialing standards for providers when they use these devices. Such credentialing also focuses on important basic skills such as basic life support and initial airway management. This process must extend beyond the care of cardiac arrest victims, who make up a small percentage of EMS systems' volume.

Interest in EMS dispatch has developed nationwide with the realization of its critical role in coordinating EMS care. Standards for dispatch of appropriate level of service and medical interrogation of the caller must be developed. Clawson and Dernocoeur[14] argue that ability to give prearrival instructions should also be a part of the dispatcher's training and duties. Authority for assessing compliance with any of these standards may not always be the prerogative of the EMS authority. Systems that use multiple PSAPs to provide medical dispatch must pay particular attention to this issue.

Credentialing must also take place for facilities and personnel that provide on-line medical direction and receive emergency patients. Providers of medical direction must have sufficient knowledge and experience regarding emergency care to provide assistance when consulted by radio. They must also be familiar with the capabilities and limitations of the prehospital care setting. For example, California requires training in a standard base station course and certification to provide on-line direction. A secondary benefit of these requirements is that they allow a concurrent review of field care by a trained provider (see Direct Medical Command later in this chapter). Guidelines must exist for an EMS medical director (EMSMD). The EMSMD must be familiar with and experienced in the provision of the entire scope of emergency care to be effective in this role.[15] The EMSMD *must* also be intimately aware of the constraints and realities of medical care in the prehospital environment.

The assurance of quality for receiving facilities often is beyond the scope of a system's authority and falls to the state health department. The EMS system, however, must have destination policies based on the capabilities of its receiving facilities and must monitor whether those facilities are capable of providing care consistent with these stated capabilities.

A prospective review of the system is the critical starting point to ensure that all components are in place to provide quality care.

Concurrent Evaluation

Review of care as it is being provided on scene is the optimal method of ensuring quality medical care. Positive behavior may be reinforced and errors corrected before patient care is affected and bad habits develop. Systems such as those in Houston, Pittsburgh, and Denver make extensive use of on-scene review.[16] This task is resource intensive, and few systems have the population density to allow frequent on-scene response by a single medical director. Delegation of this function to a field supervisor is more likely to ensure a field presence in this environment.

Alternative methods of concurrent review include review when the patient arrives at the hospital and by on-line medical direction. The value of on-line direction for patient care has come under increased scrutiny in recent years. It remains a means, however, by which a paramedic's evaluation and interpretation of a situation can be reviewed in a contemporaneous fashion. If medical direction is centralized, which often occurs in large urban or rural systems, concurrent evaluation of the system is ongoing. For decentralized systems monitoring of radio transmissions by trained medical personnel may serve as a similar, although expensive and redundant, task. This method of review depends on radio communication, which may not occur in important instances (e.g., patient refusal of care).[17]

Although not absolutely concurrent, feedback on field care rendered is best reviewed when the patient arrives at the receiving facility. Field impressions may be compared with physician evaluation and other clinical data that are available only in the emergency department. In this method the receiving physician must have the time and interest to critically review the care rendered and give feedback. The emergency department medical director should encourage the proactive participation of the emergency physicians in this review of prehospital care. Feedback of cases of good or excellent prehospital management, as well as the suboptimal managed cases, should be encouraged. Some EMS medical directors, however, argue that this method is inadequate because it does not review the process of care. For instance, a patient who has excellent cervical spine immobilization on emergency department arrival may have been told to walk to a backboard and asked to lie down. In systems with multiple receiving hospitals, a coordinated evaluation by receiving physicians is a logistic nightmare. To address this shortcoming, many systems make liberal use of EMS system review sheets, which are widely distributed and may be filled out by any person raising a concern regarding patient care. This method does not substitute for a systematic evaluation of care.

Retrospective Review

Retrospective review of care is what is typically thought of when QA is discussed. Realistically it is a small part of a QM program and is the most time-consuming and probably the least valuable. Information gathered retrospectively is most likely to be incomplete, and the greater the time gap between the review and care rendered, the more likely that important information will be lacking.

Coordinating a comprehensive review of a system with multiple providers is a daunting task and requires access to records, logistic support and, most important, political support from the providers being reviewed. Assurances must be given that findings will be treated in a confidential fashion. A baseline review must be performed to evaluate where a QM program will be most effective. Some authors advocate a 100% chart review,[18] although this is time-consuming and inefficient. Each system has preexisting areas that system members can readily identify as areas for review. A listing of areas for explicit, objective initial reviews should be constructed (Box 100-1) using standards developed locally or nationally. This inventory should be the focus of discussion throughout the system to identify issues. Identification of cases for review may be made from dispatch data (response time, scene time, and transport time), ambulance runsheet review, incident reports, or other sources. Procedure data such as intubations, field needle chest decompression, or cricothyrotomy may similarly be used. After this initial, objective, explicit screen a subjective implicit review should be performed.

Discussion must ensue regarding local system priorities to ensure appropriate use of resources and generate systemwide agreement on the value of the review. For instance, suburban EMS systems lack the volume of penetrating trauma cases that characterizes urban EMS systems and providers receive less experience with critically injured trauma patients. A review of trauma scene times and procedures might be appropriate.

The focus of retrospective review must extend beyond field care. If there are multiple providers of on-line medical direction, as is true in many communities, monitoring must occur to ensure consistency, availability, and appropriateness of medical direction.[19] This can be accomplished by on-line monitoring by the medical director or designee or by review of run tapes. Similarly, if there are multiple agencies providing medical dispatch, the accuracy and timeliness of their activities should be monitored.

Prioritization of QM activities is an important issue and requires substantial attention. Reviews should be of limited duration and not be conducted concurrently. Morale is significantly affected by a bombardment of paperwork and the perception that "big brother is always watching."

BOX 100-1

POSSIBLE EXPLICIT PARAMETERS FOR REVIEW

All Field Providers
- Trauma scenes >15 minutes duration
- Refusal of transportation
- Immediate life and limb threats
- Multicasualty incidents
- Patient deterioration en route to hospital
- Communication failure
- Equipment failure
- Cardiac arrest and automatic defibrillator use

Cognitive and Technical Skills
- Assessment compared with emergency department discharge diagnosis
- Intubation attempt
- Electrocardiogram interpretation
- Communication skills
- Time to defibrillation: paramedics and basics

Dispatch
- Time through dispatch (98% <2 minutes)*
- Identification of critical cases (those requiring transport to hospital with lights and sirens)†

On-Line Medical Control
- Availability
- Identified
- Appropriate for system
- Efficient

Administration
- Incident investigations
- Patient, healthcare provider complaints
- Ambulance accidents with injury

*Hedges JR, Joyce SM: *Prehosp Disas Med* 5:383-388, 1990.
†Cottington EM et al: *J Trauma* 29:1500-1509, 1989.

Outcome Measures

Recent efforts to evaluate EMS and all of healthcare have focused on outcome parameters to justify expense and assess benefit. Currently the measurements identified to best evaluate care are cardiac arrest and major trauma outcome data.

Cardiac Arrest. Cardiac arrest has traditionaly been used as the outcome measure to assess EMS systems. Although cardiac arrests represent only a small fraction of a system's caseload, cardiac arrest is a model condition to study for a number of reasons: (1) it is easily definable, (2) therapy is standardized, (3) a well-proven link between intervention and outcome exists, (4) survival is time dependant, and (5) outcome (dead or alive) is clearly measured.[20] Although complex and problematic, there is a wealth of published references that may be used for comparison between systems.[21-24] Cardiac arrest data may be used to assess process measures of the entire system (e.g., intubation success rates, response time, time to definitive care, and efficiency of first responders and dispatch) and their effect on outcome. Data are also increasingly available for this means of evaluation from computerized event recording modules that are present in manual and automatic defibrillators. These modules are able to precisely record critical variables such as cardiac rhythms and time intervals.

Trauma Care. The quality assurance activities of a trauma system are complex, expensive ($300,000 in one study[25]), and beyond the scope of this chapter. The review of care includes prehospital, emergency departments, and in-hospital care using both process and outcome measures. Evaluation of trauma patient outcome is an important part of the EMS systems quality activities.

Provider Quality Assurance Participation. Participation by auditors in peer review has been widely recognized as a valuable technique for educating physicians regarding important QA issues and forcing them to evaluate their own practice.[26,27] We have reviewed paramedic peer review auditing in our own system and have found it to be a valuable technique in educating paramedics regarding their own practice.[28] It also has served a valuable adjunct in an ongoing QA program, facilitating a daily review of patient care and identifying trends in field care and documentation.[29] This program has been most effective as an initial explicit review and requires the ongoing participation of the medical director to further evaluate cases and investigate issues when they are raised by paramedic auditors. Quality improvement programs in industry and healthcare use multidisciplinary teams of providers, which evaluate processes, collect problem-oriented data, and recommend and implement improvements.

Management Issues. EMS agency management must be an ongoing partner in the QM program. Management must be in agreement with program goals and must be apprised of pertinent findings and issues. Support for interventions including continuing education, clinical training, and participation in auditing must be ongoing. Management's role is primary in specific cases when disciplinary action, retraining, or outright dismissal may be contemplated. Many interventions will have been previously proscribed under employment contracts or union agreements.

EMERGENCY DEPARTMENT ROLE

Depending on the particular system structure, the emergency department or its medical director, or both, may play different roles in EMS, including the following:
- Receiving facility
- Direct medical command site (by nurses or physicians, or both)
- Direct supervisor of EMS (e.g., if an EMS system or agency is hospital based or owned)
- Member of the EMS board
- Medical director of an EMS system or agency
- Regional or state representative for an EMS council

Different combinations of the previously listed roles may be played by one or more emergency physicians from the same emergency department. It is certain that at some point the emergency department director will become involved in some sort of substantial role in EMS. For this reason, he or she should be familiar with and supportive of the EMS continuous quality improvement (CQI) process.

EMS processes are designed to facilitate patient care through the entire medical system. The emergency department director must articulate the needs and responsibilities of the emergency department within these processes. For instance, in caring for a trauma victim the EMS response should be fast, the scene times short, and the communication to the receiving facility timely and accurate. The emergency department in turn can prepare to receive this patient and can activate and allocate the necessary resources, namely, the surgeon, operating room, blood bank, radiology technicians, and so forth. A finely articulated process among EMS, the emergency department, the pharmacy, the coronary care unit, and the cardiologists provides for quality care to a patient with acute myocardial infarction. A rapid response to the scene, fast and accurate initial assessment, rapid transport, and timely communication to the emergency department result in a faster time to diagnosis, faster administration of thrombolytics, and faster definitive care.

The following sections address concepts and areas in which involvement of the emergency department is vital for QI in EMS.

Education

Traditionally education has been used to change behavior. A QM program produces an educational program with vitality because it develops material for relevant education. Tape review sessions, which are well received by EMS providers, are a classic example.[30] The National Association of EMS Physicians has advocated in a position report on dispatching that tape review sessions be a regular part of a dispatch QM program.[31] Significant obstacles exist, however, to good EMS education. In many system types the number of agencies and providers complicates efforts to ensure consistent, relevant education based on findings of QM programs. For instance, in the northern Chicago area the EMS authority coordinates more than 60 continuing education programs a month (personal communication: Stanley Zydlo, MD, Northern Chicago EMS, Chicago, June, 1990). To address this issue, innovative techniques such as systemwide computer bulletin boards and EMS continuing education cable television programs have been tested. The issue of consistent education and access to providers on a continuing basis must be addressed for a QM program to have any impact.

The involvement of the emergency department is crucial to the EMS provider's professional growth through continuing education, workshops, grand rounds, and other formal didactic activities. Regularly scheduled certification and recertification courses in Basic Cardiac Life Support and ACLS should be a part of the emergency department's academic function, especially for departments with significant EMS activity. Basic Trauma Life Support and Pediatric Advanced Life Support should also be considered for most systems. This formal didactic involvement serves as the foundation for productive clinical training through more specific clinical rotations.

Clinical Rotations

Clinical rotations are essential in the development of skills necessary for quality patient care. Compared with physicians, EMS providers have less opportunity to acquire technical and cognitive skills before they actually start delivering patient care. Depending on the particular system, their exposure to the clinical situations necessary to develop expertise varies immensely. Therefore it is crucial that the emergency department be a consistent source of this clinical experience. The department must not only be "available" but also should provide an organized, formal, and well-described clinical rotation(s) suitable to and commensurate with the level of provider. The emergency department should also provide the link with and procure commitment from other areas of the hospital that are needed to provide to the EMS provider with the necessary clinical experience. For instance, anesthesia and operating room rotations are extremely important for proper clinical exposure to airway management skills. Many systems have a low frequency of intubations per provider per year. Others even prohibit EMS providers from performing intubations in the field, except for certain selected indications. EMS systems may also frequently have problems finding adequate commitment for anesthesia and operating room training for EMS providers.

Other low-volume EMS experiences such as obstetric and neonatal care are also areas in which prehospital providers obtain little formal education and experience. In the Pittsburgh EMS system Verdile and others[32] found that only 70 emergency deliveries were performed by EMS providers in a 5-year period, with a significant rate of perinatal complications (such as preeclampsia, gestational diabetes, premature delivery, and circumnuchal umbilical cords). These clinical data are of particular interest to EMS systems in highly populated urban areas. Obstetrics and labor and delivery room commitment for emergency delivery skills, as well as neonatal resuscitation training of EMS providers, should be procured. Providers should also have in-hospital clinical exposure to high-volume EMS-like patient experiences that pose unique problems, such as management of psychiatric or violent patients. Emergency department directors are a critical resource for the EMS system in obtaining this type and other types of clinical education.

For the above mentioned educational process and clinical rotations to be effective and successful, all levels of healthcare providers (e.g., nurses, physician assistants, emergency technicians, operating room technicians, EMTs' instructors and coordinators, and phlebotomists) within the emergency department and the hospital should be actively involved. Nevertheless, since EMS is the extension of medical practice into the streets, it is paramount that physicians be involved.

Through active engagement and participation in EMS activities, the relationship of the hospital and the emergency physician with the EMS provider strengthens and grows healthy, resulting in smooth, high-quality teamwork that ultimately improves the quality of EMS care delivery.

Direct Medical Command

Direct medical command, alone or in any combination with other functions, is one of the most common types of emergency department involvement in EMS. Direct medical command is usually accomplished by emergency physicians or Certified Emergency Nurses, depending on the particular system and the governing state and local rules and laws.

It is the responsibility of the emergency department director or his or her designee to make sure that all persons giving on-line medical direction are competent and qualified.

There should be a formal training process, often called "command physician course," covering such aspects as systems structure, level of providers, and scope of practice of these providers as dictated by medical protocols, governing laws, and system capabilities. The direct medical command professional should be knowledgeable in the standard operating procedures for the system (commonly referred to as SOPs), as well as the diversion ("bypass") policies. A copy of these two documents should be kept beside the radio or telephone communication device that is used at all times, for "on-the-spot" reference.

A basic knowledge of radio equipment and communications skills is highly desirable. The operator should also be familiar with the providers themselves and the environment in which they practice. A good way of doing so is to be actively involved in the previously discussed training process of the providers. This will give the physician a sense of what that particular provider in that particular situation is capable of doing. Another way that has been discussed by some authors is to engage in "hands-on experience as a paramedic" or "ride-along" work.[16,18] Although somewhat difficult to implement for attending emergency physicians, it is a good method for exposing physicians in training to EMS patient care.

Although direct medical command is a clinical aspect of EMS practice, it is essential that QI audits be performed on a regular and timely basis. The emergency department director may and should delegate to those giving direct medical command some of the functions of CQI, such as daily run-sheet review and identification of problems and needs of the system.

Administrative Support and Emergency Department Involvement

The emergency department director should be aware of the level of administrative support required by the QI program in the EMS system. If not otherwise provided, the emergency department should provide clerical or secretarial support, protected time for CQI activities, equipment, and office space for such EMS-related activities.

Fundamental to the EMS system's QI activities is the need for outcome data from the receiving emergency department. Provision should be made and confidentiality agreements negotiated to supply these data. Communication between the administrative arms of the EMS system and the hospital are also facilitated by the emergency department. Mundane but necessary issues such as identification of exposure to infectious diseases, exchange of EMS equipment, and facilitation of EMS turnaround at the emergency department must also be addressed.

Legal Issues

An unfortunate constraint of prehospital QA activities is that activities may not be protected by statute. Although individual providers and hospitals are protected by statutes in all states, the EMS lead agencies may not be defined in statute as being a healthcare entity entitled to the protection of QA laws.[33] Few states (six by one count) have protection for EMS organizations; others have provided immunity for providers and physicians who are involved in QA activities. Major issues that must be clarified are discoverability of QA deliberations and reports generated, liability protection for providers and physicians acting in good faith, and appropriate handling of patient care records and reviews.

SUMMARY

Quality assurance activities in an EMS system are severely hampered unless a central agency exists to coordinate data collection, funding, and communication between agencies and field providers. Systems must successfully address these issues to maximize their efforts. Some regions (San Francisco, King County, Wash., and Burbank, Calif.) have developed organizations for the evaluation of prehospital care. These organizations greatly reduce the logistic impediments to evaluating EMS care and initiating improvements.

A clear goal of any program is improved patient care. This noble goal by itself will not move an EMS system to embrace needed changes. Improved efficiency with resultant decreased costs is a compelling reason for organizations to support QM activities. Improved provider morale as a result of excellent clinical performance, participation in moving toward excellence, and pride in work well done are all reasons that members of EMS systems participate in changes. An improved sense of teamwork as found in one survey[34] is another reason for initiating these programs.

Patients must receive quality emergency medical care from the moment they enter the healthcare *system.* Leadership by the medical community is crucial if this goal is to be realized.

REFERENCES

1. Saunders CE: EMS quality management: implementing an operationally integrated quality control program, *Prehosp Disas Med* 6(3):383, 1991 (abstract).
2. Donabedian A: The quality of care: how can it be assessed? *JAMA* 260(12):1743-1748, 1988.
3. Berwick D: Sounding board: continuous improvement as an ideal in health care, *N Engl J Med* 320:53-56, 1989.
4. Berwick DM, Godfrey AB, Roessner J: *Curing health care: new strategies for quality improvement,* San Francisco, 1990, Jossey-Bass.
5. Walton M: *The Deming management method,* New York, 1986, Putnam.
6. Boyd DR: The history of emergency medical services systems in the United States of America. In Boyd DR, Edlich RF, Micik S: *Systems approach to emergency medical care,* Norwalk, Conn, 1983, Appleton-Century Croft.
7. Braun O, McCallion R, Fazackerley J: Characteristics of midsized urban EMS systems, *Ann Emerg Med* 19(5):536-546, 1990.
8. Joyce SM, Witzke D, Brown D et al: Development of an optically scanned EMS reporting form and database for statewide use, *Ann Emerg Med* 16:508, 1987 (abstract).
9. Hedges JR, Joyce SM: Minimim data set for EMS report form: historical development and future implications, *Prehosp Disas Med* 5(4):383-388, 1990.
10. Stout JL: Measuring your system, *J Emerg Med Serv* 8(1):84-91, 1983.
11. Stout JL: Stout's standard's of excellence for prehospital care systems, *J Emerg Med Serv* 8:84-91, 1983.
12. Soler JM, Montes MF, Egol AB et al: The ten-year malpractice experience of a large urban EMS system, *Ann Emerg Med* 14(10):982-985, 1985.
13. American College of Emergency Physicians: System Audit Appendix to Trauma System Guidelines for Trauma Care System In: Trauma Care Systems Quality Assurance Guidelines, Dallas, April 1990, ACEP.

14. Clawson JJ, Dernocoeur K: *Principles of emergency medical dispatch,* Englewood Cliffs, NJ, 1988, Brady.
15. American College of Emergency Physicians: Position summary, medical control of EMS: the role of physicians, Dallas, 1991, ACEP.
16. Pepe PE, Stewart RD: Role of the physician in the prehospital setting, *Ann Emerg Med* 15:1480-1483, 1986.
17. Zehnder WJ, Davidson SR, Kelly JJ et al: Non-transports of prehospital patients: is stronger medical control needed? *Ann Emerg Med* 20(4):446, 1991 (abstract).
18. Ryan J: Quality assurance in emergency medical services. In Kuehl AE: *EMS Medical directors handbook,* St Louis, 1989, Mosby.
19. Pointer J: The advanced life support base hospital audit for medical control in an emergency medical services system, *Ann Emerg Med* 16:557-560, 1987.
20. Eisenberg M: *Quality assurance: is it possible?* EMS Forum, American College of Emergency Physicians Scientific Assembly, San Francisco, November 1987.
21. Cummins RO, Chamberlain DA, Abramson NS et al: Recommended guidelines for uniform reporting of data from out-of-hospital cardiac arrest: the Ustein style, *Ann Emerg Med* 20:861-874, 1991.
22. Eisenberg MS, Horwood BT, Cummins RO et al: Cardiac arrest and resuscitation: a tale of 29 cities, *Ann Emerg Med* 19(2):179-186, 1990.
23. Eisenberg MS, Bergner L, Hearne T: Out-of-hospital cardiac arrest: a review of major studies and a proposed uniform reporting system, *Am J Public Health* 70:236-240, 1980.
24. Eisenberg MS, Cummins RO, Damon S et al: Survival rates from out-of-hospital cardiac arrest: recommendations for uniform definitions and data to report, *Ann Emerg Med* 19:1249-1259, 1990.
25. Shackford SR, Cooper GF, Eastman AB: Quality in a trauma system: medical audit committee: composition, cost and results, *J Trauma* 27:866-875, 1987.
26. Overton DT: A computer-assisted emergency department chart audit, *Ann Emerg Med* 16(1):68-72, 1987.
27. Stair TO: Quality assurance, *Emerg Clin North Am* 5(1):41-54, 1987.
28. Swor RA, Bocka JJ: A Paramedic Peer Review Audit, *Prehosp Disas Med* 6(3):321-327, 1991.
29. Swor RA, Hoelzer MH: A computer-assisted quality assurance audit in a multiprovider EMS system, *Ann Emerg Med* 19(3):286-290, 1990.
30. Rottman, SJ, Fitzgerald-Westby K: A method for reviewing radiotelemetry paramedic calls, *Ann Emerg Med* 10:36-38, 1981.
31. National Association of Emergency Medical Physicians: Position paper on emergency medical dispatching, Pittsburgh, 1990, The Association.
32. Verdile VP, Tutsock G, Paris PM et al: Out-of-hospital deliveries: a five-year experience, *Prehosp Disas Med* 10:10-13, 1995.
33. Abrahamsen M: QA and the Law. In Swor RA, Pirrallo RG, Rottman S et al, editors: *Quality management in prehospital care,* St Louis, 1993, Mosby.
34. Maio RF, Bronken T: Quality assurance in emergency medical services: report of a survey. Presentation at Michigan EMS Exposition, Lansing, Mich, 1990.

ADDITIONAL READINGS

Becker LB, Ostrander MP, Barret J et al: Outcome of CPR in a large metropolitan area; where are the survivors? *Ann Emerg Med* 20(4):355-361, 1991.

Bergner L, Eisenberg M, Hallstrom J et al: Evaluation of paramedic services for cardiac arrest. National Center for Health Services Research Report Series, Pub No. PHS 82-3310, Washington, DC, 1981, Department of Health and Human Services.

Cales RH et al: Trauma registries, *Trauma Quart* 5(3):1-8, 1989.

Cayten CG: Evaluation of emergency medical services systems. In Kuehl AE: *EMS Medical directors handbook,* St Louis, 1989, Mosby.

Champion HR et al: MTOS: establishing national norms for trauma care, *J Trauma* 3(11):1356, 1990.

Champion HR, Copes WS, Sacco WJ et al: The major trauma outcome study: establishing national norms for trauma care, *J TRAUMA* 11:1356-1365, 1990.

Cobb LA, Alaveraz H III, Copass MK: A rapid response system for out-of-hospital cardiac emergencies, *Med Clin North Am* 60:283-290, 1976.

Committee on Injury Scaling: *Abbreviated injury scale: 1990 revision,* Arlington Heights, Ill, 1985, American Association for Automotive Medicine.

Curka PA, Pepe PE, Ginger VF: Computer-aided EMS priority dispatch: ability of a computerized triage system to safely spare paramedics from responses not requiring advanced life support, *Ann Emerg Med* 20(4):446, 1991 (abstract). (*Ann Emerg Med* October 1993.)

Eitel DR et al: Out-of-hospital cardiac arrest: a six-year experience in a suburban-rural system, *Ann Emerg Med* 17(8):808-812, 1988.

Kallsen GW: *The nuts and bolts of EMS quality assurance.* Presented at the American College of Emergency Physicians Scientific Assembly, New Orleans, 1988.

Kallsen G, Nabors MD: The use of priority medical dispatch to distinguish between high- and low-risk patients, *Ann Emerg Med* 19(4):458-459, 1990 (abstract).

Lilja GP, Swor RA: Emergency medical services. In Tintinalli JE: *Emergency medicine: a comprehensive study guide,* ed 2, New York, 1988, McGraw-Hill.

MacKenzie EJ, Steinwachs DM, Ramzy AI: Evaluation performance of statewide regionalized systems of trauma care, *J Trauma* 30(6):681-687, 1990.

Maio RF, Burney RE: Improving reliability of abstracted prehospital care data: use of decision rules, *Prehosp Disas Med* 6(1):15-20, 1991.

Pantridge JF, Geddes JS: A mobile intensive care unit in the management of myocardial infarction, *Lancet* 2:271-273, 1967.

Polnitsky CA, Capone RJ, Gagon DE et al: Prehospital coronary care: proposal for a uniformed reporting system, *JAMA* 237:134-139, 1977.

Pepe et al: The impact of intense physician supervision on the effectiveness of an EMS system, *Ann Emerg Med* 17(7):752, 1988 (abstract).

Pons PT, Dinerman N, Rosen P et al: The field instructor program: quality control of prehospital care—the first step, *J Emerg Med* 2:421-427, 1985.

Pories SE, Gamelli RL, Pilcher DB et al: Practical evaluation of trauma deaths, *J TRAUMA* 12:1607-1610, 1989.

Stewart RD: Medical direction in emergency medical services: The role of the physician, *Emerg Med Clin North Am* 5(1):119-132, 1987.

Stewart R et al: A computer-assisted quality assurance system for an emergency medical service, *Ann Emerg Med* 14(1):25-29, 1985.

Stout JL: System financing. In Roush WR: *Principles of EMS systems: a comprehensive text for physicians,* Dallas, 1989, American College of Emergency Physicians.

Stout JL: Measuring response time performance, *J Emerg Med Serv* 12(9):106-111, 1987.

Valenzuela TD, Criss EA, Spaite DW et al: Cost-effectiveness analysis of paramedic emergency medical services in the treatment of prehospital cardiopulmonary arrest, *Ann Emerg Med* 19:1407-1411, 1990.

101 The Role of Air Medical Services in Out-of-Hospital Care

Luis F. Eljaiek, Jr. and Thom A. Mayer

OUTLINE

Type of air medical service
Geographic service area
Type of transport
Staffing level of ground and air transport systems
Closest appropriate facility versus closest facility
Weather conditions
Additional considerations
Summary

Air medical services in the out-of-hospital civilian experience have had steady growth since they were first used in the early 1970s. Air transport of ill and injured patients has been a controversial issue in emergency medicine for many years (Figure 101-1). However, when helicopter transport is restricted to patients with conditions of sufficient severity, it has proven to be an effective adjunct in out-of-hospital care environments throughout the country. Such programs have effectively helped extend the reach of regional trauma and critical care centers through outlying areas and in the case of interhospital transports have helped ensure that a tertiary critical care network is available to outlying centers. The net result has been nearly 200 helicopter programs currently operating in the United States. Most of these are hospital based at major trauma and tertiary care centers, but others are public safety–based programs. Among these public safety programs, the majority are operated by state or local police, but some fire Emergency Medical Services (EMS) systems also operate helicopter programs. The integration of air medical and ground transport systems has several goals, including the following:

- To provide critical care interventions for selected patients with severe illnesses or injuries
- To provide transport to critical care centers for definitive therapy, particularly when surgical or procedural interventions may reduce morbidity or mortality
- To allow ground-based EMS units to remain in service when long transport times could potentially affect the care of other patients in the primary service area
- To provide the preceding conditions in as efficient and cost-effective a fashion as possible

In the early stages of out-of-hospital air transport there were no clear-cut criteria for the use of helicopters. The decision to use the helicopter for air medical transport was largely based on the availability of the service and the activation chosen by the local EMS providers on the scene. As the experience in using helicopter transport system has grown, there has been a concomitant increase in the literature relating to appropriate use of helicopters. Initially criteria were set forth by the American College of Surgeons Committee on Trauma.[1] These criteria provided parameters for the field triage of patients with traumatic injuries. Suggestions regarding candidates for air transport were also included. The Association of Air Medical Services has also provided a position paper on criteria that were somewhat broader, including both trauma and nontrauma patients who would benefit from air transport.[2] These criteria defined the patient populations ranging from the traumatically injured to adult, pediatric, neonatal, and perinatal patients with critical illnesses. Most recently the National Association of Emergency Medical Services Physicians has published several position papers that provide additional guidelines on the transport of traumatically injured patients, as well as nontrauma and pediatric patients.[3-4]

Although many excellent resource documents provide guidelines regarding which patients could potentially benefit from the helicopter transport, each individual program must develop its own dispatch guidelines to meet the mission profile of its air medical service. Figure 101-2 and Box 101-1 list the guidelines developed for Inova Medical AirCare, which have undergone repeated and substantial revision, based on Quality Improvement (QI) review of a need for medical transport, patient outcomes, and financial criteria defined by third-party carriers. It is extremely important to ensure that patients are selected for helicopter transport in a prospective and carefully reasoned fashion. Safety is the most important reason for ensuring that only patients who will benefit from air transport are flown. The safety records of out-of-hospital air medical services have generally been excellent; nonetheless, the use of rotor-wing aircraft should always be considered a high-risk operation that should be restricted to those patients who will benefit specifically from the goals of the air transport program. In addition, as healthcare costs have risen, increased scrutiny has been placed on operations such as air medical programs that have extraordinarily high fixed costs and overhead. As reimbursement for the care of ill and injured patients has been further scrutinized, so, too, has it been necessary to ensure that patients flown by air medical services meet certain thresholds of severity of illness or injury. In this regard, it is critically important to look carefully at how best to implement and integrate helicopter service into an existing ground transport system.

Among the most important factors to consider for seamless integration are the following:

- Type of air medical service (public safety or private model)

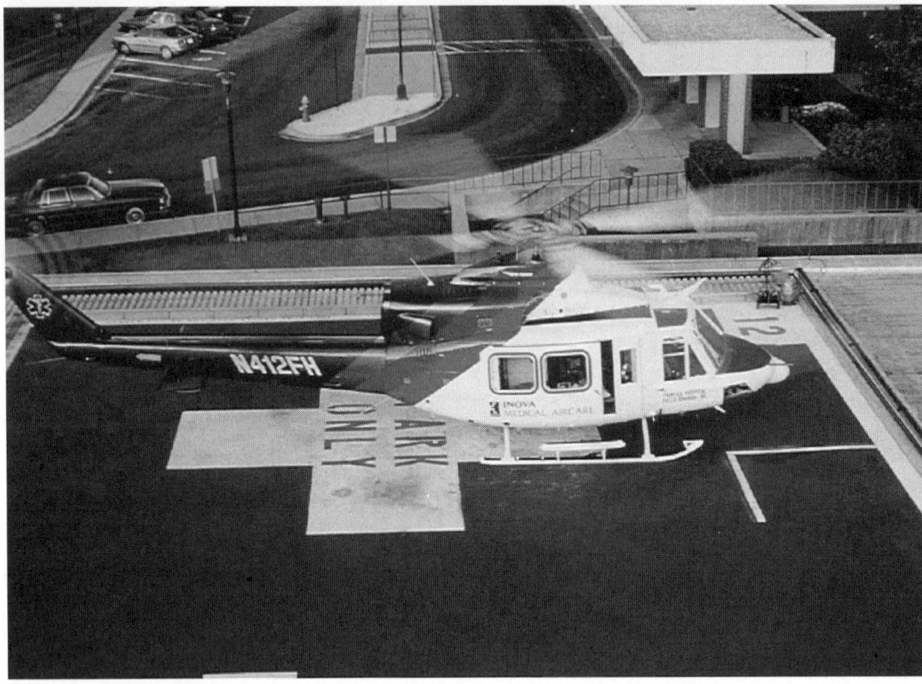

FIGURE 101-1 Inova Health System's Medical AirCare, a critical care medically configured Bell 412 HP, arrives at Fairfax Hospital.

- Urban or rural geographic area
- Scene or interfacility helicopter transports
- Level of care and personnel staffing ground and air transport systems
- Closest appropriate facility (e.g., trauma, cardiac, pediatric, perinatal, neonatal, burn, or transplant)
- Weather
- Time, distance, and traffic considerations

TYPE OF AIR MEDICAL SERVICE

As previously stated, the vast majority of helicopter air medical programs in the United States are of the private model. These usually consist of a hospital or consortium of hospitals and a fee-for-service venture. In contrast, the public safety model may be supported by local or state taxes, depending on the program, and most commonly operate as part of a combined police-patient transport, dual-mission profile. In this model police officers staff the unit, with or without the input of flight nurses from local hospitals. Police missions make up a large percentage of the flight hours in such helicopters, which are truly dual-mission aircraft designed to assist ground units with the most severely ill or injured patients. However, the issue of aircraft availability, prioritization of air medical versus police missions, and other issues relating to backup status must be resolved so that patients can be assured of expert and timely transport, regardless of the presence of police missions.

There may be political and financial limitations with either type of program. The private model must charge and recapture most of its operational cost to stay viable on a long-term basis. In the past most helicopter programs operated as cost centers, as opposed to profit centers, relying on income from inpatient revenues from the patients transported to justify the program. However, increased scrutiny of the healthcare dollar has resulted in many programs making strategic moves to ensure that their services operate with a positive bottom line, independent of the contribution made by inpatient revenues.

The private program may seek or target a particular demographic area with a larger percentage of insured patients. For example, it is increasingly common for programs to analyze the payor mix from specific service areas, hospitals, and even zip codes to help ensure that the financial viability of the program can be maintained. Therefore there can be differences in how the private model is marketed and integrated with various local ground transport and EMS systems. The public safety model may be exclusionary as well, if the program is financially supported by a particular county or other governmental jurisdiction and therefore faces specified jurisdictional boundaries. A state-supported public safety model has the advantage that there are no county or city jurisdictional boundaries, but such programs still face the potential of adjacent state boundaries. In some cases private model providers have attempted to challenge the federal antitrust status of public safety air medical providers, claiming that such programs "compete" unfairly because of public subsidies.

Other important considerations are the personnel and level of care given by each type of program. In many instances the private model consists of a nurse-paramedic staffing pattern, with some programs offering nurse-nurse or physician-nurse options. The majority of public safety models consist of a paramedic-paramedic crew. However, rather than focusing on the specific composition of the flight crew, it is more important to focus on the critical care interventions authorized by the medical director. For example, the use of rapid-sequence induction (RSI) is an important adjunct for the in-

Medical Necessity Criteria for Flight* Policy 1-6-2

- Documented, persistent, physiologic instability, includeing airway, breathing, or circulatory compromise, requiring critical care support during transport.
- Adult and Pediatric cases subject to same criteria.

CRITICAL CARE

- CVA w/evidence of impending herniation
- Other need for acute intervention
- Respiratory failure not responding to initial therapy
- Seizures not responding to therapy
- Fulminant sepsis with marked instability
- Acute epiglottis

CARDIAC

- Acute myocardial infarction following TPA
- Cardiogenic shock
- Cardiac dysrhythmia despite RX therapy
- Abd & thoracic aneurysms

TRAUMA (see below)

PERINATAL, NEONATAL, ORGAN TRANSPLANT

- General criteria for above should be applied
- Oncall physician in subspecialty service has final approval

*Other non-clinical factors need to be considered in conjunction with medical necessity. See non-clinical factors list.

Medical Necessity Criteria for Flight* Policy 1-6-3

- Documented, persistent, physiologic instability, including airway, breathing, or circulatory compromise, requiring critical care support during transport.
- Adult and Pediatric cases subject to same criteria.

Trauma-*Acute injury, Emergency department referral*

- Systolic blood pressure ≤ 85 for adults
- Systolic blood pressure ≤ 80 for children ≤ 10 years
- GCS ≤ 8
- GSW to head, neck, torso
- Stab to neck or torso if abc problem*
- Major amputation (at or proximal to wrist or ankle)
- Spine fx with or without paralysis
- Demonstrated by x-ray, 2 or more long bone fxs or pelvic fx
- Demonstrated by x-ray, maxillofacial fx plus injury resulting from a
  - motor vehicle crash with patient ejected from vehicle
  - High energy crash with speed ≥ 30 mph
  - Documented fall ≥ 20 ft

*If not abc problem, call on-call Trauma surgeon

Medical Necessity Criteria for Flight* Policy 1-6-4

- Documented, persistent, physiologic instability, including airway, breathing, or circulatory compromise, requiring critical care support during transport.
- Adult and Pediatric cases subject to same criteria.

Trauma- *Inpatient referrals*

- Certain trauma inpatient referrals may require air transport. Requests of this type should be referred to the Chief of Trauma Services - pager 5775 for determination of whether flight transport is necessary.

FIGURE 101-2 Inova Medical AirCare dispatch guidelines.

BOX 101-1

DISPATCH GUIDELINES FOR AIR MEDICAL SERVICE

I. General criteria
   A. The patient requires critical care life support that is not available from the local ground ambulance service (personnel, equipment, medications)
   B. The patient's condition requires that the least amount of time spent out of the hospital is used
   C. Ground delays such as traffic and obstacles may worsen the patient's condition
   D. The patient is in an inaccessible area
   E. The patient requires timely or specific treatment that is not available at the referring facility
   F. The patient's condition requires a special transport team (neonatal, aortic balloon pump)

II. Patient criteria
   A. Trauma
      1. Airway and breathing emergencies
      2. Systolic blood pressure = 90 mm Hg or less
      3. Glasgow Coma Score = 8 or less
      4. Suspected spinal cord injury or paralysis
      5. Penetrating injuries
         a. Head
         b. Neck
         c. Torso
      6. Blunt injuries to two or more major body parts
      7. Crush: Thorax, abdomen, pelvis, upper thighs
      8. Falls: Greater than 20 feet, two stories, or 3 times the patient's height
      9. Trauma arrest occurring after medical personnel arrives
      10. Major amputations
      11. Major lacerations
      12. Loss of consciousness or altered mental status
      13. Pregnancy: Gestation of 3 months or more
      14. Ejection from vehicle
      15. Pedestrian, motor vehicle, motorcycle, or industrial accident
      16. Burns: Greater than 20% of total body surface area or greater than 10% third degree
      17. Suspected respiratory burns
      18. High level of energy dissipation or significant vehicle damage
      19. Prolonged extrication: More than 20 minutes
      20. Death of another passenger in same accident
      21. Consider age (under 5 or over 65 years) and comorbid conditions

III. Medical, surgical and pediatric patients
   A. Cardiac patients requiring acute intervention not available at referring facility (such as pacemaker, thrombolytics, bypass grafting, angioplasty, myocardial infarction, unstable angina, or cardiac failure)
   B. Patient requires continuous intravenous medications or mechanical ventilation assistance to maintain a stable cardiac output or cardiac rhythm
   C. Hypothermia and hyperthermia management
   D. Patient has significant evidence of acidosis (pH <7.20)
   E. Cardiac or respiratory arrest within past 12 hours and is not responding to initial therapy
   F. Cerebral vascular accident with deterioration and/or cerebral edema requiring acute intervention
   G. Massive pulmonary embolus
   H. Organ transplantation or procurement
   I. Suspected dissecting or leaking aneurysms
   J. Status asthmaticus or other respiratory failure
   K. Status epilepticus
   L. Decompression illness
   M. Fulminant sepsis
   N. Acute epiglottitis
   O. Near-drowning with complications
   P. Meningitis with complications
   Q. Poisoning and overdose with complications
   R. Reye's syndrome with complications
   S. Glasgow Coma Score = 8 or less
   T. Acute renal failure with complications

IV. Perinatal patients (must have prior approval by perinatologist or neonatologist)
   A. Placenta previa, abruptio placenta
   B. Eclampsia or preeclampsia
   C. Premature labor with or without ruptured membranes
   D. Ground transport of more than 1 hour or during peak traffic
   E. Perinatologist or neonatologist not available at referring hospital

V. Neonatal patients (must have prior approval by perinatologist or neonatologist)
   A. Mechanical ventilation
   B. Seizure activity
   C. Hematologic instability
   D. Cardiac or surgical emergency
   E. Gestational age less than 35 weeks
   F. Shock
   G. Cardiac or respiratory arrest
   H. No neonatologist in attendance at the referring hospital
   I. Ground time to arrival greater than 1 hour
   J. Peak traffic time that would cause ground transport time to arrival to be more than 1 hour
   K. Requests by referring physician for air transport will be taken into consideration

tegration of air medical and ground medical services, since the majority of ground medical services do not have sufficient volume of patients being intubated each year to ensure that ground providers have RSI capability. Similarly, some programs have flight crews that are trained in central venous line placement, chest tube placement, and the like. It is important for the air medical service to carefully study the service needs of the EMS community it serves, to ensure that the crew is trained in the appropriate procedures to help reduce morbidity and mortality. For example, if the majority of flights flown by an air medical service are for scene trauma patients, it is critically important to ensure that RSI, needle and chest thoracostomy, and other trauma procedures can be performed. In circumstances under which flight crews do not have additional critical care expertise or procedures available, the helicopter service simply becomes a tool for more rapid transport of the patient, as opposed to a "higher level of out-of-hospital care."

GEOGRAPHIC SERVICE AREA

The obvious advantages of a helicopter over a ground vehicle are speed, ability to navigate the shortest route, and ability to reach remote locations. These have important impacts in both urban and rural settings. In the urban setting the ground EMS units typically are the first responders to attend to ill or injured patients. The helicopter service is brought into action when the patient's "transport time" will thereby be markedly reduced, often because of traffic considerations or scene safety. As the congestion of major highways further impairs the efficient use of ground transport, helicopter services are increasingly important, both to overcome the speed problem and to ensure that patients are offered the resources of committed trauma centers.

In contrast, the rural setting may use immediate helicopter dispatch as part of the first response to specific cases of sufficient severity. There may be limited resources in covering a much larger geographic area and therefore fewer medical crews to respond to specific sites, particularly in the case of multiple-casualty incidents. In this setting the speed and ability to navigate the shortest route play important roles in establishing the helicopter service's value to the EMS provider and their patients. The ability to reach remote areas is also extremely important in the rural setting. Ground personnel may not be able to reach injured patients in some cases because of difficult terrain, lack of roads, or both. The ability of the helicopter to overcome these obstacles can be vitally important.

TYPE OF TRANSPORT

Most ground EMS systems are inherently designed to transport scene patients, whether their injury is traumatic or medical. Depending on local circumstances, some ground EMS units are also designed to handle interfacility transports. However, very few EMS systems have developed the level of critical care expertise necessary to handle complicated interfacility transports of patients. For example, cardiac patients with multiple intravenous drips or an intraaortic balloon pump generally present transport problems that ground EMS systems have not been traditionally prepared to handle. Air transport of these patients can have a dramatic and salutary impact on the EMS system, both by ensuring that the patient is cared for by a critical care team in a rapid fashion and by allowing ground Advanced Life Support (ALS) units to remain in service for their primary responsibility. In some areas of the country, hospitals have developed combined air and ground transport units, which allow a critical care team to travel in a specially equipped critical care ground unit, when air transport is not needed or available.

There are areas of the country where the majority of interfacility transports for critically ill patients are conducted by ground units, although helicopter transport is available in most areas of the country. The helicopter is used more for its time considerations than for a combination of time factors and critical care expertise.

STAFFING LEVEL OF GROUND AND AIR TRANSPORT SYSTEMS

The level of care offered by either a ground or air medical transport system must be incorporated into a step-by-step approach for proper levels of patient care. As stated earlier, most air transport systems offer a minimum of ALS staffing, with the majority offering critical care support, including in some cases the use of transport ventilators. When the ground medical service offers only Basic Life Support, an ALS helicopter system becomes more important in rendering care to a much larger patient population than when the ground system offers ALS services. The helicopter system in the latter scenario requires more precise integration into the scheme for delivering emergency medical care.

The staffing of the helicopter also plays an important role. In programs that offer expanded critical care services, including RSI protocols, ventilator support, and intraaortic balloon pump capability, the system is designed to offer a higher level of care than most EMS systems have been able to offer. Typically a greater variety of medications is used, as well as more advanced procedures. It is important for air medical programs to cooperate fully with the EMS system, to ensure that there is a careful QI program in place to determine how many patients are transported per year, as well as the interventions that are performed on these patients. As scrutiny of healthcare costs continues, it is incumbent on both the air medical and ground components of the system to cooperate to the best extent possible in sharing information with regard to frequency of use, acuity of patients and effects of critical care interventions.

CLOSEST APPROPRIATE FACILITY VERSUS CLOSEST FACILITY

Ground medical transport systems resources are usually geographically distributed to provide a predetermined response time that is medically acceptable to the community they serve. With this in mind, the eventual transport of the patient is usually to the facility closest to the patient's home or the site of illness or injury. This provides for an efficient, cost-effective accessibility to immediate medical care and allows the ground EMS system to ensure that its units are not placed out of service for long transports. If a more advanced facility is needed after the initial stabilization of the patient's condition, another transport can be effected. This can be accomplished either by ground or by air, depending on the accepted guidelines, the level of acuity of the illness or injury, and so forth. The literature, however, is replete with studies indicating that certain patients with severe illnesses or injuries have much better outcomes if they are initially taken to designated trauma or critical care centers, which have the facilities, personnel, training, and commitment to care for the most severely ill or injured patients. Using the trauma analogy, only 10% to 15% of all trauma patients require the resources of a designated trauma center but those patients clearly fare better when cared for at an appropriate institution, as opposed to the nearest facility.

The air medical transport system is a critical piece of the equation because it allows the capability of transport from the scene of the injury directly to an appropriate trauma center. Because of such factors as speed, navigational abilities, and level of care being given to the patient, the helicopter is able to transport patients to the most appropriate facility for their care in the shortest period of time. Again, it is necessary to study the data from such flights carefully, including the necessity of providing feedback to the ground EMS system, so that the helicopter can be used appropriately. As with all specialty care resources, it is important to ensure that there is a slight amount of "overtriage," as opposed to excessive "undertriage" of patients. In this sense, overtriage can represent a political and financial problem, whereas undertriage is a medical problem, which can result in unnecessary death and morbidity for the patients the system is intended to serve.[5]

WEATHER CONDITIONS

Weather conditions are the one factor that cannot be controlled by systems design. Those who design a system for the delivery of medical care must consider contingent backup systems or plans for inclement conditions. On the surface it seems obvious that this would be most important for the air medical system. Federal Aviation Administration regulations (weather minimums) and safety practices supersede the deployment of air medical resources, regardless of the acuity of the patient. What is not as obvious is how inclement weather can also hamper ground medical transports. After rain, snow, or ice storms the road conditions may be such that ground transport may be severely affected, and helicopter resources may provide the only quick and efficient method for transport of critically ill or injured patients under such circumstances. In addition, the use of an Instrument Flight Rating helicopter system can be a substantial benefit in ensuring that aircraft are available for transport even in the midst of inclement weather.

ADDITIONAL CONSIDERATIONS

As a part of the planning of the integration of air and ground EMS systems, it is important to ensure that the air medical provider be capable of training the ground units in establishment of landing zones (LZs), preplotting designated LZs at appropriate areas throughout the jurisdiction, and ensuring that there is ongoing training regarding LZ safety. It is important for the air medical system to discuss carefully with the ground system the particular circumstances that require EMS dispatch to call for an immediate launch of the helicopter. For example, out-of-hospital scoring systems and physiologic or mechanism-of-injury criteria may be used to ensure that helicopter transport is available at the earliest possible time for selected patients. In some cases automatic dispatch of the helicopter for penetrating injuries to the head, neck, or trunk can help ensure that the aircraft is available for transport at the most appropriate time.

A detailed QI program should also be a part of the integration of air medical and ground EMS systems.[6] As a part of the tertiary care center operations, air medical personnel should be involved in the routine feedback of clinical information to ground units regarding patients that have been referred for transport. Such QI programs should ensure that the right patients are flown, the right things are done to the patient before flight, the appropriate procedures are performed during flight, and the effect on outcome is quantified to the best extent possible.

SUMMARY

Regardless of the precise details of the healthcare system in the next century, it appears that air medical transport will be a critical part of that future, even if those resources are restricted to the most critically ill and injured patients. The integration of air medical services and the ground EMS system should ideally be accomplished by a multidisciplinary group consisting of medical directors, representatives of the flight program, and the leadership of ground EMS providers. Through careful, detailed study of data from the out-of-hospital and in-hospital providers, the air medical and ground units should be able to cooperate in the best possible delivery of resources to patients.

REFERENCES

1. American College of Surgeons Committee on Trauma: Resources for optimal care of the injured patient, Chicago, 1990, American College of Surgeons.
2. Association of Air Medical Services: Position paper on the appropriate use of air medical services, *J Air Med Transport* 9:29-33, 1990.
3. National Association of EMS Physicians: Position paper: air medical dispatch—guidelines for scene response, *Prehosp Disas Med* 7:75-76, 1992.
4. National Association of EMS Physicians: Position paper: criteria for prehospital air medical transport—nontrauma and pediatric considerations, *Prehosp Disas Med* 9:140-141, 1994.
5. Grossman DC, Hart LG, Rivara FP et al: From roadside to bedside: the regionalization of trauma care in a remote rural county, *J Trauma* 38:14-21, 1995.
6. Mayer TA: Industrial models of continuous quality improvement: implications for emergency medicine, *Emerg Med Clin North Am* 10(3):523-547, 1992.

ADDITIONAL READINGS

ASTM Standards on EMS Care, American Society for Testing Materials, 1916 Race St., Philadelphia, PA 19103. (215) 299-3400.

FEMA EMS Safety Standards, Federal Emergency Management Agency, Federal Center Plaza, 500 C St., SW, Washington, DC 20472. (202) 646-2500.

Index

D

E

K

L

M

N

O

Q

T